HEADACHE

HANDBOOK OF CLINICAL NEUROLOGY

Series Editors

MICHAEL J. AMINOFF, FRANÇOIS BOLLER, AND DICK F. SWAAB

VOLUME 97

ELSEVIER

EDINBURGH LONDON NEW YORK OXFORD PHILADELPHIA
ST LOUIS SYDNEY TORONTO 2011

HEADACHE

Series Editors

MICHAEL J. AMINOFF, FRANÇOIS BOLLER, AND DICK F. SWAAB

Volume Editors

GIUSEPPE NAPPI AND MICHAEL A. MOSKOWITZ

VOLUME 97

3rd Series

ELSEVIER

EDINBURGH LONDON NEW YORK OXFORD PHILADELPHIA
ST LOUIS SYDNEY TORONTO 2011

ELSEVIER B.V.
Radarweg 29, 1043 NX, Amsterdam, The Netherlands

ISBN: 978-0-444-52139-2

British Library Cataloguing in Publication Data
A catalogue record for this book is available from the British Library

Library of Congress Cataloging in Publication Data
A catalog record for this book is available from the Library of Congress

Notices

Knowledge and best practice in this field are constantly changing. As new research and experience broaden our understanding, changes in research methods, professional practices, or medical treatment may become necessary.

Practitioners and researchers must always rely on their own experience and knowledge in evaluating and using any information, methods, compounds, or experiments described herein. In using such information or methods they should be mindful of their own safety and the safety of others, including parties for whom they have a professional responsibility.

With respect to any drug or pharmaceutical products identified, readers are advised to check the most current information provided (i) on procedures featured or (ii) by the manufacturer of each product to be administered, to verify the recommended dose or formula, the method and duration of administration, and contraindications. It is the responsibility of practitioners, relying on their own experience and knowledge of their patients, to make diagnoses, to determine dosages and the best treatment for each individual patient, and to take all appropriate safety precautions.

To the fullest extent of the law, neither the Publisher nor the authors, contributors, or editors, assume any liability for any injury and/or damage to persons or property as a matter of products liability, negligence or otherwise, or from any use or operation of any methods, products, instructions, or ideas contained in the material herein.

Printed in China

For Elsevier:
Commissioning Editor: Timothy Horne
Development Editor: Michael Parkinson
Project Manager: K. Anand Kumar
Designer/Design Direction: George Ajayi

The Publisher's policy is to use paper manufactured from sustainable forests

Handbook of Clinical Neurology 3rd Series

Available titles

Vol. 79, The human hypothalamus: basic and clinical aspects, Part I, D.F. Swaab ISBN 0444513574
Vol. 80, The human hypothalamus: basic and clinical aspects, Part II, D.F. Swaab ISBN 0444514902
Vol. 81, Pain, F. Cervero and T.S. Jensen, eds. ISBN 0444519017
Vol. 82, Motor neurone disorders and related diseases, A.A. Eisen and P.J. Shaw, eds. ISBN 0444518940
Vol. 83, Parkinson's disease and related disorders, Part I, W.C. Koller and E. Melamed, eds. ISBN 9780444519009
Vol. 84, Parkinson's disease and related disorders, Part II, W.C. Koller and E. Melamed, eds. ISBN 9780444528933
Vol. 85, HIV/AIDS and the nervous system, P. Portegies and J. Berger, eds. ISBN 9780444520104
Vol. 86, Myopathies, F.L. Mastaglia and D. Hilton Jones, eds. ISBN 9780444518966
Vol. 87, Malformations of the nervous system, H.B. Sarnat and P. Curatolo, eds. ISBN 9780444518965
Vol. 88, Neuropsychology and behavioural neurology, G. Goldenberg and B.C. Miller, eds. ISBN 9780444518972
Vol. 89, Dementias, C. Duyckaerts and I. Litvan, eds. ISBN 9780444518989
Vol. 90, Disorders of Consciousness, G.B. Young and E.F.M. Wijdicks, eds. ISBN 9780444518958
Vol. 91, Neuromuscular Junction Disorders, A.G. Engel, ed. ISBN 9780444520081
Vol. 92, Stroke – Part I: Basic and epidemiological aspects, M. Fisher, ed. ISBN 9780444520036
Vol. 93, Stroke – Part II: Clinical manifestations and pathogenesis, M. Fisher, ed. ISBN 9780444520043
Vol. 94, Stroke – Part III: Investigations and management, M. Fisher, ed. ISBN 9780444520050
Vol. 95, History of Neurology, S. Finger, F. Boller and K.L. Tyler, eds. ISBN 9780444520081
Vol. 96, Bacterial Infections of the Central Nervous System, K.L. Roos and A.R. Tunkel, eds. ISBN 9780444520159

Foreword

Migraine and other headaches are among the most frequent symptoms encountered in medicine. It has been estimated that at least 40% of neurological consultations are triggered by headache-related problems. The very high frequency of headache has made some physicians wonder whether one should call a condition that affects so many people a "disease." Headache sufferers, however, know better and have been relying for centuries on the knowledge of physicians to alleviate their symptoms. The editors of the previous series of the *Handbook of Clinical Neurology* certainly recognized the importance of the problem and, following four volumes dealing with neurological functions and their disturbances, they dedicated the first nosological volume (volume 5 of the first series) to headaches. They commented that the volume reflected the extent of our knowledge and ignorance about headache at that time (1968). As the reader will see, we have come a long way since then. In the second series, a volume on headaches was published in 1985, and the preface to that volume stated that this Cinderella of academic neurology had been transformed into an attractive princess courted by a growing circle of admirers. This is even truer today.

The present volume is part of the third series of the *Handbook*, for which we have editorial responsibility. In order to provide insight into physiological and pathogenetic mechanisms, and a basis for new therapeutic strategies for neurological disorders, we have specifically ensured that the neurobiological aspects of the nervous system in health and disease are covered, as well as more clinical aspects of neurological disease. During the last half-century, dramatic advances in the clinical and basic neurosciences have occurred, and these are emphasized in each volume of the *Handbook*. The present volume deals with various aspects of headaches. Until a few years ago, relatively little could be done in terms of therapeutic intervention and prevention of headaches, and in the headache volumes in the earlier series only few chapters dealt with therapy. Advances in our understanding of the biochemical background of headaches coupled with advances in fields as diverse as pharmacology, epidemiology, genetics, neuroimaging, interventional radiology, surgery, and even clinical psychology have profoundly altered our approach to headache. In the present volume, for example, no less than 15 chapters cover therapy, including prevention and management. Our goal is to provide basic researchers with the foundations for new investigative studies. We also intend to give clinicians a source reference to enable them to gain a thorough knowledge and understanding of the clinical features and management of the many manifestations of headaches.

As series editors, we reviewed all the chapters and made suggestions for improvement, but we were delighted to read such scholarly and comprehensive accounts of different aspects of headaches. We are grateful to the two volume editors, Professor Giuseppe Nappi and Professor Michael Moskowitz, for their untiring effort in the preparation of this work. Our gratitude extends to all those who contributed their time and expertise to summarize developments in their field and helped put together this outstanding volume. In addition to the print form, the series is now available electronically on Elsevier's ScienceDirect site. This makes the *Handbook* more accessible to readers and will also facilitate search for specific information. As always, we are especially grateful to the team at Elsevier for their unfailing and expert assistance in the development and production of this volume.

Michael J. Aminoff
François Boller
Dick F. Swaab

Preface

Significant advances in the basic and applied brain sciences have led to a veritable revolution in the headache field over the past 25 years. This revolution was generated in part by the recognition that headache disorders are among the most burdensome health-care problems worldwide. Not only do they impact unfavorably on the finances of medical care, but they also reduce the quality of life of headache sufferers and their families. It is difficult to overstate the need to expand our knowledge base in this field and to continue our quest for better treatments in order to reduce the monetary and human cost of headaches; hence the motivation for this volume.

It may be hard for the reader to comprehend how far we have advanced over the past 25–30 years without mentioning just a few of the seminal developments in the headache field. These include the headache classification system, the discovery of the trigeminovascular system, and the introduction of the triptans for acute treatment. Moreover, developments in other fields such as genetics and genomics have contributed to the emergence of migraine genetics, which has identified specific genes causing mutated ion channels and ion pumps that underlie familial hemiplegic migraine. It is fair to say that many of the tools used to advance our understanding of headache were merely in the mind's eye of the field when the predecessor to this volume, volume 48 in the *Handbook of Clinical Neurology*, was published in 1985. For example, the blood oxygen level-dependent (BOLD) technique to assess functional activation was discovered in the 1990s and used shortly thereafter to confirm the importance of cortical spreading depression to migraine aura and to identify activated cortical and brainstem regions during headache. The design and analysis of large epidemiological studies and the methodologies for clinical trials have been highly refined over the past 20 years, and the value of evidence-based medicine and translational research is now widely accepted, even demanded by the headache community.

This volume is an exhaustive and up-to-date account of the cultural developments and the scientific advances that, in the period since the publication (in 1985) of the previous volume on headache in the *Handbook*, have revolutionized understanding of both migraine and other headaches. The evolution of the concept of primary headache can be charted, essentially, through three important milestones: 1982, the year in which the International Headache Society (IHS) was founded in London; 1988, the year that saw the publication of the first IHS classification of headaches, a ground-breaking development in the field as it was the first time that precise criteria for diagnosing the various forms of headache had been formulated on the basis of empirical data (evidence-based diagnostic criteria) or, in areas where the literature lacked sufficient data, on the basis of expert consensus; and finally, 2004, the year that, in the wake of more than 15 years of intense work aimed at validating and expanding the first version, brought us the second edition of the IHS classification (*International Classification of Headache Disorders*, 2nd edn: ICHD-II).

Headache classification is a dynamic and ongoing process and, immediately after the publication of ICHD-II, it proved necessary to revise the classifications of medication-overuse headache (MOH) and chronic migraine (CM). These changes also highlighted the need for a standardization of the general diagnostic criteria for secondary headaches. According to ICHD-IIR, MOH cannot be diagnosed with certainty as long as the putative cause – medication overuse – continues to be present.

Many of the authors who have contributed to this book have been both witnesses to and protagonists on the front line of headache science. Its contents, rigorous and completely up to date, ranges from nosographical categorizations, based on the explicit recording of the classic signs and symptoms, to the emerging concept of migraine as a model of a complex, polygenic disease characterized by an environmental component and by heterogeneity as regards clinical phenotype, age at onset, gender, severity, comorbidities, and outcomes.

The book includes chapters dealing with general aspects of headache (socioeconomic, in particular), the contribution made by the biological sciences to furthering understanding of the pathophysiology of headache, and the management of headache and related problems. The main body of the book is devoted to primary and secondary headaches. The book ends with chapters intended to clarify a series of controversial issues: pathogenetic (chronobiological, endocrinological, and neuroimaging correlates), nosographic (i.e., migraine, vertigo, and headache in children), and treatment-related (new advances).

We are deeply appreciative of the invaluable contributions of Giorgio Sandrini (Pavia) and Gabriella Buzzi (Rome) to this volume. Without their efforts, the volume would never have been realized.

Giuseppe Nappi
Michael A. Moskowitz

Dedication

For my wife Emilia, my children Rossella and Roberto, and in memory of my parents Rosinella and Rubino Nappi. Their love and patience have constantly given me confidence and strength.

Giuseppe Nappi

To my Cherished Family: Mary, Jenna, Mattia, Jacob, and especially my mother Clara

Michael A. Moskowitz

List of contributors

M. Allena
University Center for Adaptive Disorders and Headache (UCADH), IRCCS "C. Mondino Institute of Neurology" Foundation, Pavia, Italy

J. Alvarez-Linera
Neuroradiology Department, Hospital Ruber Internacional, Madrid, Spain

A. Ambrosini
Headache Clinic, INM Neuromed, IRCCS, Pozzilli (Isernia), Italy

F. Antonaci
University Centre for Adaptive Disorders and Headache (UCADH) Pavia, Headache Medicine Centre, Department of Neurology Policlinic of Monza, Monza, Italy

M. Ashina
Danish Headache Center and Department of Neurology, Glostrup Hospital, Faculty of Health Sciences, University of Copenhagen, Copenhagen, Denmark

S.K. Aurora
Swedish Headache Center, Seattle, WA, USA

L. Bendtsen
Danish Headache Center, Department of Neurology, Glostrup Hospital, University of Copenhagen, Copenhagen, Denmark

S.L. Berga
Department of Gynecology and Obstetrics, Emory University School of Medicine, Atlanta, GA, USA

M.E. Bigal
Departments of Neurology, Epidemiology and Population Health, Albert Einstein College of Medicine, New York, NY, USA

J. Boivie
Department of Neurology, University Hospital, Uppsala, Sweden

H. Bolay
Department of Neurology, Gazi Hospital and Neuropsychiatry Centre, Gazi University, Besevler, Ankara, Turkey

L.H. Bonamico
Neurological and Pain Department, FLENI Neurological Institute, Buenos Aires, Argentina

G. Bono
University Center for Adaptive Disorders and Headache (UCADH) and Department of Clinical Medicine, Neurology Unit, University of Insubria, Varese, Italy

C.A. Bordini
Department of Neurology, Ribeirão Preto Medical School, São Paulo, Brazil

J.L. Brandes
Department of Neurology, Vanderbilt University Medical Center, Nashville Neuroscience Group, St Thomas Health Services and Department of Neurology, Vanderbilt University School of Medicine, Nashville, TN, USA

T. Brandt
Institute of Clinical Neurosciences and Integrated Center for Research and Treatment of Vertigo, Dizziness and Ocular Motor Disorders, Ludwig-Maximilians University, Münich, Germany

K.C. Brennan
Headache Research and Treatment Program, Department of Neurology, David Geffen School of Medicine at UCLA, Los Angeles, CA, USA

G. Broggi
Department of Neurosurgery, Fondazione IRCCS Istituto Nazionale Neurologico "Carlo Besta", Milan, Italy

T.M. Buchanan
Department of Neurology, University of Utah, Salt Lake City, UT, USA

R. Burstein
Departments of Anesthesia and Program in Neuroscience, Beth Israel Deaconess Medical Center and Harvard Medical School, Boston, MA, USA

G. Bussone
Clinical Neurosciences Department, C. Besta National Neurological Institute, Milan, Italy

M.G. Buzzi
Headache Center, IRCCS Santa Lucia Foundation, Rome, Italy

A. Carolei
Department of Neurology, University of L'Aquila, L'Aquila, Italy

T. Catarci
University Centre for Adaptive Disorders and Headache (UCADH), IRCCS, "C. Mondino Institute of Neurology" Foundation, Pavia, Italy

A. Charles
Headache Research and Treatment Program, Department of Neurology, David Geffen School of Medicine at UCLA, Los Angeles, CA, USA

A. Craven
European Headache Alliance and Migraine Association of Ireland, Dublin, Ireland

G. Cruccu
Department of Neurological Sciences, La Sapienza University, Rome, Italy

F.M. Cutrer
Department of Neurology, Mayo Clinic, Rochester, MN, USA

H-C. Diener
Department of Neurology, University of Duisburg-Essen, Essen, Germany

D.W. Dodick
Department of Neurology, Mayo Clinic Arizona, Phoenix, AZ, USA

A. Ducros
Emergency Headache Center, Lariboisière Hospital, Paris, France

P. Durham
JVIC Center for Biomedical and Life Sciences, Missouri State University, Springfield, MO, USA

G. Egli
Kopfweh- & Schmerzabteilung, Neurologische Klinik/ Unispital, Poliklinik, Zürich, Switzerland

S. Evers
Department of Neurology, University of Münster, Münster, Germany

M.D. Ferrari
Department of Neurology, Leiden University Medical Center, Leiden, The Netherlands

P. Ferroli
Department of Neurosurgery, Fondazione IRCCS Istituto Nazionale Neurologico "Carlo Besta", Milan, Italy

R.R. Frants
Department of Human Genetics, Leiden University Medical Center, Leiden, The Netherlands

A. Franzini
Department of Neurosurgery, Fondazione IRCCS Istituto Nazionale Neurologico "Carlo Besta", Milan, Italy

L. Friberg
Department of Clinical Physiology and Nuclear Medicine, Bispebjerb Hospital, Copenhagen, Denmark

A. Fumal
Headache Research Unit, Neurology and Neuroanatomy Departments, University of Liège, Liège, Belgium

F. Galli
Department of Child and Adolescent Neurology, Psychiatry and Rehabilitation, "Sapienza", University of Rome, Rome, Italy

N. Ghiotto
University Center for Adaptive Disorders and Headache (UCADH), IRCCS "C. Mondino Institute of Neurology" Foundation, Pavia, Italy

Contents

SECTION 6 Special issues

Section 1

General aspects

Handbook of Clinical Neurology, Vol. 97 (3rd series)
Headache
G. Nappi and M.A. Moskowitz, Editors

Chapter 1

Epidemiology of headache

GIAN CAMILLO MANZONI [1]* AND LARS JACOB STOVNER [2]

[1] *Headache Centre, Department of Neuroscience, University of Parma, Parma, Italy*

[2] *Department of Neuroscience, Norwegian University of Science and Technology and St. Olavs Hospital, Trondheim, Norway*

INTRODUCTION

Headache epidemiological studies may be performed for several reasons. For a disorder which has often not been taken seriously, the main aim has often been to assess prevalence and incidence in order to estimate the magnitude of the problem, and likewise to convince the public and decision-makers that headache is not only a nuisance for some individuals, but constitutes a large public health problem. In later years, several such studies have also included items relevant for determining the burden of headache in the population and for health economic calculations. Other aims of headache epidemiological studies have been to collect data outside the clinical setting on the various features of headache disorders (e.g., pain characteristics, associated symptoms), trigger factors, consequences of headache (e.g., for quality of life, professional career and family life), comorbid diseases, and possibly on causes and risk factors for headache. The present chapter will mainly focus on the first of these aims, reviewing the available evidence on the distribution of headache in various parts of the world, and among the two sexes, the different races, and in different age and socioeconomic groups. However, since it is generally accepted that the results obtained in headache epidemiological studies are highly dependent on the methods used, we will first consider some methodological issues pertinent to all headache epidemiological studies, whatever their purpose.

METHODOLOGICAL CONSIDERATIONS

Case definition

To define a case, i.e., who has headache, or who has one of the different subtypes, is problematic since the most prevalent primary headaches are all diagnosed on the basis of purely subjective experiences, without objective signs or markers. For diagnosing the headache subtypes, the criteria published by the International Headache Society (IHS) in 1988 (Headache Classification Committee of the International Headache Society, 1988), revised in 2004 (Headache Classification Subcommittee of the International Headache Society, 2004), the International Classification of Headache Disorders, 2nd edition (ICHD-II), have provided a foundation for headache epidemiology that was lacking in earlier research. They are not very different with regard to the most prevalent primary headaches, making it meaningful to compare results obtained with studies using the two versions (Eriksen et al., 2005).

However, the way in which these criteria are interpreted and applied varies greatly between studies. The only method of making headache diagnoses which formally fulfills the diagnostic criteria is personal interview and examination by a neurologist (Olesen, 1994). This "gold-standard" method is expensive (Olesen, 1994) and has been used in only a few population studies, usually with some modifications (Rasmussen et al., 1991a; Rasmussen and Olesen, 1992a; Stewart et al., 1996; Zwart et al., 2003b; Lantéri-Minet et al., 2005; Patel et al., 2004; Lyngberg et al., 2005; Stovner et al., 2006). Expert diagnosis has the advantage of assessing unlimited coexisting headache types, diagnosing rare headache syndromes as well as secondary causes of headache (Rasmussen et al., 1991b; Rasmussen, 1995; Wittrock et al., 1996; Launer et al., 1999; Scher et al., 1999). It is a particular problem for headache epidemiology that many individuals have more than one headache type, e.g., with the gold-standard method it has been demonstrated that >90% of migraineurs also have tension-type headache (TTH) (Lyngberg et al., 2005). In the

*Correspondence to: Dr. G.C. Manzoni, Headache Centre, Department of Neuroscience, University of Parma, Parma, Italy, Tel: 39 0521 704125, Fax: 39 0521 704105, E-mail: giancamillo.manzoni@unipr.it

ICHD classification it is required that each headache occurring in the same individual gets a separate diagnosis and that secondary causes of headache are excluded. There have been different ways to handle the problem of multiple headache types in population studies. Screening instruments by lay interviewers have been shown to be accurate when the aim is to identify only the most common headache types (e.g., migraine and TTH) (Stewart et al., 1996). A "recognition-based" questionnaire has also been used for mass screening of headache in adolescents. In this technique, descriptions of migraine and TTH based on the IHS criteria were read to the pupils in connection with a clinical examination, and the pupils with recurrent headaches were then asked to indicate which headache most closely resembled their own headache (Zwart et al., 2003b).

Questionnaires to be filled in by the participants at home may be an unreliable method of diagnosing headache subtypes (Rasmussen et al., 1991a), and with this method it is probably not possible to diagnose more than the dominant or most bothersome headache disorder in each individual. Secondary causes of headache are quite uncommon in the general population (Rasmussen and Olesen, 1992a), so relatively little information is missed by omitting the examination. Hence, telephone interviews by trained interviewers may be acceptable for screening purposes.

The number of headache subtypes considered may also have a great influence on the prevalence estimates. In studies from the USA (Patel et al., 2005) and France (Lantéri-Minet et al., 2005), the 1-year prevalence of migraine nearly doubled if those fulfilling the diagnosis of probable migraine (ICHD-II 1.6) was added to those with strict migraine, i.e., fulfilling all criteria for either migraine without (ICHD-II 1.1) or with (ICHD-II 1.2) aura. In other studies, the majority of those with probable migraine are most likely considered as suffering from TTH.

The term "headache" is not defined in the ICHD classification, but one may suspect that the term may have different connotations in other languages, which may be important when the term is translated. One may also surmise that there are cultural differences in the threshold for reporting pain, which may contribute to variation in headache prevalence in different regions. In addition, it has been shown that the way questions about headache are posed can greatly influence results. For example, much higher headache prevalences will be found in answer to a neutral question ("do you have headache?") compared to questions involving some specification of headache severity ("do you suffer from headache?", "do you have severe headache?" or "do you have recurrent headaches?") (Stovner et al., 2006).

Since headaches often affect individuals during certain life phases, for many reasons it is of most interest to define the proportion of the population with a current headache problem. For this reason, in most headache epidemiological studies the participants are asked about their headache during a defined period. However, it is obvious that many tend to forget about their pain problems, and one study showed that some persons who answered negatively to a direct question on whether they had headache had relatively frequent headache when asked to keep a headache diary (Wittrock et al., 1996). This is also important when a question about headache is used to screen out non-headache sufferers before the more specific questions about the features of the various headache subtypes are posed. It has been found that those who answered "no" to the screening question about headache may nevertheless suffer from migraine, and that migraine prevalence will increase considerably after including screen-negative respondents (Launer et al., 1999).

It is likely that the quality of recall will be biased towards the most recent and severe headaches (Rasmussen, 1995). For this reason, it has been found that there is generally not much difference between, e.g., the 1-year and the 3-month period prevalences (Stovner et al., 2006). For many purposes, it is most interesting to determine the part of the population that has an active headache problem by specifying a relatively limited period prevalence, the most commonly used being the 1-year prevalence. However, recall bias probably explains the fact that the results in studies using a 1-year or 3-month period prevalences are not very different (Stovner et al., 2006), and it probably also explains the apparent paradox in one study that the lifetime prevalence of migraine decreased with increasing age (Rasmussen et al., 1991b). Lifetime prevalences are often used for severe headaches like cluster headache (CH) which are probably more readily remembered, and whose prevalence would hardly be detectable in surveys using short period prevalences. Lifetime prevalence is also the most relevant for genetic studies.

Source population, sampling, and participation

The source population, i.e., the population from which study participants are drawn, is often a country, region, or city. A representative sample may be obtained by drawing a relatively large random sample from the source population, but sometimes a stratified sampling strategy is used to ensure that the study population resembles the source population with regard to some important features such as age, gender, race, or socioeconomic status.

Representativeness of the study population is also very dependent on the participation rate, i.e., the proportion of the sampled population that actively participates in the study. Overestimation of the headache prevalence may occur if headache is the main object of the study, since headache sufferers will be more likely to participate than those without headache. Likewise, if one sex or certain age or socioeconomic groups have a higher non-participation rate than the average, this may distort the results since headache prevalence is highly dependent on these factors (Stewart et al., 1992; Scher et al., 1999; Hagen et al., 2002). A high participation rate is therefore important, but if participation is found to vary substantially by demographic characteristics, prevalence rates can be adjusted to compensate for differential participation.

Validation of method

If other methods than the gold-standard method is used, a validation study of the method should be performed by comparing the diagnoses made in the study with the diagnoses made in a subsample after interview and examination by a neurologist. Relatively few studies have been validated by this method (Laínez et al., 1994; Russell et al., 1995; Hagen et al., 2000a; Zwart et al., 2003b; Laurell et al., 2004). The validation interview should be done in close temporal proximity to the main study so that any variation is due to method and not to a change in the headache condition itself. In addition, the validation sample must be drawn from the source population and not in a clinic-based sample for example, since the latter population may differ from the general population with regard to headache type and severity, and with regard to knowledge of their headache. In different validation studies, the degree of correspondence between the main study and the validation study is usually given by the sensitivity, specificity, positive and negative predictive values, and the chance-adjusted agreement rate (kappa value) (Hagen et al., 2000a).

HEADACHE PREVALENCE

Since the biology, the causes, and the consequences may differ between migraine and TTH, most headache epidemiological studies attempt to differentiate at least between these two subtypes. Most of these studies do also report the prevalence of headache in general, which usually almost equals the sum of these disorders, or exceeds it (if more than one headache type is diagnosed in one and the same individual). Some studies only report the prevalence of headache in general, which also has certain advantages, the main one being that the intricacies related to making multiple headache diagnoses in one individual are avoided. Another is that the questionnaire or interview can be made much shorter and less time-consuming. This is particularly true for those with so-called chronic daily headache (CDH), which is not a diagnosis in the ICHD classification, but which is nevertheless a frequently used term in the scientific literature. "Chronicity" in this context is usually defined as in chronic TTH (ICHD-II), as headache occurring on more than 14 days per month during the last 3 months.

In a recent survey of all headache epidemiological studies published till the end of 2005 (Stovner et al., 2007), it was found that, for headache in general, the prevalence was on average 46% based on 35 different studies from all over the world, but the variation was immense, between 1% and 87%. The lifetime prevalence was much as expected – 64%, varying between 8% and 96% in 14 studies. For current chronic headache, the average of 10 studies was 3.4%, varying between 1.7% and 7.3%.

Prevalences related to sex, age, region, and socioeconomic status

In adults, female sex is related to a higher prevalence of headache in general (Figure 1.1) and TTH, but this tendency is much more marked for migraine (Figure 1.2). In the global survey of headache epidemiology, the average headache prevalence was 52% in women and 37% in men, but for current chronic headache the difference was much larger (4.9% and 1.9%). Among children, the prevalences of headache and migraine are similar in the two sexes (Figures 1.1 and 1.2).

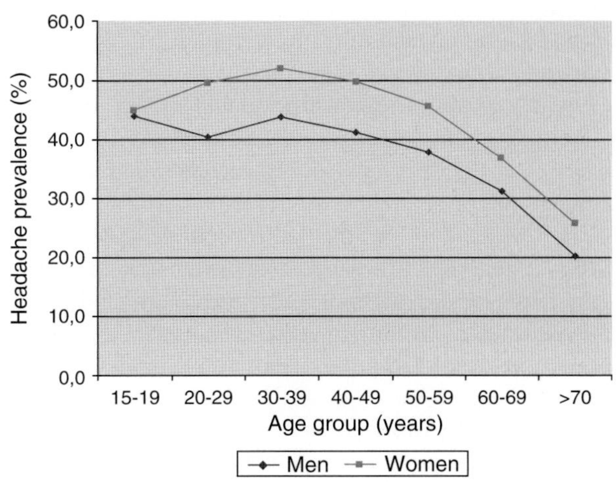

Fig. 1.1. Headache prevalence related to age in men and women. (Reproduced from Stovner et al., 2007, by courtesy of Cephalalgia.)

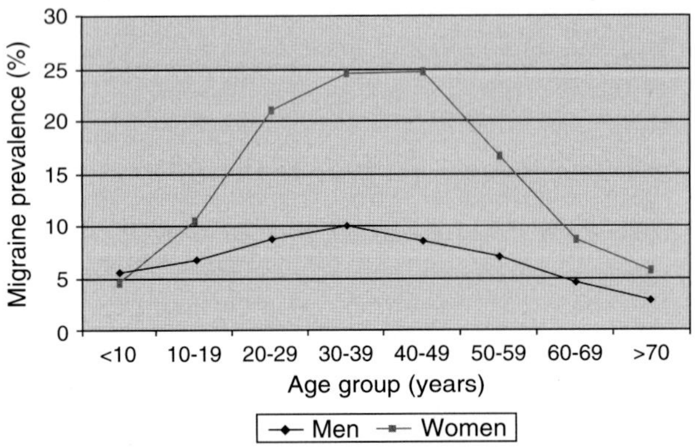

Fig. 1.2. Migraine prevalence related to age in men and women. (Reproduced from Stovner et al., 2007, by courtesy of Cephalalgia.)

There is also a clear effect of age on headache prevalence. Averaged data from three European studies showed that the prevalence in both men and women dropped markedly after the age of 60 (Figure 1.1) (Stovner et al., 2006). The effect of age is much more dramatic among women with migraine, in whom there is a dramatic increase in prevalence after puberty and a similarly dramatic decrease after menopause (Figure 1.2).

Only a few studies have addressed the effect of race on headache prevalence. In the USA, migraine seems to be most prevalent among Caucasians, followed by the African-American and Asian-American populations (Stewart et al., 1996). Non-white race also seemed to protect against chronification of the headache (Scher et al., 2003). In Singapore, the non-Chinese seemed to suffer from more severe headache and more migrainous headache than the Chinese population (Ho and Ong, 2001).

As to socioeconomic status, several studies from North America have shown that headache and migraine are more prevalent in those with lower income. This trend has been found in some, but not all, studies from Europe.

With regard to region, the global survey of headache epidemiological studies (Stovner et al., 2007) indicated that the prevalence of current headache and current migraine was lower in Africa (21% and 5% respectively) than in the other continents (Central/South America: 40% and 9%; Asia: 47% and 9%; Australia: 50%, migraine not investigated; Europe: 53% and 15%; North America: 54% and 13%) (Scher et al., 1999). For TTH, data from Africa and Australia/Oceania are lacking, and the studies are so few that comparisons between continents seem futile. A meta-analysis of headache and migraine epidemiological studies published in 1999 showed that geographic location was the most important variable accounting for age- and gender-specific estimates for migraine prevalences, and that female gender was a more important determinant of migraine than of headache in general (Scher et al., 1999).

EPIDEMIOLOGY OF DIFFERENT HEADACHE DISORDERS

In epidemiology, the way the cases are defined will have a great influence on the prevalence figures. Hence, in the following review, only studies that have used the ICHD-I or ICHD-II criteria will be considered. In addition, we have included only studies of a supposedly representative sample of the population, i.e., mostly community-based studies, and for children and youth also school-based studies.

Epidemiology of migraine

Few studies have been published so far in the medical literature on migraine incidence. Of these, two are retrospective studies (Stewart et al., 1991; Rasmussen, 1995) and therefore carry all the limitations inherent in recall of age at migraine onset, such as telescoping, failing to report real symptoms, and incorrectly reporting symptoms not actually experienced. These retrospective studies and another study (Stang et al., 1992) conducted through the linked medical record system show incidence rates that are not much different (in the under-30 age group, about 1.5–2 per 1000 person-years for men, and about 3–6 per 1000 person-years for women). The only two longitudinal studies point to higher rates. The study conducted on people of the same age group by Breslau et al. (1996) shows a rate of 6 per 1000 person-years for men, and 24 per 1000 person-years for women, while the study by Lyngberg et al. (2005) reports a rate of 8.1 per 1000 person-years with a male-to-female ratio (M/F) of 1:6. The latter study was based on a 2001 review of 453 subjects in the Copenhagen general population who had been found free of migraine in a previous epidemiological survey conducted in 1989 (Rasmussen et al., 1991b). However, this study population belonged to a higher age group (25–64 years at the time of the first survey, and 37–76 years at the time of the second study). If we consider only subjects that in 1989 were aged 25–34, the incidence rate turns out to be 13.8 per 1000 person-years.

Studies on migraine prevalence are far more numerous. Especially after the publication in 1988 of the first edition of the IHS classification, a large number of studies have been conducted throughout the world.

Most of the studies on migraine prevalence so far have investigated migraine in general; very few have investigated migraine without aura (MO) and migraine with aura (MA) separately, and a few have considered migrainous disorder (MD) or probable migraine (PM), which the first (1988) and the second (2004) edition of the International Classification of Headache Disorders (ICHD-I, ICHD-II: Headache Classification Committee of the International Headache Society, 1988, 2004) describe, respectively, as a form of headache fulfilling all diagnostic criteria for migraine but one.

Prevalence rates for migraine in general are shown in Tables 1.1–1.3. For a more consistent case definition, only post-1988 studies are reported.

Prevalence rates for western countries are fairly homogeneous. Most studies conducted in the adult general population of western Europe and North America indicate rates between 5% and 9% for men, and between 12% and 25% for women. These rates are much different from those reported by Göbel et al. (1994a) in Germany (22% for males and 32% for females). However, the German study considered as migraineurs also patients with MD.

Non-western countries report lower figures (Table 1.1). For example, in Africa's adult population, rates vary between 2% and 5% for men and between 4% and 9% for women, while in Asia they vary between 1% and 6% for men and between 4% and 13% for women. The only exception is a Korean study (Roh et al., 1998), which surprisingly shows rates higher than 20% with no significant differences between males and females. The epidemiological studies conducted in South American countries indicate widely differing rates, ranging from 2% in Chile (Lavados and Tenhamm, 1997) to 14% in Brazil (Queiroz et al., 2006) for men, and from 6% in Argentina (Morillo et al., 2005) to 29% in Brazil (Queiroz et al., 2006) for women.

Table 1.1

Studies on migraine prevalence in adults using International Headache Society modified criteria (duration of attacks between 30 min and 72 h instead of 4 h and 72 h)

Country	Reference	Time frame	Method	*n*	Age range (years)	Migraine M	Migraine F	Migraine Total
Africa								
Ethiopia	Tekle Haimanot et al. (1995)	1 year	P.i.	15 000	≥20	1.7	4.2	3.0
Nigeria	Osuntokun et al. (1982)	N.s.	P.i.	903	0–60+	4.6	8.8	6.7
Nigeria	Longe and Osuntokun (1988)	N.s.	P.i.	2925	0–99			6.3
Nigeria	Osuntokun et al. (1992)	L.t.	P.i.	18 954	0–70+	5.0	5.6	5.3
Tanzania	Dent et al. (2004)	1 year	P.i.	3351	≥11	2.5	7.0	5.0
Tunisia	Attia Romdhane et al. (1993)	N.s.	T.i.	34 874	0–100	2.5	4.5	3.4
Asia								
China	Wang et al. (1997)	1 year	P.i.	1533	≥65	0.7	4.7	3
Hong Kong	Wong et al. (1995)	N.s.	Q	2240	≥15	0.6	1.5	1
Hong Kong	Cheung (2000)	N.s.	T.i.	1436	≥15	3.0	6.2	4.7
Japan	Sakai and Igarashi (1997)	1 year	T.i.	4029	≥15	3.6	13.0	8.4
Japan	Takeshima et al. (2004)	1 year	Q	4795	≥15	2.3	9.1	6.0
Japan	Ando et al. (2007)	N.s.	Q	6470	12–15	3.3	6.5	4.8
Korea	Roh et al. (1998)	1 year	T.i.	5556	≥15	20.2	24.3	22.3
Malaysia	Alders et al. (1996)	1 year	Q	561	≥5	6.7	11.3	9
Oman	Deleu et al. (2002)	1 year	Q	1158	≥10			10.1
Singapore	Ho and Ong (2003)	L.t.	Q	2096	≥12	2.4	3.6	3.1
Taiwan	Wang et al. (2000b)	1 year	Q	3377	≥15	3.4	11.2	7.7
Europe								
Austria	Lampl et al. (2003)	1 year	P.i.	997	≥15	6.1	13.8	10.2
Croatia	Zivadinov et al. (2001)	1 year	P.i.	3794	15–65	13	20.2	16.7
Croatia	Zivadinov et al. (2001, 2003)	L.t.	P.i.	3794	15–65	14.8	22.9	19
Denmark	Rasmussen et al. (1991a)	1 year	P.i.	740	25–64	6	15	10
Denmark	Rasmussen et al. (1991b)	L.t.	P.i.	740	25–64	8	25	16.1
Denmark	Russell et al. (1995)	L.t.	Q	4061	40	12	24	18
Denmark	Lyngberg et al. (2005)	1 year	P.i.	207	25–36	5.4	23.5	15.5
Denmark	Russell et al. (2006)	1 year	Q	28 195	12–45	13.9	24.3	
France	Henry et al. (1992)	L.t.	Q	4204	5–65	6.1	17.6	12.1
France	Michel et al. (1996)	3 months	Q	9411	>18	8	18	15

(Continued)

Table 1.1

Continued

Country	Reference	Time frame	Method	*n*	Age range (years)	Migraine		
						M	F	Total
France	Henry et al. (2002)	N.s.	Q	10 585	≥15	10	23	17
France	Lantéri-Minet et al. (2005)	N.s.	Q	10 532	≥18	6.3	15.7	11.2
Germany	Göbel et al. (1994a)	L.t.	Q	4061	≥18	22	32	27.5
Germany	Fendrich et al. (2007)	3 months	Q	3324	12–15	1.6	3.5	2.6
						4.4*	9.3*	6.9*
Hungary	Bank and Marton (2000)	1 year	Q	813	15–80	2.7	6.9	9.6
Italy	Prencipe et al. (2001)	1 year	P.i.	833	≥65	7.4	13.8	11
Italy	Camarda and Monastero (2003)	1 year	P.i.	1031	≥65	2.3	6.4	4.6
Netherlands	Launer et al. (1999)	1 year	Q	6491	20–65	7.5	25	16.3
Netherlands	Launer et al. (1999)	L.t.	Q	6491	20–65	13.3	33	23.2
Norway	Hagen et al. (2000b)	1 year	Q	51 383	≥20	7.5	15.6	11.6
Serbia	Milovanović et al. (2007)	L.t.	P.i.	1259	7–12	2.1	4.6	3.3
Spain	Laínez et al. (1994)	L.t.	P.i.	2231	16–65	8	17	12
Sweden	Mattsson et al. (2000)	L.t.	Q	722	40–74		31	
Sweden	Mattsson et al. (2000b)	1 year	Q	728	40–74		18	
Sweden	Dahlöf and Linde (2001)	1 year	Q	1668	18–74	9.5	16.7	13.2
Switzerland	Merikangas et al. (1994)	1 year	P.i.	379	29–30			24.6
Turkey	Kececi and Dener (2002)	L.t.	P.i.	947	≥7	7.9	17.1	12.5
Turkey	Boru et al. (2005)	L.t	P. i	1835	15–45		15.8	
Turkey	Celik et al. (2005)	L.t.	P.i.	386	>14	9.3	29.3	19.9
Turkey	Bugdayci et al. (2005)	N.s.	P.i.	5777				10.4
Turkey	Karlı et al. (2006)	1 year	P.i.	2387	12–17			14.5
UK	Steiner et al. (2003)	1 year	T.i.	4007	16–65	7.6	18.3	14.3
North America								
Canada	Pryse-Phillips et al. (1992)	N.s.	T.i.	2737	≥15			16.2
Canada	O'Brien et al. (1994)	1 year	T.i.	2922	>18	7.4	21.9	
Canada	O'Brien et al. (1994)	L.t.	T.i.	2922	>18	7.8	24.9	17.1
USA	Stewart et al. (1992)	1 year	Q	20 468	12–80	5.7	17.6	
USA	Kryst and Scherl (1994)	1 year	T.i.	653	>20	4.5	9.8	8.5
USA	Stewart et al. (1996)	1 year	T.i.	12 328	18–65	8.9	19.0	
USA	Schwartz (1997)	1 year	T.i.	13 343	18–65			13.3
USA	Lipton et al. (2001)	1 year	Q	29 727	>12	6.2	18.2	
USA	Lipton et al. (2002)	1 year	T.i.	4804	18–65	6.0	17.2	
USA	Carson et al. (2004)	L.t.	P.i.	12 750	48–73			8
USA	Patel et al. (2004)	1 year	T.i.	8579	18–55	6.6	19.2	14.7
Central/South America								
Argentina	Morillo et al. (2005)	1 year	Q	> 500	≥15	3.8	6.1	5.0
Brazil	Wiehe et al. (2002)	L.t	P.i.	1174	≥18	10.1	22.5	16.3
Brazil	Morillo et al. (2005)	1 year	Q	> 500	≥15	7.8	17.4	12.6
Chile	Lavados and Tenhamm (1997)	1 year	Q	1385	≥15	2.0	11.9	7.3
Colombia	Morillo et al. (2005)	1 year	Q	> 500	≥15	4.8	13.8	9.3
Ecuador	Cruz et al. (1995)	N.s.	P.i.	2723	All ages	5.6	7.9	6.9
Ecuador	Morillo et al. (2005)	1 year	Q	> 500	≥15	2.9	13.5	8.2
Mexico	Morillo et al. (2005)	1 year	Q	> 500	≥15	3.9	12.1	10.0
Peru	Jaillard et al. (1997)	1 year	P.i.	3246	≥15	2.3	7.8	5.3
Puerto Rico	Miranda et al. (2003)	1 year	T.i.	1610	All ages	6.0	16.7	13.5
Venezuela	Morillo et al. (2005)	1 year	Q	> 500	≥15	4.7	12.2	8.5

Q, questionnaire; P.i., personal interview; T.i., telephone interview; L.t., lifetime; n.s., not specified.

*Modified IHS criteria.

Table 1.2

Studies on migraine prevalence in children/youths using International Headache Classification modified criteria (duration of attacks between 30 min and 72 h instead of 4 h and 72 h)

Country	Reference	Time frame	Method	*n*	Age range (years)	Migraine M	Migraine F	Migraine Total
Africa								
Nigeria	Orji and Iloeje (1997)	N.s.	Q	4398	6–13	6.4	7.2	6.8
Asia								
China	Kong et al. (2001)	1 year	Q	2120	5–16			0.5
China	Wang et al. (2005)	1 year	Q	13 426	13–15	4.9	8.9	6.8
India	Shivpuri et al. (2003)	N.s.	Q	1305	11–15	9.0	14.0	11
Taiwan	Lu et al. (2000)	L.t.	Q	4064	13–15	5.7	7.8	6.8
United Arab Emirates	Bener et al. (1998)	1 year	Q	1159	6–14			3.8
Europe								
Finland	Metsähonkala and Sillanpää (1994)	L.t.	Q	3580	8–9	3	2.3	2.7
Greece	Mavromichalis et al. (1999)	1 year	Q	3509	4–15	5.2	7.3	6.2
Italy	Raieli et al. (1995)	1 year	P.i.	1445	11–14	2.7	3.3	3.0
Sweden	Laurell et al. (2004)	1 year	Q	1850	7–15	9.8	12.2	11.0
Turkey	Zencir et al. (2004)	N.s.	Q	2490	11–18	6.7	11.0	8.8
UK	Abu-Arefeh and Russell (1994)	1 year	Q	2165	5–15	9.7	11.5	10.6
Central/South America								
Brazil	Barea et al. (1996)	1 year	P.i.	538	10–18	9.6	10.3	9.9

N.s., not specified; Q, questionnaire; L.t., lifetime; P.i., personal interview.

Table 1.3

Studies on migraine prevalence in the elderly using International Headache Society modified criteria (duration of attacks between 30 min and 72 h instead of 4 h and 72 h)

Country	Reference	Time frame	Method	*n*	Age range (years)	Migraine M	Migraine F	Migraine Total
Asia								
China	Wang et al. (1997)	1 year	P.i.	1533	>65	0.7	4.7	3
Europe								
Italy	Prencipe et al. (2001)	1 year	P.i.	833	≥65	7.4	13.8	11
Italy	Camarda and Monastero (2003)	1 year	P.i.	1031	≥65	2.3	6.4	4.6

P.i., personal interview.

Even though worldwide differences in migraine prevalence may be due to methodological considerations, it cannot be ruled out that cultural and environmental factors may play a role.

Still unclear is the role, if any, played in migraine prevalence by the sociocultural background and the economic status of the subjects studied.

The results of a study conducted by Stewart et al. (1996) suggest that race-related differences in genetic vulnerability to migraine may also be important. Indeed, migraine prevalence seems to be higher among Caucasians, followed by African-Americans and Asian-Americans in Baltimore county, Maryland.

As regards sociocultural background, classical medical literature reports a higher prevalence of migraine in subjects with a higher level of education. In 1992 Stewart and Lipton's group reported just the opposite (Stewart et al., 1992), but in 2002 they no longer found any such difference (Lipton et al., 2002).

With respect to economic status, the American Migraine Study (Stewart et al., 1992) demonstrated that the prevalence of migraine increased as household income decreased, but no such correlation was found in studies conducted in Denmark (Rasmussen, 1992), Germany (Koehler et al., 1992), France (Henry et al., 1992), and Canada (O'Brien et al., 1994), nor in two other later USA studies (Kryst and Scherl, 1994; Lipton et al., 2002).

A number of studies on migraine prevalence have been conducted on populations of children and adolescents (Table 1.2), but they were mostly concentrated in Europe and Asia. Only two studies of this kind (one each) were ever conducted in Africa and South America, in Nigeria (Orji and Iloeje, 1997) and Brazil (Barea et al., 1996), respectively. Oddly enough, there is no such study for North America.

In Europe, prevalence rates in those under 18 years of age vary according to the different age groups of the study population. Among comparable age groups, there seem to be higher rates in northern countries – around 10–11% in England (Abu-Arefeh and Russell, 1994) and Sweden (Laurell et al., 2004 – than in southern countries – around 3–6% in Italy (Raieli et al., 1995) and Greece (Mavromichalis et al., 1999).

In Asia, if we do not consider the two values at the extremes of the range, i.e., 0.5% reported in China by Kong et al. in 2001 and 11% found in India by Shivpuri et al. in 2003, the rates are fairly homogeneous and vary between 3.8% and 6.8% (Table 1.2).

On average, the predominance of the female gender is less marked in young people than in adults. In the lower age groups, there is even a slight male predominance; thus, for example, in a 1994 survey of 7–8-year-old Finnish children, Metsähonkala and Sillanpää found a lifetime migraine prevalence of 3.0% in males and of 2.3% in females.

It is well known that migraine prevalence rates tend to decrease after age 50 (Figure 1.2).

The studies specially conceived to investigate migraine prevalence in the elderly are very few, though. The rates found in a study conducted in China (Wang et al., 1997) and in two other studies carried out in Italy (Prencipe et al., 2001; Camarda and Monastero, 2003) do not differ much from those reported for children.

It is very important to make as clear as possible the question as to whether or not the epidemiological data currently available can be considered reliable and, therefore, definitive.

Indeed, the availability of reliable data about prevalence is important, not only *per se*, but also as a starting point to be taken as reference for studies on the risk running in families and on the risk of developing other diseases, as well as for studies on the social and economic impact of migraine. If today epidemiological research could not provide unquestionable evidence supporting migraine prevalence rates, studies on clinical genetics, comorbidity, and disability would lack a viable basis.

In this regard, three elements can be inferred from an analysis of the various prevalence studies. These elements are prevalence of MA, prevalence of MD (1.6 ICHD-I: Headache Classification Committee of the International Headache Society, 1988) or PM (1.8 ICHD-II: Headache Classification Committee of the International Headache Society, 2004), and the frequency of migraine attacks.

If we analyze post-1988 prevalence studies of MA in the general population, we find that prevalence rates are fairly comparable, varying from 1% to 4% in men and from 3% to 10% in women (Rasmussen et al., 1991b; Sakai and Igarashi, 1997; Launer et al., 1999; Bank and Marton, 2000; Mattsson et al., 2000; Dahlöf and Linde, 2001; Zivadinov et al., 2001; Kececi and Dener, 2002; Lipton et al., 2002). However, these percentage figures are definitely, and rather surprisingly, higher than those reported in pre-1988 studies.

According to these figures, about one-third of migraineurs suffer from MA. In other words, for every 2 patients with MO there seems to be 1 with MA. Rasmussen and Olesen (1992b) report that this ratio would even be close to 1:1. These figures are fairly consistent among the different authors, but, if we proceed to examine the results of the studies that considered migraine prevalence rates separately for MO, MA, and the coexistence of MA and MO, we find differences that may be very marked. Indeed, only 13% of subjects with MA studied by Rasmussen and Olesen (1992b) versus as many as 58% of the subjects with MA studied by Lipton et al. (2002) also suffered from MO.

To try to assess how reliable prevalence data on MA can be, it could be useful to evaluate the methods used by authors. Only four (Rasmussen et al., 1991b; Bank and Marton, 2000; Zivadinov et al., 2001; Kececi and Dener, 2002) of the post-1988 studies reported in the literature comply strictly with the IHS diagnostic criteria, while the others (Stewart et al., 1996; Launer et al., 1999; Mattsson et al., 2000; Lipton et al., 2002) introduce substantial changes to those criteria with the aim – clearly stated by the authors themselves – of increasing their validity. In this connection, it is interesting to note what Sakai and Igarashi (1997) state in their report: "Diagnosis of aura based on the IHS criteria was difficult in our questionnaire study because a significant number of answers to the question about aura symptoms were not sufficiently clear to determine whether they were truly indicative of 'focal cerebral dysfunction' as defined by the IHS criteria."

For that reason, when they had to analyze the subjects' answers to the mail questionnaire strictly based on the 1988 IHS criteria, these authors chose to consider as MA sufferers only those patients whose headache phase had the same characteristics as MO. Unfortunately, this occurs only in a proportion that varies between a little over one-third of MA cases, as Mattsson et al. (2000) showed in a Swedish study, and about half the cases, as found by Eriksen et al. (2005) in a Danish clinical case series of 362 MA patients evaluated by applying the 2004 ICHD-II diagnostic criteria.

The findings by Henry et al. (1992, 2002) appear to raise further, more serious, reservations about the validity of IHS criteria for MA in prevalence studies in the general population. Both in their first epidemiological study of the French general population published in 1992 and in a similar study published in 2002, Henry et al. applied the 1988 IHS diagnostic criteria for MO and for MA. Nonetheless, the authors stated: "No attempt was made to divide cases into those with and those without aura as this differentiation was found by the validation study to be non-reliable, because migraine sufferers often cannot distinguish unilateral sensory disturbances from nocturnal acroparesthesia, and scintillating scotoma from photophobia."

The 1988 IHS diagnostic criteria for MA are not only difficult to translate for use in a questionnaire or an interview, but they are also too loose. Indeed, if these criteria were applied strictly, what about people who report a few scintillating scotomas or paresthesias lasting as little as a few seconds (the 1988 IHS classification does not indicate any low-end limit for aura duration), who perhaps experience these scotomas during the headache phase and not before it (the 1988 IHS classification does not exclude this possibility at point 4), and who have a headache without the characteristics typical of the migraine form (the 1988 IHS classification contains no reference to the characteristics of the headache phase)? Well, these people would be coded to the MA group, but this is wrong from the clinical viewpoint. The resulting risk is that the prevalence of MA may be overestimated in an epidemiological study.

The changes introduced by the 2004 ICHD-II to the diagnostic criteria for MA of the 1988 ICHD-I are certainly welcome, but their use in future epidemiological studies will help overcome only two of the three major obstacles encountered so far: the indication that aura should last a minimum of 5 min, which makes it possible to exclude patients with MA attacks accompanied by visual symptoms lasting only a few seconds; and the possible presence of a typical aura with non-migraine headache (point 1.2.2). However, perhaps even more so than ICHD-I, ICHD-II does not address the difficult question of how to describe the focal neurological symptoms typical of this type of migraine – as listed in the diagnostic criteria of ICHD-II – using terms that can be easily understood by subjects studied through a questionnaire in an epidemiological survey.

No studies on MA prevalence have ever been published after the publication of ICHD-II. For that reason and for the above considerations, the only rates that can be taken as reference are those of the 1991 Danish study (5.1% in women and 3.7% in men), which used the method of the direct examination of subjects (Rasmussen et al., 1991b). However, further studies are needed to confirm these data.

In MD and PM, there is even greater discordance than in MA (Henry et al., 1992, 2002; Göbel et al., 1994b; Russell et al., 1995). In studies conducted by applying the diagnostic criteria of the 1998 ICHD-I, 1-year prevalence rates for MD vary from 16.2%, as reported by Göbel et al. (1994b) in the German population over 18 years of age, to 1.4%, as reported by Russell et al. (1995) the following year in the Danish population aged 40, and up to 18.2%, as reported by Queiroz et al. in a 2000 study of the Brazilian population published in 2006. More recent studies, conducted using the 2004 ICHD-II diagnostic criteria, indicate PM prevalence rates that are just as variable, ranging from a 3-month prevalence of 12.6% among adolescents aged 12–15 years in Germany (Fendrich et al., 2007) and from a 1-year prevalence of 14.6% in a USA population of over-18 adults (Bigal et al., 2006), to a 1-year prevalence as low as 4.5% in another USA population aged over 12 (Silberstein et al., 2007). In the latter study, PM prevalence was significantly higher in African-Americans than in whites (7.4% versus 4.8% for females; 4.8% versus 3.7% for males) and inversely related to household income.

Other differences that can hardly be explained are found in the frequency of migraine attacks. These appear to occur once or more than once a month in very few cases (16%) in the Danish study (Rasmussen et al., 1991b), in most cases (between 60% and 63%) in various USA studies (Stewart and Lipton, 1994; Lipton et al., 2001, 2002), and in all or almost all cases in studies conducted in France (83%) (Henry et al., 1992), Hungary (100%) (Bank and Marton, 2000), and Turkey (90%) (Kececi and Dener, 2002). What appears most striking is that there are marked differences also in studies – such as the Danish study (Rasmussen et al., 1991b) compared with the USA studies (Stewart and Lipton, 1994; Lipton et al., 2001, 2002) – that report very comparable migraine prevalence rates (Table 1.1).

A review of the existing literature on migraine prevalence points to the conclusion that currently available data on the prevalence of migraine in general, on the gender ratio, and on the variations in prevalence in the different age ranges, can be regarded as very close to reality. Conversely, much less close to reality may be data on the prevalence of the different migraine subtypes.

Epidemiology of tension-type headache

Compared to migraine, relatively few studies have been performed on TTH; the majority of these studies are from Europe (9/17), but some are also from the Americas, and East and South Asia (Table 1.4). There is a large variation in prevalence, from 11.5% lifetime prevalence in Singapore to an almost eight times higher 86.5% 1-year prevalence in Denmark. However, in the former study the figure is almost four times higher (42%) if TTH not fulfilling all criteria is also counted. It is noticeable that the highest figures are found in studies where a personal interview has been employed, in countries as different as Brazil and Denmark. This probably indicates that the prevalence of this headache type is particularly sensitive to the method of data collection, possibly because the recall of a minor headache problem is much easier to elicit by a personal interview than by a questionnaire or even telephone interview. The variation in prevalence between studies of the most severe form, chronic TTH, is somewhat less, but nevertheless quite considerable.

Epidemiology of cluster headache

Even if CH has very distinctive clinical features, there are very few data available on CH epidemiology, in particular in the general population. The reasons that may explain why epidemiological studies on CH are so few probably have to do with its low frequency. When a disease is fairly rare, for a variety of reasons it does not raise interest among private and public sponsors. In addition, a fairly rare disease presents investigators with methodological problems in epidemiological studies, mainly due to the need to investigate very large samples that are representative of the general population.

Prevalence in the general population

Six studies have been conducted to date on CH prevalence in the general population (Table 1.5). Ekbom et al. (1978) investigated a sample of 10 400 18-year-old men, who were seen by a doctor for their pre-draft physical examination between October 1975 and May 1976. During the month preceding the mandatory medical visit for military recruitment, the young men received a questionnaire that they had to fill in and send back within a week. Overall, 9610 subjects (92.4%) sent back the first questionnaire. Those who did not reply to the questionnaire were nonetheless investigated for the presence of headache during the medical visit. Data were collected for a total of 9803 subjects. The diagnostic criteria applied for CH diagnosis were those set up by Ekbom himself a few years earlier (Ekbom, 1970). Among the 436 subjects with recurrent headache, 9 fulfilled the diagnostic criteria for CH – including 8 with episodic CH and 1 with chronic CH – and their diagnosis was confirmed through a direct interview. The estimated lifetime prevalence was 90/100 000. The method used by the authors was such that CH cases could not be easily missed; realistically, the 90/100 000 prevalence rate in males of that age is very close to the present one.

However reliable this figure is, though, it cannot be made to apply to the general population, when one considers that only 20% of patients in large case series (Kudrow, 1980; Manzoni et al., 1983) developed CH in the first and second decade of life. The prevalence rate found in the San Marino studies in a population of over 20 000 inhabitants was 56–69/100 000 (D'Alessandro et al., 1986; Tonon et al., 2002) – remarkably lower than that calculated in the studies conducted in Italy, Norway, and Sweden (Sjaastad and Bakketeig, 2003; Torelli et al., 2005b; Ekbom et al., 2006). The San Marino authors used four different methods to identify suspected sufferers, namely: (1) they reviewed all clinical records of patients seen in the 15 years preceding the study by the neurologists, ophthalmologists, and ear, nose, and throat specialists practicing in San Marino; (2) they asked all 15 San Marino general practitioners (GPs) to indicate how many of their patients had CH; (3) they mailed all San Marino inhabitants a circular letter illustrating the features of CH and asking those who thought they had experienced a similar headache to call the study center; (4) they reviewed the clinical records of San Marino citizens who sought treatment at the University Headache Center in nearby Bologna, the nearest referral center to San Marino. A total of 15 CH cases (14 men and 1 woman) were detected in the first study (D'Alessandro et al., 1986) and another 15 cases (all male) in the second study (Tonon et al., 2002). Analyzing the distribution of detected CH cases with respect to the different detection methods, it appears that the most effective method by far was the review of the clinical records of the San Marino neurologists. The suspicion that

Table 1.4

Studies on the prevalence of tension-type headache (TTH)

Country	Reference	Time frame	Method	*n*	Age range (years)	TTH M	TTH F	TTH Total	Chronic TTH M	Chronic TTH F	Chronic TTH Total
ADULTS											
Asia											
Japan	Takeshima et al. (2004)	1 year	Q	4795	≥15	16.2	26.4	21.7	1.5	2.1	1.8
Malaysia	Alders et al. (1996)	1 year	Q	561	≥5	23.3	29.6	26.5			1.5
Singapore	Ho and Ong (2003)	L.t.	Q	2096	≥12	11.1	11.8	11.5	0.9	1.8	1.4
Europe											
Croatia	Zivadinov et al. (2001, 2003)	L.t.	P.i.	3794	15–65	32.3	37.1	34.8			
Denmark	Rasmussen et al. (1991b)	1 year	P.i.	740	25–64	63	86	74			
Denmark	Rasmussen et al. (1991b)	L.t.	P.i.	740	25–64	69	88	78			3.0
Denmark	Lyngberg et al. (2005)	1 year	P.i.	207	25–36	81.5	90.4	86.5			4.8
Denmark	Russell et al. (2006)	1 year	Q	28 195	12–45	78.9	92.5	86.0	0.5	1.3	0.9
Germany	Göbel et al. (1994a)	L.t.	Q	4061	≥18	37	39	38	3.0	3.0	3.0
Turkey	Koseoglu et al. (2003)	1 year	P.i.	1146	45–64		18.8				6.3
North America											
Canada	Pryse-Phillips et al. (1992)	N.s.	T.i.	2737	≥15			20.4			
USA	Schwartz et al. (1998)	1 year	T.i.	13 345	18–65	37.7	44.8	40.3	1.4	2.8	2.2
Central/South America											
Brazil	Wiehe et al. (2002)	L.t	P.i.	1174	≥18	61.5	70.9	66.2	5.2	9.3	6.8
Chile	Lavados and Tenhamm (1998)	1 year	Q	1385	≥15	18.1	35.2	26.9	1.1	3.9	2.6
CHILDREN/YOUTH											
Asia											
Taiwan	Wang et al. (2006)	1 year	P.i.	7900	12–14						1.0*
Europe											
Germany	Fendrich et al. (2007)	3 months	Q	3324	12–15	4.6	4.3	4.5	0.1	0.2	0.2
Norway	Zwart et al. (2004)	1 year	Q	8255	13–19	12.5	23.2	18.0			
Serbia	Milovanović et al. (2007)	L.t.	P.i.	1259	7–12	0.9	1.7	1.3			
Sweden	Laurell et al. (2004)	1 year	Q	1850	7–15	7.9	11.8	9.8			
Turkey	Bugdayci et al. (2005)	N.s.	P.i.	5777	8–16			24.7			1.5
Turkey	Karlı et al. (2006)	1 year	P.i.	2387	12–17			26.4			1.7
Central/South America											
Brazil	Barea et al. (1996)	1 year	P.i.	538	10–18	68.3	76.7	72.3			

*Chronic or probable chronic tension-type headache (CTTH).

Table 1.5

Cluster headache prevalence: studies conducted in the general population

Author	Year	Sample (*n*)	Age	Sex	Cluster headache cases (*n*)	Prevalence *n*/100 000 (95% CI)
Ekbom et al.	1978	9803	18 years	Male	9	90 (42–174)
D'Alessandro et al.	1986	21 792	All ages	Both	15	69 (39–114)
Tonon et al.	2002	26 628	All ages	Both	15	56 (31.3–92.4)
Sjaastad and Bakketeig	2003	1838	18–65 years	Both	6	326 (153–783)
Torelli et al.	2005b	10 071	> 14 years	Both	21	279 (173–427)
Ekbom et al.	2006	31 750	41–67 years	Both	48	151 (108–194)

CI: confidence interval.

the investigators may have missed a considerable number of cases arises from the following considerations: (1) it is simply not possible that nearly all subjects with CH in the general population were seen by a neurologist; (2) it is very odd that only 1 woman with CH – in a chronic form, no less – was found in the first study and no woman at all out of a total of 13 000 women was found in the second study; (3) the thorough screening of the population was done using a method – sending a letter to all inhabitants – that was as unreliable as it was deceptive. The San Marino studies merely indicate a CH prevalence rate in the general population of at least 56–69/100 000, but, based on the above considerations, this figure may be much lower than expected.

In an extensive epidemiological study conducted on the population of a small Norwegian county, the authors investigated a sample of 2065 dalesmen aged 18–65, living in Vågå county (Sjaastad and Bakketeig, 2003). Of them, 1838 (88.6%) were interviewed through a specially designed face-to-face questionnaire. Headache diagnosis was established according to the criteria of the first edition of the IHS classification. The survey enabled investigators to identify 6 subjects with CH (1 woman and 5 men), indicating a lifetime prevalence rate of 326/100 000 (558/100 000 in men and 106/100 000 in women). The study was accurate, but it was conducted in a limited sample.

Torelli et al. (2005b) calculated CH lifetime prevalence in a sample representative of the Italian general population aged over 14 years. "Possible CH" cases according to the 1988 IHS classification diagnostic criteria were investigated in 10 071 patients of seven GPs in the city of Parma using a previously validated, specially designed self-questionnaire. A total of 7522 people (74.7%) responded to the questionnaire in their GP's office ($n = 3338$) or at home by mail ($n = 1914$) or by phone ($n = 2270$). Of the 111 identified "suspected cases," 105 were seen by a neurologist and 6 were contacted by telephone. The diagnosis of CH was confirmed in 21 (9 female and 12 male). The lifetime prevalence rate (279/100 000, 95% confidence interval (CI) 173–427) found in this study for an over-14 population seems a reliable figure, for the following reasons: the initial sample was large and representative enough of the Parma general population aged over 14; the 74.7% rate of responders allows for results that are truly representative of the entire population; the questionnaire used for population screening had been validated and proved reliable in detecting cases with suspected CH (Torelli et al., 2005a); and the final diagnosis of CH was made according to the IHS criteria using a direct interview by a headache neurologist. Moreover, several studies conducted on large case series have shown that onset of CH is not frequent under 14 years of age.

Ekbom et al. (2006) calculated the lifetime prevalence of CH in a twin sample representative of the Swedish general population. The authors assessed CH as defined by the ICHD-II (2004) in 31 750 registered twins born from 1935 to 1958. Structured lay screening interviews were followed by neurologist interviews of possible cases. Co-twins of affected index twins were follow-up interviewed regardless of their screening outcome. A total of 250 screen-positives (0.8%) were found, of which 218 (88%) were follow-up interviewed. Forty-five (21%) had the CH diagnosis verified. Among screen-negatives, hospitalization records pointed to two more verified cases and index twins to one more verified case. A total of 48 CH cases provided a crude lifetime prevalence of 151 per 100 000 (95% CI: 108–194), indicating that as many as 1 per 500 of the general population is affected by CH.

Incidence

So far, only three studies have evaluated the incidence of CH in the general population (Swanson et al., 1994; Tonon et al., 2002; Black et al., 2005). In two American studies, the incidence of medically recognized CH within Olmsted county, Minnesota (from 1979 through 1981 and from 1989 through 1990), was determined by using modified IHS criteria. The overall age- and sex-adjusted incidence decreased from 9.8/100 000 person-years in 1979–1981 to 2.07/100 000 person-years in 1989–1990. In the San Marino study – the first prospective survey on the incidence of CH – the incidence rate was comparable to that calculated in 2005 in Minnesota (2.5/100 000/year).

Gender Ratio

CH is a disease that occurs more frequently in men than in women. The higher prevalence of CH in males has been demonstrated by several studies conducted on large patient samples (Kudrow, 1980; Ekbom and Waldenlind, 1981; Manzoni et al., 1988). The markedly higher prevalence of CH in males is even more apparent in chronic CH versus episodic CH. In his case series of 425 patients, Kudrow (1980) found a gender ratio of 4.8:1 for episodic CH and of 6.3:1 for chronic CH. This finding was confirmed by Manzoni et al. (1983), who reported a higher prevalence of males among chronic CH sufferers. Manzoni (1998) investigated changes in the M/F ratio of CH over the years through a comparative analysis of the distribution of the disease by sex and decade of onset in 482 patients. The M/F ratio has fallen from 6.2:1 for patients with CH onset before 1960, to 5.6:1, 4.3:1, 3.0:1, and 2.1:1 for patients with CH onset in the 1960s, 1970s, 1980s, and 1990s, respectively. Correspondingly, the M/F ratio has fallen from 2.6:1 to 2.4:1, 2.2:1, and 1.7:1 for the employment rate, and from 8.6:1 to 7.8:1, 3.3:1, 2.5:1, and 1.9:1 for the smoking habit, respectively. Such a close correlation suggests that the significant changes that have occurred over the last few decades in the lifestyle of both sexes – particularly women – may have played a major role in altering the gender ratio of CH. These data were confirmed by Ekbom et al. (2002) in a sample of 554 patients.

Epidemiology of other primary headaches

To date, there are very few epidemiological data on the eight clinical entities listed in this chapter of the 2004 ICHD-II.

Here is an overview of what the literature reports about their prevalence in the general population.

For primary stabbing headache, Rasmussen (1995), in an important epidemiological survey conducted on 740 subjects from the Copenhagen, Denmark, general population, found a prevalence rate of 2%. By contrast, Monteiro (1995) reported a rate as low as 0.2% in Portugal's population.

More recently, Sjaastad et al. (2001) found a lifetime prevalence rate of 35.2% in 1838 adults (aged 18–65) living in the Norwegian fjord area of Vågå (an F/M ratio of 1.49).

This is obviously a huge difference, but a close scrutiny of the methodologies used, and especially of the original working hypotheses of the different studies, reveals that the Norwegian rate is more reliable.

While there are no sure data in the literature about the prevalence of primary cough headache (coded as 4.2 of ICHD-II) and of primary headache associated with sexual activity (coded as 4.4 of ICHD-II), we do have reliable population-based data for primary exertional headache (coded as 4.3 of ICHD-II). Sjaastad and Bakketeig (2002) found a 12.3% prevalence rate for this form of headache in the same Norwegian population studied by their fellow authors (an F/M ratio of 1.38).

The literature does not offer any indications about the prevalence of hypnic headache (coded as 4.5 of ICHD-II) in the general population. This is considered a rare condition today. At the Headache Division of the Mayo Clinic in Rochester (USA), only 0.07% of all patients suffer from it (Dodick et al., 1998). At the headache outpatient clinic of Münster University (Germany), Evers et al. (2003) reported 4 cases of hypnic headache, accounting for 0.1% of all patients seen over a 4-year period.

The F/M ratio in 71 cases studied in a literature review by Evers and Goadsby in 2003 was 1.7/1.

For primary thunderclap headache (coded as 4.6 of ICHD-II), too, there are no prevalence data yet for the general population. A survey conducted in the general practice of 252 GPs in the USA over 5 years may give a vague idea of its frequency (Linn et al., 1999): 93 cases of idiopathic thunderclap headache were 93 of 1 800 000 patients seen every year, i.e., about 1 case in 100 000. Therefore, even though its prevalence is not known with certainty, there is no doubt that primary thunderclap headache is a very rare clinical entity.

Hemicrania continua (coded as 4.7 of ICHD-II) was investigated by Castillo et al. in an epidemiological survey conducted in Spain in 1999 in order to detect the presence of the various CH forms in the general population. The authors found no cases of hemicrania continua in the 1833 subjects under study. On the other hand, Peres et al. (2001) claimed that hemicrania continua is not so rare. Their assumption has recently been corroborated by evidence from Norwegian studies

(Sjaastad and Bakketeig, 2007) reporting 18 cases (11 women and 7 men) out of 1838 subjects aged 18–65 years, with a prevalence rate of about 1%.

Lastly, for new daily persistent headache (coded as 4.8 of ICHD-II), the only evidence available for the general population (Castillo et al., 1999) suggests a prevalence rate around 1‰ (2 cases out of 1883 subjects), although this should be considered a conservative estimate given the small size of the sample studied.

As regards other primary headaches (coded as 4 of ICHD-II), while there is no indication that may lead to any reliable estimates about the prevalence rates of primary cough headache and primary headache associated with sexual activity, the sparse data in the literature suggest that primary stabbing headache and primary exertional headache are rather frequent, whereas hypnic headache, primary thunderclap headache, hemicrania continua, and new daily persistent headache are rare or very rare.

Epidemiology of chronic daily headache

About a quarter-century ago, more or less simultaneously in different parts of the world, Mathew et al. (1982), Nappi and Savoldi (1985) and Sjaastad (1985) became intrigued with the large number of headache clinic patients who had been reporting headache attacks every day or almost every day for many months or even many years on end. To describe these patients, they introduced the term "chronic daily headache."

In spite of the fact that a long time has passed from that first description and a huge amount of literature has been published on this subject, there is no consensus yet on how to classify this form of headache and whether to recognize it as an autonomous entity hence, the difficulties encountered in the systematic organization of the different CDH subtypes within the framework of ICHD-II (Headache Classification Subcommittee of the International Headache Society, 2004).

Before dealing briefly with CDH prevalence, we should first recapitulate the characteristics of this disorder on which all investigators agree: (1) it is a primary headache; (2) often it represents an evolution over time of migraine without aura, which worsens to the point that there are no longer any symptom-free intervals between attacks; and (3) it is often associated with symptomatic drug overuse. On the other hand, there is no agreement as yet on: (1) how many days per month the headache must be present in order for a CDH diagnosis to be made; (2) how many months the patient must have been suffering from it; and, (3) the number and type of clinical entities that constitute it. Certainly, chronic TTH is part of CDH.

Today we have some interesting epidemiological data to rely on, especially for CDH prevalence in the general population.

Oddly enough, despite the methodological inconsistencies of the various epidemiological studies conducted so far, which are obviously the result of different investigational approaches, prevalence rates are fairly comparable, suggesting that about 4% of the adult population suffers from CDH.

Scher et al. (1998) found a prevalence rate of 4.1% in a US population of 13 343 subjects aged 18–65 years, Castillo et al. (1999) a rate of 4.7% in a Spanish population of 1883 subjects over 14 years of age, Hagen et al. (2000b) a rate of 2.4% in 51 383 Norwegian adults over 20, Lantéri-Minet et al. (2003) a rate of 3.0% in a French population of 10 585 subjects over 15, and Wiendels et al. (2006) a rate of 3.7% in a Dutch population of 16 232 subjects aged 25–55 years.

Data about eastern populations are fairly similar. Two studies, conducted on 3377 Taiwanese over 15 (Lu et al., 2001) and on 2096 Singaporeans over 12 (Ho and Ong, 2001), showed rates of 3.2% and 3.3%, respectively.

Through the various studies, women appear to be affected about 2½ times as much as men: the F/M ratio varies from a minimum of 1.6 (Hagen et al., 2002) to a maximum of 2.6 (Lantéri-Minet et al., 2003). The only remarkable evidence to the contrary was reported by Castillo et al. (1999), who found a gender ratio of 8.7.

A recent Brazilian study (Queiroz et al., 2006) conducted on 625 subjects aged 15–64 showed a higher CDH prevalence than in previous studies: 6.4% (10.1% in women and 2.1% in men).

Analgesic overuse was found in 25–34% of CDH patients (Castillo et al. 1999; Lu et al., 2001 respectively).

CDH is also frequent in adolescents. Wang et al. (2006) found a prevalence rate of 1.5% (three times as high in women as in men) among 7900 Taiwanese students aged 12–14.

Prevalence rates in the elderly are fairly similar to those in middle-aged adults. Wang et al. (2000) reported a 3.9% rate among 1533 Chinese over 65 (F/M ratio of 3.1), while Prencipe et al. (2001) found a rate of 4.4% in 833 65-plus Italians (F/M ratio of 2.4).

Epidemiology of secondary headaches

For these headaches, defined in chapters 4–11 of the ICHD-II, even less is known about the prevalence compared to the primary headaches. Furthermore, almost nothing is known about important features such as their frequency, intensity, duration, and consequences for functioning on a population scale, so that the contribution of these headaches to the total headache burden can be estimated. In a Danish population-based study (Rasmussen and Olesen, 1992a), hangover and fever headache were by far the most common secondary headaches, with a lifetime prevalence of 72% and 63%, respectively, followed by headache related to metabolic disorders (mostly due to fasting without hypoglycemia), disorders of the nose and sinuses (15%), head trauma (4%), use of substances and their withdrawal, excluding hangover 3%, eye disorders 3%, and vascular disorders and disorders of the neck 1% each, and non-vascular intracranial disorders 0.5%. Since these figures are lifetime prevalences, and the study contains no data on frequency or duration of the headaches, some of them possibly being single occurrences, the study gives no indication of the total headache burden caused by these disorders.

A main obstacle in determining the prevalence of the secondary headaches is that they are not usually defined on the basis of special headache features; in fact, for most of them special features are lacking. In general, the diagnosis is based on the demonstration that: (1) the patient has headache; (2) some disorder is known to be able to cause headache; (3) headache occurs in close temporal relationship to the other disorder, or there is other evidence of causal relationship; and (4) headache is greatly reduced or disappears after successful treatment or spontaneous remission of the causative disorder. These criteria may function reasonably well in the clinic, where a thorough clinical interview and examination, aided by ancillary investigations, treatment, and follow-up may give relatively clear evidence for an underlying cause or condition. A similar approach is virtually impossible in population-based studies of some size. Using less rigorous criteria for the diagnosis, e.g., by just asking individuals about causes of their headache, may reflect widespread beliefs among patients and possibly their doctors about headache causation rather than the real prevalence of secondary headaches. For example, in a large headache epidemiological study in the USA, approximately 40% of ICHD-I-defined migraineurs indicated that they had received a physician diagnosis of sinus headache, a disorder that is believed to be greatly overdiagnosed in the USA, often in cases that more correctly should be diagnosed as migraine (Diamond, 2002).

Since the diagnosis of secondary headaches usually requires a proper work-up and follow-up, which is usually lacking in population-based epidemiological studies, some studies report the prevalences of a "possible secondary headache," i.e., where the causative agent and the headache are present, but where other confirmatory evidence is lacking. One example is medication overuse headache (ICHD-II 8.2). In population-based studies, it has been demonstrated that approximately 1% of the adult population (Castillo et al., 1999; Zwart et al., 2003a; Colás et al., 2004), and somewhat less than 0.5% of adolescents (Dyb et al., 2006; Wang et al., 2006) have headache $\geq$ 15 days per month and medication overuse; hence they are possibly suffering from medication overuse headache. However, in none of these studies has it been possible to verify that worsening of headache developed in connection with the medication overuse, and that the headache resolves or reverts to the previous pattern within 2 months after discontinuation of acute medicines, so these figures are obviously maximal for the prevalence of this disorder.

Whereas robust knowledge about the prevalence of the secondary headaches is mostly lacking, there are quite good epidemiological data on some of the more well-defined underlying disorders, and there are also several patient-based studies reporting the proportion with the underlying disorder that will develop headache. For example, the annual incidence of temporal arteritis is 3–9 cases per 100 000 (Hauser et al., 1971; Bengtsson and Malmvall, 1982), and of subarachnoid hemorrhage 11%, with 90% of patients having headache (van Gijn and Rinkel, 2001). For carotid artery dissection the annual incidence is around 3 per 100 000, with 65–90% having pain. For these and many other secondary headaches, the causal relation between the headache and the underlying disorder is quite evident and unequivocal, and it is relatively easy to demonstrate the underlying disorder, but most of the morbidity is not related to the headache *per se* but rather to other complications of the underlying disorder. In addition, these disorders are very rare compared to the primary headaches, so their contribution to the total headache burden of the population is probably minimal.

Some of the alleged causes of headache mentioned in the ICHD-II are very prevalent, and could contribute considerably to the total headache burden. However, for some secondary headaches the causal relation is far from firmly established, a fact that is acknowledged in the ICHD-II classification where it is generally stated that the headache is "attributed to" the other disorder (Headache Classification Subcommittee of the International Headache Society, 2004). For some secondary headaches, the causative factor is usually established by patients' own reports, the diagnosis thereby depending not only on patients' recall, but also on the patients' attributions of causes for their complaints. One area where this is particularly relevant is headache related to relatively mild injuries (acute and chronic headache attributed to mild headache injury, ICHD-II 5.1.2 and 5.2.2, and acute and chronic headache attributed to whiplash injury, ICHD-II 5.3 and 5.4). The incidence of compensated insurance claims for whiplash-associated disorder, which usually includes head and neck pain, in Quebec, Canada, was 70 per 100 000 inhabitants in 1987. In clinic-based series, i.e., among patients who contact an emergency ward or a doctor some time after whiplash, the proportion with headache after less than 1 month is between 50% and 80%, and after $\geq$ 6 months it falls to between 8% and 30% (Stovner, 1996). In the few studies that are not based on patients but on unselected individuals who had been involved in rear-end traffic accidents these figures are much lower, and in the chronic stage the prevalence and severity of headache among those who have been involved in such accidents are no higher than in a control group (Berglund et al., 2001; Schrader et al., 2006). Hence, it seems possible that only the acute pain can be said to have the whiplash incidence as a cause, and that these events, although frequent, contribute little or nothing to the total headache burden of headache. The same reservations may be raised for headache after concussion (Mickeviciene et al., 2002, 2004).

CONCLUSION

Primary headaches are among the most prevalent disorders of humanity, the 1-year prevalence of migraine being around 10–14% and of tension headache above 40%. Other primary headaches probably contribute less to the total headache burden due to their much lower prevalence. Little is known about the contribution of the secondary headaches to the total headache burden, both because of difficulties with making these diagnoses in population-based epidemiological studies, and because it is very incompletely known how often the underlying conditions cause headache. There are still severe limitations in our knowledge about the headache prevalence and burden in large and populous regions of the world, and there are also many unresolved methodological problems connected with headache epidemiological studies. Nevertheless, from the present body of evidence it seems well documented that headaches, and particularly migraine and TTH, constitute large public health problems throughout the world.

References

Abu-Arefeh I, Russell G (1994). Prevalence of headache and migraine in schoolchildren. BMJ 309: 765–769.

Alders EE, Hentzen A, Tan CT (1996). A community-based prevalence study on headache in Malaysia. Headache 36: 379–384.

Ando N, Fujimoto S, Ishikawa T et al. (2007). Prevalence and features of migraine in Japanese junior high school students aged 12-15 yr. Brain Dev 29: 482–485.

Attia Romdhane N, Ben Hamida M, Mrabet A et al. (1993). Prevalence study of neurologic disorders in Kelibia (Tunisia). Neuroepidemiology 12: 285–299.

Bank J, Marton S (2000). Hungarian migraine epidemiology. Headache 40: 164–169.

Barea LM, Tannhauser M, Rotta NT (1996). An epidemiologic study of headache among children and adolescents of southern Brazil. Cephalalgia 16: 545–549.

Bener A, Swadi H, Qassimi EMA et al. (1998). Prevalence of headache and migraine in schoolchildren in the United Arab Emirates. Ann Saudi Med 18: 522–524.

Bengtsson BA, Malmvall BE (1982). Giant cell arteritis. Acta Med Scand Suppl 658: 1–102.

Berglund A, Alfredsson L, Jensen I et al. (2001). The association between exposure to a rear-end collision and future health complaints. J Clin Epidemiol 54: 851–856.

Bigal ME, Liberman JN, Lipton RB (2006). Age-dependent prevalence and clinical features of migraine. Neurology 67: 246–251.

Black DF, Swanson JW, Stang PE (2005). Decreasing incidence of cluster headache: a population-based study in Olmsted County, Minnesota. Headache 45: 220–223.

Boru UT, Kocer A, Luleci A et al. (2005). Prevalence and characteristics of migraine in women of reproductive age in Istanbul, Turkey: a population based survey. Tohoku J Exp Med 206: 51–59.

Breslau N, Chilcoat HD, Andreski P (1996). Further evidence on the link between migraine and neuroticism. Neurology 47: 663–667.

Bugdayci R, Ozge A, Sasmaz T et al. (2005). Prevalence and factors affecting headache in Turkish schoolchildren. Pediatr Int 47: 316–322.

Camarda R, Monastero R (2003). Prevalence of primary headaches in Italian elderly: preliminary data from the Zabut Aging Project. Neurol Sci 24 (Suppl.2): S122–S124.

Carson AL, Rose KM, Sanford CP et al. (2004). Lifetime prevalence of migraine and other headaches lasting 4 or more hours: the Atherosclerosis Risk in Communities (ARIC) study. Headache 44: 20–28.

Castillo J, Munoz P, Guitera V et al. (1999). Epidemiology of chronic daily headache in the general population. Headache 39: 190–196.

Celik Y, Ekuklu G, Tokuc B et al. (2005). Migraine prevalence and some related factors in Turkey. Headache 45: 32–36.

Cheung RT (2000). Prevalence of migraine, tension-type headache, and other headaches in Hong Kong. Headache 40: 473–479.

Colás R, Muñoz P, Temprano R et al. (2004). Chronic daily headache with analgesic overuse: epidemiology and impact on quality of life. Neurology 62: 1338–1342.

Cruz ME, Cruz I, Preux PM et al. (1995). Headache and cysticercosis in Ecuador, South America. Headache 35: 93–97.

D'Alessandro R, Gamberini G, Benassi G et al. (1986). Cluster headache in the Republic of San Marino. Cephalalgia 6: 159–162.

Dahlöf C, Linde M (2001). One-year prevalence of migraine in Sweden: a population-based study in adults. Cephalalgia 21: 664–671.

Deleu D, Khan MA, Al Shehab TA (2002). Prevalence and clinical characteristics of headache in a rural community in oman. Headache 42: 963–973.

Dent W, Spiss H, Helbok R et al. (2004). Prevalence of migraine in a rural area in South Tanzania: a door-to-door survey. Cephalalgia 24: 960–966.

Diamond ML (2002). The role of concomitant headache types and non-headache co-morbidities in the underdiagnosis of migraine. Neurology 58: S3–S9.

Dodick DW, Mosek AC, Campbell JK (1998). The hypnic ("alarm clock") headache syndrome. Cephalalgia 18: 152–156.

Dyb G, Holmen TL, Zwart JA (2006). Analgesic overuse among adolescents with headache: the Head-HUNT-Youth Study. Neurology 66: 198–201.

Ekbom K (1970). A clinical comparison of cluster headache and migraine. Acta Neurol Scand 46 (Suppl. 41): 1–44.

Ekbom K, Waldenlind E (1981). Cluster headache in women: evidence of hypofertility(?). Headaches in relation to menstruation and pregnancy. Cephalalgia 1: 167–174.

Ekbom K, Ahlborg B, Schele R (1978). Prevalence of migraine and cluster headache in Swedish men of 18. Headache 18: 9–19.

Ekbom K, Svensson DA, Träff H et al. (2002). Age at onset and sex ratio in cluster headache: observations over three decades. Cephalalgia 22: 94–100.

Ekbom K, Svensson DA, Pedersen NL et al. (2006). Lifetime prevalence and concordance risk of cluster headache in the Swedish twin population. Neurology 67: 798–803.

Eriksen MK, Thomsen LL, Olesen J (2005). Sensitivity and specificity of the new international diagnostic criteria for migraine with aura. J Neurol Neurosurg Psychiatry 76: 212–217.

Evers S, Goadsby PJ (2003). Hypnic headache. Clinical features, pathophysiology, and treatment. Neurology 60: 905–910.

Evers S, Rahmann A, Schwaag S et al. (2003). Hypnic headache – the first German cases including polysomnography. Cephalalgia 23: 20–23.

Fendrich K, Vennemann M, Pfaffenrath V et al. (2007). Headache prevalence among adolesents – the German DMKG headache study. Cephalalgia 27: 347–354.

Göbel H, Petersen-Braun M, Soyka D (1994a). The epidemiology of headache in Germany: a nationwide survey of a representative sample on the basis of the headache classification of the International Headache Society. Cephalalgia 14: 97–106.

Göbel H, Petersen-Braun M, Soyka D (1994b). Headache in Germany. A nationwide survey of a representative sample on the basis of the headache classification of the International Headache Society. In: J Olesen (Ed.), Headache Classification and Epidemiology. Raven Press, New York, pp. 255–261.

Hagen K, Zwart JA, Vatten L et al. (2000a). Head-HUNT: validity and reliability of a headache questionnaire in a large population-based study in Norway. Cephalalgia 20: 244–251.

Hagen K, Zwart JA, Vatten L et al. (2000b). Prevalence of migraine and non-migrainous headache-head-HUNT, a large population-based study. Cephalalgia 20: 900–906.

Hagen K, Vatten L, Stovner LJ et al. (2002). Low socio-economic status is associated with increased risk of frequent headache: a prospective study of 22718 adults in Norway. Cephalalgia 22: 672–679.

Hauser WA, Ferguson RH, Holley KE et al. (1971). Temporal arteritis in Rochester, Minnesota, 1951 to 1967. Mayo Clin Proc 46: 597–602.

Headache Classification Committee of the International Headache Society (1988). Classification and diagnostic criteria for headache disorders, cranial neuralgias and facial pain. Cephalalgia 8 (Suppl. 7): 1–96.

Headache Classification Subcommittee of the International Headache Society (2004). The international classification of headache disorders, 2nd edn. Cephalalgia 24: 1–160.

Henry P, Michel P, Brochet B et al. (1992). A nationwide survey of migraine in France: prevalence and clinical features in adults. Cephalalgia 12: 229–237.

Henry P, Auray JP, Gaudin AF et al. (2002). Prevalence and clinical characteristics of migraine in France. Neurology 59: 232–237.

Ho KH, Ong BK (2001). Headache characteristics and race in Singapore: results of a randomized national survey. Headache 41: 279–284.

Ho KH, Ong BK (2003). A community-based study of headache diagnosis and prevalence in Singapore. Cephalalgia 23: 6–13.

Jaillard AS, Mazetti P, Kala E (1997). Prevalence of migraine and headache in a high-altitude town of Peru: a population-based study. Headache 37: 95–101.

Karli N, Akis N, Zarifoglu M et al. (2006). Headache prevalence in adolescents aged 12 to 17: a student-based epidemiological study in Bursa. Headache 46: 649–655.

Kececi H, Dener S (2002). Epidemiological and clinical characteristics of migraine in Sivas, Turkey. Headache 42: 275–280.

Koehler T, Buck-Emden E, Dulz K (1992). Frequency of migraine among an unselected group of employees and variation of prevalence according to different diagnostic criteria. Headache 32: 79–83.

Kong CK, Cheng WW, Wong LY (2001). Epidemiology of headache in Hong Kong primary-level schoolchildren: questionnaire study. Hong Kong Med J 7: 29–33.

Koseoglu E, Nacar M, Talaslioglu A et al. (2003). Epidemiological and clinical characteristics of migraine and tension type headache in 1146 females in Kayseri, Turkey. Cephalalgia 23: 381–388.

Kryst S, Scherl E (1994). A population-based survey of the social and personal impact of headache. Headache 34: 344–350.

Kudrow L (1980). Cluster Headache. Mechanism and Management. Oxford University Press, New York.

Laínez MJA, Vioque J, Hernández-Aguado I et al. (1994). Prevalence of migraine in Spain. An assessment of the questionnaire's validity by clinical interview. In: J Olesen (Ed.), Frontiers in Headache Research:

Headache Classification and Epidemiology, Vol. 4. Raven Press, New York, pp. 221–225.

Lampl C, Buzath A, Baumhackl U et al. (2003). One-year prevalence of migraine in Austria: a nation-wide survey. Cephalalgia 23: 280–286.

Lantéri-Minet M, Auray JP, El Hasnaoui A et al. (2003). Prevalence and description of chronic daily headache in the general population in France. Pain 102: 143–149.

Lantéri-Minet M, Valade D, Géraud G et al. (2005). Migraine and probable migraine – results of FRAMIG 3, a French nationwide survey carried out according to the 2004 IHS classification. Cephalalgia 25: 1146–1158.

Launer LJ, Terwindt GM, Ferrari MD (1999). The prevalence and characteristics of migraine in a population-based cohort: the GEM study. Neurology 53: 537–542.

Laurell K, Larsson B, Eeg-Olofsson O (2004). Prevalence of headache in Swedish schoolchildren, with a focus on tension-type headache. Cephalalgia 24: 380–388.

Lavados PM, Tenhamm E (1997). Epidemiology of migraine headache in Santiago, Chile: a prevalence study. Cephalalgia 17: 770–777.

Lavados PM, Tenhamm E (1998). Epidemiology of tension-type headache in Santiago, Chile: a prevalence study. Cephalalgia 18: 552–558.

Linn FHH, Rinkel GJE, Algra A et al. (1999). Follow-up of idiopathic thunderclap headache in general practice. J Neurol 246: 946–948.

Lipton RB, Stewart WF, Diamond S et al. (2001). Prevalence and burden of migraine in the United States: data from the American Migraine Study II. Headache 41: 646–657.

Lipton RB, Scher AI, Kolodner K et al. (2002). Migraine in the United States: epidemiology and patterns of health care use. Neurology 58: 885–894.

Longe AC, Osuntokun BO (1988). Prevalence of neurological disorders in Udo, a rural community in southern Nigeria. Trop Geogr Med 65: 36–40.

Lu SR, Fuh JL, Juang KD et al. (2000). Migraine prevalence in adolescents aged 13–15: a student population-based study in Taiwan. Cephalalgia 20: 479–485.

Lu SR, Fuh JL, Chen WT et al. (2001). Chronic daily headache in Taipei, Taiwan: prevalence, follow-up and outcome predictors. Cephalalgia 21: 980–986.

Lyngberg AC, Rasmussen BK, Jørgensen T et al. (2005). Has the prevalence of migraine and tension-type headache changed over a 12-year period? A Danish population survey. Eur J Epidemiol 20: 243–249.

Manzoni GC (1998). Gender ratio of cluster headache over the years: a possible role of changes in lifestyle. Cephalalgia 18: 138–142.

Manzoni GC, Terzano MG, Bono G et al. (1983). Cluster headache – clinical findings in 180 patients. Cephalalgia 3: 21–30.

Manzoni GC, Micieli G, Granella F et al. (1988). Cluster headache in women: clinical findings and relationship with reproductive life. Cephalalgia 8: 37–44.

Mathew NT, Stubits E, Nigam MP (1982). Transformed or evolutive migraine. Headache 22: 66–68.

Mattsson P, Svardsudd K, Lundberg PO et al. (2000). The prevalence of migraine in women aged 40–74 years: a population-based study. Cephalalgia 20: 893–899.

Mavromichalis I, Anagnostopoulos D, Metaxas N et al. (1999). Prevalence of migraine in schoolchildren and some clinical comparisons between migraine with and without aura. Headache 39: 728–736.

Merikangas KR, Whitaker AE, Isler H et al. (1994). The Zurich study: XXIII. Epidemiology of headache syndromes in the Zurich cohort study of young adults. Eur Arch Psychiatry Clin Neurosci 244: 145–152.

Metsähonkala L, Sillanpää M (1994). Migraine in children – an evaluation of the IHS criteria. Cephalalgia 14: 285–290.

Michel P, Pariente P, Duru G et al. (1996). MIG ACCESS: a population-based, nationwide, comparative survey of access to care in migraine in France. Cephalalgia 16: 50–55.

Mickeviciene D, Schrader H, Nestvold K et al. (2002). Controlled historical cohort study on the post-concussion syndrome. Eur J Neurol 9: 581–587.

Mickeviciene D, Schrader H, Obelieniene D et al. (2004). A controlled prospective inception cohort study on the post-concussion syndrome outside the medicolegal context. Eur J Neurol 11: 411–419.

Milovanović M, Jarebinski M, Martinovic Z (2007). Prevalence of primary headaches in children from Belgrade, Serbia. Eur J Pediatr Neurol 11: 136–141.

Miranda H, Ortiz G, Figueroa S et al. (2003). Prevalence of headache in Puerto Rico. Headache 43: 774–778.

Monteiro JM (1995). Cefaleias. Estudio epidemiologico e clinico de una populacao urbana. Thesis. Porto.

Morillo LE, Alarcon F, Aranaga N et al. (2005). Prevalence of migraine in Latin America. Headache 45: 106–117.

Nappi G, Savoldi F (1985). Headache. Diagnostic System and Taxonomic Criteria. John Libbey Eurotext, London.

O'Brien B, Goeree R, Streiner D (1994). Prevalence of migraine headache in Canada: a population-based survey. Int J Epidemiol 23: 1020–1026.

Olesen J (1994). Discussion summary. In: Frontiers in Headache Research: Headache Classification and Epidemiology, Vol. 4. Raven Press, New York, pp. 227–228.

Orji GI, Iloeje SO (1997). Childhood migraine in Nigeria – I: a community-based study. West Afr J Med 16: 208–217.

Osuntokun BO, Schoenberg BS, Nottidge V et al. (1982). Migraine headache in a rural community in Nigeria: results of a pilot study. Neuroepidemiology 1: 31–39.

Osuntokun BO, Adeuja AO, Nottidge VA et al. (1992). Prevalence of headache and migrainous headache in Nigerian Africans: a community-based study. East Afr Med J 69: 196–199.

Patel NV, Bigal ME, Kolodner KB et al. (2004). Prevalence and impact of migraine and probable migraine in a health plan. Neurology 63: 1432–1438.

Peres M, Silberstein SD, Nahmias S (2001). Hemicrania continua is not that rare. Neurology 57: 948–951.

Prencipe M, Casini AR, Ferretti C et al. (2001). Prevalence of headache in an elderly population: attack frequency, disability, and use of medication. J Neurol Neurosurg Psychiatry 70: 377–381.

Pryse-Phillips W, Findlay H, Tugwell P et al. (1992). A Canadian population survey on the clinical, epidemiologic and societal impact of migraine and tension-type headache. Can J Neurol Sci 19: 333–339.

Queiroz LP, Barea LM, Blank N (2006). An epidemiological study of headache in Florianopolis, Brazil. Cephalalgia 26: 122–127.

Raieli V, Raimondo D, Cammalleri R et al. (1995). Migraine headaches in adolescents: a student population-based study in Monreale. Cephalalgia 15: 5–12.

Rasmussen BK (1992). Migraine and tension-type headache in a general population: psychosocial factors. Int J Epidemiol 21: 1138–1143.

Rasmussen BK (1995). Epidemiology of headache. Cephalalgia 15: 45–68.

Rasmussen BK, Olesen J (1992a). Symptomatic and nonsymptomatic headaches in a general population. Neurology 42: 1225–1231.

Rasmussen BK, Olesen J (1992b). Migraine with aura and migraine without aura: an epidemiological study. Cephalalgia 12: 221–228.

Rasmussen BK, Jensen R, Olesen J (1991a). Questionnaire versus clinical interview in the diagnosis of headache. Headache 31: 290–295.

Rasmussen BK, Jensen R, Schroll M et al. (1991b). Epidemiology of headache in a general population – a prevalence study. J Clin Epidemiol 44: 1147–1157.

Roh JK, Kim JS, Ahn YO (1998). Epidemiologic and clinical characteristics of migraine and tension-type headache in Korea. Headache 38: 356–365.

Russell MB, Rasmussen BK, Thorvaldsen P et al. (1995). Prevalence and sex-ratio of the subtypes of migraine. Int J Epidemiol 15: 612–618.

Russell MB, Levi N, Saltyte-Benth J et al. (2006). Tension-type headache in adolescents and adults: a population based study of 33,764 twins. Eur J Epidemiol 21: 153–160.

Sakai F, Igarashi H (1997). Prevalence of migraine in Japan: a nationwide survey. Cephalalgia 17: 15–22.

Scher AI, Stewart WF, Liberman J et al. (1998). Prevalence of frequent headache in a population sample. Headache 38: 497–506.

Scher AI, Stewart WF, Lipton RB (1999). Migraine and headache: a meta-analytic approach. In: Epidemiology of Pain. IASP Press, Seattle, pp. 159–170.

Scher AI, Stewart WF, Ricci JA et al. (2003). Factors associated with the onset and remission of chronic daily headache in a population-based study. Pain 106: 81–89.

Schrader H, Stovner LJ, Obelieniene D et al. (2006). Examination of the diagnostic validity of 'headache attributed to whiplash injury': a controlled, prospective study. Eur J Neurol 13: 1226–1232.

Schwartz BS, Stewart WF, Lipton RB (1997). Lost workdays and decreased work effectiveness associated with headache in the workplace. J Occup Environ Med 39: 320–327.

Schwartz BS, Stewart WF, Simon D et al. (1998). Epidemiology of tension-type headache. JAMA 279: 381–383.

Shivpuri D, Rajesh MS, Jain D (2003). Prevalence and characteristics of migraine among adolescents: a questionnaire survey. Indian Pediatr 40: 665–669.

Silberstein S, Loder E, Diamond S et al. (2007). Probable migraine in the United States: results of the American Migraine Prevalence and Prevention (AMPP) study. Cephalalgia 27: 220–229.

Sjaastad O (1985). "Chronic daily headache" ("cefalea cronica quotidiana"). Cephalalgia 5 (Suppl. 2): 191–193.

Sjaastad O, Bakketeig LS (2002). Exertional headache. I. Vågå study of headache epidemiology. Cephalalgia 22: 784–790.

Sjaastad O, Bakketeig LS (2003). Cluster headache prevalence. Vågå study of headache epidemiology. Cephalalgia 23: 528–533.

Sjaastad O, Bakketeig LS (2007). The rare, unilateral headaches. Vågå study of headache epidemiology. J Headache Pain 8: 19–27.

Sjaastad O, Pettersen H, Bakketeig LS (2001). The Vågå study; epidemiology of headache I: the prevalence of ultrashort paroxysms. Cephalalgia 21: 207–215.

Stang PE, Yanagihara PA, Swanson JW et al. (1992). Incidence of migraine headache: a population-based study in Olmsted County, Minnesota. Neurology 42: 1657–1662.

Steiner TJ, Scher AI, Stewart WF et al. (2003). The prevalence and disability burden of adult migraine in England and their relationships to age, gender and ethnicity. Cephalalgia 23: 519–527.

Stewart WF, Linet MS, Celentano DD et al. (1991). Age- and sex-specific incidence rates of migraine with and without visual aura. Am J Epidemiol 134: 1111–1120.

Stewart WF, Lipton RB (1994). Migraine epidemiology in the United States. In: J Olesen (Ed.), Headache Classification and Epidemiology. Raven Press, New York, pp. 239–246.

Stewart WF, Lipton RB, Celentano DD et al. (1992). Prevalence of migraine headache in the United States. Relation to age, income, race, and other sociodemographic factors. JAMA 267: 64–69.

Stewart WF, Lipton RB, Liberman J (1996). Variation in migraine prevalence by race. Neurology 47: 52–59.

Stovner LJ (1996). The nosologic status of the whiplash syndrome: a critical review based on a methodological approach. Spine 21: 2735–2746.

Stovner LJ, Zwart JA, Hagen K et al. (2006). Epidemiology of headache in Europe. Eur J Neurol 13: 333–345.

Stovner L, Hagen K, Jensen R et al. (2007). The global burden of headache: a documentation of headache prevalence and disability worldwide. Cephalalgia 27: 193–210.

Swanson JW, Yanagihara T, Stang PE et al. (1994). Incidence of cluster headaches: a population-based study in Olmsted County, Minnesota. Neurology 44: 433–437.

Takeshima T, Ishizaki K, Fukuhara Y et al. (2004). Population-based door-to-door survey of migraine in Japan: the Daisen study. Headache 44: 8–19.

Tekle Haimanot R, Seraw B, Forsgren L et al. (1995). Migraine, chronic tension-type headache, and cluster headache in an Ethiopian rural community. Cephalalgia 15: 482–488.

Tonon C, Guttmann S, Volpini M et al. (2002). Prevalence and incidence of cluster headache in the Republic of San Marino. Neurology 58: 1407–1409.

Torelli P, Beghi E, Manzoni GC (2005a). Validation of a questionnaire for the detection of cluster headache. Headache 45: 644–652.

Torelli P, Beghi E, Manzoni GC (2005b). Cluster headache prevalence in the Italian general population. Neurology 64: 469–474.

van Gijn J, Rinkel GJ (2001). Subarachnoid haemorrhage: diagnosis, causes and management. Brain 124: 249–278.

Wang SJ, Liu HC, Fuh JL et al. (1997). Prevalence of headaches in a Chinese elderly population in Kinmen: age and gender effect and cross-cultural comparisons. Neurology 49: 195–200.

Wang SJ, Fuh JL, Lu SR et al. (2000a). Chronic daily headache in Chinese elderly: prevalence, risk factors, and biannual follow-up. Neurology 54: 314–319.

Wang SJ, Fuh JL, Young YH et al. (2000b). Prevalence of migraine in Taipei, Taiwan: a population-based survey. Cephalalgia 20: 566–572.

Wang SJ, Fuh JL, Juang KD et al. (2005). Rising prevalence of migraine in Taiwanese adolescents aged 13–15 years. Cephalalgia 25: 433–438.

Wang SJ, Fuh JL, Lu SR et al. (2006). Chronic daily headache in adolescents. Prevalence, impact, and medication overuse. Neurology 66: 193–197.

Wiehe M, Fuchs SC, Moreira LB et al. (2002). Migraine is more frequent in individuals with optimal and normal blood pressure: a population-based study. J Hypertens 20: 1303–1306.

Wiendels NJ, Knuistingh Neven A, Rosendaal FR et al. (2006). Chronic frequent headache in the general population: prevalence and associated factors. Cephalalgia 26: 1434–1442.

Wittrock DA, Ficek SK, Cook TM (1996). Headache-free controls? Evidence of headaches in individuals who deny having headaches during diagnostic screening. Headache 36: 416–418.

Wong TW, Wong KS, Yu TS et al. (1995). Prevalence of migraine and other headaches in Hong Kong. Neuroepidemiology 14: 82–91.

Zencir M, Ergin H, Sahiner T et al. (2004). Epidemiology and symptomatology of migraine among school children: Denizli urban area in Turkey. Headache 44: 780–785.

Zivadinov R, Willheim K, Jurjevic A et al. (2001). Prevalence of migraine in Croatia: a population-based survey. Headache 41: 805–812.

Zivadinov R, Willheim K, Sepic-Grahovac D et al. (2003). Migraine and tension-type headache in Croatia: a population-based survey of precipitating factors. Cephalalgia 23: 336–343.

Zwart JA, Dyb G, Hagen K et al. (2003a). Analgesic use: a predictor of chronic pain and medication overuse headache: the Head-HUNT study. Neurology 61: 160–164.

Zwart JA, Dyb G, Stovner LJ et al. (2003b). The validity of 'recognition-based' headache diagnoses in adolescents. Data from the Nord-Trondelag Health Study 1995–97, Head-HUNT-Youth. Cephalalgia 23: 223–229.

Zwart JA, Dyb G, Holmen TL et al. (2004). The prevalence of migraine and tension-type headaches among adolescents in Norway. The Nord-Trondelag Health Study (Head-HUNT-Youth), a large population-based epidemiological study. Cephalalgia 24: 373–379.

Handbook of Clinical Neurology, Vol. 97 (3rd series)
Headache
G. Nappi and M.A. Moskowitz, Editors

Chapter 2

The social impact and burden of headache

RICHARD B. LIPTON* AND MARCELO E. BIGAL
Departments of Neurology, Epidemiology and Population Health, Albert Einstein College of Medicine, New York, NY, USA

INTRODUCTION

Headache disorders are among the most common afflictions of humankind. These disorders are usually associated with recurrent attacks of head pain and associated symptoms (Raskin, 1998; Headache Classification Subcommittee of the International Headache Society, 2004). The burden of headache is determined by the frequency, severity, and duration of attacks and the symptoms associated with the attack. To some degree, burden also depends upon the etiology. In this chapter we focus on the primary headache disorders and not the secondary disorders attributable to an underlying cause, such as an infection, brain tumor, or stroke (Headache Classification Subcommittee of the International Headache Society, 2004).

Of the primary headache disorders, tension-type headache (TTH) is the most common in population studies, but migraine is most common among patients who seek medical care for headache. The most important forms of migraine are migraine with and without aura, as well as a condition termed probable migraine (Rasmussen, 1995; Raskin, 1998; Scher et al., 1999). Migraine is a chronic disease with episodic manifestations that sometimes progress, giving rise to the chronic daily headaches (CDH).

In terms of its impact on individual patients, migraine is one of the most burdensome of the primary headache disorders. Epidemiological data help to describe the burden of migraine as well as its scope and distribution (Lipton and Silberstein, 1994; Lipton et al., 1994; Rasmussen, 1995; Scher et al., 1999). In exploring the burden of migraine, we distinguish clinical and public health perspectives. Clinicians are concerned with the diagnosis of individual patients as a prelude to effective treatment. From a public health perspective, it is the distribution of diagnoses in a defined population that is of importance. While clinicians are interested in the burden of headache disorders imposed on each individual patient, from a societal perspective the direct and indirect costs of illness are priorities.

In this chapter, we will review the social burden of migraine and of the CDH, emphasizing the population-based studies that used standardized diagnostic criteria. We focus on migraine because this is probably the most important primary headache disorder from the perspective of societal burden (Rasmussen et al., 1991; Henry et al., 1992; Stewart et al., 1992; Gobels et al., 1994; Stang et al., 1994; Lipton et al., 2001a). We briefly discuss the impact of TTH. The impact of the other primary headache disorders will be discussed under the specific chapters.

THE BURDEN OF MIGRAINE TO THE INDIVIDUAL

The disability imposed by migraine

The burden of migraine is significant both to the individual sufferer and to society (Gobels et al., 1994; Launer et al., 1999). The World Health Organization (WHO) defines disability in terms of the consequences of illness on ability to work and function in other roles such as household work and non-work activities (e.g., recreation, social, family). Among migraineurs, the level of disability is a major determinant of satisfaction therapies (Leonardi et al., 2005).

*Correspondence to: Richard B. Lipton, MD, Professor and Vice-Chairman, Department of Neurology, Epidemiology and Population Health, Albert Einstein College of Medicine, 1165 Morris Park Avenue, Rousso Bldg. Rm. 330, Bronx, New York, NY, 10461, USA, Tel: 718-430-3886, Fax: 718-430-3857, E-mail: rlipton@aecom.yu.edu

Within the USA, the American Migraine Study II estimates that 28 million US residents had severe migraine headaches in the year of 1999 (Lipton et al., 2001b). Nearly one in four US households had someone with migraine. Twenty-five percent of women in the USA who had migraine experienced four or more severe attacks a month; 35% experienced one to four severe attacks a month; 38% experienced one or fewer severe attacks a month. Similar frequency patterns were observed for men. In that study, 92% of women and 89% of men with severe migraine had some headache-related disability (Lipton et al., 2001b, 2007). About half were severely disabled or needed bed rest.

In addition to the attack-related disability, many migraineurs live in fear, knowing that at any time an attack could disrupt their ability to work, care for their families, or meet social obligations. Abundant evidence indicates that migraine reduces health-related quality of life (QoL).

The results of the American Migraine Study II were confirmed by the American Migraine Prevalence and Prevention (AMPP) study (Lipton et al., 2007). As a part of the AMPP, more than 160 000 individuals were interviewed. Around 37% of the migraineurs had five or more headache days per month (Table 2.1). During migraine attacks, most migraineurs reported severe impairment or the need for bed rest (53.7%); just 7.2% reported no attack-related impairment. Over a 3-month period, 35.1% of the migraineurs had at least one day of activity restriction related to headache.

The WHO has released a report on burden of diseases (Leonardi et al., 2005). The WHO report defines the "burden" of a disease to include the economic and emotional difficulties that a family experiences as a result of migraine, as well as the lost opportunities – the adjustments and compromises that prevent other family members from achieving their full potential in work, social relationships, and leisure. The global burden of disease (GBD) is an analysis of the onset of disorders and the disability caused by them. Using the GBD methodology, migraine is estimated to account for 2.0% years of life lost due to a disability in women of all ages. In both sexes of all ages, migraine is responsible for 1.4% of total years of life lost due to a disability and ranks within the top 20 most disabled studied disorders (Table 2.2) (Olesen and Leonardi, 2003).

Table 2.1

Migraine frequency and impact: the American Migraine Prevalence and Prevention Study

Variable	*n* (%)
Monthly headache frequency	
<1	4279 (23.4%)
1–4	11 481 (62.7%)
5–9	1761 (9.6%)
9–14	777 (4.2%)
Headache-related impairment during severe headache	
Function normally	1336 (7.2%)
Some impairment	7299 (39.1%)
Severe impairment or bed rest required	10 035 (53.7%)
Days of activity restriction per headache	
0	3113 (16.8%)
<1	8909 (48.1%)
1–2	5556 (30.0%)
3–5	779 (4.2%)
≥6	171 (0.9%)
School/work/social impact in previous 3 months	
Missed at least 1 day of work/school	4790 (25.3%)
Work/school productivity reduced by at least 50%	5311 (28.1%)
Did no household work	9050 (47.7%)
Household productivity reduced by at least 50%	6512 (34.3%)
Missed family or social activity	5519 (29.1%)
Migraine Disability Assessment (MIDAS) grade	
1	12 078 (63.7%)
2	2719 (14.3%)
3	2032 (10.7%)
4	2139 (11.3%)

The impact of migraine on the health-related quality of life

The concept of QoL proposes that health is defined not only by the absence of disease, but by the presence of physical, mental, and social well-being. Health-related QoL (HRQoL) is a subset of overall QoL that encompasses individuals' health state, functional status (both physical and mental), and overall well-being (Turner-Bowker et al., 2003). A body of research now demonstrates that migraine poses a substantial and unique HRQoL burden on its sufferers (Freitag, 2007). Not only do patients with migraine experience diminished HRQoL compared to normal, healthy individuals, they experience decreased HRQoL comparable to or in some cases greater than that experienced by individuals with more serious diseases. For example, Turner-Bowker and colleagues compared the burden of migraine with other conditions and found that the health-related impact of migraine was comparable to that experienced by patients with congestive heart failure, hypertension, or diabetes (Turner-Bowker et al., 2003).

Table 2.2

Global burden of migraine: leading causes of years of life lost due to a disability according to the global burden of disease initiative

	Females all ages	% Total	Both sexes all ages	% Total
1	Unipolar depressive disorders	1	Unipolar depressive disorders	11.9
2	Iron-deficiency anemia	2	Hearing loss, adult-onset	4.6
3	Hearing loss, adult-onset	3	Iron-deficiency anemia	4.5
4	Osteoarthritis	4	Chronic obstructive pulmonary disease	3.3
5	Chronic obstructive pulmonary disease	5	Alcohol use disorders	3.1
6	Schizophrenia	6	Osteoarthritis	3.0
7	Bipolar affective disorder	7	Schizophrenia	2.8
8	Falls	8	Falls	2.8
9	Alzheimer's and other dementias	9	Bipolar affective disorder	2.5
10	Obstructed labor	10	Asthma	2.1
11	Cataracts	11	Congenital abnormalities	2.1
12	**Migraine**	12	Perinatal conditions	2.0
13	Congenital abnormalities	13	Alzheimer's and other dementias	2.0
14	Asthma	14	Cataracts	1.9
15	Perinatal conditions	15	Road traffic accidents	1.8
16	*Chlamydia*	16	Protein-energy malnutrition	1.7
17	Cerebrovascular disease	17	Cerebrovascular disease	1.7
18	Protein-energy malnutrition	18	HIV/AIDS	1.5
19	Abortion	**19**	**Migraine**	**1.4**
20	Panic disorder	20	Diabetes mellitus	1.4

HIV: human immunodeficiency virus; AIDS: acquired immune deficiency syndrome.
Modified from Lipton et al. (2001b).

Several population-based studies have examined the effect of migraine on HRQoL. Using the SF-36, Terwindt and colleagues showed that migraine has a significant negative impact on HRQoL in the Dutch population (Figure 2.1). They further showed that this impact increased with frequency of migraine attacks (Terwindt et al., 2000). In a population study, both the physical and mental component scores of the SF-12 were reduced in migraineurs; this effect was independent of the influence of depression (Lipton et al., 2000). These data were supported by an additional study showing that, in a matched sample survey of migraineurs and controls, migraineurs had substantial, statistically significant reductions in eight of nine HRQoL domains. This was associated with significant work-related disability (Lipton et al., 2003a). These studies and others confirm that migraine is a disabling condition that leads to compromised HRQoL.

The interictal burden of migraine

The burden of migraine to the individual is not restricted to the attack. In a study that assessed 145 consecutive migraineurs seen in a headache clinic using three self-administered standardized questionnaires, migraineurs perceived more symptoms and greater emotional distress as well as disturbed contentment, vitality, and sleep. It was suggested that the general well-being of the migraine patient is impaired, even between attacks (Dahlöf and Dimenäs, 1995). Because migraine is comorbid with disorders that also impact the HRQoL, such as depression and anxiety, it may be suggested that the interical burden of migraine would be indirectly mediated through the comorbidity. However, recent evidence suggests that the ictal burden of migraine predisposes to anticipatory anxiety and fear of new attacks. Accordingly, the ictal burden drives a true interictal impact (Buse et al., unpublished data), and effectively treating the attacks may also be associated with improvement on the overall HRQoL.

THE IMPACT OF MIGRAINE BEYOND THE INDIVIDUAL

The impact of migraine on the family

The impact of migraine extends to household partners and other family members. A Canadian study reported that 90% of people with migraine reported postponing their household work because of headaches, 30% had

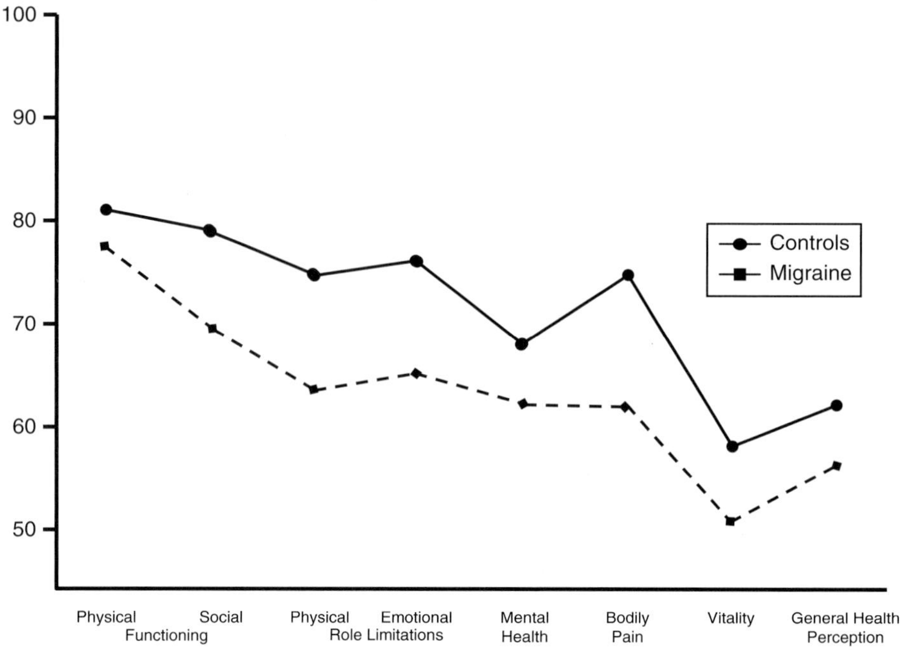

Fig. 2.1. SF-36 Health-related quality of life (HRQoL) of migraineurs versus controls. (Adapted from Terwindt et al., 2000.)

cancelled family and social activities during their last migraine attack, and two-thirds feared letting others down because of their headaches (Edmeads et al., 1993). Other studies (Smith, 1998) found that migraine attacks brought significant disruption to family life, with impact on spouses, children, and friends.

In a population study conducted in the USA and UK, migraine sufferers reported a substantial negative impact on participation in family life, family relationships, and satisfaction with work. Many respondents reported that they were less able to communicate and more likely to argue with their children, felt less involved with home and school, and spent less time with the children. Almost half felt they could be better parents if they did not have migraine. These feelings were more common among women than among men with migraine. Many also felt less able to communicate and more likely to argue with their partners, and that they could be a better partner if they did not have headaches. In this study, interviews with partners support the views of those with migraine and suggest that migraine disrupts family life (Lipton et al., 2003b). Partners reported that, from their viewpoint, headaches negatively influenced their relationships. Compared with subjects who did not have migraine, regarding their work performance, a statistically significantly higher proportion of migraine partners were unsatisfied with work demands placed on them, with their level of responsibilities and duties, and with their ability to perform. Results from this study show that the impact of migraine extends to household partners and other family members (impact beyond the individual).

Societal impact of migraine

Migraine has an enormous impact on society. Studies have evaluated both the indirect costs of migraine as well as the direct costs (D'Alessandro et al., 1988; Centers for Disease Control, 1991; Celentano et al., 1992; Edmeads et al., 1993; Stang and Osterhaus, 1993; Fry, 1996; Stang et al., 1996; Stewart et al., 1996, 1999; Michel et al., 1997; Lipton et al., 1998; Von-Korff et al., 1998; Hu et al., 1999). Direct costs are those related to the use of medical resources, including physician visits for diagnosis and/or treatment, emergency room visits, diagnostic procedures, and medication. Indirect costs are generally assessed in terms of temporary disability, reduced functionality, lost productivity, and associated costs to employers.

Direct costs

A few studies have quantified the overall direct medical costs associated with migraine. Hu and colleagues (1999) used 1994 data to estimate the economic burden of migraine in the USA. Their findings indicated that annual US migraine-related direct costs were approximately $1 billion. In a 1999–2000 matched comparison of migraineurs and healthy cohorts using inpatient, outpatient, and prescription drug databases, both adult and child migraineurs had significantly higher total direct medical costs compared to non-migraineurs. Costs for adults were $7089 for migraineurs versus $2923 for non-migraineurs, and for children were $4272 versus $1400 (Pesa and Lage, 2004). Hu and colleagues (1999) also isolated the cost of prescription drugs for migraine treatment, and found that drugs accounted for 24–30% of annual treatment costs. Prescription drug costs amounted to $46.2 million in total costs for males and $254 million in total costs for females.

Physician visits make up a large proportion of total migraine-related direct costs. In a study using 1990–1998 National Ambulatory Medical Care Survey data, Gibbs and colleagues (2003) identified 35.5 million physician visits for migraine over the study period (14 visits per 1000 persons per year) (Pesa and Lage, 2004). Hu and colleagues (1999) estimated that the cost of physician office visits represented 54% and 69% of total migraine-associated direct costs for women and men, respectively.

Indirect costs

Even though the direct costs of migraine in the USA are substantial, overall health-care utilization costs may be underestimated given the existing level of migraine underdiagnosis and undertreatment (Dhopesh et al., 1979; Lipton et al., 1997). Furthermore, direct medical costs of migraine are only a fraction of the disease's overall cost to society. Hu and colleagues (1999) found that indirect costs of migraine in the USA could be conservatively estimated at $13.3 billion, and concluded that indirect costs make up approximately 93% of the total economic burden of migraine. Most of the indirect costs of migraine are due to presenteeism, not to absenteeism.

Estimates of actual numbers of lost work days associated with migraine vary. Using lost work day equivalents (LWDE), researchers found that 51.1% of women and 38.1% of men with migraine experienced 6 or more LWDEs annually (Dhopesh et al., 1979; Solomon et al., 1993; Lipton et al., 1997, 2001c; Consumer Healthcare Products Association, 2000; Stewart et al., 2003). Other studies have estimated that migraine sufferers experience the equivalent of 4.2–12 lost work days per year. In addition, these estimates of the importance of lost work days and decreased productivity are confirmed by a 2003 cross-sectional analysis ($n = 28\,902$) applying data from the American Productivity Audit. In this study, Stewart and colleagues found that headache-related absenteeism and reduced work productivity cost approximately $19.6 billion dollars each year (Stewart et al., 2003).

Using 1986 estimates of US median earnings, the costs of migraine to employers due to reduced productivity and missed work days ranged from $5.6 billion to $17.2 billion, depending on prevalence (Osterhaus et al., 1992). Furthermore, indirect cost assessments often do not quantify the value of lost homeworker time, or time lost when workers care for family members with migraine. Nor do these data measure the burden of unemployment or underemployment due to migraine. Therefore, the true indirect cost burden of the disease may be considerably underestimated (Hu et al., 1999).

THE IMPACT OF PROBABLE MIGRAINE

Most epidemiological studies focus on the two common forms of migraine: migraine without aura (1.1) and migraine with aura (1.2). Clinic and some population-based studies show that a large number of patients with migrainous features fulfill all criteria but one for migraine with or without aura. This condition is termed probable migraine.

The impact of probable migraine is not to be neglected. In a health plan study, among 8579 respondents, the 1-year prevalence for migraine with and without aura (strict migraine) was 14.7% (19.2% in women and 6.6% in men); for probable migraine it was 14.5% (19.6% in women, 13.1% in men); pooling strict migraine and probable migraine, the prevalence of all migraine was 29.2% (38.8% in women and 19.6% in men). The prevalence of strict migraine and probable migraine was higher in females, Caucasians, and in early middle life relative to controls. HRQoL was reduced in the probable migraine, strict migraine, and all migraine groups, compared to controls (mental health scores respectively 50.2, 48.2, 50.9, and 53.1; $P < 0.0001$; physical health scores respectively 46.8, 48.8, 47.8, and 51.2; $P < 0.0001$). The proportion of subjects with high disability relative to control was elevated in probable migraine, strict migraine, and all migraine groups (Migraine Disability Assessment Scale III and IV: 13%, 31%, 22%, and 3.7%, respectively; $P < 0.0001$). Strict migraine and probable migraine were associated with an increased risk of depression (Patel et al., 2004; Bigal et al., 2006).

In the AMPP study, among probable migraine sufferers identified from the population, most (58.2%) had 1–4 days of severe headache per month. During their headaches, 48.2% had at least some impairment, while 22.1% were severely disabled. Although, over a 3-month period, the impact of probable migraine was low for most, 13.1% had missed 1 or more days of activity due to their headaches. Finally, probable migraine was amazingly undertreated. Although most probable migraine sufferers (52.8%) never used a migraine-preventive treatment and only 7.9% were current users, according to expert panel guidelines prevention should be offered (16.9%) or considered (11.5%) for 28.4% of the probable migraine sufferers in the survey (Silberstein et al., 2007).

THE IMPACT OF CHRONIC OR TRANSFORMED MIGRAINE

Evidence suggests that a subgroup of migraine sufferers may have a clinically progressive disorder (Bigal and Lipton, 2006). Chronic migraine (CM), sometimes referred to as transformed migraine (TM), is the consequence of this process of migraine chronification. Nosologically, TM/CM are subtypes of the CDH of long duration, a clinical syndrome that also includes chronic TTH, new daily persistent headache, and hemicrania continua (Scher et al., 2003; Bigal et al., 2004).

TM/CM responds to nearly half of the CDHs in the population, with a prevalence around 2% (Scher et al., 2003). Clinic-based studies show, however, that they are the most common CDH subtype in the specialty care (Bigal et al., 2004).

Although prevalent, the burden of TM is incompletely understood, in contrast to the burdens of episodic migraine, which are very well documented. We have recently conducted a study, measuring the impact of TM in individuals participating in a clinical trial of the disease. Subjects had an average of 23.6 headache days per month, with an average pain rating of 6.4 on a 10-point scale. A total of 75.2% of patients were severely disabled. Compared to norms from the population, the impact of TM on the HRQoL was substantial, with the greatest differences observed in the role physical domain (53 points) (Figure 2.2). The least difference was observed in the mental health domain (about 10 points). Other differences ranged from 14 to 36 points. Although most (53.9%) were at least somewhat satisfied with the effectiveness of the acute medications (used to treat the exacerbations of TM), just 23.6% were satisfied with their preventive treatment. Subjects made an average of 1.2 emergency department visits for headache in the previous year. Interestingly, those who used these services at least once made 4.9 visits, suggesting that the burden is disproportionably distributed (Bigal et al., unpublished data).

The disability of CM/TM is higher than the disability of migraine. In population studies, the disability scores of episodic migraine, as assessed by the Migraine Disability Assessment (MIDAS) questionnaire, usually range from 16.5 to 20.7. The scores of TM range from 34.9 to 64.8 (Tepper, 2002).

BURDEN OF TENSION-TYPE HEADACHE

TTH is the most prevalent form of primary headache in the general population (Rasmussen and Olesen, 1994; Lavados and Tenhamm, 1998; Schwartz et al., 1998). A Danish population study conducted in 1979 showed that the lifetime prevalence of episodic TTH

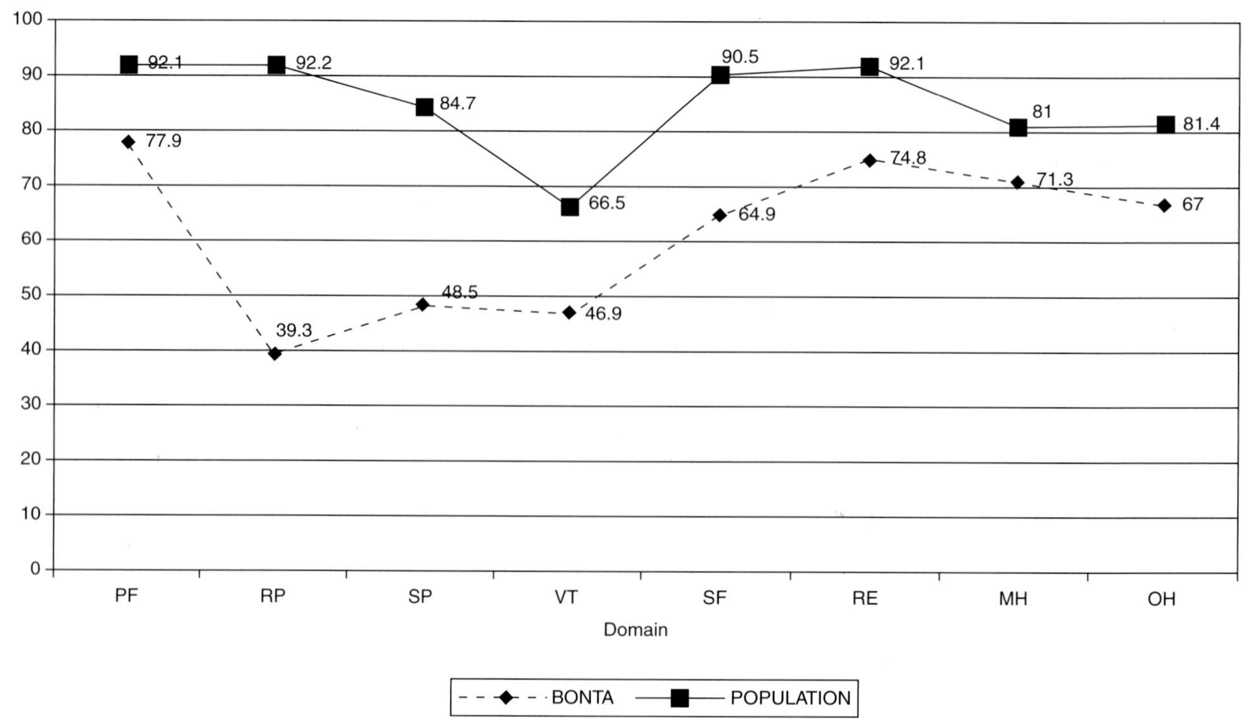

Fig. 2.2. Health-related quality of life (HRQoL) of individuals with transformed migraine participating in a clinical trial, compared with US population norms. BoNTA, onabotulinum toxin A.

(ETTH) was 79%, being 69% in men and 88% in women (Scher et al., 1999). Interestingly, when the same group replicated the study 12 years later, they found that the overall prevalence of TTH (87%), especially of what they called frequent TTH (37%), had increased significantly (Rasmussen and Olsen, 1994). In the USA, a study conducted in 1995 showed that the overall 1-year prevalence of ETTH was 38.3% (Schwartz et al., 1998). Women had slightly higher 1-year ETTH prevalence than men in all age, race, and education groups, with an overall prevalence ratio of 1.16. Prevalence peaked in the 30–39-year-old age group in both men (42.3%) and women (46.9%). Caucasians had a higher prevalence than African Americans in both men (40.1% versus 22.8%) and women (46.8% versus 30.9%). Prevalence increased with increasing educational levels in both sexes, reaching a peak in subjects with graduate school education of 48.5% for men and 48.9% for women.

In the same study, the 1-year period prevalence of chronic TTH (CTTH) was 2.2%. The prevalence of CTTH was higher in women and declined with increasing education. Of subjects with ETTH, 8.3% reported lost work days because of their headaches, while 43.6% reported decreased effectiveness at work, home, or school (Schwartz et al., 1998). Subjects with CTTH reported more lost work days (mean of 27.4 days versus 8.9 days for those reporting lost work days) and reduced-effectiveness days (mean of 20.4 versus 5.0 days for those reporting reduced effectiveness) compared with subjects with ETTH. The burden of TTH, although not as important as migraine, is well established (Lavados and Tenhamm, 1998).

The burden of TTH is far less studied than the burden of migraine. In most studies where headaches other than migraine are studied, TTH is not listed as a separate diagnosis and, when it is, its episodic and chronic forms are not usually separated. Nonetheless, functional impairment and abolished working capacities are reported in up to 60% of persons with TTH.

Studies show that the medical needs for TTH are not as significant as those of migraine. Only 16% of patients with TTH have been in contact with their general practitioner for headache. However, considering the high prevalence of TTH, the costs of this disease are likely to be significant. In Chile, consultation rates in TTH sufferers were 39% compared to 63% in migraineurs, and younger age or moderate to severe pain intensity increased the likelihood of medical consultation (Schwartz et al., 1998). TTH also has a measurable impact on the QoL. In a workplace study, individuals with ETTH had lower scores than controls in all domains of the SF-36; in vitality and bodily pain the difference reached statistical significance.

The burden of CTTH is significant, but in most studies, CTTH is studied as a part of the CDH syndrome.

MEASURING AND REDUCING THE BURDEN OF MIGRAINE

Understanding the burden of migraine should be a prelude to effective treatment designed to reduce that burden. Prior reports have identified the following barriers to migraine diagnosis and treatment: (1) underrecognition of migraine by headache sufferers themselves; (2) underconsultation among migraine sufferers who need medical care; (3) failure to diagnose all who consult; (4) failure to initiate appropriate therapy among all who are diagnosed; and (5) lack of ongoing assessment of the benefits of treatment (Lipton et al., 1994). Tools that screen for migraine and assess disability have been proposed as strategies for surmounting some of these barriers. In this final section we briefly discuss tools for screening and assessing the impact of migraine. Tools that measure comorbidities and satisfaction with treatment are also available and may be used.

Screening for migraine

Reducing the burden of migraine requires appropriate diagnosis as a prelude to effective treatment. Recently, a three-item migraine screener (ID-Migraine) was found to be a valid and reliable screening instrument for migraine headaches in primary care (Centers for Disease Control, 1991). The study was conducted at 26 primary care practice sites – the setting of intended use of ID-Migraine. Eligible subjects were making a primary care visit for any reason and had headaches that interfered with their lives, or wanted to talk to a doctor about their headaches. Eligible subjects ($n = 563$) completed a self-administered screening questionnaire that consisted of nine questions regarding headache characteristics, associated migraine symptoms, and disability. Study subjects then underwent independent diagnostic evaluations performed by headache specialists, who completed semistructured diagnostic questionnaires and examined the patients. Using the International Headache Society (IHS) criteria (Headache Classification Subcommittee of the International Headache Society, 2004), a gold-standard diagnosis of migraine was made (Lipton et al., 2003c).

The sensitivities and specificities of each item from the nine-item screener were computed. Logistic regression was used to identify the combination of items from the screener that best predicted a gold-standard migraine diagnosis. The three items independently associated with migraine included photophobia, inability to function (missing 1 or more days in the previous 3 months due to headache), and nausea. These items

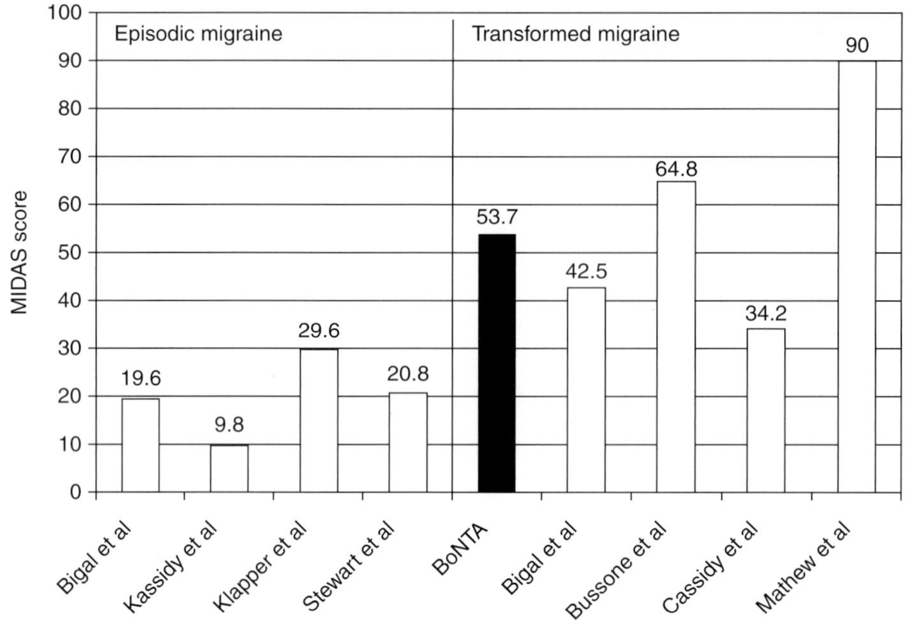

Fig. 2.3. Migraine Disability Assessment (MIDAS) scores in studies of migraine and transformed migraine. BoNTA, onabotulinum toxin A.

can be remembered using the acronym "PIN." Individuals with at least two of these three features were said to screen positive for migraine. ID-Migraine had a sensitivity of 0.81, a specificity of 0.75, and a positive predictive value of 93% for a clinical diagnosis of IHS migraine. In other words, of patients with two of three items, 93% have migraine. Using this screener should help improving the recognition of migraine. In individuals who screen positive, once the diagnosis of migraine is confirmed, disability should be assessed.

Assessing migraine disability

Measuring the burden of migraine should be a prelude to effective treatment designed to reduce that burden. The most frequently used disability instrument in migraine research is the MIDAS questionnaire (Stewart and Lipton, 2002). The MIDAS questionnaire consists of five questions that focus on lost time in three domains: school work or work for pay; household work or chores; and family, social, and leisure activities (Jacobson et al., 1995). All questions ask about either days of missed activity or days where productivity was reduced by at least half. If productivity is decreased to 50% or below, the day is considered missed. The MIDAS score is derived as the sum of missed days due to a headache over a 3-month period in the three domains. Two additional questions on the MIDAS questionnaire are not included in MIDAS score, assessing frequency and intensity of pain. The four-point grading system for the MIDAS questionnaire is as follows:

- Grade 1 (scores ranging from 0 to 5): little or no disability
- Grade 2 (scores ranging from 6 to 10): mild disability
- Grade 3 (scores ranging from 11 to 20): moderate disability
- Grade 4 (21 or greater): severe disability.

Other disability measures include the Headache Disability Inventory and the Headache Impact Test (Stewart et al., 2000; Pryse-Phillips, 2002). The Headache Disability Inventory is a 25-item with good internal consistency reliability, robust long-term test–retest stability, and good construct validity. The Headache Impact Test is a six-item (HIT-6) paper questionnaire that was recently developed and validated. An interactive version of HIT-6 is available over the internet.

Figure 2.3 provides a schematic view of how screening and assessing disability may be used to provide appropriate treatment, in accordance with the US Headache Consortium Guidelines (Lipton et al., 1998).

CONCLUSIONS

Headache disorders impose burdens on individual headache sufferers both during and between attacks. For example, migraine sufferers may experience intermittent headaches over several decades. Migraine parallels other chronic illnesses, such as asthma, hypertension, high blood pressure, and seizure disorder, in terms of impact of disease and requirement for long-term management. Recent evidence supports the concept that, at least in a subgroup of patients, migraine may be a progressive disorder. Therefore, untreated migraine may lead not only to a substantial burden, but also to progression to a more severe spectrum of the disease (CDH). Identifying and screening migraine, establishing a disease management plan for the patient, based on a stratified care treatment approach, and ongoing assessment of illness severity and disease impact are likely to improve long-term outcomes, including patient satisfaction and treatment success, and eventually to avoid disease progression. This effort must be part of a broader strategy which includes effective assessment and follow-up, patient education, behavioral approaches, and preventive treatments.

References

Bigal ME, Lipton RB (2006). When migraine progresses: transformed or chronic migraine. Expert Rev Neurother 6: 297–306.

Bigal ME, Rapoport AM, Sheftell FD et al. (2004). Transformed migraine and medication overuse in a tertiary headache centre – clinical characteristics and treatment outcomes. Cephalalgia 24: 483–490.

Bigal M, Kolodner K, Lafata J et al. (2006). Patterns of medical diagnosis and treatment of migraine and probable migraine in a health plan. Cephalalgia 26: 43–49.

Celentano DD, Stewart WF, Lipton RB et al. (1992). Medication use and disability among migraineurs: a national probability sample. Headache 32: 223–228.

Centers for Disease Control (1991). Prevalence of chronic migraine headaches – United States, 1980–89. MMWR Morb Mortal Wkly Rep 40: 331–338.

Consumer Healthcare Products Association (2000). OTC Sales Statistics – 1995–1999. AC Neilsen, Ascot.

D'Alessandro R, Benassi G, Lenzi PL et al. (1988). Epidemiology of headache in the Republic of San Marino. J Neurol Neurosurg Psychiatry 51: 21–27.

Dahlöf CG, Dimenäs E (1995). Migraine patients experience poorer subjective well-being/quality of life even between attacks. Cephalalgia 15: 31–36.

Dhopesh V, Anwar R, Herring C (1979). A retrospective assessment of emergency department patients with complaint of headache. Headache 19: 37–42.

Edmeads J, Findlay H, Tugwell P et al. (1993). Impact of migraine and tension-type headache on life-style, consulting behavior, and medication use: a Canadian population survey. Can J Neurol Sci 20: 131–137.

Freitag FG (2007). The cycle of migraine: patients' quality of life during and between migraine attacks. Clin Ther 29: 939–949.

Fry J (1996). Profiles of Disease. Livingstone: Edinburgh.

Gibbs TS, Fleischer AB, Feldman SR et al. (2003). Health care utilization in patients with migraine: demographics and patterns of care in the ambulatory setting. Headache 43: 330–335.

Gobels H, Petersen-Braun M, Soyka D (1994). The epidemiology of headache in Germany: a nationwide survey of a representative sample on the basis of the headache classification of the International Headache Society. Cephalalgia 14: 97–106.

Headache Classification Subcommittee of the International Headache Society (2004). The international classification of headache disorders, 2nd edn. Cephalalgia 24 (Suppl. 1): 1–15.

Henry P, Michel P, Brochet B et al. (1992). A nationwide survey of migraine in France: prevalence and clinical features in adults. Cephalalgia 12: 229–237.

Hu XH, Markson LE, Lipton RB et al. (1999). Burden of migraine in the United States: disability and economic costs. Arch Intern Med 159: 813–818.

Jacobson GP, Ramadan NM, Norris L et al. (1995). Headache disability inventory (HDI): short-term test–retest reliability and spouse perceptions. Headache 35: 534–549.

Launer LJ, Terwindt GM, Ferrari MD (1999). The prevalence and characteristics of migraine in a population-based cohort: the GEM study. Neurology 53: 537–542.

Lavados PM, Tenhamm E (1998). Epidemiology of tension-type headache in Santiago, Chile: a prevalence study. Cephalalgia 18: 552–558.

Leonardi M, Steiner TJ, Scher AT et al. (2005). The global burden of migraine: measuring disability in headache disorders with WHO's classification of functioning, disability and health (ICF). J Headache Pain 6: 429–440.

Lipton RB, Silberstein SD (1994). Why study the comorbidity of migraine? Neurology 44: 4–5.

Lipton RB, Amatniek JC, Ferrari MD et al. (1994). Migraine: identifying and removing barriers to care. Neurology 44 (Suppl. 6): 56–62.

Lipton RB, Stewart WF, von Korff M (1997). Burden of migraine: societal costs and therapeutic opportunities. Neurology 48 (Suppl. 3): 4–9.

Lipton RB, Stewart WF, Simon D (1998). Medical consultation for migraine: results from the American Migraine Study. Headache 38: 87–96.

Lipton RB, Hamelsky SW, Kolodner KB et al. (2000). Migraine, quality of life, and depression: a population-based case-control study. Neurology 55: 629–635.

Lipton RB, Diamond S, Reed M et al. (2001a). Migraine diagnosis and treatment: results from the American Migraine Study II. Headache 41: 638–645.

Lipton RB, Stewart WF, Diamond S et al. (2001b). Prevalence and burden of migraine in the United States: data from the American Migraine Study II. Headache 41: 646–657.

Lipton RB, Hamelsky SW, Stewart WF (2001c). Epidemiology and impact of migraine. In: SD Silberstein, RB Lipton, DJ Dalessio (Eds.), Wolff's Headache and Other Head Pain. Oxford University Press, New York, pp. 85–107.

Lipton RB, Liberman JN, Kolodner KB et al. (2003a). Migraine headache disability and health-related quality-of-life: a population-based case-control study from England. Cephalalgia 23: 441–450.

Lipton RB, Bigal ME, Kolodner K et al. (2003b). The family impact of migraine: population-based studies in the USA and UK. Cephalalgia 23: 429–440.

Lipton RB, Dodick D, Sadovsky R et al. (2003c). A self-administered screener for migraine in primary care: the ID Migraine validation study. Neurology 61: 375–382.

Lipton RB, Bigal ME, Diamond M et al. (2007). Migraine prevalence, disease burden, and the need for preventive therapy. Neurology 68: 343–349.

Michel P, Dartigues JF, Lindousli A et al. (1997). Loss of productivity and quality of life in migraine sufferers among French workers: results from the GAZEL cohort. Headache 37: 71–78.

Olesen J, Leonardi M (2003). The burden of brain diseases in Europe. Eur J Neurol 10: 471–477.

Osterhaus JT, Gutterman DL, Plachetka JR (1992). Health care resources and lost labor costs of migraine headaches in the United States. Pharmacoeconomics 2: 67–76.

Patel NV, Bigal ME, Kolodner KB et al. (2004). Prevalence and impact of migraine and probable migraine in a health plan. Neurology 63: 1432–1438.

Pesa J, Lage MJ (2004). The medical costs of migraine and comorbid anxiety and depression. Headache 44: 562–570.

Pryse-Phillips W (2002). Evaluating migraine disability: the headache impact test instrument in context. Can J Neurol Sci 29 (Suppl. 2): 11–15.

Raskin NH (1998). Headache. 2nd edn. Churchill Livingstone, New York.

Rasmussen BK (1995). Epidemiology of headache. Cephalalgia 15: 45–68.

Rasmussen BK, Olesen J (1994). Epidemiology of migraine and tension-type headache. Curr Opin Neurol 7: 264–271.

Rasmussen BK, Jensen R, Schroll M et al. (1991). Epidemiology of headache in a general population – a prevalence study. J Clin Epidemiol 44: 1147–1157.

Scher AI, Stewart WF, Lipton RB (1999). Migraine and headache: a meta-analytic approach. In: IK Crombie (Ed.), Epidemiology of Pain. IASP Press, Seattle, Washington, pp. 159–170.

Scher AI, Stewart WF, Ricci JA et al. (2003). Factors associated with the onset and remission of chronic daily headache in a population-based study. Pain 106: 81–89.

Schwartz BS, Stewart WF, Simon D et al. (1998). Epidemiology of tension-type headache. JAMA 279: 381–383.

Silberstein S, Loder E, Diamond S et al. (2007). Probable migraine in the United States: results of the American Migraine Prevalence and Prevention (AMPP) study. Cephalalgia 273: 220–234.

Smith R (1998). Impact of migraine on the family. Headache 38: 423–426.

Solomon GD, Skobieranda FG, Graff LA (1993). Quality of life and well-being of headache patients: measurement by the Medical Outcomes Study Instrument. Headache 33: 351–358.

Stang PE, Osterhaus JT (1993). Impact of migraine in the United States: data from the National Health Interview Survey. Headache 33: 29–35.

Stang PE, Osterhaus JT, Celentano DD (1994). Migraine: patterns of health care use. Neurology 44 (Suppl. 4): 47–55.

Stang PE, Sternfeld B, Sidney S (1996). Migraine headache in a pre-paid health plan: ascertainment, demographics, physiological and behavioral factors. Headache 36: 69–76.

Stewart WF, Lipton RB (2002). Need for care and perceptions of MIDAS among headache sufferers study. CNS Drugs 16 (Suppl. 1): 5–11.

Stewart WF, Lipton RB, Celentano DD et al. (1992). Prevalence of migraine headache in the United States. JAMA 267: 64–69.

Stewart WF, Lipton RB, Simon D (1996). Work-related disability: results from the American Migraine Study. Cephalalgia 16: 231–238.

Stewart WF, Lipton RB, Kolodner K et al. (1999). Reliability of the migraine disability assessment score in a population-based sample of headache sufferers. Cephalalgia 19: 107–113.

Stewart WF, Lipton RB, Kolodner K et al. (2000). Validity of the Migraine Disability Assessment (MIDAS) score in comparison to a diary-based measure in a population sample of migraine sufferers. Pain 88: 41–52.

Stewart WF, Ricci JA, Chee E et al. (2003). Lost productive time and cost due to common pain conditions in the US workforce. JAMA 290: 2443–2454.

Tepper SJ (2002). Debate: analgesic overuse is a cause, not consequence, of chronic daily headache. Analgesic overuse is a cause of chronic daily headache. Headache 42: 543–547.

Terwindt GM, Ferrari MD, Tijhuis M et al. (2000). The impact of migraine on quality of life in the general population: the GEM study. Neurology 55: 624–629.

Turner-Bowker DM, Bayliss MS, Ware JE Jr et al. (2003). Usefulness of the SF-8 Health Survey for comparing the impact of migraine and other conditions. Qual Life Res 12: 1003–1012.

Von-Korff M, Stewart WF, Simon DJ et al. (1998). Migraine and reduced work performance: a population-based diary study. Neurology 50: 1741–1745.

Section 2

Biological science of headache

Handbook of Clinical Neurology, Vol. 97 (3rd series)
Headache
G. Nappi and M.A. Moskowitz, Editors

Chapter 3

Biological sciences related to headache

TOSHIHIKO SHIMIZU* AND NORIHIRO SUZUKI
Department of Neurology, School of Medicine, Keio University, Tokyo, Japan

Headache can occur as a result of activation of pain-sensitive cranial structures, such as the dura mater, vasculature, and the cranial and cervical muscles and ligaments, which are innervated by primary afferent neurons originating from the trigeminal and dorsal root ganglia of the upper cervical spinal nerves. In relation to nociception in cases of headache, two types of nerve fiber are considered to be important: the small-caliber, unmyelinated, slow-conducting fibers called C fibers, and the small-diameter, lightly myelinated, more rapid-conducting fibers called Aδ fibers. Findings from nerve stimulation studies indicate that C fibers transmit aching, throbbing, or burning pain that builds up slowly, whereas the Aδ fibers conduct sharper initial pain sensation (Basbaum and Jessell, 2000). These primary afferent neurons transmit nociceptive information from the pain-sensitive endings in the cranial structures through the trigeminal and first and second spinal dorsal root ganglia to the brainstem at the pontine level. The nociceptive fibers then project to the central pain-conducting pathways at the spinal trigeminal nucleus. In this chapter, we shall discuss the anatomy in relation to headache, including the meninges, blood vessels, cranial and neck muscles, and the central pain-conducting pathways.

THE SCALP AND SKULL

The brain is encased in several protective layers called the scalp. As shown in Figure 3.1A, the scalp is composed of five layers: (1) the skin; (2) subcutaneous connective tissue; (3) galea aponeurotica; (4) loose areolar connective tissue; and (5) periosteum (Blumenfeld, 2002). The galea aponeurotica is a sturdy layer of dense fibrous tissue that runs between the frontal and occipital bellies of the occipitofrontal muscles. Ray and Wolff (1940) have reported that the skin, galea aponeurotica, and the fascia covering the temporal and occipital muscles are all sensitive to pain. They receive sensory innervation from the greater and lesser occipital nerves or the supraorbital nerve. The periosteum shows regional variability in the sensitivity to pain. In general, while the regions just over the eyebrows are highly sensitive to pain, the temporal and occipital regions are relatively insensitive. The cranial bones, including the diploic and emissary veins passing through them, are insensitive to pain (Ray and Wolff, 1940).

THE MENINGES

The meninges represent several layers of membranes situated between the skull and the brain to protect the brain from physical damage. The concept that the meninges may serve as one of the sources of headache originated from the results of intraoperative experiments in which electrical, mechanical, thermal, and chemical stimulation of the dural and large intracerebral arteries elicited a painful sensation (Penfield and McNaughton, 1940; Ray and Wolff, 1940).

Structure of the meninges

The meninges consist of three layers called, from the inside to the outside, the pia mater, arachnoid mater, and dura mater (Figure 3.1A). The dura mater is divided into two layers: the outer periosteal layer which is adherent to the inner surface of the skull, and an inner layer which is fused to the outer layer of the dura mater in most regions, except some, where the inner layer is folded to descend far into the cranial cavity. One of these regions is the interhemispheric fissure, in which the falx cerebri, a flat sheet of dura mater that is suspended from the top of the cranium, runs to separate the right and left cerebral hemispheres.

*Correspondence to: Toshihiko Shimizu, Department of Neurology, School of Medicine, Keio University, 35 Shinanomachi, Shinjuku-ku, Tokyo 160-8582, Japan, Tel: +81-3-5363-3788, Fax: +81-3-3353-1272, E-mail: shimizu-toshi@umin.ac.jp

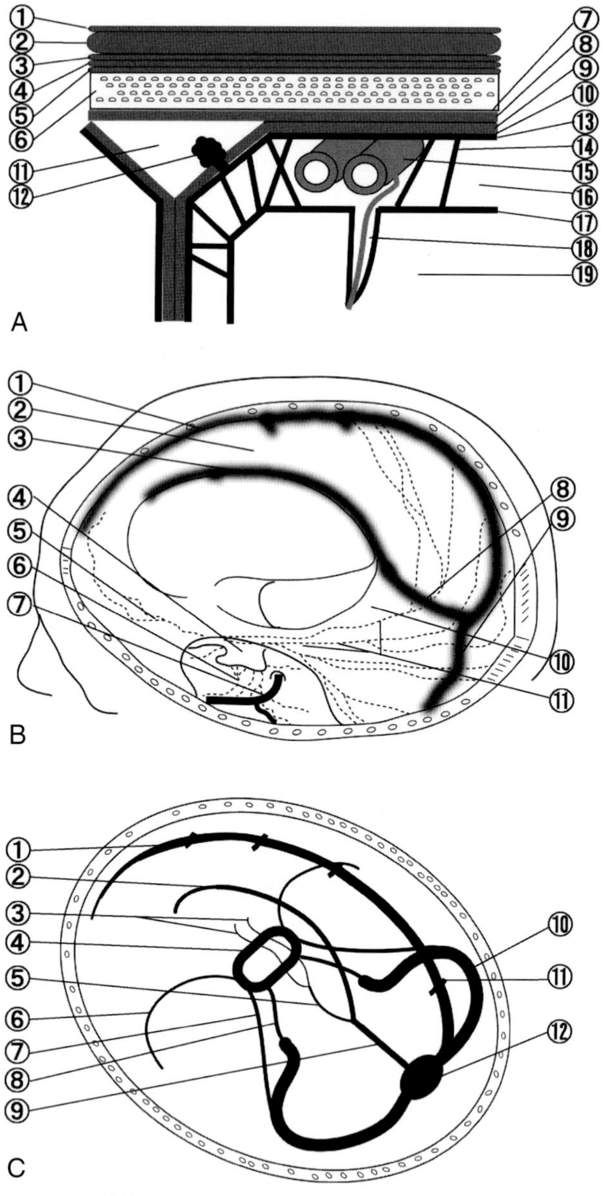

Fig. 3.1. (A) The scalp, skull, and meninges. 1, Skin; 2, subcutaneous connective tissue; 3, galea aponeurotica; 4, loose areolar connective tissue; 5, pericranium (periosteum); 6, skull; 7, epidural space; 8, dura mater (periosteal layer); 9, dura mater (meningeal layer); 10, subdural space; 11, superior sagittal sinus; 12, arachnoid granulations; 13, arachnoid mater; 14, arachnoid trabecula; 15, cerebral artery; 16, subarachnoid space; 17, pia mater; 18, perivascular space (Virchow–Robin space); 19, cerebral cortex.
(B) Falx cerebri and tentorium cerebelli with an illustration of the typical distribution of the dural nerves in the anterior and middle fossae on the left side. 1, Superior sagittal sinus; 2, falx cerebri; 3, inferior sagittal sinus; 4, trigeminal ganglion; 5, branches of the anterior and posterior ethmoidal nerves; 6, nervus meningeus medius; 7, middle meningeal artery; 8, straight sinus; 9, transverse sinus; 10, tentorium cerebelli; 11, tentorial nerves. (Modified from Penfield and McNaughton, 1940.)
(C) Dural venous sinuses. 1, Superior sagittal sinus; 2, inferior sagittal sinus; 3, internal cerebral veins; 4, cavernous sinus; 5, great vein (Galen); 6, sphenoparietal sinus; 7, superior petrosal sinus; 8, inferior petrosal sinus; 9, straight sinus; 10, transverse sinus; 11, superior cerebral vein; 12, confluence of sinuses (torcular herophili).

Another such region is the tentorium cerebelli, which represents a sheet of dura mater covering the upper surface of the cerebellum (Blumenfeld, 2002).

The arachnoid is a meningeal layer adherent to the inner surface of the dura. The innermost meningeal layer is a very thin layer of cells called the pia mater. Unlike the arachnoid, the pia is closely adherent to the surface of the brain and follows into the depths of the sulci. The pia also surrounds the initial portion of each blood vessel as it penetrates the brain surface, forming a perivascular space (Virchow–Robin space), to fuse with the blood vessel wall.

The meninges separate three spaces called the epidural space, subarachnoid space, and the subdural space. Each of these spaces contains some important blood vessels, rupture of which can cause headache. The epidural space is a potential space located between the inner surface of the skull and the tightly adherent dura. The middle meningeal artery enters the skull through the foramen spinosum and runs between the dura and the skull. Injury to this artery can result in an acute epidural hematoma.

The subdural space is also a potential space between the inner layer of the dura and the loosely adherent arachnoid mater. The bridging veins traverse the subdural space to drain into the several large dural venous sinuses. Disruption of the bridging veins is the principal cause of subdural hematoma.

The space between the arachnoid and pia is called the subarachnoid space, which is filled with cerebrospinal fluid. In addition, the major arteries of the brain also run within the subarachnoid space, and rupture of an aneurysm of these major arteries in the subarachnoid space may cause subarachnoid hemorrhage.

Innervation of the dura mater

The dura mater is innervated by afferent nerve fibers, most of which originate in the ipsilateral trigeminal ganglion (Steiger et al., 1982; Mayberg et al., 1984; Andres et al., 1987; Uddman et al., 1989). The afferent nerve fibers in the dura mater have been implicated in neurogenic inflammation, a phenomenon putatively linked to the development of migrainous pain (Moskowitz, 1984).

The dura mater in the middle cranial fossa and the middle meningeal vessels are supplied mainly by nerve fibers rising from the second and third divisions of the trigeminal ganglion (Penfield and McNaughton, 1940). A branch of the third division, the nervus spinosus, which runs along the middle meningeal artery, carries the entire trigeminal supply to the middle cranial fossa along with the nervus meningeus medius, a branch of the second division of the trigeminal nerve. Occasionally, one or more fine nerves from the first division of the trigeminal nerve run along the anterior branch of the middle meningeal artery. The dura of the anterior cranial fossa also contains a few perivascular nerves running along branches of the middle meningeal artery. They are joined by some fine nerve fibers from the anterior and posterior ethmoidal nerves, both branches of the first division of the trigeminal nerve. The tentorium cerebelli, the dura of the parieto-occipital region, the falx, and the adjacent sinuses are innervated by the tentorial nerve of Arnold, a recurrent branch of the first division of the trigeminal nerve (Figure 3.1B). It arises from the proximal ophthalmic division of the nerve within the lateral wall of the cavernous sinus just before this division enters the superior orbital fissure. It immediately turns posteriorly within the most anterior portion of the free tentorial edge and courses along close to the trochlear nerve. On reaching the tentorium, the tentorial nerves spread out, forming an abundant plexus. The nerve supply of the dura mater in the posterior cranial fossa is still unclear. The most prominent nerve supply is represented by the sensory fibers arising from the cells of the upper cervical ganglion, that run through the hypoglossal canal (Keller et al., 1985). These meningeal afferent nerve fibers show positive immunoreactivity for substance P (SP), neurokinin A, and calcitonin gene-related peptide (CGRP) (Messlinger et al., 1993). In addition to its supply from the afferent nervous system, the dura mater is also innervated by sympathetic fibers containing neuropeptide Y (NPY) arising from the superior cervical ganglion (Edvinsson and Uddman, 1981; von During et al., 1990), and comparatively sparse parasympathetic fibers containing vasoactive intestinal polypeptide (VIP) and nitric oxide synthase (NOS) (Keller and Marfurt, 1991; Berger et al., 1994).

Referred pain from the dura mater

The main trunks of all the dural arteries and the smaller branches arising from the main divisions of the middle meningeal artery have been demonstrated to be sensitive to pain (Ray and Wolff, 1940). Furthermore, according to studies conducted by the aforementioned authors, the dura covering the convexities of the cerebrum and cerebellar hemispheres and the middle fossa floor are entirely insensitive to pain except for that in regions along the margins of the dural sinuses or along the meningeal artery. The falx is also devoid of nociception, unless the margins of the superior sagittal sinus are displaced or encroached upon. On the other hand, the entire dural covering of the floor of the anterior fossa and posterior fossa is believed to be uniformly sensitive to pain. Pain transmitted by the former is referred to the ipsilateral head and eye, and that transmitted by the latter is referred to the occiput near the midline (Table 3.1). The superior surface of the tentorium cerebelli is also reported to be sensitive to pain.

Table 3.1

The regions of referred pain from intracranial structures

Region	Anatomy
The eyes and forehead	Dura of the anterior fossa Anterior middle meningeal arteries Structures innervated by the tentorial nerve (superior surface of the tentorium, transverse and straight sinuses, and the posterior half of the superior sagittal sinus) Sylvian vein Intracranial portion of the internal carotid artery Vessels of the circle of Willis and proximal portion of the larger cerebral branches First division of the fifth nerve
The temporal and parietal regions	Middle meningeal arteries Union of the inferior cerebral vein of the temporal lobe with the venous sinuses Anterior portion of the superior sagittal sinus
The occipital and suboccipital regions	In or behind the ear Inferior surface of the wall of the confluence of sinus, straight sinus, and the transverse sinus Wall of the sigmoid sinus Branches of the basilar artery
The occiput near the midline	Part of the dura of the posterior fossa Posterior meningeal arteries Proximal portion of the posterior inferior cerebellar arteries Vertebral artery Basilar artery

Innervation of and referred pain from the dural sinuses

Dural sinuses are large venous channels that lie enclosed within the two layers of dura (Figure 3.1C). Penfield and McNaughton (1940) reported that the superior sagittal sinus is supplied in its anterior aspect by branches of the ethmoidal nerve, and in its posterior aspect by nerve fibers derived from the tentorial nerve. The origin of the nerve fibers innervating the inferior sagittal sinus is obscure; however, these fibers are probably derived from the tentorial nerve. The transverse sinus, straight, and superior petrosal sinuses are crossed by many branches of the tentorial nerve. The superior petrosal sinus may also receive fibers from the third division of the trigeminal nerve or the trigeminal ganglion. The origin of the nerve supply to the vein of Galen is uncertain, although some of the fibers supplying it may arise from the tentorial nerve. According to Ray and Wolff (1940), the superior sagittal sinus, transverse sinus, straight sinus, sigmoid sinus, occipital sinus, and superior petrosal sinus are sensitive to pain. In contrast, the inferior sagittal sinus, superior cerebral vein, and inferior cerebral vein are insensitive to pain.

The cavernous sinus is a large plexus of veins bordered by the sphenoid bone and temporal bones of the skull. The sinus envelops portions of the internal carotid artery and some cranial nerves, namely the oculomotor nerve, trochlear nerve, and ophthalmic nerve, all of which are located, in descending order toward the sinus floor, in the lateral wall of the cavernous sinus, and the abducens nerve, which exists in the vicinity of the carotid artery (Blumenfeld, 2002). The cavernous sinus receives venous blood from the eyes and superficial cerebral cortex and drains into the transverse sinus via the superior petrosal sinus, or the internal jugular vein via the inferior petrosal sinus (Figure 3.1C). Sympathetic nerve fibers run around the internal carotid artery as the carotid plexus. In addition, the parasympathetic ganglion, called the cavernous ganglion, is also located between the internal carotid and abducens nerve in the cavernous sinus and contributes to parasympathetic innervation of the cerebral arteries (Suzuki and Hardebo, 1991a; Figure 3.2A). Furthermore, Bleys et al. (2001a) have reported that the cavernous ganglion has nerve fiber connections with the sympathetic and sensory nerves in the cavernous sinus, which may explain a variety of symptoms associated with injury or disease of the cavernous sinus. According to the report by Ray and Wolff (1940), stimulation of the cavernous sinus causes pain in the ipsilateral ophthalmic and maxillary nerve region. The maxillary nerve often runs through the lateral wall of the cavernous sinus for a short distance (Blumenfeld, 2002). Hence, direct stimulation of these trigeminal branches can cause pain arising from this portion of the sinus. If the internal carotid artery ruptures within the cavernous sinus, an arteriovenous fistula is created, and pain arising from the sinus is referred to the region shown in Table 3.1.

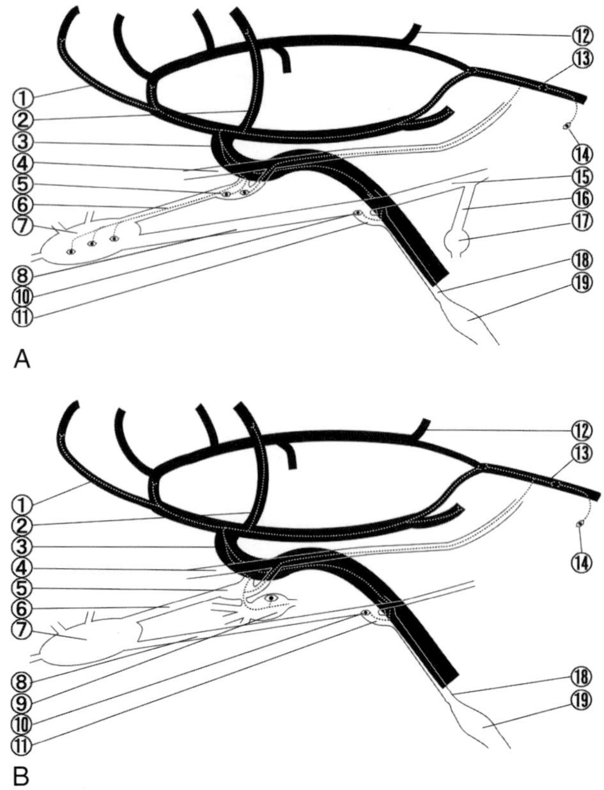

Fig. 3.2. Possible origins and pathways of the postganglionic parasympathetic (A) and sensory (B) fibers in the extrinsic innervation system of the human cerebral arteries. 1, Anterior cerebral artery; 2, middle cerebral artery; 3, internal carotid artery; 4, abducens nerve; 5, cavernous ganglion; 6, rami orbitales; 7, sphenopalatine ganglion; 8, vidian nerve; 9, trigeminal ganglion; 10, internal carotid ganglion; 11, deep petrosal nerve; 12, posterior cerebral artery; 13, basilar artery; 14, dorsal root ganglion; 15, greater superficial petrosal nerve; 16, lesser superficial petrosal nerve; 17, otic ganglion; 18, internal carotid nerve; 19, superior cervical ganglion. (Modified from Suzuki and Hardebo, 1991a.)

CEREBRAL ARTERIES

It is well known that there are two cerebral arterial innervation systems: the extrinsic and intrinsic innervation systems. The extrinsic innervation system originates from the extracranial ganglia, and mainly innervates the vessels of the circle of Willis and their penetrating cerebral branches. When they enter the brain parenchyma, the cerebral arteries lose their peripheral nerve supply from the extrinsic innervation system. After the cerebral arteries leave the Virchow–Robin space, they receive neural input from neurons located within the brain itself, represented by the intrinsic innervation system.

Extrinsic innervation system

The extrinsic innervation system of the cerebral blood vessels is composed of sympathetic, parasympathetic, and sensory neurons (Uddman and Edvinsson, 1989). Although the sensory nerve fibers may contribute to pain, the sympathetic and parasympathetic nerve fibers are presumably relevant to a considerable degree to the pathophysiology of migraine (Edvinsson and Uddman, 2005).

Extrinsic sympathetic innervation

The sympathetic nerve fibers originate from the superior cervical ganglion and contain norepinephrine and NPY as the neurotransmitters (Nielsen and Owman, 1967; Uddman and Edvinsson, 1989). The nerve fibers from the superior cervical ganglion run along the internal carotid artery, to be distributed to the circle of Willis and the basilar artery (Handa et al., 1990).

Extrinsic parasympathetic innervation

The parasympathetic nerve fibers mainly contain acetylcholine (ACh), VIP, and NOS as the neurotransmitters, and originate from the sphenopalatine, otic, internal carotid, or cavernous ganglia (Suzuki et al., 1988, 1990, 1993; Nozaki et al., 1993). The postganglionic fibers from the sphenopalatine ganglion climb up in a fine membranous structure and run through the ethmoidal foramen to enter the cranial cavity. They have then been shown to reach the cerebral blood vessels in the rat (Suzuki et al., 1988; Hara et al., 1993).

In monkeys and humans, postganglionic nerve fibers from the sphenopalatine ganglion reach the internal carotid artery in the cavernous sinus region, run along the rami orbitales, and subsequently join the orbitociliary nerve, which is a recurrent branch of the maxillary nerve (Figure 3.2A; Ruskell and Simons, 1987; Suzuki and Hardebo, 1991a). Some fibers climb along the internal carotid artery to be distributed to the anterior portion of the circle of Willis, and other fibers run along the abducens nerve and are distributed to the basilar artery, as shown in Figure 3.2A.

The otic ganglion also sends parasympathetic nerve fibers to the cerebral arteries via the lesser superficial petrosal nerve to join the greater superficial petrosal nerve. They then reach the greater deep petrosal nerve and ascend along the internal carotid artery to be distributed to the cerebral blood vessels (Suzuki and Hardebo, 1991b; Shimizu, 1994).

The cavernous ganglion is a small ganglion located between the abducens nerve and the internal carotid artery in the rostral half of the cavernous sinus region in humans. The preganglionic fibers presumably run along the rami orbitales to reach the cavernous ganglion. The pathways to the cerebral arteries of the postganglionic parasympathetic fibers originating from the cavernous ganglion are almost identical to those originating from the sphenopalatine ganglion in monkeys and humans (Ruskell and Simons, 1987; Hardebo et al., 1991). It has been revealed that the cavernous ganglion of the rat also contributes to cerebrovascular parasympathetic nervous innervation (Bleys et al., 2001b).

The internal carotid ganglion is located close to the junction between the greater superficial petrosal nerve and the deep petrosal nerve. In rats, monkeys, and humans, the majority of the cells forming the distal group of the ganglion contain the parasympathetic nerve markers VIP and ACh, whereas those forming the proximal group contain the pain fiber transmitters SP and CGRP (Suzuki et al., 1988; Hardebo et al., 1991; Suzuki and Hardebo, 1991a). Nerve section and retrograde axonal tracing experiments using True blue in rats and monkeys have revealed that parasympathetic VIP/Ach-positive nerve and sensory SP/CGRP-positive nerve fibers originating in these ganglia innervate the intracranial segment of the internal carotid artery and its intracranial ramifications.

Extrinsic sensory innervation

The trigeminal ganglion is the main origin of the cerebrovascular sensory nerve fibers. The anterior portion of the circle of Willis receives nerve fibers from the ipsilateral ophthalmic branch of the trigeminal nerve. In monkeys and humans, the sensory fibers from the ophthalmic nerve along with the autonomic fibers form the cavernous plexus in the cavernous sinus and run on to the internal carotid artery (Figure 3.2B; Ruskell and Simons, 1987; Suzuki and Hardebo, 1991a). The posterior vessels are also supplied by the trigeminal source. Branches of the ophthalmic nerve course backwards with the abducens nerve, leaving it at the level of the pons to join the basilar artery, from which they are distributed to the posterior circle of Willis and vertebral arteries. The other source of nerve supply to the posterior circulation is the upper dorsal root ganglia; however, the exact pathway to the posterior circulation of fibers arising from these ganglia remains obscure.

In rats, the majority of the fibers originate from the ophthalmic division of the trigeminal ganglion and run in the nasociliary nerve through the ethmoidal foramen. From here, the fibers can be traced along the dura mater of the frontal skull base before they reach the internal ethmoidal artery to enter the rostral half of the circle of Willis and its branches (Suzuki et al., 1989).

Referred pain from the cerebral arteries

Just like the dura mater, the internal segment of the internal carotid artery, proximal middle cerebral artery, and anterior cerebral artery is also sensitive to pain. Vessels of the posterior circulation, such as the vertebral artery, posterior inferior cerebellar artery, basilar artery, and their branches, are also reported to be sensitive to pain. Pain originating from the cerebral arteries is referred to the regions shown in Table 3.1. The pial arteries and veins over the superior and lateral convexities of the cerebrum and cerebellum are devoid of nociception (Ray and Wolff, 1940).

Intrinsic innervation

The main intrinsic neural pathways projecting to the cortical microvessels are those originating from the nucleus basalis, locus coeruleus, or raphe nucleus, and contain ACh (Hamel, 2004), norepinephrine (Hartman et al., 1972) or serotonin (Reinhard et al., 1979; Cohen et al., 1996) as the neurotransmitter, respectively. Anatomical, molecular, and pharmacological studies have revealed that these neurons send projection fibers directly to the cortical microvessels and control the vascular response. Furthermore, the vascular responses of the cortical microvessels are also believed to be regulated by the perivascular astrocytes or local cortical interneurons. These ideas are consistent with the findings that local cortical interneurons innervating the microvessels receive inputs from the intrinsic brain neurons, and that specific receptors for the vasoactive mediators are also found on astrocytes (Hamel, 2006).

TEMPOROMANDIBULAR APPARATUS

The temporomandibular apparatus is composed of the temporomandibular joints and muscles. Disturbances of the temporomandibular apparatus can be responsible for headache.

Structure of the temporomandibular joint

The temporomandibular joint is a diarthrosis joint that connects the mandible to the temporal bone on the side of the skull (Griffin et al., 1975; Piette, 1993). The zygomatic process of the temporal bone has a concavity called the articular fossa, which receives the convex condyle of the mandible. There is a fibrous articular disc between these two bones. The upper and lower laminae of the articular disc are attached separately either to the temporal bone or to the mandibular condyle (Schmolke, 1994). These structures enable the mandible to undertake gliding movements as a modified hinge joint. Furthermore, not only does the temporomandibular joint enable the lower jaw to open and close, but it also enables it to move forward and backward as well as laterally. Although the jaw can open under gravity, some temporomandibular muscles, such as the mylohyoideus and the lateral pterygoids, assist in opening the jaw. Conversely, the other temporomandibular muscles, namely the masseter, medial pterygoids, and temporalis, work to close the jaw. The medial pterygoid muscles of either side also move the mandible to produce a grinding movement of the teeth.

Innervation of the temporomandibular joint

The nerve fibers innervating the temporomandibular joint are derived from the auriculotemporal and masseteric branches of the mandibular nerve. In addition to the free nerve endings involved in nociception, there are also mechanoreceptors, such as the Ruffini endings, Vater–Pacini corpuscles, and Golgi tendon organs (Griffin and Harris, 1975; Dreessen et al., 1990). Temporomandibular muscles are innervated by the mandibular division of the trigeminal nerve.

THE MUSCLES OF THE UPPER CERVICAL SPINE

Disturbances of the muscles of the upper cervical spine may play an important role in the pathogenesis of tension-type headache. The intrinsic posterior neck muscles are composed of several muscle layers and are used for extension of the neck. The outer layer of neck muscles is composed of the trapezius and sternocleidomastoid, with the splenius capitis lying underneath these muscles. Deep to the splenius capitis are two muscles, the semispinalis capitis and the longissimus capitis. The semispinalis capitis, which is the largest and most prominent of the posterior neck muscles, arises from the transverse process of the upper thoracic spines and is inserted into the occiput below the superior nuchal line. Under the semispinalis capitis and longissimus capitis are four muscles: (1) rectus capitis posterior minor; (2) rectus capitis posterior major; (3) obliquus capitis superior; and (4) obliquus capitis inferior. These muscles connect the skull, atlas, and axis.

These muscles are mostly innervated by nerve fibers originating from the dorsal root of the upper cervical ganglia (Bogduk and Jensen, 2000). The C1–C3 spinal nerves are divided into ventral and dorsal rami. The ventral rami form the cervical plexus with the rami of C4, and the muscular branches of this plexus innervate the prevertebral muscles. On the other hand, the

Table 3.2

The muscles of the upper cervical spine

Muscle	Origin	Insertion	Innervation
Trapezius	External occipital protuberance, medial third of the superior nuchal line of the occipital bone, ligamentum nuchae and the corresponding portion of the supraspinal ligament, spinous process of the seventh cervical vertebra, spinous processes of all the thoracic vertebrae	Posterior border of the lateral third of the clavicle, medial margin of the acromion, superior lip of the posterior border of the spine of the scapula	Accessory nerve, the dorsal rami of C2–C4
Sternocleidomastoid	Medial head: upper part of the anterior surface of the manubrium sterni Lateral head: medial third of the clavicle	Lateral surface of the mastoid process	Accessory nerve, the dorsal rami of C2–C3
Splenius capitis	Lower half of the ligamentum nuchae, spinous process of the seventh cervical vertebra, spinous processes of the upper three or four thoracic vertebrae	Mastoid process of the temporal bone, lateral third of the superior nuchal line of the occipital bone	The dorsal rami of C1–C5
Semispinalis capitis	Transverse processes of the upper sixth or seventh thoracic and the seventh cervical vertebrae	Between the superior and inferior nuchal lines of the occipital bone	The dorsal rami of C1–C4
Longissimus capitis	Transverse processes of the upper four or five thoracic vertebrae and the articular processes of the lower three or four cervical vertebrae	Posterior margin of the mastoid process between the splenius capitis and sternocleidomastoid	The dorsal rami of C1–Th5
Rectus capitis posterior major	Spinous process of the axis	Lateral part of the inferior nuchal line of the occipital bone	The dorsal ramus of C1
Rectus capitis posterior minor	Tubercle on the posterior arch of the atlas	Medial part of the inferior nuchal line of the occipital bone	The dorsal ramus of C1
Obliquus capitis superior	Lateral mass of the atlas bone	Lateral half of the inferior nuchal line	Suboccipital nerve and the dorsal ramus of C1
Obliquus capitis inferior	Apex of the spinous process of the axis	Lower and back part of the transverse process of the atlas	The dorsal ramus of C1

dorsal rami of C1–C4 innervate the muscles of the upper cervical spine, as shown in Table 3.2. The large medial branch of the C2 dorsal ramus becomes the greater occipital nerve.

PAIN TRANSMISSION IN THE CENTRAL NERVOUS SYSTEM

The trigeminal–brainstem complex

The trigeminal primary afferents from the pain-sensitive structures terminate in sensory nuclei at the pontine level, which are referred to, as a whole, as the trigeminal–brainstem complex. The trigeminal–brainstem complex is composed of the principal sensory nucleus and the spinal trigeminal nucleus. Most of the large-diameter, non-nociceptive afferents of the trigeminal nerve terminate in the principal sensory nucleus. Both the large- and small-diameter fibers descend in the spinal trigeminal tract to extend into the spinal trigeminal nucleus (Messlinger et al., 2006). Olszewski (1950) subdivided the spinal trigeminal nucleus into three subnuclei: the spinal trigeminal nucleus oralis, interpolaris and caudalis. The caudal subnucleus is also called trigeminal nucleus caudalis (TNC). Although the TNC is thought to be primarily responsible for processing nociceptive and temperature information from the face and head, there is evidence that neurons in the oralis and interpolaris nuclei are also responsible for nociception (Messlinger and Burstein, 2000).

Because of its anatomic and physiological similarities to the spinal dorsal horn, TNC is often called the medullary dorsal horn. TNC was initially divided into three histologically distinct regions: (1) an outer marginal region; (2) the substantia gelatinosa; and (3) a deep magnocellular region. Furthermore, it was proposed that lamina I corresponds to the outer marginal layer, lamina II to the substantia gelatinosa, and lamina III and IV to the magnocellular region (Rexed, 1952). The trigeminovascular afferents containing neuropeptides such as SP and CGRP terminate within the superficial lamina I and II, where many of them synapse with projection neurons to other brain regions, including the thalamus (Strassman et al., 1994; Schaible et al., 1997; Uddman et al., 2002). Within the trigeminal–brainstem complex, there are connections between the various subnuclei, which allow information transfer within the trigeminal system (Stewart and King, 1963; Jacquin et al., 1990).

Projections from trigeminal nuclei

As shown in Figure 3.3A, the neurons within the TNC project on to and transmit nociceptive information to numerous subcortical sites, e.g., the hypothalamus (Malick and Burstein, 1998), the midbrain, and the pontine parabrachial nuclei (Bernard et al., 1989; Hayashi and Tabata, 1990), ipsilateral cerebellum (Huerta et al., 1983; Mantle-St John and Tracey, 1987), nucleus of the solitary tract (Marfurt and Rajchert, 1991), and brainstem reticular formation (Renehan et al., 1986).

Among these regions, projection to parabrachial nuclei is thought to be among the most important for the transmission of nociception, because most of the somatosensory neurons in the parabrachial nuclei respond exclusively to noxious stimuli (Hayashi and Tabata, 1990; Feil and Herbert, 1995). In addition, since this projection is part of the trigeminopontoamygdaloid pathway, the affective, behavioral, and autonomic reactions accompanying severe headaches can also be explained (Bernard et al., 1989).

The hypothalamus is also one of the important regions, because neurons in the TNC projecting to the hypothalamus have been reported to respond preferentially or exclusively to noxious stimulation of the dura mater (Burstein et al., 1998).

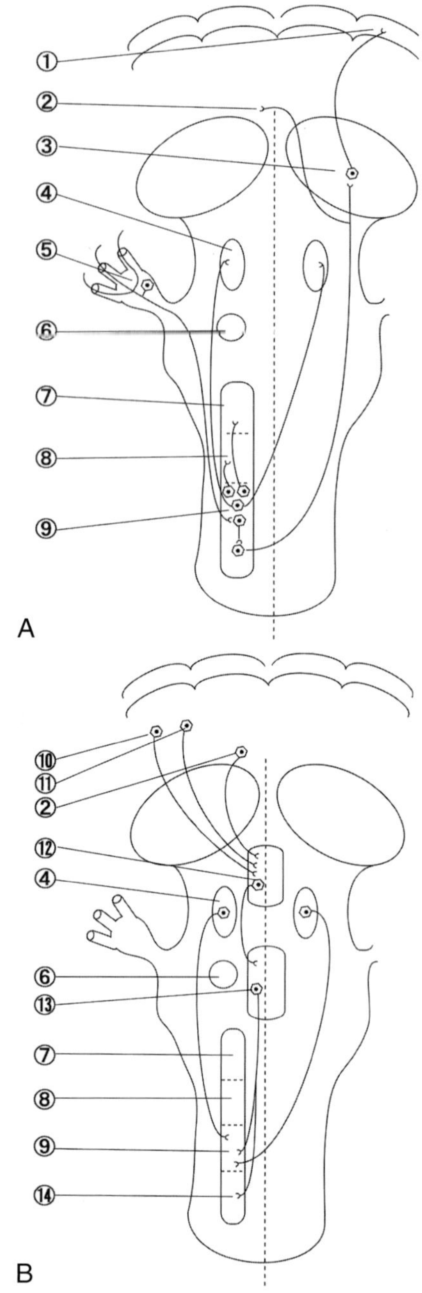

Fig. 3.3. Schematic drawing of the ascending central pathways of trigeminal nociception (A) and central pain-modulating pathways related to trigeminal nociception (B). 1, Primary somatosensory cortex; 2, hypothalamus; 3, thalamus; 4, parabrachial nucleus; 5, trigeminal ganglion; 6, trigeminal principal sensory nucleus; 7, spinal trigeminal nucleus oralis; 8, spinal trigeminal nucleus interpolaris; 9, spinal trigeminal nucleus caudalis (trigeminal nucleus caudalis); 10, amygdala; 11, insular cortex; 12, periaqueductal gray matter; 13, rostral ventromedial medulla; 14, spinal dorsal horn. (Modified from Messlinger and Burstein, 2000.)

The thalamus receives contralateral input from the trigeminal–brainstem complex (Mantle-St John and Tracey, 1987; Kemplay and Webster, 1989). The majority of the TNC neurons send fibers to the ventroposteromedial thalamus, posterior ventromedial thalamus, and ventrocaudal medialis dorsalis (Messlinger et al., 2006).

In regard to the cerebral cortex, the primary somatosensory cortex, the insular and the anterior cingulated cortex have been reported to be activated by experimental painful stimulation of the forehead (May et al., 1998; DaSilva et al., 2002).

Central inhibitory modulation of trigeminal nociception

The trigeminal–brainstem complex has been shown to receive monoaminergic, enkephalinergic, and other peptidergic projections from regions modulating the nociceptive systems (Fields et al., 2006). Within the TNC, the signals of nociception are controlled by the descending inhibitory system, the most powerful of which may be the pathway from the insular cortex and hypothalamus through the periaqueductal gray (PAG), and that from the rostral ventromedial medulla (RVM) to the superficial lamina of the TNC and the spinal dorsal horn (Figure 3.3B; Messlinger and Burstein, 2000; Cutrer, 2001). Stimulation of the PAG (Morgan et al., 1992), RVM (Lovick and Wolstencroft, 1979), and hypothalamus (Rhodes and Liebeskind, 1978) has been shown to suppress nociceptive responses. The RVM includes the nucleus raphe magnus and the adjacent reticular formation. The PAG receives projections from the amygdala, and microinjection of opioids into the amygdala has been shown to have an antinociceptive effect mediated through the PAG–RVM system (Helmstetter et al., 1998). Nuclei of the parabrachial area also have direct and bilateral projections to all the subnuclei of the trigeminal–brainstem complex (Yoshida et al., 1997). Electrical stimulation of the parabrachial area in the rat exerted inhibitory effects on the activity of the nociceptive neurons in the TNC (Chiang et al., 1994).

Inhibitory mechanisms

Within lamina II of the TNC, there are inhibitory interneurons containing gamma-aminobutyric acid (GABA), which probably act on neurons projecting to the ascending pathways of the central trigeminal system and exert nociceptive inhibition (Cutrer, 2001). These GABAergic neurons also act on the terminals of primary afferent neurons containing glutamate to influence presynaptic inhibition (Iliakis et al., 1996). These inhibitory interneurons within lamina II of the TNC are likely to receive excitatory input from serotonin-containing descending neurons from the PAG and the RVM system. Morphine has been shown to increase the release of serotonin in superficial layers of the TNC and to inhibit the presynaptic release of SP in the rabbit (Yonehara et al., 1990).

References

Andres KH, von During M, Muszynski K et al. (1987). Nerve fibres and their terminals of the dura mater encephali of the rat. Anat Embryol (Berl) 175: 289–301.

Basbaum AI, Jessell TM (2000). The perception of pain. In: ER Kandel, JH Schwartz, TM Jessell (Eds.), Principles of Neural Science. 4th edn. McGraw-Hill, New York, pp. 472–491.

Berger RJ, Zuccarello M, Keller JT (1994). Nitric oxide synthase immunoreactivity in the rat dura mater. NeuroReport 5: 519–521.

Bernard JF, Peschanski M, Besson JM (1989). A possible spino (trigemino)-ponto-amygdaloid pathway for pain. Neurosci Lett 100: 83–88.

Bleys RL, Janssen LM, Groen GJ (2001a). The lateral sellar nerve plexus and its connections in humans. J Neurosurg 95: 102–110.

Bleys RL, Thrasivoulou C, Cowen T (2001b). Cavernous sinus ganglia are sources for parasympathetic innervation of cerebral arteries in rat. J Cereb Blood Flow Metab 21: 149–156.

Blumenfeld H (2002). Neuroanatomy Through Clinical Cases. Sinauer, Sunderland, Massachusetts, pp. 120–210.

Bogduk N, Jensen R (2000). Anatomy and pathology of tension-type headache. In: J Olesen, P Tfelt-Hansen, KMA Welch (Eds.), The Headache. 2nd edn. Lippincott Williams & Wilkins, Philadelphia, pp. 551–559.

Burstein R, Yamamura H, Malick A et al. (1998). Chemical stimulation of the intracranial dura induces enhanced responses to facial stimulation in brain stem trigeminal neurons. J Neurophysiol 79: 964–982.

Chiang CY, Hu JW, Sessle BJ (1994). Parabrachial area and nucleus raphe magnus-induced modulation of nociceptive and nonnociceptive trigeminal subnucleus caudalis neurons activated by cutaneous or deep inputs. J Neurophysiol 71: 2430–2445.

Cohen Z, Bonvento G, Lacombe P et al. (1996). Serotonin in the regulation of brain microcirculation. Prog Neurobiol 50: 335–362.

Cutrer FM (2001). Pain-sensitive cranial structures: Chemical anatomy. In: SD Silberstein, RB Lipton, DJ Dalessio (Eds.), Wolff's Headache and Other Pain. 7th edn. Oxford University Press, New York, pp. 50–56.

DaSilva AF, Becerra L, Makris N et al. (2002). Somatotopic activation in the human trigeminal pain pathway. J Neurosci 22: 8183–8192.

Dreessen D, Halata Z, Strasmann T (1990). Sensory innervation of the temporomandibular joint in the mouse. Acta Anat (Basel) 139: 154–160.

Edvinsson L, Uddman R (1981). Adrenergic, cholinergic and peptidergic nerve fibres in dura mater – involvement in headache? Cephalalgia 1: 175–179.

Edvinsson L, Uddman R (2005). Neurobiology in primary headaches. Brain Res Brain Res Rev 48: 438–456.

Feil K, Herbert H (1995). Topographic organization of spinal and trigeminal somatosensory pathways to the rat parabrachial and Kolliker–Fuse nuclei. J Comp Neurol 353: 506–528.

Fields HL, Basbaum AI, Heinricher MM (2006). Central nervous system mechanisms of pain modulation. In: SB McMahon, M Koltzenburg (Eds.), Wall and Melzack's Textbook of Pain. 5th edn. Elsevier/Churchill Livingstone, Philadelphia, pp. 125–142.

Griffin CJ, Harris R (1975). Innervation of the temporomandibular joint. Aust Dent J 20: 78–85.

Griffin CJ, Hawthorn R, Harris R (1975). Anatomy and histology of the human temporomandibular joint. Monogr Oral Sci 4: 1–26.

Hamel E (2004). Cholinergic modulation of the cortical microvascular bed. Prog Brain Res 145: 171–178.

Hamel E (2006). Perivascular nerves and the regulation of cerebrovascular tone. J Appl Physiol 100: 1059–1064.

Handa Y, Caner H, Hayashi M et al. (1990). The distribution pattern of the sympathetic nerve fibers to the cerebral arterial system in rat as revealed by anterograde labeling with WGA-HRP. Exp Brain Res 82: 493–498.

Hara H, Zhang QJ, Kuroyanagi T et al. (1993). Parasympathetic cerebrovascular innervation: an anterograde tracing from the sphenopalatine ganglion in the rat. Neurosurgery 32: 822–827.

Hardebo JE, Arbab M, Suzuki N et al. (1991). Pathways of parasympathetic and sensory cerebrovascular nerves in monkeys. Stroke 22: 331–342.

Hartman BK, Zide D, Udenfriend S (1972). The use of dopamine-hydroxylase as a marker for the central noradrenergic nervous system in rat brain. Proc Natl Acad Sci U S A 69: 2722–2726.

Hayashi H, Tabata T (1990). Pulpal and cutaneous inputs to somatosensory neurons in the parabrachial area of the cat. Brain Res 511: 177–179.

Helmstetter FJ, Tershner SA, Poore LH et al. (1998). Antinociception following opioid stimulation of the basolateral amygdala is expressed through the periaqueductal gray and rostral ventromedial medulla. Brain Res 779: 104–118.

Huerta MF, Frankfurter A, Harting JK (1983). Studies of the principal sensory and spinal trigeminal nuclei of the rat: projections to the superior colliculus, inferior olive, and cerebellum. J Comp Neurol 220: 147–167.

Iliakis B, Anderson NL, Irish PS et al. (1996). Electron microscopy of immunoreactivity patterns for glutamate and gamma-aminobutyric acid in synaptic glomeruli of the feline spinal trigeminal nucleus (subnucleus caudalis). J Comp Neurol 366: 465–477.

Jacquin MF, Chiaia NL, Haring JH et al. (1990). Intersubnuclear connections within the rat trigeminal brainstem complex. Somatosens Mot Res 7: 399–420.

Keller JT, Marfurt CF (1991). Peptidergic and serotoninergic innervation of the rat dura mater. J Comp Neurol 309: 515–534.

Keller JT, Saunders MC, Beduk A et al. (1985). Innervation of the posterior fossa dura of the cat. Brain Res Bull 14: 97–102.

Kemplay S, Webster KE (1989). A quantitative study of the projections of the gracile, cuneate and trigeminal nuclei and of the medullary reticular formation to the thalamus in the rat. Neuroscience 32: 153–167.

Lovick TA, Wolstencroft JH (1979). Inhibitory effects of nucleus raphe magnus on neuronal responses in the spinal trigeminal nucleus to nociceptive compared with non-nociceptive inputs. Pain 7: 135–145.

Malick A, Burstein R (1998). Cells of origin of the trigeminohypothalamic tract in the rat. J Comp Neurol 400: 125–144.

Mantle-St John LA, Tracey DJ (1987). Somatosensory nuclei in the brainstem of the rat: independent projections to the thalamus and cerebellum. J Comp Neurol 255: 259–271.

Marfurt CF, Rajchert DM (1991). Trigeminal primary afferent projections to "non-trigeminal" areas of the rat central nervous system. J Comp Neurol 303: 489–511.

May A, Kaube H, Buchel C et al. (1998). Experimental cranial pain elicited by capsaicin: a PET study. Pain 74: 61–66.

Mayberg MR, Zervas NT, Moskowitz MA (1984). Trigeminal projections to supratentorial pial and dural blood vessels in cats demonstrated by horseradish peroxidase histochemistry. J Comp Neurol 223: 46–56.

Messlinger K, Burstein R (2000). Anatomy and central nervous system pathways related to head pain. In: J Olesen, P Tfelt-Hansen, KMA Welch (Eds.), The Headache. 2nd edn. Lippincott Williams & Wilkins, Philadelphia, pp. 77–86.

Messlinger K, Hanesch U, Baumgartel M et al. (1993). Innervation of the dura mater encephali of cat and rat: ultrastructure and calcitonin gene-related peptide-like and substance P-like immunoreactivity. Anat Embryol (Berl) 188: 219–237.

Messlinger K, Dostrovsky JO, Strassman AM (2006). Anatomy and physiology of head pain. In: J Olesen, PJ Goadsby, NM Ramadan et al. (Eds.), The Headache. 3rd edn. Lippincott Williams & Wilkins, Philadelphia, pp. 95–109.

Morgan MM, Heinricher MM, Fields HL (1992). Circuitry linking opiod-senitive nociceptive modulatory systems in periaqueductal gray and spinal cord with rostral ventromedial medulla. Neuroscience 47: 863–871.

Moskowitz MA (1984). The neurobiology of vascular head pain. Ann Neurol 16: 157–168.

Nielsen KC, Owman C (1967). Adrenergic innervation of pial arteries related to the circle of Willis in the cat. Brain Res 6: 773–776.

Nozaki K, Moskowitz MA, Maynard KI et al. (1993). Possible origins and distribution of immunoreactive nitric oxide synthase-containing nerve fibers in cerebral arteries. J Cereb Blood Flow Metab 13: 70–79.

Olszewski J (1950). On the anatomical and functional organization of the spinal trigeminal nucleus. J Comp Neurol 92: 401–413.

Penfield W, McNaughton F (1940). Dural headache and innervation of the dura mater. Arch Neurol Psychiatry 44: 43–75.

Piette E (1993). Anatomy of the human temporomandibular joint. An updated comprehensive review. Acta Stomatol Belg 90: 103–127.

Ray BS, Wolff HG (1940). Experimental studies on headache. Pain-sensitive structures of the head and their significance in headache. Arch Surg 41: 813–856.

Reinhard JF Jr, Liebmann JE, Schlosberg AJ et al. (1979). Serotonin neurons project to small blood vessels in the brain. Science 206: 85–87.

Renehan WE, Jacquin MF, Mooney RD et al. (1986). Structure–function relationships in rat medullary and cervical dorsal horns. II. Medullary dorsal horn cells. J Neurophysiol 55: 1187–1201.

Rexed B (1952). The cytoarchitectonic organization of the spinal cord in the cat. J Comp Neurol 96: 414–495.

Rhodes DL, Liebeskind JC (1978). Analgesia from rostral brain stem stimulation in the rat. Brain Res 143: 521–532.

Ruskell GL, Simons T (1987). Trigeminal nerve pathways to the cerebral arteries in monkeys. J Anat 155: 23–37.

Schaible HG, Ebersberger A, Peppel P et al. (1997). Release of immunoreactive substance P in the trigeminal brain stem nuclear complex evoked by chemical stimulation of the nasal mucosa and the dura mater encephali – a study with antibody microprobes. Neuroscience 76: 273–284.

Schmolke C (1994). The relationship between the temporomandibular joint capsule, articular disc and jaw muscles. J Anat 184: 335–345.

Shimizu T (1994). Distribution and pathway of the cerebrovascular nerve fibers from the otic ganglion in the rat: anterograde tracing study. J Auton Nerv Syst 49: 47–54.

Steiger HJ, Tew JM Jr, Keller JT (1982). The sensory representation of the dura mater in the trigeminal ganglion of the cat. Neurosci Lett 31: 231–236.

Stewart WA, King RB (1963). Fiber projections from the nucleus caudalis of the spinal trigeminal nucleus. J Comp Neurol 121: 271–286.

Strassman AM, Mineta Y, Vos BP (1994). Distribution of fos-like immunoreactivity in the medullary and upper cervical dorsal horn produced by stimulation of dural blood vessels in the rat. J Neurosci 14: 3725–3735.

Suzuki N, Hardebo JE (1991a). Anatomical basis for a parasympathetic and sensory innervation of the intracranial segment of the internal carotid artery in man. Possible implication for vascular headache. J Neurol Sci 104: 19–31.

Suzuki N, Hardebo JE (1991b). The pathway of parasympathetic nerve fibers to cerebral vessels from the otic ganglion in the rat. J Auton Nerv Syst 36: 39–46.

Suzuki N, Hardebo JE, Owman C (1988). Origins and pathways of cerebrovascular vasoactive intestinal polypeptide-positive nerves in rat. J Cereb Blood Flow Metab 8: 697–712.

Suzuki N, Hardebo JE, Owman C (1989). Origins and pathways of cerebrovascular nerves storing substance P and calcitonin gene-related peptide in rat. Neuroscience 31: 427–438.

Suzuki N, Hardebo JE, Owman C (1990). Origins and pathways of choline acetyltransferase-positive parasympathetic nerve fibers to cerebral vessels in rat. J Cereb Blood Flow Metab 10: 399–408.

Suzuki N, Fukuuchi Y, Koto A et al. (1993). Cerebrovascular NADPH diaphorase-containing nerve fibers in the rat. Neurosci Lett 151: 1–3.

Uddman R, Edvinsson L (1989). Neuropeptides in the cerebral circulation. Cerebrovasc Brain Metab Rev 1: 230–252.

Uddman R, Hara H, Edvinsson L (1989). Neuronal pathways to the rat middle meningeal artery revealed by retrograde tracing and immunocytochemistry. J Auton Nerv Syst 26: 69–75.

Uddman R, Tajti J, Hou M et al. (2002). Neuropeptide expression in the human trigeminal nucleus caudalis and in the cervical spinal cord C1 and C2. Cephalalgia 22: 112–116.

von During M, Bauersachs M, Bohmer B et al. (1990). Neuropeptide Y- and substance P-like immunoreactive nerve fibers in the rat dura mater encephali. Anat Embryol (Berl) 182: 363–373.

Yonehara N, Shibutani T, Imai Y et al. (1990). Involvement of descending monoaminergic systems in the transmission of dental pain in the trigeminal nucleus caudalis of the rabbit. Brain Res 508: 234–240.

Yoshida A, Chen K, Moritani M et al. (1997). Organization of the descending projections from the parabrachial nucleus to the trigeminal sensory nuclear complex and spinal dorsal horn in the rat. J Comp Neurol 383: 94–111.

Handbook of Clinical Neurology, Vol. 97 (3rd series)
Headache
G. Nappi and M.A. Moskowitz, Editors

Chapter 4

Pharmacology

HAYRUNNISA BOLAY[1]* AND PAUL DURHAM[2]

[1]*Department of Neurology, Gazi Hospital and Neuropsychiatry Centre, Gazi University, Besevler, Ankara, Turkey*
[2]*JVIC Center for Biomedical and Life Sciences, Missouri State University, Springfield, MO, USA*

INTRODUCTION

Complex players such as genetic predisposition, environmental and intrinsic factors mediate headache, yet the exact sites and mechanisms of interaction remain obscure. Susceptibility genes for primary headache syndromes is a challenging research area that is likely to help identify specific targets for novel treatment strategies and facilitate our understanding of the interplay between genetic and environmental factors.

The trigeminovascular system plays a fundamental role in headache (Ray and Wolff, 1940; Mayberg et al., 1981, 1984) in regard to peripheral sensitization (Strassman et al., 1996) and neurogenic inflammation in the meninges (Dimitriadou et al., 1992; Johnson and Bolay, 2006), and is also a predominant site of action for pharmaceutical agents such as triptans, ergots, neuropeptide antagonists, and non-steroidal anti-inflammatory drugs (NSAIDs) (Buzzi et al., 1989, 1992; Kaube et al., 1993; Durham and Russo, 2002). Recent findings suggest that synaptic transmission between primary sensory trigeminal ganglia neurons and trigeminal nucleus caudalis (TNC) neurons within the brainstem is a primary target of triptans and calcitonin gene-related peptide (CGRP) antagonists (Levy et al., 2004, 2005). Neurogenic inflammation is currently considered to be a phenomenon secondary to sensitization and/or activation of nociceptive neurons within the TNC (Kaube et al., 1993; Goadsby and Hoskin, 1996). Sensitization not only occurs in the peripheral structures but also develops in the brainstem and more rostral structures such as the thalamus and cerebral cortex (Burstein et al., 2000). Early administration of abortive treatments before central sensitization and cutaneous allodynia development has been reported to be most effective in treating migraine (Burstein and Jakubowski, 2004). Prostanoids, their receptors and terminal prostaglandin (PG) E synthases, particularly microsomal PGE synthase-1 (mPGES-1) along with cyclooxygenase-2 (COX-2) enzymes, are all important players in pain sensitization in both the peripheral and the central nervous system (CNS) (Zeilhofer, 2007). After COX-2 inhibitors were withdrawn from the market due to undesired side-effects, such as cardiovascular toxicity (Bresalier et al., 2005), investigations have been directed to prostanoid receptors and mPGESs as new potential targets (Zeilhofer and Brune, 2006). The effect of pharmaceutical agents commonly used for abortive and prophylactic treatment other than NSAIDs on the development of sensitization has yet to be elucidated.

Cortical spreading depression (CSD), which is a pathophysiological correlate of aura, has stimulated a growing interest in regard to recent genetic and experimental findings. In familial hemiplegic migraine (FHM), hemiplegia is seen as an aura and inherited dominantly. Investigation of those families has shown that ion channels or transporters such as CACNA1A and SCNA1 or Na^{+}/K^{+}ATPase are mutated (Ophoff et al., 1996; De Fusco et al., 2003; Dichgans et al., 2005) in a way that results in release of excessive glutamate from neurons, reduced uptake of glutamate from the synaptic cleft into glia, and/or reduced buffering capacity of potassium ions (Moskowitz et al., 2004). The common result of all three identified mutations is hyperexcitability and a reduced threshold for CSD induction, which all probably contribute to the vulnerability of the brain to migraine attacks (Moskowitz et al., 2004). From the therapeutic perspective, the efficacy of certain antiepileptic drugs in migraine patients and their action on excitability or even on CSD are noteworthy.

*Correspondence to: Hayrunnisa Bolay, MD, PhD, Professor of Neurology, Director of Neuropsychiatry Centre, Department of Neurology, Gazi Hospital and Neuropsychiatry Centre, Gazi University, Besevler, Ankara 06510, Turkey, Tel: 90-312-2025307, Fax: 90-312-2124647, E-mail: hbolay@gazi.edu.tr

When administered chronically, several drugs currently used to treat epilepsy and migraines have been shown to be capable of reducing CSD frequency in rodents (Ayata et al., 2006). CSD is known to be a sufficient stimulus to activate the trigeminovascular system, leading to activation of TNC neurons, and neurogenic edema and increased blood flow in the meninges (Bolay et al., 2002). With regard to treatment, the efficacy of abortive or prophylactic medication does not differ in migraine patients whether they have an aura or not. Therefore, the hypothesis that "CSD may also underlie migraine without aura" is worthy of testing in clinical trials.

Headache treatment has been based primarily on experiences with non-specific drugs such as analgesics, NSAIDs, or drugs that were originally developed to treat other diseases, such as beta-blockers and anticonvulsant medications. Somewhat surprisingly, we still do not fully understand their mode of action in alleviating migraine headache. Understanding the basic pathophysiological mechanisms of migraine has led to the development over the past two decades of target-specific drugs such as triptans and CGRP antagonists. However, given the limitations and side-effects of many drugs it is obvious that there is still a need to develop more specific and effective medications to treat migraine and other headache disorders.

Another concept that has changed for migraine treatment is the emphasis on prevention. Since recent evidence suggests that migraine is a chronic progressive disorder (Lipton and Pan, 2004), administration of prophylactic medication is now considered a necessary treatment option for more patients and for longer durations (Silberstein et al., 2004). Currently, the advantages or disadvantages of such an approach are not well defined.

Recent developments regarding the main groups of drugs effectively used in treating headaches are briefly summarized in the following sections. The pharmacology of selected serotonergic drugs, CGRP and other neuropeptide antagonists, prostanoids beyond cyclooxygenase inhibition, noradrenergic system and receptor blockade, and antiepileptic drugs will be discussed.

SEROTONERGIC AGONISTS

Triptans

It was thought that migraine sufferers had a hereditary systemic perturbation of serotonin (5-hydroxytryptamine, 5-HT) metabolism and neurotransmission (Humphrey, 1991; Ferrari and Saxena, 1993). Earlier clinical evidence clearly demonstrated that the vasoconstrictors 5-HT and ergotamine, acting primarily through 5-HT receptors, were effective in aborting most migraine attacks. However, their therapeutic benefit was tempered by severe systemic side-effects caused by these treatments. Thus, it was thought that design of a more selective drug that would selectively activate only 5-HT receptors in the cerebrovasculature would be even more effective in aborting migraine headache but would be without the negative systemic effects. The presence of mRNA and protein for the $5\text{-HT}_{1B/1D}$ class of 5-HT receptors has been demonstrated for human meningeal blood vessels and trigeminal ganglia neurons (Hamel et al., 1993; Longmore et al., 1997). Specifically, immunolocalization studies have shown that the 5-HT_{1B} receptor, but not the 5-HT_{1D} receptor, is expressed on meningeal smooth-muscle cells (Longmore et al., 1997). Based on the current models of migraine pathology (Pietrobon, 2005; Hargreaves, 2007), activation of the 5-HT_{1B} receptors would cause vasoconstriction and, thus, could help restore normal vascular tone of these vessels during migraine. In contrast, although mRNA and protein for both 5-HT_{1B} and 5-HT_{1D} receptors was detected in the cell bodies of human trigeminal ganglia (Bouchelet et al., 1996; Longmore et al., 1997), only the 5-HT_{1D} receptors appear to be expressed on peripheral and central projecting trigeminal nerve fibers (Longmore et al., 1997). Thus, activation of the human 5-HT_{1D} receptor is thought to be primarily responsible for mediating repression of stimulated neuropeptide release from human trigeminal nerve terminals and activation of second-order neurons. These inhibitory effects on trigeminal nerve activity would promote normalization of blood vessel diameter and also inhibit release of neuropeptides that are responsible for transmitting nociceptive stimuli to the CNS.

Sumatriptan (3-[2-dimethylamino]ethyl-*N*-methyl-^{1}H indole-5-methane sulfonamide) (GlaxoSmithKline) was the first selective $5\text{-HT}_{1B/1D}$ agonist that was specifically designed for the acute treatment of migraine headache. At least 14 different subtypes comprising seven subfamilies of distinct serotonergic receptors have been identified (Boess and Martin, 1994; Barnes and Sharp, 1999). Based on numerous animal and clinical studies, the 5-HT_1 class of receptors is now regarded as the most relevant for migraine therapy (Longmore et al., 1999). Data generated from extensive pharmacological studies have demonstrated that sumatriptan is a potent agonist of the human $5\text{-HT}_{1B/1D/1F}$ receptors (Beattie and Connor, 1995; Longmore et al., 1999). It exhibits highest affinity for the 5-HT_{1B} and 5-HT_{1D} receptors, with slightly lower affinity for the 5-HT_{1F} receptors, while showing only weak affinity for the 5-HT_{1A} and 5-HT_{1E} receptors. Importantly, sumatriptan displays only weak affinity at other 5-HT receptors ($5\text{-HT}_{2A/3/4/5/7}$) and other non-5-HT_1 receptors, such as the adrenergic, dopamine, and muscarinic receptors. Based on the success of sumatriptan in migraine therapy, several other drugs, collectively now known as the triptans, were designed with selectivity towards the $5\text{-HT}_{1B/1D}$ receptors that could overcome some of the potential shortcomings of sumatriptan (Ferrari, 1998; Longmore et al., 1999). For example, the newer drugs offer greater bioavailability, longer plasma half-life, faster absorption, and increased lipophilicity, leading to greater brain penetration than reported for sumatriptan. The new so-called second-generation triptan drugs include naratriptan (GlaxoSmithKline), zolmitriptan (Zeneca), rizatriptan (Merck), eletriptan (Pfizer), frovatriptan (Vanguard Medica), almotriptan (Almirall/Pharmacia & Upjohn), and avitriptan (Bristol-Meyers Squibb). Basically, the triptans are similar with respect to their pharmacology, efficacy, and safety. The drug LY-334370 (Eli Lilly) is reported to be highly selective for the 5-HT_{1F} receptor and to cause inhibition of dural protein plasma extravasation (Johnson et al., 1997). However, the effectiveness of this drug in migraine therapy was never established in larger clinical trials due to its withdrawal after adverse events were noted in dogs.

While clinical data clearly support the effectiveness of the triptans in aborting migraine, there is still much debate focused on which triptan should be used to treat other types of headache such as cluster headaches and menstrual migraine. Despite the success of these drugs as acute treatments of migraine, not all patients are responsive to the triptan drugs. In addition, since all triptan drugs are known to have vasoconstrictor activity, they are contraindicated in patients with vascular disease (Longmore et al., 1999). This practice is highly recommended because of the possibility of serious cardiovascular events, such as myocardial infarction (Mueller et al., 1996), cardiac arrhythmia (Ottervanger et al., 1994), and stroke (Luman and Gray, 1993; Cavazos et al., 1994). Thus, although the triptans are superior to other drugs for the acute treatment of migraine, there remains a significant number of migraineurs who are unable to be treated successfully with these drugs.

The effectiveness of sumatriptan and other triptans as acute antimigraine therapies has been proposed to be due to three separate pharmacological actions at distinct sites within the trigeminovascular system (Ferrari, 1998; Hargreaves and Shepheard, 1999). These actions include vasoconstriction of meningeal and cerebral blood vessels, inhibition of neuropeptide release from perivascular trigeminal nerves, and central effects involving decreased pain transmission (Bolay and Moskowitz, 2005; Pietrobon, 2005). In addition, a potential fourth site of action has been suggested that involves triptan inhibition of release of CGRP and possibly other neuropeptides from trigeminal neuron cell bodies that are localized in the ganglia (Zhang et al., 2007). After much research, the most important site of triptan action remains unknown but may very well function at some degree at all four levels along the trigeminovascular system to abort the pain and associated symptoms of migraine.

The vascular mechanism of the triptans has been shown to involve constriction of painfully distended intracranial blood vessels via activation of 5-HT_{1B} receptors on vascular smooth-muscle cells (Friberg et al., 1991; Humphrey and Feniuk, 1991). In a study utilizing angiography, sumatriptan was also shown to cause constriction of human meningeal (dural) blood vessels (Henkes et al., 1996). The neurogenic mechanism of triptan action is mediated by inhibiting the secretion of the vasoactive neuropeptides CGRP and substance P from perivascular trigeminal nerves via activation of the $5\text{-HT}_{1B/1D}$ receptors (Moskowitz, 1992; MacLeod et al., 1997; Williamson et al., 2001) and possibly 5-HT_{1F} receptors (Johnson et al., 1997). The central mechanism by the brain-penetrant triptan drugs involves inhibition of nociceptive activity in the brainstem trigeminal sensory nuclei (Goadsby and Edvinsson, 1994b; Shepheard et al., 1995; Goadsby and Hoskin, 1996; Cumberbatch et al., 1997). This central action is likely to be mediated by an inhibition of neuropeptide and/or glutamate release from central-projecting trigeminal afferent fibers (Cumberbatch et al., 1998) at the level of the TNC (Jenkins et al., 2004; Levy et al., 2004). Consistent with this proposed mechanism, expression of the immediate early gene c-*fos*, a marker of neuronal activation within the cephalic nociceptive system, is attenuated by triptan drugs in the TNC following noxious meningeal stimulation (Nozaki et al., 1992).

A very interesting finding was that the effect of triptans involves the activation of 5-HT_{1D} receptors on pain-responsive trigeminal primary afferents (Ahn and Basbaum, 2006). In this way, membrane expression of 5-HT_{1D} receptors on trigeminal nerves is increased under pathological conditions, making them more readily available for triptan activation. Hence, based on these findings, it is likely that the therapeutic benefit of triptans involves modulation of the 5-HT_{1D} receptors. Finally, recently published findings support the notion that triptans can function at the level of the cell body of trigeminal ganglia neurons by blocking autocrine regulation of CGRP synthesis. While it is known that CGRP can be released from neuronal cell bodies in response to inflammatory stimuli, it was not known how CGRP might function at the level of the ganglia. In a recent study, evidence was provided to demonstrate that activation of CGRP receptors expressed on trigeminal neurons leads to increased CGRP synthesis (Zhang et al., 2007). Thus, the release of CGRP from cell bodies localized within the ganglia would be able to promote further production of CGRP. Treatment with triptans would likely block this effect since 5-HT_{1D} receptors are known to be expressed on the cell body of trigeminal neurons.

Based on pharmacological data, sumatriptan and other currently used triptan antimigraine drugs exhibit potency and selectivity primarily towards the 5-HT_{1B} and 5-HT_{1D} receptors. The 5-HT_{1B} receptors were first identified in rat brain by 5-HT-binding studies (Pedigo et al., 1981). However, data from binding studies in humans, dogs, and guinea pigs clearly demonstrated the existence of another class of 5-HT_1 receptors, termed 5-HT_{1D} receptors, and found to be quite distinct pharmacologically from the 5-HT_{1B} receptors (Heuring and Peroutka, 1987; Hoyer et al., 1988; Hoyer and Middlemiss, 1989). While both humans and rats are known to express the 5-HT_{1B} and 5-HT_{1D} receptor genes, the pharmacology of these receptors is reported to be very similar in humans, but quite distinct in the rat (Boess and Martin, 1994).

All of the identified 5-HT receptors, with the exception of 5-HT_3 receptors, are known to be G-protein-coupled receptors that contain seven membrane-spanning hydrophobic segments and specific recognition domains (Boess and Martin, 1994). The G-protein-coupled receptor family is the largest and most complex group of integral membrane proteins involved in signal transduction. These receptors are activated by a diverse array of external stimuli that includes growth factors, vasoactive peptides, neurotransmitters, and hormones (Wess, 1997). Traditionally, activation of 5-HT_1 receptors involved in migraine therapy has been viewed as being coupled to an inhibition of adenylate cyclase via pertussis toxin-sensitive Gi/o-proteins, leading to a decrease in intracellular cyclic adenosine monophosphate (cAMP) levels (Boess and Martin, 1994). However, data from studies using cultured trigeminal ganglia neurons showed that sumatriptan could not inhibit forskolin-stimulated adenylate cyclase activity or forskolin-induced cAMP accumulation (Durham and Russo, 1998). In this study, the same cultures assayed for cAMP were shown to exhibit sumatriptan-mediated repression of CGRP release (Durham et al., 1997). Thus, these data provide evidence that cultured trigeminal neurons express functional 5-HT_1 receptors, as demonstrated by their response to sumatriptan, but do not couple to cAMP.

In agreement, other investigators have also reported that terminal hippocampal neuron 5-HT_1 receptors may not be coupled to Gi/o-proteins and decreased cAMP levels (Blier, 1991). Activation of human 5-HT_1 receptors has also been reported to couple to increases in intracellular Ca^{2+} levels (Adham et al., 1993; Zgombick et al., 1993). Since the increase in Ca^{2+} levels observed in these studies was blocked by pertussis toxin treatment, recruitment of Gi/o-proteins was likely involved in mediating the Ca^{2+} increases. More recently, activation of 5-HT_1 receptors has been shown to couple to increased Ca^{2+} levels, but by a different mechanism and with very different kinetics than previously reported. Rather than causing a transient Ca^{2+} increase, activation of 5-HT_1 receptors in cultured trigeminal neurons was shown to cause a prolonged submicromolar increase in intracellular Ca^{2+} levels (Durham and Russo, 1998). Importantly, the increase in intracellular Ca^{2+} was shown to block the stimulated release of CGRP from trigeminal neurons. Together, there is evidence that activation of 5-HT_1 receptors can lead to changes in cAMP and intracellular calcium levels, which are likely involved in mediating the inhibitory affects of antimigraine drugs that bind 5-HT_1 receptors.

Ergots

The ergot alkaloids, ergotamine and its derivative dihydroergotamine (DHE), are effective for the treatment of moderate to severe migraine but suffer from lack of poor bioavailability. A unique characteristic of DHE and other ergot alkaloids is that their biological activity does not directly correlate with their plasma concentrations. DHE exhibits affinity for several types of receptor, including 5-HT, adrenergic, and dopamine receptors (Saper and Silberstein, 2006). While the exact mechanism of action of DHE in treating migraine is not known, it is thought to involve its ability to bind and activate 5-HT_{1D} receptors present on trigeminal nerves. Although sumatriptan was shown to be superior to DHE in the acute relief of the headache associated with migraine, headache recurrence was reported twice as often with sumatriptan use (Winner et al., 1996). This beneficial effect of DHE is likely due to its long duration of pharmacological activity as compared to the triptans.

CALCITONIN GENE-RELATED PEPTIDE RECEPTOR ANTAGONISTS

The neuropeptide CGRP is implicated in the underlying pathology of migraine and cluster headache. In humans, CGRP exists in two forms, α-CGRP and β-CGRP, which differ by three amino acids yet exhibit similar biological functions (Amara et al., 1985; Steenbergh et al., 1985). The 37-amino-acid neuropeptide α-CGRP arises from alternative processing of the primary transcript to yield the hormone calcitonin in thyroid C cells and CGRP in a large number of neurons of the peripheral nervous system and CNS (Rosenfeld et al., 1983; Fischer and Born, 1985; Steenbergh et al., 1985). β-CGRP is encoded by a different gene that is highly homologous to the calcitonin CGRP gene.

Immunohistological studies have demonstrated that α-CGRP is preferentially expressed in sensory neurons and its concentration is three- to sixfold higher than that of β-CGRP (Mulderry et al., 1988). The role of α-CGRP will be the focus of this discussion since this isoform is predominant in trigeminal ganglia (Amara et al., 1985). Furthermore, dilation of human cerebral arteries is largely mediated by α-CGRP (Jansen-Olesen et al., 1996). For convenience, α-CGRP will simply be referred to as CGRP.

The important role of CGRP in migraine pathology is supported by both clinical and experimental evidence. CGRP is the most potent vasodilatory peptide in the cerebral circulation (Brain et al., 1985; McCulloch et al., 1986) and it is expressed in trigeminal ganglia neurons that innervate all the major cerebral blood vessels, as well as the pain-sensing meningeal blood vessels (O'Conner and Van der Kooy, 1988; van Rossum, et al., 1997). Functional studies have demonstrated that exogenous CGRP causes vasodilation of cerebral arteries *in vitro* and *in situ* (Jansen-Olesen et al., 1996). In addition to causing vasodilation, CGRP has been reported to cause dural mast cell degranulation and release of histamine, and may be involved in mediating neurogenic inflammation by facilitating plasma leakage from meningeal vessels (Ottosson and Edvinsson, 1997). In addition, CGRP is likely involved in the transmission of painful stimuli from intracranial vessels to the CNS (Cumberbatch et al., 1998). In animal models of neurogenic inflammation, CGRP levels have also been shown to be elevated in the sagittal sinus following chemical or electrical stimulation of the trigeminal ganglion nerve in the rat (Buzzi et al., 1991; Knyihar-Csillik et al., 1995) and the cat (Zagami et al., 1990).

Furthermore, excitation of afferent perivascular nerve fibers was shown to cause elevations in rat plasma CGRP levels (Buzzi et al., 1991) that are comparable with increases reported in migraine patients during an attack (Goadsby and Edvinsson, 1993). Thus, release of CGRP and other neuropeptides from trigeminal nerves is thought to mediate within the meninges neurogenic inflammation that contributes to generation of the severe cerebral pain experienced during migraine attacks. Interestingly, chemical and electrical stimulation of dural afferents was reported to cause a significant increase in the amount of CGRP, but not substance P, released from trigeminal nerves (Ebersberger et al., 1999). Thus, although other neuropeptides, such as substance P and neurokinin A, are involved in regulation of the cerebrovasculature, their roles in migraine are not clear (Edvinsson and Goadsby, 1994; Buzzi et al., 1995).

Data from clinical studies have shown that serum levels of CGRP, obtained from the external jugular vein, are elevated in patients during migraine with and without aura as well as cluster headaches (Goadsby and Edvinsson, 1993, 1994a; Edvinsson and Goadsby, 1994; Fanciullacci et al., 1995). Further evidence for a role of CGRP in migraine comes from clinical studies in which sumatriptan was shown to decrease elevated CGRP levels in migraine patients, coincident with relief of headache pain (Goadsby and Edvinsson, 1991). Furthermore, these data provide evidence that receptor antagonist molecules, which selectively bind to CGRP receptors to prevent their function, should be effective in migraine treatment by blocking the pathophysiological activities of CGRP.

The physiological effects of CGRP are mediated via activation of CGRP receptors, which are divided into two classes, CGRP1 and CGRP2 (Amara et al., 1985; Poyner et al., 2002). Functional CGRP receptors are composed of the calcitonin-like receptor (CL receptor) and a single transmembrane domain protein called receptor activity-modifying protein type 1 (RAMP1). The first CGRP receptor antagonists were C-terminal truncated fragments of the CGRP peptide (Chiba et al., 1989). The CGRP1 receptors are reported to be more sensitive to the peptide antagonist $CGRP_{8-37}$ than CGRP2 (Quirion et al., 1992). $CGRP_{8-37}$, which includes all but the first seven amino acids of normal CGRP, functions as an antagonist of CGRP receptors by blocking binding of endogenous full-length CGRP. Although $CGRP_{8-37}$ has been demonstrated to inhibit vasodilation and neurogenic inflammation in animal models, it has not proven clinically effective due to its short half-life and lack of potency *in vivo*. Other truncated CGRP analogs that exhibit higher affinity for CGRP1 receptors than $CGRP_{8-37}$ have been developed but have also not proven useful in clinical studies because of the same limitations (Rist et al., 1999). However, results from physiological studies using truncated forms of CGRP have provided evidence that blockage of CGRP receptors by small non-peptide molecules should be beneficial in treating migraine.

The introduction of the antimigraine drug sumatriptan not only changed the way in which migraine patients were managed, but also provided valuable insight into the underlying mechanisms involved in migraine pathology (Mathew, 2001; Goadsby et al., 2002a). Sumatriptan, which was specifically designed for migraine therapy, remains a standard by which other drugs for acute treatment of migraine, including the newer triptan drugs, are evaluated. Triptan-induced activation of 5-HT_1 receptors inhibits vasodilation of intracranial vessels, and blocks neurogenic inflammation and central transmission of nociceptive stimuli by inhibiting the release of CGRP, other neuropeptides, and glutamate from trigeminal nerves (Hargreaves, 2007). Unfortunately, the vasoconstrictor action of triptans is a serious, unwanted side-effect that precludes their use in some migraine patients (Visser et al., 1996). In fact, all triptans are contraindicated in patients with established cardiovascular disease and are to be used cautiously in patients in whom unrecognized coronary artery disease is likely. In addition, about one-third of patients do not respond to sumatriptan treatment, and there is a high recurrence rate associated with all triptans (Geraud et al., 2003). To offer an improved safety profile over the triptans, a drug would need to decrease CGRP release effectively from trigeminal neurons, thus inhibiting vasodilation of meningeal vessels and nociceptive transmission, but lack coronary vasoconstrictor activity.

The rationale for developing novel CGRP receptor antagonists to treat migraine was based on data obtained from studies on the mechanisms of triptans and evidence that administration of human CGRP can induce migraine-like symptoms in susceptible individuals. Doods and colleagues (2000) identified a potent and highly specific antagonist to human CGRP receptors termed olcegepant (Boehringer Ingelheim). Results from a phase II clinical trial for the treatment of migraine have been published (Olesen et al., 2004). Compounds 1 and 2, truncated analogs of olcegepant, also exhibit high affinity for human CGRP receptors, but exhibit lower potencies than olcegepant (Mallee et al., 2002). The specific affinities of these three antagonist molecules are dependent on residues within the extracellular region of RAMP1 rather than the receptor protein CL. Thus, it appears that the non-peptide antagonists function by directly competing for the binding site of the endogenous ligand, CGRP. Blockage of CGRP1 receptors expressed on cerebral arteries, meningeal blood vessels, and second-order sensory neurons would inhibit the vasodilatory and nociceptive effects of CGRP.

The ability of olcegepant to function as an antimigraine agent was supported by results suggesting that the drug could inhibit the vasodilatory effect of CGRP released following stimulation of the trigeminal ganglion (Doods et al., 2000). Data from a published clinical proof-of-concept study by Olesen and Jansen-Olesen (2000) demonstrated the effectiveness and safety of olcegepant for acute treatment of migraine. The response rate of >60% (pain-free at 2 h) is similar to values reported for oral triptans (Ferrari et al., 2001). It is likely that even higher response rates, as recently reported for the triptans, can be achieved if olcegepant is administered during the mild phase of a migraine attack before trigeminal nerve activation (Burstein et al., 2004). Notably, no cardiovascular side-effects, for example changes in basal blood pressure or heart rate, have been reported following administration of olgecepant (Kapoor et al., 2003). The lack of vasoconstrictor activity may prove to be a major advantage for using CGRP receptor antagonists to treat migraine. Clinically, it is important to determine whether patients who fail to respond to triptans might be successfully treated by olcegepant. This may be doubtful if the antimigraine effect of triptans is primarily mediated through inhibition of CGRP release from trigeminal nerves, and olcegepant blocks CGRP receptor function.

Although olcegepant has been shown to be effective in treating migraine attacks, a severe limitation is that this compound has to be delivered via intravenous injection. It is encouraging that potent oral CGRP receptor antagonists are now under investigation for the treatment of migraine. In particular, the CGRP receptor antagonist MK-0974, reported to exhibit good oral bioavailability, is a promising candidate (Paone et al., 2007). MK-0974, telcagepant, was shown in a phase II clinical study to be effective and generally well tolerated for treating moderate to severe migraine attacks with a primary endpoint of pain relief at 2 h (Ho et al., 2008b). Generally, the effective MK-0974 doses were comparable to those of rizatriptan (Ho et al., 2008a). The incidence of the most often reported adverse events for MK-0974, which included nausea, dizziness, and somnolence, were similar to that in the placebo group. Pharmacological studies have provided evidence that MK-0974 is a highly selective, potent, oral antagonist of the human CGRP receptor (Salvatore et al., 2008). In the same study, MK-0974 was shown to inhibit capsaicin-induced dermal vasodilation mediated by CGRP in rhesus monkey pharmacodynamic assay. Phase III clinical studies are under way to evaluate further the effectiveness of this novel class of CGRP receptor antagonist molecules.

There are several potential sites of action for CGRP antagonists along the trigeminovascular pathway. Since human cerebral vessels have been demonstrated to express functional CL receptor and RAMP1 proteins (Moreno et al., 1999; Oliver et al., 2002), blockage of these CGRP receptors on smooth-muscle cells would inhibit the dilation of major cerebral vessels. Indeed, olcegepant reportedly reversed the effects of CGRP-induced dilation of human middle cerebral and middle meningeal arteries (Moreno et al., 2002a, b). In addition, CGRP antagonists may block neurogenic inflammation within the meninges by inhibiting dilation of meningeal vessels, a key initiating event proposed in migraine. The drug should also be able to inhibit mast cell degranulation and subsequent release of histamine and other proinflammatory agents. Another likely target for a CGRP antagonist is CGRP receptors on second-order sensory neurons within trigeminal nuclei in the caudal brainstem and upper cervical spinal cord (Levy et al., 2004).

Competitive inhibition of these receptors would prevent the activation of nociceptive neural pathways and thus block sensitization of second-order neurons during migraine, which contribute to the intensification of pain reported during an attack. In addition, inhibition of the trigeminovascular system would also be expected to diminish the allodynic effects and autonomic-mediated symptoms commonly associated with migraine (Malick and Burstein, 2000).

Results from a randomized clinical trial of olcegepant demonstrated the effectiveness of the drug at decreasing or alleviating migraine pain, but also importantly reported patient improvement with respect to nausea, photophobia, phonophobia, and functional capacity (Olesen et al., 2004). Finally, it will be of importance to determine whether a CGRP antagonist could function at the level of the trigeminal ganglia to inhibit peripheral sensitization since trigeminal ganglia neurons and satellite glial cells are reported to express functional CGRP receptors (Thalakoti et al., 2007; Zhang et al., 2007).

In summary, based on experimental and clinical studies, CGRP is believed to play an important role in the generation of pain during migraine attacks. The CGRP receptor antagonist olcegepant has been demonstrated to be effective in treating migraine attacks. The apparent lack of coronary vasoconstrictor activity would be a major advantage of using this drug instead of triptans for the acute treatment of migraine, especially in patients with a history of cardiovascular disease. A major challenge will be to provide a more easily administered formulation of the antagonist, preferably an oral tablet or nasal spray, as has been developed for the delivery of triptans. The therapeutic potential of olcegepant, telcagepant, and possibly other CGRP receptor antagonists appears favorable for treating migraine as well as cluster headache since serum CGRP levels are greatly elevated in cluster headache patients.

PROSTANOIDS AND INFLAMMATION

NSAIDs are the most commonly used drugs worldwide for mild and moderate pain, including headache. A well-known member of this group, acetylsalicyclic acid (ASA), was first synthesized in 1899 by Felix Hoffman. However it took 80 years before it was discovered that aspirin acts as an inhibitor of COX, preventing the formation of PGs from arachidonic acid (Vane, 1971).

Prostanoids are a group of lipid mediators that consist of the PGs and thromboxanes, and derive from membrane phospholipids. Phospholipase A_2 releases arachidonic acid from membrane phospholipids in response to cell stimulation. Arachidonic acid is then subsequently converted to PG endoperoxidases in a two-step reaction, first to PGG_2 and then PGH_2 by the action of COX enzymes. PGH_2 is converted to various PGs by tissue-specific PG synthases, as determined by cell type (Garavito and Dewitt, 1999; Smith et al., 2000b). Platelets catalyze the formation of thromboxane A_2 from endoperoxide, whereas vascular endothelium produces prostacyclin (PGI_2). Once formed, prostanoids are immediately released from the cells and act in the vicinity of their sites of production via activation of G-protein-coupled receptors (Narumiya et al., 1999).

NSAIDs, which inhibit COX enzymes and thus prevent the synthesis of PGs, are known to exhibit various analgesic, anti-inflammatory, and antipyretic properties. The analgesic and anti-inflammatory properties of NSAIDs do not necessarily show correlation, as in the case of acetaminophen (McCormack and Brune, 1994).

Cyclooxygenases

COXs have different types of isoform. COX-1 and COX-2 are about 60% identical in terms of molecular structure but differ in terms of temporal and spatial expression and function. COX-1 is a constitutively expressed enzyme present in most cells involved in physiological reactions like vascular endothelium, platelets, and epithelial cells of the renal tubules (O'Neill and Ford-Hutchinson, 1993; Smith et al., 2000b). PGs formed by COX-1 are important in protecting the gastric mucosa and in maintaining the platelet and renal function. COX-2 expression is almost undetectable in most tissues under normal physiological conditions but can be induced 10–80-fold by inflammation. Various factors, including neurotransmitters, growth hormones, proinflammatory cytokines, and lipopolysaccharide, induce COX-2 expression (O'Banion, 1999; Smith et al., 2000b). However, there are exceptions to the expression pattern of the COX enzymes. For example, COX-1 levels are typically quite stable but can be induced under stressful conditions, and in the absence of inflammation COX-2 is constitutively expressed in the CNS and renal cortex, serving normal physiological functions (Morteau, 2000; Schwab et al., 2000; Yaksh et al., 2001). Acetaminophen (paracetamol in Europe) has long been considered to mediate analgesic and antipyretic actions centrally through COX-3 isoenzyme, a splice variant of COX-1, and to be devoid of significant inhibition of peripheral prostanoids (Botting, 2000; Chandrasekharan et al., 2002; Schwab et al., 2003). Recent studies failed to exhibit the existence of centrally acting COX-3 isoenzyme and demonstrated peripheral anti-inflammatory action of acetaminophen that displays an fourfold selectivity for inhibition of COX-2 both *in vitro* and *in vivo* (Hinz et al., 2008; Li et al., 2008).

Generally, NSAIDs are considered to be competetive reversible inhibitors of COX, with the exception being ASA, which inhibits all isoforms irreversibly.

Based on their inhibitory effects on COX, NSAIDs can be classified as (Samad et al., 2002; Botting, 2003):

1. Non-specific COX inhibitors: inhibit both COX-1 and COX-2 (most NSAIDs, naproxen, ibuprofen, meclofenamate)
2. Selective COX-1 inhibitors: indomethacin, piroxicam, sulindac
3. Selective COX-2 inhibitors: inhibit COX-2 in clinical therapeutic doses, also inhibit COX-1 in higher doses (meloxicam, diclofenac, nimesulid, etodolac)
4. Specific COX-1 inhibitors: inhibit COX-1 without inhibiting COX-2 (no available drug except low doses of aspirin)
5. Specific COX-2 inhibitors: inhibit COX-2 without inhibiting COX-1, coxibs (celecoxib, rofecoxib, valdecoxib, etoricoxib, parecoxib, acetaminophen).

Specific COX-2 inhibitors seemed to be better tolerated analgesics, having similar therapeutic efficacy to conventional NSAIDs, but with reported lower gastric side-effects (Katori and Majima, 2000). Rofecoxib and lumiracoxib reduced the incidence of gastrointestinal bleeds and ulceration by approximately 60% compared to non-selective NSAIDs. However, a few years ago, clinical studies suggested that rofecoxib had higher cardiovascular and renal toxicity compared to naproxen (Bombardier et al., 2000). Thereafter, rofecoxib was withdrawn from the market due to the doubled risk of myocardial infarction following long-term administration (Bresalier et al., 2005). It was proposed that there might be a slight tendency towards a drug-induced hypercoagulable state (Solomon et al., 2004). Subsequently, research has focused on new therapeutic targets in the prostanoid production (Zeilhofer and Brune, 2006), including 10 different terminal PG synthases and at least eight different prostanoid receptors activating various signal cascades in different types of cell.

Prostaglandin synthases

Recent studies indicate PG synthases are an important therapeutic target for both inflammation and pain, since at least 10 different types of enzyme have been discovered to convert PG precursors into biologically active prostanoids. Regarding its pivotal role in pain, PGE_2 synthases have received much recent attention compared to the others (Murakami et al., 2000).

PGE synthases have several forms – two membrane-bound forms, mPGES-1 and mPGES-2, and one cytosolic form, cPGES. mPGES-1 is associated with COX-2, and its expression is induced by inflammatory stimuli in both peripheral and central nervous systems (Murakami et al., 2000; Zeilhofer and Brune, 2006). mPGES-2 and cPGES are constitutively expressed and, whereas the first one is associated with both COX isoenzymes, the latter shows preferential coupling to COX-1. In accordance with preferential association of mPGES-1 with COX-2, mPGES-1 knockout mice displayed no PGE_2 increase after induction of COX-2 with lipopolysaccaride, and significantly reduced pain-associated behavior, indicating the important role of mPGES-1 in inflammation and pain response (Kamei et al., 2004). Hence, inhibition of mPGES-1, which is responsible for the synthesis of PGE_2, might be an effective analgesic with lower cardiovascular and renal side-effects comparable with coxibs. Therefore PG synthases seem to be appropriate targets for novel and potentially better-tolerated analgesics.

Prostanoid receptors

Both desired and unwanted effects of NSAIDs are mediated by prostanoid receptors, though the types of receptor as well as its tissue and cell distribution are major determinants of their ultimate function.

Prostanoid metabolites of arachidonic acid, PGD_2, PGE_2, PGF_2, PGI_2, and thromboxane A_2 exert their actions via interaction with specific plasma membrane G-protein-coupled receptors, called DP, EP, FP, IP, and TP respectively (Narumiya et al, 1999; Tsuboi et al., 2002; Sugimoto and Narumiya, 2007). EP receptors are classified further into EP_1, EP_2, EP_3, and EP_4 subtypes, each having different pharmacological properties. Various tissues and cell types express prostanoid receptors, and activation of receptor subtype influences the function (Sugimoto and Narumiya, 2007). For example, in smooth-muscle cells DP and IP receptors mediate relaxation whereas FP and TP receptors are functionally associated with contractile responses. While EP_1 and EP_2 receptors are present in the stomach, kidney, uterus, and nervous system, EP_3 and EP_4 are widely expressed in the body (Tsuboi et al., 2002; Sugimoto and Narumiya, 2007). Consistent with the role of PGE_2 in peripheral sensitization, EP_1, EP_3, and EP_4 receptor mRNAs are expressed in primary sensory neurons and trigeminal ganglia (Southall and Vasco, 2001). Postreceptor events are determined according to the G-protein subtype to which each prostanoid receptor is coupled. Stimulation of adenyl cyclase via Gs proteins leads to increases in cAMP (EP_2, EP_4, $EP_{3C,D}$, DP, and IP) while activation of Gi leads to a decrease in intracellular cAMP (EP1, $EP3_A$, FT, and TP). EP_1 and EP_3 receptors mediate smooth-muscle contraction by inhibition of cAMP via Gq/Gi proteins (Negishi et al., 1995). In contrast, EP_2 and EP_4 receptors mediate relaxation in the vascular smooth muscle (Tsuboi et al., 2002; Sugimoto and Narumiya, 2007).

Among the PGE_2 receptors, EP_1 is the main receptor responsible for mucosal protection. Recent data from EP receptor-deficient mice suggest that reduced activation of EP_1 and EP_3 receptors underlies the ulcerogenic effects of COX inhibitors (Suzuki et al., 2001). Cardiovascular risk of COX-2-selective agents (Tegeder and Geisslinger, 2006) might arise due to the alteration of thromboxane and PGI_2, where the first one is notable with vasoconstrictive and proaggregatory properties, while the latter has vasodilating and antiaggregatory properties (Audoly et al., 1999). It should be kept in mind that an increase in blood pressure that is seen with almost all COX inhibitors may predispose patients with a risk for cardiovascular complications. Although renal function abnormalities are basically associated with prostacyclin synthase (PGIS) knockout mice, EP_2 and EP_4 receptor-deficient mice also display dysregulation of blood pressure (Kennedy et al., 1999).

EP receptors have been shown to be localized in trigeminal ganglion neurons where the stimulation results in CGRP release (Vasco et al., 1994; Jenkins et al., 2001). Moreover, EP_4 receptors mediate PGE_2-induced dilation of middle cerebral artery (Davis et al., 2004). It is likely that PGs, particularly PGE_2, may be involved in the pathology of migraine headache and sensitization of neurons by stimulating CGRP release from trigeminal afferents and also by mediating vascular responses.

Prostanoids and pain

Prostanoids produced in both the peripheral structures and in the CNS, particularly in the spinal cord, play a role in the development of pain. The PGs such as PGE_1 and PGE_2 do not directly activate nociceptor and mediate pain transmission but they contribute to hyperalgesia peripherally by sensitizing nociceptive sensory nerve endings to other mediators (like histamine and bradykinin) and by sensitizing nociceptors to respond to non-nociceptive stimuli (allodynia) (Woolf and Salter, 2000; Bolay and Moskowitz, 2002). Prostanoids play a significant role in peripheral sensitization through EP receptor-coupled postreceptor events such as protein kinase A-mediated phosphorylation of the tetrodotoxin-resistant $Na_V1.8$ sodium channel (Waxman et al., 1999; Villarreal et al., 2005; Meves, 2006) and transient receptor potential vanilloid-1 (TRPV1) non-selective cation channels (Moriyama et al., 2005), which are directly involved in depolarization of nociceptor terminals (Figure 4.1). Thereby prostanoids function to reduce the firing threshold and increase excitability to consecutive nociceptive stimuli such as heat, protons, bradykinin, and prostanoid itself. PGs also have direct actions on the spinal cord to enhance nociception, notably at the terminals of sensory neurons in the dorsal horn (Reinold et al., 2005; Zeilhofer, 2007). This effect is mediated by increasing the release of glutamate and substance P from primary nociceptive afferents (Hingtgen and Vasco, 1994; Southall and Vasco, 2001), which depolarize second-order nociceptive neurons in the dorsal horn, and by inhibiting the glycine-mediated

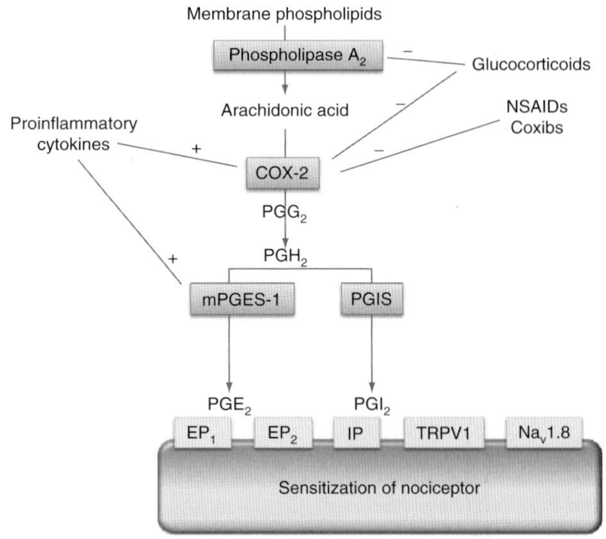

Fig. 4.1. Schematic representation of prostanoid formation and peripheral sensitization. Arachidonic acid released from membrane phospholipids by phospholipases A_2 is a substrate for cyclooxygenase-2 (COX-2), generating prostaglandin G_2 (PGG_2) and then PGH_2. PGH_2 is the substrate for most terminal prostaglandin synthases, including microsomal PGE synthase-1 (mPGES-1) and prostacyclin synthase (PGIS). Inflammatory cytokines induce both COX-2 and mPGES-1 in the periphery and in the central nervous system. Although prostaglandins do not directly activate nociceptors, PGE_2 binds to prostaglandin E (EP) receptors, activates phosphokinases intracellularly, and increases sodium channel permeability through postreceptor events that sensitize nociceptive sensory nerve endings to other mediators (like histamine and bradykinin) and by sensitizing nociceptors to respond to non-nociceptive stimuli (allodynia). Prostanoids mediate pain sensitization through mainly EP_1, EP_2, and IP. PGE_2 and PGI_2 also indirectly potentiate transient receptor potential vanilloid-1 (TRPV1) channel and $Na_V1.8$ sodium channel activation by phosphorylation via PKA and PKC. Those events lead to an elevation of the resting membrane potential and a reduction in the firing threshold of trigeminal nerves. In the spinal cord, PGE_2 acts on EP_2 receptors on the second-order nociceptive neurons, resulting in inhibition of glycine receptors through PKA-dependent phosphorylation. Glucocorticoids and non-steroidal anti-inflammatory drugs (NSAIDs) have the ability to block phospholipase A and COX enzymes.

inhibition (Baba et al., 2001; Ahmadi et al., 2002). Inhibition of glycine receptor occurs through EP_2 receptor-coupled PKA phosphorylation of glycine receptor isoform containing α_3 subunit, which is specifically expressed in superficial nociceptive layers (Harvey et al., 2004). Prostanoids, as briefly mentioned above, modulate other receptors involved in depolarization, such as tetrodotoxin Na^+ channels, TRPV1 channels, or strichnine-sensitive glycine receptors in a way that enhances nociception.

PGs have both pro- and anti-inflammatory properties. The specific response is determined by prostanoid produced, specific receptor, cell type, and the time course of inflammatory signal (Zeilhofer, 2007). For example, PGE_2 is generally considered as a proinflammatory molecule acting on EP_2 receptor coupled to cAMP increase (Samad et al., 2002; Zeilhofer, 2007). Prostanoids may alternatively modulate anti-inflammatory action by binding to peroxisome proliferator-activated receptor (PPAR)γ nuclear hormone receptor (Rotondo and Davidson, 2002). Depending on the time course of inflammation, prostanoid production has two distinct phases (Balsinde and Dennis, 1996). The first phase of arachidonic acid and prostanoid release occurs within minutes of stimulation. However, the late phase requires synthesis of new proteins such as phospholipase A_2, COX-2, and PGES. While arachidonic acid generated during the initial phase is metabolized by constitutively expressed COX-1/COX-2 enzymes, it is a main substrate for COX-2 in the delayed-phase response, yielding prostanoids such as PGE_2 (Tegeder et al., 2001; Samad et al., 2002).

COX-2 is upregulated following inflammation and direct neural input, and also humoral factors play a role in this process. Inflammatory proteins, cytokines released into the circulation such as interleukin 6 (IL-6), trigger the formation of IL-1β, and the production of COX-2 and PGE_2 in the CNS (Samad et al., 2001). COX-2 expression seen throughout the CNS, including the thalamus and cerebral cortex bilaterally, is a humoral response and cannot be prevented by dissection of the nerves carrying the pain from the affected site (Samad et al., 2001). COX-2 is produced in several cells such as neurons and glial cells, and vascular endothelial cells. Although some studies suggest that COX-1 plays a role in spinal transmission of pain, a much greater body of evidence is available supporting the concept that COX-2 is more responsible for PGs involved in hyperalgesia in the peripheral and CNS (Samad et al., 2002). Compounds specifically blocking COX-1 fail to reduce hyperalgesia, but COX-2 and mixed COX-1/COX-2 inhibitors are antihyperalgesic.

NSAIDs prevent prostanoid production and the sensitizing action of PGE_2 by inhibiting the COX enzyme (Vane, 1971). NSAIDs have been shown in animals to reduce hyperalgesia, reversing the inhibition of the descending opioid-mediated noradrenergic pathways. There is also evidence suggesting the roles of 5-HT and nitric oxide (NO) in the production of analgesia by NSAIDs (Bjorkman, 1995). They exert antipyretic effects centrally by inhibiting pyretic cytokines such as IL-1, TNF-α, and PGE_2 released from the hypothalamic thermoregulatory center (Bjorkman, 1995; Botting, 2003). NSAIDs have some other central effects but their mode of action is still not known. However, some data suggest that they might interfere with prostanoid synthesis and catecholamine and 5-HT turnover in the brain. NSAIDs could also mediate peripheral analgesic actions in a COX-independent way, by inhibiting dorsal root acid-sensing ion channels (ASICs) located on sensory nerve terminals (Voilley et al., 2001).

Migraine and inflammation

Migraine is associated with neurogenic inflammation in meninges characterized by CGRP and other neuropeptide release from perivascular trigeminal afferents resulting in vasodilation and plasma protein extravasation within the dura mater (Moskowitz, 1993). This process leads to release of inflammatory molecules, such as 5-HT, histamine, bradykinin, and prostanoids, that are all capable of further stimulating trigeminal afferent fibers to cause peripheral and central sensitization in headache (Strassman et al., 1996; Burstein, 2001). A cocktail of those inflammatory mediators has been shown both to sensitize meningeal nociceptors peripherally and to decrease the firing threshold of central trigeminal neurons in rodents. NO is a vasoactive and pronociceptive molecule that is implicated in migraine headache (Van der Kuy, 2003). The NO donor, glyceryl trinitrate (GTN), induces delayed migraine headache and therefore the GTN-induced headache model is now being used for both human and animal studies (Olesen et al., 1994; Iversen, 2001). In rodents it has been shown that GTN infusion triggered inducible NO synthase expression in dural macrophages accompanied by mast cell degranulation and IL-6 expression, which led to plasma protein extravasation (Reuter et al., 2001, 2002). Those inflammatory events in the dura mater are preceded by the activation of NF-$\kappa\beta$ and induction of IL-1β (Reuter et al., 2002). During headache attacks, proinflammatory cytokines are released in close proximity to trigeminal nerve fibers.

It is highly probable that the aura phase of migraine is also accompanied by proinflammatory molecules. During CSD, potassium ions, protons, NO, adenosine, and arachidonic acid are released into the extracellular space and under certain conditions can cause depolarization of trigeminal perivascular nerve fibers (Bolay et al., 2002). CSD has been shown to induce neurogenic inflammation in the dura mater and be a noxious stimulus that is capable of activating second-order trigeminal neurons in the brainstem (Bolay et al., 2002). Matrix metalloproteinase 9, which is inducible by cytokines, has been shown to be activated shortly after CSD, which implies that the aura is also capable of inducing the release of inflammatory molecules (Gursoy-Ozdemir et al., 2004). In addition, PGE_2 levels are found to be elevated in the plasma during headache attacks, and migraine-like symptoms can be induced by infusion of PGE_2 in migraineurs (Peatfield et al., 1981; Sarchielli et al., 2000). Therefore, it is likely that inflammatory molecules and prostanoids are important mediators of migraine headache.

NSAIDs are widely used and effective drugs for both acute remedy and prophylactic treatment of migraine and tension-type headache, which highlights the importance of prostanoids and their receptors in headache. Aspirin and acetaminophen are the most frequently used drugs for abortive treatment (Prior et al., 2002; Diener et al., 2006). Whether the action of NSAIDs on platelet aggregation may also account for their effectiveness in migraine prophylaxis is controversial. NSAIDs and ASA may exert more specific effects on the trigeminal and antinociceptive system in the brainstem and thalamus (Jurna and Brune, 1990; Kaube et al., 1993). The selective COX-2 inhibitor rofecoxib was found to be effective in pain relief (57%) compared to placebo control (Silberstein et al., 2004), though this drug, among other coxibs, was withdrawn from the market due to undesired effects on the cardiovascular system.

Remarkably, prednisolone infusion could be effective for status migrainosus when the attack is prolonged and refractory to usual abortive medication. Glucocorticoids are also useful for management of cluster headache (Mir et al., 2003; Antonaci et al., 2005; May et al., 2006). Bearing in mind that an important mechanism of glucocorticoids is blocking arachidonic acid release from membrane phospholipids by inhibiting phospholipase A_2, those clinical applications support the notion that prostanoids are involved in headache in some way.

Despite being the most commonly administered group of drugs, the mode of action of NSAIDs in headache syndromes is still not fully understood and future drug developments should focus on better-tolerated COX-2 inhibitors, blockade of specific prostanoid receptors such as EP_1, EP_2, and/or EP_4, inhibition of inducible mPGES-1 enzyme, or more upsteam molecules such as IL-1β.

NORADRENERGIC SYSTEM AND OTHER BIOGENIC AMINES

Central biogenic amine systems using norepinephrine, dopamine, and 5-HT as neurotransmitters play a significant role in headache syndromes (Johnson et al., 1998; D'Andrea et al., 2007), besides regulating various vital functions in the cardiovascular and endocrine systems, emotional states, and energy balance (Nelson and Gehlert, 2006). Histamine, 5-HT and dopamine, and norepinephrine are derived from three different amino acids – respectively histidine, tryptophan, and tyrosine. Biogenic amines exert their effects primarily through G-protein-coupled receptors (Strader et al., 1989; Hoyer et al., 2002).

β–Adrenoreceptor blockers

Norepinephrine is the catecholamine synthesized by the action of dopamine B hydroxylase in locus coeruleus neurons that project widely throughout the CNS. The noradrenergic system has predominant innervations to all cortical layers, with the highest density in the primary sensorimotor areas and limbic cortices and vascular structures in the brain (Gaspar et al., 2004). Norepinephrine mediates a diverse range of responses through α or β adrenoreceptors located on both neuronal and non-neuronal cells (Hieble, 2007). Alpha receptors are widely distributed in skin vessels, mucosa, and kidney, where their stimulation leads to vasoconstriction. Beta-receptor subtypes all stimulate adenylate cyclase via Gs proteins and are abundant in the myocardium, skeletal muscle, and bronchi, where they function in myocardial excitation, broncodilation, and vasodilation (Brede et al., 2004; Owen et al., 2007; Shin and Johnson, 2007).

Non-selective beta-blocking drugs that have equal affinity to β_1 and β_2 receptors are at present the first-choice preventive medication in migraine (Linde and Rossnagel, 2004; Evers et al., 2006). Propranolol is a non-selective drug which has a purely antagonistic action without any intrinsic sympathomimetic activity on β receptors (Shanks, 1991). However metoprolol, another effective agent, has greater affinity to β_1 receptors. Propranolol, alprenolol, and metoprolol are extremely lipophilic and readily penetrate into the CNS. On the other hand, atenolol, a hydrophilic drug with poor penetration into the CNS, is also efficient in migraine prophylaxis (Tfelt-Hansen and Rolan, 2006). Therefore, it is still not clear which property of a beta-blocking drug determines the efficacy in migraine, since penetration through the blood–brain barrier, cardioselectivity, and membrane-stabilizing activity are not common properties. Recent data indicate that beta-blockers could also be effective through central mechanisms. That is supported by Shields and Goadsby (2005), who reported that the preventive action of propranolol is partially mediated by β_1-adrenoreceptor inhibition of third-order trigeminovascular nociceptive neurons in the thalamus. Propranolol has also been shown to influence cortical excitability and significantly reduced the number of potassium-evoked CSDs in rodent cerebral cortex (Ayata et al., 2006). Whether those effects are epiphenomena and how they relate to CSD have to be elucidated by further investigations (Alemdar et al., 2007). It is noteworthy that Na^+/K^+ ATPase activity of cerebral microvessels, and the consequent transport of Na^+ and K^+ across the blood–brain barrier, is probably modulated by noradrenergic innervations from the locus coeruleus (Harik, 1986) and by this means by beta-blocker agents, though its significance for headache remains indistinct.

Reuptake inhibitors of serotonin and norepinephrine

Serotonergic neurons are principally located in the raphe nucleus, where extensive axonal projections innervate almost all regions in the CNS. The action of 5-HT within the synaptic cleft is terminated by an active reuptake via serotonin transporter (SERT) into serotonergic neurons. Most of the 5-HT is then degraded by an enzyme named monoamine oxidase to its major metabolite, 5-hydroxyindole acetaldehyde. There are at least 14 different 5-HT receptor subtypes defined in both pre- and postsynaptic locations mediating a diverse range of actions (Boess and Martin, 1994; Barnes and Sharp, 1999). All 5-HT receptors belong to the G-protein-coupled receptor family except 5-HT_3 receptors, which are ligand-gated ion channels (Hoyer et al., 2002; Kroeze et al., 2002).

5-HT is known to play a pivotal role in migraine pathophysiology since acute remedy medications such as triptans and ergots activate 5-HT_1 receptors, particularly 5-HT_{1B}, 5-HT_{1D}, and 5-HT_{1F} subtypes (Beattie and Connor, 1995; Longmore et al., 1999). In addition, 5-HT_2 antagonism provided by methysergide and cyproheptadine (which is also an antihistaminic and blocks Ca^{2+} channels) mediates prophylaxis in migraine headache (Mylecharane, 1991; Silberstein, 1998).

Selective serotonin reuptake inhibitors (SSRIs) potently block the active reuptake via 5-HT transporter located on serotoninergic neurons that leads to an increased probability of 5-HT interacting with its pre- and postsynaptic receptors. SSRIs exert antinociceptive effects via descending serotonergic fibers and primarily spinal 5-HT_{2A} or 5-HT_{2C} receptors (Honda et al., 2006). Fluoxetine-induced antinociception seems to involve central opioid pathways, since it is shown to be sensitive to blockade by naloxone and naltrexone (Singh et al., 2001). On the other hand, the efficacy of SSRIs for migraine prevention is controversial (Adly et al., 1992) and SSRIs are found to be no more efficacious than placebo in patients with migraine (Saper et al., 1994; Moja et al., 2005). SSRIs are useful in patients with chronic tension-type headache, though they are less efficacious than tricyclic antidepressants (Moja et al., 2005).

Serotonin norepinephrine reuptake inhibitors (SNRI), venlafaxine, duloxetine, and milnacipran, block both norepinephrine and 5-HT reuptake, and thus have dual-action mechanisms. Similar to 5-HT, norepinephrine is also implicated in modulating descending inhibitory pain pathways in the CNS, and therefore SNRIs are used for pain syndromes. Duloxetine is a selective and balanced serotonergic and noradrenergic reuptake inhibitor, and may be efficacious in the treatment of persistent and/or inflammatory pain states at doses that have modest or no effect on acute nociception or motor performance (Iyengar et al., 2004). Venlafaxine has a favorable efficacy and side-effect profile when compared to amitriptyline and was found to be effective for both migraine and tension-type headache prophylaxis (Ozyalcin et al., 2005; Zissis et al., 2007). SNRIs seem to be more effective than SSRIs for headache, and further studies with newer drugs are required to delineate their exact role in headache.

Mirtazapine, which causes reduced neuronal norepinephrine and 5-HT reuptake by selectively blocking central α_2 autoreceptors and postsynaptic 5-HT_2 and 5-HT_3 receptors, has been reported to be effective in headache prevention (Bendtsen and Jensen, 2004).

Drugs such as amitriptyline, imipramine, clomipramine, desipramine, nortriptyline, and maprotiline are classified as trycyclic antidepressants due to their three-ringed organic chemical structure. Their mode of action is mainly through the inhibition of reuptake of 5-HT, norepinephrine, and dopamine. Tricyclic antidepressant drugs are 50–150-fold more potent at inhibiting transport of norepinephrine than 5-HT. Tricyclic antidepressants also exert their effect by blocking sodium channels (in the heart and brain), 5-HT_{2A} receptors, muscarinic and cholinergic receptors, histamine H1 receptors, and adrenergic α_1 receptors (Dick et al., 2007; Paudel et al., 2007). Blockade of the neurotransmitter reuptake pumps is thought to account for the therapeutic actions, and the other mechanisms are thought to account for their wide range of unwanted clinical side-effects. Tricyclic antidepressants bind to an allosteric site close to the neurotransmitter transporter so that the binding, and reuptake, of the neurotransmitter is blocked. Amitriptyline is the only tricyclic antidepressant drug with established efficacy in migraine prophylaxis (Couch and Hassanein, 1979;

Evers et al., 2006); however, its effect does not seem to depend on its antidepressant action since the usual dosage of amitriptyline is lower (up to 75 mg/day) than that used in depression and beneficial effects usually begin within the first week.

MODULATORS OF EXCITABILITY AND ION CHANNEL FUNCTIONS

Data acquired from various studies are consistent with the notion that general cortical dysfunction that leads to increased neuronal hyperexcitability exists in migraineurs (Welch, 2005). Whether increased excitability is relevant for other headache syndromes has not been established. Glutamate mediates excitatory neurotransmission principally through *N*-methyl-D-aspartate (NMDA) receptors that also play critical roles in the generation and propagation of CSD (Vikelis and Mitsikostas, 2007), in addition to other diverse functions such as neuronal plasticity, learning and memory, and neuronal growth (Rao and Finkbeiner, 2007). NMDA receptors are cation-specific ion channels that can be blocked by magnesium in a voltage-dependent manner. Glycine, polyamines, Zn^{2+}, and redox agents all have modulatory sites in NMDA receptors (Scatton, 1993). In the brain, magnesium has a stabilizing role on Na^{+}/K^{+}ATPase beside physiological blockade of NMDA receptors. A strategy to block excitability and/or CSD could be achieved through NR2B subtype inhibition (Gogas, 2006), augmenting Mg^{2+} site blockade, glycine site modulators, or sigma R receptor agonism.

Presynaptic P/Q-type Ca^{2+} channels and voltage-gated Na^{+} channels play pivotal roles in vesicular release of neurotransmitters, particularly of glutamate (Moskowitz et al., 2004). CSD is associated with increased excitability of the cerebral cortex, as shown by mutations that lead to FHM (Moskowitz et al., 2004). In that sense mutations uncovered studying FHM are related to either vesicular glutamate release directly from presynaptic terminals (FHM1 and FHM3) (Ophoff et al., 1996; Dichgans et al., 2005) or glutamate reuptake into perisynaptic astrocytes, or indirectly through affecting Na^{+}/K^{+} ATPase (FHM2) (De Fusco et al., 2003). The P/Q-type channel is expressed throughout the brain and influences the transmission of nociceptive impulses through the TNC (Knight et al., 2002). Presynaptic $Ca_v2.1$ and $Ca_v2.2$ channels are implicated in excessive glutamate release in FHM1 (Qian and Noebels, 2001), which accounts for decreased threshold for CSD along with accompanied cerebellar symptoms. The development of new drugs that focus on the $Ca_v2.1$ and 2.2 channels provides hope for the treatment of migraine without aura.

Besides the P/Q-type calcium channels, the L-type calcium channel blockers (e.g., verapamil) may have some role in headache prevention. They may exert their effect by potentiating opioid and acetaminophen analgesia (Weizman et al., 1999). Verapamil is one of the most efficient drugs used as a preventive medication for cluster headache (May et al., 2006), though its efficacy in migraine is controversial. On the other hand, flunarizine is the most effective calcium antagonist for migraine prevention (Evers et al., 2006) and likely interacts with the release of NO from perivascular nerve fibers (Ayajiki et al., 1997). The N-type calcium channel blocker (ziconotide) that is not available for oral administration has been studied for pain (Wermeling, 2005), but its efficacy for headache syndromes has to be investigated.

Tonabersat (SB-220453) is a novel benzopyran compound reported to block propagation of spreading depression and inhibit neurogenic inflammation and trigeminal ganglion stimulation-induced carotid vasodilation (Smith et al., 2000a; Parsons et al., 2001). In addition, tonabersat has been reported to attenuate trigeminal nerve-induced neurovascular reflexes in the cat (Parsons et al., 2001). Particularly with the property of blocking CSD, SB-220453 has entered clinical trials in migraine. Though the preliminary results are promising, with approximately 62% decrease in headache frequency reported (Goadsby et al., 2009), further clinical studies are warranted.

The most important drugs that directly work on excitabiliy are antiepileptic drugs that are used as migraine-preventive medications (Welch, 2005; Calabresi et al., 2007). Among antiepileptic drugs, sodium valproate and topiramate are acclaimed. Sodium valproate is the first anticonvulsant drug that was approved by the National Institutes of Health for migraine prophylaxis. Sodium valproate is an effective drug for migraine prevention and has the ability to inhibit neurogenic plasma protein extravasation in dura mater (mediated by $GABA_A$ receptors) and block the central transmission within the TNC (Cutrer et al., 1995). It probably blocks voltage-dependent sodium channels and T-type calcium currents, and augments the action of a GABA-synthesizing enzyme, glutamic acid decarboxylase (GAD). Further studies displayed the potential of valproic acid to interfere with multiple regulatory mechanisms, including histone deacetylases, GSK3 α and β, Akt, the ERK pathway, the phosphoinositol pathway, and the tricarboxylic acid cycle (Kostrouchova et al., 2007).

Valproic acid has been shown to influence CSD generation in a dose- and time-dependent way (Ayata et al., 2006). Topiramate has the ability to suppress CSD (Ayata et al., 2006) and cortical neuronal excitability via inhibiting the AMPA/kainate glutamate receptor, potentiating the modulatory effect on the

GABAergic neurotransmission (Simeone et al., 2006), influencing intracellular phosphorylation mechanisms, and blocking presynaptic voltage-gated sodium and calcium channels. It has been shown to inhibit trigeminovascular nociceptive impulses, though the efficacy in models of neurogenic inflammation is yet to be determined (Storer and Goadsby, 2004).

Lamotrigine, which inhibits presynaptic voltage-gated Na^+ channels and thereby reduces glutamate release (Leach et al., 1986), is probably effective on migraine auras but did not reduce the frequency of migraine attacks (Evers et al., 2006). Gabapentin is among the third-choice drugs for migraine prevention and showed a significant efficacy in one placebo-controlled trial in doses between 1200 and 1600 mg (Evers et al., 2006). Gabapentin basically prevents intracellular calcium entry through voltage-gated calcium channels and is believed to modulate various glutamate transporters.

The angiotensin-converting enzyme inhibitor, lisinopril, and angiotensin receptor type 1 (AT1) inhibitor, candesartan, have demonstrated efficacy in migraine prophylaxis, though their mechanism of action is poorly understood (Schrader et al., 2001; Tronvik et al., 2003). Angiotension II regulates cerebral blood flow response via AT1 receptors that inhibit GABA release in the brain (Zhu et al., 1998). AT1 receptor colocalization with glutamate and GABA receptors in the brainstem nociceptive structures implicates their modulatory role in nociception.

Specific types of K^+ channels, such as G-protein-activated, adenosine triphosphate-sensitive inward rectifier or Ca^{2+}-activated K^+ channels, are implicated in the antinociceptive actions of several drugs (Galeotti et al., 2001; Ocana et al., 2004). Potassium ion channels potentially modulate neuronal excitability of trigeminal neurons (Spigelman and Puil, 1989). It is noteworthy that meclofenamic acid and diclofenac, two related molecules widely prescribed as anti-inflammatory drugs, have been demonstrated to act as novel potassium channel openers, resulting in decreased neuronal excitability (Peretz et al., 2005). K^+ channel opening may also play a role in antinociception mediated by G-protein-coupled receptors in the trigeminovascular system, such as $GABA_B$ or opioid receptors (Takeda et al., 2004).

ASICs belong to ligand-gated non-voltage-dependent Na^+ channels and are activated by a decrease of pH in the extracellular milieu (Krishtal, 2003). ASIC3 is colocalized with CGRP in rat trigeminal ganglia neurons and its expression is upregulated with inflammatory mediators, leading to altered firing properties of neurons (Ichikawa and Sugimoto, 2002). NSAIDs can prevent inflammation-induced ASIC upregulation (Voilley et al., 2001) and activation of ASICs is modulated by protein kinase C and can be blocked by the drug amiloride.

TRPV1 is a non-selective cation channel that is activated by noxious stimuli such as capsaicin, heat, or protons. TRPV1 channels are colocalized with CGRP in trigeminal neurons and probably mediate neurogenic inflammation in the dura mater in response to capsaicin (Ichikawa and Sugimoto, 2001). Since TRPV1 channels play a significant role in the generation of nociception, its antagonism could have a therapeutic potential for headache. A clinical trial with small-molecule TRPV1 antagonists has been continuing in migraine patients. Activation of prejunctional adenosine A1 receptors mediates antinociception, and A1 receptor agonist, GR79236, blocks CGRP release and, neurogenic dural vasodilation, and reduces trigeminal nerve firing in human subjects (Goadsby et al., 2002b; Honey et al., 2002; Giffin et al., 2003).

The purinergic system has two main receptors, ionotropic P2X receptor and G-protein-coupled P2Y receptor family, that are both activated in response to extracellular ATP (Chizh and Illes, 2001). P2X3-type purinergic receptors have become more important compared to others in regard to headache development. P2X3 receptors mediate sensitization and hyperalgesia and their effect is augmented in the presence of inflammatory mediators (North, 2003). Trigeminal nerve terminals possess a high density of P2X3 receptors where CGRP potentiates their response to ATP (Ichikawa and Sugimoto, 2004). Therefore purinergic receptors are also an important target for new drug development.

OTHER TREATMENTS AND NEW TARGETS

Botulinum toxin type A

Botulinum neurotoxin type A (BoNT) has been increasingly utilized to treat migraine, tension-type headache, and other primary headache disorders. BoNT has been used clinically for the treatment of neuromuscular disorders, including focal dystonias and relief of pain associated with cervical dystonia and oromandibular dystonias. It is well established that BoNT blocks the presynaptic release of the neurotransmitter acetylcholine at neuromuscular junctions by cleaving the vesicle docking protein SNAP-25, a member of the soluble *N*-ethylmaleimide-sensitive factor attachment receptor (SNARE) proteins. However, blockage of acetylcholine release is not likely the primary mechanism by which BoNT functions as a prophylactic treatment of migraine and other headaches, since reduction in pain is often noted by patients before muscle changes. Rather, the clinical benefits of BoNT may involve regulation of neuropeptide release from trigeminal ganglia neurons (Durham et al., 2004). Recent animal studies have provided evidence that BoNT can block the stimulated release of CGRP, glutamate, and substance P from trigeminal neurons as well as reduce c-*fos* gene expression in second-order neurons. In addition, data from inflammatory pain models have clearly demonstrated an antinociceptive effect of BoNT. Taken together, it is likely that the therapeutic benefit of BoNT involves inhibition of peripheral sensitization, which results in a reduction in central sensitization and blockage of pain transmission.

Oxygen treatment of cluster headache

Inhalation of 100% oxygen, which is used therapeutically for cluster headache, has been reported to reduce the level of CGRP in blood from the external jugular vein to near-normal levels. The therapeutic benefit of inhaling 100% oxygen is thought to involve vasoconstriction of cerebral blood vessels and inhibition of the trigeminovascular system. Towards this end, in recent animal studies, hyperoxia was shown to inhibit dural protein plasma extravasation caused by electrical stimulation of the rat trigeminal ganglion. Thus, the beneficial effect of oxygen treatment is thought to involve inhibition of trigeminal nerve activity that results in decreased pain transmission.

Non-inhaled intranasal CO_2 delivery

Data from phase II clinical trials presented at scientific meetings have provided evidence that a new therapeutic approach provides relief of migraine headache (Spierings, 2005). The method involves 100% carbon dioxide (CO_2), administered at a flow rate of 10 ml/s through one nostril while holding the breath or breathing through the mouth. The exact cellular mechanism by which CO_2 mediates these quite different physiological events is currently unknown, but is likely to occur by a mechanism different from oxygen treatment of cluster headache. Based on results from a recent *in vitro* animal study (Vause et al., 2007), CO_2 treatment of cultured trigeminal ganglia neurons blocked the stimulated release of CGRP. This inhibitory effect of CO_2 on trigeminal nerve activation is thought to involve a decrease in intracellular pH and inhibition of calcium channel activity, which prevents release of neuropeptides such as CGRP. In contrast to oxygen therapy, CO_2 treatment involves non-inhaled intranasal delivery and thus would not be expected to cause a significant change in arterial CO_2 levels. However, despite the differences in delivery methods, both CO_2 and oxygen treatments have been shown to inhibit trigeminal nerve activity. It will be of interest to determine whether CO_2 treatment can inhibit protein plasma extravasation following trigeminal nerve stimulation and whether exposure to 100% CO_2 would be effective in treating cluster headache.

Gap junction inhibitors

Drugs that target gap junction activity are now being tested for their ability to treat migraine. Gap junctions are protein channels that occur between cells and allow for diffusion of small molecules to pass from one cell to the other. Gap junctions are known to increase in number in neurological diseases and are thought to be involved in the initiation and propagation of CSD as well as playing a role in peripheral sensitization of trigeminal neurons. Although its mechanism of action is not known, the compound tonabersat is thought to inhibit gap junction communication between neurons and glia. Interestingly, communication between neurons and glia is thought to be involved in CSD (Smith et al., 2000a) as well as contributing to peripheral sensitization of trigeminal nerves within the trigeminal ganglia (Thalakoti et al., 2007). Further animal and clinical studies are needed to determine the exact mechanism of action, efficacy, and safety profile of tonabersat.

CONCLUDING COMMENTS AND FUTURE DIRECTIONS

Though effective abortive and prophylactic treatments for migraine and other types of headache are available (Table 4.1), there is still a need for improvement since many of the currently used drugs cause unwanted side-effects or are not selective for the trigeminovascular system (Tables 4.1–4.3). However, a better understanding of the pathophysiology and genetic basis of migraine is directing the development of a new generation of drugs that will bind to specific cellular targets. Drugs with increased selectivity and specificity for the 5-HT_{1D} or 5-HT_{1F} receptors may replace currently available triptans. The development of oral forms of a CGRP antagonist would be very exciting.

Since inflammation plays a central role in headache syndromes, research for future studies should include inhibition of inducible mPGES-1 enzyme, prostanoid receptors implicated in headache, and the inflammatory molecules such as leukotrienes, NF-κB, IL-1β, and matrix metallopeptidase 9. Given the emerging evidence for CSD and hyperexcitability in headache disorders, targeting agents that reduce excitability of both cerebral cortical neurons leading to increased threshold for CSD and brainstem nociceptive neurons directly generating and transmitting pain perception will be more important clinically. Potential inhibition of CSD can be provided by targeting presynaptic

Table 4.1

Currently available drugs for headache treatment

Drugs	Indication	Efficacy	Dose (daily)	Precautions/contraindications
Abortive medication				
NSAIDs				
Paracetamol	All types of primary headache (except for cluster, SUNCT)	A	1000 mg	Liver, kidney disease, bleeding disorder, peptic ulcer, gastrointestinal complications. Caution for MOH
Acetylsalicylic acid		A	1000 mg	
Ibuprofen		A	200–800 mg	
Naproxen		A	500–1000 mg	
Triptans				
Sumatriptan	Migraine attack, cluster attack (parenteral forms)	A	6 mg (subcutaneous), 20 mg (nasal), 50–100 mg (oral)	Chest discomfort, nausea, distal paresthesia, fatigue. Uncontrolled hypertension, ischemic heartcerebrovascular/ peripheral vascular disease, pregnancy, lactation, <18 years, >65 years.
Zolmitriptan		A	2.5–5 mg (nasal/oral)	
Naratriptan		A	2.5 mg	
Rizatriptan		A	10 mg	
Almotriptan		A	12.5 mg	
Eletriptan		A	20–40 mg	
Frovatriptan		A	2.5 mg	
Ergot alkaloids	Migraine attack, cluster attack (parenteral forms)	A		Nausea, vomiting, paresthesia, ergotism. Uncontrolled hypertension, ischemic heart disease, cerebrovascular disease, peripheral vascular disease, pregnancy, lactation. Caution for MOH
Metoclopramide	Migraine attack	B	10–20 mg	Dyskinesia, lactation, childhood
Oxygen 100%	Cluster attack	A	>7 l/min (nasal)	
Preventive medication				
Beta-blockers				
Propranolol	Migraine (+ hypertension)	A	40–240 mg	Fatigue, insomnia, dizziness, depression, asthma, heart failure, atrioventricular block
Metoprolol		A	50–200 mg	
Antiepileptics				
Valproic acid	Migraine (+ epilepsy)	A	500–1800 mg	Sedation, nausea, weight gain, tremor, hair loss, liver toxicity
Topiramate		A	25–100 mg	Paresthesia, fatigue, weight loss, dysgeusia, cognitive impairment, depression
Gabapentin		C	1200–1600 mg	Dizziness, drowsiness, giddiness
Lamotrigine	Migraine with aura	C	50–100 mg	Skin rash
Antidepressants				
Amitriptyline	Migraine, tension-type headache	B/A	25–75 mg	Dry mouth, drowsiness, weight gain, constipation, arrhythmias, glaucoma

Table 4.1

Continued

Drugs	Indication	Efficacy	Dose (daily)	Precautions/contraindications
Calcium channel blockers				
Verapamil	Cluster	A	240–360 mg	Dizziness, constipation, distal edema, bradycardia, heart block
Flunarizine	Migraine (childhood)	A	5–10 mg	Weight gain, depression, sedation, extrapyramidal symptoms
Indomethacin	Paroxysmal hemicrania, hemicrania continua	A	150 mg	Gastrointestinal complications, peptic ulcer, nausea, purpura
Prednisolone	Cluster	A	60–100 mg	Gastrointestinal symptoms, ulcer disease, diabetes, hypertension
Angiotension blockade				
Lisinopril	Migraine (+ hypertension)	C	10–20 mg	Cough, lightheadedness, blurred vision, pregnancy
Candesartan		C	16 mg	

NSAIDs: non-steroidal anti-inflammatory drugs; SUNCT: short-lasting unilateral neuralgiform headache attacks with conjuntival injection and tearing; MOH: medication overuse headache.
A: effective; B: probably effective; C: possibly effective (Evers et al., 2006; May et al., 2006; Fumal & Schoenen, 2008).

Table 4.2

Summary of mechanisms that mediate the action of currently used drugs for aborting and preventing migraine

Abortive medications	Preventive medications
Serotonin 5-HT 1B, D, F agonists	β-adrenoreceptor antagonism
CGRP receptor antagonism	Inhibition reuptake of both norepinephrine and 5-HT
COX-2, COX-3 inhibition	Voltage-gated Na^+, Ca^{2+} channel inhibition
Oxygen therapy (cluster headache)	K^+ channel opening
Dopamine D_2 receptor antagonism	$GABA_A$ agonistic activation
	AT1 receptor antagonism
	$5\text{-}HT_2$ antagonism
	Carbonic anhydrase inhibition
	Suppression of CSD
	Increased GABA level
	Inhibition of prostaglandin synthesis

CGRP: calcitonin gene-related peptide; COX: cyclooxygenase; AT1: angiotensin receptor type 1; CSD: cortical spreading depression; GABA: gamma-aminobutyric acid.

Table 4.3

Therapeutics in development for treating headache disorders

Selective $5\text{-}HT_{1D}$ or $5\text{-}HT_{1F}$ agonist activity
Selective $mPGE_1$ inhibition
EP_1, EP_2, EP_4 inhibition
P/Q-type presynaptic Ca^{2+} modulation
Na^+/K^+ ATPase 2 modulation
GAP junction blockade (Connexin 43)
NR2B blockade
iGlu5/AMPA inhibition
TRPV1 inhibition
ASICs blockade
iNOS inhibition
MMP9 inhibition
PAR2 antagonism
IL-1β inhibition
NF-κB inhibition
CO_2 treatment

See text for definitions of abbreviations.

P/Q-type Ca^{2+} and SCNA1 Na^+ channels, ionotropic glutamate receptors (iGlu5/AMPA), NR2B subunit and sigma R receptors as well as gap junctions. Sensory neuron-specific sodium channel ($Na_v1.8$, $Na_v1.7$) inhibition, K^+ channel opening, antagonisms of purinergic

P2X3 receptors, TRPV1 receptors, ASIC3 channels, and proteinase-activated receptors are prime targets for providing antinociception.

Dopamine has gained importance and its possible therapeutic action and receptor subtypes involved other than D_2 receptor need to be explored further (Akcali et al., 2008). Whether disturbances in tyrosine metabolism such as dopamine and other trace amines contribute to the underlying pathology of cluster and migraine attacks needs to be investigated.

The effects of newer antiplatelet and possibly anticoagulant agents have to be tested in migraineurs, since migraine patients were shown to have an increased risk for thromboembolic events and they may have silent brain lesions in which convergence of vascular factors and the neurogenic mechanisms are largely unrevealed.

References

Adham N, Borden LA, Schechter LE et al. (1993). Cell-specific coupling of the cloned human 5-HT1F receptor to multiple signal transduction pathways. Naunyn Schmiedebergs Arch Pharmacol 348: 566–575.

Adly C, Straumanis J, Chesson A (1992). Fluoxetine prophylaxis of migraine. Headache 32: 101–104.

Ahmadi S, Lippross S, Neuhuber WL et al. (2002). PGE_2 selectively blocks inhibitory glycinergic neurotransmission onto rat superficial dorsal horn neurons. Nat Neurosci 5: 34–40.

Ahn A, Basbaum A (2006). Tissue injury regulates serotonin 1D receptor expression: implications for the control of migraine and inflammatory pain. J Neurosci 26: 8332–8338.

Akcali DT, Doganay-Aydin H, Bolay H (2008). Metoclopramide inhibits trigeminovascular activation: evidence for effective acute attack treatment in migraine. Cephalalgia 28: 464.

Alemdar M, Akman O, Selekler H et al. (2007). Does metoprolol inhibit the cortical spreading depression? Acute effects of systematic metropol on CSD in rats. Cephalalgia 27: 1010–1013.

Amara S, Arriza J, Leff S et al. (1985). Expression in brain of a messenger RNA encoding a novel neuropeptide homologous to calcitonin gene-related peptide. Science 229: 1094–1097.

Antonaci F, Costa A, Candeloro E et al. (2005). Single high-dose steroid treatment in episodic cluster headache. Cephalalgia 25: 290–295.

Audoly LP, Rocca B, Fabre JE et al. (1999). Identification of specific EP receptors responsible for the hemodynamic effects of PGE_2. Am J Physiol 277: H924–H930.

Ayajiki K, Okamura T, Toda N (1997). Flunarizine, an anti-migraine agent, impairs nitroxidergic nerve function in cerebral arteries. Eur J Pharmacol 329: 49–53.

Ayata C, Jin H, Kudo C et al. (2006). Suppression of cortical spreading depression in migraine prophylaxis. Ann Neurol 59: 652–661.

Baba H, Kohno T, Moore KA et al. (2001). Direct activation of rat spinal dorsal horn neurons by prostaglandin E_2. J Neurosci 21: 1750–1756.

Balsinde J, Dennis EA (1996). Distinct roles in signal transduction for each of the phospholipase A_2 enzymes present in P388D1 macrophages. J Biol Chem 271: 6758–6765.

Barnes N, Sharp T (1999). A review of central 5-HT receptors and their function. Neuropharmacology 38: 1083–1152.

Beattie D, Connor H (1995). The pre- and postjunctional activity of CP-122,288, a conformationally restricted analogue of sumatriptan. Eur J Pharmacol 276: 271–276.

Bendtsen L, Jensen R (2004). Mirtazapine is effective in the prophylactic treatment of chronic tension-type headache. Neurology 62: 1706–1711.

Bjorkman R (1995). Central antinociceptive effects of non-steroidal anti-inflammatory drugs and paracetamol. Experimental studies in the rat. Acta Anaesthesiol Scand Suppl 103: 1–44.

Blier P (1991). Terminal serotonin autoreceptor function in the rat hippocampus is not modified by pertussis and cholera toxins. Naunyn Schmiedebergs Arch Pharmacol 344: 160–166.

Boess F, Martin I (1994). Molecular biology of 5-HT receptors. Neuropharmacology 33: 275–317.

Bolay H, Moskowitz MA (2002). Mechanism of pain modulation in chronic syndromes. Neurology 59 (Suppl. 2): S2–S7.

Bolay H, Moskowitz M (2005). The emerging importance of cortical spreading depression in migraine headache. Rev Neurol 161: 655–657.

Bolay H, Reuter U, Dunn AK et al. (2002). Intrinsic brain activity triggers trigeminal meningeal afferents in a migraine model. Nat Med 8: 136–142.

Bombardier C, Laine L, Reicin A et al. (2000). Comparison of upper gastrointestinal toxicity of rofecoxib and naproxen in patients with rheumatoid arthritis. VIGOR Study Group. N Engl J Med 343: 1520–1528.

Botting R (2000). Mechanism of action of acetaminophen: Is there a cylooxygenase 3? Clin Infect Dis 31: S202–S210.

Botting R (2003). COX-1 and COX-3 inhibitors. Thromb Res 110: 269–272.

Bouchelet I, Cohen Z, Casae B et al. (1996). Differential expression of sumatriptan-sensitive 5-hydroxytryptamine receptors in human trigeminal ganglia and cerebral blood vessels. Mol Pharmacol 50: 219–223.

Brain S, Williams T, Tippins JR et al. (1985). Calcitonin gene-related peptide is a potent vasodilator. Nature 313: 54–56.

Brede M, Philipp M, Knaus A et al. (2004). Alpha2-adrenergic receptor subtypes – novel functions uncovered in gene-targeted mouse models. Biol Cell 96: 343–348.

Bresalier RS, Sandler RS, Quan H et al. (2005). Cardiovascular events associated with rofecoxib in a colorectal adenoma chemoprevention trial. N Engl J Med 352: 1092–1102.

Burstein R (2001). Deconstructing migraine headache into peripheral and central sensitization. Pain 89: 107–110.

Burstein R, Jakubowski M (2004). Analgesic triptan action in an animal model of intracranial pain: a race against the development of central sensitization. Ann Neurol 55: 27–36.

Burstein R, Yarnitsky D, Goor-Areyh I (2000). An association between migraine and cutaneous allodynia. Ann Neurol 47: 614–624.

Burstein R, Collins B, Jakubowski M et al. (2004). Defeating migraine pain with triptans: a race against the development of cutaneous allodynia. Ann Neurol 55: 19–26.

Buzzi MG, Sakas DE, Moskowitz MA (1989). Indomethacin and acetylsalicylic acid block neurogenic plasma protein extravasation in rat dura mater. Eur J Pharmacol 165: 251–258.

Buzzi M, Carter W, Shimizu T et al. (1991). Dihydroergotamine and sumatriptan attenuate levels of CGRP in plasma in rat superior saggital sinus during electrical stimulation of the trigeminal ganglia. Neuropharmacology 30: 1193–1200.

Buzzi MG, Dimitriadou V, Theoharides TC et al. (1992). 5-Hydroxytryptamine receptor agonists for the abortive treatment of vascular headaches block mast cell, endothelial and platelet activation within the rat dura mater after trigeminal stimulation. Brain Res 583: 137–149.

Buzzi M, Bonamini M, Moskowitz M et al. (1995). Neurogenic model of migraine. Cephalalgia 15: 277–280.

Calabresi P, Galletti F, Rossi C et al. (2007). Antiepileptic drugs in migraine: from clinical aspects to cellular mechanisms. Trends Pharmacol Sci 28: 188–195.

Cavazos JE, Caress JB, Chilukuri VR et al. (1994). Sumatriptan-induced stroke in sagittal sinus thrombosis. Lancet 343: 1105–1106.

Chandrasekharan NV, Dai H, Roos KL et al. (2002). COX-3, a cyclooxygenase-1 variant inhibited by acetaminophen and other analgesic/antipyretic drugs: cloning, structure, and expression. Proc Natl Acad Sci U S A 99: 13926–13931.

Chiba T, Yamaguchi A, Yamatani T et al. (1989). Calcitonin gene-related peptide receptor antagonist human CGRP-(8–37). Am J Physiol 256: E331–E335.

Chizh BA, Illes P (2001). P2X receptors and nociception. Pharmacol Rev 53: 553–568.

Couch JR, Hassanein RS (1979). Amitriptyline in migraine prophylaxis. Arch Neurol 36: 695–699.

Cumberbatch M, Hill R, Hargreaves RJ et al. (1997). Rizatriptan has central antinociceptive effects against durally evoked responses. Eur J Pharmacol 328: 37–40.

Cumberbatch M, Hill R, Hargreaves RJ et al. (1998). The effects of 5-HT1A, 5-HT1B and 5-HT1D receptor agonists on trigeminal nociceptive neurotransmission in anaesthetized rats. Eur J Pharmacol 362: 43–46.

Cutrer FM, Limmroth V, Ayata G et al. (1995). Attenuation by valproate of c-fos immunoreactivity in trigeminal nucleus caudalis induced by intracisternal capsaicin. Br J Pharmacol 116: 3199–3204.

D'Andrea G, Nordera GP, Perini F et al. (2007). Biochemistry of neuromodulation in primary headaches: focus on anomalies of tyrosine metabolism. Neurol Sci 28 (Suppl. 2):S94–S96.

Davis RJ, Murdoch CE, Ali M et al. (2004). EP4 prostanoid receptor-mediated vasodilatation of human middle cerebral arteries. Br J Pharmacol 141: 580–585.

De Fusco M, Marconi R, Silvestri L et al. (2003). Haploinsufficiency of *ATP1A2* encoding the Na-,K-pump -2 subunit gene is responsible for familial hemiplegic migraine type 2. Nat Genet 33: 192–196.

Dichgans M, Freilinger T, Eckstein G et al. (2005). Mutation in the neuronal voltage-gated sodium channel SCN1A in familial hemiplegic migraine. Lancet 366: 371–377.

Dick IE, Brochu RM, Purohit Y et al. (2007). Sodium channel blockade may contribute to the analgesic efficacy of antidepressants. J Pain 8: 315–324.

Diener HC, Lampl C, Reimnitz P et al. (2006). Aspirin in the treatment of acute migraine attacks. Expert Rev Neurother 6: 563–573.

Dimitriadou V, Buzzi MG, Theoharides TC et al. (1992). Ultrastructural evidence for neurogenically mediated changes in blood vessels of the rat dura mater and tongue following antidromic trigeminal stimulation. Neuroscience 48: 187–203.

Doods H, Hallermayer G, Wu D et al. (2000). Pharmacological profile of BIBN4096BS, the first selective small molecule CGRP antagonist. Br J Pharmacol 129: 420–423.

Durham P, Russo A (1998). Serotonergic repression of mitogen-activated protein kinase control of the calcitonin gene-related peptide enhancer. Mol Endocrinol 12: 1002–1009.

Durham PL, Russo AF (2002). New insights into the molecular actions of serotonergic antimigraine drugs. Pharmacol Ther 94: 77–92.

Durham P, Sharma R, Russo AF et al. (1997). Repression of the calcitonin gene-related peptide promoter by 5-HT1 receptor activation. J Neurosci 17: 9545–9553.

Durham PL, Cady R, Cady R (2004). Regulation of calcitonin gene-related peptide secretion from trigeminal nerve cells by botulinum toxin type A: implications for migraine therapy. Headache 44: 35–43.

Ebersberger A, Averbeck B, Messlinger K et al. (1999). Release of substance P, calcitonin gene-related peptide and prostaglandin E_2 from rat dura mater encephali following electrical and chemical stimulation in vitro. Neuroscience 89: 901–907.

Edvinsson L, Goadsby P (1994). Neuropeptides in migraine and cluster headache. Cephalalgia 14: 320–327.

Evers S, Afra J, Frese A et al. (2006). EFNS guideline on the drug treatment of migraine – report of an EFNS task force. Eur J Neurol 13: 560–572.

Fanciullacci M, Alessandri M, Figini M et al. (1995). Increase in plasma calcitonin gene-related peptide from the extracerebral circulation during nitroglycerin-induced cluster headache attack. Pain 60: 119–123.

Ferrari MD (1998). Migraine. Lancet 351: 1043–1051.

Ferrari M, Saxena P (1993). On serotonin and migraine: a clinical and pharmacological review. Cephalalgia 13: 151–165.

Ferrari M, Roon K, Lipton RB et al. (2001). Oral triptans (serotonin 5-HT(1B/1D) agonists) in acute migraine treatment: a meta-analysis of 53 trials. Lancet 358: 1668–1675.

Fischer J, Born W (1985). Novel peptides from the calcitonin gene: expression, receptors and biological function. Peptides 6: 265–271.

Friberg L, Olesen J, Iversen HK et al. (1991). Migraine pain associated with middle cerebral artery dilatation: reversal by sumatriptan. Lancet 338: 13–17.

Fumal A, Schoenen J (2008). Current migraine management – patient acceptability and future approaches. Neuropsychiatr Dis Treat 4: 1043–1057.

Galeotti N, Ghelardini C, Bartolini A (2001). Involvement of potassium channels in amitriptyline and clomipramine analgesia. Neuropharmacology 40: 75–84.

Garavito RM, Dewitt DL (1999). The cyclooxygenase isoforms: structural insights into the conversion of arachidonic acid to prostaglandins. Biochim Biophys Acta 1441: 278–287.

Gaspar P, Berger B, Febvret A et al. (2004). Catecholamine innervation of the human cerebral cortex as revealed by comparative immunohistochemistry of tyrosine hydroxylase and dopamine-beta-hydroxylase. J Comp Neurol 279: 249–271.

Geraud G, Keywood C, Senard JM et al. (2003). Migraine headache recurrence: relationship to clinical, pharmacological, and pharmacokinetic properties of triptans. Headache 43: 376–388.

Giffin JJ, Kowacs F, Libri V et al. (2003). Effect of the adenosine A1 receptor agonist GR79236 on trigeminal nociception with blink reflex recording in healthy human subjects. Cephalalgia 23: 287–292.

Goadsby P, Edvinsson L (1991). Sumatriptan reverses the changes in calcitonin gene-related peptide seen in the headache phase of migraine. Cephalalgia 11: 3–4.

Goadsby P, Edvinsson L (1993). The trigeminovascular system and migraine: studies characterizing cerebrovascular and neuropeptide changes seen in humans and cats. Ann Neurol 33: 48–56.

Goadsby P, Edvinsson L (1994a). Human in vivo evidence for trigeminovascular activation in cluster headache. Neuropeptide changes and effects of acute attacks therapies. Brain 117: 427–434.

Goadsby P, Edvinsson L (1994b). Peripheral and central trigeminovascular activation in cat is blocked by the serotonin (5HT)-1D receptor agonist 311C90. Headache 34: 394–399.

Goadsby PJ, Hoskin KL (1996). Inhibition of trigeminal neurons by intravenous administration of the serotonin (5HT) 1B/D receptor agonist zolmitriptan (311C90): are brain stem sites therapeutic target in migraine? Pain 67: 355–359.

Goadsby P, Lipton R, Ferrari M et al. (2002a). Migraine – current understanding and treatment. N Engl J Med 346: 257–270.

Goadsby PJ, Hoskin KL, Storer RJ et al. (2002b). Adenosine A(1) receptor agonists inhibit trigeminovascular nociceptive transmission. Brain 125: 1392–1401.

Goadsby PJ, Ferrari MD, Csanyi A et al. (2009). Randomized, double-blind, placebo-controlled, proof-of-concept study of the cortical spreading depression inhibiting agent tonabersat in migraine prophylaxis. Cephalalgia 29: 742–750.

Gogas KR (2006). Glutamate-based therapeutic approaches: NR2B receptor antagonists. Curr Opin Pharmacol 6: 68–74.

Gursoy-Ozdemir Y, Qiu J, Mastuoka N et al. (2004). Cortical spreading depression activates and upregulates MMP-9. J Clin Invest 113: 1447–1455.

Hamel E, Fan E, Linville D et al. (1993). Expression of mRNA for the serotonin 5-hydroxytryptamine1D beta receptor subtype in human and bovine cerebral arteries. Mol Pharmacol 44: 242–246.

Hargreaves R (2007). New migraine and pain research. Headache 47: S26–S43.

Hargreaves R, Shepheard S (1999). Pathophysiology of migraine – new insights. Can J Neurol Sci 26: S12–S19.

Harik SI (1986). Blood–brain barrier sodium/potassium pump: modulation by central noradrenergic innervation. Proc Natl Acad Sci U S A 83: 4067–4070.

Harvey RJ, Depner UB, Waissle H et al. (2004). Glyr alpha3: an essential target for spinal PGE_2-mediated inflammatory pain sensitization. Science 304: 884–887.

Henkes H, May A, Kühne D et al. (1996). Sumatriptan: vasoactive effect on human dural vessels, demonstrated by subselective angiography. Cephalalgia 16: 224–230.

Heuring R, Peroutka S (1987). Characterization of a novel ^{3}H-5-hydroxytryptamine binding site subtype in bovine brain membranes. J Neurosci 7: 894–903.

Hieble JP (2007). Subclassification and nomenclature of alpha- and beta-adrenoceptors. Curr Top Med Chem 7: 129–134.

Hingtgen CM, Vasko MR (1994). The phosphatase inhibitor, okadaic acid, increases peptide release from rat sensory neurons in culture. Neurosci Lett 178: 135–138.

Hinz B, Cheremina O, Brune K (2008). Acetaminophen (paracetamol) is a selective cyclooxygenase-2 inhibitor in man. FASEB J 22: 383–390.

Honda M, Uchida K, Tanabe M et al. (2006). Fluvoxamine, a selective serotonin reuptake inhibitor, exerts its antiallodynic effects on neuropathic pain in mice via 5-HT2A/2C receptors. Neuropharmacology 51: 866–872.

Honey AC, Bland-Ward PA, Connor HE et al. (2002). Study of an adenosine A1 receptor agonist on trigeminally evoked dural blood vessel dilation in the anaesthetized rat. Cephalalgia 22: 260–264.

Ho TW, Ferrari MD, Dodick DW et al. (2008a). Efficacy and tolerability of MK-0974 (telcagepant), a new oral antagonist of calcitonin gene-related peptide receptor, compared with zolmitriptan for acute migraine: a randomised, placebo-controlled, parallel-treatment trial. Lancet 372: 2115–2123.

Ho TW, Mannix LK, Fan X et al. (2008b). MK-0974 Protocol 004 study group. Randomized controlled trial of an oral CGRP receptor antagonist, MK-0974, in acute treatment of migraine. Neurology 70: 1304–1312.

Hoyer D, Middlemiss DN (1989). Species differences in the pharmacology of terminal 5-HT autoreceptors in mammalian brain. Trends Pharmacol Sci 10: 130–132.

Hoyer D, Waeber C, Pazos A et al. (1988). Identification of a 5-HT1 recognition site in human brain membranes different from 5-HT1A, 5-HT1B and 5-HT1C sites. Neurosci Lett 85: 357–362.

Hoyer D, Hannon JP, Martin GR (2002). Molecular, pharmacological and functional diversity of 5-HT receptors. Pharmacol Biochem Behav 71: 533–554.

Humphrey P (1991). 5-Hydroxytryptamine and the pathophysiology of migraine. J Neurol 238: S38–S44.

Humphrey P, Feniuk W (1991). Mode of action of the antimigraine drug sumatriptan. Trends Pharmacol Sci 12: 444–446.

Ichikawa H, Sugimoto T (2001). VR1-immunoreactive primary sensory neurons in the rat trigeminal ganglion. Brain Res 890: 184–188.

Ichikawa H, Sugimoto T (2002). The co-expression of ASIC3 with calcitonin gene-related peptide and parvalbumin in the rat trigeminal ganglion. Brain Res 943: 287–291.

Ichikawa H, Sugimoto T (2004). The co-expression of P2X3 receptor with VR1 and VRL-1 in the rat trigeminal ganglion. Brain Res 998: 130–135.

Iversen HK (2001). Human migraine models. Cephalalgia 21: 781–785.

Iyengar S, Webster AA, Hemrick-Luecke SK et al. (2004). Efficacy of duloxetine, a potent and balanced serotonin–norepinephrine reuptake inhibitor in persistent pain models in rats. J Pharmacol Exp Ther 311: 576–584.

Jansen-Olesen I, Mortensen A, Edvinsson L et al. (1996). Calcitonin gene-related peptide is released from capsaicin-sensitive nerve fibres and induces vasodilatation of human cerebral arteries concomitant with activation of adenylyl cyclase. Cephalalgia 16: 310–316.

Jenkins DW, Feniuk W, Humphrey PP (2001). Characterization of the prostanoid receptor types involved in mediating calcitonin gene-related peptide release from cultured rat trigeminal neurones. Br J Pharmacol 134: 1296–1302.

Jenkins D, Langmead C, Parsons AA et al. (2004). Regulation of calcitonin gene-related peptide release from rat trigeminal nucleus caudalis slices in vitro. Neurosci Lett 366: 241–244.

Johnson K, Bolay H (2006). Neurogenic inflammatory mechanisms in migraine. In: J Olesen, P Goadsby, N Ramadan et al. (Eds.), The Headaches. 3rd edn. Lippincott Williams & Wilkins, Philadelphia, pp. 309–319.

Johnson K, Schaus J, Durkin MM et al. (1997). 5-HT1F receptor agonists inhibit neurogenic dural inflammation in guinea pigs. Neuroreport 8: 2237–2240.

Johnson KW, Phebus LA, Cohen ML (1998). Serotonin in migraine: theories, animal models and emerging therapies. Prog Drug Res 51: 219–244.

Jurna I, Brune K (1990). Central effect of the non-steroid anti-inflammatory agents, indomethacin, ibuprofen, and diclofenac, determined in C fibre-evoked activity in single neurones of the rat thalamus. Pain 41: 71–80.

Kamei D, Yamakawa K, Takegoshi Y et al. (2004). Reduced pain hypersensitivity and inflammation in mice lacking microsomal prostaglandin E synthase-1. J Biol Chem 279: 33684–33695.

Kapoor K, Arulmani U, Heiligers JPC et al. (2003). Effects of BIBN4096BS on cardiac output distribution and on CGRP-induced carotid haemodynamic responses in the pig. Eur J Pharmacol 475: 69–77.

Katori M, Majima M (2000). Cyclooxygenase-2: its rich diversity of roles and possible application of its selective inhibitors. Inflamm Res 49: 367–392.

Kaube H, Hoskin KL, Goadsby PJ (1993). Intravenous acetylsalicylic acid inhibits central trigeminal neurons in the dorsal horn of the upper cervical spinal cord in the cat. Headache 33: 541–544.

Kennedy CR, Zhang Y, Brandon S et al. (1999). Salt-sensitive hypertension and reduced fertility in mice lacking the prostaglandin EP2 receptor. Nat Med 5: 217–220.

Knight YE, Bartsch T, Kaube H et al. (2002). P/Q-type calcium-channel blockade in the periaqueductal gray facilitates trigeminal nociception: a functional genetic link for migraine? J Neurosci 22: RC213.

Knyihar-Csillik E, Tajti J, Csillik EA et al. (1995). Electrical stimulation of the Gasserian ganglion induces structural alterations of calcitonin gene-related peptide-immunoreactive perivascular sensory nerve terminals in the rat cerebral dura mater: a possible model of migraine headache. Neurosci Lett 184: 189–192.

Kostrouchova M, Kostrouch Z, Kostrouchova M (2007). Valproic acid, a molecular lead to multiple regulatory pathways. Folia Biol (Praha) 53: 37–49.

Krishtal O (2003). The ASICs: signaling molecules? Modulators? Trends Neurosci 26: 477–483.

Kroeze WK, Kristiansen K, Roth BL (2002). Molecular biology of serotonin receptors structure and function at the molecular level. Curr Top Med Chem 2: 507–528.

Leach MJ, Marden CM, Miller AA (1986). Pharmacological studies on lamotrigine, a novel potential antiepileptic drug: II. Neurochemical studies on the mechanism of action. Epilepsia 27: 490–497.

Levy D, Jakubowski M, Burstein R (2004). Disruption of communication between peripheral and central trigeminovascular neurons mediate the antimigraine action of 5HT1B/1D receptor agonists. Proc Natl Acad Sci U S A 101: 4274–4279.

Levy D, Burstein R, Strassman AM (2005). Calcitonin gene-related peptide does not excite or sensitize meningeal nociceptors: implications for the pathophysiology of migraine. Ann Neurol 58: 698–705.

Li S, Doub W, Tang Y et al. (2008). Acetaminophen: antipyretic or hypothermic in mice? In either case, PGHS-1b (COX-3) is irrelevant. Prostaglandins Other Lipid Mediat 85: 89–99.

Linde K, Rossnagel K (2004). Propranolol for migraine prophylaxis. Cochrane Database Syst Rev 2: CD003225.

Lipton RB, Pan J (2004). Is migraine a progressive brain disease? JAMA 28: 493–494.

Longmore J, Dowson A et al. (1999). Advances in migraine therapy – 5-HT receptor subtype-specific agonist drugs. Curr Opin CPNS Invest Drugs 1: 39–53.

Longmore J, Shaw D, Smith D et al. (1997). Differential distribution of 5HT1D- and 5HT1B-immunoreactivity within the human trigemino-cerebrovascular system: implications for the discovery of new antimigraine drugs. Cephalalgia 17: 833–842.

Luman W, Gray R (1993). Adverse reactions associated with sumatriptan. Lancet 341: 1091–1092.

MacLeod A, Street L, Reeve AJ et al. (1997). Selective, orally active 5-HT1D receptor agonists as potential antimigraine agents. J Med Chem 40: 3501–3503.

Malick A, Burstein R (2000). Peripheral and central sensitization during migraine. Funct Neurol 15: S28–S35.

Mallee J, Salvatore C, LeBourdelles B et al. (2002). Receptor activity-modifying protein 1 determines the species selectivity of non-peptide CGRP receptor antagonists. J Biol Chem 277: 14294–14298.

Mathew N (2001). Pathophysiology, epidemiology, and impact of migraine. Clin Cornerstone 4: 1–17.

May A, Leone M, Afra J et al. (2006). EFNS guidelines on the treatment of cluster headache and other trigeminal-autonomic cephalalgias. Eur J Neurol 13: 1066–1077.

Mayberg M, Langer RS, Zervas NT et al. (1981). Perivascular meningeal projections from cat trigeminal ganglia: possible pathway for vascular headaches in man. Science 213: 228–230.

Mayberg MR, Zervas NT, Moskowitz MA (1984). Trigeminal projections to supratentorial pial and dural blood vessels in cats demonstrated by horseradish peroxidase histochemistry. J Comp Neurol 223: 46–56.

McCormack K, Brune K (1994). Dissociation between the antinociceptive and antiinflammatory drugs and the dissociation between their antiinflammatory and analgesic effects. Drugs 47: 28–45.

McCulloch J, Uddman R, Kingman TA et al. (1986). Calcitonin gene-related peptide: functional role in cerebrovascular regulation. Proc Natl Acad Sci U S A 83: 5731–5735.

Meves H (2006). The action of prostaglandins on ion channels. Curr Neuropharmacol 4: 41–57.

Mir P, Alberca R, Navarro A et al. (2003). Prophylactic treatment of episodic cluster headache with intravenous bolus of methylprednisolone. Neurol Sci 24: 318–321.

Moja PL, Cusi C, Sterzi RR et al. (2005). Selective serotonin re-uptake inhibitors (SSRIs) for preventing migraine and tension-type headaches. Cochrane Database Syst Rev 3: CD002919.

Moreno M, Cohen Z, Stanimirovic DB et al. (1999). Functional calcitonin gene-related peptide type 1 and adrenomedullin receptors in human trigeminal ganglia, brain vessels, and cerebromicrovascular or astroglial cells in culture. J Cereb Blood Flow Metab 19: 1270–1278.

Moreno M, Abounader R, Lantin S et al. (2002a). Efficacy of the non-peptide CGRP receptor antagonist BIBN4096BS in blocking CGRP-induced dilations in human and bovine cerebral arteries: potential implications in acute migraine treatment. Neuropharmacology 42: 568–576.

Moreno M, Terron J, Stanimirovic D et al. (2002b). Characterization of calcitonin gene-related peptide (CGRP) receptors and their receptor-activity-modifying proteins (ramps) in human brain microvascular and astroglial cells in culture. Neuropharmacology 42: 270–280.

Moriyama T, Higashi T, Togashi K et al. (2005). Sensitization of TRPV1 by EP1 and IP reveals peripheral nociceptive mechanism of prostaglandins. Mol Pain 1: 3.

Morteau O (2000). Prostaglandins and inflammation: the cyclooxygenase controversy. Arch Immunol Ther Exp 48: 473–480.

Moskowitz MA (1992). Neurogenic versus vascular mechanisms of sumatriptan and ergot alkaloids in migraine. Trends Pharmacol Sci 13: 307–311.

Moskowitz MA (1993). Neurogenic inflammation in the pathophysiology and treatment of migraine. Neurology 43 (Suppl. 3): S16–S20.

Moskowitz MA, Bolay H, Dalkara T (2004). Deciphering migraine mechanisms: clues from familial hemiplegic migraine genotypes. Ann Neurol 55: 276–280.

Mueller L, Gallagher R, Ciervo CA et al. (1996). Vasospasm-induced mycocardial infarction with sumatriptan. Headache 36: 329–331.

Mulderry P, Ghatei M, Spokes RA et al. (1988). Differential expression of alpha-CGRP and beta-CGRP by primary sensory neurons and enteric autonomic neurons of the rat. Neuroscience 25: 195–205.

Murakami M, Naraba H, Tanioka T et al. (2000). Regulation of prostaglandin E_2 biosynthesis by inducible membrane-associated prostaglandin E_2 synthase that acts in concert with cyclooxygenase-2. J Biol Chem 275: 32783–32792.

Mylecharane EJ (1991). 5-HT_2 receptor antagonists and migraine therapy. J Neurol 238 (Suppl. 1): S45–S52.

Narumiya S, Sugimoto Y, Ushikubi F (1999). Prostanoid receptors: structures, properties, and functions. Physiol Rev 79: 1193–1226.

Negishi M, Sugimoto Y, Ichikawa A (1995). Molecular mechanisms of diverse actions of prostanoid receptors. Biochim Biophys Acta 1259: 109–119.

Nelson DL, Gehlert DR (2006). Central nervous system biogenic amine targets for control of appetite and energy expenditure. Endocrine 29: 49–60.

North RA (2003). The P2X3 subunit: a molecular target in pain therapeutics. Curr Opin Investig Drugs 4: 833–840.

Nozaki K, Boccalini P, Moskowitz MA et al. (1992). Expression of c-fos-like immunoreactivity in brainstem after meningeal irritation by blood in the subarachnoid space. Neuroscience 49: 669–680.

O'Banion MK (1999). Cyclooxygenase-2: molecular biology, pharmacology, and neurobiology. Crit Rev Neurobiol 13: 45–82.

O'Conner T, Van der Kooy D (1988). Enrichment of a vasoactive neuropeptide (calcitonin gene related peptide) in the trigeminal sensory projection to the intracranial arteries. J Neurosci 8: 2468–2476.

O'Neill GP, Ford-Hutchinson AW (1993). Expression of mRNA for cyclooxygenase-1 and cyclooxygenase-2 in human tissues. FEBS Lett 330: 156–160.

Ocana M, Cendan CM, Cobos EJ et al. (2004). Potassium channels and pain: present realities and future opportunities. Eur J Pharmacol 500: 203–219.

Olesen J, Jansen-Olesen I (2000). Nitric oxide mechanisms in migraine. Pathol Biol (Paris) 48: 648–657.

Olesen J, Thomsen LL, Iversen H (1994). Nitric oxide is a key molecule in migraine and other vascular headaches. Trends Pharmacol Sci 15: 149–153.

Olesen J, Diener H, Husstedt IW et al. (2004). Calcitonin gene-related peptide receptor antagonist BIBN 4096 BS for the acute treatment of migraine. N Engl J Med 350: 1104–1110.

Oliver KR, Wainwright A, Edvinsson L et al. (2002). Immunohistochemical localization of calcitonin receptor-like receptor and receptor activity-modifying proteins in the human cerebral vasculature. J Cereb Blood Flow Metab 22: 620–629.

Ophoff RA, Terwindt GM, Vergouwe MN et al. (1996). Familial hemiplegic migraine and episodic ataxia type-2 are caused by mutations in the calcium channel gene CACNL1A4. Cell 87: 543–552.

Ottervanger J, van Witsen T, Valkenburg HA et al. (1994). Adverse reactions attributed to sumatriptan. A postmarketing study in general practice. Eur J Clin Pharmacol 47: 305–309.

Ottosson A, Edvinsson L (1997). Release of histamine from dural mast cells by substance P and calcitonin gene-related peptide. Cephalalgia 17: 166–174.

Owen SF, Giltrow E, Huggett DB et al. (2007). Comparative physiology, pharmacology and toxicology of beta-blockers: mammals versus fish. Aquat Toxicol 82: 145–162.

Ozyalcin SN, Talu GK, Kiziltan E et al. (2005). The efficacy and safety of venlafaxine in the prophylaxis of migraine. Headache 45: 144–152.

Paone D, Shaw A, Nguyen D et al. (2007). Potent, orally bioavailable calcitonin gene-related peptide receptor antagonists for the treatment of migraine: discovery of N-[(3R,6S)-6-(2,3-difluorophenyl)-2-oxo-1-(2,2,2-trifluoroethyl)azepan-3-yl]-4-(2-oxo-2,3-dihydro-1H-imidazo[4,5-b]pyridin-1-yl) piperidine-1-carboxamide (MK-0974). J Med Chem 50: 5564–5567.

Parsons AA, Bingham S, Raval P et al. (2001). Tonabersat (SB-220453) a novel benzopyran with anticonvulsant properties attenuates trigeminal nerve-induced neurovascular reflexes. Br J Pharmacol 132: 1549–1557.

Paudel KR, Das BP, Rauniar GP et al. (2007). Antinociceptive effect of amitriptyline in mice of acute pain models. Indian J Exp Biol 45: 529–531.

Peatfield RC, Gawel MJ, Rose FC (1981). The effect of infused prostacyclin in migraine and cluster headache. Headache 21: 190–195.

Pedigo N, Schoemaker H, Morelli M et al. (1981). Benzodiazepine receptor binding in young, mature and senescent rat brain and kidney. Neurobiol Aging 2: 83–88.

Peretz A, Degani N, Nachman R et al. (2005). Meclofenamic acid and diclofenac, novel templates of KCNQ2/Q3 potassium channel openers, depress cortical neuron activity and exhibit anticonvulsant properties. Mol Pharmacol 67: 1053–1066.

Pietrobon D (2005). Migraine: new molecular mechanisms. Neuroscientist 11: 373–386.

Poyner D, Sexton P, Marshall I et al. (2002). International Union of Pharmacology. XXXII. The mammalian calcitonin gene-related peptides, adrenomedullin, amylin, and calcitonin receptors. Pharmacol Rev 54: 233–246.

Prior MJ, Cooper KM, May LG et al. (2002). Efficacy and safety of acetaminophen and naproxen in the treatment of tension-type headache. A randomized, double-blind, placebo-controlled trial. Cephalalgia 22: 740–748.

Qian J, Noebels JL (2001). Presynaptic Ca^{2+} channels and neurotransmitter release at the terminal of a mouse cortical neuron. J Neurosci 21: 3721–3728.

Quirion R, Van Rossum D, Dumont Y et al. (1992). Characterization of CGRP1 and CGRP2 receptor subtypes. Ann N Y Acad Sci 657: 88–105.

Rao VR, Finkbeiner S (2007). NMDA and AMPA receptors: old channels, new tricks. Trends Neurosci 30: 284–291.

Ray BS, Wolff HG (1940). Experimental studies on headache: pain-sensitive structures of the head and their significance in headache. Arch Surg 41: 813–856.

Reinold H, Ahmadi S, Depner UB et al. (2005). Spinal inflammatory hyperalgesia is mediated by prostaglandin E receptors of the EP2 subtype. J Clin Invest 115: 673–679.

Reuter U, Bolay H, Jansen-Olesen I et al. (2001). Delayed inflammation in rat meninges: implications for migraine pathophysiology. Brain 124: 2490–2502.

Reuter U, Chiarugi A, Bolay H et al. (2002). Nuclear factor-kappaB as a molecular target for migraine therapy. Ann Neurol 51: 507–516.

Rist B, Lacroix J, Entzeroth M et al. (1999). CGRP 27–37 analogues with high affinity to the CGRP1 receptor show antagonistic properties in a rat blood flow assay. Regul Pept 79: 153–158.

Rosenfeld M, Mermod JJ, Amara SG et al. (1983). Production of a novel neuropeptide encoded by the calcitonin gene via tissue-specific RNA processing. Nature 304: 129–135.

Rotondo D, Davidson J (2002). Prostaglandin and PPAR control of immune cell function. Immunology 105: 20–22.

Salvatore C, Hershey J, Corcoran H et al. (2008). Pharmacological characterization of MK-0974 [N-[(3R,6S)-6-(2,3-difluorophenyl)-2-oxo-1-(2,2,2-trifluoroethyl)azepan-3-yl]-4-(2-oxo-2,3-dihydro-1H-imidazo[4,5-b]pyridin-1-yl)piperidine-1-carboxamide], a potent and orally active calcitonin gene-related peptide receptor antagonist for the treatment of migraine. J Pharmacol Exp Ther 324: 416–421.

Samad TA, Moore KA, Sapirstein A et al. (2001). Interleukin-1beta-mediated induction of Cox-2 in the CNS contributes to inflammatory pain hypersensitivity. Nature 410: 471–475.

Samad TA, Sapirstein A, Woolf CJ (2002). Prostanoids and pain: unraveling mechanisms and revealing therapeutic targets. Trends Mol Med 8: 390–396.

Saper J, Silberstein S (2006). Pharmacology of dihydroergotamine and evidence for the efficacy and safety in migraine. Headache 46: S171–S181.

Saper JR, Silberstein SD, Lake AE et al. (1994). Double-blind trial of fluoxetine: chronic daily headache and migraine. Headache 34: 497–502.

Sarchielli P, Alberti A, Codini M et al. (2000). Nitric oxide metabolites, prostaglandins and trigeminal vasoactive peptides in internal jugular vein blood during spontaneous migraine attacks. Cephalalgia 20: 907–918.

Scatton B (1993). The NMDA receptor complex. Fundam Clin Pharmacol 7: 389–400.

Schrader H, Stovner LJ, Helde G et al. (2001). Prophylactic treatment of migraine with angiotensin converting enzyme inhibitor (lisinopril): randomised, placebo controlled, crossover study. BMJ 322: 19–22.

Schwab JM, Brechtel K, Nguyen TD et al. (2000). Persistent accumulation of cyclooxygenase-1 (COX-1) expressing microglia/macrophages and upregulation by endothelium following spinal cord injury. J Neuroimmunol 111: 122–130.

Schwab JM, Schluesener HJ, Meyermann R et al. (2003). COX-3 the enzyme and the concept: steps towards highly specialized pathways and precision therapeutics? Prostaglandins Leukot Essent Fatty Acids 69: 339–343.

Shanks RG (1991). Clinical pharmacology of vasodilatory beta-blocking drugs. Am Heart J 121: 1006–1011.

Shepheard S, Williamson D, Williams J et al. (1995). Comparison of the effects of sumatriptan and the NK1 antagonist CP-99,994 on plasma extravasation in dura mater and c-fos mRNA expression in trigeminal nucleus caudalis of rats. Neuropharmacology 34: 255–261.

Shields KG, Goadsby PJ (2005). Propranolol modulates trigeminovascular responses in thalamic ventroposteromedial nucleus: a role in migraine? Brain 128: 86–97.

Shin J, Johnson JA (2007). Pharmacogenetics of beta-blockers. Pharmacotherapy 27: 874–887.

Silberstein SD (1998). Methysergide. Cephalalgia 18: 421–435.

Silberstein S, Tepper S, Brandes J et al. (2004). Randomized, placebo-controlled trial of rofecoxib in the acute treatment of migraine. Neurology 62: 1552–1557.

Simeone TA, Wilcox KS, White HS (2006). Subunit selectivity of topiramate modulation of heteromeric GABA (A) receptors. Neuropharmacology 50: 845–857.

Singh VP, Jain NK, Kulkarni SK (2001). On the antinociceptive effect of fluoxetine, a selective serotonin reuptake inhibitor. Brain Res 915: 218–226.

Smith MI, Read SJ, Chan WN et al. (2000a). Repetitive cortical spreading depression in a gyrencephalic feline brain: inhibition by the novel benzoylamino-benzopyran SB-220453. Cephalalgia 20: 546–553.

Smith WL, DeWitt DL, Garavito RM (2000b). Cyclooxygenases: structural, cellular, and molecular biology. Annu Rev Biochem 69: 145–182.

Solomon DH, Schneeweiss S, Glynn RJ et al. (2004). Relationship between selective cyclooxygenase-2 inhibitors and myocardial infarction in older adults. Circulation 109: 2068–2073.

Southall MD, Vasco MR (2001). Prostaglandin receptor subtypes, EP3C and EP4, mediate the prostaglandin E-2-induced cAMP production and sensitization of sensory neurons. J Biol Chem 276: 16083–16091.

Spierings G (2005). Abortive treatment of migraine headache with non-inhaled, intranasal carbon dioxide: a randomized, double-blind, placebo-controlled, parallel-group study. Headache 45: 809.

Spigelman I, Puil E (1989). K^+-channel blockade in trigeminal root ganglion neurons: effects on membrane outward currents. J Neurophysiol 62: 802–809.

Steenbergh P, Hoppener J, Zandberg J et al. (1985). A second human calcitonin/CGRP gene. FEBS Lett 183: 403–407.

Storer RJ, Goadsby PJ (2004). Topiramate inhibits trigeminovascular neurons in the cat. Cephalalgia 24: 1049–1056.

Strader CD, Sigal IS, Dixon RA (1989). Structural basis of beta-adrenergic receptor function. FASEB J 3: 1825–1832.

Strassman AM, Raymond SA, Burstein R (1996). Sensitization of meningeal sensory neurons and the origin of headaches. Nature 384: 560–564.

Sugimoto Y, Narumiya S (2007). Prostaglandin E receptors. J Biol Chem 282: 11613–11617.

Suzuki K, Araki H, Mizoguchi H et al. (2001). Prostaglandin E inhibits indomethacin-induced gastric lesions through EP-1 receptors. Digestion 63: 92–101.

Takeda M, Tanimoto T, Ikeda M et al. (2004). Activation of GABAB receptor inhibits the excitability of rat small diameter trigeminal root ganglion neurons. Neuroscience 123: 491–505.

Tegeder I, Geisslinger G (2006). Cardiovascular risk with cyclooxygenase inhibitors: general problem with substance specific differences? Naunyn Schmiedebergs Arch Pharmacol 373: 1–17.

Tegeder I, Niederberger E, Vetter G et al. (2001). Effects of selective COX-1 and -2 inhibition on formalin-evoked nociceptive behaviour and prostaglandin E(2) release in the spinal cord. J Neurochem 79: 777–786.

Tfelt-Hansen P, Rolan P (2006). Beta-adrenoceptor blocking drugs in migraine prophylaxis. In: J Olesen, P Goadsby, N Ramadan et al. (Eds.), The Headaches. 3rd edn. Lippincott Williams & Wilkins, Philadelphia, pp. 519–528.

Thalakoti S, Patil V, Damodaram S et al. (2007). Neuron–glia signaling in trigeminal ganglion: implications for migraine pathology. Headache 47: 1008–1023.

Tronvik E, Stovner LJ, Helde G et al. (2003). Prophylactic treatment of migraine with an angiotensin II receptor blocker: a randomized controlled trial. JAMA 289: 65–69.

Tsuboi K, Sugimoto Y, Ichikawa A (2002). Prostanoid receptor subtypes. Prostaglandins Other Lipid Mediat 68–69: 535–556.

Van der Kuy PH, Lohman JJ (2003). The role of nitric oxide in vascular headache. Pharm World Sci 25: 146–151.

Van Rossum D, Hanisch U, Quirion R et al. (1997). Neuroanatomical localization, pharmacological characterization and functions of CGRP, related peptides and their receptors. Neurosci Biobehav Rev 21: 649–678.

Vane JR (1971). Inhibition of prostaglandin synthesis as a mechanism of action for aspirin like drugs. Nat New Biol 231: 232–235.

Vasco MR, Campbell WB, Waite KJ (1994). Prostaglandin E (2) enhances bradykinin-stimulated release of neuropeptides from rat sensory neurons in culture. J Neurosci 14: 4987–4997.

Vause C, Bowen E, Spierings E et al. (2007). Effect of carbon dioxide on calcitonin gene-related peptide secretion from trigeminal neurons. Headache 47: 1385–1397.

Vikelis M, Mitsikostas DD (2007). The role of glutamate and its receptors in migraine. CNS Neurol Disord Drug Targets 6: 251–257.

Villarreal CF, Sachs D, Cunha FQ, Parada CA, Ferreira SH (2005). The role of $Na_V1.8$ sodium channel in the maintenance of chronic inflammatory hypernociception. Neurosci Lett 386: 72–77.

Visser W, Jaspers N, de Vriend RH et al. (1996). Chest symptoms after sumatriptan: a two-year clinical practice review in 735 consecutive migraine patients. Cephalalgia 16: 554–559.

Voilley N, de Weille J, Mamet J et al. (2001). Nonsteroid anti-inflammatory drugs inhibit both the activity and the inflammation-induced expression of acid-sensing ion channels in nociceptors. J Neurosci 21: 8026–8033.

Waxman SG, Dib-Hajj S, Cummins TR et al. (1999). Sodium channels and pain. Proc Natl Acad Sci U S A 96: 7635–7639.

Weizman R, Getslev V, Pankova IA et al. (1999). Pharmacological interaction of the calcium channel blockers verapamil and flunarizine with the opioid system. Brain Res 818: 187–195.

Welch KM (2005). Brain hyperexcitability: the basis for antiepileptic drugs in migraine prevention. Headache 45 (Suppl. 1): S25–S32.

Wermeling DP (2005). Ziconotide, an intrathecally administered N-type calcium channel antagonist for the treatment of chronic pain. Pharmacotherapy 25: 1084–1094.

Wess J (1997). G-protein-coupled receptors: molecular mechanisms involved in receptor activation and selectivity of G-protein recognition. FASEB J 11: 346–354.

Williamson D, Hill R, Goadsby PJ et al. (2001). The antimigraine 5-HT(1B/1D) agonist rizatriptan inhibits neurogenic dural vasodilation in anaesthetized guinea-pigs. Br J Pharmacol 133: 1029–1034.

Winner P, Ricalde O, Le Force B et al. (1996). A double-blind study of subcutaneous dihydroergotamine vs subcutaneous sumatriptan in the treatment of acute migraine. Arch Neurol 53: 180–184.

Woolf CJ, Salter MW (2000). Neuronal plasticity: increasing the gain in pain. Science 288: 1765–1769.

Yaksh TL, Dirig DM, Conway CM et al. (2001). The acute antihyperalgesic action of nonsteroidal, anti-inflammatory drugs and release of spinal prostaglandin E_2 is mediated by the inhibition of constitutive spinal cyclooxygenase-2 (COX-2) but not COX-1. J Neurosci 21: 5847–5853.

Zagami A, Goadsby P, Edvinsson L et al. (1990). Stimulation of the superior sagittal sinus in the cat causes release of vasoactive peptides. Neuropeptides 16: 69–75.

Zeilhofer HU (2007). Prostanoids in nociception and pain. Biochem Pharmacol 73: 165–174.

Zeilhofer HU, Brune K (2006). Analgesic strategies beyond the inhibition of cyclooxygenases. Trends Pharmacol Sci 27: 467–474.

Zgombick J, Borden L, Cochran TL et al. (1993). Dual coupling of cloned human 5-hydroxytryptamine1D alpha and 5-hydroxytryptamine1D beta receptors stably expressed in murine fibroblasts: inhibition of adenylate cyclase and elevation of intracelluar calcium concentrations via pertussis toxin-sensitive G protein(s). Mol Pharmacol 44: 575–582.

Zhang Z, Winborn C, Marquez de Prado B et al. (2007). Sensitization of calcitonin gene-related peptide receptors by receptor activity-modifying protein-1 in the trigeminal ganglion. J Neurosci 27: 2693–2703.

Zhu DN, Moriguchi A, Mikami H et al. (1998). Central amino acids mediate cardiovascular response to angiotensin II in the rat. Brain Res Bull 45: 189–197.

Zissis NP, Harmoussi S, Vlaikidis N et al. (2007). A randomized, double-blind, placebo-controlled study of venlafaxine XR in out-patients with tension-type headache. Cephalalgia 27: 315–324.

Handbook of Clinical Neurology, Vol. 97 (3rd series)
Headache
G. Nappi and M.A. Moskowitz, Editors

Chapter 5

Biological science of headache channels

DANIELA PIETROBON*
Department of Biomedical Sciences, University of Padova, Padova, Italy

ION CHANNELS AND CHANNELOPATHIES

Ion channels are membrane proteins forming pores that allow ions to move rapidly through cell membranes down their electrochemical gradients, thus producing rapid changes in membrane potential. Most ion channels are gated, i.e., capable of making transitions between conducting (open) and non-conducting (closed) conformations. Gating of ion channels can be dependent on membrane potential (voltage-gated channels), ligand binding (ligand-gated channels), mechanical stimuli, and other factors. Opening and closing of ion channels generate a complex system of electrical signaling and form the basis of cellular excitability in neurons and muscle cells. Since Ca^{2+} ions are intracellular second messengers, Ca^{2+} channels regulate a diversity of additional cellular functions, besides excitability, including secretion, gene expression, cell survival and differentiation, and muscle contraction. Moreover, ion channels are essential for transepithelial transport of salt and water, and for regulation of cellular volume and pH (Hille, 2001).

More than 40 human disorders are caused by mutations in ion channel genes and hence classified as channelopathies (Ashcroft, 2000; Cannon, 2006). Most of them are episodic neurological or muscular diseases caused by mutations in voltage-gated ion channels, including different types of epilepsy, episodic ataxia, familial hemiplegic migraine (FHM), and different types of periodic paralysis and myotonia, as well as long QT syndromes.

The superfamily of voltage-gated ion channels includes K^+, Na^+, and Ca^{2+} channels, whose pore-forming α_1 subunits share a fundamental design consisting of six membrane-spanning segments (S1–S6) that are repeated in four homologous domains in Na^+ and Ca^{2+} channels (Hille, 2001) (Figure 5.1). The four domains (or four α_1 subunits in the case of K^+ channels) are arranged in a tetrameric structure to form a transmembrane aqueous pore, whose walls and selectivity filter are thought to be formed by segments S5 and S6 and the S5–S6 loop, respectively. The S4 segments, which contain positively charged residues at every third or fourth position, play a major role in voltage sensing. Voltage-gated channels are multisubunit structures, comprising auxiliary subunits that modulate channel function and targeting. Large molecular and functional diversity of voltage-gated channels is created by multiple genes for each subunit (in the case of the α_1 subunit, at least 9, 10, and 80 genes for Na^+, Ca^{2+}, and K^+ channels, respectively) and multiple splice variants for each gene. This large diversity likely reflects the complexity of specific signaling needs, particularly in the brain where almost all the different isoforms are expressed, in a neuron-specific and subcellular-specific manner.

The types of voltage-gated (in particular, Na^+ and K^+, but also Ca^{2+}) channels expressed by a given neuron determine its specific electrical activity, i.e., shape, amplitude, and duration of action potentials and the specific temporal pattern of spontaneous and/or stimulus-evoked action potentials. In addition, neuronal voltage-gated Ca^{2+} channels play a fundamental role in neurotransmitter release, and thus shape the balance between excitatory and inhibitory synaptic inputs that is a key determinant of network behavior in neuronal circuits. Most channelopathies of the nervous system (as most of those of skeletal and cardiac muscle) are diseases of membrane and/or network excitability. The analysis of the functional consequences of disease-causing mutations has shown that even subtle changes in the biophysical properties

*Correspondence to: Daniela Pietrobon PhD, Department of Biomedical Sciences, University of Padova, Viale G. Colombo 3, 35121, Padova, Italy, Tel: 39-049-8276052, Fax: 39-049-8276049, E-mail: daniela.pietrobon@unipd.it

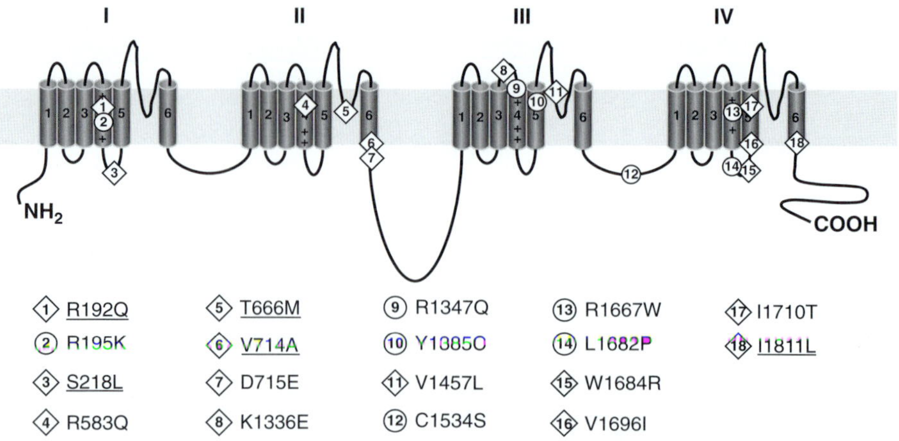

Fig. 5.1. Secondary structure of the $Ca_V2.1$ α_1 subunit and location of the familial hemiplegic migraine (FHM1) mutations identified so far. Diamonds: mutations whose functional consequences have been studied in heterologous expression systems. Underlined: mutations whose functional consequences have also been studied in transfected neurons from $Ca_V2.1^{-/-}$ mice.

of voltage-gated channels can alter membrane excitability and have important pathological consequences.

The classification of FHM as a channelopathy, following the discovery that two of its causative genes encode α_1 subunits of voltage-gated ion channels (Ophoff et al., 1996; Dichgans et al., 2005), has introduced a new perspective in headache research and has strengthened the idea of migraine as a disorder of neural excitability.

FUNCTIONAL CONSEQUENCES OF FAMILIAL HEMIPLEGIC MIGRAINE GENE MUTATIONS AND DISEASE MECHANISMS

FHM is a rare autosomal-dominant subtype of migraine with aura (MA), whose aura symptoms include motor weakness or paralysis. Apart from the obligatory motor aura, typical FHM attacks resemble MA attacks. FHM is genetically heterogeneous. Mutations in the genes *CACNA1A* at chromosome 19p13 (Ophoff et al., 1996), *ATP1A2* at 1q23 (De Fusco et al., 2003), and *SCNA1A* at 2q24 (Dichgans et al., 2005) are responsible for FHM type 1 (FHM1), type 2 (FHM2), and type 3 (FHM3), respectively.

Familial hemiplegic migraine type 1

The FHM1 gene *CACNA1A* encodes the pore-forming α_1 subunit of the neuronal voltage-gated calcium channel $Ca_V2.1$ (or P/Q-type Ca^{2+} channel). $Ca_V2.1$ channels are located in presynaptic terminals and somatodendritic membranes throughout the brain, where they play a prominent role in controlling neurotransmitter release, particularly at central excitatory synapses (Pietrobon, 2005a). The somatodendritic localization of $Ca_V2.1$ channels points to additional postsynaptic roles, e.g., in neural excitability. $Ca_V2.1$ channels are expressed in all brain structures that have been implicated in the pathogenesis of migraine, including the cerebral cortex, the trigeminal ganglia, and brainstem nuclei involved in the central control of nociception (Pietrobon and Striessnig, 2003). Their expression is particularly high in the cerebellum.

Deletion of the $Ca_V2.1\alpha_1$ mouse gene leads to severe cerebellar ataxia and dystonia together with selective progressive cerebellar degeneration (Pietrobon, 2002, 2005a). Different mouse strains with spontaneous $Ca_V2.1\alpha_1$ mutations all suffer from ataxia and exhibit reduced P/Q-type current in Purkinje cells. Moreover, null $Ca_V2.1^{-/-}$ mice and the majority of the spontaneous mutants harboring loss-of-function mutations in $Ca_V2.1$ show absence seizures (Pietrobon, 2002, 2005a). A 50% loss of $Ca_V2.1$ channels leads to reduced responses to inflammatory and neuropathic pain in heterozygous $Ca_V2.1^{-/+}$ mice, revealing an important role of these channels in central sensitization (Luvisetto et al., 2006). In humans, mutations in the *CACNA1A* gene cause, in addition to FHM1, a few autosomal-dominant neurological disorders characterized by cerebellar dysfunction, such as episodic ataxia type 2 (EA2, which may be associated with absence epilepsy in a few cases) and spinocerebellar ataxia type 6 (SCA6) (Ophoff et al., 1996; Zhuchenko et al., 1997; Imbrici et al., 2004). EA2 mutations lead to loss-of-function of recombinant human $Ca_V2.1$ channels in heterologous expression systems (Pietrobon, 2005a), whereas SCA6 mutations do not affect channel function in Purkinje cells of knockin mice expressing human $Ca_V2.1$ channels with extended polyglutamine repeats (Saegusa et al., 2006).

Eighteen different missense mutations associated with FHM1 have been described, including the Y1385C sporadic mutation (Haan et al., 2005) (Figure 5.1). All produce substitutions of conserved amino acids in important functional regions, including the pore lining and the voltage sensors. The functional studies of mutant Ca^{2+} channels support the conclusion that FHM1 mutations lead to gain-of-function of human neuronal $Ca_V2.1$ channels; the gain-of-function is mainly due to a shift to lower voltages of channel activation (Pietrobon, 2005a, b). Mutant Ca^{2+} channels open at lower voltages than wild-type (wt) channels and Ca^{2+} influx can occur in response to small depolarizations insufficient to open wt channels; moreover, in a wide range of mild depolarizations mutant channels stay open for a larger fraction of time, thus allowing more Ca^{2+} in than wt channels.

Indeed, recombinant human mutant $Ca_V2.1$ channels carrying eight different FHM1 mutations (Figure 5.1) showed an increased single-channel Ca^{2+} influx in a wide range of mild depolarizations, reflecting an increased channel open probability mainly due to a shift to lower voltages of channel activation (Tottene et al., 2002, 2005a; and our unpublished observations). A similar increase in neuronal P/Q Ca^{2+} current density in a wide range of mild depolarizations, reflecting a shift to lower voltages of $Ca_V2.1$ channel activation, was measured in cerebellar and cortical neurons of knockin mice carrying two different FHM1 mutations (R192Q and S218L) (Shapovalova et al., 2004; van den Maagdenberg et al., 2004; Pizzorusso et al., 2006). The shift to lower voltages of $Ca_V2.1$ channel activation and the gain-of-function of the neuronal $Ca_V2.1$ current were about twice as large in homozygous compared to heterozygous knockin mice, revealing an allele dosage effect consistent with dominance of the mutation in FHM1 patients (Pizzorusso et al., 2006).

While the R192Q mutation produces a pure FHM phenotype characterized by typical attacks, the S218L mutation produces a severe clinical phenotype, in which typical attacks of FHM triggered by minor head trauma are frequently followed by deep coma or profound stupor (sometimes preceded by a generalized seizure), fever, and long-lasting severe cerebral edema; other common symptoms are ataxia and cerebral and/or cerebellar atrophy (Kors et al., 2001). Accordingly, while the homozygous R192Q knockin mice appear healthy, the homozygous S218L mice are prone to sudden death for seemingly unknown reasons (probably due to severe seizures) and are ataxic (A. van den Maagdenberg, personal communication). Compared with the other FHM1 mutations analyzed, S218L is one of the mutations that produces the largest shift of activation of human $Ca_V2.1$ channels and the largest gain-of-function, especially for small depolarizations (Tottene et al., 2005a). Accordingly, at low voltages close to the threshold of activation of mutant channels, the gain-of-function of the $Ca_V2.1$ current was larger in S218L than in R192Q knockin mice (van den Maagdenberg et al., 2004; Pizzorusso et al., 2006).

As a consequence of the gain-of-function of $Ca_V2.1$ channels, the FHM1 mutations produce gain-of-function of $Ca_V2.1$-dependent neurotransmitter release. The FHM1 knockin mice showed increased neurotransmission at the neuromuscular junction in conditions of low release probability (evoked release at low Ca^{2+} and spontaneous release) (Kaja et al., 2004, 2005; van den Maagdenberg et al., 2004). The increase in spontaneous release was much larger in S218L than in R192Q knockin mice, in agreement with the lower threshold of activation of S218L compared to R192Q $Ca_V2.1$ channels. Of special interest for the pathophysiology of migraine (see below) is the finding that cortical neurons of R192Q knockin mice in microculture show an increased action potential-evoked glutamate release at physiological Ca^{2+} concentrations, due to an increased contribution of P/Q Ca^{2+} channels (Tottene et al., 2005b).

Neuroimaging findings indicate that migraine aura is due to cortical spreading depression (CSD), a wave of sustained strong neuronal depolarization that slowly progresses across the cortex, generating a transient intense spike activity that is followed by long-lasting neural suppression (Pietrobon and Striessnig, 2003). In animals, CSD can be induced by focal stimulation (electrical, mechanical, or with high K^+) of the cerebral cortex, by inhibition of the Na^+/K^+ ATPase, and by other stimuli (Somjen, 2001). In the rat, CSD can activate the meningeal trigeminal nociceptive afferents and evoke alterations in the meninges and brainstem consistent with the development of headache (Bolay et al., 2002). Moreover, a series of known antimigraine prophylactic drugs have the common property of elevating the stimulation threshold for induction of CSD after protracted administration (Ayata et al., 2006). These animal studies support the idea that CSD may initiate migraine attacks (Pietrobon and Striessnig, 2003; Pietrobon, 2005b; Sanchez-Del-Rio et al., 2006).

Interestingly, FHM1 knockin mice are more susceptible to CSD than wt mice. In both R192Q and S218L knockin mice, gain-of-function of $Ca_V2.1$ channels leads to a lower threshold for CSD induction and an increased velocity of propagation of CSD induced by electrical stimulation of the visual cortex *in vivo* (van den Maagdenberg et al., 2004; Pizzorusso et al., 2006). In correlation with the more severe clinical phenotype of the S218L mutation, the facilitation of CSD, especially its rate of propagation, was larger in S218L than

R192Q knockin mice. Moreover, S218L knockin mice showed a much higher incidence of recurrent CSDs. Recurrent CSDs might open the blood-brain barrier (Gursoy-Ozdemir et al., 2004) and they might underlie the delayed cerebral edema and severe clinical phenotype produced by the S218L mutation. The facilitation of CSD induction and propagation were about twice as large in homozygous compared to heterozygous S218L KI mice (Pizzorusso et al., 2006); the allele-dosage effect is consistent with the autosomal dominant inheritance of the mutation in FHM1 patients. These findings support a key role of CSD in the pathogenesis of FHM1.

Although the mechanisms for initiation and propagation of CSD are not completely understood, a local increase above a critical value of the K^+ concentration in the narrow space surrounding cortical neurons and the activation of a sustained net inward current in apical dendrites appear crucial for initiating the positive-feedback cycle that almost zeroes the neuronal membrane potential and ignites CSD (Somjen, 2001). Together with previous CSD data from spontaneous *Cacna1a* mutant mice, the CSD data from FHM1 knockin mice support a key role for $Ca_V2.1$ channels in the initiation and propagation of CSD. Loss-of-function of $Ca_V2.1$ channels in *leaner* and *tottering* mice leads to a higher threshold for CSD induction, a lower velocity of propagation, and a shorter duration of the CSD depolarization *in vivo* (Ayata et al., 2000). Similar inhibitory effects on CSD initiation, propagation, and duration were produced *in vivo* by *N*-methyl-D-aspartate (NMDA) antagonists in a dose-dependent manner (Marrannes et al., 1988). Moreover, a decrease in intracortical glutamate was measured by *in vivo* microdialysis during high K^+ exposure in *leaner* and *tottering* mice (Ayata et al., 2000). Thus, $Ca_V2.1$-dependent release of glutamate from cortical excitatory synapses and activation of NMDA receptors appear crucial in determining both initiation and propagation of CSD.

A possible positive-feedback mechanism for CSD induction consistent with the pivotal role played by $Ca_V2.1$ channels, NMDA receptors, and extracellular K^+ concentration is shown in Figure 5.2. In this scheme, the local buildup of K^+ above a critical value depolarizes presynaptic terminals and activates $Ca_V2.1$ channels, and also depolarizes postsynaptic membranes and reduces the Mg^{2+} block of NMDA receptors. Excessive $Ca_V2.1$-dependent release of glutamate from synaptic terminals depolarized by high K^+ and consequent activation of NMDA receptors leads to further depolarization of the postsynaptic membrane, further

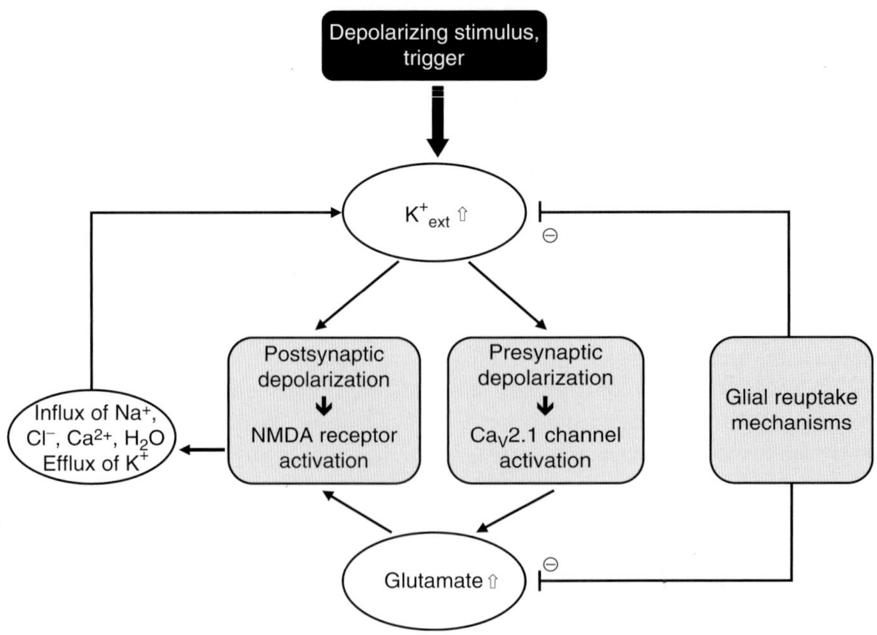

Fig. 5.2. Possible positive-feedback mechanism involved in initiation of cortical spreading depression. The mechanism is consistent with the evidence for a crucial role of $Ca_V2.1$ channels, *N*-methyl-D-aspartate (NMDA) receptors, and a local increase of the extracellular K^+ above a critical value in initiation of cortical spreading depression (CSD: see text). Gain-of-function mutations in $Ca_V2.1$ channels (familial hemiplegic migraine 1: FHM1) or $Na_V1.1$ channels (FHM3) and loss-of-function mutations in α_2 Na^+/K^+ ATPases (FHM2) may all render the brain more susceptible to CSD by causing either excessive synaptic glutamate release (FHM1) or excessive extracellular K^+ (FHM3), or decreased removal of K^+ and glutamate from the synaptic cleft (FHM2).

increase of K^+ in the extracellular space (which has narrowed, mainly as a consequence of swelling of astrocytes due to KCl uptake), further release of glutamate, further activation of the NMDA receptor, and so on (Pietrobon, 2005b). The normal brain has efficient regulatory mechanisms, among which the glial uptake mechanisms are particularly important, to keep the extracellular concentration of K^+ within the physiological range during neuronal activity. The CSD threshold is reached when the regulatory mechanisms that keep the local K^+ ion concentration in the physiological range are overwhelmed by the buildup of K^+ via positive-feedback loops (Figure 5.2). In FHM1 this might occur as a consequence of cortical hyperexcitability due to excessive release of glutamate secondary to increased Ca^{2+} influx through $Ca_V2.1$ channels. Enhanced susceptibility to CSD in FHM1 can be explained considering that, given the lowered voltage threshold for activation of mutant $Ca_V2.1$ channels, a lower increase of extracellular K^+ is necessary to activate synaptic $Ca_V2.1$ channels and to release enough glutamate to initiate the positive-feedback cycle leading to CSD. Thus, a relatively weak depolarizing stimulus, such as a minor head trauma, which is without consequences in healthy individuals, may be able to initiate CSD in FHM1 patients.

Whereas initiation of migraine pain depends on the activation and sensitization of meningeal nociceptors, its maintenance depends on self-sustained central sensitization of the trigeminovascular system (Pietrobon and Striessnig, 2003; Pietrobon, 2005b). Long-term potentiation of nociceptive synapses in the trigeminal nucleus caudalis and/or alterations of descending endogenous pain modulatory pathways appear as plausible hypothetical mechanisms of central sensitization (Knight and Goadsby, 2001; Pietrobon and Striessnig, 2003; Pietrobon, 2005b). There is evidence that $Ca_V2.1$ channels play an important role in central sensitization in the spinal cord (Vanegas and Schaible, 2000; Luvisetto et al., 2006) and that $Ca_V2.1$ channels located in the periaqueductal gray region and in the rostroventromedial medulla play a role in descending inhibitory and facilitatory pathways that regulate trigeminal and spinal pain (Knight et al., 2002; Urban et al., 2005). Moreover, $Ca_V2.1$ channels are involved in the control of neurotransmitter release from perivascular terminals of meningeal afferents and consequent neurogenic vasodilation (Akerman et al., 2003; Pietrobon and Striessnig, 2003). Thus, although the consequences of FHM1 mutations on trigeminal nociception remain unexplored, one may predict alterations that probably lead to hyperexcitability of the nociceptive trigeminovascular pathways in FHM1. This hypothesis can be investigated using the available FHM1 knockin mice.

Familial hemiplegic migraine type 2

The FHM2 gene *ATP1A2* encodes the α_2 subunit of Na^+/K^+ ATPase. Na^+/K^+ ATPase is a P-type type ion pump that utilizes the energy of adenosine triphosphate (ATP) to transport Na^+ ions out of and K^+ ions into the cell. It is usually composed of two subunits: a catalytic α subunit, which contains the binding sites for ATP and the cations, and a regulatory β subunit. The α subunit consists of ten membrane spanning segments; the large intracellular loop between segments 4 and 5 undergoes major conformational changes during the enzymatic cycle and contains the nucleotide-binding domain and the phosphorylation site (Jorgensen et al., 2003) (Figure 5.3). The Na^+/K^+ ATPase generates the ion gradients that maintain both the resting membrane potential and the cell volume and provide the driving force for nutrient and neurotransmitter uptake. Glial and neuronal Na^+/K^+ ATPases play an important role in clearance of K^+ from the extracellular space during neuronal activity and are fundamental also for the clearance of released glutamate from the synaptic cleft, since active transport of glutamate into astrocytes and neurons is driven by both Na^+ and K^+ gradients.

Four genes encoding Na^+/K^+ ATPase α subunits have been identified (Jorgensen et al., 2003). In contrast with the α_1 isoform, which maintains generalized cellular homeostasis of Na^+ and K^+ as a housekeeping role, the α_2 isoform plays more specific roles by colocalization with various ion transporters. In the murine brain, the α_2 Na^+/K^+ ATPase is expressed primarily in neurons during embryonic development and at the time of birth, and primarily in glial cells in the adult (Cholet et al., 2002; Moseley et al., 2003). Impaired clearance of neurotransmitters and enhanced neuronal excitation in the amygdala and pyriform cortex were shown in *Atp1a2*$^{-/-}$ mice at the embryonic stage (Ikeda et al., 2003). These mice die at birth because of lack of spontaneous respiratory activity due to functional impairment of the brainstem respiratory neurons, probably as a result of elevated intracellular [Cl^-], which would switch the GABA response from hyperpolarization to depolarization; the data suggest a specific coupling between the α_2 Na^+/K^+ ATPase and the neuron-specific K^+/Cl^- cotransporter, which excludes Cl^- ions from the cytosol in respiratory center neurons (Ikeda et al., 2004). A specific colocalization of the α_2 isoform of the Na^+/K^+ pump with the Na^+/Ca^{2+} exchanger in microdomains that overlie subplasmalemmal endoplasmic reticulum was demonstrated in cultured astrocytes, suggesting a specific functional role for this isoform also in the regulation of intracellular Ca^{2+}, particularly in the endoplasmic reticulum (Juhaszova and Blaustein, 1997). Indeed,

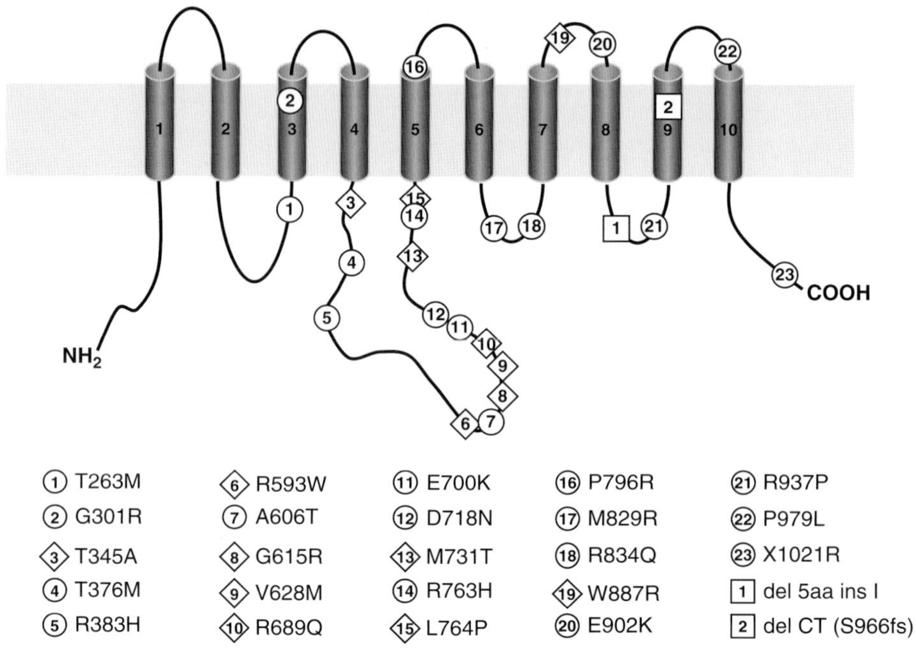

Fig. 5.3. Secondary structure of the Na^+/K^+ATPase α_2 subunit and location of the familial hemiplegic migraine 2 (FHM2) mutations identified so far. Diamonds: mutations whose functional consequences have been studied in heterologous expression systems.

elevated levels of intracellular Ca^{2+} ions as well as elevated stores of Ca^{2+} in the endoplasmic reticulum were measured in cultured astrocytes from *Atp1a2*$^{-/-}$ mice (Golovina et al., 2003). In the adult somatosensory cortex, the α_2 Na^+/K^+ ATPase isoform is located exclusively in glial cells and shows a localization virtually identical to that of the astrocytic glutamate transporters; at the ultrastructural level it appears preferentially localized in astrocytic processes around asymmetrical (glutamatergic) synaptic junctions, and not around GABAergic terminals (Cholet et al., 2002). The data are consistent with a specific functional coupling of the α_2 Na^+/K^+ ATPase with astrocytic glutamate transporters and a specific role in glutamate clearance by glial cells during neuronal activity in the adult cortex.

Twenty-three different missense mutations associated with FHM2 have been described, including the R383H sporadic mutation (Haan et al., 2005; Pierelli et al., 2006; Vanmolkot et al., 2006a, b) (Figure 5.3). All produce substitutions of conserved amino acids in important functional regions. Two additional mutations associated with FHM2 were deletions, one in-frame and one leading to a frameshift and a premature stop codon (Figure 5.3). The investigation of the functional consequences of eight FHM2 mutations in heterologous expression systems (Figure 5.3) has shown that these mutations lead to loss-of-function of Na^+/K^+ ATPase pump activity (De Fusco et al., 2003; Segall et al., 2004, 2005; Vanmolkot et al., 2006a, b). Three mutations (L764P, W887R, G615R) produced severe or complete loss-of-function of pump activity (De Fusco et al., 2003; Vanmolkot et al., 2006b). Among the milder loss-of-function mutants, the T345A had a lower affinity for extracellular K^+, which would slow removal of K^+ from the extracellular space and slow the recovery from neuronal excitation (Segall et al., 2004); the M731T and R689Q mutants had a decreased catalytic turnover and increased affinity for extracellular K^+, which would also slow extracellular K^+ clearance in the plausible hypothesis that the lower catalytic turnover overrides the effect of increased K^+ affinity, at least at high extracellular K^+ concentrations (Segall et al., 2005).

Impaired clearance of K^+ and glutamate by astrocytes during cortical neuronal activity, consequent to a decreased number of functional Na^+/K^+ ATPases or a decreased affinity for K^+ or a decreased catalytic turnover of the α_2 Na^+/K^+-ATPase pumps, would depolarize neurons and enhance glutamate concentration in the synaptic cleft, thus impairing recovery from neuronal excitation. Within the scheme in Figure 5.2, one may predict enhanced susceptibility to CSD in FHM2 considering that relatively weak depolarizing stimuli (which would be without consequences in healthy individuals whose efficient glial uptake mechanisms keep the concentration of K^+ within the physiological range) may be able to produce a local buildup of K^+

concentration above the critical value that ignites CSD in FHM2 patients with impaired K^+ and glutamate reuptake mechanisms. The generation of FHM2 knockin mice will allow testing of this prediction.

Familial hemiplegic migraine type 3

The FHM3 gene *SCN1A* encodes the α_1 subunit of the voltage-gated Na^+ channel $Na_V1.1$. $Na_V1.1$ channels are expressed primarily in the central nervous system in late postnatal stages; they are a relatively minor component of total brain Na^+ channels, but are broadly expressed in many types of neuron, including hippocampal and cortical pyramidal cells and inhibitory interneurons, where they appear specifically localized in the soma and proximal dendrites (Yu et al., 2006). The specific somatodendritic localization implies that $Na_V1.1$ channels may play a key role in mediating dendritic excitability, an important component of synaptic signal processing. Deletion of the $Na_V1.1\alpha_1$ gene had no discernible effect on Na^+ currents in hippocampal pyramidal neurons of *Scn1a*$^{-/-}$ mice, but led to 50% reduction of Na^+ currents in inhibitory interneurons of heterozygote *Scn1a*$^{-/+}$ mice; this finding suggests that $Na_V1.1$ channels may be responsible for most or all of the Na^+ current in these interneurons and for a minor fraction of the Na^+ current in pyramidal cells (Yu et al., 2006). GABAergic interneuron excitability was reduced in both *Scn1a*$^{-/-}$ and *Scn1a*$^{-/+}$ mice, a finding that might underlie the epileptic phenotype of these mice (Yu et al., 2006).

A single FHM3 mutation (Gln1489Lys), located in the cytoplasmic segment that links domain III and IV of the $Na_V1.1$ α_1 subunit, has been identified in three German families (Dichgans et al., 2005). The mutation causes accelerated recovery from fast inactivation of recombinant human $Na_V1.5$ channels expressed in tsA201 cells, an effect that is predicted to increase neuronal firing rates (Dichgans et al., 2005). Given the evidence that mutation of the same conserved residue may have different functional effects on different Na_V channels (Meisler and Kearney, 2005), it will be important to confirm this finding in human $Na_V1.1$ channels.

In a perhaps simplistic view, within the scheme in Figure 5.2 one may predict enhanced susceptibility to CSD in FHM3, considering that relatively weak depolarizing stimuli, which would be without consequences in healthy individuals, may produce excessive neuronal firing that might lead to increases in local concentrations of extracellular K^+ above the critical value that ignites CSD in FHM3 patients. The generation of FHM3 *Scn1a* knockin mice will allow testing of this prediction.

Implications for migraine mechanisms and treatment

A major, incompletely understood, issue in the neurobiology of migraine concerns the nature and mechanisms of the primary brain dysfunction that lead to activation and sensitization of the trigeminovascular system and the ensuing headache (Pietrobon and Striessnig, 2003; Pietrobon, 2005b). Much current evidence points to CSD (the phenomenon underlying migraine aura) as a key primary brain dysfunction that may initiate migraine pain, but this idea is still under debate, particularly in the case of migraine without aura (MO) (Goadsby, 2001; Pietrobon and Striessnig, 2003; Pietrobon, 2005b; Sanchez-Del-Rio et al., 2006). An alternative view considers migraine aura and headache as parallel rather than sequential processes and proposes that the primary cause of migraine headache is an episodic dysfunction in brainstem nuclei involved in the central control of nociception (May and Goadsby, 1999). The mechanisms that lead to CSD vulnerability and initiate migraine aura remain unknown. While altered cortical excitability in migraineurs has been well documented, whether the cortex is hypo- or hyperexcitable is still a matter of debate, although most of the consistent findings point to hyperexcitability (Ambrosini and Schoenen, 2003; Pietrobon and Striessnig, 2003; Welch, 2005). The mechanisms that underlie the cortical hyperexcitability and its periodicity remain unknown.

The functional studies of FHM just described support a key role for CSD in migraine pathogenesis. The available data suggest that, most likely, FHM1, FHM2, and FHM3 mutations share the ability of rendering the brain more susceptible to CSD, by causing either excessive synaptic glutamate release (FHM1) or decreased removal of K^+ and glutamate from the synaptic cleft (FHM2) or excessive extracellular K^+ (FHM3) (Figure 5.2). The remarkably overlapping headache phenotype produced by gain-of-function mutations in neuronal Ca^{2+} and Na^+ channels, and loss-of-function mutations in astrocytic Na^+/K^+ ATPases, favors the idea that CSD may initiate migraine attacks and that aura and migraine headache are causally related. The alternative possibility, that FHM1, FHM2, and FHM3 mutations alter in a similar manner trigeminovascular pain transmission and its central control, appears less likely and remains to be tested.

The FHM data point to ion transport dysfunction as a key factor in determining the brain susceptibility to CSD and to cortical hyperexcitability as the basis for vulnerability to CSD and to migraine attacks. Dysfunction of many other channels and transporters, beside $Ca_V2.1$ and $Na_V1.1$ channels and Na^+/K^+ ATPases, and also dysfunction of other proteins (e.g., involved in energy supply) may render the brain susceptible to CSD and migraine. The many different molecular mechanisms that can potentially underlie vulnerability to CSD are consistent with the large genetic variability and the complex genetics of migraine.

The FHM data support novel therapeutic strategies that consider CSD and cortical hyperexcitability as key targets of preventive migraine treatment. In this respect, it is very interesting that five migraine prophylactic drugs, belonging to distinct therapeutic classes (valproate, topiramate, amitriptyline, propranolol, and methysergide) and all effective in reducing attack frequency of both MO and MA, have the common property of inhibiting CSD susceptibility after protracted administration (Ayata et al., 2006). The need for protracted administration suggests that changes in gene expression underlie the therapeutic efficacy. In contrast, tonabersat (SB-220453), a benzopyran with anticonvulsant properties (currently in phase II clinical trial in the prevention of MA), was found to inhibit CSD after acute administration (Smith et al., 2000). The mechanisms by which these drugs inhibit CSD have not been demonstrated.

Further studies of the incompletely understood mechanisms of initiation and propagation of CSD, and of the changes in gene expression after chronic treatment with current prophylactic drugs, appear important for the development of novel preventive migraine treatment. Even though the FHM genes are probably not involved in common migraines, the study of the cellular mechanisms of enhanced susceptibility to CSD and enhanced cortical excitability in FHM knockin animal models may provide unique insights into possible molecular targets for therapeutic strategies aimed at inhibiting CSD susceptibility and cortical hyperexcitability in migraine. For example, the FHM1 functional studies suggest that drugs capable of shifting the activation range of $Ca_V2.1$ channels to more depolarized voltages would make the cortex more resistant to CSD, and may thus be able to prevent migraine attacks.

RECENT FINDINGS

After submission of this chapter, a few important novel findings regarding the functional consequences of FHM mutations have been published.

Tottene et al. (2009) investigated cortical neurotransmission both in neuronal microculture and in the context of functional neuronal circuits in brain slices from FHM1 knockin mice carrying the R192Q mutation, and revealed increased action potential evoked Ca^{2+} influx and glutamate release at cortical pyramidal cell synapses, but unaltered GABA release at fast-spiking interneuron synapses. These findings demonstrate that FHM1 mutations may differently affect synaptic transmission at different cortical synapses, and, as a consequence, very likely alter the neuronal circuits that dynamically adjust the balance between excitation and inhibition during cortical activity. Tottene et al. (2009) provided direct evidence of a causative link between gain-of-function of glutamate release at pyramidal cell synapses and facilitation of experimental CSD in FHM1 mutant mice. In fact, the facilitation of induction and propagation of experimental (K^+-induced) CSD observed in acute slices of somatosensory cortex of R192Q knockin mice was completely eliminated (both CSD threshold and velocity became similar to those in wt slices) when glutamate release at pyramidal cell synapses was brought back to wt values using subsaturating concentrations of a specific P/Q channel blocker. The synapse-specific effect of FHM1 mutations points to disruption of the balance between excitation and inhibition and consequent neuronal hyperactivity as the basis for episodic vulnerability to CSD ignition in migraine.

After confirming the facilitation of experimental CSD in FHM1 knockin mice *in vivo*, Eikermann-Haerter et al. (2009) investigated the neurological deficits in motor performance produced by one or more KCl-induced CSDs, and revealed more severe and prolonged neurological deficits in mutant than in wt mice, and in S218L than in R192Q knockin mice, in correlation with the severity of the clinical phenotype observed in FHM1 patients. Homozygous S218L mice also developed generalized seizures after a single CSD. Other interesting novel findings reported by Eikermann-Haerter et al. (2009) are: (1) the demonstration that CSD can propagate to the striatum in FHM1 but not in wt mice, suggesting that corticostriatal CSD propagation is the likely explanation for the motor deficits in FHM1; and (2) the modulation of CSD susceptibility in FHM1 knockin mice by female gonadal hormones, as shown by the larger facilitation of CSD in females than in males and the similar facilitation in old females or after ovariectomy of young females. As a whole, these findings further strengthen the link between CSD and migraine aura.

Weiss et al. (2008) and Serra et al. (2009) investigated the effect of FHM1 mutations on the G-protein-mediated inhibition of recombinant $CA_V2.1$ Ca^{2+} channels expressed in HEK293 cells, and found that both the S218L (Weiss et al., 2008) and the novel Y1245C mutation (Serra et al., 2009) reduce the G-protein-mediated channel inhibition, as previously shown by Melliti et al. (2003) for the R192Q mutation. Thus, in addition to activation at lower voltages, another common feature of mutant FHM1 $Ca_V2.1$ channels seems to be a reduced G-protein-mediated inhibition, which may lead to further gain-of-function of Ca^{2+} influx through mutant channels. If confirmed for native presynaptic $Ca_V2.1$ channels activated with physiological action potential stimuli, this feature of mutant channels may have important implications for the pathophysiology of FHM1.

At least another 33 novel FHM2 mutations have been identified (see Barrett et al., 2008, for review). Tavraz et al. (2008) investigated the functional consequences of 11 additional FHM2 mutations (in addition to those indicated in Figure 5.3), and found that all produce partial or complete loss of activity of the α_2 Na^+/K^+ ATPAse expressed in *Xenopus* oocytes. A broad range of functional abnormalities was observed in the mutant pumps that can be subdivided in two classes: (1) severe reduction or loss of catalytic activity or impairment of plasma membrane delivery; and (2) more subtle functional impairments, such as changes in apparent cation affinities, voltage dependence or kinetics, frequently occurring in parallel with a reduction in turnover number. These findings strongly support the general conclusion that FHM2 mutations lead to impairment of α_2 Na^+/K^+ ATPAse function under physiological conditions.

Cestele et al. (2008) and Kahlig et al. (2008) investigated for the first time the functional consequences of the Q1489K FHM3 mutation on recombinant human $Na_V1.1$ Na^+ channels, and revealed more complex effects than those previously reported for recombinant $Na_V1.5$ channels. The findings of the two studies support conflicting conclusions regarding the overall effect of the FHM3 mutation: a predominant gain-of-function leading to an enhanced capacity of the Na^+ channel to sustain high-frequency neuronal discharge (as shown by a decreased inactivation of the mutant Na^+ current during trains of action potentials at high frequency, and a higher frequency of action potentials recorded in cortical neurons overexpressing the mutant Na^+ channel) in Cestele et al. (2008); in contrast, a predominant loss-of-function leading to a diminished capacity to sustain high-frequency neuronal discharge (as shown by an increased inactivation of the mutant Na^+ current during trains of action potentials at high frequency) in Kahlig et al. (2008). Moreover, in the latter study, the functional consequences on recombinant human $Na_V1.1$ channels of two novel FHM3 mutations were studied: L1649Q, in S4 segment of domain IV, and L263V, in S5 segment of domain I. Gain- or loss-of-function effects, depending on the mutation, were found: in fact, L263V mutant Na^+ channels were inactivated less than wt channels during high-frequency trains of action potentials, whereas trafficking to the membrane of L1649 mutant channels was impaired (with consequent lack of significant Na^+ current in the transfected HEK293 cells). These conflicting data are difficult to reconcile with a common pathogenic mechanism, and experiments on cortical neurons of FHM3 knockin mice appear necessary to shed light on FHM3 mechanisms.

Acknowledgments

I acknowledge support from Telethon-Italy (GGP06234), the Italian Ministry of University and Research (Prin2005, FIRB2002), and the European Community (EUROHEAD (LSHM-CT-2004-504837). I gratefully thank Dr. Angelita Tottene for preparing the figures.

References

Akerman S, Williamson DJ, Goadsby PJ (2003). Voltage-dependent calcium channels are involved in neurogenic dural vasodilatation via a presynaptic transmitter release mechanism. Br J Pharmacol 140: 558–566.

Ambrosini A, Schoenen J (2003). The electrophysiology of migraine. Curr Opin Neurol 16: 327–331.

Ashcroft FM (2000). Ion Channels and Disease. Academic Press, San Diego.

Ayata C, Shimizu-Sasamata M, Lo EH et al. (2000). Impaired neurotransmitter release and elevated threshold for cortical spreading depression in mice with mutations in the α_{1A} subunit of P/Q type calcium channels. Neuroscience 95: 639–645.

Ayata C, Jin H, Kudo C et al. (2006). Suppression of cortical spreading depression in migraine prophylaxis. Ann Neurol 59: 652–661.

Barrett CF, Van den maagdenberg AMJM, Frants RR et al. (2008). Familial hemiplegic migraine. Adv Genet 63: 57–83.

Bolay H, Reuter U, Dunn AK et al. (2002). Intrinsic brain activity triggers trigeminal meningeal afferents in a migraine model. Nat Med 8: 136–142.

Cannon SC (2006). Pathomechanisms in channelopathies of skeletal muscle and brain. Annu Rev Neurosci 29: 387–415.

Cestele S, Scalmani P, Rusconi R et al. (2008). Self-limited hyperexcitability: functional effect of a familial hemiplegic migraine mutation of the Na(v)1.1 (SCN1A) Na^+ channel. J Neurosci 28: 7273–7283.

Cholet N, Pellerin L, Magistretti PJ et al. (2002). Similar perisynaptic glial localization for the Na^+, K^+-ATPase alpha 2 subunit and the glutamate transporters GLAST and GLT-1 in the rat somatosensory cortex. Cereb Cortex 12: 515–525.

De Fusco M, Marconi R, Silvestri L et al. (2003). Haploinsufficiency of ATP1A2 encoding the Na^+/K^+ pump alpha2 subunit associated with familial hemiplegic migraine type 2. Nat Genet 33: 192–196.

Dichgans M, Freilinger T, Eckstein G et al. (2005). Mutation in the neuronal voltage-gated sodium channel SCN1A in familial hemiplegic migraine. Lancet 366: 371–377.

Eikermann-Haerter K, Dilekoz E, Kudo C et al. (2009). Genetic and hormonal factors modulate spreading depression and transient hemiparesis in mouse models of familial hemiplegic migraine type 1. J Clin Invest 119: 99–109.

Goadsby PJ (2001). Migraine, aura, and cortical spreading depression: why are we still talking about it? Ann Neurol 49: 4–6.

Golovina VA, Song H, James PF et al. (2003). Na^{+} pump alpha 2-subunit expression modulates Ca^{2+} signaling. Am J Physiol Cell Physiol 284: C475–C486.

Gursoy-Ozdemir Y, Qiu J, Matsuoka N et al. (2004). Cortical spreading depression activates and upregulates MMP-9. J Clin Invest 113: 1447–1455.

Haan J, Kors EE, Vanmolkot KR et al. (2005). Migraine genetics: an update. Curr Pain Headache Rep 9: 213–220.

Hille B (2001). Ionic Channels of Excitable Membranes. Sinauer Associates, Sunderland.

Ikeda K, Onaka T, Yamakado M et al. (2003). Degeneration of the amygdala/piriform cortex and enhanced fear/anxiety behaviors in sodium pump alpha2 subunit (Atp1a2)-deficient mice. J Neurosci 23: 4667–4676.

Ikeda K, Onimaru H, Yamada J et al. (2004). Malfunction of respiratory-related neuronal activity in Na^{+}, K^{+}-ATPase alpha2 subunit-deficient mice is attributable to abnormal Cl^{-} homeostasis in brainstem neurons. J Neurosci 24: 10693–10701.

Imbrici P, Jaffe SL, Eunson LH et al. (2004). Dysfunction of the brain calcium channel cav2.1 in absence epilepsy and episodic ataxia. Brain 127: 2682–2692.

Jorgensen PL, Hakansson KO, Karlish SJ (2003). Structure and mechanism of Na,K-ATPase: functional sites and their interactions. Annu Rev Physiol 65: 817–849.

Juhaszova M, Blaustein MP (1997). Na^{+} pump low and high ouabain affinity alpha subunit isoforms are differently distributed in cells. Proc Natl Acad Sci U S A 94: 1800–1805.

Kahlig KM, Rhodes TH, Pusch M et al. (2008). Divergent sodium channel defects in familial hemiplegic migraine. Proc Natl Acad Sci U S A 105: 9799–9804.

Kaja S, van de Ven RC, Broos LA et al. (2004). Increased transmitter release at neuromuscular synapses of a novel Cacna1a S218L knock-in mouse model for familial hemiplegic migraine. Society for Neuroscience 34th Annual Meeting, Abstract 593.4.

Kaja S, van de Ven RC, Broos LA et al. (2005). Gene dosage-dependent transmitter release changes at neuromuscular synapses of CACNA1A R192Q knockin mice are non-progressive and do not lead to morphological changes or muscle weakness. Neuroscience 135: 81–95.

Knight YE, Goadsby PJ (2001). The periaqueductal grey matter modulates trigeminovascular input: a role in migraine? Neuroscience 106: 793–800.

Knight YE, Bartsch T, Kaube H et al. (2002). P/Q-type calcium-channel blockade in the periaqueductal gray facilitates trigeminal nociception: a functional genetic link for migraine? J Neurosci 22: RC213.

Kors EE, Terwindt GM, Vermeulen FL et al. (2001). Delayed cerebral edema and fatal coma after minor head trauma: role of the CACNA1A calcium channel subunit gene and relationship with familial hemiplegic migraine. Ann Neurol 49: 753–760.

Luvisetto S, Marinelli S, Panasiti MS et al. (2006). Pain sensitivity in mice lacking the $ca_v2.1\alpha1$ subunit of P/Q-type Ca^{2+} channels. Neuroscience 142: 823–832.

Marrannes R, Willems R, De Prins E et al. (1988). Evidence for a role of the *N*-methyl-D-aspartate (NMDA) receptor in cortical spreading depression in the rat. Brain Res 457: 226–240.

May A, Goadsby PJ (1999). The trigeminovascular system in humans: pathophysiologic implications for primary headache syndromes of the neural influences on the cerebral circulation. J Cereb Blood Flow Metab 19: 115–127.

Meisler MH, Kearney JA (2005). Sodium channel mutations in epilepsy and other neurological disorders. J Clin Invest 115: 2010–2017.

Melliti K, Grabner M, Seabrook GR (2003). The familial hemiplegic migraine mutation R192Q reduces G-protein-mediated inhibition of P/Q-type (Ca(V)2.1) calcium channels expressed in human embryonic kidney cells. J Physiol 546: 337–347.

Moseley AE, Lieske SP, Wetzel RK et al. (2003). The Na, K-ATPase alpha 2 isoform is expressed in neurons, and its absence disrupts neuronal activity in newborn mice. J Biol Chem 278: 5317–5324.

Ophoff RA, Terwindt GM, Vergouwe MN et al. (1996). Familial hemiplegic migraine and episodic ataxia type-2 are caused by mutations in the Ca^{2+} channel gene CACNL1A4. Cell 87: 543–552.

Pierelli F, Grieco GS, Pauri F et al. (2006). A novel ATP1A2 mutation in a family with FHM type II. Cephalalgia 26: 324–328.

Pietrobon D (2002). Calcium channels and channelopathies of the central nervous system. Mol Neurobiol 25: 31–50.

Pietrobon D (2005a). Function and dysfunction of synaptic calcium channels: insights from mouse models. Curr Opin Neurobiol 15: 257–265.

Pietrobon D (2005b). Migraine: new molecular mechanisms. Neuroscientist 11: 373–386.

Pietrobon D, Striessnig J (2003). Neurobiology of migraine. Nat Rev Neurosci 4: 386–398.

Pizzorusso T, Shapovalova M, Gherardini L et al. (2006). Facilitation of neuronal $ca_v2.1$ channels and cortical spreading depression in knockin mice with mutation S218L causing familial hemiplegic migraine and coma after minor head trauma. Society for Neuroscience 36th Annual Meeting, Abstract 727.1.

Saegusa H, Wakamori M, Matsuda Y et al. (2006). Properties of human cav2.1 channel with a spinocerebellar ataxia type 6 muttaion expressed in Purkinje cells. Mol Cell Neurosci 34: 261–270.

Sanchez-Del-Rio M, Reuter U, Moskowitz MA (2006). New insights into migraine pathophysiology. Curr Opin Neurol 19: 294–298.

Segall L, Scanzano R, Kaunisto MA et al. (2004). Kinetic alterations due to a missense mutation in the Na,K-ATPase alpha2 subunit cause familial hemiplegic migraine type 2. J Biol Chem 279: 43692–43696.

Segall L, Mezzetti A, Scanzano R et al. (2005). Alterations in the alpha2 isoform of Na,K-ATPase associated with familial hemiplegic migraine type 2. Proc Natl Acad Sci U S A 102: 11106–11111.

Serra SA, Fernandez-Castillo N, Macaya A et al. (2009). The hemiplegic migraine-associated Y1245C mutation in CACNA1A results in a gain of channel function due to its effect on the voltage sensor and G-protein-mediated inhibition. Pfluegers Arch 458: 459–502.

Shapovalova M, Matiello S, Tottene A et al. (2004). Calcium channel ($ca_v2.1$) knock-in mice with a familial hemiplegic migraine mutation show an increased calcium current density in cortical pyramidal neurons. Society for Neuroscience 34th Annual Meeting, Abstract 848.9.

Smith MI, Read SJ, Chan WN et al. (2000). Repetitive cortical spreading depression in a gyrencephalic feline brain: inhibition by the novel benzoylamino-benzopyran SB-220453. Cephalalgia 20: 546–553.

Somjen GG (2001). Mechanisms of spreading depression and hypoxic spreading depression-like depolarization. Physiol Rev 81: 1065–1096.

Tavraz NN, Friedrich T, Durr KL et al. (2008). Diverse functional consequences of mutations in the Na^+/K^+-ATPase alpha(2)-subunit causing familial hemiplegic migraine type 2. J Biol Chem 283: 31097–31106.

Tottene A, Fellin T, Pagnutti S et al. (2002). Familial hemiplegic migraine mutations increase Ca^{2+} influx through single human $ca_v2.1$ channels and decrease maximal $ca_v2.1$ current density in neurons. Proc Natl Acad Sci U S A 99: 13284–13289.

Tottene A, Pivotto F, Fellin T et al. (2005a). Specific kinetic alterations of human $ca_v2.1$ calcium channels produced by mutation S218L causing familial hemiplegic migraine and delayed cerebral edema and coma after minor head trauma. J Biol Chem 280: 17678–17686.

Tottene A, Shapovalova M, Frants RR et al. (2005b). Gain-of-function of $ca_v2.1$ calcium channels leads to increased excitatory synaptic transmission in microcultures of cortical neurons from cacna1a knockin mice with the R192Q familial hemiplegic migraine mutation. Society for Neuroscience 35th Annual Meeting, Abstract 35.1.

Tottene A, Conti R, Fabbro A et al. (2009). Enhanced excitatory transmission at cortical synapses as the basis for facilitated spreading depression in Ca(v)2.1 knockin migraine mice. Neuron 61: 762–773.

Urban MO, Ren K, Sablad M et al. (2005). Medullary N-type and P/Q-type calcium channels contribute to neuropathy-induced allodynia. Neuroreport 16: 563–566.

van den Maagdenberg AM, Pietrobon D, Pizzorusso T et al. (2004). A Cacna1a knockin migraine mouse model with increased susceptibility to cortical spreading depression. Neuron 41: 701–710.

Vanegas H, Schaible H (2000). Effects of antagonists to high-threshold calcium channels upon spinal mechanisms of pain, hyperalgesia and allodynia. Pain 85: 9–18.

Vanmolkot KR, Kors EE, Turk U et al. (2006a). Two de novo mutations in the Na,K-ATPase gene ATP1A2 associated with pure familial hemiplegic migraine. Eur J Hum Genet 14: 555–560.

Vanmolkot KR, Stroink H, Koenderink JB et al. (2006b). Severe episodic neurological deficits and permanent mental retardation in a child with a novel FHM2 ATP1A2 mutation. Ann Neurol 59: 310–314.

Weiss N, Sandoval A, Felix R et al. (2008). The S218L familial hemiplegic migraine mutation promotes deinhibition of Ca(v)2.1 calcium channels during direct G-protein regulation. Pfluegers Arch 457: 315–326.

Welch KM (2005). Brain hyperexcitability: the basis for antiepileptic drugs in migraine prevention. Headache 45 (Suppl. 1): S25–S32.

Yu FH, Mantegazza M, Westenbroek RE et al. (2006). Reduced sodium current in gabaergic interneurons in a mouse model of severe myoclonic epilepsy in infancy. Nat Neurosci 9: 1142–1149.

Zhuchenko O, Bailey J, Bonnen P et al. (1997). Autosomal dominant cerebellar ataxia (SCA6) associated with small polyglutamine expansions in the α_{1A}-voltage-dependent calcium channel. Nat Genet 15: 62–69.

Handbook of Clinical Neurology, Vol. 97 (3rd series)
Headache
G. Nappi and M.A. Moskowitz, Editors

Chapter 6

Genetics of headaches

ARN M.J.M. VAN DEN MAAGDENBERG,[1,2] GISELA M. TERWINDT,[2] JOOST HAAN,[2,3]
RUNE R. FRANTS,[1] AND MICHEL D. FERRARI[2]*

[1]*Department of Human Genetics, Leiden University Medical Center, Leiden, The Netherlands*
[2]*Department of Neurology, Leiden University Medical Center, Leiden, The Netherlands*
[3]*Rijnland Hospital, Leiderdorp, The Netherlands*

INTRODUCTION

Advances in genetic research have increased our knowledge of primary headaches considerably. For migraine a genetic component was already well established, based on family and twin studies (Russell and Olesen, 1993). In the last decade several discoveries at molecular level have further established this genetic component (de Vries et al., 2006). Recently evidence for genetic susceptibility has also been obtained for cluster headache (CH) and tension-type headache (TTH) (Russell, 2001, 2004; Pinessi et al., 2005).

In this review, genetic discoveries in primary headache syndromes will be discussed. It will also be described how genetic insight has changed the view of the pathophysiology of primary headaches.

MIGRAINE

Genetic epidemiology

Many patients have first-degree relatives who also suffer from migraine (Russell and Olesen, 1993). Population-based family studies have shown that the familial risk of migraine is increased (Russell and Olesen, 1995; Stewart et al., 1997). A moderate ~1.5-fold increased migraine risk was reported for first-degree relatives associated with the severity of the disease (Stewart et al., 1997). Although the risk of migraine (without or with aura) was moderately increased for first-degree relatives when the proband had migraine without aura, the risk of suffering from migraine with aura was almost fourfold increased when the proband also had migraine with aura (Russell and Olesen, 1995).

Studies of twin pairs are the classical method of investigating the relative importance of genetic and environmental factors. Significantly increased pairwise concordance rate among monozygotic compared to dizygotic twin pairs drawn from the general population indicates that genetic factors are important in susceptibility to migraine (Hönkasalo et al., 1995; Gervil et al., 1999; Ulrich et al., 1999; Mulder et al., 2003). As the concordance rate in these studies did not reach 100%, environmental factors besides genetic factors must be involved as well. Therefore, migraine can be regarded as a multifactorial disorder. The relative importance of genetic factors was estimated in a large population-based twin study investigating 30 000 twin pairs with migraine (Mulder et al., 2003). The heritability estimate in this study was 40–50%. It was concluded that shared environmental factors seemed a minor factor in the susceptibility of migraine, which is in accordance with the results of earlier reports on the comparison of twins raised together and apart that did not provide evidence for a role of shared rearing environment (Ziegler et al., 1998; Svensson et al., 2003).

It has been suggested that migraine with and without aura should be seen as different diseases (Russell and Olesen, 1995). However, there are clinical observations that support the view that migraine with and without aura are variants of the same disorder, since: (1) the different types of migraine share identical headache symptoms; (2) both types of attack occur frequently in the same individual or family; and (3) there is often a remarkable development in disease presentation during life. A patient can have migraine with aura as a child, lose the aura as a young adult, and have

*Correspondence to: Professor Michel D Ferrari, MD PhD, Department of Neurology, Leiden University Medical Center, PO Box 9600, 2300 RC Leiden, The Netherlands, Tel: +31-71-5262895, Fax: +31-71-5248253, E-mail: M.D.Ferrari@lumc.nl

aura without headache after age 50 (Blau, 1995; Haan et al., 2007). Therefore, one would assume some migraine susceptibility genes to be shared by the different migraine types.

Recent so-called latent class analyses on migraine characteristics from the diagnostic criteria (Headache Classification Subcommittee of the International Headache Society, 2004), including unilateral location, pulsating quality, and nausea/vomiting, in two large populations from Australia and the Netherlands support the hypothesis that migraine with and without aura are clinical presentations of the same disorder (Nyholt et al., 2004; Ligthart et al., 2006). A Finnish study of over 200 migraine families suggested that there is a continuum from pure migraine with aura at one end of the spectrum to pure migraine without aura at the other end (Kallela et al., 2001).

Finding genes for monogenic and complex disorders: the migraine highway

Identifying genes for migraine is hampered by the fact that multiple genes with a low penetrance may contribute to disease susceptibility and that the phenotypic expression is modulated by endogenous and exogenous non-genetic factors. In addition, migraine is a very prevalent disorder and the onset of disease may be at a late age (Haan et al., 2007). The most complicating factor, however, is the absence of a reliable (clinical) biomarker as the diagnosis of migraine completely depends on the patient's disease history. Several approaches have been tried to identify migraine genes.

The most successful approach until now has been linkage analysis in families with rare monogenic subtypes of migraine (de Vries et al., 2006). In traditional gene hunting studies, linkage is performed (testing hundreds of genetic markers equally spread over the chromosomes and selecting those markers, and thereby the chromosomal localization, best segregating with the disease), followed by positional cloning and identification of the causative mutation. It is hypothesized that rare monogenic subtypes and common multifactorial types of migraine share common genes and related biochemical pathways for the trigger threshold and initiation mechanisms of attacks (Haan et al., 2005). Thus, the rare monogenic variant may serve as a genetic and/or functional model for the common complex forms. In the latter case, the functional changes caused by the causative gene mutations are more relevant than the genes themselves, as they might hint at shared pathogenic pathways. So far, three genes have been identified for familial hemiplegic migraine (FHM), which can be seen as a representative at one of the extremes of the migraine spectrum or "migraine highway."

Genetics of familial hemiplegic migraine

FHM is a rare, severe, monogenic subtype of migraine with aura, characterized by at least some degree of weakness (hemiparesis) during the aura (Whitty, 1986; Headache Classification Subcommittee of the International Headache Society, 2004; Black, 2006). The hemiparesis may last from minutes to several hours or even days. Patients are frequently initially misdiagnosed with epilepsy. Attacks of FHM may be triggered by mild head trauma. Apart from the hemiparesis, the headache and aura features of the FHM attack are identical to those of attacks of migraine with aura and migraine without aura. In addition to hemiplegic attacks, the majority of FHM patients also experience attacks of "normal" migraine with or without aura (Thomsen et al., 2003a, b). Thus, from a clinical point of view, FHM seems a representative of the migraine spectrum, and a valid model to study the common forms of migraine. Major clinical differences, apart from the hemiparesis, include that FHM in 20% of cases may also be associated with cerebellar ataxia and other neurological symptoms such as epilepsy, mental retardation, brain edema, and (fatal) coma (Haan et al., 2005; Black, 2006). Thus far, three genes for FHM have been published, but, based on linkage results in several families, there are more to come.

The FHM1 *CACNA1A* gene

The first gene identified for FHM was the *CACNA1A* gene on chromosome 19p13 (Ophoff et al., 1996). The FHM1 gene encodes the pore-forming α_{1A} subunit of $Ca_v2.1$ (P/Q type), voltage-gated, neuronal calcium channels. The main function of neuronal $Ca_v2.1$ calcium channels is to modulate release of neurotransmitters, at peripheral neuromuscular junctions as well as central synapses, mainly within the cerebellum, brainstem, and cerebral cortex (Catterall, 1998). Over 50 *CACNA1A* mutations have been associated with a wide range of clinical phenotypes (de Vries et al., 2006). These include pure forms of FHM (Ophoff et al., 1996), combinations of FHM with various degrees of cerebellar ataxia (Ophoff et al., 1996; Ducros et al., 2001), or fatal coma due to excessive cerebral edema (Kors et al., 2001). *CACNA1A* mutations also cause disorders not associated with hemiplegic migraine attacks, such as episodic ataxia type 2 (Ophoff et al., 1996), progressive ataxia (Yue et al., 1997), spinocerebellar ataxia type 6 (Zhuchenko et al., 1997), and various forms of epilepsy (Jouvenceau et al., 2001; Imbrici et al., 2004). FHM is caused only by missense mutations, T666M and R583Q being the most prevalent ones (Ducros et al., 2001; Kors et al., 2003). Patients with *CACNA1A* mutations can have exclusively attacks of migraine with aura without hemiparesis, confirming that FHM mutations may also be implicated in multifactorial migraine.

The FHM2 *ATP1A2* gene

The FHM2 *ATP1A2* gene on chromosome 1q23 encodes the α_2 subunit of a Na^+/K^+ ATPase pump (De Fusco et al., 2003). This catalytic subunit binds Na^+, K^+, and ATP, and utilizes ATP hydrolysis to exchange Na^+ ions out of the cell for K^+ ions into the cell. Na^+ pumping provides the steep Na^+ gradient essential for the transport of glutamate and Ca^{2+}. *ATP1A2* is predominantly expressed in neurons in neonates and in glial cells in adults (Moseley et al., 2003). In adults, an important function of this specific ATPase is to modulate the reuptake of potassium and glutamate from the synaptic cleft into the glial cell. Mutations in the *ATP1A2* gene have been associated with pure FHM (De Fusco et al., 2003; Riant et al., 2005; Vanmolkot et al., 2006) and FHM in combination with cerebellar ataxia (Spadaro et al., 2004), alternating hemiplegia of childhood (Bassi et al., 2004; Swoboda et al., 2004), and benign focal infantile convulsions (Vanmolkot et al., 2003). In one family an *ATP1A2* gene mutation segregated with basilar-type migraine (Ambrosini et al., 2005), a subtype of migraine with aura characterized by aura symptoms attributable to the brainstem and both occipital lobes. In two non-FHM migraine families, *ATP1A2* variants were identified, suggesting that this gene may also be involved in the susceptibility to common forms of migraine (Todt et al., 2006).

The FHM3 *SCNA1* gene

The *SCNA1* gene on chromosome 2q24 encodes the α_1 subunit of neuronal voltage-gated sodium ($Na_v1.1$) channels. $Na_v1.1$ channels play an important role in the generation and propagation of action potentials. Over 100 mutations in this gene have been associated with childhood epilepsy and febrile seizures (Meisler and Kearney, 2005). Migraine has not been reported in these patients.

A Q1489K mutation was identified in three German FHM families (Dichgans et al., 2005). The three families share a common haplotype, suggesting common ancestry. Recently, an L1649Q mutation was found in a North American FHM family (Vanmolkot et al., 2007), independently confirming the relationship between *SCNA1* and FHM3. Mutation scanning of a large number of other FHM families suggested that the *SCN1A* gene is a rare cause of FHM (Dichgans et al., 2005; Thomsen et al., 2007).

Population-based study of FHM mutations

In a large Danish population-based study, 44 FHM families were identified (Thomsen et al., 2007). In three of the families a *CACNA1A* mutation was found, among which was one novel one (C1369Y). Three families had an *ATP1A2* mutation (V138A, R202Q, R763C), all of which were novel. None of the families were linked to the *SCN1A* locus or had a Q1489K mutation. The results of this study are interesting for several reasons. First, it shows that by using a population-based approach many FHM families can be identified. It must be stressed, however, that the majority of families identified were very small, consisting of two or three individuals each. Importantly, mutation-negative families had fewer affected members than those with an identified mutation, which could point to other than genetic factors in those small families (Low and Singleton, 2007). Second, in the majority of FHM families the disease is apparently not caused by a mutation in one of the known genes. Only in six of the 44 families was a *CACNA1A* or *ATP1A2* mutation found. So, there must be at least a fourth gene with a major contribution to the FHM phenotype, or a large number of additional genes with a smaller contribution. Third, the contribution of *CACNA1A* and *ATP1A2* is almost equal in this population, but the *SCN1A* gene seems to be of minor importance.

Sporadic hemiplegic migraine (SHM)

Hemiplegic migraine patients are not always clustered in families (Terwindt et al., 2002; Black, 2006). In fact, sporadic patients (without affected family members) are quite frequent and sometimes represent the first "FHM patient" (for instance, in cases with a *de novo* mutation) in a family (Vahedi et al., 2000; Thomsen et al., 2003a; Vanmolkot et al., 2006). SHM patients have a greatly increased risk of also suffering from typical migraine with aura, and their first-degree relatives have a greatly increased risk of migraine both with and without aura (Thomsen et al., 2003b). Thus, SHM is also clearly a part of the (genetic) migraine highway. In a study of the *CACNA1A* gene in SHM patients, only 2 of 27 patients carried a mutation (Terwindt et al., 2002). The genetic relationship between FHM and SHM has not been fully established yet.

Functional consequences of FHM gene mutations

Understanding the functional consequences of gene mutations is crucial to an understanding of the disease pathways. For the FHM genes, functional consequences of mutations have been studied in cellular models, in transgenic knockin mouse models carrying a human pathogenic mutation (FHM1), or in knockout mouse models (FHM2).

Cellular models for FHM1 *CACNA1A* mutations

Several FHM1 and episodic ataxia type 2 (EA2) mutations have been analyzed with electrophysiological techniques in neuronal and non-neuronal cell models (Kraus et al., 1998, 2000; Hans et al., 1999; Jouvenceau et al., 2001; Tottene et al., 2002, 2005; Cao et al., 2004; Imbrici et al., 2004). While EA2 *CACNA1A* mutations all show a dramatic decrease or even complete loss of current density (Guida et al., 2001; Jen et al., 2001; Jouvenceau et al., 2001; Wappl et al., 2002; Imbrici et al., 2004; Spacey et al., 2004; Wan et al., 2005; Jeng et al., 2006), FHM1 mutations cause different effects on channel conductance, kinetics, and/or expression in transfected cells (Kraus et al., 1998, 2000; Hans et al., 1999; Tottene et al., 2002, 2005; Cao et al., 2004). However, the consistent change found with FHM1 mutations, when tested in single-channel configuration, was a hyperpolarizing shift of about 10 mV of the activation voltage (Hans et al., 1999; Tottene et al., 2002, 2005). There are indications that the overall change in calcium influx may vary during high neuronal activity. For instance, mutant $Ca_v2.1$ channels can switch from low conductance mode to the wild-type state (for mutant T666M and V714A) or can accumulate in an inactive state (for mutant R583Q and D715E) during repetitive stimulation, which could contribute to the paroxysmal presentation of clinical symptoms (Hans et al., 1999; Kraus et al., 2000).

Observed gain-of-function effects of single channels in theory lead to an easier opening of channels in neurons. From transfected neurons one cannot reliably predict the consequence on calcium influx. For instance, evidence for reduced calcium influx at the whole-cell level has been reported in transfected, cultured, mouse hippocampal neurons (Cao et al., 2004). The *in vivo* consequences, however, are determined by a delicate interplay between the functional effects of a particular mutation, the different channel properties and density, the different auxiliary channel subunits, the different splice forms of the channel subunits, and the direct and indirect cellular environment. It seems, therefore, more appropriate to study the functional consequences of gene mutations in knockin mouse models carrying human pathogenic mutations.

Natural and knockout *CACNA1A* mouse mutants

Naturally occurring mouse mutants with *Cacna1a* missense mutations (*tottering*, *rocker*, *rolling Nagoya*) or *Cacna1a* truncation mutations (*Leaner*) display different combinations and severities of various types of epilepsy and ataxia (Pietrobon, 2005). A reduction in calcium current density appears to be the main effect of these mutated $Ca_v2.1$ channels (Dove et al., 1998; Lorenzon et al., 1998; Wakamori et al., 1998; Mori et al., 2000), accompanied by a change in channel kinetics for the *leaner* and *rolling Nagoya* mutants (Dove et al., 1998; Lorenzon et al., 1998; Mori et al., 2000).

Three *Cacna1a*-null (knockout) mouse models were generated, showing ataxia, dystonia, and lethality at a young age (Jun et al., 1999; Fletcher et al., 2001; Kaja et al., 2007). Loss of $Ca_v2.1$ channels resulted in reduced total Ca^{2+} influx in cerebellar cells and reduced neurotransmission at the neuromuscular junction (Urbano et al., 2003; Kaja et al., 2007) or unchanged level of neurotransmission in hippocampal neurons (Jun et al., 1999) with partly or complete compensation, respectively, by N- ($Ca_v2.2$), R- ($Ca_v2.3$) and/or L- (Ca_v1) type calcium channels. Moreover, *Leaner* mice showed an increased threshold for cortical spreading depression (CSD) – the phenomenon that explains the migraine aura (see below) – and reduced release of cortical glutamate (Ayata et al., 2000) and reduced transmitter release at the neuromuscular junction (Kaja et al., 2007).

FHM1 *CACNA1A* knockin mouse model

Unlike the natural *Cacna1a* mutant mouse models, transgenic knock-in mice carrying the human FHM1 R192Q mutation exhibit no overt clinical phenotype or structural abnormalities (van den Maagdenberg et al., 2004). This is very similar to the human situation: the R192Q mutation causes only mild FHM attacks, very similar to the common forms of migraine, albeit with hemiparesis, without permanent (interictal) neurological signs. Extensive functional analysis revealed consistent multiple gain-of-function effects: increased Ca^{2+} influx in cerebellar neurons, increased release of neurotransmitters at the neuromuscular junction (both spontaneous release and release upon stimulation in low Ca^{2+}), and a reduced trigger threshold for CSD that propagates with increased velocity. It seems that whole-animal studies may be better suited to dissect the effects of mutations and to understand the integrated physiology of the disease.

Cellular models for FHM2 *ATP1A2* mutations

Over 20 mutations in the *ATP1A2* gene have been associated with FHM, but only a few have been tested for their functional consequences at the molecular level. Mutations L764P and W887R resulted in non-functional proteins (Capendeguy and Horisberger, 2004; Koenderink et al., 2005), whereas other mutants showed partially active pumps with decreased (mutant T345M) or increased (mutants R689Q and M731T) K^+ affinities or reduced turnover rates (mutants R689Q and M731T) (Segall et al., 2004, 2005). Apparently FHM2 mutations have diverse functional consequences, but all seem to result in loss or diminished function of the sodium/potassium pump and thus predict reduced uptake of K^+ and glutamate into glial cells.

Atp1a2 knockout mouse models

Atp1a2-null mice that lack the α_2 subunit have a very severe phenotype and die immediately after birth because of their inability to start breathing (James et al., 1999; Ikeda et al., 2004). *Atp1a2*-null fetuses revealed selective neuronal apoptosis in the amygdala and piriform cortex in response to neural hyperactivity. When kept on a 129/Sv genetic background *Atp1a2*-null mice died within 24 h of birth after frequent generalized seizures. Remarkably, epilepsy has also been reported in several human *ATP1A2* mutation carriers. In contrast, heterozygous *Atp1a2*± mice are viable, but show several phenotypes, including a cardiac phenotype. Their heart shows a hypercontractile state with positive inotropic response and resembles what is typically seen after the administration of cardiac glycosides (James et al., 1999). In addition, heterozygous animals display enhanced fear and anxiety behaviors after conditioned fear stimuli, probably related to neuronal hyperactivity in the amygdala and piriform cortex (Ikeda et al., 2003). At present, it is not known whether the heterozygous *Atp1a2* mice may be valid models for FHM2. No *Atp1a2* knockin models have been reported.

Cellular models for the FHM3 *SCN1A* mutations

The Q1489K (Dichgans et al., 2005) and L1649Q *SCN1A* (Vanmolkot et al., 2007) mutations have been studied for their functional effects in tsA201 cells using the highly homologous SCN5A channel. Although located in very different domains, both mutations interfere with fast inactivation of the channel. Mutation Q1489K is located in the cytoplasmic linker between domains III and IV, which is critical for fast inactivation, whereas L1649Q localizes to S4 segment of domain 4, a domain that acts as a voltage sensor and is implicated in channel gating. Q1489K causes a two- to fourfold quicker recovery from fast inactivation (Dichgans et al., 2005), whereas L1649Q results in an overall slower inactivation of the channel: a depolarizing shift by ~10 mV in the voltage dependence of steady-state inactivation and an accelerated recovery from fast inactivation. These findings still await confirmation using the original SCN1A channel, but suggest a gain-of-function mechanism in FHM3 with predicted enhanced neuronal excitability and release of neurotransmitters.

Scn1a knockout mouse model

Homozygous *Scn1a*-null mice developed ataxia and died on postnatal day 15 (Yu et al., 2007). Heterozygous *Scn1a*± mice had spontaneous seizures and sporadic deaths beginning after P21. Electrophysiological analysis revealed that reduced sodium currents in GABAergic inhibitory interneurons in these mice may cause hyperexcitability, which may explain the epileptic phenotype in severe myoclonic epilepsy of infancy. No knockin mouse model for FHM3 has been reported.

Pathophysiology of migraine and its molecular basis

Cortical spreading depression in experimental animals

It is now well accepted that the migraine aura is neurally driven and most likely caused by the human equivalent of the CSD of Leão (Lauritzen, 1994). In experimental animals, CSD is a wave of neuronal and glial cell depolarization membranes that slowly spreads over the brain cortex at a rate of 2–5 mm/min and is accompanied by massive fluxes of ions (Ca^{2+}, Na^+, and K^+) followed by a longer-lasting inhibition of spontaneous and evoked neuronal activity. In experimental animals, the electrophysiological changes are associated with sequences of increased and decreased changes in cerebral blood flow (CBF). CSD appears to be a self-defense mechanism of the brain to strong stimuli and can be triggered by electrical stimulation of brain tissue, cortical trauma, cerebral ischemia, or cortical application of high concentrations of K^+ or neuroexcitatory amino acids such as glutamate (for review on CSD, see Somjen 2001).

CSD and the migraine aura

Clinical evidence supports the view that CSD is the likely basis of migraine aura. For instance, there is a good correlation of the speed of spreading of visual aura symptoms over the visual field and the propagation rate of CSD in experimental animals. The positive (e.g., scintillations, paresthesias) and negative (e.g., scotomata, paresis) phenomena of the migraine aura can be well explained by the initial transient hyperexcitation front of CSD followed by neuronal depression. Most importantly, blood oxygen level-dependent (BOLD) functional neuroimaging studies in humans have convincingly demonstrated that cerebral blood flow changes that occur during migraine aura are very similar to those observed in experimental animals during CSD (Hadjikhani et al., 2001).

Can CSD trigger the mechanisms for the headache phase?

Although CSD can explain the migraine aura, it is still controversial whether CSD can also initiate the migraine headache cascade through activation of the trigeminovascular system. Experimental evidence in rats indicated that induction of CSD was able to activate the ipsilateral trigeminal nucleus caudalis neurons, resulting in a long-lasting blood flow increase in the rat middle meningeal artery, and leakage of dural plasma protein, that can be inhibited by section of the ipsilateral trigeminal nerve (Bolay et al., 2002). An important role for CSD in migraine pathology comes from experimental evidence in rats that chronic daily, but not acute, administration of migraine prophylactic drugs, dose- and duration-dependently suppressed KCl-induced CSD frequency by 40–80%, and increased the triggering threshold for inducing CSD (Ayata et al., 2006).

Despite the experimental animal data in favor of a role for CSD in triggering the headache, the main clinical arguments against the hypothesis are that only a minority of migraine patients experience auras, headache may occur at the same side of the aura (instead of the opposite side, as expected if CSD had triggered the trigeminovascular system), aura can occur after the headache has started, and medication that aborts the aura (ketamine) does not affect the headache. Therefore, the exact role of CSD in triggering migraine headache mechanisms in humans remains unclear and needs further investigation.

A mechanism for triggering FHM attacks: evidence from genetic findings

How can we integrate *CACNA1A*, *ATP1A2,* and *SCN1A* into one (final) common pathway? As described above, CSD is an obvious candidate (Moskowitz et al., 2004). Mutant $Ca_v2.1$ calcium channels in autaptic cortical neurons isolated from FHM1 R192Q knockin mice cause increased glutamate release, which can induce, maintain, and propagate CSD. FHM2 mutations in the sodium/potassium pump predict *in vivo* reduced glial uptake of K^+ and glutamate from the synaptic cleft. FHM3 mutations in the $Na_v1.1$ sodium channel predict *in vivo* hyperexcitability and most likely enhanced neurotransmitter release. The consequence for FHM1, FHM2, and FHM3 is increased levels of glutamate and K^+ in the synaptic cleft causing an increased propensity for CSD. The propensity for CSD could well explain the aura phase of migraine attacks. As discussed above, it remains to be established whether the enhanced tendency for CSD might also be responsible for triggering the headache phase. Also, the mechanisms triggering FHM attacks are still poorly understood. This is one of the areas where transgenic mouse models might be exceptionally valuable. The identification of additional FHM genes will likely provide further insight.

Mutation in glutamate transporter supports a central role for glutamate in migraine

Additional support for a central role of glutamate in migraine came from an observation by Jen et al. (2005) that a heterozygous, *de novo*, P290R mutation in the *SLC1A3* gene resulted in a complex phenotype of episodic ataxia, hemiplegic migraine, and seizures in a 10-year-old boy. *SLC1A3* encodes the excitatory amino acid transporter (EAAT)1, which removes glutamate from the synaptic cleft. Mutation P290R caused a dramatic loss in glutamate uptake in a cellular assay. Dysfunction of glutamate transport from the synaptic cleft was also predicted for the FHM genes. Clearly, confirmation of this initial finding is needed with additional patients with EAAT1 mutations.

Migraine associated with other monogenic diseases

CADASIL

Cerebral autosomal-dominant arteriopathy with subcortical infarcts and leukoencephalopathy (CADASIL) is a non-amyloid arteriopathy caused by mutations in the *NOTCH3* gene (Joutel et al., 1996; Dichgans, 2007). The syndrome is characterized by recurrent subcortical infarcts, progressive white-matter lesions, accumulating cognitive deficits, and stroke-related disability. Most relevant here, up to 40% of mutation carriers have migraine with aura (Chabriat et al., 1995; Dichgans et al., 1998). Migraine is even among the main presenting symptoms. The *NOTCH3* gene is primarily expressed in vascular smooth-muscle cells and regulates arterial differentiation during embryonic development (Domenga et al., 2004). Why mutations in this gene would cause migraine is unclear. There is no evidence for a primary neuronal effect. However, it might be that secondary neuronal damage and ischemia facilitate the occurrence of CSD and migraine attacks. The high prevalence of aura symptoms would agree with this concept. Alternatively, there might be a primary vascular mechanism. Hemodynamic studies in transgenic mice have demonstrated an abnormal vasomotor response and disturbed autoregulation, and similar findings have been obtained in humans (Pfefferkorn et al., 2001; Lacombe et al., 2005). Studying neuronal and vascular changes in parallel in CADASIL transgenic animals may prove invaluable in dissecting the triggering mechanisms for migraine attacks.

Migraine and other cerebral angiopathies

A rare syndrome, hereditary cerebrovasculopathy, clinically characterized by a combination of cerebroretinal vasculopathy, Raynaud phenomenon, pseudotumor cerebri, and variable other forms of vascular dysfunction, has been described (Terwindt et al., 1998; Dichgans, 2007). Migraine is part of the syndrome (Hottenga et al., 2005). The disease was linked to chromosome 3p21 (Ophoff et al., 2001). Identification of the hereditary cerebrovasculopathy gene might shed light on the pathogenesis of a wide range of vascular disorders, including migraine.

An increased prevalence of migraine, in particular migraine with aura, has further been reported in another rare angiopathy that is associated with porencephaly, infantile hemiparesis, and stroke (Vahedi et al., 2003). *COL4A1*, which encodes type IV collagen, an integral component of the vascular basement membrane, has recently been identified as the causal gene (Gould et al., 2006). The association between migraine and several early-onset cerebral angiopathies is remarkable, but the mechanisms underlying this association are still poorly understood (Dichgans, 2007).

A large pedigree has been described in which patients suffer from familial aortic dissection and several other blood vessel abnormalities (Law et al., 2006). Many patients (10 of 14) carrying the causative mutation (R460H in the transforming growth factor β receptor 2 gene) also suffered from migraine.

Gene loci and genes implicated in multifactorial forms of migraine

Unlike the successes with the monogenic subtypes of migraine, there are only a few genetic breakthroughs for the multifactorial subtypes of migraine. Many studies applied affected sib-pair analysis. Using this linkage approach, chromosomal areas are identified that are shared by affected siblings with a probability greater than by chance alone. For individual genes in the area of linkage, case–control association studies need to be performed to identify the causative gene. In association studies candidate genes are tested by identifying those single nucleotide polymorphisms that statistically differ in allele frequency between cases and controls and that explain increased susceptibility to the disease.

An alternative, hypothesis-driven approach that is often used involves direct testing of prominent candidate genes in case–control association studies (i.e., without prior linkage studies, but using knowledge of the gene product). Recent technical advances have made it feasible to perform non-hypothesis-driven testing for genomewide association by scanning hundreds of thousands of single-nucleotide polymorphisms in extended and clinically homogenous populations (Hirschhorn and Daly, 2005), but such studies have not been reported for migraine.

Until now, despite huge efforts, no (definite) migraine genes have been identified for linkage studies in multifactorial migraine. Of all the significant findings in hypothesis-driven association studies, only a few have been replicated, which is considered a gold standard for this approach.

Linkage studies

Genomewide linkage studies have identified several gene regions with significant or suggestive linkage for non-hemiplegic migraine; linkage to chromosomes 6p12 and 4q24 has been replicated in independent samples. Linkage to chromosome 6p12.2–p21.1 in a large Swedish family with migraine with and without aura (Carlsson et al., 2002) was confirmed in Australian patients (Nyholt et al., 2005), albeit with low statistical evidence for linkage. Linkage to 4q24 in 50 Finnish families with migraine with aura (Wessman et al., 2002) was confirmed in a study in Icelandic patients with migraine without aura (Björnsson et al., 2003). Additional migraine loci have been mapped, but are (not yet) replicated (Table 6.1). The variety reported is probably a reflection of the genetic heterogeneity of migraine.

Linkage studies using quantitative trait and trait component analyses

Nyholt and colleagues (Lea et al., 2005a; Nyholt et al., 2005) performed a quantitative trait linkage analysis in about 800 independent sib pairs, selected from a large Australian sample of over 12 000 twins. By applying latent class analysis – a categorical analog of factor analysis for finding subtypes of related cases (latent classes) – they found significant linkage on chromosome 5q21 for a severe migraine phenotype with pulsating headache. Low evidence for linkage

Table 6.1

Gene loci for common forms of migraine

Phenotype	Sample	Method	Chromosomal region	Reference
Migraine with aura	50 families	Linkage (genomewide)	4q24	Wessman et al., 2002
	43 families	Linkage (genomewide)	11q24	Cader et al., 2003
	10 families	Linkage (candidate gene region)	15q11–13	Russo et al., 2005
Migraine without aura	1 family	Linkage (genomewide)	14q21.2–22.3	Soragna et al., 2003
	289 subjects	Linkage (genomewide)	4q21	Björnsson et al., 2003
Migraine with and without aura	2 families	Linkage (X-chromosomal)	Xq24–28	Nyholt et al., 1998
	1 family	Linkage (genomewide)	6p12.2–21.1	Carlsson et al., 2002
	83 families	Linkage (candidate gene region)	1q31	Lea et al., 2002
Migraine (special aspects)	92 families	Linkage (genomewide)	18p11*	Lea et al., 2005a
	790 sib pairs	Linkage (genomewide)	5q21†	Nyholt et al., 2005

*Severe form of migraine;
†Latent class analysis: linkage for "migrainous headache" phenotype.

was observed for specific headache characteristics; phonophobia (on chromosomes 1q21–q23 and 10), activity-prohibiting headache and photophobia (on chromosomes 6p12.2.–p21.1, 10, and 13), and nausea/vomiting (on chromosome 8).

A Finnish study used the individual clinical symptoms of migraine (trait component analysis) to determine affection status in genomewide linkage analyses of 50 migraine families (Anttila et al., 2006). The previously identified chromosome 4q24 locus (Wessman et al., 2002) was now found to link to several migraine traits. Their main findings were novel loci for pulsation on chromosome 17p13, an age at onset of migraine on chromosome 4q28, and a trait combination phenotype (full International Headache Society criteria) on chromosome 18q12. The use of symptoms of migraine rather than the full end diagnosis seems a promising novel approach to stratify samples for genetic studies.

For none of the chromosomal loci has the underlying gene been identified.

Association studies

In complex multifactorial disease, multiple genes likely interact with environmental factors while the effect sizes attributable to individual genetic variants are likely to be small. Finding such genes by using the classical linkage approach in family material with multifactorial forms of migraine may be difficult. Association-based methods are particularly suited because they are a powerful instrument to identify susceptibility genes with small relative risks. However, there are a number of important pitfalls when conducting such studies. Critical issues include the sample size, the definition of patients, adequate control samples, and, most importantly, replication in other populations. Many candidate gene association studies have investigated the relationship between migraine and genes for dopamine receptors and genes implicated in the metabolism and transportation of serotonin (Montagna et al., 2005). Until now no associations have been replicated convincingly. Those associations that have been replicated at least once are discussed in the next paragraph.

The enzyme 5,10-methylenetetrahydrofolate reductase (MTHFR) plays a role in maintaining homocysteine levels. An association between the C677T variant in the *MTHFR* gene and migraine with aura has been found in some (but not all) clinic-based (and therefore selected) study populations (Kowa et al., 2000; Kara et al., 2003; Todt et al., 2006) but also, and most importantly, in a large sample taken from the general population (Scher et al., 2006). This makes *MTHFR* the first migraine risk gene at the population level. The strength of association is enhanced in the presence of another *MTHFR* variant (A1298C) (Kara et al., 2003), and in combination with an angiotensin I-converting enzyme (ACE) DD/ID genotype (Lea et al., 2005b). If replicated, this would indicate the first gene–gene interaction to be involved in modulating the risk for migraine. As a note of caution, a recent, large, well conducted, Finnish study could not replicate an association with the *MTHFR* gene (Kaunisto et al., 2006).

Other replicated associations, but only in selected clinic-based samples, have included associations with: a progesterone receptor (PGR) Alu insertion in two independent populations (Colson et al., 2005); the estrogen receptor 1 (ESR1) in two independent populations for the G594A polymorphism (Colson et al., 2005), although Oterino and colleagues (2006) only found an association for the G325C polymorphism (threefold increased risk), but not for the G594A polymorphism; the tumor necrosis factor gene in two separate studies (Trabace et al., 2002; Rainero et al., 2004a); and variants in ACE (Paterna et al., 2000; Kowa et al., 2005; Lea et al., 2005b). Remarkably, in one study the ACE DD variant seemed to have a slightly protective effect against migraine in male patients (Lin et al., 2005). Also for ESR1 and PGR variants a synergistical effect increasing the risk for migraine has been observed (Colson et al., 2005).

CLUSTER HEADACHE

At first, CH was considered a sporadic disorder, but since the 1990s a familial occurrence has been increasingly recognized (Russell, 2004). Families were reported with three CH patients in three generations. In addition, monozygotic twin pairs with CH were described.

Family studies have shown an increased risk for CH in first- and second-degree family members of CH patients. In a clinical study among 370 Danish CH patients, Russell et al. (1995a) found a 14-fold increased risk for CH in first-degree family members of CH patients, and a twofold increased risk in second-degree family members. In a complex segregation analysis, it was found that the mode of inheritance was probably autosomal-dominant, with a higher penetrance in males (Russell et al., 1995b). These results, however, were not statistically significant. In a study of 220 Italian CH patients, 44 (20%) had a positive family history (Leone et al., 2001).

Candidate genes for CH should ideally explain all clinical features of CH, including the strictly unilateral pain, the autonomic features, and the paroxysmal occurrence. Furthermore, it should account for the periodicity and circadian rhythm of the attacks, the predominant occurrence in males, the incomplete penetrance, and the association with smoking. Obviously, a large number of possible genes can be brought up, including clock genes and genes involved in pain.

Only a few molecular genetic studies have been performed in CH thus far. A mitochondrial myopathy, encephalopathy, lactacidosis, and stroke-like episodes (MELAS) 3243-point mutation in platelet mitochondrial $tRNA^{Leu(UUR)}$ was reported in one CH patient, who had no family history of CH (Shimomura et al., 1994). After that, a patient was presented who had CH and familial chronic progressive external ophthalmoplegia, and multiple deletions of the mitochondrial DNA (Odawara et al., 1997). Both reports suggested an association of mtDNA abnormalities with CH. Subsequent studies could not confirm these findings in other patients with CH (Cortelli et al., 1995; Seibel et al., 1996). This is not very surprising as, from the reported pedigrees with multiple CH patients and our own data (see below), it is clear that an autosomal-dominant mode of inheritance (probably with a low penetrance) is more likely than maternal mitochondrial inheritance, as in several families transmission from father to offspring occurs.

The *CACNA1A* gene has been investigated in two studies in CH (Haan et al., 2001; Sjöstrand et al., 2001). Both studies were negative, indicating that the *CACNA1A* gene is unlikely to have a large impact on sporadic or familial CH. Likewise, association studies in CH with markers in nitric oxide synthase genes (Sjöstrand et al., 2001) and with the 3092 T→C clock gene (Rainero et al., 2005) were negative.

Recently, a significant association was found in Italian patients between hypocretin receptor 2 (*HCRTR2*) gene polymorphism G1246A and CH (Rainero et al., 2004b), which was replicated in a large German cohort of CH patients (Schürks et al., 2006), but not in another study (Baumber et al., 2006). Further studies are needed to confirm the involvement of the hypocretin receptor 2 gene or other genes in this chromosomal region. A recent genomewide linkage analysis in five Danish kindreds identified several chromosomal areas with weak evidence for linkage to CH (Baumber et al., 2006).

TENSION-TYPE HEADACHE

There is now also good evidence that genetic factors seem to be involved in TTH (Ulrich et al., 2004; Russell et al., 2006). In a large twin study of over 11 000 twin pairs from Denmark, both the "no tension-type headache" and the "frequent tension-type headache" phenotype were shown to have a genetic component, whereas "infrequent tension-type headache" seemed primarily caused by environmental factors. Data regarding "chronic tension-type headache" were inconclusive (Russell et al., 2006).

References

Ambrosini A, D'Onofrio M, Grieco GS et al. (2005). Familial basilar migraine associated with a new mutation in the ATP1A2 gene. Neurology 65: 1826–1828.

Anttila V, Kallela M, Oswell G et al. (2006). Trait components provide tools to dissect the genetic susceptibility of migraine. Am J Hum Genet 79: 85–99.

Ayata C, Shimizu-Sasamata M, Lo EH et al. (2000). Impaired neurotransmitter release and elevated threshold for cortical spreading depression in mice with mutations in the alpha 1A subunit of P/Q type calcium channels. Neuroscience 95: 639–645.

Ayata C, Jin H, Dalkara T et al. (2006). Suppression of cortical spreading depression in migraine prophylaxis. Ann Neurol 59: 652–661.

Bassi MT, Bresolin N, Tonelli A et al. (2004). A novel mutation in the ATP1A2 gene causes alternating hemiplegia of childhood. J Med Genet 41: 621–628.

Baumber L, Sjöstrand C, Leone M et al. (2006). A genome-wide scan and HCRTR2 candidate gene analysis in a European cluster headache cohort. Neurology 66: 1888–1893.

Björnsson A, Gudmundsson G, Gudfinnsson E et al. (2003). Localization of a gene for migraine without aura to chromosome 4q21. Am J Hum Genet 73: 986–993.

Black DF (2006). Sporadic and familial hemiplegic migraine: diagnosis and treatment. Semin Neurol 26: 208–216.

Blau JN (1995). Migraine with aura and migraine without aura are not different entities. Cephalalgia 15: 186–190.

Bolay H, Reuter U, Dunn AK et al. (2002). Intrinsic brain activity triggers trigeminal meningeal afferents in a migraine model. Nat Med 8: 136–142.

Cader ZM, Noble-Topham S, Dyment DA et al. (2003). Significant linkage to migraine with aura on chromosome 11q24. Human Mol Genet 12: 2511–2517.

Cao YQ, Piedras-Renteria ES, Smith GB et al. (2004). Presynaptic Ca^{2+} channels compete for channel type-preferring slots in altered neurotransmission arising from Ca^{2+} channelopathy. Neuron 43: 387–400.

Capendeguy O, Horisberger JD (2004). Functional effects of $Na^{+}K^{+}$-ATPase gene mutations linked to familial hemiplegic migraine. Neuromol Med 6: 105–116.

Carlsson A, Forsgren L, Nylander PO et al. (2002). Identification of a susceptibility locus for migraine with and without aura on 6p12.2-p21.1. Neurology 59: 1804–1807.

Catterall WA (1998). Structure and function of neuronal Ca^{2+} channels and their role in neurotransmitter release. Cell Calcium 24: 307–323.

Chabriat H, Tournier-Lasserve E, Vahedi K et al. (1995). Autosomal dominant migraine with MRI white-matter abnormalities mapping to the CADASIL locus. Neurology 45: 1086–1091.

Colson NJ, Lea RA, Quinlan S et al. (2005). Investigation of hormone receptor genes in migraine. Neurogenetics 6: 17–23.

Cortelli P, Zacchini A, Barboni P et al. (1995). Lack of association between mitochondrial tRNA(Leu(UUR)) point mutation and cluster headache. Lancet 345: 1120–1121.

De Fusco M, Marconi R, Silvestri L et al. (2003). Haploinsufficiency of ATP1A2 encoding the Na^{+}/K^{+} pump α_2 subunit associated with familial hemiplegic migraine type 2. Nat Genet 33: 192–196.

de Vries B, Haan J, Frants RR et al. (2006). Genetic biomarkers for migraine. Headache 46: 1059–1068.

Dichgans M (2007). Genetics of ischaemic stroke. Lancet Neurol 6: 149–161.

Dichgans M, Mayer M, Uttner I et al. (1998). The phenotypic spectrum of CADASIL: clinical findings in 102 cases. Ann Neurol 44: 735–739.

Dichgans M, Freilinger T, Eckstein G et al. (2005). Mutation in the neuronal voltage-gated sodium channel SCN1A causes familial hemiplegic migraine. Lancet 366: 371–377.

Domenga V, Fardoux P, Lacombe P et al. (2004). Notch3 is required for arterial identity and maturation of vascular smooth muscle cells. Genes Dev 18: 2730–2735.

Dove LS, Abbott LC, Griffit WH (1998). Whole-cell and single-channel analysis of P-type calcium currents in cerebellar Purkinje cells of *leaner* mutant mice. J Neurosci 18: 7687–7699.

Ducros A, Denier C, Joutel A et al. (2001). The clinical spectrum of familial hemiplegic migraine associated with mutations in a neuronal calcium channel. N Engl J Med 345: 17–24.

Fletcher CF, Tottene A, Lennon VA et al. (2001). Dystonia and cerebellar atrophy in CACNA1A null mice lacking P/Q calcium channel activity. FASEB J 15: 1288–1290.

Gervil M, Ulrich V, Kaprio J et al. (1999). The relative role of genetic and environmental factors in migraine without aura. Neurology 53: 995–999.

Gould DB, Phalan FC, van Mil SE et al. (2006). Role of COL4A1 in small-vessel disease and hemorrhagic stroke. N Engl J Med 354: 1489–1496.

Guida S, Trettel F, Pagnutti S et al. (2001). Complete loss of P/Q calcium channel activity caused by a CACNA1A missense mutation carried by patients with episodic ataxia type 2. Am J Hum Genet 68: 759–764.

Haan J, van Vliet JA, Kors EE et al. (2001). No involvement of the calcium channel gene (CACNA1A) in a family with cluster headache. Cephalalgia 21: 959–962.

Haan J, Kors EE, Vanmolkot KJ et al. (2005). Migraine genetics: an update. Curr Pain Head Rep 9: 213–220.

Haan J, Hollander J, Ferrari MD (2007). Migraine in the elderly: a review. Cephalalgia 27: 97–106.

Hadjikhani N, Sanchez del Rio M, Wu O et al. (2001). Mechanisms of migraine aura revealed by functional MRI in human visual cortex. Proc Natl Acad Sci U S A 98: 4687–4692.

Hans M, Luvisetto S, Williams ME et al. (1999). Functional consequences of mutations in the human alpha(1A) calcium channel subunit linked to familial hemiplegic migraine. J Neurosci 19: 1610–1619.

Headache Classification Subcommittee of the International Headache Society (2004). The international classification of headache disorders, 2nd edn. Cephalalgia 24: 1–160.

Hirschhorn JN, Daly MJ (2005). Genome-wide association studies for common diseases and complex traits. Nat Rev Genet 6: 95–108.

Hönkasalo M-L, Kaprio J, Winter T et al. (1995). Migraine and concomitant symptoms among 8167 adult twin pairs. Headache 35: 70–78.

Hottenga JJ, Vanmolkot KR, Kors EE et al. (2005). The 3p21.1-p21.3 hereditary vascular retinopathy locus increases the risk for Raynaud phenomenon and migraine. Cephalalgia 25: 1168–1172.

Ikeda K, Onaka T, Yamakado M et al. (2003). Degeneration of the amygdala/piriform cortex and enhanced fear/anxiety behaviors in sodium pump alpha2 subunit (Atp1a2)-deficient mice. J Neurosci 23: 4667–4676.

Ikeda K, Onimaru H, Yamada J et al. (2004). Malfunction of respiratory-related neuronal activity in Na^+ K^+-ATPase alpha2 subunit-deficient mice is attributable to abnormal Cl^- homeostasis in brainstem neurons. J Neurosci 24: 10693–10701.

Imbrici P, Jaffe SL, Eunson LH et al. (2004). Dysfunction of the brain calcium channel cav2.1 in absence epilepsy and episodic ataxia. Brain 127: 2682–2692.

James PF, Grupp IL, Grupp G et al. (1999). Identification of a specific role for the Na,K-ATPase alpha 2 isoform as a regulator of calcium in the heart. Mol Cell 3: 555–563.

Jen J, Wan J, Graves M et al. (2001). Loss-of-function EA2 mutations are associated with impaired neuromuscular transmission. Neurology 57: 1843–1848.

Jen JC, Wan J, Palos TP et al. (2005). Mutation in the glutamate transporter EAAT1 causes episodic ataxia hemiplegia and seizures. Neurology 65: 529–534.

Jeng CJ, Chen YT, Chen YW et al. (2006). Dominant-negative effects of human P/Q-type Ca^{2+} channel mutations associated with episodic ataxia type 2. Am J Physiol 290: 1209–1220.

Joutel A, Corpechot C, Ducros A et al. (1996). Notch3 mutations in CADASIL, a hereditary adult-onset condition causing stroke and dementia. Nature 383: 707–710.

Jouvenceau A, Eunson LH, Spauschus A et al. (2001). Human epilepsy associated with dysfunction of the brain P/Q-type calcium channel. Lancet 358: 801–807.

Jun K, Piedras-Renteria ES, Smith SM et al. (1999). Ablation of P/Q-type $Ca^{(2+)}$ channel currents altered synaptic transmission and progressive ataxia in mice lacking the alpha(1A)-subunit. Proc Natl Acad Sci U S A 96: 15245–15250.

Kaja S, van de Ven RC, Broos LA et al. (2007). Characterization of acetylcholine release and the compensatory contribution of non-Ca(v)2.1 channels at motor nerve terminals of *leaner* Ca(v)2.1-mutant mice. Neuroscience 144: 1278–1287.

Kallela M, Wessman M, Havanka H et al. (2001). Familial migraine with and without aura: clinical characteristics and co-occurrence. Eur J Neurol 8: 441–449.

Kara I, Sazci A, Ergul E et al. (2003). Association of the C677T and A1298C polymorphisms in the 510 methylenetetrahydrofolate reductase gene in patients with migraine risk. Mol Brain Res 111: 84–90.

Kaunisto MA, Kallela M, Hamalainen E et al. (2006). Testing of variants of the MTHFR and ESR1 genes in 1798 Finnish individuals fails to confirm the association with migraine with aura. Cephalalgia 26: 1462–1472.

Koenderink JB, Zifarelli G, Qiu LY et al. (2005). Na,K-ATPase mutations in familial hemiplegic migraine lead to functional inactivation. Biochim Biophys Acta 1669: 61–68.

Kors EE, Terwindt GM, Vermeulen FL et al. (2001). Delayed cerebral edema and fatal coma after minor head trauma: role of CACNA1A calcium channel subunit gene and relationship with familial hemiplegic migraine. Ann Neurol 49: 753–760.

Kors EE, Haan J, Giffin NJ et al. (2003). Expanding the phenotypic spectrum of the CACNA1A gene T666M mutation: a description of 5 families with familial hemiplegic migraine. Arch Neurol 60: 684–688.

Kowa H, Yasui K, Takeshima T et al. (2000). The homozygous C677T mutation in the methylenetetrahydrofolate reductase gene is a genetic risk factor for migraine. Am J Med Genet 96: 762–764.

Kowa H, Fusayasu E, Ijiri T et al. (2005). Association of the insertion/deletion polymorphism of the angiotensin I-converting enzyme gene in patients of migraine with aura. Neurosci Lett 374: 129–131.

Kraus RL, Sinnegger MJ, Glossmann H et al. (1998). Familial hemiplegic migraine mutations change alpha(1A) Ca^{2+} channel kinetics. J Biol Chem 273: 5586–5590.

Kraus RL, Sinnegger MJ, Koschak A et al. (2000). Three new familial hemiplegic migraine mutants affect P/Q-type $Ca^{(2+)}$ channel kinetics. J Biol Chem 275: 9239–9243.

Lacombe P, Oligo C, Domenga V et al. (2005). Impaired cerebral vasoreactivity in a transgenic mouse model of cerebral autosomal dominant arteriopathy with subcortical infarcts and leukoencephalopathy arteriopathy. Stroke 36: 1053–1058.

Lauritzen M (1994). Pathophysiology of the migraine aura. The spreading depression theory. Brain 117: 199–210.

Law C, Bunyan D, Castle B et al. (2006). Clinical features in a family with an R460H mutation in transforming growth factor beta receptor 2 gene. J Med Genet 43: 908–916.

Lea RA, Sheperd AG, Curtain RP et al. (2002). A typical migraine susceptibility region localizes to chromosome 1q31. Neurogenetics 4: 17–22.

Lea RA, Nyholt DR, Curtain RP et al. (2005a). A genome-wide scan provides evidence for loci influencing a severeheritable form of common migraine. Neurogenetics 6: 67–72.

Lea RA, Ovcaric M, Sundholm J et al. (2005b). Genetic variants of angiotensin converting enzyme and methylenetetrahydrofolate reductase may act in combination to increase migraine susceptibility. Brain Res Mol Brain Res 136: 112–117.

Leone M, Russell MB, Rigamonti A et al. (2001). Increased familial risk of cluster headache. Neurology 56: 1233–1236.

Ligthart L, Boomsma DI, Martin NG et al. (2006). Migraine with aura and migraine without aura are not distinct entities: further evidence from a large Dutch population study. Twin Res Hum Genet 9: 54–63.

Lin JJ, Wang PJ, Chen CH et al. (2005). Homozygous deletion genotype of angiotensin converting enzyme confers protection against migraine in man. Acta Neurol Taiwan 14: 120–125.

Lorenzon NM, Lutz CM, Frankel WN et al. (1998). Altered calcium channel currents in Purkinje cells of neurological mutant mouse leaner. J Neurosci 18: 4482–4489.

Low N, Singleton A (2007). Establishing the genetic heterogeneity of familial hemiplegic migraine. Brain 130: 312–313.

Meisler MH, Kearney JA (2005). Sodium channel mutations in epilepsy and other neurological disorders. J Clin Invest 115: 2010–2017.

Montagna P, Pierangeli G, Cevoli S et al. (2005). Pharmacogenetics of headache treatment. Neurol Sci 26: S143–S147.

Mori Y, Wakamori M, Oda S et al. (2000). Reduced voltage sensitivity of activation of P/Q-type Ca^{2+} channels is associated with the ataxic mouse mutation *rolling Nagoya* (tg(rol)). J Neurosci 20: 5654–5662.

Moseley AE, Lieske SP, Wetzel RK et al. (2003). The Na,K-ATPase alpha 2 isoform is expressed in neurons and its absence disrupts neuronal activity in newborn mice. J Biol Chem 278: 5317–5324.

Moskowitz MA, Bolay H, Dalkara T (2004). Deciphering migraine mechanisms: clues from familial hemiplegic migraine genotypes. Ann Neurol 55: 276–280.

Mulder EJ, van Baal C, Gaist D et al. (2003). Genetic and environmental influences on migraine: a twin study across six countries. Twin Res 6: 422–431.

Nyholt DR, Dawkins JL, Brimage PJ et al. (1998). Evidence for an X-linked genetic component in familial typical migraine. Hum Mol Genet 7: 459–463.

Nyholt DR, Gillespie NG, Heath AC et al. (2004). Latent class and genetic analysis does not support migraine with aura and migraine without aura as separate entities. Genet Epidemiol 26: 231–244.

Nyholt DR, Morley KI, Ferreira MA et al. (2005). Genome-wide significant linkage to migrainous headache on chromosome 5q21. Am J Hum Genet 77: 500–512.

Odawara M, Tamaoka A, Mizusawa H et al. (1997). A case of cluster headache associated with mitochondrial DNA deletions. Muscle Nerve 20: 394–395.

Ophoff RA, Terwindt GM, Vergouwe MN et al. (1996). Familial hemiplegic migraine and episodic ataxia type-2 are caused by mutations in the Ca^{2+} channel gene CACNL1A4. Cell 87: 543–552.

Ophoff RA, de Young J, Service SK et al. (2001). Hereditary vascular retinopathy cerebroretinal vasculopathy and hereditary endotheliopathy with retinopathy nephropathy and stroke map to a single locus on chromosome 3p21.1-p21.3. Am J Hum Genet 69: 447–453.

Oterino A, Pascual J, Ruiz de Alegria C et al. (2006). Association of migraine and ESR1 G325C polymorphism. Neuroreport 17: 61–64.

Paterna S, Di Pasquale P, D'Angelo A et al. (2000). Angiotensin-converting enzyme gene deletion polymorphism determines an increase in frequency of migraine attacks in patients suffering from migraine without aura. Eur Neurol 43: 133–136.

Pfefferkorn T, Stuckrad-Barre S, Herzog J et al. (2001). Reduced cerebrovascular CO_2 reactivity in CADASIL: a transcranial Doppler sonography study. Stroke 32: 17–21.

Pietrobon D (2005). Migraine: new molecular mechanisms. Neuroscientist 11: 373–386.

Pinessi L, Rainero I, Rubino E et al. (2005). Genetics of cluster headache: an update. J Head Pain 6: 234–236.

Rainero I, Grimaldi LM, Salani G et al. (2004a). Association between the tumor necrosis factor-alpha-308 G/A gene polymorphism and migraine. Neurology 62: 141–143.

Rainero I, Gallone S, Valfre W et al. (2004b). A polymorphism of the hypocretin receptor 2 gene is associated with cluster headache. Neurology 63: 1286–1288.

Rainero I, Rivoiro C, Gallone S et al. (2005). Lack of association between the 3092 T→C Clock gene polymorphism and cluster headache. Cephalalgia 25: 1078–1081.

Riant F, De Fusco M, Aridon P et al. (2005). ATP1A2 mutations in 11 families with familial hemiplegic migraine. Hum Mut 26: 281.

Russell MB (2001). Genetics of migraine without aura migraine with aura migrainous disorder head trauma migraine without aura and tension-type headache. Cephalalgia 21: 778–780.

Russell MB (2004). Epidemiology and genetics of cluster headache. Lancet Neurol 3: 279–283.

Russell MB, Olesen J (1993). The genetics of migraine without aura and migraine with aura. Cephalalgia 13: 245–248.

Russell MB, Olesen J (1995). Increased familial risk and evidence of genetic factor in migraine. BMJ 311: 541–544.

Russell MB, Andersson PG, Thomsen LL (1995a). Familial occurrence of cluster headache. J Neurol Neurosurg Psychiatry 58: 341–343.

Russell MB, Andersson PG, Thomsen LL et al. (1995b). Cluster headache is an autosomal dominantly inherited disorder in some families: a complex segregation analysis. J Med Genet 32: 954–956.

Russell MB, Saltyte-Benth J, Levi N (2006). Are infrequent episodic, frequent episodic and chronic tension-type headache inherited? A population-based study of 11 199 twin pairs. J Head Pain 7: 119–126.

Russo L, Mariotti P, Sangiorgi E et al. (2005). A new susceptibility locus for migraine with aura in the 15q11-q13 genomic region containing three GABA-A receptor genes. Am J Hum Genet 76: 327–333.

Scher AI, Terwindt GM, Verschuren WM et al. (2006). Migraine and MTHFR C677T genotype in a population-based sample. Ann Neurol 59: 372–375.

Schürks M, Kurth T, Geissler I et al. (2006). Cluster headache is associated with the G1246A polymorphism in the hypocretin receptor 2 gene. Neurology 66: 1917–1919.

Seibel P, Grunewald T, Gundolla A et al. (1996). Investigation on the mitochondrial transfer RNA(Leu)(UUR) in blood cells from patients with cluster headache. J Neurol 243: 305–307.

Segall L, Scanzano R, Kaunisto MA et al. (2004). Kinetic alterations due to a missense mutation in the Na,K-ATPase alpha 2 subunit cause familial hemiplegic migraine type 2. J Biol Chem 279: 43692–43696.

Segall L, Mezzetti A, Scanzano R et al. (2005). Alterations in the alpha2 isoform of Na,K-ATPase associated with familial hemiplegic migraine type 2. Proc Natl Acad Sci U S A 102: 11106–11111.

Shimomura T, Kitano A, Marukawa H et al. (1994). Point mutation in platelet mitochondrial tRNA Leu(UUR) in patient with cluster headache. Lancet 344: 625.

Sjöstrand C, Giedratis V, Ekbom K et al. (2001). CACNA1A gene polymorphisms in cluster headache. Cephalalgia 21: 953–958.

Somjen GG (2001). Mechanisms of spreading depression and hypoxic spreading depression-like depolarization. Physiol Rev 81: 1065–1096.

Soragna D, Vettori A, Carraro G et al. (2003). A locus for migraine without aura maps on chromosome 14q21.2-q22.3. Am J Hum Genet 72: 161–167.

Spacey SD, Hildebrand ME, Materek LA et al. (2004). Functional implications of a novel EA2 mutation in the P/Q-type calcium channel. Ann Neurol 56: 213–220.

Spadaro M, Ursu S, Lehmann-Horn F et al. (2004). A G301R Na^+/K^+-ATPase mutation causes familial hemiplegic migraine type 2 with cerebellar signs. Neurogenetics 5: 177–185.

Stewart WF, Staffa J, Lipton RB et al. (1997). Familial risk of migraine: a population-based study. Ann Neurol 41: 166–172.

Svensson DA, Larsson B, Waldenlind E et al. (2003). Shared rearing environment in migraine: results from twins reared apart and twins reared together. Headache 43: 235–244.

Swoboda KJ, Kanavakis E, Xaidara A et al. (2004). Alternating hemiplegia of childhood or familial hemiplegic migraine? A novel ATP1A2 mutation. Ann Neurol 55: 884–887.

Terwindt GM, Haan J, Ophoff RA et al. (1998). Clinical and genetic analysis of a large Dutch family with autosomal dominant vascular retinopathy migraine and Raynaud's phenomenon. Brain 121: 303–316.

Terwindt G, Kors E, Haan J et al. (2002). Mutation analysis of the CACNA1A calcium channel subunit gene in 27 patients with sporadic hemiplegic migraine. Arch Neurol 59: 1016–1018.

Thomsen LL, Ostergaard E, Olesen J et al. (2003a). Evidence for a separate type of migraine with aura: sporadic hemiplegic migraine. Neurology 60: 595–601.

Thomsen LL, Ostergaard E, Romer SF et al. (2003b). Sporadic hemiplegic migraine is an aetiologically heterogeneous disorder. Cephalalgia 23: 921–928.

Thomsen LL, Kirchmann M, Björnsson A et al. (2007). The genetic spectrum of a population-based sample of familial hemiplegic migraine. Brain 130: 346–356.

Todt U, Freudenberg J, Goebel I et al. (2006). MTHFR C677T polymorphism and migraine with aura. Ann Neurol 60: 621–622.

Tottene A, Tottene A, Fellin T et al. (2002). Familial hemiplegic migraine mutations increase Ca^{2+} influx through single human cav2.1 channels and decrease maximal cav2.1 current density in neurons. Proc Natl Acad Sci U S A 99: 13284–13289.

Tottene A, Pivotto F, Fellin T et al. (2005). Specific kinetic alterations of human cav2.1 calcium channels produced by mutation S218L causing familial hemiplegic migraine and delayed cerebral edema and coma after minor head trauma. J Biol Chem 280: 17678–17686.

Trabace S, Brioli G, Lulli P et al. (2002). Tumor necrosis factor gene polymorphism in migraine. Headache 42: 341–345.

Ulrich V, Gervil M, Kyvik KO et al. (1999). Evidence of a genetic factor in migraine with aura: a population based Danish twin study. Ann Neurol 45: 242–246.

Ulrich V, Gervil M, Olesen J (2004). The relative influence of environment and genes in episodic tension-type headache. Neurology 62: 2065–2069.

Urbano FJ, Piedras-Renteria ES, Jun K et al. (2003). Altered properties of quantal neurotransmitter release at endplates of mice lacking P/Q-type Ca^{2+} channels. Proc Natl Acad Sci U S A 100: 3491–3496.

Vahedi K, Denier C, Ducros A et al. (2000). CACNA1A gene de novo mutation causing hemiplegic migraine coma and cerebellar atrophy. Neurology 55: 1040–1042.

Vahedi K, Massin P, Guichard JP et al. (2003). Hereditary infantile hemiparesis retinal arteriolar tortuosity and leukoencephalopathy. Neurology 60: 57–63.

van den Maagdenberg AMJM, Pietrobon D, Pizzorusso T et al. (2004). A Cacna1a knock-in migraine mouse model with increased susceptibility to cortical spreading depression. Neuron 41: 701–710.

Vanmolkot KRJ, Kors EE, Hottenga JJ et al. (2003). Novel mutations in the Na^+/K^+-ATPase pump gene ATP1A2 associated with familial hemiplegic migraine and benign familial infantile convulsions. Ann Neurol 54: 360–366.

Vanmolkot KJR, Kors EE, Turk U et al. (2006). Two de novo mutations in the Na,K-ATPase gene ATP1A2 associated with pure familial hemiplegic migraine. Eur J Hum Genet 14: 555–560.

Vanmolkot KRJ, Pusch M, de Vries B et al. (2007). The novel L1649Q mutation in the SCN1A epilepsy gene is associated with familial hemiplegic migraine: genetic and functional studies. Hum Mutat 28: 522.

Wakamori M, Yamazaki K, Matsunodaira H et al. (1998). Single *tottering* mutations responsible for the neuropathic phenotype of the P-type calcium channel. J Biol Chem 273: 34857–63487.

Wan J, Khanna R, Sandusky M et al. (2005). CACNA1A mutations causing episodic and progressive ataxia alter channel trafficking and kinetics. Neurology 64: 2090–2097.

Wappl E, Koschak A, Poteser M et al. (2002). Functional consequences of P/Q-type Ca^{2+} channel Cav2.1 missense mutations associated with episodic ataxia type 2 and progressive ataxia. J Biol Chem 277: 6960–6966.

Wessman M, Kallela M, Kaunisto MA et al. (2002). A susceptibility locus for migraine with aura on chromosome 4q24. Am J Hum Genet 70: 652–662.

Whitty CWM (1986). Familial hemiplegic migraine. In: PJ Vinken, GW Bruyn, FF Clifford Rose (Eds.), Handbook of Clinical Neurology. Elsevier Science, Amsterdam, pp. 141–153.

Yu FH, Mantegazza M, Westenbroek RE et al. (2007). Reduced sodium current in gabaergic interneurons in a mouse model of severe myoclonic epilepsy in infancy. Nat Neurosci 10: 134.

Yue Q, Jen JC, Nelson SF et al. (1997). Progressive ataxia due to a missense mutation in a calcium-channel gene. Am J Hum Genet 61: 1078–1087.

Zhuchenko O, Bailey J, Donnen P et al. (1997). Autosomal dominant cerebellar ataxia (SCA6) associated with small polyglutamine expansions in the α1A-voltage-dependent calcium channel. Nat Genet 15: 62–69.

Ziegler DK, Hur YM, Bouchard TJ et al. (1998). Migraine in twins raised together and apart. Headache 38: 417–422.

Handbook of Clinical Neurology, Vol. 97 (3rd series)
Headache
G. Nappi and M.A. Moskowitz, Editors

Chapter 7

The neurobiology of migraine

ANDREW CHARLES* AND K.C. BRENNAN
Headache Research and Treatment Program, Department of Neurology, David Geffen School of Medicine at UCLA, Los Angeles, CA, USA

ANATOMICAL COMPONENTS OF MIGRAINE

Cerebral cortex

There is substantial clinical and imaging evidence for changes in cortical activity associated with migraine. Migraine is associated with a variety of symptoms that can be attributed to changes in cortical function. The most prominent among these are the visual changes associated with migraine aura that arise from altered function in the occipital lobe. Migraine patients may also experience cortical sensory, motor, language, or other cognitive dysfunction. These symptoms are typically described in the context of migraine with aura, but they may also occur with migraine that does not meet diagnostic criteria for migraine with aura. Functional imaging studies confirm that migraine is associated with dramatic changes in blood flow and metabolic activity in the cortex (Cutrer and Black, 2006). These imaging phenomena have been demonstrated primarily in patients with migraine with aura, but may also occur in patients with migraine without aura (Woods et al., 1994; Geraud et al., 2005). Migraine-related changes in blood flow and functional magnetic resonance imaging (fMRI) signal in the cortex are propagated with temporal and spatial characteristics that are remarkably similar to those of cortical spreading depression (CSD), the spreading wave of depolarization followed by suppression of electrocortical activity originally described by Leão in 1944 (Woods et al., 1994; Hadjikhani et al., 2001). The correlation between the characteristics of the clinical symptoms of migraine aura, CSD in animal models, and functional imaging has provided support for the long-standing hypothesis that CSD is a fundamental mechanism of migraine aura. A much more controversial question continues to be whether similar cortical phenomena may also occur in migraine without aura. As discussed below, distinct patterns of signaling in individual cellular compartments could underlie cortical activity that does not necessarily evoke classical aura symptoms.

Other evidence for fundamental changes in cortical excitability in migraine comes from clinical electrophysiology studies. A significant number of studies find an increased amplitude as well as a decreased habituation of cortical evoked potentials in migraine patients compared with controls during the interictal period, with normalization of these differences during the ictal period (Schoenen, 2006). Other studies also show that the threshold for generation of phosphenes by transcranial magnetic stimulation is reduced in migraine patients (Aurora et al., 1999, 2003; Gerwig et al., 2005). Migraine patients have also been reported to show reduced magnetic stimulation-induced suppression of visual accuracy (Aurora et al., 2007). These findings are consistent with an increased cortical excitability (or decreased inhibition) in patients with migraine.

However, there are also a significant number of studies that show either no differences in clinical electrophysiological parameters between migraine patients and controls, or in fact changes in the opposite direction consistent with a reduced cortical excitability in migraine patients (Ambrosini and Shoenen, 2006). The discrepancies between these studies may arise in part from methodological differences in the way the studies were performed. But another key explanation for these discrepancies is that the level of cortical excitability in migraine patients may vary substantially over time. Consistent with this idea, the thresholds for phosphene generation evoked by consecutive transcranial magnetic stimulation were found to be more

*Correspondence to: Andrew Charles MD, Headache Research and Treatment Program, Department of Neurology, David Geffen School of Medicine at UCLA, 635 Charles Young Drive, Los Angeles, CA 90095, USA, Tel: 310-206-7226, Fax: 310-206-6906, E-mail: acharles@ucla.edu

variable in migraine patients than in controls (Antal et al., 2006). This suggests that, rather than having cortical excitability that can be characterized simply as either increased or reduced, migraine patients have a dysregulation of cortical excitability (Ambrosini and Shoenen, 2006; Stankewitz and May, 2007). Abnormally wide swings in cortical excitability are an appealing explanation for the complex variety of symptoms that are experienced by migraine patients.

Brainstem

There is also strong evidence that brainstem mechanisms play a significant role in the pathophysiology of migraine. Nausea, vertigo, and autonomic symptoms are among the clinical features of migraine that may arise from an alteration of signaling in the brainstem. It has also been suggested that the pain of migraine may arise primarily from the brainstem (Weiller et al., 1995; Tajti et al., 2001). Functional imaging studies of migraine patients consistently demonstrate activation of the brainstem during migraine attacks, particularly the region of the dorsolateral pons (Bahra et al., 2001; Afridi et al., 2005; Denuelle et al., 2007). Positron emission tomography (PET) and fMRI studies suggest that metabolism and function in the brainstem may also be chronically altered in patients with chronic migraine (Welch et al., 2001; Aurora et al., 2007). There have also been multiple reports of structural lesions in the brainstem that appear to cause headache in humans (Haas et al., 1993; Goadsby, 2002; Fragoso and Brooks, 2007). Furthermore, electrical stimulation in the region of the periaqueductal gray can evoke headache (Raskin et al., 1987).

The trigeminal pathway

Although it is clear from functional imaging studies that multiple brain regions involved in nociception are activated during a migraine attack (Weiller et al., 1995; Cao et al., 1999, 2002; Bahra et al., 2001; Afridi et al., 2005; Denuelle et al., 2007), the site where the initial activation of these nociceptive pathways occurs has not been determined with certainty. The idea that dilation of cerebral vessels is a primary cause of migraine pain has been challenged by a variety of evidence. However, the "trigeminovascular system" continues to be widely accepted as an important component of the headache. This concept developed based on the early observations that stimulation of trigeminally innervated vessels evoked pain in conscious patients, whereas stimulation of the brain parenchyma did not evoke discomfort (Penfield, 1935; Ray and Wolff, 1940). A role for the trigeminovascular system was supported by the observation that calcitonin gene-related peptide (CGRP), a neuropeptide known to be involved in cerebral vasoregulation, is increased in jugular venous blood during a migraine attack (Goadsby and Edvinsson, 1994). The idea of trigeminovascular activation has been reinforced by the effects of triptans, and more recently CGRP antagonists, whose effects have been presumed to be in large part mediated by inhibition of perivascular trigeminal nociceptive input. However, the findings that activation of 5-HT1 receptors by triptans at multiple other sites was involved in trigeminal nociception, including the nucleus caudalis, periaqueductal gray, and thalamus indicate that the perivascular trigeminal nerve endings are not necessarily the only site of action of these drugs (Goadsby and Hoskin, 1996; Ellrich et al., 2001; Boers et al., 2004; Shields and Goadsby, 2006). Other migraine therapies such as ergotamines, that had initially been presumed to act primarily at the peripheral trigeminal vascular complex, have also been shown to have central mechanisms of action (Hoskin et al., 1996).

It is also important to recognize that CGRP-containing neurons are found through the central and peripheral nervous system (including the trigeminal nucleus caudalis in the brainstem) (Tajti et al., 2001; Jenkins et al., 2004; Offenhauser et al., 2005; D'Hanis, 2007), and these neurons could represent an alternative source of the CGRP that is released during a migraine attack. Thus, although there is considerable indirect evidence for trigeminovascular activation in migraine, there is as yet no direct evidence that confirms this hypothesis. This may be because there is no reasonable way of measuring such activation in humans. However, it is interesting to note that trigeminal rhizotomy, even when complete disruption of trigeminal sensory function has been achieved, is not consistently effective in the prevention of migraine or cluster headache that is experienced on the side ipsilateral to the trigeminal deafferentation (Matharu and Goadsby, 2002). This observation suggests that it is possible for nociceptive pathways responsible for headache to be activated in the absence of peripheral trigeminal input from the same side on which the headache is experienced. Further investigation regarding the sites of actions of the triptans and CGRP receptor antagonists in humans may shed important light on this issue.

Is there an anatomical sequence in migraine?

The sequence of activation of different brain regions in migraine remains uncertain. At this stage it is not clear whether changes in cortical activity activate the brainstem, or vice versa. Alternatively, changes in these brain regions could occur in parallel, without an orderly sequence from one to the next. The typical occurrence of the migraine aura before migraine headache supports the hypothesis that cortical activation precedes brainstem activation. Consistent with this concept, important studies in experimental models demonstrate that it is possible for CSD to activate neurons in the trigeminal nucleus caudalis via trigeminal afferents (Bolay et al., 2002). Conversely, it has been shown that brainstem activation can evoke changes in cortical blood flow, raising the possibility that a process beginning in the brainstem could secondarily evoke some of the cortical phenomena of migraine (Adams et al., 1989; Goadsby and Duckworth, 1989). But it is also possible that both brain regions are activated simultaneously, a concept that is supported by the observations that, in some patients, clinical symptoms may occur without any clearly defined sequence that indicates alteration in the function of one region leading to change in function of another. Regardless of the order of their activation, however, it is clear that both cortical and brainstem signaling mechanisms are involved in migraine and are appealing targets for new therapeutic approaches for migraine.

CELLULAR COMPONENTS OF MIGRAINE

The concept of migraine as a primarily vascular headache has given way to the understanding that it is an episodic disorder of brain excitability that involves coordinated changes in neuronal, glial, and vascular function. Examination of the individual cellular components of migraine identifies new potential pathophysiological mechanisms, and new targets for treatment.

Nociception

It is generally assumed that migraine pain is initiated by activation of meningeal sensory afferents that synapse in the trigeminal nucleus caudalis, although, as discussed above, this assumption has not been definitively confirmed. Trigeminal neurons that innervate the meninges have properties that are in many ways similar to other visceral sensory neurons (Strassman and Levy, 2006). The only sensation that they appear to transmit is pain. However, the specific stimuli that trigger sensory neurons to produce migraine pain are not certain. A variety have been proposed, including mechanical pressure, changes in the ionic composition of the extracellular space (e.g., increased K^+, increased osmolarity, and decreased pH), neuropeptides (e.g., bradykinin, substance P, endothelin, and CGRP), neurotransmitters (glutamate, serotonin, histamine, adenosine triphosphate, adenosine), eicosanoids, and nitric oxide. There may be subsets of trigeminal neurons that respond specifically to different stimuli with different thresholds. Individual neurons with conduction velocities consistent with A and C fibers have been identified, with different sensitivities to mechanical versus neurochemical stimuli, and different responses to repetitive or sequential combinations of stimuli (Levy and Strassman, 2002).

Peripheral trigeminal neurons, as with other neurons in the trigeminal pathway, show the phenomenon of sensitization, whereby exposure to an algesic stimulus lowers the threshold for the response of the neuron to the same stimulus, or a different stimulus (Strassman et al., 1996). For example, exposure to inflammatory mediators lowers the threshold of trigeminal neurons for responding to a mechanical stimulus (Levy and Strassman, 2002). This type of sensitization has been suggested as a mechanism whereby otherwise painless localized or diffuse changes in pressure (such as might occur with vascular pulsations) could result in the pulsating pain of migraine. It has been proposed that both peripheral and central sensitization are involved in the generation and maintenance of migraine pain, as well as the associated phenomenon of cutaneous allodynia.

Cortical waves

A complex interplay between neurons, glial cells, and vascular cells may be particularly critical in cortical mechanisms of migraine. As discussed above, the anatomical spread of migraine aura symptoms as well as the propagated changes in blood flow and metabolism observed in migraine patients has implicated the phenomenon of CSD in migraine. CSD was originally reported by Leão in 1944 as a suppression of electrical activity that spread slowly across large areas of the cortex (Leão, 1944). Subsequent recordings demonstrated that the suppression of activity was preceded by a dramatic depolarization, resulting in a "DC [direct current] shift" of the electrocortical signal, indicating that the CSD wave consists of a propagated wave of profound cortical activation followed by sustained inhibition of activity (Leão, 1947).

The clinical symptoms of migraine aura, as well as the clinical electrophysiological and transcranial magnetic stimulation responses of migraine patients, indicate a fundamental role for changes in neuronal excitability as a basis for increased cortical excitability in migraine. Other evidence comes from genetic and pharmacological studies. Mutations in neuron-specific genes have been identified as the cause of familial hemiplegic migraine in some families. These include mutations in the P/Q-type calcium channel (FHM1)

(Ophoff et al., 1996; van den Maagdenberg et al., 2004), and SCN1A voltage-gated sodium channel (Dichgans et al., 2005). In each case, the resulting alteration of function of the channel results in an increase in the excitability of the neuron.

Pharmacological studies indicate that inhibition of neuron-specific receptors or channels can inhibit CSD. Inhibition of *N*-methyl-d-aspartate (NMDA) receptors, which are expressed primarily on neurons, can inhibit the occurrence of CSD *in vitro* and *in vivo* preparations (Hernandez-Caceres et al., 1987; Peeters et al., 2007). CSD *in vitro* can also be blocked by inhibitors of P/Q-type calcium channels, which are specific to neurons (Kunkler and Kraig, 2004). Conversely, studies with a knock-in mouse model expressing a mutation of the P/Q calcium channel gene associated with familial hemiplegic migraine show that alteration in the function of this neuronal channel lowers the threshold for evoking CSD, and increases its rate of propagation (van den Maagdenberg et al., 2004). These studies indicate that neuronal hyperexcitability is involved in the triggering of CSD and its propagation.

Astrocyte waves

Glial cells may also play a key role in the changes in cortical activity associated with migraine. Direct evidence for such a role comes from the discovery that a mutation in an Na^+/K^+ ATPase that is expressed primarily in astrocytes is responsible for familial hemiplegic migraine type 2 (De Fusco et al., 2003; Vanmolkot et al., 2006). *In vitro* studies indicate that this mutation reduces the function of the enzyme (Segall et al., 2005; Vanmolkot et al., 2006), an effect that would be expected to increase excitability by increasing extracellular K^+. Astrocytes are abundant cells in the central nervous system that have been traditionally viewed as playing only a passive and supportive role in nervous system function. But recent studies demonstrate that astrocytes are capable of extensive intercellular signaling that can modulate both neuronal and vascular activity. Astrocytes express a variety of neurotransmitter receptors that allow them to respond to neuronal activity (Fellin et al., 2006). Conversely, they are capable of active release of transmitters, including glutamate and adenosine triphosphate (ATP), that can modulate neuronal function (Haydon and Carmignoto, 2006). Astrocytes are also in close contact with vascular cells via their endfeet, that enwrap blood vessels. Astrocyte signaling has been shown to modulate vascular tone directly, resulting in either vasoconstriction or vasodilation via release of eicosanoids, K^+, and ATP (Zonta et al., 2003; Mulligan and MacVicar, 2004; Filosa et al., 2006; Takano et al., 2006).

Astrocytes are capable of extensive intercellular communication via increases in intracellular calcium concentration that are propagated from cell to cell in a wave-like pattern (Charles et al., 1991). The primary mechanism for these intercellular calcium waves appears to be release of ATP into the extracellular space and activation of purinergic receptors on adjacent cells (Guthrie et al., 1999). These intercellular calcium waves in astrocytes can be triggered by chemical, electrical, or mechanical stimuli, and spread with temporal and spatial characteristics that are remarkably similar to those of CSD (Charles, 1998). In fact, recent microscopic imaging studies have shown that calcium waves in astrocytes consistently occur in association with spreading depression, both *in vitro* and *in vivo* (Peters et al., 2003; Chuquet et al., 2007). However, each phenomenon can occur independently of the other. Inhibition of astrocyte calcium waves does not block spreading depression, and astrocyte calcium waves occur in the absence of spreading depression (Peters et al., 2003; Chuquet et al., 2007). Thus, they appear to be related phenomena that occur in parallel but without a requisite interdependence.

It has been assumed for decades that spreading depression as it is observed in animal models is the physiological basis for migraine aura. But the classical electroencephalogram (EEG) changes of CSD have not been observed in migraine patients. This could be because surface EEG recordings have not been sensitive enough to detect it. However, CSD in animal models is a profound neurophysiological event. It would be expected to produce not only EEG changes, but also a greater degree of neurological impairment than is observed in most migraine patients. A speculative alternative to classical CSD as a mechanism of the propagated cortical changes in migraine is a phenomenon that involves astrocyte waves. Astrocyte calcium waves are associated with release of significant amounts of ATP, glutamate, and vasoactive mediators (Haydon and Carmignoto, 2006). Based on this function, and based on their close spatial relationship with both neurons and vascular cells, astrocytes are ideally positioned to modulate widely propagated changes in both vascular activity and neuronal activity with the pattern that is observed in migraine patients. A primary role for astrocytes could explain both the propagated changes in blood flow and metabolism that are observed with functional imaging studies, as well as the cortical symptoms that in most patients are not as profound as might be expected to result from classical CSD. Even if astrocytes do not play such a primary role, it is likely that their activity represents a substantial component of the cellular pathophysiology of migraine.

Vascular waves

In addition to the changes in neuronal and glial cell function, migraine clearly involves significant changes in the activity of vascular cells. Mutations in genes encoding proteins expressed predominantly by vascular cells have been found in families with vasculopathies that have migraine as part of the clinical phenotype. Mutations in the gene encoding Notch3, which in adult humans is expressed predominantly in vascular smooth-muscle cells, cause cerebral autosomal-dominant arteriopathy with subcortical infarcts and leukoecephelopathy (CADASIL). This condition begins with migraine with aura in approximately one-third of patients (Dichgans et al., 1998). Mutations in the gene encoding the widely expressed exonuclease TREX1 also cause a vasculopathy that may have migraine as part of the phenotype (Richards et al., 2007).

As with astrocytes, it has long been assumed that vascular cells simply respond passively to changes in neuronal function. But it is important to keep in mind that vascular cells are also capable of active intercellular signaling, and can release messengers like nitric oxide that could potentially modulate the function of surrounding neurons and glia. As mentioned above, the longstanding hypothesis that migraine pain is a direct consequence of vasodilation has been increasingly challenged by functional imaging studies in migraine patients. The classic blood flow studies by Olesen and colleagues (1990) clearly demonstrated an increase in blood flow in patients with migraine. However, they found that the onset of pain preceded the onset of increased blood flow, and in fact began during the period of hypoperfusion that was associated with migraine aura. Conversely, the phase of increased blood flow often persisted for a significant duration after the pain of migraine had stopped. These studies suggest that vasodilation and the pain of migraine are not necessarily temporally correlated.

A variety of other functional imaging studies with PET and fMRI techniques also show cortical hypoperfusion during the onset of migraine pain (Woods et al., 1994; Hadjikhani et al., 2001; Geraud et al., 2005). Still other more recent studies with pharmacologically induced migraine also demonstrate that the onset of pain is not correlated with vasodilation. Olesen and colleagues found that, with migraine induced by sildenafil, the pain of migraine did not begin until after recovery from the drug-induced cerebral vasodilation, as indicated by transcranial Doppler (Kruuse et al., 2003). Similarly, Schoonman and colleagues (2008) used magnetic resonance angiography techniques to show that migraine pain evoked by nitroglycerin did not occur until after recovery from nitroglycerin-induced cerebral vasodilation.

The complex vascular changes that are observed with CSD may provide some insight into the complex vascular phenomena seen with functional imaging studies in migraine patients. Spreading depression in mice is associated with a multiphasic vascular response. There is an initial dilation of cortical surface vessels that may be actively propagated along the vessel via an intrinsic vascular mechanism (Brennan et al., 2007b). This is followed by a profound constriction of the vessels, after which there is subsequent vasodilation and then eventual recovery to normal caliber (Ayata et al., 2004; Brennan et al., 2007b). There may be significant species-specific and methodology-related differences in the presence and extent of the vasoconstriction component of the surface arteriolar response to CSD. In humans, a significant vasoconstriction is supported by functional imaging studies that consistently show a hypoperfusion associated with migraine aura, and even in migraine without aura (Woods et al., 1994; Cao et al., 1999; Geraud et al., 2005). *In vivo* imaging studies in rodent models provide evidence that astrocyte calcium waves mediate the propagated vasoconstriction associated with CSD, indicating a primary role for glial cells in this process (Chuquet et al., 2007) (Figure 7.1).

Vasoconstriction could be involved in the generation of migraine pain via a variety of mechanisms. First, constriction is associated with the release of messengers and peptides that are believed to be involved in the generation of migraine. CGRP, widely accepted as a potentially important mediator of migraine pain, is released by perivascular neurons in response to vasoconstriction as part of a reflex arc whose purpose is to maintain vascular caliber. Nitric oxide may also be released by vascular cells in response to constriction. Vasoconstriction associated with CSD and/or astrocyte calcium waves could also result in an uncoupling of blood flow and metabolic activity. Reduced parenchymal blood flow in the face of intense neuronal and glial activity could cause the release of cellular metabolites and lower extracellular pH to trigger a nociceptive response. For example, transient receptor potential channels or acid-sensing ion channels on nociceptive trigeminal neurons could be activated under these conditions (McCleskey and Gold, 1999).

THE BLOOD–BRAIN BARRIER

In addition to changes in vascular caliber, cortical waves may be associated with changes in the permeability of the vasculature. The blood–brain barrier is a structural and functional barrier comprised of both

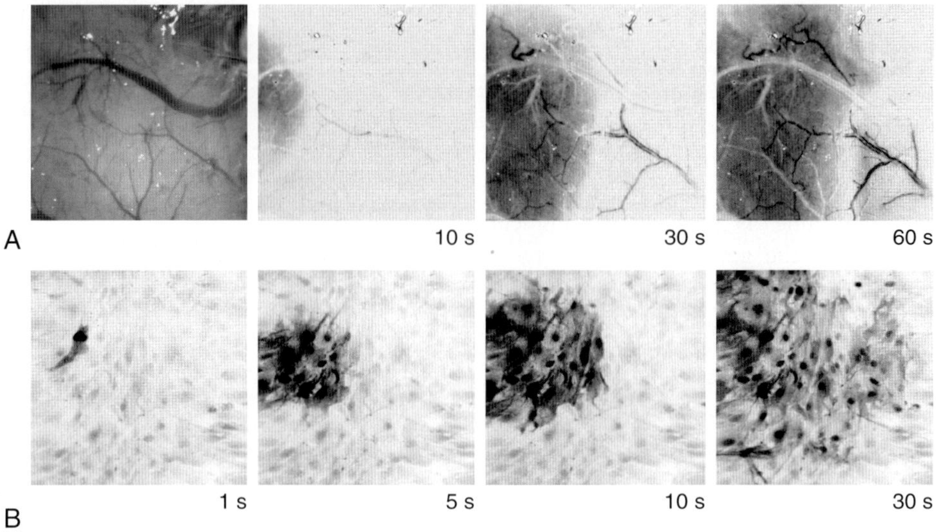

Fig. 7.1. Cortical spreading depression (CSD) and astrocyte calcium waves. (A) Optical imaging of the cortical surface in a mouse. Far left panel shows image of mouse cortex visualized through the thinned skull of an anesthetized mouse (a recording electrode is seen in the upper right of the field; image scale = 1200 × 1200 μm). Subsequent images show change in reflectance of this area of cortex over time associated with a CSD wave. A change in optical signal of the parenchyma spreads slowly across the cortex. Dilation (darkening) of surface arteries propagates ahead of the CSD wavefront, followed by constriction of these vessels accompanying the CSD wave. (B) Astrocyte calcium wave. Images show fluorescence of the calcium indicator fluo-4 with an inverse gray scale (darker gray indicates higher intracellular calcium; image scale = 400 × 400 μm). Mechanical stimulation of a single cell with a micropipette evokes a wave of increased calcium concentration that spreads from cell to cell over as many as hundreds of cells. The temporal and spatial characteristics of this wave are remarkably similar to those of CSD.

vascular and astrocytic components. Tight junctions between endothelial cells, and astrocyte endfeet that are closely apposed to the abluminal surface of the vessel, create a specialized structure with extremely limited permeability (Persidsky et al., 2006). This structure, in combination with a variety of membrane pumps and transporters, results in a barrier that allows only highly selective entry of glucose, amino acids, and other specific molecules from the vasculature into the brain. It has long been speculated that migraine is associated with a breakdown of the blood–brain barrier, partly because of temporal differences in the efficacy of abortive medications based on the phase of the migraine attack in which they are delivered (Harper et al., 1977). There are a few case reports of cortical gadolinium enhancement on MRI in migraineurs during attacks, indicating increased permeability of the blood–brain barrier (Smith et al., 2002; Dreier et al., 2005) (although this is a rare exception to the typically normal MRI studies of most migraine patients). CSD in rats has been associated with increased permeability of the blood–brain barrier as indicated by activation and upregulation of matrix metalloproteinase-9 (Gursoy-Ozdemir et al., 2004). This study provides evidence that one of the consequences of the propagated cortical activity in migraine may be an increase in blood–brain barrier permeability, and raises the possibility that leakage across the blood–brain barrier could be a mechanism for migraine pain. While inhibitors of plasma protein extravasation have not been effective in treating migraine, these agents were developed with models where the trigger for plasma extravasation was neurogenic inflammation, rather than spreading depression. Thus, they do not necessarily exclude a role for blood–brain barrier breakdown that is due to cortical waves.

GENETIC MODULATION OF MIGRAINE MECHANISMS

A wide variety of factors may influence the individual cellular components of migraine. As discussed above, genetic variations in the function of neurons, astrocytes, and vascular cells have each been implicated in different forms of migraine. It is important to note that mutations in genes expressed in multiple cell types and responsible for a variety of cellular functions all result in a similar clinical phenotype. This indicates that there are multiple points of entry to a final common pathway leading to migraine. For the FHM mutations, the resulting alterations in function are all likely to lead to an increase in cortical excitability. A knockin mouse expressing one identified mutation in the P/Q-type calcium channel associated with FHM1 provides compelling evidence for increased cortical excitability related to migraine (van den Maagdenberg et al., 2004). The threshold for evoking CSD in this mouse is significantly reduced compared with wild-type controls, and the rate of propagation of CSD is increased. For the FHM2 mutation in the astrocyte Na^+/K^+ ATPase, there is as yet no mouse model expressing this mutation. However, a reduced function of this pump, as has been shown *in vitro* in cells expressing the FHM2 mutations, would be expected to increase cortical excitability. Consistent with this concept, the Na^+/K^+ inhibitor ouabain reliably evokes CSD in rodent models (Basarsky et al., 1998). The increased excitability of neurons associated with the voltage-gated Na^+ channel mutations responsible for FHM3 would also be expected to increase cortical excitability. Thus, at least for FHM genes, an increased cortical excitability potentially predisposing to the occurrence of cortical waves may represent a common mechanism leading to the similar clinical phenotype. It will be interesting to determine if other migraine genes share this mechanism.

SEX MODULATION OF MIGRAINE MECHANISMS

Sex is another important modulator of migraine pathophysiology. The mechanisms underlying the dramatically greater prevalence of migraine in adult females are poorly understood. But as with genetic factors, sex may influence migraine through modulation of cortical excitability. We have found that the threshold for induction of CSD in mice is significantly reduced in female mice as compared with males (Brennan et al., 2007a). This result was obtained in randomly sampled mice without monitoring of the estrous cycle, such that the results cannot be easily explained by a reduced threshold for CSD occurring only at a single specific phase of the hormonal cycle. This increased susceptibility to CSD could involve changes in cortical excitability that are mediated by sustained exposure to gonadal hormones over days to months, developmental effects of hormones, chromosomal effects that are independent of hormones, or any combination of the above. Another potential mechanism for modulation of migraine by sex is alteration of sensitization of trigeminal nociceptive pathways. Martin et al. (2007) found that there was increased sensitization of nociceptive neuronal responses in the trigeminal nucleus caudalis in association with specific phases of the estrous cycle in rat, suggesting that alteration in the frequency and pattern of migraine associated with the menstrual cycle could involve changes in the sensitization of the trigeminal pathway.

AN INTEGRATED MODEL

The following is a hypothesized model for the sequence of events leading to migraine. In the cortex, a variety of different factors (genetic, neurochemical, ionic, and/or hormonal) lead to a dysregulation of excitability. This altered excitability triggers propagated waves of neuronal and glial activation, including astrocyte calcium waves, that are similar to, but not necessarily identical to, classical CSD. These cortical waves are associated with propagated changes in vascular caliber, and also breakdown of the blood–brain barrier. Cortical waves are also associated with release of a wide variety of neurotransmitters and neuromodulators, as well as changes in the ionic composition of the extracellular space that can activate nociceptive signaling pathways. These signaling pathways may also be activated by vascular constriction associated with cortical waves, through the release of messengers such as CGRP and nitric oxide that also evoke vasodilation, as well as by changes in the extracellular chemical and ionic condition resulting from vascular-metabolic uncoupling. Events occurring primarily in the cortex are then transmitted via peripheral trigeminal pathways to the brainstem, where second-order neurons are activated and eventually become sensitized. Alternatively, second-order neurons in the brainstem are activated in parallel to, or even in the absence of, cortical phenomena by changes in cellular excitability that may be similar to those described in the cortex. Third-order neurons in the thalamus and cortex are then activated and sensitized.

Specific neuronal, glial, and vascular signaling pathways may represent distinct targets for acute and preventive migraine therapies (Figure 7.2). An increased understanding of these pathways is now more accessible with advanced imaging and physiological recording techniques in combination with novel genetic models and molecular and pharmacological approaches. It is likely that there is extensive variation in the specific pathways that lead to migraine in different individuals. There may be opportunities to tailor new treatments to these specific molecular and cellular pathways in order to maximize efficacy and tolerability of therapy for this complex neurobiological disorder.

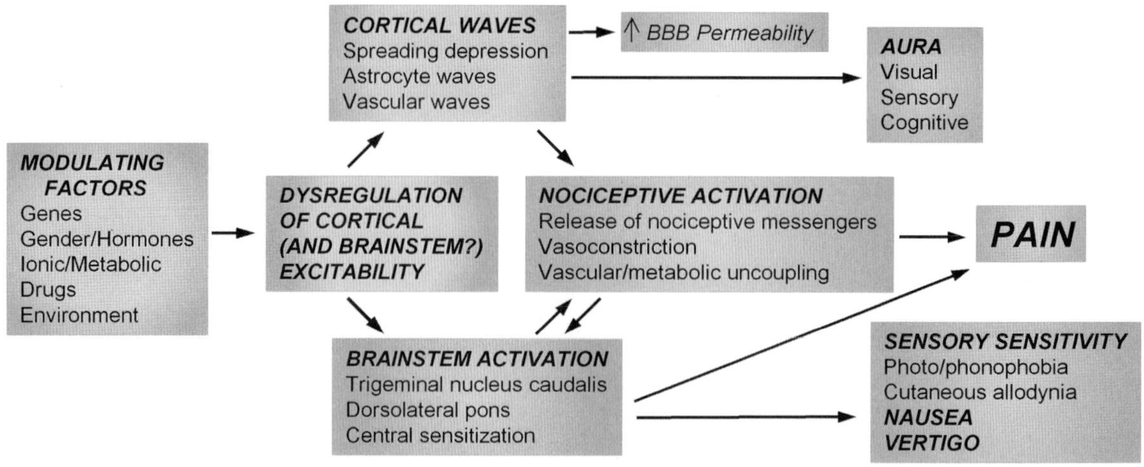

Fig. 7.2. Schematic of hypothesized sequence of events in migraine. Each step in the sequence may have discrete thresholds, and involve distinct molecular, cellular, and neurochemical pathways. This complexity may underlie the heterogeneous and variable clinical presentation of migraine. BBB, blood–brain barrier.

References

Adams RW, Lambert GA, Lance JW (1989). Stimulation of brainstem nuclei in the cat: effect on neuronal activity in the primary visual cortex of relevance to cerebral blood flow and migraine. Cephalalgia 9: 107–118.

Afridi SK, Matharu MS, Lee L et al. (2005). A PET study exploring the laterality of brainstem activation in migraine using glyceryl trinitrate. Brain 128: 932–939.

Ambrosini A, Shoenen J (2006). Electrophysiological response patterns of primary sensory cortices in migraine. J Headache Pain 7: 377–388.

Antal A, Arlt S, Nitsche MA et al. (2006). Higher variability of phosphene thresholds in migraineurs than in controls: a consecutive transcranial magnetic stimulation study. Cephalalgia 26: 865–870.

Aurora SK, Cao Y, Bowyer SM et al. (1999). The occipital cortex is hyperexcitable in migraine: experimental evidence. Headache 39: 469–476.

Aurora SK, Welch KMA, Al-Sayed F (2003). The threshold for phosphenes is lower in migraine. Cephalalgia 23: 258–263.

Aurora SK, Barrodale PM, Tipton RL et al. (2007). Brainstem dysfunction in chronic migraine as evidenced by neurophysiological and positron emission tomography studies. Headache 47: 996–1003; discussion 1004–1007.

Ayata C, Shin HK, Salomone S et al. (2004). Pronounced hypoperfusion during spreading depression in mouse cortex. J Cereb Blood Flow Metab 24: 1172–1182.

Bahra A, Matharu MS, Buchel C et al. (2001). Brainstem activation specific to migraine headache. Lancet 357: 1016–1017.

Basarsky TA, Duffy SN, Andrew RD et al. (1998). Imaging spreading depression and associated intracellular calcium waves in brain slices. J Neurosci 18: 7189–7199.

Boers P, Donaldson C, Zagami A et al. (2004). Naratriptan has a selective inhibitory effect on trigeminovascular neurones at central 5-HT1A and 5-HT1B/1D receptors in the cat: implications for migraine therapy. Cephalalgia 24: 99–109.

Bolay H, Reuter U, Dunn AK et al. (2002). Intrinsic brain activity triggers trigeminal meningeal afferents in a migraine model. Nat Med 8: 136–142.

Brennan KC, Romero-Reyes MR, Lopez-Valdes HE et al. (2007a). Reduced threshold for cortical spreading depression in female mice. Ann Neurol 61: 603–606.

Brennan KC, Beltran-Parrazal L, Lopez-Valdes HE et al. (2007b). Distinct vascular conduction with cortical spreading depression. J Neurophysiol 97: 4143–4151.

Cao Y, Welch KM, Aurora S et al. (1999). Functional MRI-BOLD of visually triggered headache in patients with migraine. Arch Neurol 56: 548–554.

Cao Y, Aurora SK, Nagesh V et al. (2002). Functional MRI-BOLD of brainstem structures during visually triggered migraine. Neurology 59: 72–78.

Charles A (1998). Intercellular calcium waves in glia. Glia 24: 39–49.

Charles AC, Merrill JE, Dirksen ER et al. (1991). Intercellular signaling in glial cells: calcium waves and oscillations in response to mechanical stimulation and glutamate. Neuron 6: 983–992.

Chuquet J, Hollender L, Nimchinsky EA (2007). High-resolution in vivo imaging of the neurovascular unit during spreading depression. J Neurosci 27: 4036–4044.

Cutrer FM, Black DF (2006). Imaging findings of migraine. Headache: J Head Face Pain 46: 1095–1107.

D'Hanis W, Linke R, Yilmazer-Hanke DM (2007) Topography of thalamic and parabrachial calcitonin gene-related peptide (CGRP) immunoreactive neurons projecting to subnuclei of the amygdala and extended amygdala. J Comp Neurol 505: 268–291.

De Fusco M, Marconi R, Silvestri L et al. (2003). Haploinsufficiency of ATP1A2 encoding the Na^+/K^+ pump alpha2 subunit associated with familial hemiplegic migraine type 2. Nat Genet 33: 192–196.

Denuelle M, Fabre N, Payoux P et al. (2007). Hypothalamic activation in spontaneous migraine attacks. Headache 47: 1418–1426.

Dichgans M, Mayer M, Uttner I et al. (1998). The phenotypic spectrum of CADASIL: Clinical findings in 102 cases. Ann Neurol 44: 731–739.

Dichgans M, Freilinger T, Eckstein G et al. (2005). Mutation in the neuronal voltage-gated sodium channel SCN1A in familial hemiplegic migraine. Lancet 366: 371–377.

Dreier JP, Jurkat-Rott K, Petzold GC et al. (2005). Opening of the blood–brain barrier preceding cortical edema in a severe attack of FHM type II. Neurology 64: 2145–2147.

Ellrich J, Messlinger K, Chiang CY et al. (2001). Modulation of neuronal activity in the nucleus raphe magnus by the 5-HT(1)-receptor agonist naratriptan in rat. Pain 90: 227–231.

Fellin T, Sul JY, D'Ascenzo M et al. (2006). Bidirectional astrocyte–neuron communication: the many roles of glutamate and ATP. Novartis Found Symp 276: 208–217; discussion 217–221, 233–207, 275–281.

Filosa JA, Bonev AD, Straub SV et al. (2006). Local potassium signaling couples neuronal activity to vasodilation in the brain. Nat Neurosci 9: 1397–1403.

Fragoso YD, Brooks JB (2007). Two cases of lesions in brainstem in multiple sclerosis and refractory migraine. Headache 47: 852–854.

Geraud G, Denuelle M, Fabre N et al. (2005). [Positron emission tomographic studies of migraine.] Rev Neurol (Paris) 161: 666–670.

Gerwig M, Niehaus L, Kastrup O et al. (2005). Visual cortex excitability in migraine evaluated by single and paired magnetic stimuli. Headache: J Head Face Pain 45: 1394–1399.

Goadsby PJ (2002). Neurovascular headache and a midbrain vascular malformation: evidence for a role of the brainstem in chronic migraine. Cephalalgia 22: 107–111.

Goadsby PJ, Duckworth JW (1989). Low frequency stimulation of the locus coeruleus reduces regional cerebral blood flow in the spinalized cat. Brain Res 476: 71–77.

Goadsby PJ, Edvinsson L (1994). Human in vivo evidence for trigeminovascular activation in cluster headache. Neuropeptide changes and effects of acute attacks therapies. Brain 117: 427–434.

Goadsby PJ, Hoskin KL (1996). Inhibition of trigeminal neurons by intravenous administration of the serotonin (5HT) 1B/D receptor agonist zolmitriptan (311C90): are brain stem sites therapeutic target in migraine? Pain 67: 355–359.

Gursoy-Ozdemir Y, Qiu J, Matsuoka N et al. (2004). Cortical spreading depression activates and upregulates MMP-9. J Clin Invest 113: 1447–1455.

Guthrie PB, Knappenberger J, Segal M et al. (1999). ATP released from astrocytes mediates glial calcium waves. J Neurosci 19: 520–528.

Haas DC, Kent PF, Friedman DI (1993). Headache caused by a single lesion of multiple sclerosis in the periaqueductal gray area. Headache 33: 452–455.

Hadjikhani N, Sanchez del Rio M, Wu O et al. (2001). Mechanisms of migraine aura revealed by functional MRI in human visual cortex. Proc Natl Acad Sci 98: 4687–4692.

Harper AM, MacKenzie ET, McCulloch J et al. (1977). Migraine and the blood–brain barrier. Lancet 1: 1034–1036.

Haydon PG, Carmignoto G (2006). Astrocyte control of synaptic transmission and neurovascular coupling. Physiol Rev 86: 1009–1031.

Hernandez-Caceres J, Macias-Gonzalez R, Brozek G et al. (1987). Systemic ketamine blocks cortical spreading depression but does not delay the onset of terminal anoxic depolarization in rats. Brain Res 437: 360–364.

Hoskin KL, Kaube H, Goadsby PJ (1996). Central activation of the trigeminovascular pathway in the cat is inhibited by dihydroergotamine. A c-Fos and electrophysiological study. Brain 119: 249–256.

Jenkins DW, Langmead CJ, Parsons AA et al. (2004). Regulation of calcitonin gene-related peptide release from rat trigeminal nucleus caudalis slices in vitro. Neurosci Lett 366: 241–244.

Kruuse C, Thomsen LL, Birk S et al. (2003). Migraine can be induced by sildenafil without changes in middle cerebral artery diameter. Brain 126: 241–247.

Kunkler PE, Kraig RP (2004). P/Q Ca^{2+} channel blockade stops spreading depression and related pyramidal neuronal Ca^{2+} rise in hippocampal organ culture. Hippocampus 14: 356–367.

Leão AAP (1944). Spreading depression of activity in the cerebral cortex. J Neurophysiol 7: 359–390.

Leão AAP (1947). Further observations on the spreading depression of activity in the cerebral cortex. J Neurophysiol 10: 409–414.

Levy D, Strassman AM (2002). Mechanical response properties of A and C primary afferent neurons innervating the rat intracranial dura. J Neurophysiol 88: 3021–3031.

Martin VT, Lee J, Behbehani MM (2007). Sensitization of the trigeminal sensory system during different stages of the rat estrous cycle: implications for menstrual migraine. Headache: J Head Face Pain 47: 552–563.

Matharu MS, Goadsby PJ (2002). Persistence of attacks of cluster headache after trigeminal nerve root section. Brain 125: 976–984.

McCleskey EW, Gold MS (1999). Ion channels of nociception. Annu Rev Physiol 61: 835–856.

Mulligan SJ, MacVicar BA (2004). Calcium transients in astrocyte endfeet cause cerebrovascular constrictions. Nature 431: 195–199.

Offenhauser N, Zinck T, Hoffmann J et al. (2005). CGRP release and c-fos expression within trigeminal nucleus caudalis of the rat following glyceryltrinitrate infusion. Cephalalgia 25: 225–236.

Olesen J, Friberg L, Olsen TS et al. (1990). Timing and topography of cerebral blood flow, aura, and headache during migraine attacks. Ann Neurol 28: 791–798.

Ophoff RA, Terwindt GM, Vergouwe MN et al. (1996). Familial hemiplegic migraine and episodic ataxia type-2 are caused by mutations in the Ca^{2+} channel gene CACNL1A4. Cell 87: 543–552.

Peeters M, Gunthorpe MJ, Strijbos PJ et al. (2007). Effects of pan- and subtype-selective NMDA receptor antagonists on cortical spreading depression in the rat: therapeutic potential for migraine. J Pharmacol Exp Ther 321: 564–572.

Penfield W (1935). A contribution to the mechanism of intracranial pain. Assoc Res Nerv Ment Dis 15: 399–416.

Persidsky Y, Ramirez S, Haorah J et al. (2006). Blood–brain Barrier: structural components and function under physiologic and pathologic conditions. J Neuroimmune Pharmacol 1: 223–236.

Peters O, Schipke CG, Hashimoto Y et al. (2003). Different mechanisms promote astrocyte Ca^{2+} waves and spreading depression in the mouse neocortex. J Neurosci 23: 9888–9896.

Raskin NH, Hosobuchi Y, Lamb S (1987). Headache may arise from perturbation of brain. Headache 27: 416–420.

Ray BS, Wolff HG (1940). Experimental studies in headache: Pain-sensitive structures of the head and their structural significance. Arch Surg 41: 813–856.

Richards A, van den Maagdenberg AMJM, Jen JC et al. (2007). C-terminal truncations in human 3[prime]-5 [prime] DNA exonuclease TREX1 cause autosomal dominant retinal vasculopathy with cerebral leukodystrophy. Nat Genet 39: 1068–1070.

Schoenen J (2006). Neurophysiological features of the migrainous brain. Neurol Sci 27(Suppl. 2): S77–S81.

Schoonman GG, van der Grond J, Kortman C et al. (2008). Migraine headache is not associated with cerebral or meningeal vasodilation – a 3T magnetic resonance angiography study. Brain 131: 2192–2200.

Segall L, Mezzetti A, Scanzano R et al. (2005). Alterations in the alpha2 isoform of Na,K-ATPase associated with familial hemiplegic migraine type 2. Proc Natl Acad Sci U S A 102: 11106–11111.

Shields KG, Goadsby PJ (2006). Serotonin receptors modulate trigeminovascular responses in ventroposteromedial nucleus of thalamus: A migraine target? Neurobiol Dis 23: 491–501.

Smith M, Cros D, Sheen V (2002). Hyperperfusion with vasogenic leakage by fMRI in migraine with prolonged aura. Neurology 58: 1308–1310.

Stankewitz A, May A (2007). Cortical excitability and migraine. Cephalalgia 27: 1454–1456.

Strassman AM, Levy D (2006). Response properties of dural nociceptors in relation to headache. J Neurophysiol 95: 1298–1306.

Strassman AM, Raymond SA, Burstein R (1996). Sensitization of meningeal sensory neurons and the origin of headaches. Nature 384: 560–564.

Tajti J, Uddman R, Edvinsson L (2001). Neuropeptide localization in the 'migraine generator' region of the human brainstem. Cephalalgia 21: 96–101.

Takano T, Tian GF, Peng W et al. (2006). Astrocyte-mediated control of cerebral blood flow. Nat Neurosci 9: 260–267.

van den Maagdenberg AMJM, Pietrobon D, Pizzorusso T et al. (2004). A Cacna1a knockin migraine mouse model with increased susceptibility to cortical spreading depression. Neuron 41: 701–710.

Vanmolkot KRJ, Kors EE, Turk U et al. (2006). Two de novo mutations in the Na,K-ATPase gene ATP1A2 associated with pure familial hemiplegic migraine. Eur J. Human Genetics 14: 555–560.

Weiller C, May A, Limmroth V et al. (1995). Brain stem activation in spontaneous human migraine attacks. Nat Med 1: 658–660.

Welch KM, Nagesh V, Aurora SK et al. (2001). Periaqueductal gray matter dysfunction in migraine: cause or the burden of illness? Headache 41: 629–637.

Woods RP, Iacoboni M, Mazziotta JC (1994). Bilateral spreading cerebral hypoperfusion during spontaneous migraine headache. N Engl J Med 331: 1689–1692.

Zonta M, Angulo MC, Gobbo S et al. (2003). Neuron-to-astrocyte signaling is central to the dynamic control of brain microcirculation. Nat Neurosci 6: 43–50.

Handbook of Clinical Neurology, Vol. 97 (3rd series)
Headache
G. Nappi and M.A. Moskowitz, Editors

Chapter 8

Experimental models of migraine

M.G. BUZZI[1] AND C. TASSORELLI[2]*

[1]*Headache Center, IRCCS Santa Lucia Foundation, Rome, Italy*

[2]*Headache Science Center, IRCCS "C. Mondino Institute of Neurology" Foundation and University Center for the Study of Adaptive Disorders and Headache (UCADH), University of Pavia, Pavia, Italy*

INTRODUCTION

In the past two decades, the availability of animal models of migraine has allowed impressive advances in understanding the mechanisms and mediators underlying migraine attacks, as well as the development of new and more specific therapeutic agents. The trigeminovascular system (TVS) has emerged as a critical efferent component, and the mediators of its activity have been identified and characterized, as have some of the receptors involved. Studies involving substances known to induce migraine-like attacks have provided interesting insights into the central nuclei probably involved in the initiation and recurrence of migraine attacks. Furthermore, new molecules, potentially effective in migraine treatment, have been screened and tested in the different experimental models so far available and, having given satisfactory results, are now in the pipeline to become commercially available antimigraine drugs (Figure 8.1).

Over the years, animal models of several types have been devised, proposed, tested, and used. These models are listed in a schematic classification in Table 8.1 (for review see also Bergerot et al., 2006).

VASCULAR MODELS

In vitro

Isolated cranial (meningeal, temporal, basilar) and coronary arteries of animals are used as *in vitro* models of migraine to characterize the receptors in these blood vessels and to study the effects of potential antimigraine molecules. However, it should be borne in mind that a species that is a good model for a certain class of drugs may be less suitable for studying other receptor systems. Blood vessels can be studied using anatomical, physiological, and pharmacological methods and studies are needed to confirm which species provides the best model.

Isolated animal vessels

Vascular segments obtained from several species are mounted in organ baths and contraction or relaxation is measured isometrically. Construction of cumulative concentration response curves is used to determine the potency (pEC_{50}) and efficacy (E_{max}) of a potential antimigraine agent. Experiments in endothelium-denuded blood vessels provide information on the localization of the receptor, while measurements of second messengers or intracellular calcium concentrations (Ishida et al., 2001) may provide information on the receptors involved. The role of endogenous neuropeptides in perivascular nerve endings was investigated in artery segments stimulated chemically (Franco-Cereceda et al., 1987) or electrically to release calcitonin gene-related peptide (CGRP) and other neuropeptides. CGRP receptors have been studied in blood vessels obtained from several species, including the pig, guinea pig, and rat (Jansen-Olesen et al., 2001; Wu et al., 2002). Instead, bovine cerebral arteries (Bouchelet et al., 2000; Roon et al., 2000) and the dog or rabbit saphenous vein have frequently been used to study contractile responses to the triptans.

Isolated human vessels

The therapeutic efficacy of antimigraine drugs is probably mediated by constriction of dilated cranial arteries (Saxena and Tfelt-Hansen, 2005). Models of isolated cranial blood vessels use three cranial arteries: the

*Correspondence to: Cristina Tassorelli, Headache Science Center, IRCCS "C. Mondino Institute of Neurology" Foundation and University Center for the Study of Adaptive Disorders and Headache (UCADH), University of Pavia, Pavia, Italy, Tel: +39(0)382-380425, Fax: +39(0)382-380448, E-mail: cristina.tassorelli@mondino.it

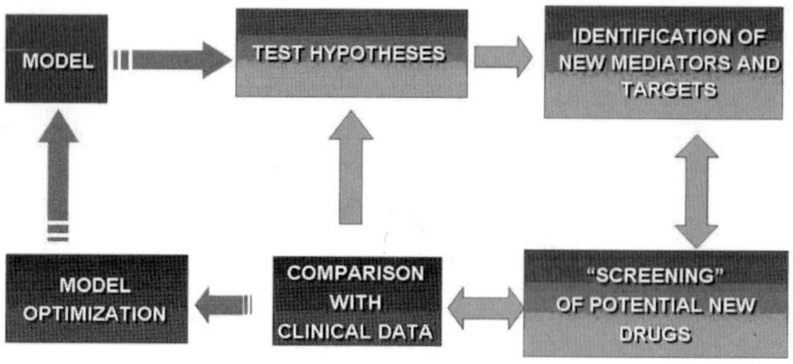

Fig. 8.1. Virtuous cycle connecting experimental models of migraine with advances in understanding based on the disease pathophysiology and treatment and with improvement of the models themselves.

middle meningeal, the basilar, and the temporal. The human middle meningeal artery, in particular, is richly innervated with afferent sensory fibers containing substance P (SP), neurokinin A (NKA), and CGRP originating from the trigeminal ganglion. The rank order of potency of serotonin (5-HT) receptor agonists in this preparation positively correlates with affinity measurements in cell lines expressing the 5-HT_{1B} receptor. Human isolated coronary arteries are used to test the effect of antimigraine drugs on vascular beds other than the cerebral one. The right epicardial coronary artery is the most commonly used segment in isolated coronary blood vessel models.

Advantages

Isolated cerebral blood vessel models offer several advantages, i.e. they make it possible to localize the receptor involved, to investigate the role of endogenous neuropeptides, to measure second messengers or intracellular calcium concentrations, and to evaluate the role of endogenous neuropeptides in perivascular nerve endings. In addition, studies of *in vitro* human models allow the assessment of receptorial cranial selectivity and the collection of reliable information regarding the behavior of these vessels in migraine headache. In particular, denudation of the cranial arteries provides information on whether the receptors are present on the endothelium or in the vascular smooth muscle of arteries. Furthermore, isolated human coronary arteries are useful in analyzing a major potential side-effect of antimigraine drugs, namely chest symptoms (chest pressure, tightness, and pain).

Limitations

These *in vitro* models study drug–receptor interactions at equilibrium without the influence of pharmacokinetic factors, central and autonomic mechanisms, or circulating hormones. In addition, they cannot reflect the complexity of the mechanisms underlying migraine pathophysiology.

Table 8.1

Animal models of migraine

Type of model	Investigated structure or function	Methodology
Vascular (vasoconstriction or vasodilatation)		
In vitro	Isolated arteries and veins	Effects of drugs, modulation of electrical stimulation
In vivo	Carotid arterial bed, arteriovenous anastomoses, pial arteries	Evaluation of vascular resistance, measurement of diameter
Neurovascular		
Plasma protein extravasation (PPE)	Trigeminovascular system	Induction or inhibition of PPE by electrical or chemical stimulation of the ganglion and evaluation of PPE with dyes or radiolabeled tracers
Activation of trigeminal nucleus caudalis (TNC)	Trigeminovascular system Central nociceptive pathways	Meningeal stimulation or electrical/ mechanical stimulation of the superior sagittal sinus
Cortical spreading depression	Vasodilatation and activation of trigeminal neurons by spreading depression	Cortical application of potassium chloride solutions, Fos expression in TNC
Effects of nitric oxide donors	Trigeminovascular system Central nociceptive pathways Autonomic–nociceptive interaction	Neurochemical, cerebrovascular, and nociceptive response to systemic or central administration of nitroglycerine

(Reproduced from Bergerot et al., 2006.)

In vivo

In vivo vascular animal models are developed to mimic cranial vasodilatation as an integral part of the pathophysiology of migraine and they are based on vascular or neurogenic theories (De Vries et al., 1999a). The species most frequently used in these models are pigs and dogs.

Constriction of carotid arteriovenous anastomoses in anaesthetized pigs and of the canine external carotid bed

Arteriovenous anastomoses are precapillary communications between the arteries and veins; they are predominantly located in the scalp, ears, nasal mucosa, eyes, and dura mater in several species, including humans and pigs (Saxena, 1995). It has been shown that several acutely acting antimigraine drugs, including ergot alkaloids and triptans, constrict porcine carotid arteriovenous anastomoses and that a dilatation of these "shunt" vessels may be involved in the pathophysiology of migraine (Heyck, 1969; Saxena, 1995; De Vries et al., 1996, 1999a). Indeed, opening of the carotid arteriovenous anastomoses during a migraine attack might cause a large quantity of oxygenated blood to be shunted directly into the veins, resulting in facial pallor, a lowering of skin temperature, and an increase in vascular pulsations (Saxena, 1995). This increase in vascular pulsations stimulates the so-called stretch receptors located in the blood vessel walls, which in turn activate peptide-containing perivascular trigeminal nerves (e.g., CGRP) (De Vries et al., 1999a; Villalón et al., 2002). Radioactive microspheres are used to measure the carotid arteriovenous anastomotic blood flow and the effects of drugs on this parameter (De Vries et al., 1999b).

Similar to the porcine model is the model of constriction of the canine external carotid bed (De Vries et al., 1999a). This model has proven its merit over the years and has been highly predictive of antimigraine activity in the clinical setting.

Advantages

The major advantage of these models is that one can simultaneously study different vascular beds in order to evaluate the cranioselectivity of antimigraine drugs (De Vries et al., 1999b; Willems et al., 2003). All acutely active antimigraine agents, including ergot alkaloids and triptans, as well as α-adrenoceptor agonists, potently constrict the porcine carotid bed and the corresponding arteriovenous anastomoses (De Vries et al., 1996, 1999b; Willems et al., 1999). These agents also provoke long-lasting vasoconstriction in the canine external carotid bed (Saxena and de Vlaam-Schluter, 1974), although the pharmacological profile of this effect is very complex (Hoyer et al., 1994) and involves subtype-selective α-adrenoceptors (Willems et al., 2003).

Limitations

Although highly predictive of antimigraine activity, these experimental models will only pick up the activity of potential antimigraine drugs that act via vascular mechanisms.

Intravital microscopy

Intravital microscopy makes it possible to study the peripheral branch of the TVS. This model uses a thinned closed cranial window and video microscopy to visualize cranial, dural, and pial blood vessels, and allows measurement of changes in their diameter (Williamson et al., 1997a, b). The cranial window is covered with mineral oil (37 °C) and a branch of the middle meningeal artery is viewed using an intravital microscope, with the image displayed on a television monitor. Electrical stimulation of the cranial window causes a reproducible dural and pial blood vessel dilatation, which involves activation of the trigeminal nerve, via the release of CGRP from presynaptic trigeminal nerve endings (Williamson et al., 1997a; Akerman et al., 2002; Petersen et al., 2004). Similarly, CGRP and nitric oxide (NO), when used in intravital microscopy, are able to cause reproducible dural blood vessel dilatation (Akerman et al., 2002), and therefore the model acts as a direct correlate of the migraine attack. Triptans, 5-$HT_{1B/1D}$ receptor agonists, dihydroergotamine, and CGRP receptor antagonists (administered intravenously) are capable of inhibiting neurogenic dural vasodilatation (Williamson et al., 1997a; Petersen et al., 2004). Other compounds found to inhibit neurogenic dural vasodilatation, and useful in antimigraine therapy, are neuronal NO synthase (NOS) inhibitors and indomethacin, a non-steroidal anti-inflammatory drug (Akerman et al., 2002). Also, cannabinoid CB1 receptor agonists (Akerman et al., 2004), P/Q-, N-, and L-type voltage-dependent calcium channel blockers (Akerman et al., 2003), nociceptin (Bartsch et al., 2002), and adenosine A1 receptor agonists (Honey et al., 2000) were tested in this model and emerged as potential targets in the clinic.

Meningeal blood flow studies using laser Doppler flowmetry

Laser Doppler flowmetry uses changes in blood flow as an indirect measure of vessel diameter. Measurements of meningeal blood flow via laser Doppler flowmetry have also proved successful in predicting antimigraine efficacy. This model was a precursor to the intravital microscopy method for directly measuring changes in dural meningeal blood vessels as an output of trigeminovascular activation, but using an open cranial window. Indeed, some methodologies have combined the two strategies to measure both meningeal and cerebral changes (Petersen et al., 2004). Electrical stimulation of dural sites causes a reproducible increase in meningeal blood flow (Kurosawa et al., 1995; Messlinger et al., 1997), and these changes are attenuated by 5-HT_1 receptor agonists and abolished by a CGRP receptor antagonist (Kurosawa et al., 1995; Messlinger et al., 1997).

Advantages

The intravital microscopy models not only help us to identify compounds that may have therapeutic value in the clinic, but are also able to help us dissect the pharmacology of the TVS, and therefore the mechanisms underlying migraine and the actions of therapeutic compounds. In addition, these models provide information about the tolerability profile of drugs and the anatomy and physiopathology of cortical spreading depression (CSD). The intravital microscopy models directly measure dural vessels rather than measuring blood flow via laser Doppler flowmetry, and measurement of dural vessel diameter may be more relevant to the mechanisms of migraine pain than measurement of dural blood flow.

Measurements of meningeal blood flow via laser Doppler flowmetry were able to predict compounds with a lack of clinical efficacy and have also assisted in dissecting the pharmacology of meningeal nociception and the TVS.

Limitations

Direct measurement of dural vessel diameter gives a direct measure of vasodilatation, while blood flow measurements are complicated by a number of factors, including blood cell velocity, cell concentration, and perfusion pressure, and increases in flow may not be due to vasodilatation alone.

NEUROVASCULAR MODELS

The neurogenic model of migraine implies that any stimulus that depolarizes trigeminal sensory fibers activates the TVS and induces blood flow changes in intra- and extracranial tissues receiving trigeminal innervation (Moskowitz, 1984). The trigeminal pain pathway, as related to migraine, is comprised of three main sites: (1) the trigeminal cells in the ganglion with their projections to the vessels (TVS) and to the brainstem; (2) the trigeminal nucleus caudalis (TNC) in the brainstem; and (3) the brain as the site of pain consciousness. Each of these sites has been suggested to play an essential role in migraine pathophysiology.

Neurogenic inflammation (vasodilatation and plasma protein extravasation) within cephalic tissues has been proposed as a possible mechanism of headache pathogenesis (Mayberg et al., 1984; Moskowitz, 1984). The main mediators of neurogenic inflammation are SP (Lembeck and Holzer, 1979), NKA, and CGRP, which are released upon depolarization of sensory fibers innervating blood vessels (Saria et al., 1985, 1986). Tachykinin (SP and NKA) receptors are located on the endothelium to mediate endothelium-dependent vasodilatation and increased permeability, whereas receptors located on vascular smooth muscle mediate CGRP-induced vasodilatation.

The dura mater is an important source of headache pain (Ray and Wolff, 1940), provides a thick covering for the brain, and contains blood vessels with fenestrated capillary endothelium (Andres et al., 1987). The dura and its attendant blood vessels are innervated by trigeminal and upper sensory nerve fibers which contain the vasoactive peptides (SP, NKA, and CGRP) (Edvinsson and Uddman, 1982; Mayberg et al., 1984; Jansen et al., 1986). Small perivascular unmyelinated C fibers reside within the adventitial layer and upon depolarization they release the above peptides to produce neurogenic plasma extravasation.

Activation and modulation of the trigeminovascular system

Trigeminal stimulation and plasma protein extravasation

Plasma protein extravasation can be elicited in the rat dura mater by unilateral electrical trigeminal ganglion stimulation (UETGS) or chemical stimulation. UETGS has been performed in rats (Markowitz et al., 1987) by means of stereotactic lowering of a bipolar electrode in the trigeminal ganglion through which an electrical stimulus was delivered at a magnitude of 1.2 mA, 5 Hz, for 5 min. Radiolabeled albumin, given intravenously prior to stimulation, served to detect the amount of plasma extravasation following the stimulus. Dura mater from the stimulated side and from the non-stimulated side were compared to detect differences in plasma protein leakage, according to counts of leaked radioactive albumin. Protein leakage also occurred in extracranial tissues (conjunctiva, eyelid, lip, and tongue) receiving trigeminal innervation (Buzzi and Moskowitz, 1990). Following UETGS, plasma protein leakage was observed in the dura mater on light microscopy by means of intravenous injection of horseradish peroxidase (HRP), which usually binds to plasma protein and can be visualized as an electron-dense HRP reaction product (Buzzi et al., 1992). Evans blue dye was concomitantly administered along with active tracers, in order to confirm the correct location of the electrode (by enhancing the blue color of the skin on the stimulated side). The effects of the antimigraine drugs, ergot derivatives and sumatriptan, were tested in this model and were found to block protein leakage effectively (Buzzi and Moskowitz, 1990). In order to verify whether their effect was mediated by vasoconstriction, ergot alkaloids and sumatriptan were tested in rats in conditions of exogenous SP-induced protein leakage and vasodilatation (Buzzi and Moskowitz, 1990). Leakage was not blocked and a mechanism of action mediated by prejunctional receptors for ergots and sumatriptan has been postulated in this model (Buzzi and Moskowitz, 1990). Pharmacological data (Humphrey et al., 1988) suggested that a 5-HT receptor subtype mediates the effects of sumatriptan in the UETGS model. Results obtained by using different 5-HT agonists and antagonists in the same experimental setting proved that the effects of sumatriptan were highly consistent with a $5\text{-HT}_{1B/D}$-mediated activity (Buzzi et al., 1991).

Activation of trigeminal sensory fibers innervating cephalic blood vessels has also been obtained by systemic administration of capsaicin (the pungent ingredient of hot pepper) and plasma protein leakage detected, as described above, in rat dura mater, eyelid, and lip of capsaicin-stimulated versus non-stimulated animals (Markowitz et al., 1987; Saito et al., 1988; Buzzi and Moskowitz, 1990). Degranulation of mast cells accompanies the plasma leakage response in the dura mater following UETGS (Dimitriadou et al., 1991), and contributes to the inflammatory reaction in this tissue during migraine attacks (Waeber and Moskowitz, 2005; Levy et al., 2006). Mast cell degranulation was inhibited by sumatriptan (Buzzi et al, 1992). A stimulation intensity-dependent increase in CGRP plasma levels was observed during UETGS in the venous blood obtained from the superior sagittal sinus (SSS) (Buzzi et al., 1991). Sumatriptan reduced this CGRP increase, confirming the activity of the drug on prejunctional receptors on trigeminal sensory fibers. The latter observation is in agreement with the increase of CGRP plasma levels in the cat following trigeminal ganglion stimulation, and in blood obtained from the jugular vein of humans during migraine attacks (Goadsby and Edvinsson, 1993). CGRP levels fell in humans following sumatriptan administration, and the migraine pain improved as well (Goadsby and Edvinsson, 1993).

Peripheral activation of trigeminal fibers is reflected in the modulation of cells receiving primary afferent inputs. As demonstrated by Nishimori and co-workers (1989), UETGS increases preproenkephalin expression in laminae I and II of the ipsilateral TNC (Figure 8.2).

Chemical stimulation of the meninges

Subarachnoid hemorrhage is one of the most predictable and dramatic causes of vascular headaches (Wolff, 1972). The pain is thought to be attributable, to a large degree, to sensitization and stimulation of perivascular afferents and to reflect increased neurotransmission within sensory fibers projecting to cephalic blood vessels (Moskowitz et al., 1989). Subarachnoid hemorrhage alters levels of tachykinins and mRNA in trigeminal ganglia and in perivascular axons (Linnik et al., 1989). SP levels increase in the trigeminal ganglion 2 days after intravenous injection. Accordingly, preprotachykinin mRNA, encoding for the peptide, increases in the trigeminal ganglion. SP increases in the trigeminal ganglion may reflect compensation for the depletion occurring in perivascular fibers.

Direct stimulation of primary sensory neurons supplying the meninges has been obtained through injection of meningeal irritants via microcatheter into the cisterna magna through the atlantooccipital membrane of anesthetized rats (Mitsikostas et al., 1998), mice

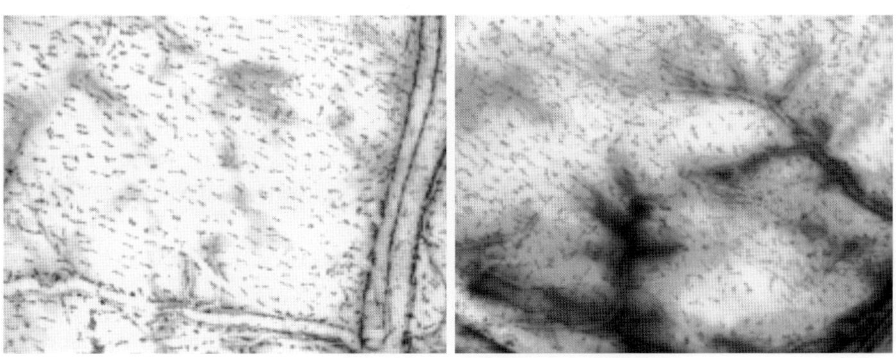

Fig. 8.2. Samples of rat dura mater obtained from the side ipsilateral to unilateral electrical trigeminal ganglion stimulation (right) and from the unstimulated side (left) after intravenous injection of horseradish peroxidase (HRP). HRP leakage from vessels is due to increased permeability following trigeminal fiber depolarization. (Reproduced from Buzzi et al., 1992.)

(Mitsikostas et al., 2002), and guinea pigs (Cutrer et al., 1999). Meningeal irritants include autologous blood (Linnik et al., 1989; Nozaki et al., 1992a), capsaicin (Mitsikostas et al., 1998), and carrageenin (Nozaki et al., 1992b). Fos protein immunoreactivity in both sides of the TNC is detected 2 h after injection. Capsaicin induces Fos protein expression in a dose-dependent manner (Mitsikostas et al., 1998), and the response is inhibited by destruction of unmyelinated fibers (Nozaki et al., 1992a). This experimental setting has limitations due to the lack of intra-animal control – it is not possible to explore lateralization of Fos protein expression within the TNC – and also due to possible damage caused by capsaicin that may alter the blood–brain barrier functioning, leading to indirect activation of central sites (Mitsikostas and Sanchez del Rio, 2001).

Stimulation of the superior sagittal sinus

The SSS is one of the sources of cephalic pain. Indeed, stimulation of this structure in humans produces pain referred to the head (Ray and Wolff, 1940). Therefore, stimulation of the SSS in animals has been considered a possible experimental model for evaluating mechanisms underlying head pain. SSS stimulation has been performed in rats, cats (Kaube et al., 1993), and nonhuman primates (Goadsby and Hoskin, 1999) in order to study trigeminovascular nociceptive afferents. Electrical stimulation of the pain-producing structures of the head, including the SSS, as well as chemical and electrical stimulation of trigeminal sensory fibers (see above), are established methods of trigeminovascular activation and they have been widely used to investigate the activation of neurons, reflected in increased Fos expression (see also paragraph on Fos expression) in the TNC following trigeminal ganglion, dural or SSS stimulation in the cat, and to evaluate the effects, on Fos, of a variety of compounds. 5-HT$_{1B/1D}$ receptor agonists zolmitriptan (Goadsby and Hoskin, 1998) and eletriptan (Goadsby and Hoskin, 1999; Knyihár-Csillik et al., 2000) have both been shown to reduce Fos immunoreactivity in the trigeminocervical complex, whereas the less lipophilic sumatriptan was unable to reduce Fos expression (Goadsby and Hoskin, 1999) unless the blood–brain barrier was disrupted (Kaube et al., 1993). *In vivo* pretreatment with CP93,129, sumatriptan, or dihydroergotamine inhibits Fos expression in the TNC induced by subarachnoid hemorrhage (Moskowitz and Macfarlane, 1993). Taken together, this evidence suggests a peripheral as well as central site of action for the triptans, a hypothesis that has now been definitively confirmed. The antagonists of the *N*-methyl-D-aspartate receptor (MK-801) and the GluR5 kainate receptor ([3S,4aR,6S,8aR]-6-[4-carboxyimidazol-1-ylmethyl] decahydroisoquinoline-3-carboxylic acid) both inhibit Fos expression in this model of trigeminovascular activation (Classey et al., 2001; Filla et al., 2002), implicating their receptor systems in the pathophysiology of migraine.

Advantages

The neurogenic inflammation model in animals has provided a simple and reproducible experimental setting for testing the effects of different compounds on the peripheral and central components of cephalic pain. This was the case, for instance of CGRP antagonists (Storer et al., 2004). The similarity of the trigeminal innervation across species has made it possible to draw conclusions on the neurophysiological responses to electrical or chemical stimulation of the trigeminal fibers (for review see Goadsby et al., 2009).

Limitations

The lack of an adequate experimental human model of induced neurogenic inflammation and the likely species differences in receptor subtypes are the main limitations preventing us from establishing the full clinical relevance of the data obtained from animal studies.

Fos expression within the trigeminal nucleus caudalis as a marker of trigeminal nociception

Fos protein is used as a marker of nociception and of neuronal activation. It is known that a peripheral noxious stimulation induces Fos immunoreactivity within laminae I and II of the spinal dorsal horns (Williams et al., 1990). Fos expression within the TNC may be induced by applying mechanical, electrical, or chemical stimuli to either extracranial or intracranial tissues innervated by the trigeminal nerve (e.g., SSS stimulation, chemical stimulation of the meninges, and trigeminal ganglion stimulation). Thus, Fos immunoreactivity offers a method for identifying subpopulations of neurons activated in response to noxious stimuli, or other types of stimuli that may be relevant to migraine (Tassorelli and Joseph, 1995), and the relative nociceptive pathways. Expression of the gene can be measured via Northern blot analysis (Ashmawi et al., 2003) or with *in situ* hybridization (Nakagawa et al., 2003), while the protein expression is usually visualized by means of immunocytochemical techniques (Benjamin et al., 2004).

Advantages

Studies based on the evaluation of *c-fos* gene activation have provided information on the neuroanatomy of the structures that may be involved in migraine pathophysiology, the timing of their activation, as well as on possible modulation of this activation by pharmacological probes.

Limitations

Fos immunhistochemistry provides information on metabolically activated pathways, but not on circuits that may be inhibited by a given stimulus. In addition, absence of Fos expression does not necessarily mean that the neuronal population was not activated; it may simply mean that the *c-fos* pathways were not activated by the stimulus.

Nitric oxide donors

Nitric oxide (NO) plays a pivotal role in the control of several physiological phenomena in the central nervous system, such as nociception, toxicity, degeneration, and memory. NO donors have been used as probes to study the role of NO in a variety of neurological diseases (Rayman et al., 2003; Kakizawa et al., 2007). A relationship between NO and migraine has been suggested since headaches are a side-effect of NO donors (Iversen and Olesen, 1996).

Nitrovasodilators, in view of their vasodilatory effect, were originally used in the treatment of ischemic cardiac disease (Parker et al., 1995) to produce NO in several body tissues (including the brain). This has favored a resurgence of scientific interest in this group of substances in the field of the neurosciences. Among the various nitrovasodilators commercially available, nitroglycerine (NTG) is a classic NO donor that acts as trigger or provoking agent in cluster headache (Ekbom, 1968). Furthermore, infusion of NTG leads to a migraine attack in migraineurs with a latency of 4–6 h (Iversen et al., 1989; Olesen et al., 1994; Sances et al., 2004) and inhibition of NOS has antimigraine activity (Lassen et al., 2003). There exists experimental evidence of an accumulation of NTG in the rat brain tissue, since the NO donor is highly lipophilic and easily crosses the blood–brain barrier (Torfgård et al., 1991). Systemic administration of this organic nitrate induces, in the rat, neuronal activation in several brain nuclei belonging to the neurovegetative, neuroendocrine, behavioral, and nociceptive systems (such as the TNC) (Tassorelli and Joseph, 1995; Tassorelli et al., 1997).

The precise mechanisms involved in NO-triggered migraine remain to be determined. The temporal profile of neuronal activation following NTG administration shows that neuronal activation begins as early as 60 min postinjection in brain areas that control the cardiovascular function, and reaches its maximum expression 3 h later in nociceptive and integrative structures (Tassorelli et al., 1997). This modulated temporal course suggests a dual mechanism of action for NTG on the brain: an initial effect on the vascular compartment followed by the involvement of integrative-nociceptive structures. This activation, which in some areas develops with a latency of hours, contrasts with the very short plasma half-life of the drug, although this longer latency may be a consequence of NTG accumulation in the brain (Torfgård et al., 1991). Reuter et al. (2001) demonstrated that NTG administration induces an up-regulation of proinflammatory genes, with a subsequent, delayed inflammatory reaction in the dura mater of the rat. Intravenous NTG increases NO production within macrophages of dura mater with a delay of hours, via the expression of the inducible isoform of NOS (iNOS) (Reuter et al., 2001, 2002). iNOS expression is preceded by a significant increase in the activity of nuclear factor kappa B (NF-κB), a transcription factor that is crucial for inflammation reaction (Reuter et al., 2002).

Co-localization studies have shown that NTG-induced neuronal activation takes place in adrenergic, nitrergic and neuropeptidergic structures (Tassorelli et al., 1999), indicating some of the possible signaling pathways involved in the phenomenon. Neuropharmacologic manipulations have suggested that NTG-induced neuronal activation probably involves exogenous (NTG-derived) NO that might act directly at both the vascular and neuronal levels, or indirectly activate neurovascular responses via multiple pathways (Greco et al., 2005; Tassorelli et al., 2007). Previous data support the idea that cyclic guanosine monophosphate is an important mediator of the NTG effect in vascular and neuronal structures (Tassorelli et al., 2004), however recently it was shown that NTG administration is capable of activating the cyclooxygenase-2 pathway within cerebral areas of the rat, explaining the pronociceptive effect of NTG described in animal and human models of pain (Tassorelli et al., 2000, 2003, 2007).

Indeed, Tassorelli et al. (2003) have shown that NTG-induced changes in central and/or peripheral neurotransmission are related to a hyperalgesic state and this is reflected in the sustained activation of nociceptive nuclei in the rat (Tassorelli and Joseph, 1995). This explanation could also account for the initiation of a spontaneous migraine-like attack in predisposed subjects following NTG administration (Iversen et al., 1989; Sances et al., 2004). This hypothesis has also been supported by other findings obtained by other groups, which strongly suggest a definite role for NTG in pain mediation. Pardutz et al. (2000) showed that NTG administration increases the number of NOS-immunoreactive cells in the rat spinal TNC, which points to the activation of second-order neurons through a presynaptic excitatory mechanism. Lambert et al. (2000) demonstrated that systemic NTG increases the firing rate of second-order trigeminal neurons, which transport inputs from cranial structures via a serotonin-mediated

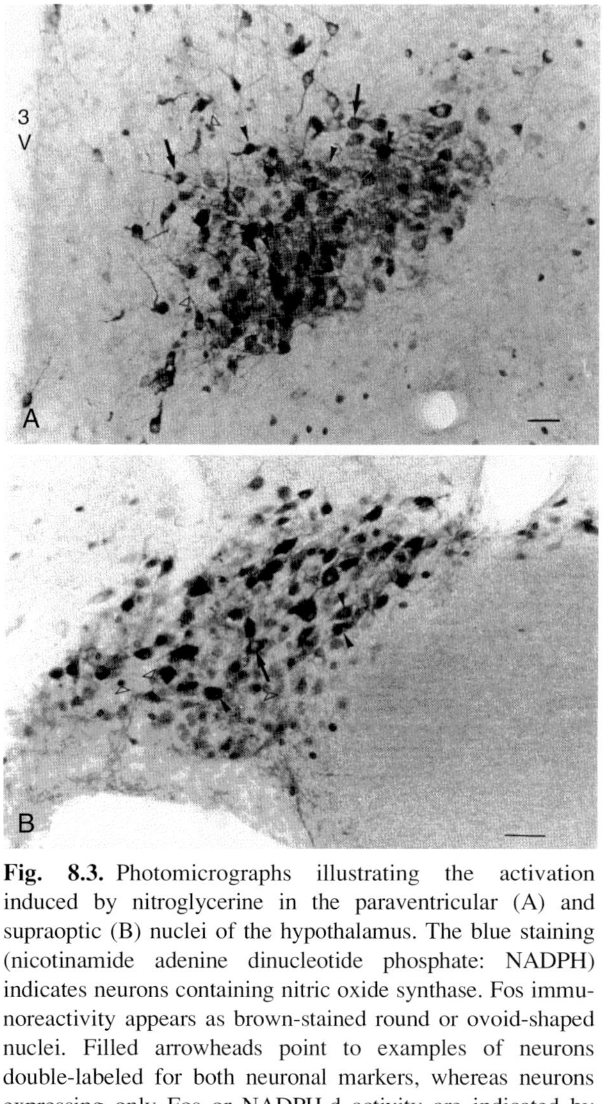

Fig. 8.3. Photomicrographs illustrating the activation induced by nitroglycerine in the paraventricular (A) and supraoptic (B) nuclei of the hypothalamus. The blue staining (nicotinamide adenine dinucleotide phosphate: NADPH) indicates neurons containing nitric oxide synthase. Fos immunoreactivity appears as brown-stained round or ovoid-shaped nuclei. Filled arrowheads point to examples of neurons double-labeled for both neuronal markers, whereas neurons expressing only Fos or NADPH-d activity are indicated by empty arrowheads and arrows, respectively. Scale bar: 60 μm. 3V, third ventricle. (Reproduced from Tassorelli et al., 1999.)

mechanism that is blocked by the administration of selective 5-$HT_{1B/1D}$ agonists (Figure 8.3).

Advantages

The data obtained using the animal methods based on the administration of NO donors have yielded an increasing body of evidence for a better understanding of migraine pathophysiology. In addition, they have provided information on potential new targets for antimigraine drugs (Greco et al., 2009; Vàmos et al., 2009).

Areas of controversy

There is some controversy, in the literature, with regard to the neurochemical effects of NTG. For instance, some investigators (Jones et al., 2001; Martin and Martin, 2001; Offenhauser et al., 2005) failed to detect NTG-induced Fos expression in the TNC. However, several possible variables must be carefully controlled when using NTG-based animal models to study the TVS: (1) the drug dose and modality of administration; (2) the drug-dissolving vehicle; (3) the chosen observation time; and (4) systems for administration of the drug. In studies where Fos expression was not detected in the rat, doses of NTG similar to those in human migraine studies were used (0.2–2 g/kg intravenously). In studies in which NTG-induced Fos expression was consistently noted, higher doses of NTG were given subcutaneously. Finally, as regards the issue of the duration of observations, it must be noted that, in order to be relevant to migraine, the effects of NTG infusion in studies using this technique will need to be observed for several hours in order to reflect the timing of the development of migraine attacks (Iversen et al., 1989).

Cortical spreading depression

Leão's (1944) hypothesis that CSD could play a role in migraine has become very credible. Functional magnetic resonance imaging data from the human visual cortex provide strong evidence that CSD underlies migraine visual aura (Hadjikhani et al., 2001), and a similar phenomenon may underlie migraine auras emanating from other brain regions. CSD can be induced in animals by chemical (superfusion with potassium chloride solution), pinprick, or electrical stimulation over the cortex surface. A reduction in the threshold for the induction of CSD has been demonstrated in female mice compared with male mice (Brennan et al., 2007; Figure 8.4).

CSD provokes the expression of Fos protein-like immunoreactivity within neurons of the TNC via trigeminovascular mechanisms (Moskowitz et al., 1993).

c-fos gene activation following unilateral spreading depression is inhibited both by sumatriptan and trigeminal denervation, suggesting a role for peripheral fibers in this model and their involvement in the mechanism of action of the drugs (Moskowitz et al., 1993).

CSD induces long-lasting blood flow enhancement within the middle meningeal artery, consistent with the consequences of a noxious stimulus within the trigeminal receptive field (Bolay et al., 2002). Vasodilatation is caused by the release of vasoactive agents from parasympathetic projections originating from parasympathetic nuclei of cranial nerve VII. Parasympathetic neurons are activated by monosynaptic connections with the TNC. CSD also causes plasma protein leakage into the ipsilateral dura mater

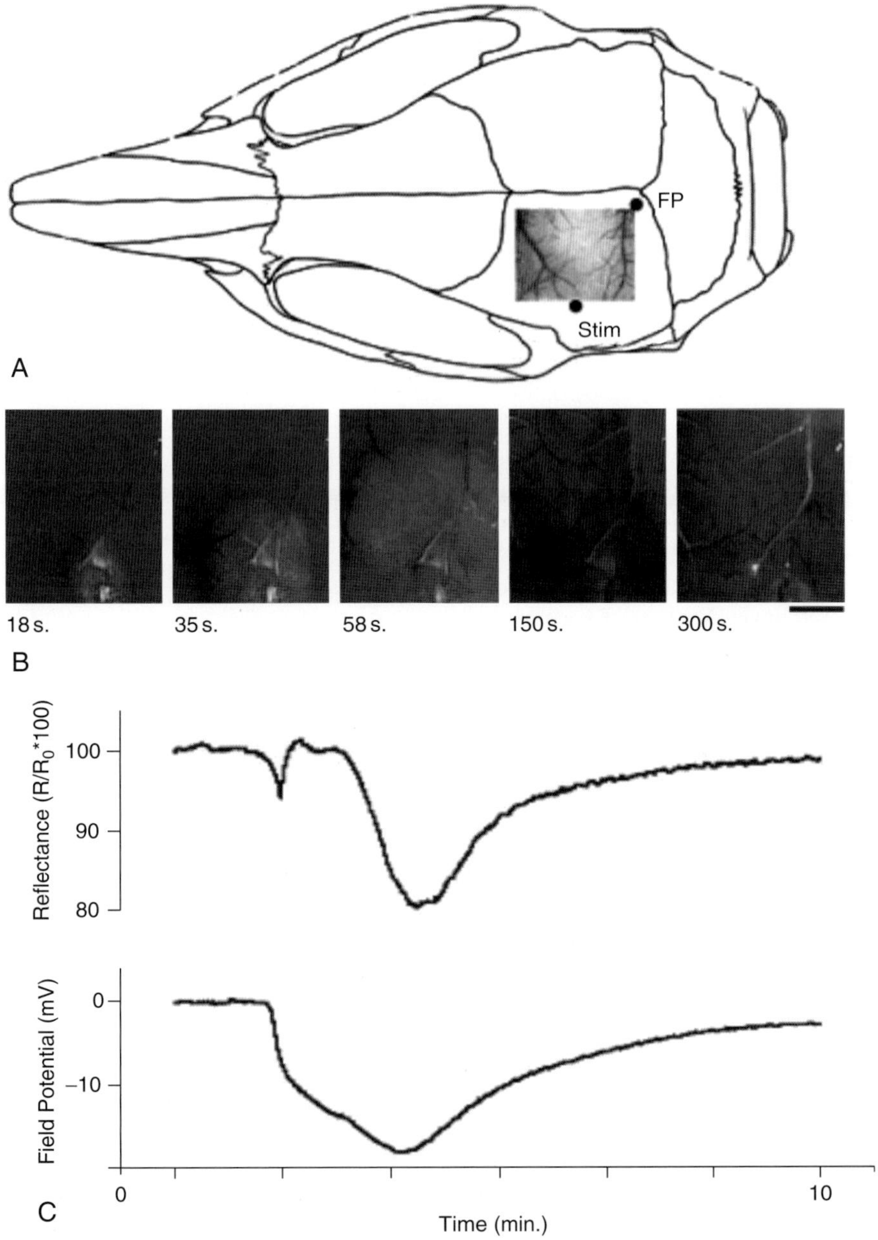

Fig. 8.4. Optical intrinsic signal imaging of cortical spreading depression (CSD) in mice. B shows the propagation of CSD, while C shows the time course of the optical signal and the field potential changes, from a region of interest immediately adjacent to the field potential electrode. FP: field potential. (Reproduced from Brennan et al., 2007.)

(Bolay et al., 2002). As detailed above, protein extravasation is mediated via release of proinflammatory peptides from trigeminal axon collaterals innervating the meninges. This finding supports the complex neuronal-neurovascular model of the migraine attack. Meningeal inflammation persists after CSD subsides, an observation which suggests that intense and transient brain activity can cause sustained meningeal events and C-fiber discharge.

Advantages

The demonstration that CSD is a mechanism underlying neurovascular events is of great interest since it creates a link between cortical and peripheral components and opens up the way for the development of adequate preventive therapies that may act centrally as inhibitors of migraine episodes. The ability of preventive therapies commonly used in the prophylaxis of migraine without aura to suppress CSD events in animal models (Ayata et al., 2006) also suggests that migraine with aura and migraine without aura may be different manifestations of the same disorder.

Limitations

It remains to be elucidated whether silent aura events occur in migraine without aura and where they take place, prior to the activation of the peripheral component of the pain.

Central pain sensitization and the trigeminal nerve

The theory of chemical activation of meningeal perivascular sensory fibers suggests that ions, protons, and inflammatory agents that activate and sensitize peripheral nociceptors are released in the vicinity of sensory fibers innervating the dura after an episode of CSD or neurogenic inflammation. Exposure of perivascular fibers to chemical agents alters their sensitivity to mechanical stimuli and leads to the sensitization observed in head pain. Application of acidic and inflammatory agents to the dura enabled peripheral fibers innervating the dura (Strassman et al., 1996) to respond to mechanical stimuli that had initially evoked minimal or no response. This phenomenon may explain the hypersensitivity of migraine patients to normally induced changes in intracranial pressure, as in bending or coughing. This hypothesis has been tested in the rat by recording changes in the responsiveness of dura-sensitive neurons in the TNC to mechanical stimulation of their dural receptive fields and to mechanical or thermal stimulation of their cutaneous receptive fields after local application of inflammatory mediators or acid agents to the dura (Burstein et al., 1998). Brief chemical stimulation induced significantly increased sensitivity to mechanical indentation of the dura as well as increased cutaneous mechanosensitivity and thermosensitivity. The role of a central mechanism has been suggested in this model, since local application of lidocaine to the dura abolished the response to dural stimulation but not to cutaneous stimulation.

According to these findings, chemical activation and sensitization of dura-sensitive peripheral nociceptors could lead to enhanced responses in central neurons, and central sensitization could therefore result in extracranial tenderness in the absence of extracranial pathology. In subsequent studies (Yamamura et al., 1998), it has been demonstrated that non-noxious stimuli in sensitized dura induce cardiovascular responses, at a magnitude similar to that observed following noxious stimuli, thus confirming that non-noxious stimuli are perceived as noxious in sensitized tissues. All the above data support the notion of peripheral and central sensitization during migraine attacks (Burstein, 2001).

Advantages

The recognition of sensitization phenomena in migraine patients may contribute to the development of targeted therapies: not only early treatments for migraine attacks, but also the development of compounds able to prevent the evolution of episodic forms of migraine into chronic pain.

Limitations

In order to develop targeted drugs that may reduce the risk of chronic pain, detailed neurophysiology and functional neuroimaging investigations are needed to demonstrate the presence of sensitization in the dura mater and central nuclei in humans.

GENETIC FACTORS AND MIGRAINE

Genetic factors play an important role in migraine pathophysiology (Kors et al., 2004), probably by lowering the threshold for migraine. Familial hemiplegic migraine (FHM) is an autosomal-dominant subtype of migraine with aura. Apart from the characteristic hemiparesis, typical attacks of FHM are identical to those of the common forms of migraine. This rare and severe form of migraine has been associated with three different mutations identified in three genes encoding subunits of a calcium channel (CACNA1A), a sodium-potassium pump (ATP1A2) and a sodium channel (SCN1A) (Ophoff et al., 1996; De Fusco et al., 2003; Dichgans et al., 2005). The *CACNA1A* gene (FHM1) encodes the pore-forming α_1-subunit of voltage-gated neuronal $Ca_v2.1$ (P/Q-type) Ca^{2+} channels; the *ATP1A2* gene (FHM2) encodes the α_2-subunit of Na^+-K^+ pumps, while the *SCN1A* gene (FHM3) encodes the α_1-subunit of neuronal sodium channels. Missense mutations of *CACNA1A* cause an increased open probability of P/Q-type calcium channels and a shift of the activation voltage range towards depolarization (Tottene et al., 2002) with an increased glutamate release in cortical neurons. Fifteen different missense mutations in the *CACNA1A* gene have been associated with FHM.

Although the consequences of *CACNA1A* gene mutations on trigeminal nociception remain undocumented, one can predict that the gain-of-function of calcium channels at synaptic level may lead to hyperexcitability of nociceptive trigeminovascular pathways due to enhanced release of vasoactive neuropeptides from perivascular nerve endings and, possibly, facilitation of sensitization of second-order central trigeminal neurons. In fact, within the TVS, P/Q-type channels, together with N-type channels, control CGRP release from capsaicin-sensitive trigeminovascular afferents (Hong et al., 1999). Some mutations cause pure FHM, whereas other mutations may cause FHM plus additional neurological symptoms such as ataxia or coma (Ducros et al., 2001). Mutations in *ATP1A2* result in either a loss of Na-K pump function or a reduced affinity of potassium for Na-K pumps (De Fusco et al., 2003; Segall et al., 2004). Consequently, extracellular K^+ levels might be expected to be higher in *ATP1A2*. FHM3 mutations in the *SCN1A* gene cause a more rapid recovery from fast inactivation of neuronal Nav1.1 sodium channels after depolarization. Because these sodium channels are crucial for the generation and propagation of action potentials, FHM3 mutations are likely to cause an increased frequency of neuronal firing and enhanced neuronal excitability and neurotransmitter release (Dichgans et al., 2005).

Genetic models

CACNA1A mouse models

Several mouse *CACNA1A* mutants, either natural or transgenic, are available, most of them with variable symptoms of ataxia and epilepsy. The most promising *CACNA1A* model for migraine mechanisms is a recently generated knock-in (KI) mouse model carrying the human FHM1 R192Q mutation in the endogenous *CACNA1A* gene (van den Maagdenberg et al., 2004). Unlike the other *CACNA1A* mice, R192Q KI mice do not exhibit any overt phenotype. The results in R192Q KI mice may explain the mechanism underlying the increased susceptibility of the migraine brain to aura and reinforce the hypothesis that migraine is associated with neuronal hyperexcitability at cortical and, possibly, brainstem level (van den Maagdenberg et al., 2004).

It has been reported that mutated Cav2.1 channels allow increased calcium influx and cause more neurotransmitter release. This might, in turn, be associated with transient neuronal hyperexcitability. Cav2.1 channels can best be studied in their native neuronal environment at their endogenous level of expression, evaluating how they affect mechanisms involved in migraine such as neurotransmission and CSD. Cav2.1 channels are expressed in all brain structures that have been implicated in the pathogenesis of migraine, including the cerebral cortex, the trigeminal ganglia, and brainstem nuclei involved in the central control of nociception (Pietrobon and Striessnig, 2003).

ATP1A2 mouse models

Transgenic mice in which the *ATP1A2* (FHM2) gene was abolished (*ATP1A2*-null mutants) have been generated, but they die immediately after birth because they cannot breathe spontaneously (Ikeda et al., 2003). Heterozygous $ATP1A2^{+/-}$ mice revealed enhanced fear and anxiety behaviors after conditioned fear stimuli, probably due to neuronal hyperactivity in the amygdala and piriform cortex (Ikeda et al., 2003). Therefore, these mice do not, as yet, seem to provide an adequate substrate for learning more about the role of the described FHM *ATP1A2* mutation in the pathogenesis of migraine.

Acknowledgment

The authors are grateful to Dr Rosaria Greco for her support in the preparation of the manuscript.

References

Akerman S, Williamson DJ, Kaube H et al. (2002). Nitric oxide synthase inhibitors can antagonize neurogenic and calcitonin gene-related peptide induced dilation of dural meningeal vessels. Br J Pharmacol 137: 62–68.

Akerman S, Kaube H, Goadsby PJ (2003). Vanilloid type 1 receptors (VR_1) on trigeminal sensory nerve fibres play a minor role in neurogenic dural vasodilatation, and are involved in capsaicin-induced dural dilation. Br J Pharmacol 140: 718–724.

Akerman S, Kaube H, Goadsby PJ (2004). Anandamide acts as a vasodilator of dural blood vessels in vivo by activating TRPV1 receptors. Br J Pharmacol 142: 1354–1360.

Andres KH, von Düring M, Muszinsky K et al. (1987). Nerve fibers and their terminals of the dura mater encephali of the rat. Anat Embryol (Berl) 175: 289–301.

Ashmawi HA, Chambergo FS, Araújo Palmeira CC et al. (2003). The effects of pyrilamine and cimetidine on mrna *c-fos* expression and nociceptive flinching behavior in rats. Anesth Analg 97: 541–546.

Ayata C, Jin H, Kudo C et al. (2006). Suppression of cortical spreading depression in migraine prophylaxis. Ann Neurol 59: 652–661.

Bartsch T, Akerman S, Goadsby PJ (2002). The ORL-1 (NOP1) receptor ligand nociceptin/orphanin FQ (N/OFQ) inhibits neurogenic dural vasodilatation in the rat. Neuropharmacology 43: 991–998.

Benjamin L, Levy MJ, Lasalandra MP et al. (2004). Hypothalamic activation after stimulation of the superior sagittal sinus in the cat: a Fos study. Neurobiol Dis 16: 500–505.

Bergerot A, Holland PR, Akerman S et al. (2006). Animal models of migraine: looking at the component parts of a complex disorder. Eur J Neurosci 24: 1517–1534.

Bolay H, Reuter U, Dunn AK et al. (2002). Intrinsic brain activity triggers trigeminal meningeal afferents in a migraine model. Nat Med 8: 136–142.

Bouchelet I, Case B, Olivier A et al. (2000). No contractile effect for 5-HT_{1D} and 5-HT_{1F} receptor agonists in human and bovine cerebral arteries: similarity with human coronary artery. Br J Pharmacol 129: 501–508.

Brennan KC, Romero Reyes M, López Valdés HE et al. (2007). Reduced threshold for cortical spreading depression in female mice. Ann Neurol 61: 603–606.

Burstein R (2001). Deconstructing migraine headache into peripheral and central sensitization. Pain 89: 107–110.

Burstein R, Yamamura H, Malick A et al. (1998). Chemical stimulation of the intracranial dura induces enhanced response to facial stimulation in brain stem trigeminal neurons. J Neurophysiol 79: 964–982.

Buzzi MG, Moskowitz MA (1990). The antimigraine drug, sumatriptan (GR43175), selectively blocks neurogenic plasma extravasation from blood vessels in dura mater. Br J Pharmacol 99: 202–206.

Buzzi MG, Carter WB, Shimizu T et al. (1991). Dihydroergotamine and sumatriptan attenuate levels of CGRP in plasma in rat superior sagittal sinus during electrical stimulation of the trigeminal ganglion. Neuropharmacology 30: 1193–1200.

Buzzi MG, Dimitriadou V, Theoharides TC et al. (1992). 5-Hydroxytryptamine receptor agonists for the abortive treatment of vascular headaches block mast cell, endothelial and platelet activation within the rat dura mater after trigeminal stimulation. Brain Res 583: 137–149.

Classey JD, Knight E, Goadsby PJ (2001). The NMDA receptor antagonist MK-801 reduces Fos-like immunoreactivity within the trigeminocervical complex following superior sagittal sinus stimulation in the cat. Brain Res 907: 117–124.

Cutrer FM, Mitsikostas DD, Ayata G et al. (1999). Attenuation by butalbital of capsaicin-induced *c-fos*-like immunoreactivity in trigeminal nucleus caudalis. Headache 39: 697–704.

De Fusco M, Marconi R, Silvestri L et al. (2003). Haploinsufficiency of ATP1A2 encoding the Na^+/K^+ pump $\alpha 2$ subunit associated with familial hemiplegic migraine type 2. Nat Genet 33: 192–196.

De Vries P, Heiligers JC, Villalón CM et al. (1996). Blockade of porcine carotid vascular response to sumatriptan by GR 127935, a selective 5-HT_{1D} receptor antagonist. Br J Pharmacol 118: 85–92.

De Vries P, Villalón CM, Saxena PR (1999a). Pharmacological aspects of experimental headache models in relation to acute antimigraine therapy. Eur J Pharmacol 375: 61–74.

De Vries P, Villalón CM, Saxena PR (1999b). Pharmacology of triptans. Emerg Drugs 4: 107–125.

Dichgans M, Freilinger T, Eckstein G et al. (2005). Mutation in the neuronal voltage-gated sodium channel SCN1A in familial hemiplegic migraine. Lancet 336: 371–377.

Dimitriadou V, Buzzi MG, Moskowitz MA et al. (1991). Trigeminal sensory fiber stimulation induces morphological changes reflecting secretion in rat dura mater mast cells. Neuroscience 44: 97–112.

Ducros A, Denier C, Joutel A et al. (2001). The clinical spectrum of familial hemiplegic migraine associated with mutations in a neuronal calcium channel. N Engl J Med 345: 17–24.

Edvinsson L, Uddman R (1982). Immunohistochemical localization and dilatatory effect of substance P on human cerebral vessels. Brain Res 232: 466–471.

Ekbom K (1968). Nitrolglycerin as a provocative agent in cluster headache. Arch Neurol 19: 487–493.

Filla SA, Winter MA, Johnson KW et al. (2002). Ethyl (3S,4ar,6S,8ar))6-(4-ethoxycarbonylimidazol)1-ylmethyl) decahydroiso-quinoline)3-carboxylic ester: a prodrug of a GluR5 kainate receptor antagonist active in two animal models of acute migraine. J Med Chem 45: 4383–4386.

Franco-Cereceda A, Rudehill A, Lundberg JM (1987). Calcitonin gene-related peptide but not substance P mimics capsaicin-induced coronary vasodilation in the pig. Eur J Pharmacol 142: 235–243.

Goadsby PJ, Edvinsson L (1993). The trigeminovascular system and migraine: studies characterizing cerebrovascular and neuropeptide changes seen in humans and cats. Ann Neurol 33: 48–56.

Goadsby PJ, Hoskin KL (1998). Serotonin inhibits trigeminal nucleus activity evoked by craniovascular stimulation through a 5HT1B/1D receptor: a central action in migraine. Ann Neurol 43: 711–718.

Goadsby PJ, Hoskin KL (1999). Differential effects of low dose CP122,288 and eletriptan on Fos expression due to stimulation of the superior sagittal sinus in cat. Pain 82: 15–22.

Goadsby PJ, Charbit AR, Andreou AP et al. (2009). Neuroscience forefront review – Neurobiology of migraine. Neuroscience 161 (2009) 327–341.

Greco R, Tassorelli C, Cappelletti D et al. (2005). Activation of the transcription factor NF-kappaB in the nucleus trigeminalis caudalis in an animal model of migraine. Neurotoxicology 26: 795–800.

Greco R, Gasperi V, Sandrini G et al. (2009). Alterations of the endocannabinoid system in an animal model of migraine: evaluation in cerebral areas of rat. Cephalalgia 2009 [Epub ahead of print].

Hadjikhani N, Sanchez Del Rio M, Wu O et al. (2001). Mechanisms of migraine aura revealed by functional MRI in human visual cortex. Proc Natl Acad Sci U S A 98: 4687–4692.

Heyck H (1969). Pathogenesis of migraine. Res Clin Stud Headache 2: 1–28.

Honey AC, Bland-Ward PA, Connor HE et al. (2000). Study of an adenosine A1 receptor agonist on trigeminally evoked dural blood vessel dilation in the anaesthetized rat. Cephalalgia 22: 260–264.

Hong KW, Kim CD, Rhim BY et al. (1999). Effect of omega-conotoxin GVIA and omega-agatoxin IVA on the capsaicin-sensitive calcitonin gene-related peptide release and autoregulatory vasodilation in rat pial arteries. J Cereb Blood Flow Metab 19: 53–60.

Hoyer D, Clarke DE, Fozard JR et al. (1994). International Union of Pharmacology classification of receptors for 5 hydroxytryptamine (serotonin). Pharmacol Rev 46: 157–203.

Humphrey PP, Feniuk W, Perren MJ et al. (1988). GR43175, a selective agonist for the 5-HT1-like receptor in dog isolated saphenous vein. Br J Pharmacol 94: 1123–1132.

Ikeda K, Onaka T, Yamakado M et al. (2003). Degeneration of the amygdala/piriform cortex and enhanced fear/anxiety behaviors in sodium pump alpha2 subunit (ATP1A2)-deficient mice. J Neurosci 23: 4667–4676.

Ishida A, Murray J, Saito C et al. (2001). Expression of vascular endothelial growth factor receptors in smooth muscle cells. J Cell Physiol 188: 359–368.

Iversen HK, Olesen J (1996). Headache induced by a nitric oxide donor (nitroglycerin) responds to sumatriptan. A human model for development of migraine drugs. Cephalalgia 16: 412–418.

Iversen HK, Olesen J, Tfelt-Hansen P (1989). Intravenous nitroglycerin as an experimental model of vascular headache. Basic characteristics. Pain 38: 17–24.

Jansen I, Uddman R, Hocherman M et al. (1986). Localization and effects of neuropeptide Y, vasoactive intestinal polypeptide, substance P, and calcitonin gene-related peptide in human temporal arteries. Ann Neurol 20: 496–501.

Jansen-Olesen I, Kaarill L, Edvinsson L (2001). Characterization of CGRP (1) receptors in the guinea pig basilar artery. Eur J Pharmacol 414: 249–258.

Jones MG, Lever I, Bingham S et al. (2001). Nitric oxide potentiates response of trigeminal neurones to dural or facial stimulation in the rat. Cephalalgia 21: 643–655.

Kakizawa H, Matsui F, Tokita Y et al. (2007). Neuroprotective effect of nipradilol, an NO donor, on hypoxic-ischemic brain injury of neonatal rats. Early Hum Dev 83: 535–540.

Kaube H, Hoskin KL, Goadsby PJ (1993). Inhibition by sumatriptan of central trigeminal neurones only after blood–brain barrier disruption. Br J Pharmacol 109: 788–792.

Knyihár-Csillik E, Tajti J, Csillik AE et al. (2000). Effects of eletriptan on the peptidergic innervation of the cerebral dura mater and trigeminal ganglion, and on the expression of *c-fos* and c-jun in the trigeminal complex of the rat in an experimental migraine model. Eur J Neurosci 12: 3991–4002.

Kors EE, Vanmolkot KR, Haan J et al. (2004). Recent findings in headache genetics. Curr Opin Neurol 17: 283–288.

Kurosawa M, Messlinger K, Pawlak M et al. (1995). Increase of meningeal blood flow after electrical stimulation of rat dura mater encephali: mediation by calcitonin gene-related peptide. Br J Pharmacol 114: 1397–1402.

Lambert GA, Donaldson C, Boers PM et al. (2000). Activation of trigeminovascular neurons by glyceryl trinitrate. Brain Res 887: 203–210.

Lassen LH, Christiansen I, Iversen HK et al. (2003). The effect of nitric oxide synthase inhibition on histamine induced headache and arterial dilatation in migraineurs. Cephalalgia 23: 877–886.

Leao AA (1944). Spreading depression of activity in the cerebral cortex. J Neurophysiol 7: 359–390.

Lembeck F, Holzer P (1979). Substance P as neurogenic mediator of antidromic vasodilation and neurogenic plasma extravasation. Naunyn Schmiedebergs Arch Pharmacol 310: 175–183.

Levy D, Burstein R, Strassman AM (2006). Mast cell involvement in the pathophysiology of migraine headache: a hypothesis. Headache 46: S13–S18.

Linnik MD, Sakas DE, Uhl GR et al. (1989). Subarachnoid blood and headache: altered trigeminal tachykinin gene expression. Ann Neurol 25: 179–184.

Markowitz S, Saito K, Moskowitz MA (1987). Neurogenically mediated leakage of plasma protein occurs from blood vessels in dura mater but not brain. J Neurosci 7: 4129–4136.

Martin RS, Martin GR (2001). Investigations into migraine pathogenesis: time course for effects of m-CPP, BW723C86 or glyceryl trinitrate on appearance of Fos-like immunoreactivity in rat trigeminal nucleus caudalis (TNC). Cephalalgia 21: 46–52.

Mayberg MR, Zervas NT, Moskowitz MA (1984). Trigeminal projections to supratentorial pial and dural blood vessels in cats demonstrated by horseradish peroxidase histochemistry. Comp Neurol 223: 46–56.

Messlinger K, Hotta H, Pawlak M et al. (1997). Effects of the 5-HT1 receptor agonists, sumatriptan and CP 93,129, on dural arterial flow in the rat. Eur J Pharmacol 332: 173–181.

Mitsikostas DD, Sanchez del Rio M (2001). Receptor systems mediating *c-fos* expression within trigeminal nucleus caudalis in animal models of migraine. Brain Res Rev 35: 20–35.

Mitsikostas DD, Sanchez del Rio M, Waeber C et al. (1998). The NMDA receptor antagonist MK-801 reduces capsaicin-induced *c-fos* expression within rat trigeminal nucleus caudalis. Pain 76: 239–248.

Mitsikostas DD, Sanchez del Rio M, Waeber C (2002). 5-Hydroxytryptamine (1B/1D) and 5-hydroxytryptamine1f receptors inhibit capsaicin-induced *c-fos* immunoreactivity within mouse trigeminal nucleus caudalis. Cephalalgia 22: 384–394.

Moskowitz MA (1984). The neurobiology of vascular head pain. Ann Neurol 16: 157–168.

Moskowitz MA, Macfarlane R (1993). Neurovascular and molecular mechanisms in migraine headaches. Cerebrovasc Brain Metab Rev 5: 159–177.

Moskowitz MA, Buzzi MG, Sakas DE et al. (1989). Pain mechanisms underlying vascular headaches. Progress report 1988. Rev Neurol (Paris) 145: 181–193.

Moskowitz MA, Nozaki K, Kraig RP (1993). Neocortical spreading depression provokes the expression of *c-fos* protein-like immunoreactivity within trigeminal nucleus caudalis via trigeminovascular mechanisms. J Neurosci 13: 1167–1177.

Nakagawa T, Katsuya A, Tanimoto S et al. (2003). Differential patterns of *c-fos* mrna expression in the amygdaloid nuclei induced by chemical somatic and visceral noxious stimuli in rats. Neurosci Lett 344: 197–200.

Nishimori T, Buzzi MG, Moskowitz MA et al. (1989). Preproenkephalin mrna expression in nucleus caudalis neurons is enhanced by trigeminal stimulation. Brain Res Mol Brain Res 6: 203–210.

Nozaki K, Boccalini P, Moskowitz MA (1992a). Expression of *c-fos*-like immunoreactivity in brainstem after meningeal irritation by blood in the subarachnoid space. Neuroscience 49: 669–680.

Nozaki K, Moskowitz MA, Boccalini P (1992b). CP-93,129, sumatriptan, dihydroergotamine block *c-fos* expression within the rat trigeminal nucleus caudalis caused by chemical stimulation of the meninges. Br J Pharmacol 106: 409–415.

Offenhauser N, Zinck T, Hoffmann J et al. (2005). CGRP release and *c-fos* expression within trigeminal nucleus caudalis of the rat following glyceryltrinitrate infusion. Cephalalgia 25: 225–236.

Olesen J, Thomsen LL, Iversen H (1994). Nitric oxide is a key molecule in migraine and other vascular headaches. Trends Pharmacol Sci 15: 149–153.

Ophoff RA, Terwindt GM, Vergouwe MN et al. (1996). Familial hemiplegic migraine and episodic ataxia type-2 are caused by mutations in the Ca^{2+} channel gene CACNL1A4. Cell 87: 543–552.

Pardutz A, Krizbai I, Multon S et al. (2000). Systemic nitroglycerin increases nnos levels in rat trigeminal nucleus caudalis. Neuroreport 11: 3071–3075.

Parker JO, Amies MH, Hawkinson RW et al. (1995). Intermittent transdermal nitroglycerin therapy in angina pectoris. Clinically effective without tolerance or rebound. Minitran Efficacy Study Group. Circulation 91: 1368–1374.

Petersen KA, Birk S, Doods H et al. (2004). Inhibitory effect of BIBN4096BS on cephalic vasodilatation induced by CGRP or transcranial electrical stimulation in the rat. Br J Pharmacol 143: 697–704.

Pietrobon D, Striessnig J (2003). Neurobiology of migraine. Nat Rev Neurosci 4: 386–398.

Ray BS, Wolff HG (1940). Experimental studies on headache. Pain sensitive structures of the head and their significance in headache. Arch Surg 41: 813–856.

Rayman G, Baker NR, Krishnan ST (2003). Glyceryl trinitrate patches as an alternative to isosorbide dinitrate spray in the treatment of chronic painful diabetic neuropathy. Diabetes Care 26: 2697–2698.

Reuter U, Bolay H, Jansen-Olesen I et al. (2001). Delayed inflammation in rat meninges: implications for migraine pathophysiology. Brain 124: 2490–2502.

Reuter U, Chiarugi A, Bolay H et al. (2002). Nuclear factor-kappab as a molecular target for migraine therapy. Ann Neurol 51: 507–516.

Roon KI, Olesen J, Diener HC et al. (2000). No acute antimigraine efficacy of CP-122,288, a highly potent inhibitor of neurogenic inflammation: results of two randomized, double-blind, placebo-controlled clinical trials. Ann Neurol 47: 238–241.

Saito K, Markowitz M, Moskowitz MA (1988). Ergot alkaloids block neurogenic extravasation in dura mater: proposed action in vascular headache. Ann Neurol 24: 732–737.

Sances G, Tassorelli C, Pucci E et al. (2004). Reliability of the nitroglycerin provocative test in the diagnosis of neurovascular headaches. Cephalalgia 24: 110–119.

Saria A, Ma RC, Dun NJ (1985). Neurokinin A depolarizes neurons of the guinea pig inferior mesenteric ganglia. Neurosci Lett 60: 145–150.

Saria A, Gamse R, Petermann J et al. (1986). Simultaneous release of several tachykinins and calcitonin gene-related peptide from rat spinal cord slices. Neurosci Lett 63: 310–314.

Saxena PR (1995). Cranial arteriovenous shunting, an *in vivo* animal model for migraine. In: J Olesen, MA Moskowitz (Eds.), Experimental Headache Models, Vol. 27. Lippincott-Raven, Philadelphia, pp. 189–198.

Saxena PR, de Vlaam-Schluter GM (1974). Role of some biogenic substances in migraine and relevant mechanism in antimigraine action of ergotamine – studies in an experimental model for migraine. Headache 3: 142–163.

Saxena PR, Tfelt-Hansen P (2005). Triptans, 5-$HT_{1B/1D}$ receptor agonists in the acute treatment of migraine. In: J Olesen, PJ Goadsby, N Ramadan et al. (Eds.), The Headaches. Lippincott Williams & Wilkins, Philadelphia, pp. 469–503.

Segall L, Scanzano R, Kaunisto MA et al. (2004). Kinetic alterations due to a missense mutation in the Na,K-atpase alpha2 subunit cause familial hemiplegic migraine type 2. J Biol Chem 279: 43692–43696.

Storer RJ, Akerman S, Goadsby PJ (2004). Calcitonin gene-related peptide (CGRP) modulates nociceptive trigeminovascular transmission in the cat. Br J Pharmacol 142: 1171–1181.

Strassman AM, Raymond SA, Burstein R (1996). Sensitization of meningeal sensory neurons and the origin of headache. Nature 384: 560–564.

Tassorelli C, Joseph SA (1995). Systemic nitroglycerin induces Fos immunoreactivity in brainstem and forebrain structures of the rat. Brain Res 682: 167–181.

Tassorelli C, Joseph SA, Nappi G (1997). Neurochemical mechanisms of nitroglycerin-induced neuronal activation in rat brain: a pharmacological investigation. Neuropharmacology 36: 1417–1424.

Tassorelli C, Joseph SA, Buzzi MG et al. (1999). The effects on the central nervous system of nitroglycerin – putative mechanisms and mediators. Prog Neurobiol 57: 607–624.

Tassorelli C, Costa A, Blandini F et al. (2000). Effect of nitric oxide donors on the central nervous system nitroglycerin studies in the rat. Funct Neurol 15: 19–27.

Tassorelli C, Greco R, Wang D et al. (2003). Nitroglycerin induces hyperalgesia in rats – a time-course study. Eur J Pharmacol 464: 159–162.

Tassorelli C, Blandini F, Greco R et al. (2004). Nitroglycerin enhances cgmp expression in specific neuronal and cerebrovascular structures of the rat brain. J Chem Neuroanat 27: 23–32.

Tassorelli C, Greco R, Armentero MT et al. (2007). A role for brain cyclooxygenase-2 and prostaglandin-E_2 in migraine: effects of nitroglycerin. Int Rev Neurobiol 82: 373–382.

Torfgård K, Ahlner J, Axelsson KL et al. (1991). Tissue levels of glyceryl trinitrate and cgmp after in vivo administration in rat, and the effect of tolerance development. Can J Physiol Pharmacol 69: 1257–1261.

Tottene A, Fellin T, Pagnutti S et al. (2002). Familial hemiplegic migraine mutations increase Ca(2+) influx through single human cav2.1 channels and decrease maximal cav2.1 current density in neurons. Proc Natl Acad Sci U S A 99: 13284–13289.

Vàmos E, Fejes A, Koch J et al. (2009). Kynurenate Derivative Attenuates the Nitroglycerin-Induced CamKIIalpha and CGRP Expression Changes. Headache [Epub ahead of print].

van den Maagdenberg AM, Pietrobon D, Pizzorusso T et al. (2004). A CACNA1A knock-in migraine mouse model with increased susceptibility to cortical spreading depression. Neuron 41: 701–710.

Villalón CM, Centurión D, Valdivia LF et al. (2002). An introduction to migraine: from ancient treatment to functional pharmacology and antimigraine therapy. Proc West Pharmacol Soc 45: 199–210.

Waeber C, Moskowitz MA (2005). Migraine as an inflammatory disorder. Neurology 64: S9–S15.

Willems EW, Trion M, De Vries P et al. (1999). Pharmacological evidence that $alpha_1$- and $alpha_2$-adrenoceptors mediate vasoconstriction of carotid arteriovenous anastomoses in anaesthetized pigs. Br J Pharmacol 127: 1263–1271.

Willems EW, Valdivia LF, Villalón CM et al. (2003). Possible role of alpha-adrenoceptor subtypes in acute migraine therapy. Cephalalgia 23: 245–257.

Williamson DJ, Hargreaves RJ, Hill RG et al. (1997a). Sumatriptan inhibits neurogenic vasodilation of dural blood vessels in the anaesthetized rat – intravital microscope studies. Cephalalgia 17: 525–531.

Williamson DJ, Hargreaves RJ, Hill RG et al. (1997b). Intravital microscope studies on the effects of neurokinin agonists and calcitonin gene-related peptide on dural vessel diameter in the anaesthetized rat. Cephalalgia 17: 518–524.

Williams S, Evan GI, Hunt SP (1990). Changing patterns of *c-fos* induction in spinal neurons following thermal cutaneous stimulation in the rat. Neuroscience 36: 73–81.

Wolff HG (1972). Headache and Other Head Pain. Oxford University Press, New York.

Wu D, Doods H, Arndt K et al. (2002). Development and potential of non-peptide antagonists for calcitonin-gene-related peptide (CGRP) receptors: evidence for CGRP receptor heterogeneity. Biochem Soc Trans 30: 468–473.

Yamamura H, Malick A, Chamberlin NL et al. (1998). Cardiovascular and neuronal response to head stimulation reflect central sensitisation and cutaneous allodynia in a rat model of migraine. J Neurophysiol 81: 479–493.

Section 3

Management of headache

Handbook of Clinical Neurology, Vol. 97 (3rd series)
Headache
G. Nappi and M.A. Moskowitz, Editors

Chapter 9

Management of headache patients

GRAZIA SANCES[1]* AND TERESA CATARCI[2]

[1]*National Institute of Neurology "C. Mondino" Foundation, IRCCS Via Mondino, Pavia, Italy*

[2]*University Centre for Adaptive Disorders and Headache (UCADH), IRCCS, "C. Mondino Institute of Neurology" Foundation, Pavia, Italy*

INTRODUCTION AND GENERAL ASPECTS

Headache is a very common complaint, in both primary care and in specialist settings. Headache patients account for around 20% of all outpatients seen in neurological practices (Linet et al., 1991; Pascual et al., 1995), and their management, particularly when they present with intractable headache, or are suspected of having secondary headaches, can be a challenge for the clinician.

It is noteworthy that, in spite of the high prevalence of the disease, relatively little time is devoted to the teaching of headache in medical schools, and only the most difficult cases are referred to specialists. In Europe, the 1-year mean prevalence in the general population has been estimated to be 51% (Stovner et al., 2006), but only 4 out of 100 patients consult their general practitioner (GP) because of headache. Moreover, 39% of all headache patients are prescribed antimigraine drugs and only 2% are referred to neurology departments by UK general practices (Latinovic et al., 2006).

The management and follow-up of patients with the most common forms of primary headache (migraine with or without aura, tension-type headache, cluster headache) should be the responsibility of GPs. Referrals to neurologists or to headache specialists is necessary when the diagnosis of primary headache is not clear-cut, when the case is complicated, difficult, or rare, or when it is not responsive to acute or preventive therapy.

The aim of this chapter is to help the clinician to approach the headache patient in the most effective way. To this end, we will discuss some of the available clinical guidelines for headache management, explain how to obtain useful personal, headache, and family histories from patients and discuss the problem of secondary headaches, including medication overuse headache. We will also look at lifestyle recommendations for headache patients, the comorbid conditions that should be looked for, and the situations in which a second opinion should be sought. Finally, a separate paragraph will be devoted to the management of headache in the elderly.

CLINICAL GUIDELINES

There are seven published sets of evidence-based guidelines, most of which are devoted solely to migraine management, such as those of the Canadian Headache Association (Pryse-Phillips et al., 1997), the US Headache Consortium (Silberstein, 2000), the French Society for the Study of Migraine (Geraud et al., 2004), and the German Society for Neurology and the German Migraine and Headache Society (www.ehf-org.org/pdf/Germany.pdf, 2006). The guidelines issued by other societies, namely the British Association for the Study of Headache (BASH) (www.bash.org.uk, 2004), the Italian Society for the Study of Headache (Ad Hoc Committee, 1993; www.sisc.it, 2002), and the European Federation of Neurological Societies (EFNS) (Evers et al., 2006; May et al., 2006), also cover the management of other headaches, such as tension-type headache, medication overuse headache, cluster headache, and other autonomic cephalalgias.

All the guidelines agree that the diagnosis of headache is merely clinical and that "testing is not recommended if the individual is not significantly more likely than anyone else in the general population to

*Correspondence to: Dr Grazia Sances, National Institute of Neurology "C. Mondino" Foundation, IRCCS Via Mondino, 2, 27100 Pavia, Italy, Tel: +39 0382 380207, Fax: +39 0382 380286, E-mail: grazia.sances@mondino.it

have a significant abnormality" (Silberstein, 2000). The other important point of consensus is that an electroencephalogram is not indicated in the routine evaluation of headache patients. The BASH recommends careful investigation of new headaches or those whose features have recently changed. Even though these headaches will be due to intracranial tumors in only 3–4% of cases, it is worth performing a funduscopic examination in all patients. It is essential, too, to distinguish headache due to meningitis, subarachnoid hemorrhage, giant cell temporal arteritis, primary angle closure glaucoma, idiopathic benign intracranial hypertension, and carbon monoxide poisoning (see below).

The BASH identifies four factors for good migraine management, applicable to all primary headaches: (1) correct and timely diagnosis; (2) explanation and reassurance; (3) identification and avoidance of predisposing factors; and (4) intervention (drug or non-drug).

The treatment of headache will be discussed elsewhere in this chapter, and it must be said that in this regard there is less agreement among the different guidelines. For example, the approach to acute treatment, namely stepped care versus stratified care, varies from country to country and, at present, is not defined. Nevertheless, most guidelines agree that the decision to treat or not to treat depends on the headache type, the severity of the attacks, and the presence of associated symptoms and disability. The type of treatment is chosen taking into account possible comorbidities and specific contraindications. Generally, acute therapy alone is suggested for patients with migraine and tension-type headache reporting a low number of attacks (1–2 per month).

Even though there is no standard indication for starting a preventive therapy, this (in cases of migraine and tension-type headache) is usually prescribed after 2 months of observation through a prospective headache diary. Thus, a preventive treatment (to be continued for at least 3 months) is suggested when the patient records more than 3 attacks per month. In the event of early withdrawal of the treatment it will be necessary to consider both drug-related adverse events and lack of efficacy (e.g., due to the patient's poor compliance with the treatment, or to symptomatic medication overuse). Even though there are no specific indications about the duration of the preventive treatment, it is advisable, when it is effective, to taper it down after 6–12 months.

Finally, all guidelines agree that preventive treatment must be prescribed immediately in patients with chronic form of cluster headache or other chronic trigeminal autonomic cephalalgias.

When the patient is a non-responder to several trials of symptomatic and preventive drugs, it is appropriate to reconsider the original diagnosis.

Figure 9.1 shows a flow chart of headache patient management that is based on clinical guidelines and on the personal, clinical experience of the authors.

HISTORY

There is no test or specific treatment response for the diagnosis of headache, and the possibility of misdiagnosis, in most cases, is reduced by careful and detailed history taking. There are obviously some rare exceptions to this rule, as in the case, for example, of the dramatic response to indomethacin seen in chronic paroxysmal hemicrania and hemicrania continua (Headache Classification Committee of the International Headache Society, 2004), and the rapid effect of oxygen inhalation seen only in cluster headache attacks (Kudrow, 1981; Fogan, 1985).

In a busy setting, it is helpful to have the patient fill in a diary card, where information can be collected about headache frequency, intensity, duration, and types of abortive medication taken. This filling-in of the diary card can be done either retrospectively, while the patient is in the waiting room, or prospectively, by asking patients, when they first fix an appointment at the clinic, to start keeping a diary of attacks (Nappi et al., 2006).

Information about headache should be collected at the beginning of the interview; doing this can reduce a patient's anxiety, provide motivation, and help to recollect events more accurately. A full history of the temporal profile of the headache should be gathered first: when it first started, the circumstances of its onset, whether it has remained the same over time, and, if not, in what way it has changed. In order to establish whether a severe headache started in childhood, a good question to ask is whether the patient remembers ever being sent home from school because of a headache. If the patient recalls experiencing a different headache in the past, it is advisable to collect the histories of the two headaches separately, beginning with the earliest one: a second headache that goes unrecognized is a frequent reason for treatment failure (Lipton et al., 2003).

The patient should be questioned carefully about frequency, duration of untreated (if any) attacks, and severity of the pain over the past 6 months. A single attack can sometimes last days, and recurrence of pain after an interruption of less than 24 h is not to be considered a separate attack. In the presence of daily headache, it is useful to ask how many completely headache-free days the patient has per month and

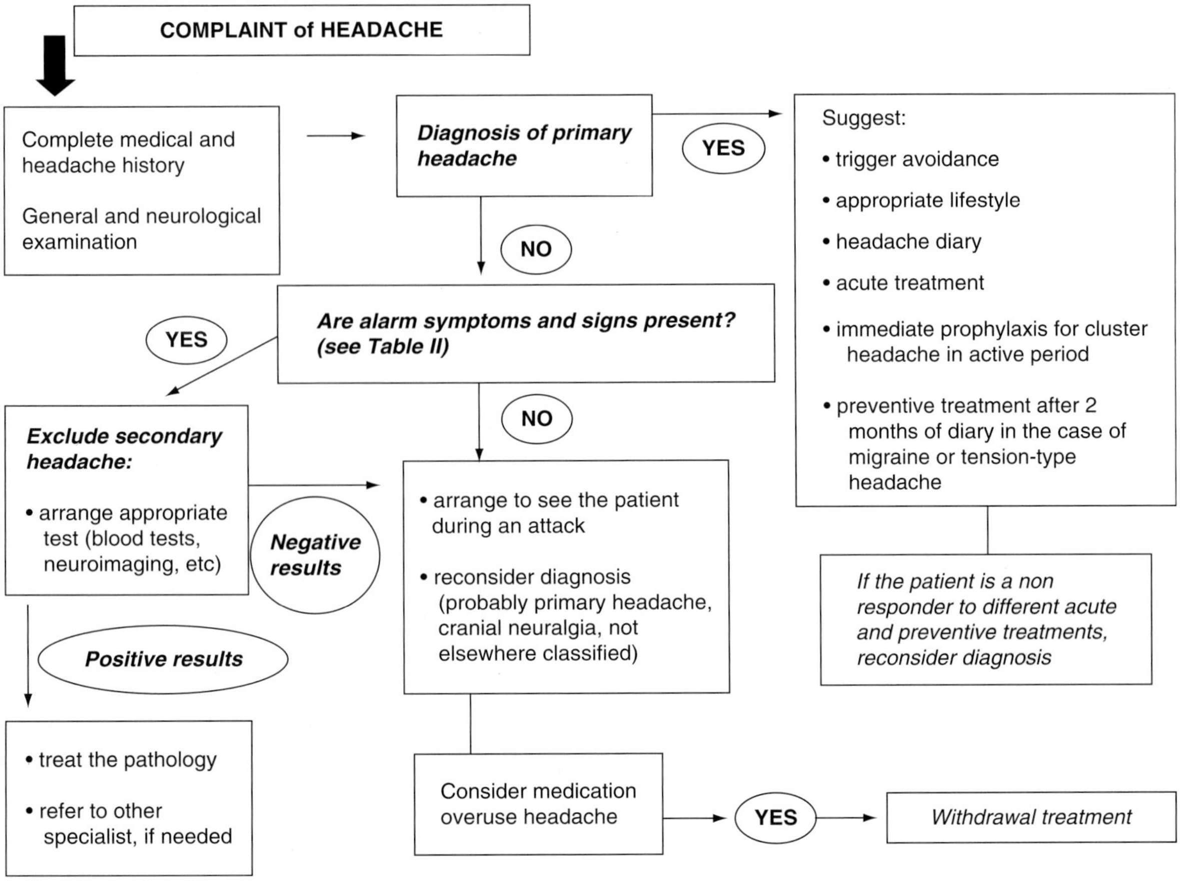

Fig. 9.1. Flow chart of the management of headache patient.

about possible variations in the intensity of the pain during the day. Severity is measured on a four-item scale, in accordance with the recommendation of the second edition of the International Classification of Headache Disorders (ICHD-II: Headache Classification Committee of the International Headache Society, 2004), where 0 = no pain, 1 = mild pain (no interference with daily activities at all), 2 = moderate pain (there is some disruption of daily activities but the patient can still work), 3 = severe pain (bed rest or inability to work). It is important to ask about the pattern of the pain intensity during the day, i.e., whether it is severe on awakening or, instead, is initially mild and then gets worse during the day, as well as about changes in intensity following light or heavy physical activity, changes of posture, sneezing or coughing, bending down, and after assuming the standing and the supine position. Then, it is necessary to establish the site, spreading pattern and type of the pain (burning, pounding, throbbing, dull, like an electric shock, pressing, tightening; it is often useful to prompt the patient with these terms). Information must be collected regarding the presence of other, non-pain symptoms occurring before (prodrome), during (accompanying symptoms), and after (postdrome) the attack, and the presence of the neurological symptoms of the aura (more likely to occur before the attack, these can also start during or, more rarely, after an attack).

It is also important to gather information about triggers or precipitating factors (dietary factors, menstruation, medications, quality and quantity of sleep, occupational and environmental factors, Valsalva maneuver), about what (other than drugs) worsens or improves the pain, and about the patient's behavior during the headache attack.

Finally, a detailed pharmacological interview should be done. This should include questions about all the kinds of medication taken by the patient (including treatments for other pathologies, hormone treatments, herbals and nutritional supplements), since headache is the most common adverse effect of various drug treatments (e.g., nitrates, calcium channel blockers, indomethacin) (Lipton et al., 2003). Subsequently, the patient should be asked about the type and number of painkillers or antimigraine drugs used, their efficacy on pain or associated symptoms, the speed and duration of the effect, and their efficacy when treating recurrence of pain. At the end of the headache interview, it is important to remember to ask about preventive medications taken in the past, and about the efficacy of and compliance with past treatments.

Personal history is also important: lifestyle factors, marital and family status, education, occupation, hobbies and sports, friendships, alcohol intake, and use of other substances and smoking. It is also necessary to establish whether there is a history of other diseases (cardiocerebrovascular pathologies, epilepsy, diabetes, obesity, gastrointestinal and allergic conditions, oromandibular dysfunction, malignancies, past operations, head and cervical trauma) and to investigate gynecological and psychological history. Details of blood tests, electrocardiogram (ECG), and any other kinds of test performed in the past should be noted, as should usual blood pressure values.

The family history is also very important: first-degree relatives of migraine with aura and of migraine without aura patients have, respectively, a fourfold and a twofold risk of developing migraine themselves (Russel, 1997). In addition, the presence of at least one first- or second-degree relative with migraine with aura, including motor weakness, is needed for a diagnosis of familial hemiplegic migraine (Headache Classification Committee of the International Headache Society, 2004). Table 9.1 summarizes the steps of the interview performed in headache patients.

Even after this detailed headache, personal, and family history taking, it is still possible that the headache characteristics will not point to a specific diagnosis: the patient may not recall or may be unable to report important details. In these cases it is advisable to ask the patient to fill in a headache diary; sometimes, direct medical observation of the patient during a typical attack may also be useful.

GENERAL AND NEUROLOGICAL EXAMINATION

History alone allows a diagnosis of probable primary headache. Signs of a possible secondary headache must be carefully sought in all patients, even in apparently clear-cut cases. In fact, the ICHD-II criteria for all the primary headache forms clearly state that the headache "is not attributed to another disorder," on the basis of history and physical and neurological examination (Headache Classification Committee of the International Headache Society, 2004). In a busy neurology setting, the examination needs to be quick but effective; therefore, the general physical examination should concentrate on: (1) measurement of blood pressure and heart rate, including auscultation over the neck and orbits (presence of vascular alarm symptoms); (2) checking for disorders of the face and skull, considering nasal sinuses, temporomandibular joint, temporal arteries, trigger points, and possible hypersensitivity of the scalp; and (3) checking for disorders of the neck, considering pain trigger points and vertical (flexion and extension) and horizontal (lateral) movements of the neck.

Table 9.1

The steps in the headache patient interview

Family history	**Personal history**	**Specific headache history**
Affected family members	Birth	Age at onset
Other familial diseases	Type/rhythms of work	Changes in the course of life
Substance abuse-related disorders	Marital status	Situations accompanying changes in frequency or severity
	Lifestyle habits (diet, sleep)	Specific characteristics of pain (location, type, intensity, duration)
	Presence of stressful situations	Presence of accompanying symptoms, aura, prodromes, postdromes
	Obstetric and gynaecological history (menstrual cycles, pregnancies, deliveries, menopause, specific illnesses, use of hormone therapies)	Trigger/precipitating/alleviating factors
	Remote pathological history (cardio-cerebrovascular diseases, traumas, affective-behavioural disorders, endocrine diseases, substance abuse, other)	Use of drugs (abortive and preventive), number per month, effectiveness, side effects
	Use of specific drugs	If chronic, length of chronic pattern/previous detoxification treatments
		Previous diagnostic tests

A complete neurological examination, to exclude secondary headache or establish the presence of concomitant diseases, should include: (1) cranial nerve examination; (2) funduscopic examination (to exclude papilledema or hemorrhage); (3) clinical visual field; (4) power, tone, coordination, sensation, deep tendon reflexes, and plantar responses; (5) gait and equilibrium; and (6) mental status, speech.

DIAGNOSIS OF PRIMARY AND SECONDARY HEADACHE

The priority of a clinician confronted with a new patient with headache is to establish whether the headache is primary, or secondary to a life-threatening condition. It is helpful to bear in mind that most headaches in the community are either primary or due to mild systemic infections: the lifetime prevalence of brain tumors has been reported to be only 0.1% in the general population (Rassmussen, 1995). The differential diagnosis between primary and secondary headache is based, in the first instance, on the headache history: obviously, a new-onset headache merits much more attention than a long-standing one, as does a headache with onset after the age of 40 years. Severity is not an issue, whereas a sudden change in the features of a headache is rather worrying. The possible presence of epilepsy is another important consideration. Of a series of 897 patients with migraine fulfilling the International Headache Society criteria and a normal neurological examination, 4 had abnormal computed tomography scans, and, of these 4, 2 had experienced seizures (Quality Standard Subcommittee of the American Academy of Neurology, 1994). Other important symptoms like fever, worsening of the pain after sneezing, coughing, or sexual intercourse, and the presence of focal neurological signs, obviously point towards a diagnosis of secondary headache (Table 9.2). It is worth mentioning that a migraine aura can be a cause of concern when it shows atypical features, such as fast progression of the symptoms, prolonged or very short duration, presence of negative features (e.g., hemianopia), and has onset after the age of 40 years. In the same way, any changes in the aura or headache characteristics or in the timing of the aura onset are important and may require further investigation (differential diagnosis versus transient ischemic attack, vascular malformations, and occipital epilepsia).

Table 9.2

Alarm symptoms and signs in headache patients

- new-onset headache
- headache with onset after the age of 40 years
- sudden change in the headache features
- strictly unilateral pain
- worsening of the pain after sneezing, coughing, sexual intercourse or in clinostatic/orthostatic position
- concomitant fever, neck stiffness, rash,
- presence of focal neurological signs (other than aura)
- papilloedema
- association with confusion, loss of consciousness, seizures

According to the BASH guidelines (www.bash.org.uk, 2004), there are seven serious secondary headache scenarios to look out for:

1. Intracranial tumors: failure to respond to treatment or development of a new headache in patients already known to have a cancer elsewhere or a suppressed immune system
2. Meningitis: progressive headache for hours accompanied by nausea and disturbed consciousness
3. Subarachnoid hemorrhage: worst headache ever in a patient with a history of uncomplicated headache, in whom the present headache is clearly different from previous ones
4. Temporal arteritis: must be suspected in all patients aged over 50 years at headache onset; unreliable signs are: localization of pain to the temples, objective inflammation of the temporal artery, erythrocyte sedimentation rate (ESR) >50 mm/h; more reliable signs are: jaw claudication, scalp tenderness, patient systemically unwell
5. Primary-angle glaucoma: non-specific severe headache localized to one eye, with nausea and vomiting, associated with impaired vision, or episodic mild eye pain with visual symptoms in a middle-aged patient
6. Idiopathic (benign) intracranial hypertension: most common in young obese females, it should be suspected even in cases of normal optic fundi, especially in children; these patients must be referred for cerebrospinal fluid pressure measurement, after brain imaging, to avoid serious complications like visual loss
7. Carbon monoxide (CO) poisoning: symptoms of subacute intoxication include headache, nausea, vomiting, giddiness, muscular weakness, dimness of vision, and double vision; when symptoms are present in a number of members of a single household, during the cold season, CO poisoning should always be suspected.

A less serious cause of secondary headache, but equally important to diagnose, is medication overuse in patients with a previous diagnosis of primary headache (Headache Classification Committee, 2006). This is a chronic headache, often unresponsive to any kind of prophylaxis, that can last for many years and, for the patient, may result in social isolation and unemployment. Withdrawal of the overused medications and restoration of headache prophylaxis is the only treatment. There are no established guidelines about the withdrawal of overused medications and clinicians have different approaches: inpatient or outpatient program, abrupt withdrawal, various treatments during the start of drug withdrawal. However, inpatient treatment is advisable in the following circumstances: disease lasting for more than 5 years; failure of previous outpatient management; withdrawal or overuse of drugs containing barbiturates or opioids or tranquilizers; concomitant depression or anxiety; and signs of ergotism, peptic ulcers, diarrhea, anemia. The association of behavioral techniques and adequate medical support (for the patient and the family) is very important for a positive outcome. Timely diagnosis and treatment are important, since the effects of medication overuse could become permanent and thus not reversible after discontinuation (Zeeberg et al., 2006).

Finally, headaches that occur on awakening can be due to sleep-disordered breathing or to a specific sleep disorder (e.g., upper-airway resistance syndrome, obstructive sleep apnea, primary insomnia, circadian phase abnormalities), even when they show characteristics typical of a primary headache (Rains and Poceta, 2006).

One of the dilemmas facing the neurologist is when to scan a patient with primary headache. According to the most recent EFNS clinical guidelines (Evers et al., 2006), magnetic resonance imaging (MRI) is recommended when:

1. The neurological examination is not normal
2. Typical migraine attacks occur for the first time after the age of 40 years
3. The frequency, or intensity, of migraine attacks continuously increases
4. The accompanying symptoms of migraine attacks change
5. New psychiatric symptoms occur in relation to the attacks.

For cluster headache and trigeminal autonomic cephalalgias, the guidelines are less clearly defined. It is our opinion that brain imaging is warranted in all atypical cases and in cases with onset of headache in middle age.

Unfortunately, there exist no systematic studies that have sought to identify the causes of secondary headache. An interesting clinical approach to the dilemma "to scan or not to scan" is to investigate all headache patients who have a troublesome headache that is not clearly migraine (Goadsby, 2004) or cluster headache, even when red flags are absent and neurological examination is normal.

LIFESTYLE AND COMORBID CONDITIONS

Once a secondary headache has been reasonably ruled out, it can help the patient to investigate possible comorbid pathologies and suggest appropriate lifestyle changes.

The most serious comorbidity is ischemic stroke in migraine patients, and particularly in young women with migraine with aura (Kurth et al., 2005). It has also been demonstrated that migraine is a risk factor for subclinical stroke determined by MRI; patients at greatest risk are those with migraine with aura and with a frequency of more than one attack per month (Kruit et al., 2004). Another population study revealed that migraine with aura patients had several cardiovascular risk factors, like high cholesterol, high blood pressure, and a positive family history of myocardial infarction (Scher et al., 2005). These data strongly support the clinical value of checking all migraine patients for cardio- and cerebrovascular risk factors and of suggesting lifestyle changes and treatment accordingly.

Psychiatric comorbidity is also frequent in migraine patients: depression has been found to show a bidirectional association with migraine (Breslau et al., 2003) and anxiety with headache (Zwart et al., 2003).

Therefore, the lifestyle of a migraineur should, first of all, include standard measures to prevent vascular events, such as regular exercise, a low-salt and low-fat diet, and no cigarette smoking. It is also important to recognize the first symptoms of depression and anxiety, which could, setting up a vicious cycle, lead to increased attack frequency and a higher risk of vascular events or acute medication overuse.

Trigger factors should also be considered when helping migraine patients to modify their lifestyle. Although most of these factors seem to trigger headache only occasionally and not consistently (Wober et al., 2006), it can still be useful, for an individual patient, to keep a "trigger diary" and to try to avoid as many triggers as possible.

The most frequently reported avoidable factors are: relaxation after stress (www.bash.org.uk, 2004; Wober et al., 2006), change of routine, skipping meals or sleep, sleeping too much, certain alcoholic drinks, some types of cheese, possibly chocolate, strenuous unaccustomed exercise, and menstruation (www.bash.org.uk, 2004).

Cluster headache attacks can be triggered by fewer but better defined factors, such as afternoon naps and alcohol consumption. Cigarette smoking can also be associated with the onset of a cluster hadache period, even though its avoidance produces less immediate effects.

more epidemiological and nosological research in this underinvestigated field.

As another major innovation, code-numbering included World Health Organization (WHO) *International Classification of Diseases,* 10th edition, neurological adaptation, codes (Tables 11.1 and 11.2). The reason was that these codes are widely used in daily practice.

USING ICHD-II IN PRACTICE

A number of rules guide the practical application of ICHD-II. Some of these, relevant to implementation, are listed here:

- Patients receive a diagnosis according to the headache phenotypes that they currently present or that they have presented within the last year.
- Each distinct type of headache that the patient has must be separately diagnosed and coded (this multiple-diagnosis system inherited from ICHD-I has proven valuable in pointing out the need for appropriately differentiated treatments).
- When a patient receives more than one diagnosis these should be listed in the order of importance to the patient.
- Fulfillment of the diagnostic criteria for *migraine, TTH, or cluster headache and other trigeminal autonomic cephalalgias*, or any of their subtypes, always trumps fulfillment of criteria for the *probable* diagnostic categories of each, which are last described in the respective groups. For example, headache fulfilling criteria for both *probable migraine and infrequent episodic TTH* is correctly diagnosed as the latter. (Nevertheless, there is always the possibility that two headache types coexist, so that some attacks meet one set of criteria whilst others meet another set. In such cases, two diagnoses should be made.)
- A *new* headache occurring for the first time in close temporal relation to another disorder that is a known cause of headache is diagnosed as a secondary headache attributed to the causative disorder. This is so even when the headache has the characteristics of migraine, TTH, cluster headache, or one of the other trigeminal autonomic cephalalgias.
- When a *pre-existing* primary headache is made worse in close temporal relation to another disorder that is a known cause of headache, there are two possibilities and judgment is required. The patient can either be given only the diagnosis of the pre-existing primary headache or be given both the primary headache diagnosis and a secondary headache diagnosis according to the other disorder. Factors that support adding the secondary headache diagnosis are: a very close temporal relation to the causative disorder, a marked worsening of the primary headache, very good evidence that the causative disorder can aggravate the primary headache in the manner observed, and, finally, improvement or disappearance of the headache after relief from the presumed causative disorder.
- The last criterion for most of the secondary headaches – that the headache greatly improves or resolves within a specified period after relief from the causative disorder – is part of the evidence for a causal relationship. The diagnosis before this disorder is treated, or before the result of treatment is known, is *headache probably attributed to [the disorder].* Once the treatment results are known, the diagnosis becomes *headache attributed to [the disorder]*, or is changed if the criterion is not fulfilled. (The few exceptions to this rule include *posttraumatic headache, headache attributed to whiplash injury,* and *chronic postbacterial meningitis headache.*)

Implementation

Like its 1988 predecessor, ICHD-II is intended equally for research and for clinical practice. No research studies should be accepted in scientific journals without adhering to this classification, and it is unlikely that they will be. However, the classification is equally important in the pursuit of better headache management and, therefore, for clinicians. Accordingly, ICHD-II is perhaps the single most important document for doctors with an interest in the diagnosis and management of headache patients.

Yet there is often a huge and highly visible gap between researchers and clinicians. It has been suggested that there should be two classifications, one for research and one for clinical use. That would, however, be highly problematic: translation of findings from research, conducted according to a special research classification, could not be applied directly to clinical practice, which would use a different classification. There must be one classification only, but it must recognize that the needs and interests of clinicians *are* different from those of researchers. The solution lies in the way the classification is constructed, so that it can be used at different levels of specialization – in particular, in the hierarchical system already adopted by ICHD-I, which is unchanged in ICHD-II. All headache disorders are classified into major groups, with each group then subdivided one, two, or three times into headache types, subtypes, and subforms. For example, 1. *Migraine* is a group consisting of one headache type (migraine), and the subtypes of migraine such as 1.2 *Migraine with aura* are described at the next level (second digit). Migraine with aura is again divided into subforms, for example 1.2.1 *Typical aura with migraine headache.* The Appendix shows other examples.

Primary-care practitioners (who treat most headache) may need to diagnose only at the first level, e.g., migraine, in order to select appropriate treatment. Neurologists and headache specialists may diagnose at any level that suits their interests, whilst researchers may have reason to focus on the precise subform of migraine with aura at the third level.

Three challenges

When ICHD-I was published in 1988, it was highly uncertain how it would be received by the clinical and the research communities. Fortunately, it was rapidly accepted throughout the world. Amongst those who gave it their endorsement was the WHO, so that the main principles of ICHD-I were included in ICD-10.

Following in its path, ICHD-II was therefore, on the surface, a predictable immediate success, put to use throughout the world by headache clinical experts and by headache researchers. Promulgation has been greatly assisted by modern communication technology not available to ICHD-I: in particular, the internet. ICHD-II was first published in IHS's journal *Cephalalgia* (Headache Classification Subcommittee of the International Headache Society, 2004), but immediately afterwards on IHS's own website at www.i-h-s.org. Subsequently it was presented at www.ihs-classification.org, in a format developed by H Göbel that made effective use of website capabilities to facilitate reference. International adoption has been greatly aided by translations published in more than 15 languages, and there are others in preparation.

It is probably true that it has been far more of a success than is visible on the surface. Yet, there are three recognizable areas of difficulty. One is geographical, perhaps cultural. Another is a possible systemic fault in the definition of secondary headache disorders. The third reflects the divide between specialist and primary care.

Chronic migraine

The one country in the world where the penetration of ICHD-II is not completely successful is, unfortunately, the world's most powerful. Behind this challenge is another, which has politicocultural roots: the USA has never adopted ICD-10. This contains a much more modern headache classification than ICD-8 or ICD-9, in which headache classification is obsolete and without detail.

One consequence is that TTH is not identified in the USA as a specific neurological disorder. This means that reimbursement problems can arise in that country when the diagnosis of TTH is given by a neurologist, and it may be one explanation for the relative lack of interest in TTH in the USA. The pharmaceutical industry and the general public in the USA are, on the contrary, very interested in it, as is illustrated by the many TV advertisements recommending painkillers for headache. A related consequence is that patients with frequent headache because they have a mixture of migraine and TTH are not diagnosed with the latter; this brings into being a group of people who have headache on most days but are diagnosed with migraine only. ICHD-II introduced a new entity, *chronic migraine*, but the strict diagnostic criteria for this are fulfilled by very few of the patients in this group. The situation is further complicated by the fact that medication usage tends to be high amongst such patients, bringing the possibility of MOH also into play. A diagnosis of this disorder can also lead to reimbursement problems.

There is an underlying debate here that sets purists against pragmatists, and this debate will probably continue for a long time. Meanwhile it has been recognized that a group of patients were not being well served by ICHD-II. The process of change is not helped by genuine disagreement about the phenotype(s) these patients express, and a lack of research to elucidate it. Pending the latter, including the publication of results from work in progress, new appendix criteria (which means they are proposed but *not* formally adopted) have relaxed the definitions of chronic migraine and MOH (Headache Classification Committee, 2006).

Headache probably attributed to ...

We stated earlier that the need, specified by criterion D for most secondary headaches, for recovery following removal of the presumed cause sometimes means the diagnosis cannot be made. This criterion was seen as essential to complete the evidence for a causal relationship. Diagnosis before the presumed causative disorder is treated, or before the result of treatment is known, can only be *headache probably attributed to [the disorder]*. Once the treatment results are known, the diagnosis becomes *headache attributed to [the disorder]*, or is changed if the criterion is not fulfilled.

The underlying rationale here was good, but the consequences have been problematic for two main reasons. First, in many cases, when a secondary headache cannot be diagnosed until later – when it is greatly improved or has disappeared – at that time the diagnosis is not interesting. In essence, the headache cannot in these cases be diagnosed until it has gone, which is clinically unhelpful. A good example of this is MOH, where correct diagnosis directs treatment – withdrawal of the causative medication – but (theoretically) cannot be made prior to treatment. Second, when the presumed causative disorder cannot be treated, and does not resolve spontaneously, it appears the headache can *never* be diagnosed. In practice this is less of a problem than might be expected, and it was partly anticipated so that exceptions include *posttraumatic headache, headache attributed to whiplash injury*, and *postbacterial meningitis headache*, all of which were recognized to be likely to progress from acute to chronic headache. In other cases, however, which may not be common but nonetheless must be catered for, patients may never fulfill the criteria for a secondary headache because, rather than improving, they develop chronic headache which itself cannot be diagnosed by ICHD-II criteria.

Revision of the standard criteria for secondary headache is necessary. The process has been begun. The likely solution will involve a more case-by-case approach that recognizes other evidence of causation specific to each. More research may well be needed before the solution is complete.

The primary-care physician in Peru

ICHD-II, perfect or not, sets out the best diagnostic criteria we have. Therefore, they should be used everywhere if the diagnosis of headache disorders is to be made accurately throughout the world as the necessary basis of best treatment. If this is true in secondary (specialist) care, it must be true also in primary care. When ICHD-II is scrutinized with this object in mind, it is not so easy to see how to get it into the routine clinical practice of the primary-care physician in, for example, Peru (Steiner, 2004a). ICHD-II occupies 160 pages to cover some 200 headache disorders in 13 categories. They are published in English in a specialist journal or on websites that no primary-care physicians, anywhere, are likely to access. True, there are translations, but it cannot be denied that these aspects of ICHD-II erect substantial barriers to its implementation by the primary-care physician in Peru who might wish to improve diagnosis of headache disorders.

To achieve implementation in primary care around the world, ICHD-II first needs translating, into many more languages than the 20 achieved by ICHD-I. If this task is left wholly to national headache societies, there will be no penetration wherever there is no society, which is most of the world. IHS needs also to work on this with agencies such as the pharmaceutical industry and WHO, both of whom have an interest in seeing this done.

Second, ICHD-II needs distributing far and wide, a process requiring more money and better networks than IHS commands. Again the pharmaceutical industry can help, given that they have good distribution networks in many countries, and again they should wish to. It is also possible to use the Global Campaign (Steiner, 2004b) as it develops national and regional initiatives.

Third, ICHD-II needs simplifying. This does not mean that a different classification should be considered – we have already argued strongly against that – but ICHD-II has far too many entities for the practicing physician because it is serving the purposes of everybody. Even specialists will not, in daily practice, use most of the diagnostic categories that still need to be classified. Unfortunately for the primary-care physician in Peru, ICHD-II gives no prominence to those that are common or important.

The Global Campaign has prepared a "core version" of ICHD-II, to which national or regional groups can add according to local variation. It is set out at the end of this chapter (Appendix). It includes just seven primary headache disorders, and if every primary-care physician became familiar with and could correctly diagnose each of these, the lives of their headache patients would be transformed. It also includes eight other headaches, six secondary and two neuralgias, making 15 in all. If primary-care physicians mastered these as well, they would probably have done all that they reasonably could in this field.

CONCLUSIONS

ICHD-II, like its predecessor, has been well received and widely adopted by headache specialists and scientists working in the field. A small (and only small) number of issues have arisen, which is inevitable when usage is worldwide. These are being addressed, as will others as they develop in consequence of future nosological research.

More problematic is to bring ICHD-II into the routine working practice of health-care practitioners who treat most patients with headache – those in primary care. ICHD-II needs some adaptation to achieve this, but not such as to change in any way its fundamental principles. Rather, it needs simplification, and wider distribution.

References

Ad Hoc Committee on Classification of Headache (1962). Classification of headache. JAMA 179: 717–718.

Granella F, D'Alessandro R, Manzoni GC et al. (1994). International Headache Society classification: interobserver reliability in the diagnosis of primary headache. Cephalalgia 14: 16–20.

Headache Classification Committee (2006). New appendix criteria open for a broader concept of chronic migraine. Cephalalgia 26: 742–746.

Headache Classification Committee of the International Headache Society (1988). Classification and diagnostic criteria for headache disorders, cranial neuralgias and facial pain. Cephalalgia 8 (Suppl. 7): 1–96.

Headache Classification Subcommittee of the International Headache Society (2004). International classification of headache disorders, 2nd edition. Cephalalgia 24 (Suppl. 1): 1–160.

Leone M, Filippini G, D'Amico D et al. (1994). Assessment of International Headache Society diagnostic criteria: a reliability study. Cephalalgia 14: 280–284.

Michel P, Dartigues JF, Henry P et al. (1993). Validity of the International Headache Society criteria for migraine. Neuroepidemiology 12: 51–57.

Olesen J (1996). The International Headache Society classification and diagnostic criteria are valid and extremely useful. Cephalalgia 16: 293–296.

Steiner TJ (2004a). National and international action plans for improving headache diagnosis. In: J Olesen (Ed.), Classification and Diagnosis of Headache Disorders. Oxford University Press, Oxford, pp. 265–271.

Steiner TJ (2004b). Lifting the burden: the global campaign against headache. Lancet Neurol 3: 204–205.

World Federation of Neurology Research Group on Migraine and Headache (1969). J Neurol Sci 9: 202.

World Health Organization (1997). Application of the International Classification of Diseases to Neurology (ICD-NA). World Health Organization, Geneva.

Appendix

ICHD-II diagnostic criteria for headache disorders in primary care (developed by the global campaign to reduce the burden of headache worldwide; Steiner, 2004b)

INTRODUCTION

ICHD distinguishes between *primary headaches*, which have no other underlying causative disorder, and *secondary headaches*, which are attributed to some other disorder.

Set out in this adaptation of ICHD specifically for primary care are the criteria for the 15 headache disorders that are important in primary care. These include the headache disorders most likely to be seen, and those that are important because they are symptomatic of another serious underlying disorder requiring treatment. They are numbered below as in the classification; WHO ICD-10 codes, used in some countries, are given in parentheses.

PRIMARY HEADACHES

The last diagnostic criterion for all primary headaches is "not attributed to another disorder." This means that history and physical and neurological examinations do not suggest any underlying and possibly causative disorder, or history and/or examination do suggest such a disorder but it is ruled out by appropriate investigations, or such a disorder is present but attacks do not occur for the first time in close temporal relation to it.

1.1. [G43.0] Migraine without aura

Diagnostic criteria

A. At least five attacks fulfilling criteria B–D
B. Headache attacks lasting 4–72 h (untreated or unsuccessfully treated)
C. Headache has at least two of the following characteristics:
   1. Unilateral location
   2. Pulsating quality
   3. Moderate or severe pain intensity
   4. Aggravation by or causing avoidance of routine physical activity (e.g., walking or climbing stairs)
D. During headache at least one of the following:
   1. Nausea and/or vomiting
   2. Photophobia and phonophobia
E. Not attributed to another disorder

1.2. [G43.1] Migraine with aura

1.2.1. [G43.10] Typical aura with migraine headache

Diagnostic criteria

A. At least two attacks fulfilling criteria B–D
B. Aura consisting of at least one of the following, but no motor weakness:
   1. Fully reversible visual symptoms including positive features (e.g., flickering lights, spots, or lines) and/or negative features (loss of vision)
   2. Fully reversible sensory symptoms including positive features (pins and needles) and/or negative features (numbness)
   3. Fully reversible dysphasic speech disturbance
C. At least two of the following:
   1. Homonymous visual symptoms and/or unilateral sensory symptoms
   2. At least one aura symptom develops gradually over $\geq$5 min and/or different aura symptoms occur in succession over $\geq$5 min
   3. Each symptom lasts $\geq$5 and $\leq$60 min
D. Headache fulfilling criteria B–D for 1.1 *migraine without aura* begins during the aura or follows aura within 60 min
E. Not attributed to another disorder

1.2.3. [G43.104] Typical aura without headache

Diagnostic criteria

A. At least two attacks fulfilling criteria B–D
B. Aura consisting of at least one of the following, with or without speech disturbance but no motor weakness:
   1. Fully reversible visual symptoms including positive features (e.g., flickering lights, spots, or lines) and/or negative features (loss of vision)
   2. Fully reversible sensory symptoms including positive features (pins and needles) and/or negative features (numbness)

C. At least two of the following:
   1. Homonymous visual symptoms and/or unilateral sensory symptoms
   2. At least one aura symptom develops gradually over $\geq$5 min and/or different aura symptoms occur in succession over $\geq$5 min
   3. Each symptom lasts $\geq$5 and $\leq$60 min
D. Headache does not occur during aura nor follow aura within 60 min
E. Not attributed to another disorder

2.2. [G44.2] Frequent episodic tension-type headache

Diagnostic criteria

A. At least 10 episodes occurring on $\geq$1 but $<$15 days per month for at least 3 months ($\geq$12 and $<$180 days per year) and fulfilling criteria B–D
B. Headache lasting from 30 min to 7 days
C. Headache has at least two of the following characteristics:
   1. Bilateral location
   2. Pressing/tightening (non-pulsating) quality
   3. Mild or moderate intensity
   4. Not aggravated by routine physical activity such as walking or climbing stairs
D. Both of the following:
   1. No nausea or vomiting (anorexia may occur)
   2. No more than one of photophobia or phonophobia
E. Not attributed to another disorder

2.3. [G44.2] Chronic tension-type headache

Diagnostic criteria

A. Headache occurring on $\geq$15 days per month on average for $>$3 months ($\geq$180 days per year) and fulfilling criteria B–D
B. Headache lasts hours or may be continuous
C. Headache has at least two of the following characteristics:
   1. Bilateral location
   2. Pressing/tightening (non-pulsating) quality
   3. Mild or moderate intensity
   4. Not aggravated by routine physical activity such as walking or climbing stairs
D. Both of the following:
   1. No more than one of photophobia, phonophobia, or mild nausea
   2. Neither moderate or severe nausea nor vomiting
E. Not attributed to another disorder[1]

Note

1. When medication overuse is present, the diagnosis may be 8.2 *medication overuse headache*. This will remain uncertain until 2 months after medication has been withdrawn.

3.1. [G44.0] Cluster headache

Cluster headache is one of a group of disorders (trigeminal autonomic cephalalgias) sharing the clinical features of short-duration headache and prominent cranial parasympathetic autonomic features. It should be recognized because the pain of cluster headache is excruciating.

It is unusual amongst primary headaches in being more common in men than in women.

Diagnostic criteria

A. At least five attacks fulfilling criteria B–D
B. Severe or very severe unilateral orbital, supraorbital, and/or temporal pain lasting 15–180 min if untreated
C. Headache is accompanied by at least one of the following:
   1. Ipsilateral conjunctival injection and/or lacrimation
   2. Ipsilateral nasal congestion and/or rhinorrhea
   3. Ipsilateral eyelid edema
   4. Ipsilateral forehead and facial sweating
   5. Ipsilateral miosis and/or ptosis
   6. A sense of restlessness or agitation
D. Attacks have a frequency from 1 every other day to 8 per day
E. Not attributed to another disorder

3.1.1. [G44.01] Episodic cluster headache

Diagnostic criteria

A. Attacks fulfilling criteria A–E for 3.1 *cluster headache*
B. At least two cluster periods lasting 7–365 days and separated by pain-free remission periods of $\geq$1 month

3.1.2. [G44.02] Chronic cluster headache

Diagnostic criteria

A. Attacks fulfilling criteria A–E for 3.1 *cluster headache*
B. Attacks recur over $>$1 year without remission periods or with remission periods lasting $<$1 month

SECONDARY HEADACHES

A new headache occurring with another disorder recognized to be capable of causing it is always diagnosed as secondary.

General diagnostic criteria for secondary headaches

A. Headache [with the following listed characteristics] fulfilling criteria C and D
B. Another disorder known to be able to cause headache has been demonstrated
C/D. Evidence of a causal relationship

Criteria B–D may require tests or procedures to be carried out that cannot be undertaken in primary care. In such cases, the diagnosis cannot be confirmed in primary care. The crucial role of primary care is to recognize the possibility of the diagnosis.

5.2.1. [G44.30] Chronic posttraumatic headache attributed to moderate or severe head injury

Chronic posttraumatic headache is often part of the posttraumatic syndrome, which includes symptoms such as equilibrium disturbance, poor concentration, decreased work ability, irritability, depressive mood, and sleep disturbances.

Diagnostic criteria

A. Headache, no typical characteristics known, fulfilling criteria C and D
B. Head trauma with at least one of the following:
   1. Loss of consciousness for >30 min
   2. Glasgow Coma Scale (GCS) <13
   3. Posttraumatic amnesia for >48 h
   4. Imaging demonstration of a traumatic brain lesion (cerebral hematoma, intracerebral and/or subarachnoid hemorrhage, brain contusion, and/or skull fracture)
C. Headache develops within 7 days after head trauma or after regaining consciousness following head trauma
D. Headache persists for >3 months after head trauma

6.2.2. [G44.810] Headache attributed to subarachnoid hemorrhage (SAH)

SAH can occur in anyone, including patients already diagnosed as having a primary headache of any type. Physicians must be alert to the occurrence of new or different headache. SAH is a neurosurgical emergency: it is fatal in 50% of cases whilst 50% of survivors are left disabled.

Diagnostic criteria

A. Severe headache of sudden onset fulfilling criteria C and D
B. Neuroimaging (computed tomography (CT) or magnetic resonance imaging (MRI) T_2 or fluid-attenuated inversion recovery (FLAIR)) or cerebrospinal fluid (CSF) evidence of non-traumatic subarachnoid hemorrhage, with or without other clinical signs
C. Headache develops simultaneously with hemorrhage
D. Headache resolves within 1 month

6.4.1. [G44.812] Headache attributed to giant cell arteritis (GCA)

Giant cell arteritis is conspicuously associated with headache, but its characteristics are variable. Any persisting headache with recent onset in a patient over 60 years of age should suggest GCA.

GCA must be recognized. The major risk is of blindness, preventable by immediate steroid treatment. The time interval between visual loss in one eye and in the other is usually less than 1 week.

Diagnostic criteria

A. Any new persisting headache fulfilling criteria C and D
B. At least one of the following:
   1. Swollen tender scalp artery with elevated erythrocyte sedimentation rate (ESR) and/or C-reactive protein (CRP)
   2. Temporal artery biopsy demonstrating giant cell arteritis
C. Headache develops in close temporal relation to other symptoms and signs of giant cell arteritis
D. Headache resolves or greatly improves within 3 days of high-dose steroid treatment

7.2. [G44.820] Headache attributed to low CSF pressure

The three subtypes of this disorder are distinguished by etiology. The key diagnostic criteria are similar for all three.

Diagnostic criteria

A. Headache that worsens within 15 min after sitting or standing and improves within 15 min after lying, with at least one of the following and fulfilling criteria C and D:
   1. Neck stiffness
   2. Tinnitus

   3. Hypacusia
   4. Photophobia
   5. Nausea
B. One of the following:
   1. Dural puncture has been performed
   2. Persistent CSF leakage (CSF fistula) has been caused by another procedure or by trauma, or low CSF pressure has developed spontaneously,[1] with at least one of the following:
      a) Evidence of low CSF pressure on MRI (e.g., pachymeningeal enhancement)
      b) Evidence of CSF leakage on conventional myelography, CT myelography, or cisternography
      c) CSF opening pressure <60 mmH_2O in sitting position
C. Headache develops in close temporal relation to B1[2] or B2
D. Headache resolves either spontaneously within 1 week[3] or after intervention to seal the spinal fluid leak

Notes

1. A history of trivial increase in intracranial pressure (e.g., on vigorous coughing) is often elicited. In other cases a sudden drop in atmospheric pressure has occurred.
2. Headache may develop up to 5 days after lumbar puncture.
3. Post-lumbar puncture headache often resolves spontaneously within 1 week. Persistence of headache beyond a week is likely to require specialist intervention whatever the etiology.

7.4.1. [G44.822] Headache attributed to increased intracranial pressure or hydrocephalus caused by neoplasm

A history indicating raised intracranial pressure should first suggest intracranial neoplasm.

Diagnostic criteria

A. Diffuse non-pulsating headache with at least one of the following characteristics and fulfilling criteria C and D:
   1. Associated with nausea and/or vomiting
   2. Worsened by physical activity and/or maneuvers known to increase intracranial pressure (such as Valsalva maneuver, coughing, or sneezing)
   3. Occurring in attack-like episodes
B. Space-occupying intracranial tumor demonstrated by CT or MRI and causing hydrocephalus
C. Headache develops and/or deteriorates in close temporal relation to the hydrocephalus
D. Headache improves within 7 days after surgical removal or volume reduction of tumour

8.2. [G44.41 or G44.83] Medication overuse headache (MOH)

Patients with this disorder will not improve without withdrawal of the offending medication.

Diagnostic criteria

A. Headache present on ≥15 days/month fulfilling criteria C and D
B. Regular overuse[1] for >3 months of one or more drugs that can be taken for acute and/or symptomatic treatment of headache[2]
C. Headache has developed or markedly worsened during medication overuse
D. Headache resolves or reverts to its previous pattern within 2 months after discontinuation of overused medication

Notes

1. Intake on ≥15 days/month for simple analgesics alone and *in all other cases* on ≥10 days/month.
2. Drugs may be ergotamine, one or more triptans, simple analgesics, opioids, combination analgesics, or any combination of these.

CRANIAL NEURALGIAS, CENTRAL AND PRIMARY FACIAL PAIN

13.1.1. [G44.847] Classical trigeminal neuralgia

Diagnostic criteria

A. Paroxysmal attacks of unilateral pain lasting from a fraction of a second to 2 min, affecting one or more divisions of the trigeminal nerve and fulfilling criteria B and C
B. Pain has at least one of the following characteristics:
   1. Intense, sharp, superficial, or stabbing
   2. Precipitated from trigger areas[1] or by trigger factors[2]
C. Attacks are stereotyped in the individual patient
D. There is no clinically evident neurological deficit
E. Not attributed to another disorder

Notes

1. Small areas in the nasolabial fold and/or chin may be particularly susceptible to the precipitation of pain (trigger areas).

2. Pain frequently occurs spontaneously, but is commonly evoked by trivial stimuli (trigger factors) such as washing, shaving, smoking, talking, and/or brushing the teeth.

13.18.4. [G44.847] Persistent idiopathic facial pain

Diagnostic criteria

A. Pain in the face, present daily and persisting for all or most of the day, fulfilling criteria B and C
B. Pain is confined at onset to a limited area on one side of the face,[1] and is deep and poorly localized
C. Pain is not associated with sensory loss or other physical signs
D. Investigations including X-ray of face and jaws do not demonstrate any relevant abnormality

Note

1. Pain at onset is commonly in the nasolabial fold or side of the chin, and may spread to the upper or lower jaw or a wider area of the face and neck.

Handbook of Clinical Neurology, Vol. 97 (3rd series)
Headache
G. Nappi and M.A. Moskowitz, Editors

Chapter 12

Triggers of migraine and tension-type headache

CHRISTIAN WÖBER [1]* AND ÇIÇEK WÖBER-BINGÖL [2]
[1]*Department of Neurology, Medical University of Vienna, Vienna, Austria*
[2]*Department of Psychiatry of Childhood and Adolescence, Medical University of Vienna, Vienna, Austria*

INTRODUCTION

Primary headaches are one of the most common disorders, showing a lifetime prevalence of up to 90%. The 1-year prevalence of migraine ranges between 10% and 15%, whereas that of frequent episodic tension-type headache (TTH) is between 24% and 43%. Recurrent headaches are frequently related to a considerable impairment in quality of life and require adequate therapy (Wessely and Wöber, 2003).

Identification of trigger factors or precipitants is frequently recommended as a basic strategy in the treatment of primary headaches. Trigger factors increase the probability of headache in the short term. Potential trigger factors have been examined most frequently in migraine and less often in TTH. Many of these factors are related to migraine as well as to TTH, but their prevalence may differ in the two headache types (Rasmussen, 1993; Scharff et al., 1995; Fernandez and Sheffield, 1996; Spierings et al., 2001; Holzhammer and Wöber, 2006a, b). Menstruation, environmental and psychological factors, sleep disturbances, fatigue, alcohol, and nutrition are mentioned most frequently.

The vast majority of studies on trigger factors are based on retrospectively recorded, subjective patient information. Accordingly, the validity of these data is reduced by recall bias, selective memory, and the patients' need for causal explanations. In addition, only a few studies, such as those of Kelman (2007) and Wöber et al. (2006), differentiated whether a trigger factor was present consistently or only occasionally. Controlled studies are rare and frequently restricted to single trigger factors such as menstruation, chocolate, and alcohol (Littlewood et al., 1988; Marcus et al., 1997; MacGregor and Hackshaw, 2004). In one prospective diary study, migraine patients recorded a wide spectrum of possible trigger factors daily over a period of 3 months irrespective of the presence of headache (Wöber et al., 2007).

In this chapter, we will review the findings of retrospective as well as of prospective and controlled studies. The details of papers including multiple trigger factors are summarized in Table 12.1.

NUTRITIONAL FACTORS

Missing meals

Avoiding irregular meals and longer periods of hunger is a major element of lifestyle modification in migraine. The percentage of patients giving hunger as trigger of headaches ranges between <30% and >75%. Both patients with migraine and those with TTH have reported such experience (Table 12.2). The effect of 19 h of food deprivation in 56 students with frequent migraine or TTH confirms these retrospective observations (Martin and Seneviratne, 1997). The biological pathway remains unclear, however. Hypoglycemia seems not to explain the occurrence of headache after skipping meals (Clifford Rose, 1997).

Insufficient fluid intake

Blau (2005) has stressed the importance of insufficient fluid intake. The author found that more than one-third of 95 patients with migraine experienced attacks precipitated by fluid deficiency. In 2004 Blau et al. reported improvement of headache in 33 of 34 patients within 3 h of intake of 500–750 ml water.

Food and alcohol in general

Certain foods and alcoholic beverages are frequently related to the occurrence of headache. The proportion of patients reporting headache associated with the

*Correspondence to: Professor Christian Wöber, Head of the Headache Group, Department of Neurology, Medical University of Vienna, Währinger Gürtel 18-20, 1090 Vienna, Austria, Tel: +43-1-40400-3441 or -3117, Fax: +43-1-40400-3141, E-mail: christian.woeber@meduniwien.ac.at

Table 12.1

Methods of studies including $\geq$4 trigger factors of migraine, migraine without aura (MoA), migraine with aura (MA), tension-type headache (TTH), and other headaches (other HA)

Reference	Number of triggers	Design	Patient recruitment	Number of patients	Headache diagnoses (number of patients)				
					Migraine	MoA	MA	TTH	Other HA
Bánk and Márton (2000)	7	Retro	Population	78	78	(62)	(16)	–	–
Chabriat et al. (1999)	22	Pro	Population	535	366	–	–	–	169
Cologno et al. (1999)	7	Retro	Clinic	77	–	–	77	–	–
Fernandez and Sheffield (1996)	15	Retro	Newspaper	261	111	–	–	123	87
Henry et al. (2002)	45	Retro	Population	880	880	–	–	–	–
Kelman (2007)	15	Retro	Clinic	1750	1207	?	?	–	–
Peatfield et al. (1984)	9	Retro	Clinic	494	494	–	–	–	–
Peatfield (1995)	4	Retro	Clinic	556	429	–	–	86	39
Rasmussen & Olesen (1992)	7	Retro	Population	96	96	58	38	–	–
Rasmussen (1993)	7	Retro	Population	286	119	–	–	167	–
Robbins (1994)	13	Retro	Clinic	494	494	–	–	–	–
Russell et al. (1996)	8	Retro	Population	333	333	222	111	–	–
Scharff et al. (1995)	16	Retro	Clinic	172	69	69	–	52	53
Spierings et al. (2001)	18	Retro	Clinic	55	38	–	–	17	–
Turner et al. (1995)	12	Retro	Population	132	132	–	–	–	–
Ulrich et al. (1996)	8	Retro	Population	332	288	192	96	332	
Ulrich et al. (2000)	4	Retro	Population	169	169	–	169	–	–
Van den Bergh et al. (1987)	27	Retro	Newspaper	217	217	–	–	–	–
Wöber et al. (2006)	25	Retro	Clinic	120	71	–	–	49	
Wöber et al. (2007)	81	Pro	Newspaper	327	327	–	–	–	–
Zivadinov et al. (2003)	16	Retro	Population	2039	720	462	258	1319	–

Retro: retrospective; Pro: prospective.

Table 12.2

Nutritional trigger factors of migraine and tension-type headache in retrospective studies. The figures given for each trigger factor are the numbers of studies reporting a particular percentage

	Migraine				Tension-type headache			
Trigger factor	<10%	10–25%	26–50%	>50%	<10%	10–25%	26–50%	>50%
Skipping meals	–	–	5	3	–	–	2	3
Food, alcohol (in general)	–	3	1	–	1	2	–	–
Food	1	3	2	1	1	–	1	–
Alcohol	2	4	5	2	–	1	5	–
Beer/spirits	1	3	–	–	3	1	–	–
Red wine	–	1	1	–		1	1	–
Red wine/cheese	–	1	1	–	1	2	–	–
Cheese	2	3	–	–	3	–	–	–
Chocolate	2	4	–	–	2	2	–	–
Caffeine	2	2	–	–	2	1	–	–
Aspartame	2	–	–	–	–	1	–	–
Monosodium glutamate	1	1	–	–	–	1	–	–
Vegetables	2	–	–	–	1	–	–	–
Citrus fruits	1	1	–	–	–	–	–	–
Milk, dairy products	2	–	–	–	–	–	–	–
Sugar	1	–	–	–	1	–	–	–
Ice cream	1	–	–	–	1	–	–	–
Fatty meals	–	1	–	–	–	–	–	–
Meat	2	–	–	–	–	–	–	–
Fish	1	–	–	–	–	–	–	–

intake of food or alcohol ranges between 12% and 58% in migraine and between 0% and 35% in TTH (Table 12.2). Studies comparing the two headache types found either a higher prevalence in migraine or no difference (Rasmussen, 1993; Peatfield, 1995; Chabriat et al., 1999; Spierings et al., 2001). A shortcoming of almost all studies is the lack of recording the amount of intake and the time between intake and onset of headache. According to a study by Peatfield (1995), more than 50% of patients with migraine change their diet or avoid certain foods. However, there are no prospective data on the usefulness of this strategy.

In a comprehensive prospective diary study which covered more than 28 000 patient days and differentiated 13 types of food or food additives as well as five types of alcoholic beverage, not one of the foods or drinks was related to headache, even though chocolate and cheese, for example, were consumed on more than 40% of the days and red wine on almost 10%. Surprisingly, beer even decreased the risk of occurrence of migraine (Wöber et al., 2007).

Alcohol

In numerous papers, alcoholic drinks in general and red wine in particular are considered as possible trigger factors of headache (Holzhammer and Wöber, 2006a). The percentage of patients giving alcohol as a headache trigger ranges between <10% and >50% (Table 12.2) and seems to depend on the type of headache as well as on the type of drink.

In an epidemiological study (Rasmussen and Olesen, 1992), wine, beer, or spirits were reported to precipitate headache by 28% in patients with migraine without aura, but by only 8% in patients with migraine with aura. Peatfield (1995) found that >10% of patients with migraine were sensitive to red wine but not to white wine. Russell et al. (1996) and Ulrich et al. (1996) compared the cumulative sensitivity of red wine/overmatured cheese and beer/spirits and found higher rates for the former (16–28%) than for the latter (6–11%).

Further information is provided by a prospective study (Nicolodi and Sicuteri, 1999) in 307 persons with migraine without aura who kept a headache diary for 14 months recording also the type and amount of alcoholic beverages and details of the lifestyle. As an overall result, it was observed that low amounts of alcohol did not induce a significant increase in the frequency of migraine attacks. A statistically significant relationship between alcohol and migraine attacks was only found for the intake of alcohol during stressful periods.

Data on the consumption of alcohol in subjects with headache are limited. In two retrospective studies

(Mannix et al., 1997; Ulrich et al., 2000) alcohol use did not differ in patients with headache and headache-free controls. The proportion of patients with migraine drinking no alcohol at all was <5% in a population-based study and >40% in a headache clinic (Peatfield et al., 1984; Ulrich et al., 2000). Among these clinic patients, 28% reported that alcohol had no effect on their migraine.

The mechanism underlying headache or migraine precipitated by alcohol is unknown. Ethanol, biogenic amines (histamine, tyramine, phenylethylamine, and others), sulfites, phenolic flavonoids, release of serotonin from thrombocytes, and dehydration have been discussed (Holzhammer and Wöber, 2006a). The relevance of ethanol is questioned by a controlled study suggesting that red wine but not vodka provokes headache in migraineurs (Littlewood et al., 1988). However, in an animal model, ethanol caused vasodilation of meningeal vessels by activation of transient receptor potential vanilloid 1 (TRPV1) and calcitonin G-related peptide release, and this finding may be relevant to the mechanism by which alcohol ingestion triggers migraine attacks (Nicoletti et al., 2008).

Cheese

Among foods, (ripened) cheese is frequently suspected to precipitate migraine attacks. Cheese contains various biogenic amines that theoretically could provoke headache (Finn, 1992). The number of patients reporting headache or migraine triggered by cheese ranges between 0% and 19% (Table 12.2). Peatfield et al. (1984) have found that 15% of patients with migraine avoid the consumption of cheese. There is not one controlled study supporting the importance of cheese as a precipitant of migraine or headache.

Chocolate

Similar to cheese, chocolate is traditionally mentioned as an important alimentary trigger of migraine attacks. However, the agent that might provoke headache is unknown (Littlewood et al., 1982; Finn, 1992) and it has been seriously doubted that chocolate triggers headache or migraine at all (Marcus et al., 1997). Possible precipitating agents include theobromine, caffeine, and biogenic amines such as phenylethylamine and a deficiency in platelet phenolsulfotransferase (Littlewood et al., 1982; Holzhammer and Wöber, 2006a).

Asking for headache triggers, up to 20% of patients with migraine and TTH reported that chocolate precipitates their headache (Table 12.2). Double-blind placebo-controlled studies revealed controversial findings. Gibb et al. (1991) found in patients with migraine who believed that chocolate provoked their attacks that ingestion of chocolate was followed by a typical migraine episode in 5 out of 12 patients, while none of 8 patients challenged with placebo had an attack. In a similar study, Moffett et al. (1974) found no difference between chocolate and placebo. Marcus et al. (1997) published a prospective, double-blind, placebo-controlled trial with a very strict study design. This study showed that chocolate was no more likely to provoke headache than placebo in any of the diagnostic groups. Interestingly, these results were independent of the subjects' beliefs regarding the role of chocolate in the instigation of headache.

Another aspect qualifying the importance of chocolate as a headache trigger is the observation that some patients experience craving for sweets during the premonitory phase of a migraine attack. Thus, intake of chocolate could be the first symptom and not the precipitant of an attack.

Biogenic amines

Biogenic amines such as histamine, tyramine, phenylethylamine, putrescine, cadaverine, and spermidine are found in certain foods and play a role as regulatory agents in human metabolism. Histamine, tyramine, and phenylethylamine have been related most frequently to migraine and headache (Holzhammer and Wöber, 2006a). Histamine was shown to provoke headache after intravenous and subcutaneous administration, and after inhalation (Headache Classification Subcommittee, 2004). Headaches precipitated by foods containing histamine were related to a deficiency in diaminoxidase which is competitively inhibited by alcohol (Jarisch and Wantke, 1996). However, adequate, double-blind, placebo-controlled studies supporting the hypothesis that dietary histamine precipitates migraine or TTH are lacking up to now. Similarly, there is no evidence for headache triggered by tyramine and phenylethylamine (Headache Classification Subcommittee, 2004). However, increased plasma levels of biogenic amines in patients with migraine and cluster headache (D'Andrea et al., 2004) demonstrate that further studies are required to clarify the role of biogenic amines in primary headache disorders.

Caffeine

In two retrospective studies, caffeine use did differ in patients with headache and headache-free controls (Guarnieri et al., 1990; Mannix et al., 1997). An epidemiological study (Rasmussen, 1993) failed to demonstrate that the intake of coffee was related to the prevalence of migraine and TTH. Among patients with

Table 12.3

Non-nutritional trigger factors of migraine and tension-type headache in retrospective studies. The figures given for each trigger factor are the numbers of studies reporting a particular percentage

	Migraine				Tension-type headache			
Trigger factor	<10%	10–25%	26–50%	>50%	<10%	10–25%	26–50%	>50%
Menstruation/hormones	–	2	7	[a]6	–	1	5	1
Ovulation	1	–	–	–	–	–	–	–
Oral contraceptives	–	1	3	–	–	–	2	–
Weather	2	4	4	4	1	1	4	1
Wind	1	–	1	–	1	–	–	–
Heat	1	–	2	–	–	–	1	–
Sun	–	2	2	–	–	1	–	–
Bright lights, glare	2	2	7	–	3	3	3	–
Computer screen	–	1	–	–	–	–	–	–
Neon lights	–	1	–	–	–	–	–	–
Noise	2	–	1	1	1	–	2	1
Lights, noise	–	–	1	–	–	–	1	–
Odors, perfume	2	–	5	2	2	1	1	1
Smoke, smoking	5	1	3	2	4	–	2	1
Stress, tension	–	–	7	6	–	1	2	4
Relaxation after stress	–	2	–	1	–	–	–	1
Anxiety	–	–	–	1	–	–	–	–
Irritation	–	–	1	–	–	–	–	–
Worrying	1	–	1	–	1	–	–	–
Emotions	2	–	1	–	2	–	–	–
Depression, frustration	–	–	2	–	–	–	–	–
Discomfort	1	–	–	–	[b]1	–	–	–
Psychological	–	–	1	–	–	–	–	–
Sleep disturbances	–	–	2	–	–	–	–	–
Change in sleeping habits	–	–	1	1	–	1	–	1
Getting up late	–	2	–	–	–	1	–	–
Lack of sleep	–	–	2	2	–	–	–	2
Sleeping	–	–	1	1	–	–	1	1
Fatigue, exhaustion	1	1	3	2	–	1	2	3
Physical or sexual activity	3	5	4	–	3	2	2	–
Overwork	–	–	2	–	–	1	–	–
Posture, particular	1	2	–	–	1	–	–	–
Sneezing, coughing	1	–	–	–	–	1	–	–
Neck problems	1	–	1	–	2	–	–	–
Head trauma	1	–	–	–	–	–	–	–
Infectious diseases	–	1	–	–	–	1	–	–
Traveling, driving	1	–	1	1	1	1	1	1
Vacation	–	1	–	–	–	–	–	–
Cinema	–	–	–	–	–	1	–	–
Reading	–	1	–	–	–	1	1	–
Shopping	–	–	–	–	–	1	–	–
No trigger	–	1	2	–	–	–	–	–

headache, 6–14% experienced attacks provoked by caffeine (Table 12.2). Shirlow and Mathers (1985) found a statistically significant correlation between headache and caffeine use. In subjects with a daily consumption of 240 mg caffeine, the relative risk of headache was 1.3 compared with that in caffeine abstainers.

In contrast to the conflicting findings for caffeine intake, headache attributed to the withdrawal of caffeine has been confirmed by placebo-controlled studies and included in the second edition of the International Classification of Headache Disorders (ICHD-II) (Hughes et al., 1991; Headache Classification Subcommittee,

2004). In a study by Silverman et al. (1992), for example, more than half of the subjects with an average consumption of 235 mg caffeine per day developed moderate or severe headache after administration of placebo.

Aspartame

Aspartame is an artificial sweetener. Its sweetness is 150–200 times that of sucrose. Among numerous complaints which have been related to aspartame there are many neurological symptoms, in particular headache. The proportion of patients reporting headache precipitated by aspartame ranges between 4% and 12% (Table 12.2) and seems to be similar in migraine and TTH (Scharff et al., 1995). The findings of double-blind placebo-controlled trials are controversial (Holzhammer and Wöber, 2006a). Three studies with fewer than 20 subjects each found some relation between aspartame and headache. Three other studies (with 12, 40, and 108 participants) failed to demonstrate any relation. The daily dose administered was usually 30 mg/kg body weight. In the largest study with negative results the dose was even 75 mg/kg body weight (equivalent to 10 liters of a "light" drink). A review published by the manufacturer concludes that aspartame is safe, and that there are no unresolved questions regarding its safety under conditions of intended use (Butchko et al., 2002).

Monosodium glutamate

In western countries, the daily intake of monosodium glutamate (MSG) averages between 0.3 and 1 g; in single cases 5 g may be reached. MSG has been related to the "Chinese restaurant syndrome" characterized by headache, flush, a sensation of pressure and burning in the face, neck, shoulders and thorax, dizziness, and abdominal discomfort. Regarding the precipitation of primary headaches (Table 12.2), Scharff et al. (1995) reported that 13% of patients with migraine and 15% of those with TTH related some of their headaches to MSG. In another study the proportion was <5% (Van den Bergh et al., 1987). In patients with mixed headache, a restrictive diet free of MSG was associated with a marked decrease in headache frequency (Scopp, 1991). However, there are no controlled studies supporting the usefulness of this diet. According to a double-blind placebo-controlled study in self-identified subjects sensitive to MSG, there is an apparent threshold dose for the occurrence of symptoms of 2.5 g MSG (Yang et al., 1997).

Nitrite and nitrate

The essential role of nitric oxide (NO) in the pathogenesis of primary headaches has been confirmed in a series of studies (Thomsen and Olesen, 2001). NO is synthesized endogenously from arginine and oxygen by nitric oxide synthase. Organic nitrates such as glyceryl trinitrate (nitroglycerine), isosorbide dinitrate, and isosorbide mononitrate are NO donors. It has been shown that the majority of healthy persons as well as patients with migraine, TTH, and cluster headache develop a NO-donor headache (Headache Classification Subcommittee, 2004).

Regarding headaches precipitated by foods containing nitrites or nitrates, there is only one paper, published in 1972 (cited by Scher and Scher, 1992). Accordingly, the importance of dietary nitrates and nitrites as trigger factors of migraine and TTH remains unclear.

Fruits and vegetables

Similarly, there are no controlled studies on the potential role of fruits and vegetables as precipitants of headache. Citrus fruits, bananas, tomatoes, and beans have been related to headache, postulating that octopamine, a biogenic amine, might explain headaches triggered by citrus fruits (Finn, 1992).

Considering that fruits and vegetables are generally recommended as the basis of a healthy diet, there is every indication that fruits or vegetables should only be avoided if there is no doubt that their consumption is related to the occurrence of headache (or another disorder).

Further nutritional factors

Apart from the factors discussed above, nuts, milk, and dairy products, ice cream, sugar, and fatty diet have been suspected to trigger headaches, but none of them has been examined in controlled studies (Table 12.2; Holzhammer and Wöber, 2006a).

HORMONES

Menstruation

The relation between migraine and menstruation has been confirmed in several papers. In two epidemiological studies (Dzoljic et al., 2002; Couturier et al., 2003) the prevalence of menstrually related migraine was 8.0% and 6.1%, respectively, and that of pure menstrual migraine was 0.85% and 1.5%, respectively.

There is evidence for an association between estrogen withdrawal and attacks of migraine without aura, as well as evidence for an association between high estrogen states and attacks of migraine with aura (Russell et al., 1996; MacGregor, 2004). Women with an onset of migraine during the time of menarche seem to be affected more often by menstrual migraine than women without an onset at that time (Russell et al., 1996).

In studies recruiting participants from the general population or via newspapers, the proportion of patients reporting a relation between menstruation and migraine ranges between 16% and 68% (Table 12.3). In a prospective study over 3 months (Chabriat et al., 1999), menstruation was related to headache in 32% of patients with migraine and in 19% of migraine-free controls. In two other prospective studies, migraine was up to 1.7 times more likely to occur during the 2 days before menstruation, up to 2.5 times more likely to occur during the first 3 days of menstruation, and up to 1.4 times more likely to occur on the remaining days of menstruation (MacGregor and Hackshaw, 2004; Wöber et al., 2007).

Fewer studies are available regarding the relation between menstruation and TTH (Table 12.3). In two large epidemiological studies (Rasmussen, 1993; Zivadinov et al., 2003), the proportion of subjects reporting headache related to menstruation did not differ between patients with migraine and those with TTH.

Menstrual migraine is most probably related to falling estrogen concentrations and abnormal reactions of neurotransmitters such as serotonin or beta-endorphin (Marcus, 1995; MacGregor, 2004). The effect of hormones on migraine and TTH may explain, at least in part, the higher prevalence of these disorders in women compared to men (Rasmussen, 1993).

Ovulation

In prospective studies, there is no evidence for ovulation favoring the occurrence of migraine attacks (MacGregor and Hackshaw, 2004). On the contrary, ovulation seems to reduce the risk of headache (Stewart et al., 2000).

Oral contraceptives

The influence of oral contraception on the course of migraine is highly variable. Headaches that worsen in frequency or severity have been reported in 18–50% of cases, with most attacks occurring during the drug-free interval of the cycle. Migraine improvement has been reported in 3–35% of women and there has been no change in 39–65% (Massiou and MacGregor, 2000). The variability of these findings can be explained by differences in the ethinylestradiol content of combined oral contraceptives, a lack of definition of worsening and improvement of headache, and use of International Headache Society criteria in more recent studies only. Asking the patients themselves, approximately 30% related a worsening of migraine to the pill (Table 12.3).

Similar to migraine, there are controversial findings regarding the effect of oral contraceptives on TTH. In two studies, patients reported a worsening; in one they did not (Mraz et al., 1993; Scharff et al., 1995; Zivadinov et al., 2003).

Little research has been undertaken on the possible mechanisms for the adverse changes in migraine that are associated with the use of oral contraceptives. Headaches occurring during the pill-free interval are probably triggered by estrogen withdrawal (Massiou and MacGregor, 2000).

Hormone replacement therapy

Several studies have shown that hormonal replacement therapy is associated with higher migraine prevalence or may affect the course of migraine unfavorably (Facchinetti et al., 2002; Aegidius et al., 2007). Accordingly, it is recommended to observe women with migraine on hormone replacement therapy closely regarding headache frequency, duration, and severity.

ENVIRONMENTAL FACTORS

Weather

In a study on weather sensitivity, headache was the most common symptom reported by more than 60% of participants (von Mackensen et al., 2005). On the other hand, many headache patients experience headache related to (changes in) the weather. The proportion of patients ranges between 8% and 86% (Table 12.3). This marked variability may be explained by differences in patient recruitment, headache diagnoses, study design, and formulation of questions as well as by geographical, social, and cultural differences. In a population-based and in a clinic-based study, patients with migraine reported more often headache precipitated by weather changes than those with TTH (Chabriat et al., 1999; Spierings et al., 2001). In another epidemiological study (Rasmussen, 1993), the result was the opposite way around.

Studies relating meteorological data to headache showed controversial findings. In two studies (Wilkinson and Woodrow, 1979; De Matteis et al., 1994), there was no relation between migraine attacks and meteorological parameters (air temperature, air pressure, humidity, velocity and direction of wind). A study from Germany found a clear but small correlation between headache and a bio-weather categorization system during summer (Walach et al., 2002). Another group from Germany investigated very low frequency sferics and other weather phenomena (Vaitl et al., 2001). Sferics are pulse-shaped electromagnetic fields originating from atmospheric discharges. They move faster than wind and therefore may act 1–2 days before a weather change. The study showed that migraine was related to sferics activity during the fall, but not during summer (when the thunderstorm activity had been very intense), and that TTH was associated with temperature and vapor pressure during summer.

A Canadian study (Cooke et al., 2000) focused on chinook weather conditions in the southern part of Alberta. Chinooks are warm westerly winds specific to the region. Among 75 clinic patients the probability of migraine onset was increased on both prechinook days (odds ratio 1.24) and on days with chinook winds (odds ratio 1.19) compared with non-chinook days. In contrast to this small increase, 79% of patients indicated that chinooks adversely influenced their migraine.

A prospective diary study in eastern Austria (Wöber et al., 2007) showed that some meteorological factors (daily sunshine duration >3 h, low pressure over the UK, air advection from the north) increase and others (maximum air pressure >1000 hPa, small pressure gradient) decrease the risk of headache or migraine in migraineurs.

Sensory stimuli

Photophobia, phonophobia, and osmophobia are frequently associated with migraine attacks. Only few studies in patients with migraine and TTH have examined the sensitivity to sensory stimuli and the potential of these stimuli in precipitating headache. Vingen et al. (1999) investigated the sensitivity to light, sound, smell, and other stimuli in patients with different headache types. Without headache, migraineurs differed from the other headache patients and controls mainly in their increased sensitivity to light. Kelman (2004) found perfume or odor trigger of acute migraine in more than 45% of 724 patients (22.7% occasional, 10.2% frequent, and 12.6% very frequent). In the study by Wöber et al. (2007), odors (but not bright lights and noise) were related to a small increase in the risk of headache in migraineurs. According to Hay et al. (1994) women with classical migraine express greater disability than those with common migraine or controls, both in respect of number of visual sensitivities reported and severity of consequences of such stimuli. Women with classical migraine related visual stimuli to migraine in 75%, to visual disturbances and nausea in 50%, and to non-migrainous headache in one-third. The effect of visual stimuli was less pronounced in patients with common migraine and least in healthy controls. Studies using the International Headache Society criteria confirm that visual stimuli are more important in migraine with aura than in migraine without aura (Table 12.3). Interestingly, visual stimuli seem to precipitate TTH more often in patients suffering also from migraine with aura than in those with pure TTH or additional migraine without aura (Ulrich et al., 1996).

It remains unclear, however, whether it is useful to avoid sensory stimuli precipitating migraine, as there may be a risk of establishing an insidious sensitization process, thereby increasing headache frequency (Wilkins et al., 2002; Martin et al., 2006). Based on a review of the literature Martin and MacLeod (2009) argue that the philosophy of "avoidance of triggers" should be replaced with "coping with triggers," as the latter includes both avoidance and approach/confront strategies involving exposure to triggers.

Smoking and passive smoking

The proportion of patients considering (passive) smoking as a trigger factor of headache varies between 1% and 61% (Table 12.3). Patients suffering from migraine without aura experience headaches triggered by (passive) smoking more often than those suffering from migraine with aura (Rasmussen and Olesen, 1992; Russell et al., 1996). In prospective studies there was only little or no evidence for smoke or smoking precipitating a migraine (Chabriat et al., 1999; Wöber et al., 2007).

STRESS AND OTHER PSYCHOLOGICAL FACTORS

Many patients with migraine and TTH relate their headache to stress (Table 12.3). In cross-sectional epidemiological studies, stress was given by 30–90% of patients. In the study with the smallest percentage (Henry et al., 2002), a number of other psychological factors was included. Anxiety and irritation were reported to trigger headache by 50% of patients, worrying by 44%, and feeling depressed by 27%. The differentiated questions may explain the low percentage for stress.

Comparing the prevalence of self-reported stress in patients with migraine and TTH, the findings are controversial. In some studies, migraineurs reported stress more frequently, and in others less frequently, than patients with TTH (Rasmussen, 1993; Chabriat et al., 1999; Zivadinov et al., 2003). In a prospective study (Holm et al., 1997), single stress parameters showed a statistically significant temporal relation to migraine attacks in 50–70% of female migraineurs. A controlled study showed no evidence of a specific serotonergic, sympathoadrenomedullary, or cerebrovascular response of migraine patients to mental stress as compared to non-migraineurs (Stronks et al., 1998). Similarly, Schoonman et al. (2007) failed to detect any objective evidence for a biological stress response before or during migraine attacks in 17 patients. In contrast, a prospective study including 327 patients (Wöber et al., 2007) showed that stress in private life and psychic tension are related to a small increase in the risk of headache on the subsequent day.

In a study investigating the role of major stressful life events versus daily hassles (De Benedittis and Lorenzetti, 1992), headache patients reported a significantly higher frequency and density of daily hassles, but not of major life events, than controls. Furthermore, daily hassles were significantly correlated with headache frequency. Significant differences between headache subgroups were found, with TTH and mixed headache sufferers reporting a higher incidence and density of daily hassles than migrainous patients.

SLEEP, FATIGUE, EXHAUSTION

Sleep

Sleep disorders are commonly seen and affect about one-quarter of the population older than 15 years of age (Zeitlhofer et al., 2000). Beside many other disorders, pain and headaches may cause sleep disturbances. In contrast, sleep disorders such as narcolepsy, sleep apnea syndrome, or habitual snoring can lead to headaches (Neau et al., 2002; Dahmen et al., 2003; Scher et al., 2003).

The proportion of patients reporting sleeping habits and sleeping problems as triggers of migraine or TTH varies considerably. Headaches precipitated by sleeping too long, or getting up late, were reported by 24% of sufferers and lack of sleep by 31–74% of patients with migraine and by up to 71% of those with TTH (Table 12.3). In an epidemiological prospective study (Chabriat et al., 1999), fatigue and sleeping problems were identified as triggers by 80% of patients with migraine and by 57% of those with other forms of headache. Wöber et al. (2007) found that tiredness is related to a small increase in the risk of occurrence of migraine and non-migrainous headache in migraineurs.

Interpreting sleep and headache diaries (Niederberger et al., 1998) showed that the mean duration of sleep was shorter in nights before the onset of a migraine attack due to awakening earlier because of headache. In addition, sleep quality was significantly reduced and sleep was restless and often interrupted. Patients with various chronic headaches reported reduced quality of sleep, more problems falling asleep, and awakening during the night more often than healthy controls (Paiva et al., 1994). In an epidemiological study (Rasmussen, 1993), sleeping problems were related to TTH, whereas lack of relaxation by sleeping was specifically associated with migraine.

Fatigue and exhaustion

Fatigue and exhaustion were related to headache by 16–79% of migraineurs and by 21–65% of patients with TTH (Table 12.3). In a prospective study using electronic diaries, feeling tired and weary was identified as the most common premonitory symptom of migraine attacks, reported by 72% of patients (Giffin et al., 2003). Furthermore, migraine was related to higher prevalence of morning fatigue (Wacogne et al., 2003). More than 80% of patients with chronic migraine showed increased scores in the Fatigue Severity Scale and two-thirds of them fulfilled all criteria of the chronic fatigue syndrome (Peres et al., 2002). It remains open, however, whether sleep disorders, fatigue, and exhaustion are triggers or symptoms of migraine, or whether they are caused by a comorbid condition such as a depressive disorder.

WEEKENDS

Some patients experience migraine or headaches particularly during weekends. Most frequently, weekend migraine has been explained by relaxation and relief from stress after work (Morrison, 1990; Couturier et al., 1992; Hering et al., 1992). In addition, changes in lifestyle at weekends compared with working days, such as longer duration of sleep, skipping breakfast, caffeine withdrawal, and more frequent use of alcohol and nicotine have been discussed (Couturier et al., 1992; Hering et al., 1992; Torelli et al., 1999a). Finally, marital conflicts and loss of day structure during weekends and dissatisfaction at work have been related to weekend headaches (Nattero et al., 1989; Torelli et al., 1999a).

In retrospective studies (Torelli et al., 1999b; Vaitl et al., 2001), up to 35% of patients experienced weekends as a trigger factor for headache. Data from a migraine clinic (Couturier et al., 1992) suggested that patients with headache occurring predominantly during the weekend consume significantly more caffeine and awake later than those whose headaches are not focused on weekends.

Prospective studies do not provide evidence for weekends as triggers of headaches. Nattero et al. (1989) found migraine attacks independent of the week day in 58 patients and attacks occurring merely on weekends in 46. Studies by Morrison (1990) and Wöber et al. (2007), however, failed to show any relation. The latter showed that the risk of migraine is not increased on Saturdays and Sundays and that holidays and days off reduce the risk by approximately 15%.

PHYSICAL ACTIVITY

Physical activities may trigger primary headaches (Table 12.3), but are also able to reduce frequency and intensity of headaches (Köseoglu et al., 2003). Phenomenologically, headaches triggered by physical activity are most frequently migraine or TTH. Primary exertional headache and primary headache associated with sexual activity are coded as separate entities in ICHD-II (Headache Classification Subcommittee, 2004).

In studies on trigger factors of primary headaches, physical exhaustion and physical activity were experienced as trigger by up to 44% of patients with migraine and by up to 35% of those with TTH (Table 12.3). In daily practice, it is important to clarify whether physical activity is an obligatory or a facultative trigger factor and it is crucial to assess further details such as lack of fluid intake, heat, and/or high altitude.

FURTHER TRIGGER FACTORS

In single studies, various other factors such as overwork, sexual activity, (head) posture, certain movements, neck problems, coughing and sneezing, head trauma, infectious diseases, traveling, driving, vacation, cinema, reading, and shopping have been included. Some details are summarized in Table 12.3.

CONCLUDING COMMENTS

Taken together, virtually all aspects of life have been suspected to trigger migraine or TTH, but scientific evidence for many of these triggers is poor. Menstruation has a prominent unfavorable role in migraine and possibly in TTH. There is at least some evidence that migraine and TTH may be precipitated by environmental factors such as weather, lights, noise, and odors, stress and other psychological factors, sleeping problems, fatigue, and tiredness. In addition, intake of alcohol, caffeine withdrawal, skipping meals, and possibly dehydration may trigger migraine and TTH in some patients, whereas scientific evidence is lacking that any other food or food additive plays a relevant role as trigger factor of headaches.

References

Aegidius KL, Zwart JA, Hagen K et al. (2007). Hormone replacement therapy and headache prevalence in postmenopausal women. The Head-HUNT study. Eur J Neurol 14: 73–88.

Bánk J, Márton S (2000). Hungarian migraine epidemiology. Headache 40: 164–169.

Blau JN (2005). Water deprivation: a new migraine precipitant. Headache 45: 757–759.

Blau JN, Kell CA, Sperling JM (2004). Water-deprivation headache: a new headache with two variants. Headache 44: 79–83.

Butchko HH, Stargel WW, Comer CP et al. (2002). Aspartame: review of safety. Regul Toxicol Pharmacol 35: S1–S93.

Chabriat H, Danchot J, Michel P et al. (1999). Precipitating factors of headache. A prospective study in a national control-matched survey in migraineurs and nonmigraineurs. Headache 39: 335–338.

Clifford Rose F (1997). Food and headache. Headache Q 8: 319–329.

Cologno D, Torelh P, Manzoni CC (1999). Possible predictive factors in the prognosis of migraine with aura. Cephalalgia 19: 824–830.

Cooke LJ, Rose MS, Becker WJ (2000). Chinook winds and migraine headache. Neurology 54: 302–307.

Couturier EGM, Hering R, Steiner TJ (1992). Weekend attacks in migraine patients: caused by caffeine withdrawal? Cephalalgia 12: 99–100.

Couturier EG, Bomhof MA, Neven AK et al. (2003). Menstrual migraine in a representative Dutch population sample: prevalence, disability and treatment. Cephalalgia 23: 302–308.

Dahmen N, Kasten M, Wieczorek S et al. (2003). Increased frequency of migraine in narcoleptic patients: a confirmatory study. Cephalalgia 23: 14–19.

D'Andrea G, Terrazzino S, Leon A et al. (2004). Elevated levels of circulating trace amines in primary headaches. Neurology 62: 1701–1705.

De Benedittis G, Lorenzetti A (1992). The role of stressful life events in the persistence of primary headache: major events vs. daily hassles. Pain 51: 35–42.

De Matteis G, Vellante M, Marrelli A et al. (1994). Geomagnetic activity, humidity, temperature and headache: is there any correlation? Headache 34: 41–43.

Dzoljic E, Sipetic S, Vlajinac H et al. (2002). Prevalence of menstrually related migraine and nonmigraine primary headache in female students of Belgrade University. Headache 42: 185–193.

Facchinetti F, Nappi RE, Tirelli A et al. (2002). Hormone supplementation differently affects migraine in postmenopausal women. Headache 42: 924–929.

Fernandez E, Sheffield J (1996). Descriptive features and causal attributions of headache in an Australian community. Headache 36: 246–250.

Finn R (1992). Food allergy – fact or fiction: a review. J R Soc Med 85: 560–564.

Gibb CM, Davies PT, Glover V et al. (1991). Chocolate is a migraine-provoking agent. Cephalalgia 11: 93–95.

Giffin NJ, Ruggiero L, Lipton RB et al. (2003). Premonitory symptoms in migraine: an electronic diary study. Neurology 60: 935–940.

Guarnieri P, Radnitz CL, Blanchard EB (1990). Assessment of dietary risk factors in chronic headache. Biofeedback Self Regul 15: 15–25.

Hay KM, Mortimer MJ, Barker DC et al. (1994). 1044 women with migraine: the effect of environmental stimuli. Headache 34: 166–168.

Headache Classification Subcommittee of the International Headache Society (2004). The international classification of headache disorders, 2nd edition. Cephalalgia 24: 1–151.

Henry P, Auray JP, Gaudin AF et al. (2002). Prevalence and clinical characteristics of migraine in France. Neurology 59: 232–237.

Hering R, Couturier EGM, Steiner TJ (1992). Weekend migraine in men. Lancet 339: 67.

Holm JE, Lokken C, Myers TC (1997). Migraine and stress: a daily examination of temporal relationships in women migraineurs. Headache 37: 553–558.

Holzhammer J, Wöber Ch (2006a). Alimentäre Triggerfaktoren bei Migräne und Kopfschmerz vom Spannungstyp. Schmerz 20: 151–159.

Holzhammer J, Wöber Ch (2006b). Nichtalimentäre Triggerfaktoren bei Migräne und Kopfschmerz vom Spannungstyp. Schmerz 20: 226–237.

Hughes JR, Higgins ST, Bickel WK et al. (1991). Caffeine self-administration, withdrawal, and adverse effects among coffee drinkers. Arch Gen Psychiatry 48: 611–617.

Jarisch R, Wantke F (1996). Wine and headache. Int Arch Allergy Immunol 110: 7–12.

Kelman L (2004). Osmophobia and taste abnormalities in migraineurs: a tertiary care study. Headache 44: 1019–1023.

Kelman L (2007). The triggers or precipitants of the acute migraine attack. Cephalalgia 27: 394–402.

Köseoglu E, Akboyraz A, Soyuer A et al. (2003). Aerobic exercise and plasma beta endorphin levels in patients with migrainous headache without aura. Cephalalgia 23: 972–976.

Littlewood J, Glover V, Sandler M et al. (1982). Platelet phenolsulphotransferase deficiency in dietary migraine. Lancet i: 983–986.

Littlewood JT, Gibb C, Glover V et al. (1988). Red wine as a cause of migraine. Lancet i: 558–559.

MacGregor EA (2004). Oestrogen and attacks of migraine with and without aura. Lancet Neurol 3: 354–361.

MacGregor EA, Hackshaw A (2004). Prevalence of migraine on each day of the natural mentrual cycle. Neurology 63: 351–353.

Mannix LK, Frame JR, Solomon GD (1997). Alcohol, smoking and caffeine use among headache patients. Headache 37: 572–576.

Marcus DA (1995). Interrelationships of neurochemicals, estrogen, and recurring headache. Pain 62: 129–139.

Marcus DA, Scharff L, Turk D et al. (1997). A double-blind provocative study of chocolate as a trigger of headache. Cephalalgia 17: 855–862.

Martin PR, Seneviratne HM (1997). Effects of food deprivation and a stressor on head pain. Health Psychol 16: 310–318.

Martin PR, Reece J, Forsyth M (2006). Noise as a trigger for headaches: relationship between exposure and sensitivity. Headache 46: 962–972.

Martin PR, MacLeod C (2009). Behavioral management of headache triggers: avoidance of triggers is an inadequate strategy. Clin Psychol Rev 29: 483–495.

Massiou H, MacGregor EA (2000). Evolution and treatment of migraine with oral contraceptives. Cephalalgia 20: 170–174.

Moffett AM, Swash M, Scott DF (1974). Effect of chocolate in migraine: a double-blind study. J Neurol Neurosurg Psychiatry 37: 445–448.

Morrison DP (1990). Occupational stress in migraine – is weekend headache a myth or reality? Cephalalgia 10: 189–193.

Mraz M, Aull S, Feucht M et al. (1993). Spannungskopfschmerz – neue Bewertung auf Basis der Kriterien der International Headache Society. Wien Klin Wochenschr 105: 42–52.

Nattero G, De Lorenzo C, Biale L et al. (1989). Psychological aspects of weekend headache sufferers in comparison with migraine patients. Headache 29: 93–99.

Neau JP, Paquereau J, Bailbe M et al. (2002). Relationship between sleep apnoea syndrome, snoring and headaches. Cephalalgia 22: 333–339.

Nicoletti P, Trevisani M, Manconi M et al. (2008). Ethanol causes neurogenic vasodilation by TRPV1 activation and CGRP release in the trigeminovascular system of the guinea pig. Cephalalgia 28: 9–17.

Nicolodi M, Sicuteri F (1999). Wine and migraine: compatibility or incompatibility? Drugs Exp Clin Res 25: 147–153.

Niederberger U, Gerber WD, Schiffer N (1998). Migräne und Schlaf. Retrospektive und prospektive Analyse anhand von Kopfschmerz- und Schlafprotokollen. Schmerz 12: 389–395.

Paiva T, Martins P, Batista A et al. (1994). Sleep disturbances in chronic headache patients: a comparison with healthy controls. Headache Q 5: 135–141.

Peatfield RC (1995). Relationships between food, wine and beer-precipitated migrainous headaches. Headache 35: 355–357.

Peatfield RC, Glover V, Littlewood JT et al. (1984). The prevalence of diet-induced migraine. Cephalalgia 4: 179–183.

Peres MF, Zukerman E, Young WB et al. (2002). Fatigue in chronic migraine patients. Cephalalgia 22: 720–724.

Rasmussen BK (1993). Migraine and tension-type headache in a general population: precipitating factors, female hormones, sleep pattern and relation to lifestyle. Pain 53: 65–72.

Rasmussen BK, Olesen J (1992). Migraine with aura and migraine without aura: an epidemiological study. Cephalalgia 12: 221–228.

Robbins L (1994). Precipitating factors in migraine: a retrospective review of 494 patients. Headache 34: 214–216.

Russell MB, Rasmussen BK, Fenger K et al. (1996). Migraine without aura and migraine with aura are distinct clinical entities: a study of four hundred and eighty-four male and female migraineurs from the general population. Cephalalgia 16: 239–245.

Scharff L, Turk DC, Marcus DA (1995). Triggers of headache episodes and coping responses of headache diagnostic groups. Headache 35: 397–403.

Scher AI, Lipton RB, Stewart WF (2003). Habitual snoring as a risk factor for chronic daily headache. Neurology 60: 1366–1368.

Scher W, Scher BM (1992). A possible role for nitric oxide in glutamate (MSG)-induced Chinese restaurant syndrome, glutamate-induced asthma, "hot-dog headache", pugilistic Alzheimer's disease, and other disorders. Med Hypotheses 38: 18518.

Schoonman GG, Evers DJ, Ballieux BE et al. (2007). Is stress a trigger factor for migraine? Psychoneuroendocrinology 32: 532–538.

Scopp AL (1991). MSG and hydrolyzed vegetable protein induced headache: review and case studies. Headache 31: 107–110.

Shirlow MJ, Mathers CD (1985). A study of caffeine consumption and symptoms; indigestion, palpitations, tremor, headache and insomnia. Int J Epidemiol 14: 239–248.

Silverman K, Evans SM, Strain EC et al. (1992). Withdrawal syndrome after the double-blind cessation of caffeine consumption. N Engl J Med 327: 1109–1114.

Spierings ELH, Ranke AH, Honkoop PC (2001). Precipitating and aggravating factors of migraine versus tension-type headache. Headache 41: 554–558.

Stewart WF, Lipton RB, Chee E et al. (2000). Menstrual cycle and headache in a population sample of migraineurs. Neurology 55: 1517–1523.

Stronks DL, Tulen JHM, Verheij R et al. (1998). Serotonergic, catecholaminergic, and cardiovascular reactions to mental stress in female migraine patients. A controlled study. Headache 38: 270–280.

Thomsen LL, Olesen J (2001). Nitric oxide in primary headaches. Curr Opin Neurol 14: 315–321.

Torelli P, Cologno D, Manzoni GC (1999a). Weekend headache: a possible role of work and life-style. Headache 39: 398–408.

Torelli P, Cologno D, Manzoni GC (1999b). Weekend headache: a retrospective study in migraine without aura and episodic tension-type headache. Headache 39: 11–20.

Turner LC, Molgaard CA, Gardner CH et al. (1995). Migraine trigger factors in a non-clinical Mexican-American population in San Diego county: implications for etiology. Cephalalgia 15: 523–530.

Ulrich V, Russell MB, Jensen R et al. (1996). A comparison of tension-type headache in migraineurs and in non-migraineurs: a population-based study. Pain 67: 501–506.

Ulrich V, Olesen J, Gervil M et al. (2000). Possible risk factors and precipitants for migraine with aura in discordant twin-pairs: a population-based study. Cephalalgia 20: 821–825.

Vaitl D, Propson N, Stark R et al. (2001). Headache and sferics. Headache 41: 845–853.

Van den Bergh V, Amery WK, Waelkens J (1987). Trigger factors in migraine: a study conducted by the Belgian Migraine Society. Headache 27: 191–196.

Vingen JV, Sand T, Stovner LJ (1999). Sensitivity to various stimuli in primary headaches: a questionnaire study. Headache 39: 552–558.

von Mackensen S, Hoeppe P, Maarouf A et al. (2005). Prevalence of weather sensitivity in Germany and Canada. Int J Biometeorol 49: 156–166.

Wacogne C, Lacoste JP, Guillibert E et al. (2003). Stress, anxiety, depression and migraine. Cephalalgia 23: 451–455.

Walach H, Schweickhardt A, Bucher K (2002). Hat das Wetter Einfluss auf Kopfschmerzen? Schmerz 16: 1–8.

Wessely P, Wöber C (Hrsg) (2003). Behandlung von Kopf- und Gesichtsschmerzen. Therapieempfehlungen der Österreichischen Kopfschmerzgesellschaft. Facultas, Vienna.

Wilkins AJ, Patel R, Adjamian P et al. (2002). Tinted spectacles and visually sensitive migraine. Cephalalgia 22: 711–719.

Wilkinson M, Woodrow J (1979). Migraine and weather. Headache 19: 375–378.

Wöber Ch, Holzhammer J, Zeitlhofer J et al. (2006). Trigger factors of migraine and tension-type headache: experience and knowledge of the patients. J Headache Pain 7: 188–195.

Wöber Ch, Brannath W, Schmidt K et al. (2007). Prospective analysis of factors related to migraine attacks: the PAMINA study. Cephalalgia 27: 304–314.

Yang WH, Drouin MA, Herbert M et al. (1997). The monosodium glutamate symptom complex: assessment in a double-blind, placebo-controlled, randomized study. J Allergy Clin Immunol 99: 757–762.

Zeitlhofer J, Schmeiser-Rieder A, Tribl G et al. (2000). Sleep and quality of life in the Austrian population. Acta Neurol Scand 102: 249–257.

Zivadinov R, Willheim K, Sepic-Grahovac D et al. (2003). Migraine and tension-type headache in Croatia: a population-based survey of precipitating factors. Cephalalgia 23: 336–343.

Handbook of Clinical Neurology, Vol. 97 (3rd series)
Headache
G. Nappi and M.A. Moskowitz, Editors

Chapter 13

Acute headache in the emergency department

DOMINIQUE VALADE* AND ANNE DUCROS
Emergency Headache Center, Lariboisière Hospital, Paris, France

INTRODUCTION

Headache is an extremely common complaint in the emergency department, accounting for 1–16% of all visits according to studies (Dhopesh et al., 1979; Dickman and Masten, 1979; Leicht, 1980; Fodden et al., 1989; Silberstein, 1992; Luda et al., 1995; Ramirez-Lassepas et al., 1997; Morgenstern et al., 1998; Newman and Lipton, 1998; Stevenson et al., 1998; Cortelli et al., 2004). Emergency department patients with headache are mostly young adults, with a female preponderance. While primary headaches are the most frequent, serious and sometimes potentially life-threatening conditions are disclosed in 5–15% of cases. The top priority is thus to establish a precise etiological diagnosis and to distinguish between primary headaches, benign secondary headaches – such as headache due to influenza – and serious secondary headaches requiring emergent investigations and treatment (subarachnoid hemorrhage (SAH), meningitis, intracranial hypertension).

The crucial part of the diagnostic procedure is the interview, further completed by the physical examination. This clinical evaluation determines the management, i.e., administration of specific acute headache treatments usually conducted on an outpatient basis for primary headaches, investigations if needed followed by treatment on an outpatient basis for benign secondary headaches, and, finally, emergent investigations and treatment in the hospital setting for secondary headaches with serious underlying causes. The treatment of secondary headaches requires the treatment of the underlying cause, for example, embolization or surgery of a ruptured intracranial aneurysm, antibiotics for bacterial meningitis, or steroids in temporal arteritis. It is useful to administer symptomatic treatment to patients suffering from acute unusual headaches; however, physicians should be aware that headaches might be alleviated even when they are symptomatic of a serious cause. A good response should not be a reason for postponing etiological investigations.

STEPS IN THE INITIAL DIAGNOSIS OF A HEADACHE SEEN IN THE EMERGENCY ROOM

Obtaining a detailed history of present and previous headaches

The first step of the diagnosis procedure is to obtain a history from the patient by interview. This can be difficult for a patient suffering from an intense headache, but can be manageable in a quiet, dark room. Interviewing the patient's family or friends is often useful. When the patient and the physician do not speak the same language, and if there is no available translator, severe headaches should be considered and investigated as potential secondary headaches symptomatic of a serious cause: a cerebral computed tomography (CT) scan and cerebrospinal fluid (CSF) analysis are mandatory.

MODE OF ONSET AND TIME COURSE OF THE HEADACHE

Primary headaches account for the vast majority of emergency department visits for headache. The most important part of the interview is thus to ascertain if the patient is affected by a definite primary headache disorder – the most frequent being migraine, episodic or chronic tension-type headache, and cluster headache – or not. The patient should be questioned as to whether the headache is acute or chronic and whether it is unusual for the patient or a new attack of a known headache pattern.

According to the responses to these two questions, there are three different situations. Firstly, the patient

*Correspondence to: Dr Dominique Valade, Emergency Headache Center, Lariboisière Hospital, 2 rue Ambroise, Pare, 75010 Paris, France, Tel: 33 1 49 95 89 53, Fax: 33 1 49 95 24 81, E-mail: dominique.valade@lrb.aphp.fr

is able to say that he or she has already suffered from several similar headaches for months or years. In such cases, a primary headache disorder is the most likely cause and the description of headache characteristics – age of onset, duration of headache attacks, pain location, associated signs and symptoms, trigger factors – will help to make a precise diagnosis. Secondly, the patient denies a previous headache history and reports having headaches for the first time. In such cases, a secondary headache has to be excluded and investigations must be performed. Finally, the patient reports a history of definite primary headaches but states that this acute headache is different from usual headache attacks. In such cases, a secondary headache has to be suspected and investigations are noteworthy. In both latter cases of acute unusual headaches, additional questions have to be asked:

- How did the headache begin? (sudden or progressive onset)
- How has the pain changed since its onset? (improvement, worsening, or stability).

Unusual headaches with a sudden onset may reveal a wide range of serious conditions, including mainly vascular disorders such as SAH. Unusual progressive headaches are the mode of presentation of multiple conditions, including intracranial hypertension, meningitis, or meningoencephalitis, local cranial disorders, and temporal arteritis.

Characteristics of the headache

The intensity of the pain does not help to distinguish between a primary and a secondary headache. Nevertheless any sudden and severe headache (thunderclap headache) must be regarded as secondary and further explored in the emergency department. It is important to consider the concordance between the intensity of the pain described by the patient and the consequences of the pain on the patient's attitude (e.g., does the patient require bed rest, does the patient have difficulty in expressing him- or herself). A wide range of pain types may be described (pulsatile, continuous, "electric shock," crushing, pressure, discomfort) but none is specific for a peculiar etiology. Topography may sometimes be an element in favor of a peculiar etiology, such as the temporal pain in temporal arteritis; however, it is usually not specific for a particular etiology.

Circumstances of onset

The circumstances surrounding the onset of a headache can sometimes guide the physician to an immediate diagnosis: cranial trauma (hemorrhage or cerebral contusion), medication or drugs recently taken, recent lumbar puncture, peridural (epidural) or spinal anesthesia causing CSF hypotension, and fever associated with general disease. However, the circumstances surrounding onset can also be misleading: an exertional headache can be benign but also a symptom of a subarchnoid hemorrhage; a headache after lumbar puncture is generally caused by a low CSF pressure but can sometimes reveal a cerebral venous thrombosis (Benzon et al., 2003).

Medical history

The patient's medical history must be obtained in a systematic way because it may guide the diagnosis. Cardiovascular disease and hypertension (strokes), postpartum or previous history of venous thrombosis of the lower limbs (cerebral venous thrombosis), cancer (cranial metastases), known human immunodeficiency virus (HIV) seropositivity (cerebral toxoplasmosis), anxiety and depression (decompensation with tension-type headache), and consumption of psychotropic drugs can all affect headache diagnosis.

Associated symptoms

Any recent and unusual headache associated with a neurological symptom, such as consciousness impairment, epileptic seizures, or focal signs, should always be assumed to be due to an intracranial lesion until proven otherwise. A headache with deterioration of health or claudication of the jaw in a patient of more than 60 years of age should immediately point to a possible diagnosis of temporal arteritis. On the other hand nausea, vomiting, photophobia, and phonophobia are non-specific symptoms that may be part of a meningeal syndrome but are also associated with migraine. The absence of any associated symptom does not eliminate a secondary headache and should not postpone the initiation of investigations if the headache is recent, unusual, and persistent.

Physical examination

The first step is to assess blood pressure, pulse rate, and body temperature. An elevated blood pressure is often the consequence and not the cause of a severe head pain. Headache associated with fever immediately points to an infectious disorder. Skin has to be examined in all febrile headache patients suspected of bacterial meningitis in order to search for purpuric lesions. The rest of the clinical examination should include a neurological as well as a local (head and neck) physical examination. Any abnormality in either the neurological or physical examination indicates the need for further evaluation. On the other hand, a strictly normal clinical examination does not eliminate the possibility of a serious cause and should not preclude investigations.

Neurological examination

The first step is to assess the state of consciousness and to search for a meningeal syndrome. Then, the physician should check for a focal neurological deficit that the interview could have missed. Eyelids and pupils are crucial to examine. A painful Horner's sign points to a dissection of the homolateral internal carotid artery. Headaches associated with unilateral mydriasis or a complete third cranial nerve paralysis point to an aneurysm of the posterior communicating artery or the termination of the internal carotid artery compressing the third nerve. Patients have to be checked for a static or kinetic cerebellar syndrome that may be overlooked in a patient lying down with severe headache, and who is vomiting and reluctant to move. Moreover, the visual field also has to be carefully ascertained, even in patients who do not complain of visual problems. Indeed, a right-handed patient with a right occipital lesion may have a left-sided homonymous hemianopia and complain only about headaches because of being anosognosic of the visual deficit. Finally, a fundoscopic examination will search for papillary edema indicating intracranial hypertension or for hypertensive retinopathy possibly indicating hypertensive encephalopathy.

Local physical examination

The local cranial examination should include inspection for redness of the eyes, exophthalmy or swelling of the eyelids, palpation of the temporal arteries, of the eyeballs, and of the cranial sinuses to search for an unusual sensitivity to pressure, and, finally, auscultation for cervical or cranial murmurs. It is also important to palpate the cervical and chewing muscles which are very often contracted and painful in the case of a tension-type headache.

Identifying headache emergencies and urgencies

The golden rule is to consider all recent and unusual headaches as secondary to an organic cerebral cause and to perform adequate investigations. In all patients with an acute brutal headache (thunderclap headache) and in all patients with an acute progressive and persistent headache, investigations have to be started in the emergency room (Table 13.1). Hospitalization is necessary when a serious underlying cause is rapidly found and has to be treated, but is also often necessary when the first investigations have not permitted a firm diagnosis and additional investigations are required. When a benign secondary headache is obvious after the clinical interview and examination (for example, headache due to influenza), the patient can be managed as an outpatient. Finally, primary headaches or idiopathic facial neuralgias may show acute exacerbations with intractable pain and impossibility in eating or drinking, with a risk of dehydration. These are pain emergencies that may require hospitalization for a few days to give parenteral treatment.

Table 13.1

Clinical features in favor of a secondary headache requiring investigations

Recent *de novo* headache (either acute or progressive)
Unusual headache in a subject suffering from primary headaches
Thunderclap headache
Focal neurological deficit (except typical migrainous aura in a patient)
Consciousness impairment or confusion
Abnormal neurological examination
Papillary edema
Neck stiffness
Fever
Serious general disorder
Severe elevated blood pressure
Painful and inflammatory temporal arteries

STRATEGY OF THE DIAGNOSTIC EVALUATIONS

The usual blood examinations are seldom conclusive, except for an increased erythrocyte sedimentation rate, which indicates temporal arteritis or an infectious state. Any recent headache which is unusual and persistent, whether of sudden or progressive onset, requires two basic examinations to be carried out in a systematic way: a CT scan without contrast injection and a lumbar puncture (Boulan et al., 2004).

CT scan

A cerebral CT scan is the first investigation to perform. Images have to be carefully examined for the presence of abnormal hyperdensities indicating blood either in the subarachnoid spaces or in the cerebral or cerebellar parenchyma, for dilation of the ventricules indicating hydrocephalus, for a localized hypodensity (ischemia), or a localized mass effect indicating an expansive lesion (tumor, abscess, infarct with edema). Those abnormalities will then have to be further investigated later by CT scan with injection or better with magnetic resonance imaging (MRI) (Prager and Mikulis, 1991). If there is a possibility of acute sinusitis, a scan of the sinuses is the procedure of choice. A normal CT scan does not preclude an organic cause:

5–10% of meningeal hemorrhages, 30–50% of cerebral venous thrombosis, most cervical arterial dissections with isolated headaches and local signs, and the vast majority of cases of meningitis present with a normal CT scan and require futher investigations.

Lumbar puncture

Lumbar puncture (LP) should be performed in all patients with unusual and persistent headache, whether the onset was sudden or progressive. Analyzing the CSF is the only way to diagnose meningitis. Moreover, the LP permits the diagnosis of subarchnoid hemorrhage in the 5% of patients who have a normal CT scan. In headache patients, the LP has to be performed after brain imaging (CT scan or MRI) to rule out a contraindication, i.e., a space-occupying lesion with mass effect and risk of brain herniation. Rarely, LP may be indicated without previous brain imaging when the patient is highly supected of bacterial meningitis and has normal consciousness and no focal neurological signs. It is essential to measure the CSF pressure. Intracranial hypertension with normal CT scan requires check for a cerebral venous thrombosis or a dural fistula.

Cervical and transcranial ultrasound examination

This examination must be conducted when the clinical picture is in favor of a carotid or a vertebral artery dissection. Isolated headache may reveal a cervical arterial disscetion (Arnold et al., 2006). Echography can visualize a hematoma in the arterial wall, and cervical and transcranial duplex scanning can evaluate the hemodynamic repercussion. However, both examinations can be strictly normal when the dissection affects an intracranial portion of the artery or when the hematoma does not produce a significant arterial stenosis. In such cases, investigations have to be continued with MRI (cervical and cranial axial sequences with Fat Sat) and cervical and cerebral MR angiography (MRA).

Magnetic resonance imaging

MRI is much more sensitive than CT scan for a number of disorders that may be revealed by isolated headaches. Cerebral MRI has to be performed in all patients with an unusual severe and persistent headache, even after a normal CT scan and a normal or near-normal LP. Indeed, several conditions revealed by an acute headache may present with a normal CT scan and a normal LP. A large number of sequences are necessary: diffusion-weighted sequences (acute ischemic lesions), fluid-attenuated inversion recovery (FLAIR: small cortical subarchnoid hemorrhage, pituitary necrosis, posterior leukoencephalopathy), Fat Sat axial cervical and cerebral sequences (arterial dissection), T1- and T2*-weighted sequences as well as MR venography (cerebral venous thrombosis). T1-weighted sequences with gadolinium enhancement are needed to search for a pachymeningeal enhancement when an idiopathic low CSF pressure syndrome is suspected. MRA may disclose an arterial aneurysm, a dissection, or segmental spasms consistent with cerebral vasoconstriction syndroms. If MR apparatus is not available, CT venography and angiography are helpful.

Conventional cerebral angiography

Conventional cerebral angiography is indicated in the event of acute headaches in only two cases. First, if CT or MRA is doubtful, some patients with a SAH must have a conventional angiogram in order to search for a ruptured aneurysm. Second, a conventional angiogram may be discussed in some patients with a sudden and severe headache, if all preceding investigations are normal and the headaches persist or worsen. Indeed, MR or CT angiography may sometimes be insufficient to exclude a cerebral venous thrombosis, an arterial dissection, especially a vertebral dissection, or a cerebral vasoconstriction syndrome.

DIAGNOSIS AND MANAGEMENT OF THE MOST FREQUENT CAUSES OF HEADACHE

Epidemiological studies on headaches in the emergency room are rare (Bourrier et al., 2001). Patients are characterized by a female preponderance and a mean age of around 35–40 years. Most patients are affected by primary headache and benign secondary headache (upper tract respiratory infections, general viral syndromes). Among primary headaches, tension-type headaches and migraine are the two most frequently seen. However, 5–15% of patients have a serious secondary cause. The following sections deal with the most frequent serious and benign non-traumatic causes (Figure 13.1). Patients with a severe acute posttraumatic headache, with focal neurological signs and/or consciousness impairment, need an emergency CT scan. Patients with an epidural hematoma or a traumatic subdural hematoma require immediate neurosurgery.

Thunderclap headache

A thunderclap headache is a severe and explosive headache that reaches maximal intensity in less than 1 min (Schwedt et al., 2006). Every thunderclap headache has to be considered as symptomatic of an organic cause and immediately investigated. Indeed, 30–80% of thunderclap headaches reveal an underlying disorder, the most frequent being vascular disorders.

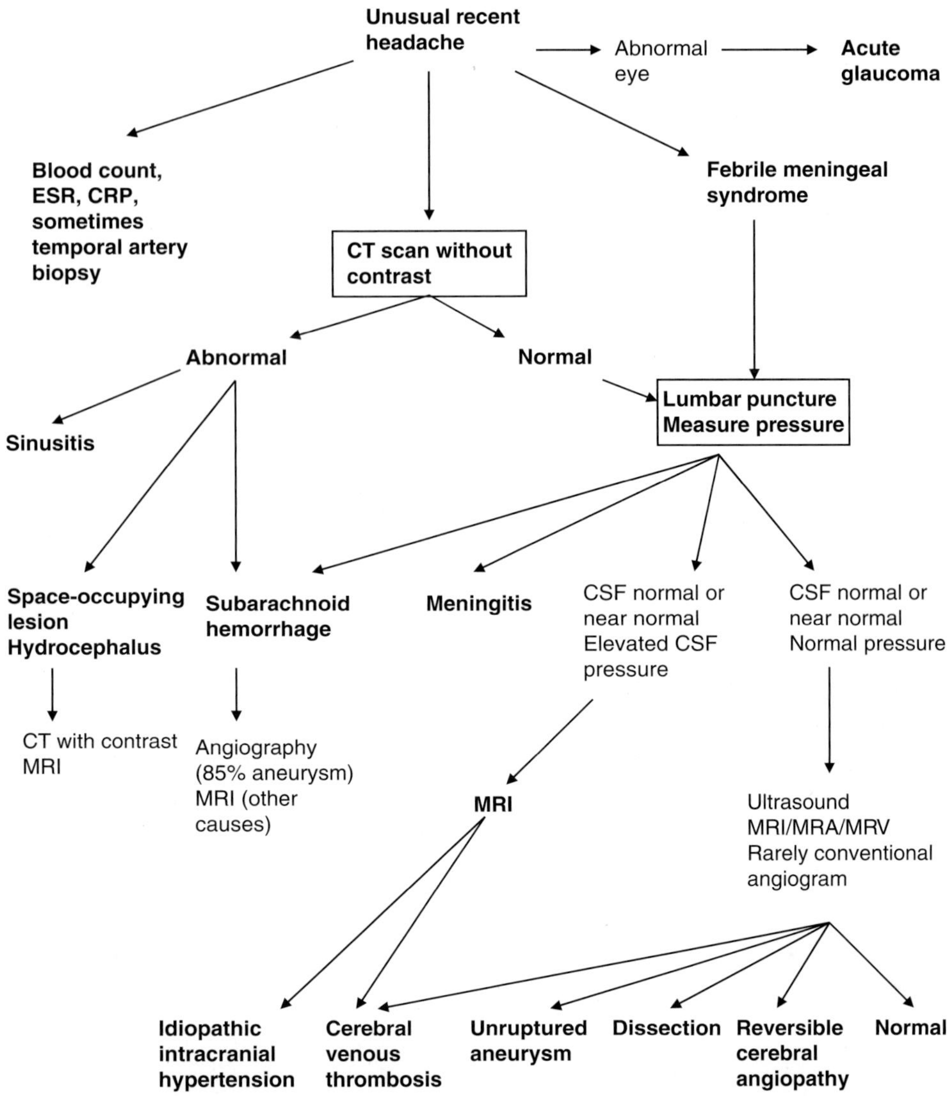

Fig. 13.1. Strategy of investigations in an acute headache patient with a suspicion of an organic cause. ESR: erythrocyte sedimentation rate; CRP: C-reactive protein; CT: computed tomography; CSF: cerebrospinal fluid; MRI: magnetic resonance imaging; MRA: magnetic resonance angiography; MRV: magnetic resonance venography.

The location and the type of thunderclap headache are not specific to a particular cause. Duration may range according to the various causes from some minutes to several days. A thunderclap headache may be isolated or be recurrent over a few days. It may start spontaneously or be triggered by Valsalva maneuvers, physical effort, or sexual intercourse. The first cause to search for is a SAH: 11–33% of thunderclap headaches are due to SAH (Linn et al., 1994; Lledo et al., 1994; Landtblom et al., 2002) and 70% of SAH present with isolated headaches consistent with a thunderclap headache in 50% of cases (Linn et al., 1998).

CT scan has to be performed immediately, followed by LP if the CT is normal. Patients must be hospitalized to undergo a conventional angiogram. In 85% of cases a ruptured aneurysm is the cause, and the definitive treatment requires neurosurgical intervention or an intra-arterial embolization. Other intracranial hemorrhages account for 5–10% of thunderclap headaches (Fodden et al., 1989; Lledo et al., 1994; Landtblom et al., 2002). Isolated headaches are frequent in cerebellar or intraventricular hemorrhages that mimic a SAH. They are rare but possible in some supratentorial parenchymal hematomas, especially right frontal or temporal hematomas in right-handed persons. Finally, a thunderclap headache exceptionally reveals a subdural hematoma.

CT scan easily diagnoses these cerebral hemorrhages. Ischemic infarcts with the same topography may also be revealed by isolated brutal headaches

(Schwedt and Dodick, 2006). The initial CT scan may be normal, MRI being much more sensitive (diffusion) (Schwedt and Dodick, 2006). Patients with cerebellar infarcts or hemorrhages have to be hospitalized in intensive care units close to a neurosurgery department because they may deteriorate acutely if a compression of the fourth ventricle provokes an acute hydrocephalus and a brain hernia. Numerous other vascular disorders may present with isolated thunderclap headaches, including about 5% of cervical or intracranial artery dissections, 2–3% of cerebral venous thromboses, some pituitary necrosis, rare cases of temporal arteritis, and most reversible cerebral vasoconstriction syndromes (also known as reversible or benign cerebral angiopathy) (Dodick and Wijdicks, 1998; Cumurciuc et al., 2005; Arnold et al., 2006; Chen et al., 2006). In all these causes, CT scan and LP may be normal, so MRI with MRA and MR venography (MRV) is mandatory. When these diagnoses are confirmed, patients have to be hospitalized in a stroke unit (if possible) to receive specific treatment: heparin for cerebral venous thrombosis, blood pressure control and heparin for cervical artery dissection, and nimodipine for cerebral vasoconstriction syndromes.

Finally, the existence of thunderclap headaches due to an unruptured aneurysm is still debated. The rule that a systematic MRI/MRA/MRV is to be performed in all patients with one or several thunderclap headaches will permit the disclosure of most aneurysms with a diameter of at least 2–3 mm and further address the patient to specialized neurovascular teams.

An isolated thunderclap headache may also reveal a non-vascular condition: acute blocked sinusitis, parenchymal or intraventricular tumors with hydrocephalus (colloid cyst of the third ventricle), some meningitis, and some cases of low CSF pressure syndrome. Indeed, about 15% of cases of idiopathic low CSF pressure syndrome are revealed by a thunderclap headache. Diagnosis is made on the postural character of the headache (alleviated by lying down) and the typical MRI features (meningeal enhancement, craniocaudal displacement of the brain structures, subdural collections). If bed rest for a few days does not improve the headache, an autologous epidural blood patch may represent the treatment of choice (Berroir et al., 2004).

Unusual headaches with progressive onset

The list of etiologies is long, including all causes of thunderclap headache that may also provoke progressive headaches, all causes of intracranial hypertension, all causes of meningitis and meningoencephalitis, temporal arteritis, and all extracerebral head and neck lesions (eyes, ears, teeth, oropharyngeal tract, skull).

Intracranial hypertension

An intracranial hypertension is suspected when a patient describes progressive worsening headaches increased by cough, effort, or lying down, associated with nausea or vomiting, bilateral papillary edema, sometimes with horizontal diplopia due to sixth nerve paralysis and visual eclipses. However, headaches may be isolated, especially at the initial phase. CT scan discloses hydrocephalus (stenosis of the sylvian aqueduct) and most of the space-occupying lesions sufficiently important to cause an intracranial hypertension. A CT scan with contrast enhancement and/or cerebral MRI are needed when there is a suspicion of posterior fossa lesion. If neuroimaging rules out a hydrocephalus or a space-occupying lesion, LP with measurement of CSF pressure is mandatory. A high opening CSF pressure (above 20 cmH_2O) indicates intracranial hypertension and the need to search for a vascular cause not seen on the CT scan, such as cerebral venous thrombosis or dural fistula. The LP also permits a CSF subtraction in order to alleviate the headache. If the CT scan, CSF analysis, and MRI/MRA/MRV are normal, it will be concluded that the patient has a "benign" intracranial hypertension, which may be due to drugs (steroids, vitamin A) or be idiopathic, mostly in young obese women.

Meningitis and meningoencephalitis

A febrile headache with neck stiffness, nausea/vomiting, and photophobia points to infectious meningitis. LP is the only way to confirm the diagnosis and guide the choice of treatment. However, fever may be absent (use of over-the-counter antipyretics) and the meningeal syndrome may be absent. This favors the rule of systematically performing LP in patients complaining of recent headache and having a normal CT scan. In some meningoencephalitides, headache may be the presenting symptom before the onset of focal deficits, consciousness impairment, or seizures. In a case of lymphocytic meningoencephalitis, herpes zoster treatment must be started without awaiting viral confirmation (polymerase chain reaction on the CSF).

Temporal arteritis

Every patient aged above 50–60 years and complaining of unusual headaches is suspected of temporal arteritis. Diagnosis is made on an elevated erythrocyte sedimentation rate (and C-reactive protein) and a temporal artery biopsy. When the clinical suspicion is strong (fatigue, febricula, inflammatory signs on temporal arteries, jaw claudication, girdle pain, loss of vision), steroids must be initiated before the results of the temporal artery biopsy. The efficacy of steroids on headache in cases of temporal arteritis is so conclusive that the persistence of headaches after 4 days should lead to consideration of an alternative diagnosis.

Local cranial lesions

Where there is an unusual recent headache without any neurological signs or symptoms, two main causes have to be considered: acute sinusitis and acute glaucoma. Acute sinusitis often provokes severe acute headaches, increased by putting the head down or lying down. Pain may be isolated in blocked sinusitis and especially in sphenoid sinusitis (Gordon-Bennett et al., 2006). Indeed purulent rhinorrhea and fever are not constant. Diagnosis requires a cranial CT scan of the sinuses. Antibiotic and anticongestant therapy is required and, if appropriate, sinus drainage may be carried out. An acute angle-closure glaucoma should be suspected where there is severe periorbital pain with a red eye and unilateral visual loss. However, the clinical features are sometimes misleading (Gordon-Bennett et al., 2006). Examination may disclose an areactive semimydriasis. Diagnosis requires measurement of intraocular pressure. Treatment is based on miotics such as systemic acetazolamide, pilocarpine, or eye drops of beta-blockers.

Carbon monoxide poisoning

Carbon monoxide (CO) is a colorless and odorless gas. Most intoxications are due to dysfunctions of heating or cooking apparatus, where the combustion systems produce CO. Headache is the most frequent symptom and the most frequent presenting symptom (90%) of chronic or acute CO intoxication. Headaches have no specific characteristics. They usually precede other symptoms, including dizziness, syncope, visual problems, and general weakness. Severe symptoms such as seizures, coma, dysrhythmias, and cardiac ischemia occur later (Kao and Nanagas, 2006). The intensity of symptoms is correlated with the level of blood carboxyhemoglobin (HbCO). From 10% to 20%, headache is generally isolated. Above 20%, headache is associated with nausea, vomiting, fatigue, and irritability. Above 30%, headaches become intractable; the patient becomes confused and than comatose. Blood has to be drawn as soon as possible, if possible at the place of intoxication, because the level of HbCO immediately decreases when exposure to CO stops and may even be normal if the test is performed too late. Diagnosis is easier when intoxication is collective, affecting persons living in the same place. Some characteristics indicate diagnosis: headache during the night that improves in the morning, headaches that improve when the patient is outside. Treatment consists of oxygen therapy, supportive care, and, in selected cases, hyperbaric oxygen therapy. Eradication of the source of contamination is crucial to prevent recurrences.

Primary headaches in the emergency room

The most important step is to make an exact diagnosis: is it a migraine attack? An exacerbation of tension-type headaches in the setting of stress, anxiety, or depression? Or a cluster headache? The patient should be carefully interviewed because the diagnosis is based on the description of the characteristics of headache attacks and on a normal physical and neurological examination. As a result, emergency physicians have to be familiar with the diagnostic criteria of these primary headaches.

Management of migraine attacks in the emergency room

Treatment of the attack, adjusted to previous therapies, to contraindications, and to any excessive use of medicinal products, will be offered to the patient (Valade, 2006). In the aftermath of the attack, the patient should be managed and in particular should consult his or her family doctor or a neurologist or a headache specialist. The risk of medication overuse should be systematically explained to the patient. If medication overuse is present, withdrawal should be planned and the advice of a headache specialist on preventive migraine treatment is crucial.

It frequently occurs that a patient comes to the emergency department without having taken any treatment, and then it may be sufficient to initiate therapy with a single 1-g oral dose of aspirin or even with a non-steroidal anti-inflammatory drug (NSAID), either by the oral route or, where there is nausea, in suppository form. Metoclopramide or metopimazine in suppositories or by intravenous administration is given in combination with the above-mentioned drugs if serious vomiting is present.

If the patient has already taken aspirin, a NSAID, or acetaminophen, possibly combined with caffeine, codeine, or dextropropoxyphene, the use of specific antimigraine therapy is indicated, preferably by nasal or subcutaneous route (20 mg sumatriptan nasal spray or 6 mg/0.5 ml subcutaneous sumatriptan).

Where there is a known allergy or contraindication to triptans, it is possible to use dihydroergotamine (DHE) by either the nasal route (spray) or the injectable route (intramuscular, subcutaneous, or intravenous): DHE 1 mg/ml. Either metoclopramide or metopimazine in suppository form or by injectable route must always be administered in combination with therapy.

When specific antimigraine drugs are not effective, preference should be given to the parenteral route of administration. Depending on individual habits and types of medication previously taken by the patient to treat the attack, the following can be administered:

- 1 g acetaminophen as a short 20-min intravenous infusion in the absence of previous excessive self-medication with acetaminophen
- Ketoprofen (100 mg) infusion under the same conditions
- Nefopam in infusion under the same conditions.

A 20- or 50-mg ampoule of clorazepate can be added to the intravenous infusion depending on the patient's anxiety condition; if there is nausea or vomiting, a 10-mg ampoule of metoclopramide can also be added.

In the event of failure of the above-mentioned infusions, or when there is excessive use of medications preventing the use of the above-mentioned drugs, 50 mg amitriptyline and 1 mg/ml clonazepam can be administered, especially if the acute attack is accompanied by tension-type headache. Amitriptyline and clonazepam are infused slowly over approximately 2 h, after informing the patient that, as a result of the sedative effect of these drugs, it will be necessary for them to be escorted home by another person.

In status migrainosus, the patient should be hospitalized to continue this treatment. When there is medication overuse, withdrawal should be planned in a second phase.

For pregnant or nursing women, intravenous acetaminophen may be used as first-line therapy in the absence of contraindication (previous excessive oral intake). Oxygen delivered via face mask at a rate of 10 l/min for 30 min may be administered.

For young children, the recommended first-line therapies are as follows:

- 20 mg/ml ibuprofen: 0.5 ml/kg, i.e., 10 mg/kg body weight, for children over 6 months of age
- Diclofenac 25-mg suppositories starting at 16 kg body weight, i.e., children over 4 years of age
- 275 mg naproxen starting at 25 kg body weight, i.e., children over 6 years of age
- Acetaminophen alone or in combination with metoclopramide under the same conditions as described above
- Ergotamine tartrate 1 tablet in children over 10 years of age, never exceeding 6 tablets/week
- Sumatriptan 20 mg nasal spray starting at 35 kg body weight, i.e., over 12 years of age.

The rectal route or nasal spray should be given preference in the event of nausea/vomiting.

A child presenting with migraine should receive relaxation therapy as soon as possible.

Management of cluster headache in the emergency room

Even if the cluster headache attacks are short-lived, patients very often visit the emergency room, for various reasons. First, patients may have cluster headache and the diagnosis has not been made before. The delay between the first attacks of cluster headache and the diagnosis is often several years. These patients come because they have very severe pain and no effective treatment. If they are seen during an attack, the only two effective acute treatments are subcutaneous sumatriptan (6 mg/ml) and oxygen therapy (10 l/min for 20–30 min via face mask).

Patients known to be affected by episodic or chronic cluster headache may visit the emergency department for other reasons: the urgent need for a prescription because they used their last subcutaneous sumatriptan the previous night; an increase in the number of daily attacks for a few days; a fear of adverse reactions because they have treated 6 or 7 attacks with sumatriptan in the same day (contraindicated), or accentuation of the number of attacks over a number of days. When there is an increase in the number of attacks, oxygen should always be tried because it may represent a good option in patients having more than 2 attacks a day. A preventive treatment with high doses of verapamil should be initiated. Sometimes intranasal lidocaine may be effective and, finally, 1 g hydrocortisone intravenously may be tried.

Management of tension-type headaches in the emergency room

Patients with episodic or chronic tension-type headache visit the emergency room when the intensity of pain has increased, often in the setting of stress, anxiety, or sometimes depression, and when they can no longer cope. They often have an intense fear of having a cerebral lesion such as a brain tumor or an aneurysm, and ask for brain imaging. A careful interview and clinical examination are necessary to make the appropriate diagnosis. If there is no doubt about the diagnosis, investigations are not necessary and it is important to provide patients with explanations about tension-type headaches. A treatment with tranquilizers such as lorazepam, or muscle relaxants such as clonazepam, may be initiated. In frequent episodic or chronic tension-type headache, a follow-up with a neurologist or a headache specialist must be recommended.

References

Arnold M, Cumurciuc R, Stapf C et al. (2006). Pain as the only symptom of cervical artery dissection. J Neurol Neurosurg Psychiatry 77: 1021–1024.

Benzon HT, Iqbal M, Tallman MS et al. (2003). Superior sagittal sinus thrombosis in a patient with postdural puncture headache. Reg Anesth Pain Med 28: 64–67.

Berroir S, Loisel B, Ducros A et al. (2004). Early epidural blood patch in spontaneous intracranial hypotension. Neurology 63: 1950–1951.

Boulan P, Ducros A, Berroir S et al. (2004). Les céphalées aiguës. In: P Amarenco, P Niclot (Eds.), Urgences Neurologiques. Da Te Be Editions, Puteaux, pp. 13–26.

Bourrier P, Perroux D, Lannehoa Y et al. (2001). Epidémiologie des céphalées de l'adulte dans les services d'urgences. In: P Bourrier (Ed.), Céphalées en Urgence. Masson, Paris, pp. 3–10.

Chen SP, Fuh JL, Lirng JF et al. (2006). Recurrent primary thunderclap headache and benign CNS angiopathy: spectra of the same disorder? Neurology 67: 2164–2169.

Cortelli P, Cevoli S, Nonino F et al. (2004). Evidence-based diagnosis of nontraumatic headache in the emergency department: a consensus statement on four clinical scenarios. Headache 44: 587–595.

Cumurciuc R, Crassard I, Sarov M et al. (2005). Headache as the only neurological sign of cerebral venous thrombosis: a series of 17 cases. J Neurol Neurosurg Psychiatry 76: 1084–1087.

Dhopesh V, Anwar R, Herring C (1979). A retrospective assessment of emergency department patients with complaint of headache. Headache 19: 37–42.

Dickman RL, Masten T (1979). The management of non-traumatic headache in a university hospital emergency room. Headache 19: 391–396.

Dodick DW, Wijdicks EF (1998). Pituitary apoplexy presenting as a thunderclap headache. Neurology 50: 1510–1511.

Fodden DI, Peatfield RC, Milsom PL (1989). Beware the patient with a headache in the accident and emergency department. Arch Emerg Med 6: 7–12.

Gordon-Bennett P, Ung T, Stephenson C et al. (2006). Misdiagnosis of angle closure glaucoma. BMJ 333: 1157–1158.

Kao LW, Nanagas KA (2006). Toxicity associated with carbon monoxide. Clin Lab Med 26: 99–125.

Landtblom AM, Fridriksson S, Boivie J et al. (2002). Sudden onset headache: a prospective study of features, incidence and causes. Cephalalgia 22: 354–360.

Leicht MJ (1980). Non-traumatic headache in the emergency department. Ann Emerg Med 9: 404–409.

Linn FH, Wijdicks EF, van der Graaf Y et al. (1994). Prospective study of sentinel headache in aneurysmal subarachnoid haemorrhage. Lancet 344: 590–593.

Linn FH, Rinkel GJ, Algra A et al. (1998). Headache characteristics in subarachnoid haemorrhage and benign thunderclap headache. J Neurol Neurosurg Psychiatry 65: 791–793.

Lledo A, Calandre L, Martinez-Menendez B et al. (1994). Acute headache of recent onset and subarachnoid hemorrhage: a prospective study. Headache 34: 172–174.

Luda E, Comitangelo R, Sicuro L (1995). The symptom of headache in emergency departments. The experience of a neurology emergency department. Ital J Neurol Sci 16: 295–301.

Morgenstern LB, Luna-Gonzales H, Huber JC Jr et al. (1998). Worst headache and subarachnoid hemorrhage: prospective, modern computed tomography and spinal fluid analysis. Ann Emerg Med 32: 297–304.

Newman LC, Lipton RB (1998). Emergency department evaluation of headache. Neurol Clin 16: 285–303.

Prager JM, Mikulis DJ (1991). The radiology of headache. Med Clin North Am 75: 525–544.

Ramirez-Lassepas M, Espinosa CE, Cicero JJ et al. (1997). Predictors of intracranial pathologic findings in patients who seek emergency care because of headache. Arch Neurol 54: 1506–1509.

Schwedt TJ, Dodick DW (2006). Thunderclap stroke: embolic cerebellar infarcts presenting as thunderclap headache. Headache 46: 520–522.

Schwedt TJ, Matharu MS, Dodick DW (2006). Thunderclap headache. Lancet Neurol 5: 621–631.

Silberstein SD (1992). Evaluation and emergency treatment of headache. Headache 32: 396–407.

Stevenson RJ, Dutta D, MacWalter RS (1998). The management of acute headache in adults in an acute admissions unit. Scott Med J 43: 173–176.

Valade D (2006). Headache in the emergency room. In: J Olesen, PJ Goadsby, NM Ramadan et al. (Eds.), The Headaches. Lippincott Williams & Wilkins, Philadelphia, pp. 1133–1138.

Table 14.2

Continued

Finding	Recommendation
Butorphanol nasal spray	
The clinical efficacy of butorphanol specifically in migraine has been documented in two published reports	Clinical experience and expert consensus concur that butorphanol represents a treatment option for some patients with migraine. Specifically, butorphanol may be considered when other medications cannot be used or as a rescue medication when significant sedation would not jeopardize the patient. Clinical concerns regarding the use of butorphanol lie in the fact that it is widely used despite the established risk of overuse and dependence. In patients for whom use might be indicated, special attention should be given to these clinical concerns
Opiates: oral combination	
Studies demonstrated the effectiveness of oral opiate combination agents in terms of pain relief	Oral opiate combinations may be considered for use in acute migraine when sedation side-effects will not put the patient at risk and/or the risk for abuse has been addressed
Opiates IM/IV	
To date, only one placebo-controlled study has been published for methadone IM, and meperidine IM. This study demonstrated the effectiveness of opiates for pain relief	Parenteral opiates may be considered for rescue therapy in a supervised setting for acute migraine when sedation side-effects will not put the patient at risk and when the risk for abuse has been addressed
Triptans (5-$HT_{1B/1D}$ receptor agonists)	
Naratriptan, rizatriptan, sumatriptan, zolmitriptan	The triptans are an appropriate treatment choice and may be considered for use in patients with moderate to severe migraine who have no contraindications for their use
Triptans are effective and relatively safe for the acute treatment of migraine headaches. To date, no evidence supports their use during the aura phase of a migraine attack. (Published case reports of cardiovascular ischemic events with this class of drug are found in the literature and are included in the product label)	
Isometheptene and isometheptene combination agents	
Isometheptene-containing compounds were superior to placebo, with a small but statistically significant effect	Based on clinical evidence and favorable tolerability, isometheptene-containing compounds may be a reasonable choice for patients with mild to moderate headache
Dexamethasone or hydrocortisone	
No good-quality studies support or refute the effectiveness of steroids for acute migraine	Corticosteroids may be considered as a treatment choice for rescue therapy for patients with status migrainosus
Lidocaine intranasal	
Limited studies reported lidocaine superior to placebo in relieving acute migraine headache at 15 min. The incidence of recurrence has been reported with mixed results	Evidence is insufficient at this time to establish a defined role for intranasal lidocaine in the management of acute migraine headache
Lidocaine IV	
A few small studies suggested that lidocaine IV is not significantly better than placebo and is less effective than other parenteral therapies for treatment of acute migraine	Evidence is insufficient to support the role for lidocaine IV in the management of acute migraine

*Currently not available in the USA.
IM: intramuscularly; IV: intravenously; PR: per rectum; PO: orally; NSAIDs: non-steroidal anti-inflammatory drugs; DHE: dihydroergotamine; SC: subcutaneously.
(Adapted from Matchar et al., 1999.)

to be effective for the acute treatment of migraine? The complete list of findings and recommendations is summarized in Table 14.2.

Based on the results of the evidence review, acute migraine medications have been grouped according to proven efficacy, possible efficacy, or lack of efficacy, and are shown in Table 14.3. Since the original guideline, additional medications have been assessed for the acute treatment of migraine, such as frovatriptan and almotriptan, among others. These large,

Table 14.3

Acute therapies for migraine

Group 1: Proven pronounced statistical and clinical benefit *(at least two double-blind, placebo-controlled studies + clinical impression of effect)*	**Group 2: Moderate statistical and clinical benefit** *(one double-blind, placebo-controlled study + clinical impression of effect)*	**Group 3: Statistically but not clinically proven or clinically but not statistically proven to be effective** *(conflicting, inconsistent, insufficient evidence)*	**Group 4: Proven to be statistically or clinically ineffective or not tolerated** *(failed efficacy versus placebo)*
Acetaminophen, aspirin, plus caffeine PO Almotriptan PO[†] Aspirin PO Butorphanol IN* DHE SC, IM, IV, IN DHE IV plus antiemetic Eletriptan PO[†] Frovatriptan PO[†] Ibuprofen PO Naproxen sodium PO Naratriptan PO Prochlorperazine IV Rizatriptan PO Sumatriptan SC, IN, PO Zolmitriptan PO, IN Sumatriptan plus naproxen[†]	Acetaminophen plus codeine PO* Butalbital, aspirin, caffeine plus codeine PO* Butorphanol IM* Chlorpromazine IV Diclofenac K PO Ergotamine plus caffeine plus pentobarbital plus Bellafoline PO Flurbiprofen PO Isometheptene PO[†] Lidocaine IN Meperidine IM, IV Methadone IM Metoclopramide IV Naproxen PO Prochlorperazine IM, PR	Butalbital, aspirin plus caffeine PO* Dexamethasone IV Ergotamine PO Ergotamine plus caffeine PO Hydrocortisone IV Metoclopramide IM, PR	Acetaminophen PO Chlorpromazine IM Granisetron IV Lidocaine IV Ondansetron IV[†] Ketorolac IM[†]

*Opiates, barbiturates and narcotics are proven clinically effective for pain relief, and some specifically in migraine, but their use should be highly restricted due to the risk of dependency.
PO: orally; IN: intranasally; SC: subcutaneously; IM: intramuscularly; IV: intravenously; PR: per rectum.
(Adapted and updated from Matchar et al., 1999. [†]Indicates a change or update from original guideline.)

randomized, double-blind, placebo-controlled trials need to be considered within the review of evidence-based treatment options for the acute treatment of migraine. Based on the evidence published in the literature, these new agents have been included and are noted in Table 14.3.

Recent studies also show that specific approaches to managing an acute attack improve the efficacy and response to selected migraine therapies. Several class I studies show that early intervention or treatment when pain is mild may improve response to acute treatment (Brandes et al., 2004, 2005; Cady et al., 2004; Mathew et al., 2004). Stratified care is a treatment approach that specifically assesses illness severity and matches to treatment according to need. The results of a single class II study suggest that stratified care is probably an effective strategy for the acute treatment of migraine (Lipton et al., 2000). Combinations of different classes of acute therapies have also been studied in class I prospective, randomized, controlled trials in order to address the need for additional therapeutic benefit. Specifically, triptans given in combination with longer-acting NSAIDs (e.g., naproxen sodium) provide additional therapeutic benefit over monotherapeutic approaches (Krymchantowski, 2000; Krymchantowski and Barbosa, 2002; Smith et al., 2005; Brandes et al., 2007).

Recommendations for acute treatment strategies for migraine

- Acute treatment choice should probably be based on attack-related disability, which encompasses the severity, duration, presence of associated symptoms, and frequency of migraine attacks.
- Patients should treat migraine early in the course of the pain phase of an attack. Treatment of migraine with triptans when pain is mild confers therapeutic benefits.

- Combination of triptans (i.e., sumatriptan or rizatriptan) plus naproxen sodium should be used in the acute treatment of migraine and offers improved clinical response over either treatment given as monotherapy.

MIGRAINE PREVENTION

The results of a recent validated self-administered headache questionnaire to 162 576 participants found that only 12.4% of migraineurs use a migraine-preventive medication, suggesting that this treatment strategy is likely underutilized in patients with migraine (Diamond et al., 2007). Importantly, assessment of the efficacy and safety of this group of medications is needed in order to help treat this group of headache suffers optimally. With this aim, the AAN has reviewed the available evidence published in the literature that addresses the clinical question: what pharmacological therapies are effective for migraine prevention? (Ramadan et al., 1999; Silberstein, 2000). The results of this guideline are summarized herein and additional findings from newly available clinical evidence are noted in Table 14.4. Since the publication of the original guideline, based on clinical evidence available in the literature, there are sufficient data to make clinical recommendations for the following eight pharmacological agents for migraine prevention: topiramate, divalproex sodium, sodium valproate, amitriptyline, metoprolol, propranolol, timolol, and *Petasites* (Ramadan et al., 1999; Silberstein et al., 2000; Grossman and Schmidramsl, 2001; Newman et al., 2001; Freitag et al., 2002; Brandes et al., 2004; Bulut et al., 2004; Diener et al., 2004; Lipton et al., 2004).

In a recently completed assessment of botulinum neurotoxin in the treatment of autonomic disorders and pain by the Therapeutics and Technology Subcommittee of the AAN, two class I (Silberstein et al., 2000; Evers et al., 2004) and two class II (Elkind et al., 2006; Relja et al., 2007) studies were reviewed. The committee concluded that there was insufficient evidence to support or refute the benefit of these injections for the prevention of migraine. Consequently, it may be concluded that, based upon the current evidence, it appears that botulinum toxin injections are not effective for the treatment of episodic migraine headache, and clinical studies are assess efficacy in chronic migraine.

Non-pharmacological therapies have been used for years for migraine prevention, although published class I studies are limited. The original AAN guideline reviewed the literature on non-pharmacological interventions for migraine prevention and found sufficient evidence to make recommendations for selected non-pharmacological therapies, including the use of relaxation therapy, biofeedback, and cognitive-behavioral therapy for migraine prevention (Campbell et al., 1999; Silberstein, 2000).

Recommendations for cognitive and behavioral therapies

- Relaxation training, thermal biofeedback combined with relaxation training, electromyographic biofeedback, and cognitive-behavioral therapy may be considered as treatment options for prevention of migraine. Specific recommendations regarding which of these to use for specific patients cannot be made.
- Behavioral therapy may be combined with preventive drug therapy to achieve additional clinical improvement for migraine relief.
- Evidence-based treatment recommendations regarding the use of hypnosis, acupuncture, transcutaneous electrical nerve stimulation, chiropractic or osteopathic cervical manipulation, occlusal adjustment, and hyperbaric oxygen as preventive or acute therapy for migraine are not yet possible.

PEDIATRIC AND ADOLESCENT HEADACHE

Treatment of children and adolescents with migraine should follow the same basic principles as in adults, recognizing differences between adults and children regarding diagnosis, triggers, and use of medication. The general principles of treatment are similar to those for adults, recognizing that children are not just little adults.

For acute treatment of migraine:

- Treat attacks rapidly and consistently.
- Minimize the use of back-up and rescue medications.
- Be cost-effective with overall management.
- Restore the patient's ability to function.
- Optimize self-care and reduce subsequent use of resources.
- Have minimal or no adverse events.

For preventive therapy, the goals are:

- Decrease attack frequency, severity, and duration.
- Reduce disability and improve quality of life.
- Improve responsiveness to treatment of acute attacks.

There are some features of migraine in children that differ from those in adults. Attacks may be shorter than in adults, lasting 1–4 hours. Because of this, not all attacks will require pharmacological intervention.

Table 14.4

List of migraine-preventive treatments based on proven efficacy based on clinical studies

Group 1: Medications with proven high efficacy based on two class I trials	**Group 2:** Medications are probably effective based on one class I or two class II studies	**Group 3:** Medication use is possibly effective based on one class II or two class III studies or conflicting studies	**Group 4:** Medication use cannot be recommended based on inadequate or conflicting data with no class I, II, or III trials (class IV studies or no studies)	**Group 5:** Medications probably ineffective (based on one class I or two class II studies)
Antiepileptic drugs	**ACE inhibitors**	**Alpha-agonists**	**Anticoagulants**	**Antiepileptic drugs**
Divalproex sodium†	Candesartan*	Clonidine*	Acenocoumarol*	Clonazepam*
Sodium valproate*	Lisinopril*	Guanfacine*	Coumadin*	Oxycarbamazepine*
Topiramate*	**Antiepileptic drugs**	Mirtazapine	Picotamide*	**Other**
Antidepressants	Gabapentin	**Antiepileptic drugs**	**Antiepileptic drugs**	Acetazolamide*
Amitriptyline	**Antidepressants**	Carbamazepine*	Lamotrigine*	Botulinum toxin A
Beta-blockers	***SSRI/SSNRI***	**Ca^{2+} blockers**	Tiagabine	Indomethacin
Metoprolol*	Fluoxetine	Diltiazem	**Antidepressants**	Lanipitant*
Propranolol	Venlafaxine*	Nicardipine*	***SSRI/SSNRI***	Montelukast*
Timolol	**Antihistamines/**	Nifedipine*	Clomipramine	Nabumetone
Other	**leukotriene**	Nimodipine*	Fluvoxamine	Omega-3*
*Petasites**	**antagonists**	Verapamil *	Paroxetine*	Vitamin E*
Serotonin agonists	Cyproheptadine*	**Other**	S-fluoxetine	
(MRM)	Histamine*	Bupropion	Sertraline	
Frovatriptan*‡	**Beta-blockers**	Trazodone	***TCAs***	
Serotonin antagonists	Atenolol		Doxepin	
Methysergide	Nadolol		Imipramine	
	NSAIDs		Nortriptyline	
	Aspirin‡		Protriptyline	
	Fenoprofen		**Beta-blockers**	
	Flurbiprofen		Acebutolol	
	Ibuprofen*		Bisoprolol	
	Ketoprofen		Pindolol	
	Mefenamic acid‡		**MAOIs**	
	Naproxen		Phenylzine	
	Naproxen sodium		**Other**	
	Other		Mirtazapine	
	Coenzyme Q10*		***Serotonin antagonists***	
	MIG-99 (feverfew)		Methylergonovine	
	Magnesium		(methylergometrine	
	Vitamin B_2		***Serotonin agonists***	
	Serotonin agonists		DHE (oral)	
	(MRM)			
	Naratriptan*			

*Indicates a change or update in recommendation since the original guideline. (Silberstein 2000; Ramadan et al., 1999)

†Weight gain as a side-effect.

‡For short-term prophylaxis of menstrually related migraine (MRM).

ACE: angiotensin-converting enzyme; SSRI: selective serotonin reuptake inhibitor; SSNRI: selective serotonin and norepinephrine reuptake inhibitor; NSAIDs: non-steroidal anti-inflammatory drugs; TCAs: tricyclic antidepressants; MAOIs: monoamine oxidase inhibitors; DHE: dihydroergotamine.

(Adapted from Ramadan et al., 1999.)

In addition, the presence of associated symptoms may be difficult to elicit by history because of the child's inability to recognize and articulate symptoms. Symptoms such as photophobia, phonophobia, and nausea may be inferred by behavior, such as voluntarily going into a dark room, lack of desire to watch television or play video games, requiring other family members to be quiet or leave the house, or refusal to eat. There are other infectious, allergic, or gastrointestinal disorders of childhood that may have similar symptoms or trigger migraine. Other paroxysmal disorders of childhood that have a link to migraine may lead physicians away from the migraine diagnosis. These include cyclic vomiting syndrome and abdominal migraine. Often, these diagnoses are not considered until exhaustive testing for gastrointestinal, metabolic, or systemic illnesses has been pursued. Even after a correct diagnosis has been made, there is often hesitancy to use acute or preventive medications by the children, their parents, and at times physicians due to the limited safety and efficacy data for migraine medications in children and adolescents as well as a general reluctance to give children medications for what is often erroneously perceived as a not very disabling condition.

The AAN Quality Standards Subcommittee and the Practice Committee of the Child Neurology Society reviewed the relevant literature and developed a practice parameter for pharmacological treatment of migraine in children and adolescents (Lewis et al., 2004). Since the original guideline, additional published studies have addressed the high placebo rates noted in adolescent studies in order to assess more accurately the efficacy of triptans. Lewis and colleagues (2007) found that zolmitriptan 5 mg nasal spray was effective for the acute treatment of migraine in adolescents. This study used a single-blind "placebo challenge" to eliminate placebo responders from each attack. Ahonen and colleagues (2006) found that rizatriptan tablets were effective over placebo in a three-attack crossover trial.

Recommendations for acute treatment of pediatric and adolescent migraine

- Ibuprofen is effective for the acute treatment of migraine in children.
- Sumatriptan nasal spray is effective and zolmitriptan nasal spray is possibly effective for the acute treatment of migraine in adolescents.
- There are inadequate data to make a judgment on the efficacy of subcutaneous sumatriptan in children.
- Rizatriptan oral tablets are probably effective for the acute treatment of adolescent migraine, but there is no consistent evidence that the other oral triptans are effective in this population.
- Acetaminophen is probably effective and should be considered for the acute treatment of migraine in children.

The available data regarding migraine prevention in children and adolescents are even more limited than for acute treatment (Lewis et al., 2004). Since publication of the practice parameter in children and adolescents, three studies have assessed the efficacy of topiramate in adolescent migraine. All three studies reported positive findings, and two studies reported positive efficacy for their primary endpoints (Lewis et al., 2009; Lakshmi et al., 2007; Winner et al., 2005).

Recommendations for prevention of pediatric and adolescent migraine

- Based on the results from three clinical studies, topiramate is likely effective for migraine prevention in adolescents.
- Based on limited or conflicting studies, propranolol and trazodone are possibly effective for migraine prevention.
- Nimodipine and clonidine are not effective for the prevention of migraine.
- There was insufficient evidence to make recommendations regarding the use of cyproheptadine, amitriptyline, divalproex sodium, or levetiracetam.

Migraine has a significant impact on children and adolescents and warrants treatment. While the evidence supporting medication use is limited, treating physicians should use the evidence that is available along with clinical judgment and personal experience to devise treatment strategies for children and adolescents. Treatment choices should be based on those that will have the highest likelihood of success based on evidence and have a tolerability profile and dosing regimen that are acceptable to the child and the parents.

CLUSTER HEADACHE AND OTHER TRIGEMINAL AUTONOMIC CEPHALALGIAS

The European Federation of Neurological Sciences Expert Consensus Panel evaluated the evidence surrounding the treatment of cluster headache, paroxysmal hemicrania, and short-lasting unilateral neuralgiform headache attacks with conjunctival injection and tearing (SUNCT) syndrome (May et al., 2006). The objective of this panel was to provide evidence-based recommendations for the treatment of these headache disorders based on an exhaustive review of the literature and consensus amongst a panel of experts where evidence was lacking or incomplete.

Table 14.5

Treatment of cluster and other autonomic cephalalgias

	Treatment of choice		
Therapy	Cluster headache	Paroxysmal hemicrania	SUNCT syndrome
Acute	100% oxygen, 15 l/min (A) Sumatriptan 6 mg SC (A) Sumatriptan 20 mg nasal (A) Zolmitriptan 5 mg nasal (A/B) Zolmitriptan 10 mg nasal (A/B) Zolmitriptan 10 mg oral (B) Zolmitriptan 5 mg oral (B) Lidocaine intranasal (B) Octreotide (B)	None	None
Preventive	Verapamil (A) Steroids (A) Lithium carbonate (B) Methysergide (B) Topiramate (B) Ergotamine tartrate (B) Valproic acid (C) Melatonin (C) Baclofen (C)	Indomethacin (A) Verapamil (C) NSAIDs (C)	Lamotrigine (C)

A: proven effective; B: probably effective; C: possibly effective.
SUNCT: short-lasting unilateral neuralgiform headache attacks with conjunctival injection and tearing; SC: subconjunctival; NSAIDs: non-steroidal anti-inflammatory drugs.
(Reproduced from May et al., 2006.)

The findings in these studies were evaluated according to the recommendations of the European Federation of Neurological Societies, resulting in recommendations and good practice points, and are shown in Table 14.5.

Recommendations for cluster and other autonomic cephalalgias

- For the acute treatment of cluster headache attacks, oxygen (100%) with a flow of at least 7 l/min over 15 min and 6 mg subcutaneous sumatriptan are drugs of first choice.
- Prophylaxis of cluster headache should be performed with verapamil at a daily dose of at least 240 mg (maximum dose depends on efficacy or tolerability).
- Although no class I or II trials are available, steroids are clearly effective in cluster headache. Therefore, the use of at least 100 mg methylprednisone (or equivalent corticosteroid) given orally or up to 500 mg intravenously per day over 5 days (then tapering down) is recommended.
- Methysergide, lithium, and topiramate are recommended as alternative treatments. Surgical procedures, although in part promising, require further scientific evaluation.
- For paroxysmal hemicranias, indomethacin at a daily dose of up to 225 mg is the drug of choice.
- For treatment of SUNCT syndrome, large series suggest that lamotrigine is the most effective preventive agent, with topiramate and gabapentin also being useful.
- Intravenous lidocaine may also be helpful as an acute therapy when patients are extremely distressed and disabled by frequent attacks.

CONCLUSION

The therapeutic and diagnostic guidelines presented in this chapter represent the most exhaustive, rigorous, and recent in the field of headache. They represent a systematic evaluation of the evidence base for the acute and prophylactic treatment of migraine and trigeminal autonomic cephalalgias generated by international experts in the field of headache medicine. The variability in diagnosis and appropriate treatment of primary headache disorders is wide and it is the intention that these specific guidelines, if systematically and appropriately implemented in clinical practice, will improve the quality, appropriateness, and cost-effectiveness of the care of patients with headache.

References

Ahonen K, Hämäläinen ML, Eerola M et al. (2006). A randomized trial of rizatriptan in migraine attacks in children. Neurology 67: 1135–1140.

Audet AM, Greenfield S, Field M (1990). Medical practice guidelines: current activities and future directions. Ann Intern Med 30: 709–714.

Brandes JL, Saper JR, Diamond M et al; MIGR-002 Study Group (2004). Topiramate for migraine prevention: a randomized controlled trial. JAMA 291: 965–973.

Brandes JL, Kudrow D, Cady R et al. (2005). Eletriptan in the early treatment of acute migraine: influence of pain intensity and time of dosing. Cephalalgia 25: 735–742.

Brandes JL, Kudrow D, Stark SR et al. (2007). Sumatriptan-naproxen for acute treatment of migraine: a randomized trial. JAMA 297: 1443–1454.

Bulut S, Berilgen MS, Baran A et al. (2004). Venlafaxine versus amitriptyline in the prophylactic treatment of migraine: randomized, double-blind, crossover study. Clin Neurol Neurosurg 107: 44–48.

Cabana MD, Rand CS, Powe NR et al. (1999). Why don't physicians follow clinical practice guidelines? A framework for improvement. JAMA 282: 1458–1465.

Cady R, Elkind A, Goldstein J et al. (2004). Randomized, placebo-controlled comparison of early use of frovatriptan in a migraine attack versus dosing after the headache has become moderate or severe. Curr Med Res Opin 20: 1465–1472.

Cala LA, Mastaglia FL (1976). Computerized axial tomography findings in a group of patients with migrainous headaches. Proc Aust Assoc Neurol 13: 35–41.

Campbell JK, Penzien DB, Wall EM (1999). Evidence-based guidelines for migraine headache: behavioral and physical treatments. Available online at: http://www.aan.com/professionals/practice/pdfs/gl0089.pdf (accessed March 20, 2008).

Carrera GF, Gerson DE, Schnur J et al. (1977). Computed tomography of the brain in patients with headache or temporal lobe epilepsy: findings and cost-effectiveness. J Comput Assist Tomogr 1: 200–203.

Chassin MR (1990). Practice guidelines: best hope for quality improvement in the 1990s. J Occup Med 32: 1199–1206.

Diamond S, Bigal ME, Silberstein S et al. (2007). Patterns of diagnosis and acute and preventive treatment for migraine in the United States: results from the American Migraine Prevalence and Prevention Study. Headache 47: 355–363.

Diener HC, Tfelt-Hansen P, Dahlöf C et al. (2004). Topiramate in migraine prophylaxis – results from a placebo-controlled trial with propranolol as an active control. J Neurol 251: 943–950.

Duarte J, Sempere AP, Delgado JA et al. (1996). Headache of recent onset in adults: a prospective population-based study. Acta Neurol Scand 94: 67–70.

Elkind AH, O'Carrol P, Blumenfeld A et al. (2006). A series of three sequential, randomized, controlled studies of repeated treatments with botulinum toxin type A for migraine prophylaxis. J Pain 7: 688–696.

Evers S, Vollmer-Haase J, Schwaag S et al. (2004). Botulinum toxin A in the prophylactic treatment of migraine – a randomized, double-blind, placebo-controlled study. Cephalalgia 24: 838–843.

Field MJ, Lohr MJ (1990). Clinical Practice Guidelines: Directions for a New Program. National Academy Press, Washington, DC.

Freitag FG, Collins SD, Carlson HA et al. (2002). A randomized trial of divalproex sodium extended-release tablets in migraine prophylaxis. Neurology 58: 1652–1659.

Frishberg B, Rosenberg JH, Matchar DB et al. (1999). Evidence-based guidelines in the primary care setting: neuroimaging in patients with nonacute headache. Available online at:http://www.aan.com/professionals/practice/pdfs/gl0088.pdf (accessed March 20, 2008).

Gozke E, Osgul O, Dortcan N et al. (2004). Cranial magnetic resonance imaging finding in patients with migraine. Headache 44: 166–169.

Grossman W, Schmidramsl H (2001). An extract of *Petasites hybridus* is effective in the prophylaxis of migraine. Altern Med Rev 6: 303–310.

Jordan JE, Ramirez GF, Bradley WG et al. (2000). Economic and outcomes assessment of magnetic resonance imaging in the evaluation of headache. J Natl Med Assoc 92: 573–578.

Kahn CE Jr, Sanders GD, Lyons EA et al. (1993). Computed tomography for nontraumatic headache: current utilization and cost-effectiveness. Can Assoc Radiol J 44: 189–193.

Kruit MC, van Buchem MA, Hofman PA et al. (2004). Migraine as a risk factor for subclinical brain lesions. JAMA 291: 427–434.

Kruit MC, Lenore J, Launer MD et al. (2005). Infarcts in the posterior circulation territory in migraine: the population-based MRI Camera Study. Brain 128: 2068–2077.

Kruit MC, Launer LJ, Ferrari MD et al. (2006). Brain stem and cerebellar hyperintense lesions in migraine. Stroke 37: 1109–1112.

Krymchantowski AV (2000). Naproxen sodium decreases migraine recurrence when administered with sumatriptan. Arq Neuropsiquiatr 58: 428–430.

Krymchantowski AV, Barbosa JS (2002). Rizatriptan combined with rofecoxib vs. rizatriptan for the acute treatment of migraine: an open label pilot study. Cephalalgia 22: 309–312.

Lakshmi CV, Singhi P, Malhi P et al. (2007). Topiramate in the prophylaxis of pediatric migraine: a double-blind placebo-controlled trial. J Child Neurol 22: 829–835.

Larson EB, Omenn GS, Lewis H (1980). Diagnostic evaluation of headache. Impact of computerized tomography and cost-effectiveness. JAMA 243: 359–362.

Lewis DW, Winner P, Hershey AD et al. (2007). Adolescent Migraine Steering Committee. Efficacy of zolmitriptan nasal spray in adolescent migraine. Pediatrics 120: 390–396.

Lewis D, Ashwal S, Hershey A et al. (2004). American Academy of Neurology Quality Standards Subcommittee; Practice Committee of the Child Neurology Society. Practice parameter: pharmacological treatment of migraine headache in children and adolescents: report of the American Academy of Neurology Quality Standards Subcommittee and the Practice Committee of the Child Neurology Society. Neurology 63(12): 2215–2224.

Lipton RB, Stewart WF, Stone AM et al. (2000). Disability in Strategies of Care study group. Stratified care vs step care strategies for migraine: the Disability in Strategies of Care (DISC) study: a randomized trial. JAMA 284: 2599–2605.

Lipton RB, Gobel H, Einhaupl KM et al. (2004). *Petasites hybridus* root (butterbur) is an effective preventive treatment for migraine. Neurology 63: 2240–2244.

Lomas J, Anderson GM, Domnick-Pierre K et al. (1989). Do practice guidelines guide practice? The effect of a consensus statement on the practice of physicians. N Engl J Med 321: 1306–1311.

Matchar D, Young W, Rosenberg R et al. (1999). Evidence-based guidelines for migraine in the primary care setting. Pharmacological management of acute attacks. Available at http://www.aan.com/professionals/practice/pdfs/gl0087.pdf (accessed March 20, 2008).

Mathew NT, Kailasam J, Meadors L (2004). Early treatment of migraine with rizatriptan: a placebo-controlled study. Headache 44: 669–673.

May A, Leone M, Afra J et al. (2006). EFNS guidelines on the treatment of cluster headache and other trigeminal-autonomic cephalalgias. Eur J Neurol 13: 1066–1077.

Mitchell CS, Osborn RE, Grosskreutz SR (1993). Computed tomography in the headache patient: is routine evaluation really necessary? Headache 33: 82–86.

Newman L, Mannix LK, Landy S et al. (2001). Naratriptan as short-term prophylaxis of menstrually associated migraine: a randomized, double-blind, placebo-controlled study. Headache 41: 248–256.

Paemeleire K, Proot P, De Keyzer K et al. (2005). Magnetic resonance angiography of the circle of Willis in migraine patients. Clin Neurol Neurosurg 107: 301–305.

Quality Standards Subcommitte of the AAN (1995). Practice parameter: the electroencephalogram in the evaluation of headache (summary statement). Neurology 45: 1411–1413.

Ramadan NM, Silberstein SD, Freitag FG et al. (1999). Evidence-based guidelines for migraine headache in the primary care setting: pharmacological management for prevention of migraine. Available online at: http://www.aan.com/professionals/practice/pdfs/gl0090.pdf (accessed March 22, 2008).

Relja M, Poole A, Schoenen J et al. (2007). A multicentre, double-blind, randomized, placebo-controlled, parallel group study of multiple treatments of botulinum toxin type A (BoNTA) for the prophylaxis of episodic migraine headaches. Cephalalgia 27: 492–503.

Sargent JD, Solbach P (1983). Medical evaluation of migraineurs: review of the value of laboratory and radiologic tests. Headache 23: 62–65.

Sempere AP, Porta-Etessam J, Medrano V et al. (2005). Neuroimaging in the patient with non-acute headache. Cephalalgia 25: 30–35.

Shaneyfelt TM, Mayo-Smith MF, Rothwangl J (1999). Are guidelines following guidelines? The methodological quality of clinical practice guidelines in the peer-reviewed medical literature. JAMA 281: 1900–1905.

Silberstein SD (2000). Practice parameter: evidence-based guidelines for migraine headache (an evidence-based review): report of the Quality Standards Subcommittee of the American Academy of Neurology. Neurology 26: 754–762.

Silberstein S, Mathew N, Saper J et al. (2000). Botulinum toxin type A as a migraine preventive treatment. For the BOTOX Migraine Clinical Research Group (comment). Headache 40: 445–450.

Smith TR, Sunshine A, Stark SR et al. (2005). Sumatriptan and naproxen sodium for the acute treatment of migraine. Headache 45: 983–991.

Swartz RH, Kern RZ (2004). Migraine is associated with magnetic resonance imaging white matter abnormalities: a meta-analysis. Arch Neurol 61: 1366–1368.

Tsushima Y, Endo K (2005). MRI imaging in the evaluation of chronic or recurrent headache. Radiology 235: 575–579.

Valenca MM, Valenca LP, Menezes TL (2002). Computed tomography scan of the head in patients with migraine or tension-type headache. Arq Neuropsiquiatr 60: 542–547.

Wang H, Simonsen T (2001). Brain MR imaging in the evaluation of chronic headache in patients without other neurologic symptoms. Acad Radiol 8: 405–408.

Winner P, Pearlman EM, Linder SL et al. (2005). Topiramate Pediatric Migraine Study investigators. Topiramate for migraine prevention in children: a randomized, double-blind, placebo-controlled trial. Headache 45: 1304–1312.

Woolf SH (1993). Practice guidelines: a new reality in medicine, III: impact on patient care. Arch Intern Med 153: 2646–2655.

Handbook of Clinical Neurology, Vol. 97 (3rd series)
Headache
G. Nappi and M.A. Moskowitz, Editors

Chapter 15

The role of prevention

STEWART J. TEPPER*

Cleveland Clinic Lerner College of Medicine, Department of Neurology, Headache Center, Cleveland Clinic, Cleveland, OH, USA

BASIC SCIENCE AND MECHANISMS OF ACTION FOR PREVENTIVE MEDICATIONS IN MIGRAINE

Pathophysiology

The initiation of migraine remains controversial. Migraine is usually an inherited disorder of neuronal hyperexcitability, and the genesis of an attack is linked to neuronal activation. Debate continues as to whether the onset of migraine occurs as a result of cortical spreading depression (CSD) or is precipitated by a central brainstem generator.

CSD is characterized by a slow activation of neurons and glia with associated hyperemia suggesting spreading activation, and can be precipitated by trauma, embolus, electrical or chemical (e.g., postassium ion) stimulation. The initial activation is followed by a wave of decreased brain activity with oligemia. The wave of activation and then depression spreads at a rate of about 3 mm/min and can occur in cortex, cerebellum, or hippocampus. CSD is the basis for human aura, and it can initiate meningeal migraine pain mechanisms in the form of neurogenic inflammation, vasodilation, and plasma protein extravasation, and activate meningeal trigeminovascular nociceptive afferents. In addition, CSD alters the blood–brain barrier by activating brain matrix metalloproteinases (MMPs), such as MMP-9, and this opening of the blood–brain barrier is a hallmark of migraine pain (Gursoy-Ozdemir et al., 2004).

CSD is associated with increased transmission at cortical glutamatergic (excitatory) synapses. In three forms of familial hemiplegic migraine (FHM), facilitation of CSD is explained by increased glutamatergic tone.

FHM1 mutations are in the *CACNA1A* gene located on chromosome 19p13. *CACNA1A* codes for the alpha1A subunit of the $Ca_V2.1$ P/Q calcium channel located on presynaptic neuronal membranes. Action potentials provoke calcium influx at presynaptic membranes necessary to trigger synaptic vesicle fusion and subsequent glutamate release into the synapse via these P/Q calcium channels. The gain of function seen with FHM1 mutations leads to increased presynaptic calcium transport at glutamatergic synapses, resulting in more glutamate release, and this excitatory excess results in lower thresholds for, and faster propagation of, CSD (Ophoff et al., 1986).

FHM2 mutations are in the *ATP1A2* gene located on chromosome 1q21. *ATP1A2* codes for the alpha2 subunit of the sodium/potassium (Na/K) ATPase pump located on astrocyte membranes, a pump which maintains ionic gradient across astrocytic plasma membranes, providing energy for passive astrocyte membrane transporters. The glutamate transporter excitatory amino acid transporter (EAAT1) or glutamate aspartate transporter (GLAST) is a passive transporter that removes excess glutamate out of the synapse after release from neuronal presynaptic membranes. In FHM2, there is a loss of function of the Na/K ATPase pump, the passive astrocyte membrane transporters such as EAAT1/GLAST transporters function inadequately, more glutamate then becomes available to reach postsynaptic glutamate receptors as there is reduced glutamate reuptake, and the increased excitation that results facilitates CSD.

FHM3 mutations occur in the *SCN1A* gene on chromosome 2q24. *SCN1A* codes for the neuronal voltage-gated Na channels located on axonal membranes, channels necessary for propagation of action potentials along axons. A gain of function occurs when FHM3 mutations lead to faster recovery of the Na channels after axonal depolarization, allowing more action potentials to be propagated per unit time, and thereby increasing glutamate release into the synapses.

*Correspondence to: Stewart J. Tepper, MD, Cleveland Clinic Lerner College of Medicine, Department of Neurology, Headache Center, Cleveland Clinic, T33, 9500 Euclid Ave, Cleveland, OH 44195, USA, Tel: 216-636-5549, Fax: 216-445-1696, E-mail: teppers@ccf.org

The unresolved issue for CSD migraine genesis is the fact that aura occurs in only a minority of migraineurs, requiring CSD to be documented in those without aura, presumably in silent areas of the brain, or at subclinical intensity. In one classic case report, changes consistent with bilateral CSD were found in a patient with migraine without aura experiencing a migraine while undergoing positron emission tomography (PET) for cognitive testing (Woods et al., 1994), so it is possible that CSD does in fact occur in non-aura migraineurs as an initiating event (Pietrobon and Striessnig, 2003). However, the failure of a large, prospective trial of a CSD blocker or gap junction inhibitor, tonabersat, in migraine prophylaxis, announced in a press release but not published or presented at the time of this writing, makes CSD as a generator for migraine less likely.

The evidence for a midbrain/periaqueductal gray/dorsal raphe/locus coeruleus unilateral generator for migraine stems from observation that stimulation of this region produces headaches with characteristics of migraine in non-migraine patients (Raskin et al., 1987) and that this area showed regional cerebral blood flow increases contralateral to the migraine pain in a PET study (Weiller et al., 1995).

Following initiation of migraine by either CSD or a brainstem generator, meningeal pain mechanisms are triggered by trigeminovascular activation. These pain mechanisms include release of neuroinflammatory peptides such as substance P, inflammatory cytokines, and calcitonin gene-related peptide (CGRP), the latter of which causes vasodilation, plasma extravasation, and mast cell degranulation with further release of the same chemicals, and repetitive pathology. This neurogenic inflammation and vasodilation, in turn, sensitizes trigeminovascular nociceptive sensory afferents that carry pain signals via the trigmeminal ganglion to the trigeminal nucleus caudalis (TNC) in the caudal brainstem. Activation of this peripheral nociceptor is referred to as peripheral sensitization, while activation of the TNC and rostral brain structures involved in the integration of the migraine pain signals is associated with central sensitization (Moskowitz, 1990; Bolay et al., 2002; Burstein and Jakubowski, 2004; Burstein et al., 2004).

Mechanisms of action of preventive medications in migraine include inhibition of CSD through various mechanisms (Ayata et al., 2006), including blocking Na and Ca channels (Cohen, 2005), inhibition of MMPs, as well as blocking gap junctions used in conveying the CSD signals themselves (Read et al., 2001; Theis et al., 2005), although, as noted above, the gap junction/connexin inhibitor tonabersat failed in migraine prevention studies.

Ayata et al. (2006) induced CSD in animal models and evaluated several migraine-preventive medications. Their hypothesis was that effective migraine-preventive drugs elevate CSD threshold, thereby reducing migraine attacks. They studied six medications: topiramate, valproate, amitriptyline, DL-propranolol, D-propranolol (inactive isomer), and methysergide. A reduction in propagation speed of CSD was observed in animals medicated with topiramate, valproate, DL-propranolol, and amitriptyline. Topiramate reduced CSD propagation speed after a single dose. Susceptibility to CSD was suppressed with treatment of topiramate, valproate, propranolol, and amitriptyline. The inactive D-propranolol behaved as a placebo, and neither had an effect on CSD.

Different preventive medications have multiple mechanisms of action in prophylaxis of migraine, but no medications have been successfully designed for migraine prevention since the synthesis of methysergide. Thus, preventive medications have been found by serendipity, and their disparate modes of prophylaxis implied by back deduction.

The mechanisms of action of prevention are not mutually exclusive. Glutamate inhibition (by reduced synthesis, reduced release, increased uptake, or receptor blockade) decreases central excitability and propensity to aura. Pro-gamma-aminobutyric acid (GABA) activity (by increased synthesis, reduced uptake, increased GABA responsiveness, or GABA-mimetic activity), is inhibitory and decreases tendency to neuronal firing. Preventive medications often have modulatory effects on serotonin (5-HT) and monoamines, generally resulting in further inhibitory effects on central neuronal hyperexcitability. Preventive medications which alter ionic channels often interfere with excitatory tone as well.

Mechanisms of action of specific classes of prevention

Tricyclic antidepressants

Tricyclic antidepressants (TCAs) vary by type and class, but all inhibit, to a lesser or greater extent, norepinephrine and 5-HT high-affinity uptake. TCAs downregulate beta-adrenergic receptors, and thus change excitatory tone (Heninger and Charney, 1987). It is by no means clear that these actions alone have prophylactic action, because migraine can be thought of as a condition in which excitatory influences mediated by 5-HT_2 receptors are in excess of inhibitory influences mediated by 5-HT_1 receptors. Some TCAs such as amitriptyline do block 5-HT_2 receptors or downregulate 5-HT_2 receptor binding over time, and blocking 5-HT_2, in addition to being inhibitory, may also prevent the stimulation of arachidonic acid metabolism at the onset of a migraine attack, preventing neurogenic inflammation (Peroutka, 1990).

In addition, TCAs upregulate GABA-B receptors. GABA is a major inhibitory neurotransmitter, and increasing inhibitory tone in the excitatory migrainous state can reduce the likelihood of neuronal firing. As noted, amitriptyline also decreases propagation speed of CSD, and susceptibility to CSD (Ayata et al., 2006). Finally, TCAs inhibit neuronal reuptake of adenosine, with resultant agonist effect at adenosine A1 receptors, which appears to work against pain mechanisms (Taiwo and Levine, 1991).

Beta-blockers

Beta-blockers probably exert their antimigraine effects by reducing adrenergic tone overall. They do this via a variety of mechanisms, including blockade of presynaptic noradrenergic receptors with resultant reduction in norepinephrine release, a reduction of norepinephrine synthesis via a block of tyrosine hydroxylase, inhibition of central beta-adrenergic receptors, and a resultant reduction in firing of the adrenergic locus coeruleus (Ablad and Dahlof, 1986). In addition, beta-blockers may prevent CSD, via a blocking effect on both antikainate and anti-*N*-methyl-D-aspartic acid (NMDA) glutamate receptors (Ramadan, 2004). Propranolol clearly reduces both speed of propagation of CSD and CSD susceptibility (Ayata et al., 2006).

Calcium channel blockers

Suppression of CSD may also play a role in the preventive effects of calcium channel blockers. The discovery of the calcium channelopathy of FHM1 and the suggestion that calcium channelopathies may be present in other more common forms of migraine make the blocking of calcium influx and reduction of glutamate release a probable mode of action for calcium channel blockers (Ambrosini et al., 2001; Sandor et al., 2001). In addition, since calcium calcium channel blockers inhibit 5-HT release, they may also inhibit the consequences of that release (Wauquier et al., 1985; Miljanich and Ramachandran, 1995).

Angiotensin-converting enzyme inhibitors and angiotensin receptor blockers

There are two small, positive, randomized controlled trials (RCTs) for lisinopril and candesartan in the prevention of migraine. How these medications would work in migraine prevention is unknown, but angiotensin II modulates both potassium channels and calcium activity in cells and increases the level of the main 5-HT metabolite, 5- hydroxyindoleacetic acid (5-HIAA) (Tronvik et al., 2003).

Antiepilepsy drugs

Three antiepilepsy drugs have RCT data proving effectiveness in preventing migraine, but their mechanisms of action differ (valproate, topiramate, gabapentin).

Valproate

Valproate is an inhibitory antiepilepsy drug and increases brain GABA. Valproate suppresses neurogenic inflammation via GABA-A receptors and directly attenuates nociceptive neurotransmission. Valproate enhances GABA synthesis, inhibits GABA degradation, and increases responsiveness to GABA by hyperpolarizing postsynaptic membranes through increased potassium conductance (Welch et al., 1975; Cutrer and Moskowitz, 1996; Cutrer et al., 1997). The GABAergic central effects may in addition modulate 5-HT, as valproate helps suppress the rostral brainstem generator or modulator (Moskowitz, 1992a).

Valproate also inhibits NMDA depolarization, and thus reduces glutamate responses, suppressing CSD (Zeise et al., 1991). This antiglutamate effect may play a role in the noted decrease in CSD susceptibility and propagation speed with valproate (Ayata et al., 2006).

Topiramate

Topiramate has multiple actions, all of which may prevent migraine. Topiramate blocks both voltage-gated Na and Ca channels, enhances GABAergic inhibitory activity through GABA-A receptors similar to valproate, and inhibits excitatory glutamatergic receptors such as α-amino-3-hydroxy-5-methylisoxazole-4-propionic acid (AMPA)/kainate receptors (Shank et al., 2000); all of these mechanisms can reduce CSD. This is reflected in both decreased susceptibility to and speed of CSD propagation, seen after a single dose in laboratory animals (Ayata et al., 2006).

Topiramate also inhibits central activation of the TNC and upper spinal cord (Storer and Goadsby, 2004). Topiramate is a carbonic anhydrase inhibitor, although the significance of this action has not been explained in antimigraine effect.

Gabapentin

Gabapentin blocks voltage-gated Ca, but not Na channels (Cohen, 2005). Gabapentin, as with valproate, raises brain GABA concentrations, and probably increases GABA synthesis. Gabapentin increases 5-HT concentrations in human whole blood, which may have inhibitory effects on migraine. In some pain conditions, central sensitization may optimize gabapentin antinociceptive efficacy, and gabapentin may also inhibit glutamate synthesis (Petroff et al., 1996; Taylor et al., 1998).

Antiserotonin drugs

The antiserotonin medications include the ergots methysergide and methylergonovine (methylergometrine), as well as cyproheptadine and pizotifen. All of these medications block 5-HT_{2B} and 5-HT_{2C} excitatory receptors (Moskowitz, 1992b, c), implicated in migrainous vasodilation via a CGRP/nitric oxide mechanism. The ergots also have agonist effects at 5-HT_{1B} and 5-HT_{1D} receptors (Muller, 1992), which antagonize migraine via presynaptic inhibition of the release of neuroinflammatotory peptides, postsynaptic vasoconstriction, and inhibition of the transduction of peripheral nociceptive signals to the brainstem.

Herbs, minerals, vitamins, and supplements

Magnesium

Since magnesium blocks the NMDA glutamate receptor, low magnesium is associated with increased NMDA glutamate activation and CSD. Magnesium supplementation and administration have been found helpful in patients with low brain ionized magnesium and in migraine with aura (Ramadan et al., 1989; Mauskop et al., 1993; Peikert et al., 1996; Bigal et al., 2002).

Riboflavin, coenzyme Q10

A low phosphorylation ratio of adenosine diphosphate/adenosine triphosphate has been reported in migraine brain, and mitochondropathy is implicated in some forms of migraine. Flavinoids are a cofactor in the Krebs cycle, and riboflavin is a precursor for flavin mononucleotides in the electron transport chain in mitochondria. Coenzyme Q10 transfers electrons in the electron transport chain, and is thus critical for mitochondrial function. Both supplements have been reported to prevent migraine in RCTs, presumably by treating mitochondropathy (Schoenen et al., 1998; Sandor et al., 2005).

Petasites

The extract of the *Petasites hybridus* root, the butterbur root, has anti-inflammatory properties and blocks leukotriene synthesis. Leukotrienes are released in migrainous neurogenic inflammation (Sheftell et al., 2000). Two RCTs have reported efficacy for *Petasites* root extract in migraine prevention (Grossman and Schmidramsl, 2000; Lipton et al., 2004).

EVIDENCE OF EFFECTIVENESS

The US Headache Consortium published guidelines and technical reports on preventive medications in 2000 (Ramadan et al., 2000; Silberstein, 2000). These reports evaluated preventive agents by strength of evidence, scientific effect measures, and clinical impression of effect. Also, the medications were placed in groups, as shown in Table 15.1.

Since that time, additional RCTs have been published that change the position and evidence on a number of important preventive agents, and these will be covered below under clinical use.

THE PREVENTIVE AGENTS: CLINICAL USE, DOSING, AND SIDE-EFFECTS

Goals of and circumstances warranting preventive treatment

The US Headache Consortium lists the following goals for preventive treatment: (1) decrease attack frequency (by 50%), and decrease intensity and duration; (2) improve responsiveness to acute treatment; (3) improve function and decrease disability; and (4) intervene to prevent transformation into chronic daily headache, medication overuse headache, or rebound (Ramadan et al., 2000).

The guidelines consider the following circumstances as warranting daily preventive medications: (1) recurring migraine that significantly interferes with the patient's daily routine despite acute treatment (e.g., two or more attacks a month that produce disability that lasts at least 3 days or headache attacks that are infrequent but produce profound disability); (2) failure, contraindication to, or troublesome side-effects from acute medications; (3) overuse of acute medications; (4) special circumstances, such as hemiplegic migraine or attacks with a risk of permanent neurological injury; (5) very frequent headaches (more than two a week), or a pattern of increasing attacks over time, with the risk of developing medication overuse headache or rebound with acute attack medicines; or (6) patient preference, i.e., the desire to have as few acute attacks as possible (Ramadan et al., 2000).

There is a direct relationship between frequency, disability or impact, and need for migraine prevention. As frequency of headache days per month rises, the risk for transformation from episodic into daily headache rises as well. The odds ratio for transformation to daily headache over a year is 6.2 when comparing patients who start off the year with 0–4 headache days/month, compared with those who start off with 5–9 headache days per month. The odds ratio for this feared chronification over a year is 20.1 when patients with 0–4 headache days/month at the beginning of the year are compared

Petroff OA, Rothman DL, Behar KL et al. (1996). The effect of gabapentin on brain gamma-aminobutyric acid in patients with epilepsy. Ann Neurol 39: 95–99.

Pietrobon D, Striessnig J (2003). Neurobiology of migraine. Nat Rev Neurosci 4: 386–398.

Ramadan NM (2004). Prophylactic migraine therapy: mechanisms and evidence. Curr Pain Headache Rep 8: 91–95.

Ramadan NM, Halvorson H, Vande-Linde A et al. (1989). Low brain magnesium in migraine. Headache 29: 590–593.

Ramadan NM, Silberstein SD, Freitag FG et al. (2000). Multispecialty consensus on diagnosis and treatment of headache: pharmacological management for prevention of migraine. Neurology serial online, available online at: http://www.aan.com/professionals/practice/pdfs/gl0090.pdf.

Raskin NH, Hosobuchi Y, Lamb S (1987). Headache may arise from perturbation of brain. Headache 27: 416–420.

Read SJ, Hirst WD, Upton N et al. (2001). Cortical spreading depression produces increased cGMP levels in cortex and brain stem that is inhibited by tonabersat (SB-220453) but not sumatriptan. Brain Res 891: 69–77.

Sandor PS, Mascia A, Seidel L et al. (2001). Subclinical cerebellar impairment in the common types of migraine: a three-dimensional analysis of reaching movements. Ann Neurol 49: 668–672.

Sandor PS, DiClemente L, Coppola G et al. (2005). A randomized controlled trial of coenzyme Q10 in migraine prophylaxis. Neurology 64: 713–715.

Scher AI, Stewart WF, Ricci JA et al. (2003). Factors associated with the onset and remission of chronic daily headache in a population-based study. Pain 106: 81–89.

Schoenen J, Jacquy J, Lanaerts M (1998). Effectiveness of high-dose riboflavin in migraine prophylaxis. Neurology 50: 466–470.

Schrader H, Stovner LJ, Helde G et al. (2001). Prophylactic treatment of migraine with angiotensin converting enzyme inhibitor (lisinopril): randomised, placebo controlled, crossover study. BMJ 322: 19–22.

Shank RP, Gardocki JF, Streeter AJ et al. (2000). An overview of the preclinical aspects of topiramate: pharmacology, pharmacokinetics, and mechanism of action. Epilepsia 41 (Suppl. I): S3–S9.

Sheftell F, Rapoport A, Weeks R et al. (2000). Montelukast in the prophylaxis of migraine: a potential role for leukotriene modifiers. Headache 40: 158–163.

Silberstein SD (2000). Practice parameter: evidence-based guidelines for migraine headache (an evidence-based review): report of the Quality Standards Subcommittee of the American Academy of Neurology. Neurology 55: 754–762.

Silberstein SD, Goadsby PJ (2002). Migraine: preventive treatment. Cephalalgia 22: 491–512.

Silberstein SD, Lipton RB, Goadsby PJ (2000). Headache in Clinical Practice. 2nd edn. Martin Dunitz, Oxford, pp. 91–92.

Silberstein SD, Neto W, Schmitt J et al. (2004). Topiramate in migraine prevention: results of a large controlled trial. Arch Neurol 61: 490–495.

Silberstein S, Loder E, Diamond S et al. (2007). Probable migraine in the United States: results of the American Migraine Prevalence and Prevention (AMPP) study. Cephalalgia 27: 220–234.

Steiner TJ, Findley LJ, Yuen AW (1997). Lamotrigine versus placebo in the prophylaxis of migraine with and without aura. Cephalalgia 17: 109–112.

Storer RJ, Goadsby PJ (2004). Topiramate inhibits trigeminovascular neurons in the cat. Cephalalgia 24: 1049–1056.

Taiwo YO, Levine JD (1991). Further confirmation of the role of adenyl cyclase and of cAMP-dependent protein kinase in primary afferent hyperalgesia. Neuroscience 44: 131–135.

Taylor CP, Gee NS, Su TZ et al. (1998). A summary of mechanistic hypotheses of gabapentin pharmacology. Epilepsy Res 29: 233–248.

Theis M, Sohl G, Eiberger J et al. (2005). Emerging complexities in identity and function of glial connexins. Trends Neurosci 28: 188–195.

Tronvik E, Stovner LJ, Helde G et al. (2003). Prophylactic treatment of migraine with an angiotensin II receptor blocker: a randomized controlled trial. JAMA 289: 65–69.

Wauquier A, Ashton D, Marranes R (1985). The effects of flunarizine in experimental models related to the pathogenesis of migraine. Cephalalgia 5: 119–120.

Weiller C, May A, Limmroth V et al. (1995). Brain stem activation in spontaneous human migraine attacks. Nat Med 1: 658–660.

Welch KMA, Chabi E, Bartosh K et al. (1975). Cerebrospinal fluid gamma aminobutyric acid levels in migraine. BMJ 3: 516–517.

Woods RP, Iacoboni M, Mazziotta JC (1994). Brief report: bilateral spreading cerebral hypoperfusion during spontaneous migraine headache. N Engl J Med 331: 1689–1692.

Zeise ML, Kasparow S, Zieglgansberger W (1991). Valproate suppresses *N*-methyl-D-aspartate-evoked, transient depolarizations in the rat neocortex *in vitro*. Brain Res 544: 345–348.

Ziad el K, Rahi AC, Hamdan SA et al. (2005). Age, dose, and environmental temperature are risk factors for topiramate-related hyperthermia. Neurology 65: 1139–1140.

Handbook of Clinical Neurology, Vol. 97 (3rd series)
Headache
G. Nappi and M.A. Moskowitz, Editors

Chapter 16

Managing migraine associated with sensitization

RAMI BURSTEIN* AND MOSHE JAKUBOWSKI
Departments of Anesthesia and Program in Neuroscience, Beth Israel Deaconess Medical Center and Harvard Medical School, Boston, MA, USA

Among the common symptoms of peripheral sensitization during migraine are the throbbing of the headache and its aggravation during routine physical activities that increase intracranial pressure, such as coughing and bending over (Blau and Dexter, 1981; Rasmussen et al., 1991). Such intracranial hypersensitivity involves the sensitization of nociceptors that innervate the meninges (Strassman et al., 1996). Accordingly, fluctuations in intracranial pressure (Daley et al., 1995) associated with normal vascular pulsation (4–10 mmHg), as well as those associated with bending over or coughing (4–25 mmHg), effectively activate meningeal nociceptors during migraine, when they are sensitized, but not in the absence of migraine, when they are not sensitized.

Among the common symptoms of central sensitization during migraine is the phenomenon of allodynia, where patients become irritated by mundane mechanical and thermal stimulation of the scalp and facial skin (Liveing, 1873; Selby and Lance, 1960; Tfelt-Hansen et al., 1981; Lous and Olesen, 1982; Waelkens, 1985; Blau, 1987; Drummond, 1987; Jensen et al., 1988, 1993; Gobel et al., 1992; Jensen, 1993; Burstein et al., 2000a). This hypersensitivity is manifested in response to activities such as combing, shaving, breathing cold air, and wearing eyeglasses, contact lenses, earrings, or necklaces. Such allodynia involves the sensitization of nociceptive trigeminovascular neurons of the medullary dorsal horn that receive converging sensory input from the dura and skin (Burstein et al., 1998). Accordingly, innocuous skin stimuli evoke dramatic activity in central trigeminovascular neurons during migraine, when they are sensitized, but produce little or no response in the absence of migraine, when they are not sensitized.

PERIPHERAL SENSITIZATION

Peripheral sensitization is thought to be a major contributor to hypersensitivity in many painful syndromes, including migraine headaches (Strassman et al., 1996; Andrew and Greenspan, 1999; Levine and Reichling, 1999). It generally refers to a state where primary afferent nociceptive neurons exhibit increased responsiveness to external mechanical or thermal stimuli at the original site of inflammation or injury. Such changes can be manifested as a novel response to previously ineffective stimulus intensities, indicating decreased activation thresholds (Martin et al., 1987; Schaible and Schmidt, 1988; Davis et al., 1993; Wang et al., 1996; Levy and Strassman, 2002), and increased response magnitude to suprathreshold stimuli either with or without a noticeable change in threshold (Cooper et al., 1991; Su and Gebhart, 1998; Andrew and Greenspan, 1999; Halata et al., 1999). In addition to marked changes in their stimulus response properties, peripheral sensitization can also be manifested as an increased level of ongoing discharge (i.e., spontaneous activity) in the absence of externally applied stimuli.

Inflammatory mediators of peripheral sensitization

A large number of chemical mediators produced at the site of tissue injury and inflammation can promote the excitation and sensitization of nociceptors. Mediators such as bradykinin, histamine, serotonin (5-HT), and prostaglandin E_2 (PGE_2) have been shown to produce both excitation and mechanical sensitization of somatic (Steen et al., 1992) and meningeal nociceptors (Strassman et al., 1996; Levy and Strassman, 2002). Other inflammatory mediators known to promote peripheral

*Correspondence to: Rami Burstein, Departments of Anesthesia and Program in Neuroscience, Beth Israel Deaconess Medical Center and Harvard Medical School, Boston, MA, USA, Tel: (617) 735-2832, Fax: (617) 735-2833, E-mail: rburstei@bidmc.harvard.edu

sensitization are cytokines, most notably interleukins 1, 6, and 8 (IL-1, IL-6, IL-8) and tumor necrosis factor-alpha (TNF-alpha) (Obreja et al., 2002; Sachs et al., 2002). These mediators are believed to promote nociceptor sensitization through the endogenous release of eicosanoids and sympathetic amines (Sachs et al., 2002). Additional inflammatory mediators proposed to promote peripheral sensitization include protons, proteases, and nitric oxide. Increased levels of protons (acidic pH) found in inflamed tissues not only produce activation and sensitization of meningeal nociceptors (Strassman et al., 1996), but also enhance the effects of other inflammatory mediators (Steen et al., 1992). Inflammatory proteases, especially tryptase and trypsins, activate protease-activated receptors (PARs) on nociceptors, most notably PAR-2 (Hoogerwerf et al., 2001). Nitric oxide has been shown to produce local inflammation within the meninges (Reuter et al., 2001), sensitize meningeal nociceptors (Levy and Strassman, 2004), and induce headache or migraine in patients (Olesen et al., 1994).

Cellular mechanisms of peripheral sensitization

Most sensitizing agents activate receptors that are coupled to second-messenger cascades which, in turn, modulate voltage-gated ion channels. Other potential targets for the actions of sensitizing agents on nociceptors may also include direct action on sensory transduction elements. Mechanical and thermal sensitivity can be modulated independently in individual nociceptors, suggesting the existence of separate, possibly multiple, transduction mechanisms (Belmonte et al., 1991; Pozo et al., 1992). For example, increased thermal skin sensitivity can be mediated by the transient receptor potential ion channel 1 (TRPV1), a transducer of noxious heat (Tominaga et al., 1998; Premkumar and Ahern, 2000), when its threshold is lowered by bradykinin, PAR-2 agonist, and protons (Sugiura et al., 2002; Ryu et al., 2003; Dai et al., 2004). The mechanism underlying increased mechanical sensitivity remains largely unknown as transducers of noxious mechanical stimuli are yet to be identified.

Peripheral sensitization can also be promoted by changes in the properties of voltage-gated ion channels, such as the tetrodotoxin (TTX)-resistant sodium channel (TTX-R). Inflammatory agents such as PGE_2 and 5-HT are thought to sensitize sensory neurons by modulating TTX-R sodium currents (Gold, 1999) through activation of the cyclic adenosine monophosphate (cAMP)-protein kinase A (PKA) second-messenger cascade (Gold et al., 1998). Such action may be involved in sensitization of mechanosensitive meningeal nociceptors, as they express the TTX-R channels (Strassman and Raymond, 1999) and are sensitized by the cAMP-PKA cascade (Levy and Strassman, 2002). The cAMP-PKA is also likely to be involved in mechanical sensitization through the suppression of the sustained (delayed rectifier) outward K^+ current that is thought to modulate the firing threshold (England et al., 1996; Evans et al., 1999) and the enhancement of I_h, the hyperpolarization-activated cation current that is thought to facilitate repetitive firing (Ingram and Williams, 1996). Another second-messenger cascade that may promote mechanical sensitization is the cyclic guanosine monophosphate (cGMP)-dependent protein kinase (PKG), cascade that is activated by nitric oxide. The sensitizing action of nitric oxide on meningeal nociceptors may involve the activation of this cascade, probably through the facilitation of Ca^{2+}-activated potassium (BK) channels (Klyachko et al., 2001).

The proximate factors that cause local release of sensitizing chemicals during migraine remain unknown. One presumed factor is cortical spreading depression – a slowly propagating wave of neural inhibition and excitation associated with extracellular release of excitatory agents such as potassium and glutamate. Bolay et al. (2002) have shown that cortical spreading depression activates the trigeminovascular system. One of the potential consequences of sensory fiber activation is the release of neuropeptides such as substance P and calcitonin gene-related peptide (CGRP) from the peripheral terminals of meningeal nociceptors which, in turn, promotes vasodilation and plasma extravasation (Shepheard et al., 1993; Kurosawa et al., 1995; Carmody et al., 1996). CGRP and substance P are thought to sensitize nociceptors indirectly by inducing the release of sensitizing inflammatory mediators such as histamine, 5-HT, BK, TNF-alpha, and nitric oxide from other immune cells, especially mast cells, in a process known as mast cell degranulation (Yano et al., 1989; Reynier-Rebuffel et al., 1994; Suzuki et al., 1999).

CENTRAL SENSITIZATION

Physiological properties of central sensitization

Central sensitization in somatosensory pain pathways was first discovered in the rat spinal cord, where it was shown to play a role in postinjury pain hypersensitivity (Woolf, 1983), and later documented in several animal models and in humans (Simone et al., 1991; Hu et al., 1992; Torebjork et al., 1992; Ren and Dubner, 1993; Koltzenburg et al., 1994; Magerl et al., 1998). Central sensitization refers to a condition where nociceptive neurons in the dorsal horn of the spinal cord exhibit increased excitability, increased synaptic strength, and enlargement of their receptive fields beyond the original site of inflammation or injury (McMahon et al., 1993; Woolf and Doubell, 1994; Woolf, 1995). Central sensitization is triggered by sensory input arriving from sensitized nociceptors that supply the affected site. Once initiated, central sensitization may remain dependent on incoming input (i.e., activity-dependent) or become self-sufficient altogether (i.e., activity-independent). Sensitized dorsal horn nociceptors become responsive to innocuous (previously subthreshold) sensory signals that arrive from areas outside the affected site, resulting in expansion of their receptive fields. Clinically, central sensitization is manifested as decreased pain threshold and exaggerated pain response that is referred outside the original pain site.

There is good evidence that central sensitization can also be produced in trigeminovascular neurons in the deep laminae of the medullary dorsal horn, and that these sensitized neurons may play a role in the pathogenesis of migraine headache (Burstein, 2001). Topical application of inflammatory agents on the exposed rat dura, which activates the trigeminovascular pathway for many hours (Ebersberger et al., 1997; Burstein et al., 1998; Schepelmann et al., 1999), induces long-lasting sensitization in medullary dorsal horn neurons that receive convergent intracranial input from the dura and extracranial input from the periorbital skin. This neuronal sensitization is manifested as increased responsiveness to mechanical stimulation of the dura; increased responsiveness to mechanical and thermal stimulation of the skin; decreased response thresholds and increased response magnitude to dural and skin stimulation; and expansion of dural and cutaneous receptive fields (Burstein et al., 1998).

Cellular mechanisms of central sensitization

Central sensitization can be divided into two distinct phases, the initiation phase and the maintenance phase, each mediated by different mechanisms.

Initiation of sensitization in the spinal cord depends on the input nociceptive neurons of the dorsal horn receive from C-fiber nociceptors that contain the excitatory amino acid glutamate and neuropeptides such as substance P and CGRP (Willis and Coggeshall, 1991). Once activated from the periphery (leading to action potential invasion of the central terminals), calcium inflow into the central terminals of C-fiber nociceptors causes them to release a number of neuropeptides in the superficial layers of the medullary dorsal horn. Consequently, activation of C-fibers elicits slow synaptic potentials (Murase et al., 1986; Sivilotti et al., 1993), leading to cumulative depolarization of dorsal horn neurons. C-fiber input can also contribute to the progression and establishment of sustained depolarization in dorsal horn neurons by recruiting L-type calcium plateau currents (Morisset and Nagy, 2000).

Maintenance of sensitization in spinal cord neurons can be activity-dependent or activity-independent (Ji et al., 2003). The activity-dependent form of central sensitization is the consequence of neurotransmitter (glutamate) and neuromodulator (substance P, brain-derived neurotrophic factor, ephrin-B ligand)-induced activation of multiple intracellular signaling pathways in dorsal horn neurons by virtue of activation of ligand-gated ion channels (*N*-methyl-D-aspartate (NMDA), α-amino-3-hydroxy-5-methyl-4-isoxazolepropionic acid (AMPA)/kainate), G-protein-coupled metabotropic receptors (NK-1, mGluR), and tyrosine kinase receptors (TrkB, EphR). Enhanced neuronal excitability in this form of central sensitization involves phosphorylation of intracellular (PKA, PKC) and extracellular (ERK) kinases and enhanced production of cyclooxygenase in the spinal cord. PKA and PKC activation leads to the phosphorylation of ionotropic glutamate receptors (NMDA and AMPA), which increases synaptic efficacy by altering channel open time and promoting the trafficking of receptors to the synaptic membrane (Malmberg et al., 1997; Woolf and Salter, 2000). ERK phosphorylation increases A-type K^+ current via $K_v4.2$ channel regulation (Hu and Gereau, 2003). Increased cyclooxygenase level in the dorsal horn activates prostaglandin receptors to facilitate transmitter release from nociceptor central terminals (Vasko, 1995), produce a direct depolarization of dorsal horn neurons (Baba et al., 2001), and reduce glycine receptor activity (Ahmadi et al., 2002). Activity-dependent central sensitization is displayed by many cells in both the superficial and deep laminae of the dorsal horn, but its contribution to pain sensitivity appears to be mediated by lamina I neurons, particularly those expressing the NK1 receptor (Mantyh et al., 1997; Ikeda et al., 2003).

The activity-independent form of central sensitization develops slowly over several hours and lasts for prolonged periods. This form of sensitization, like the activity-dependent form, is initiated by intense activity in nociceptors (Ji et al., 2002), which induces activation of NMDA, mGlu, NK-1 and trkB receptors in the central neurons. This, in turn, activates PKA, PKC, and ERK, as described above, but it also increases production of the cytokine IL-1β in endothelial cells and spinal microglia (DeLeo and Yezierski, 2001). Central sensitization shifts from activity-dependent mode to activity-independent mode upon widespread increase in expression of transcription factor genes such as cAMP-response element (CRE)-binding protein (Ji and Rupp, 1997; Ji and Woolf, 2001), immediate early genes such as c-fos and COX-2 (Hunt et al., 1987; Samad et al., 2001), and late-response genes encoding prodynorphine, NK-1 and trkB (Iadarola et al., 1988; McCarson and Krause, 1994; Mannion et al., 1999; Ji et al., 2002). Interestingly, these genes share CRE sites in their promoter region (Ji et al., 2002; Seybold et al., 2003).

Clinical symptoms of central sensitization

Assuming that migraine in humans is associated with sensitization of medullary dorsal horn neurons, as observed in the rat, it is reasonable to predict that it should also be associated with allodynia in the periorbital skin. Using quantitative sensory testing technique, it was shown that 79% of patients developed mechanical and/or thermal allodynia on the facial skin ipsilateral to the migraine pain 1–2 h after onset of the attack (Burstein et al., 2000b). By 4 h, allodynia frequently extended outside the referred pain area to the skin over the contralateral head and both arms (Burstein et al., 2000b). A standardized questionnaire can now be used to identify patients reliably as allodynic or non-allodynic (Jakubowski et al., 2005b; Ashkenazi et al., 2007).

The history of migraine literature is dotted with accounts of increased skin sensitivity during migraine. In 1873, Edward Liveing quoted Tissot in his seminal book *On Megrim* as saying: "so painful is this hyperasthesia in a certain stage of the seizure with some people that, he [the patient] could not bear anything to touch his head." In 1953, Harold Wolff (Wolff et al., 1953) found that, in cranial tissue, deep-pain thresholds were high during the headache-free period and low during the headache, that the zone of low threshold expanded to include areas on the non-painful side of the head, that deep-pain threshold began to decrease several hours after the onset of headache, and that, commonly, this hypersensitivity outlasted the headache for hours and even days. In 1960, James Lance (Selby and Lance, 1960) found that two-thirds (317/500) of migraine patients experienced scalp tenderness during migraine.

Implications for migraine therapy

Acute or chronic pain is generally more complicated to treat with triptans in the presence of allodynia. Patients who do not exhibit allodynia during migraine are highly responsive to triptans; they are typically rendered pain-free within 2 h of treatment (Burstein and Jakubowski, 2004). Patients whose migraine headache is accompanied by cutaneous allodynia become increasingly resistant to triptan therapy with the progression of the attack (Burstein and Jakubowski, 2004). These patients are highly likely to be rendered pain-free by triptan treatment early in the attack, when they have not yet exhibited signs of allodynia, or even in the early presence of allodynia. The same patients, however, would fail to respond to triptans if treatment were delayed until they had fully developed allodynia over a period of several hours (Burstein and Jakubowski, 2004). These observations can be explained by the effects of triptans on central trigeminovascular neurons that mediate allodynia during migraine.

In the rat, sensitization in central trigeminovascular neurons induced by topical application of inflammatory soup to the dura is blocked by coadministration of sumatriptan (i.e., early treatment paradigm). In contrast, sumatriptan intervention several hours after inflammatory soup application (i.e., late treatment paradigm) could not reverse the ongoing sensitization in the central neurons (Burstein and Jakubowski, 2004). Therefore, central trigeminovascular neurons appear to be unequipped to respond to triptans directly. A similar experimental paradigm showed that early triptan treatment cannot prevent the induction of sensitization in meningeal nociceptors, and that late treatment has no effect on the ongoing state of peripheral sensitization (Levy and Strassman, 2004). Collectively, these data suggest that triptan action in the dorsal horn is mainly mediated by presynaptic inhibition of signal transmission between peripheral (first-order) and central (second-order) trigeminovascular neurons (Figure 16.1). This conclusion is consistent with the selective presence of presynaptic 5-HT_{1D} receptors on central terminals of peripheral nociceptors in the dorsal horn (Potrebic et al., 2003). Accordingly, termination of migraine headache and the associated allodynia using triptan treatment is possible as long as the excitability of the central neurons remains driven by incoming signals from the meninges, but not after they developed autonomous activity (Burstein and Jakubowski, 2004).

Most patients testify that triptans are much more likely to render them painfree when taken early rather than late, but routinely delay treatment until attacks are fully developed or the pain is severe. Justifying the delayed treatment are concerns about side-effects, addiction, limits on supply imposed by prescribers, cost, and, most commonly, waiting to see if headache develops into a severe migraine attack (Foley et al., 2005). For these patients, one way to terminate migraine with allodynia and fully developed central sensitization is parenteral administration of cyclooxygenase-1 (COX-1)/COX-2 inhibitors (Jakubowski et al., 2005a). Infusion of the COX-1/COX-2 inhibitor ketorolac in allodynic patients who had already missed the critical period for triptan therapy terminated both

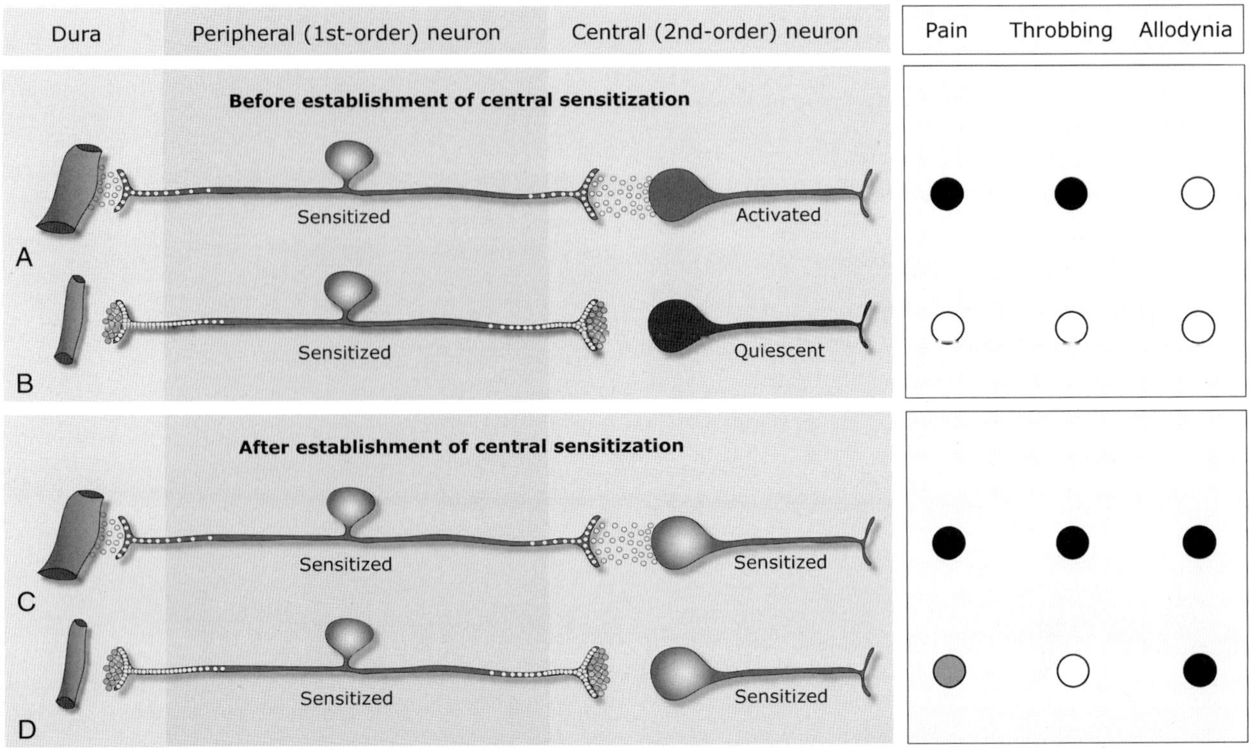

Fig. 16.1. Proposed mechanism of action for $5HT_{1B/1D}$ agonists during migraine. (A) Peripheral sensitization begins with release of neuropeptides that promote local vasodilation and plasma extravasation through their peripheral branch in the meninges, and activation of central trigeminovascular neurons through their central branch in the dorsal horn. Consequently, rhythmic pulsation of the meninges generates bursts of action potentials that activate the central trigeminovascular neuron and the pain (●) begins to throb (●). (B) Systemically administered triptan molecules bind to presynaptic $5HT_{1B/1D}$ receptors on terminals of both the peripheral and central branches of the meningeal nociceptor; this blocks neuropeptide release from the peripheral terminal, but has no effect on the hyperexcitability of the meningeal nociceptor. However, blockade of neuropeptide release from the central terminal of meningeal nociceptor renders the central trigeminovascular neuron inactive, resulting in termination of pain (○) and throbbing (○). (C) After the establishment of central sensitization, the pain continues to throb (●) and the skin becomes allodynic (●). (D) At this stage, blockade of neuropeptide release from the central terminals of the meningeal nociceptor cannot reverse the hyperexcitability of the central trigeminovascular neuron because its activity no longer depends on input from the meningeal nociceptor. In the face of the autonomous activity of the central trigeminovascular neuron, this blockade of synaptic transmission provides partial pain relief (◉), terminates the throbbing (○), and does not resolve the allodynia (●).

the headache and the allodynia provided that the patient had no history of using opioids to treat migraine. In the rat, infusion of COX-1/COX-2 inhibitors blocked sensitization in meningeal nociceptors and suppressed ongoing sensitization in spinal trigeminovascular neurons, suggesting that parenteral non-steroidal anti-inflammatory drug (NSAID) administration acts in the dorsal horn to inhibit the central neurons directly and reduce the synaptic input from the peripheral trigeminovascular neuron (Jakubowski et al., 2005a, 2007; Figure 16.2).

Though impractical as a routine migraine therapy, parenteral NSAID administration should be useful as a non-narcotic rescue therapy for migraine in the setting of the emergency department. Patients who use an opioid therapy over extended periods of time are at high risk of developing medication overuse headache and low response to non-narcotic drugs. The rationale for recommending against the use of opioids in allodynic migraine patients is based on evidence that opioids can facilitate sensitization in the dorsal horn (Mayer et al., 1999; Ozawa et al., 2001; Raith and Hochhaus, 2004; Watkins et al., 2005) through: (1) upregulation of NMDA receptor function; (2) down-regulation of glutamate transporters; (3) production of nitric oxide; (4) activation of spinal glia; and (5) increased extracellular level of prostaglandins.

Acknowledgment

This study was supported by NIH grant NS051484 and NS35611 from NINDS.

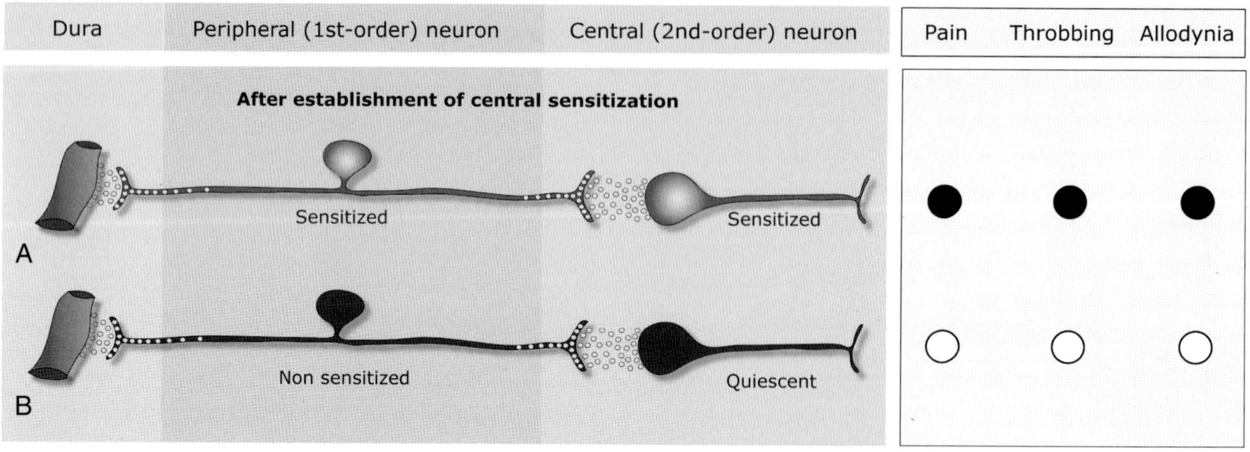

Fig. 16.2. Proposed mechanism of action for cyclooxygenase-1 (COX-1)/COX-2 inhibitors during migraine. (A) After the establishment of central sensitization, the pain throbs (●) and the skin is allodynic (●). (B) At this stage, COX-1/COX-2 inhibitors reverse the sensitization of both the peripheral and central trigeminovascular neurons, resulting in termination of pain, throbbing, and allodynia (○).

References

Ahmadi S, Lippross S, Neuhuber WL et al. (2002). PGE(2) selectively blocks inhibitory glycinergic neurotransmission onto rat superficial dorsal horn neurons. Nat Neurosci 5: 34–40.

Andrew D, Greenspan JD (1999). Mechanical and heat sensitization of cutaneous nociceptors after peripheral inflammation in the rat. J Neurophysiol 82: 2649–2656.

Ashkenazi A, Silberstein S, Jakubowski M et al. (2007). Improved identification of allodynic migraine patients using a questionnaire. Cephalalgia 27: 325–329.

Baba H, Kohno T, Moore KA et al. (2001). Direct activation of rat spinal dorsal horn neurons by prostaglandin E2. J Neurosci 21: 1750–1756.

Belmonte C, Gallar J, Pozo MA et al. (1991). Excitation by irritant chemical substances of sensory afferent units in the cat's cornea. J Physiol (Lond) 437: 709–725.

Blau JN (1987). Adult migraine: the patient observed. In: JN Blau (Ed.), Migraine – Clinical, Therapeutic, Conceptual and Research Aspects. Chapman and Hall, Cambridge.

Blau JN, Dexter SL (1981). The site of pain origin during migraine attacks. Cephalalgia 1: 143–147.

Bolay H, Reuter U, Dunn AK et al. (2002). Intrinsic brain activity triggers trigeminal meningeal afferents in a migraine model. Nat Med 8: 136–142.

Burstein R (2001). Deconstructing migraine headache into peripheral and central sensitization. Pain 89: 107–110.

Burstein R, Jakubowski M (2004). Analgesic triptan action in an animal model of intracranial pain: a race against the development of central sensitization. Ann Neurol 55: 27–36.

Burstein R, Yamamura H, Malick A et al. (1998). Chemical stimulation of the intracranial dura induces enhanced responses to facial stimulation in brain stem trigeminal neurons. J Neurophysiol 79: 964–982.

Burstein R, Yarnitsky D, Goor-Aryeh I et al. (2000a). An association between migraine and cutaneous allodynia. Ann Neurol 47: 614–624.

Burstein R, Cutrer FM, Yarnitsky D (2000b). The development of cutaneous allodynia during a migraine attack: clinical evidence for the sequential recruitment of spinal and supraspinal nociceptive neurons in migraine. Brain 123: 1703–1709.

Carmody J, Pawlak M, Messlinger K (1996). Lack of a role for substance P in the control of dural arterial flow. Exp Brain Res 111: 424–428.

Cooper BY, Ahlquist M, Friedman RM et al. (1991). Properties of high-threshold mechanoreceptors in the goat oral mucosa. II. Dynamic and static reactivity in carrageenan-inflamed mucosa. J Neurophysiol 66: 1280–1290.

Dai Y, Moriyama T, Higashi T et al. (2004). Proteinase-activated receptor 2-mediated potentiation of transient receptor potential vanilloid subfamily 1 activity reveals a mechanism for proteinase-induced inflammatory pain. J Neurosci 24: 4293–4299.

Daley ML, Pasupathy H, Griffith M et al. (1995). Detection of loss of cerebral vascular tone by correlation of arterial and intracranial pressure signals. IEEE Trans Biomed Eng 42: 420–424.

Davis KD, Meyer RA, Campbell JN (1993). Chemosensitivity and sensitization of nociceptive afferents that innervate the hairy skin of monkey. J Neurophysiol 69: 1071–1081.

DeLeo JA, Yezierski RP (2001). The role of neuroinflammation and neuroimmune activation in persistent pain. Pain 90: 1–6.

Drummond PD (1987). Scalp tenderness and sensitivity to pain in migraine and tension headache. Headache 27: 45–50.

Ebersberger A, Ringkamp M, Reeh PW et al. (1997). Recordings from brain stem neurons responding to chemical stimulation of the subarachnoid space. J Neurophysiol 77: 3122–3133.

England S, Bevan S, Docherty RJ (1996). PGE2 modulates the tetrodotoxin-resistant sodium current in neonatal rat dorsal root ganglion neurones via the cyclic AMP-protein kinase A cascade. J Physiol (Lond) 495: 429–440.

Evans AR, Vasko MR, Nicol GD (1999). The cAMP transduction cascade mediates the PGE2-induced inhibition of potassium currents in rat sensory neurones. J Physiol (Lond) 516: 163–178.

Foley KA, Cady R, Martin V et al. (2005). Treating early versus treating mild: timing of migraine prescription medications among patients with diagnosed migraine. Headache 45: 538–545.

Gobel H, Ernst M, Jeschke J et al. (1992). Acetylsalicylic acid activates antinociceptive brain-stem reflex activity in headache patients and in healthy subjects. Pain 48: 187–195.

Gold MS (1999). Tetrodotoxin-resistant Na^+ currents and inflammatory hyperalgesia. Proc Natl Acad Sci U S A 96: 7645–7649.

Gold MS, Levine JD, Correa AM (1998). Modulation of TTX-R INa by PKC and PKA and their role in PGE2-induced sensitization of rat sensory neurons *in vitro*. J Neurosci 18: 10345–10355.

Halata Z, Cooper BY, Baumann KI et al. (1999). Sensory nerve endings in the hard palate and papilla incisiva of the goat. Exp Brain Res 129: 218–228.

Hoogerwerf WA, Zou L, Shenoy M et al. (2001). The proteinase-activated receptor 2 is involved in nociception. J Neurosci 21: 9036–9042.

Hu HJ, th Gereau RW (2003). ERK integrates PKA and PKC signaling in superficial dorsal horn neurons. II. Modulation of neuronal excitability. J Neurophysiol 90: 1680–1688.

Hu JW, Sessle BJ, Raboisson P et al. (1992). Stimulation of craniofacial muscle afferents induces prolonged facilitatory effects in trigeminal nociceptive brain-stem neurones. Pain 48: 53–60.

Hunt SP, Pini A, Evan G (1987). Induction of c-fos-like protein in spinal cord neurons following sensory stimulation. Nature 328: 632–634.

Iadarola MJ, Douglass J, Civelli O et al. (1988). Differential activation of spinal cord dynorphin and enkephalin neurons during hyperalgesia: evidence using cDNA hybridization. Brain Res 455: 205–212.

Ikeda H, Heinke B, Ruscheweyh R et al. (2003). Synaptic plasticity in spinal lamina I projection neurons that mediate hyperalgesia. Science 299: 1237–1240.

Ingram SL, Williams JT (1996). Modulation of the hyperpolarization-activated current (Ih) by cyclic nucleotides in guinea-pig primary afferent neurons. J Physiol 492: 97–106.

Jakubowski M, Levy D, Goor-Aryeh I et al. (2005a). Terminating migraine with allodynia and ongoing central sensitization using parenteral administration of COX1/COX2 inhibitors. Headache 45: 850–861.

Jakubowski M, Silberstein S, Ashkenazi A et al. (2005b). Can allodynic migraine patients be identified interictally using a questionnaire? Neurology 65: 1419–1422.

Jakubowski M, Levy D, Kainz V et al. (2007). Sensitization of central trigeminovascular neurons: blockade by intravenous naproxen infusion. Neuroscience 148: 573–583.

Jensen K (1993). Extracranial blood flow, pain and tenderness in migraine. Clinical and experimental studies. Acta Neurol Scand Suppl 147: 1–27.

Jensen K, Tuxen C, Olesen J (1988). Pericranial muscle tenderness and pressure-pain threshold in the temporal region during common migraine. Pain 35: 65–70.

Jensen R, Rasmussen BK, Pedersen B et al. (1993). Prevalence of oromandibular dysfunction in a general population. J Orofac Pain 7: 175–182.

Ji RR, Rupp F (1997). Phosphorylation of transcription factor CREB in rat spinal cord after formalin-induced hyperalgesia: relationship to c-fos induction. J Neurosci 17: 1776–1785.

Ji RR, Woolf CJ (2001). Neuronal plasticity and signal transduction in nociceptive neurons: implications for the initiation and maintenance of pathological pain. Neurobiol Dis 8: 1–10.

Ji RR, Befort K, Brenner GJ et al. (2002). ERK MAP kinase activation in superficial spinal cord neurons induces prodynorphin and NK-1 upregulation and contributes to persistent inflammatory pain hypersensitivity. J Neurosci 22: 478–485.

Ji RR, Kohno T, Moore KA et al. (2003). Central sensitization and LTP: do pain and memory share similar mechanisms? Trends Neurosci 26: 696–705.

Klyachko VA, Ahern GP, Jackson MB (2001). cGMP-mediated facilitation in nerve terminals by enhancement of the spike afterhyperpolarization. Neuron 31: 1015–1025.

Koltzenburg M, Torebjork HE, Wahren LK (1994). Nociceptor modulated central sensitization causes mechanical hyperalgesia in acute chemogenic and chronic neuropathic pain. Brain 117: 579–591.

Kurosawa M, Messlinger K, Pawlak M et al. (1995). Increase of meningeal blood flow after electrical stimulation of rat dura mater encephali: mediation by calcitonin gene-related peptide. Br J Pharmacol 114: 1397–1402.

Levine JD, Reichling DB (1999). Peripheral mechanisms of inflammatory pain. In: PD Wall, R Melzak (Eds.), Textbook of Pain. Churchill Livingstone, New York, pp. 59–84.

Levy D, Strassman AM (2002). Distinct sensitizing effects of the cAMP-PKA second messenger cascade on rat dural mechanonociceptors. J Physiol 538: 483–493.

Levy D, Strassman AM (2004). Modulation of dural nociceptor mechanosensitivity by the nitric oxide – cyclic GMP signaling cascade. J Neurophysiol 92: 766–772.

Liveing E (1873). On Megrim, Sick Headache. Arts & Boeve, Nijmegen.

Lous I, Olesen J (1982). Evaluation of pericranial tenderness and oral function in patients with common migraine, muscle contraction headache and 'combination headache'. Pain 12: 385–393.

Magerl W, Wilk SH, Treede RD (1998). Secondary hyperalgesia and perceptual wind-up following intradermal injection of capsaicin in humans. Pain 74: 257–268.

Malmberg AB, Chen C, Tonegawa S et al. (1997). Preserved acute pain and reduced neuropathic pain in mice lacking PKCgamma. Science 278: 279–283.

Mannion RJM, Costigan I, Decosterd F et al. (1999). Neurotrophins: peripherally and centrally acting modulators of tactile stimulus-induced inflammatory pain hypersensitivity. Proc Natl Acad Sci U S A 96: 9385–9390.

Mantyh PW, Rogers SD, Honore P et al. (1997). Inhibition of hyperalgesia by ablation of lamina I spinal neurons expressing the substance P receptor [see comments]. Science 278: 275–279.

Martin HA, Basbaum AI, Kwait GC et al. (1987). Leukotriene and prostaglandin sensitization of cutaneous high threshold C- and A-delta mechanonociceptors in the hairy skin of rat hindlimb. Neuroscience 22: 651–659.

Mayer DJ, Mao J, Holt J et al. (1999). Cellular mechanisms of neuropathic pain, morphine tolerance, and their interactions. Proc Natl Acad Sci U S A 96: 731–736.

McCarson KE, Krause JE (1994). NK-1 and NK-3 type tachykinin receptor mrna expression in the rat spinal cord dorsal horn is increased during adjuvant or formalin-induced nociception. J Neurosci 14: 712–720.

McMahon SB, Lewin GR, Wall PD (1993). Central hyperexcitability triggered by noxious inputs. Curr Opin Neurobiol 3: 602–610.

Morisset V, Nagy F (2000). Plateau potential-dependent windup of the response to primary afferent stimuli in rat dorsal horn neurons. Eur J Neurosci 12: 3087–3095.

Murase K, Ryu PD, Randic M (1986). Substance P augments a persistent slow inward calcium-sensitive current in voltage-clamped spinal dorsal horn neurons of the rat. Brain Res 365: 369–376.

Obreja O, Schmelz M, Poole S et al. (2002). Interleukin-6 in combination with its soluble IL-6 receptor sensitises rat skin nociceptors to heat, in vivo. Pain 96: 57–62.

Olesen J, Thomsen LL, Iversen H (1994). Nitric oxide is a key molecule in migraine and other vascular headaches. Trends Pharmacol Sci 15: 149–153.

Ozawa T, Nakagawa T, Shige K et al. (2001). Changes in the expression of glial glutamate transporters in the rat brain accompanied with morphine dependence and naloxone-precipitated withdrawal. Brain Res 905: 254–258.

Potrebic S, Ahn AH, Skinner K et al. (2003). Peptidergic nociceptors of both trigeminal and dorsal root ganglia express serotonin 1D receptors: implications for the selective antimigraine action of triptans. J Neurosci 23: 10988–10997.

Pozo MA, Gallego R, Gallar J et al. (1992). Blockade by calcium antagonists of chemical excitation and sensitization of polymodal nociceptors in the cat's cornea. J Physiol (Lond) 450: 179–189.

Premkumar LS, Ahern GP (2000). Induction of vanilloid receptor channel activity by protein kinase C. Nature 408: 985–990.

Raith K, Hochhaus G (2004). Drugs used in the treatment of opioid tolerance and physical dependence: a review. Int J Clin Pharmacol Ther 42: 191–203.

Rasmussen BK, Jensen R, Olesen J (1991). A population-based analysis of the diagnostic criteria of the International Headache Society. Cephalalgia 11: 129–134.

Ren K, Dubner R (1993). NMDA receptor antagonists attenuate mechanical hyperalgesia in rats with unilateral inflammation of the hindpaw. Neurosci Lett 163: 22–26.

Reuter U, Bolay H, Jansen-Olesen I et al. (2001). Delayed inflammation in rat meninges: implications for migraine pathophysiology. Brain 124: 2490–2502.

Reynier-Rebuffel AM, Mathiau P, Callebert J et al. (1994). Substance P, calcitonin gene-related peptide, and capsaicin release serotonin from cerebrovascular mast cells. Am J Physiol 267: R1421–R1429.

Ryu S, Liu B, Qin F (2003). Low pH potentiates both capsaicin binding and channel gating of VR1 receptors. J Gen Physiol 122: 45–61.

Sachs D, Cunha FQ, Poole S et al. (2002). Tumour necrosis factor-alpha, interleukin-1beta and interleukin-8 induce persistent mechanical nociceptor hypersensitivity. Pain 96: 89–97.

Samad TA, Moore KA, Sapirstein A et al. (2001). Interleukin-1beta-mediated induction of Cox-2 in the CNS contributes to inflammatory pain hypersensitivity. Nature 410: 471–475.

Schaible HG, Schmidt RF (1988). Excitation and sensitization of fine articular afferents from cat's knee joint by prostaglandin E2. J Physiol (Lond) 403: 91–104.

Schepelmann K, Ebersberger A, Pawlak M et al. (1999). Response properties of trigeminal brain stem neurons with input from dura mater encephali in the rat. Neuroscience 90: 543–554.

Selby G, Lance JW (1960). Observations on 500 cases of migraine and allied vascular headache. J Neurol Neurosurg Psychiatry 23: 23–32.

Seybold VS, McCarson KE, Mermelstein PG et al. (2003). Calcitonin gene-related peptide regulates expression of neurokinin1 receptors by rat spinal neurons. J Neurosci 23: 1816–1824.

Shepheard SL, Williamson DJ, Hill RG et al. (1993). The non-peptide neurokinin1 receptor antagonist, RP 67580, blocks neurogenic plasma extravasation in the dura mater of rats. Br J Pharmacol 108: 11–12.

Simone DA, Sorkin LS, Oh U et al. (1991). Neurogenic hyperalgesia: central neural correlates in responses of spinothalamic tract neurons. J Neurophysiol 66: 228–246.

Sivilotti LG, Thompson SW, Woolf CJ (1993). Rate of rise of the cumulative depolarization evoked by repetitive stimulation of small-caliber afferents is a predictor of action potential windup in rat spinal neurons *in vitro*. J Neurophysiol 69: 1621–1631.

Steen KH, Reeh PW, Anton F et al. (1992). Protons selectively induce lasting excitation and sensitization to mechanical stimulation of nociceptors in rat skin, in vitro. J Neurosci 12: 86–95.

Strassman AM, Raymond SA (1999). Electrophysiological evidence for tetrodotoxin-resistant sodium channels in slowly conducting dural sensory fibers. J Neurophysiol 81: 413–424.

Strassman AM, Raymond SA, Burstein R (1996). Sensitization of meningeal sensory neurons and the origin of headaches. Nature 384: 560–564.

Su X, Gebhart GF (1998). Mechanosensitive pelvic nerve afferent fibers innervating the colon of the rat are polymodal in character. J Neurophysiol 80: 2632–2644.

Sugiura T, Tominaga M, Katsuya H et al. (2002). Bradykinin lowers the threshold temperature for heat activation of vanilloid receptor 1. J Neurophysiol 88: 544–548.

Suzuki R, Furuno T, McKay DM et al. (1999). Direct neurite-mast cell communication *in vitro* occurs via the neuropeptide substance P. J Immunol 163: 2410–2415.

Tfelt-Hansen P, Lous I, Olesen J (1981). Prevalence and significance of muscle tenderness during common migraine attacks. Headache 21: 49–54.

Tominaga M, Caterina MJ, Malmberg AB et al. (1998). The cloned capsaicin receptor integrates multiple pain-producing stimuli [see comments]. Neuron 21: 531–543.

Torebjork HE, Lundberg LE, LaMotte RH (1992). Central changes in processing of mechanoreceptive input in capsaicin-induced secondary hyperalgesia in humans. J Physiol (Lond) 448: 765–780.

Vasko MR (1995). Prostaglandin-induced neuropeptide release from spinal cord. Prog Brain Res 104: 367–380.

Waelkens J (1985). Warning symptoms in migraine: characteristics and therapeutic implications. Cephalalgia 5: 223–228.

Wang JF, Khasar SG, Ahlgren SC et al. (1996). Sensitization of C-fibres by prostaglandin E2 in the rat is inhibited by guanosine 5′-O-(2-thiodiphosphate), 2′,5′-dideoxyadenosine and Walsh inhibitor peptide. Neuroscience 71: 259–263.

Watkins LR, Hutchinson MR, Johnston IN et al. (2005). Glia: novel counter-regulators of opioid analgesia. Trends Neurosci 28: 661–669.

Willis WD, Coggeshall RE (1991). Sensory Mechanisms of the Spinal Cord. Plenum Press, New York.

Wolff HG, Tunis MM, Goodell H (1953). Studies on migraine. Arch Intern Med 92: 478–484.

Woolf CJ (1983). Evidence for a central component of post-injury pain hypersensitivity. Nature 306: 686–688.

Woolf CJ (1995). Somatic pain – pathogenesis and prevention. Br J Anaesth 75: 169–176.

Woolf CJ, Doubell TP (1994). The pathophysiology of chronic pain – increased sensitivity to low threshold A beta-fibre inputs. Curr Opin Neurobiol 4: 525–534.

Woolf CJ, Salter MW (2000). Neuronal plasticity: increasing the gain in pain. Science 288: 1765–1769.

Yano H, Wershil BK, Arizono N et al. (1989). Substance P-induced augmentation of cutaneous vascular permeability and granulocyte infiltration in mice is mast cell dependent. J Clin Invest 84: 1276–1286.

Handbook of Clinical Neurology, Vol. 97 (3rd series)
Headache
G. Nappi and M.A. Moskowitz, Editors

Chapter 17

Botulinum neurotoxin in the treatment of headache disorders

ALEXANDER MAUSKOP*

New York Headache Center and Downstate Medical Center, State University of New York, New York, NY, USA

Botulinum toxin (BoNT) has been investigated for the prophylactic treatment of several headache disorders. This chapter will present a discussion of the clinical pharmacology, the physical characteristics of the available formulations, the injection techniques and protocols, and the clinical efficacy and safety of BoNT in the prophylactic treatment of headache disorders.

BOTULINUM NEUROTOXIN

BoNT is a purified protein produced by the bacterium *Clostridium botulinum*. It is a member of the family of Gram-positive bacilli (Shukla and Sharma, 2005), and the toxin exists as seven distinct serotypes (A–G), which have distinct properties and differing clinical effects (Aoki and Guyer, 2001). The human nervous system is susceptible to five toxin serotypes (A, B, E, F, G) and unaffected by two (C, D) (Huang et al., 2000). BoNTA is commercially available in some countries as Botox (BoNTA; Allergan, Irvine, CA, USA) and Dysport (BoNTA; Ipsen Pharmaceuticals, Slough, UK), and BoNTB is commercially available as Myobloc and NeuroBloc (BoNTB; Solstice Neurosciences, South San Francisco, CA, USA/Solstice Neurosciences, Dublin, Ireland). BoNT has several unique features: high degree of potency; nanogram quantities are utilized effectively; focal delivery by injection; and long duration of action (months) after a single treatment. BoNTA and to a lesser extent BoNTB have been used for various forms of dystonia, hyperhydrosis, blepharospasm, glabellar lines, spastic bladder, and gastrointestinal disorders. The beneficial effect of BoNTA treatment for migraine was first noted in patients who were given the protein for the treatment of facial wrinkles and reported relief from their migraine headaches (Binder et al., 2000). Multiple open-label and randomized, placebo (PBO)-controlled trials have investigated the safety and efficacy of BoNTA in the treatment of several headache disorders.

MECHANISM OF ACTION

One of the main sites of action for BoNT is the neuromuscular junction. By interfering with acetylcholine release from the presynaptic axon terminal at this site, BoNT causes dose-dependent and reversible muscle relaxation (Dolly, 2003). Axonal sprouting, which occurs following BoNT entrance into the cell, causes termination of the toxin-induced effect in 2–4 months (de Paiva et al., 1999; Dolly, 2003). The eventual disappearance of the toxin-induced effect allows the return of neuromuscular transmission and regression of sprouts (Dolly, 2003; Aoki, 2005a).

Local muscle paralysis and reduction in overall muscle contraction do not fully explain the pain relief mechanism of BoNT. Recent studies have discovered that BoNTA inhibits release of glutamate (Cui et al., 2004) and calcitonin gene-related peptide (Meng et al., 2007) in sensory nerve terminals, thereby possibly resulting in reduction of inflammatory pain and causing indirect inhibition of central sensitization (Aoki, 2005b).

PRODUCT VARIATION

There are currently three BoNT products available for clinical use. The indications listed below are approved in some countries, but not others. Botox (BoNTA; Allergan, Irvine, CA, USA), the most widely used BoNT in clinical practice, is approved for the treatment of glabellar lines, cervical dystonia, blepharospasm, strabismus, hyperhidrosis, adult spasticity, and juvenile cerebral palsy. Dysport (BoNTA; Ipsen Pharmaceuticals, Slough, UK) is approved for the treatment of blepharospasm, glabellar lines, hyperhydrosis, hemifacial

*Correspondence to: Alexander Mauskop, MD, New York Headache Center and Downstate Medical Center, State University of New York, 30 East 76th Street, New York, NY 10021, USA, Tel: (212) 794-3550, Fax: (212) 794-0591, E-mail: DrMauskop@nyheadache.com

spasm, spasmodic torticollis, arm spasticity due to stroke, and dynamic equinus foot deformity. Myobloc or Neurobloc (BoNTB; Solstice Neurosciences, South San Francisco, CA) formulation is approved for the treatment of cervical dystonia.

All available BoNTs determine their unit activities using mouse lethality assays to establish the intraperitoneal dose that results in lethality of 50% of a population of mice; however, no standardized methodology has been applied throughout the industry (Huang et al., 2000). Botox and Dysport vary regarding the strains of toxin-producing organisms used in fermentation, methods of purification, excipients, and formulation, which results in distinct properties regarding potency, diffusion, and antigenicity. Thus, Botox and Dysport (both BoNTA) should not be regarded as generic equivalents and, as cited in the product inserts of the commercially available toxin products, biological activity units are unique to each BoNT preparation and cannot be compared or converted into another.

The term "botulinum toxin" is being replaced by specific names that better describe various commercial toxin products. OnabotulinumtoxinA is the name for the product marketed as Botox or Botox Cosmetic, abobotulinumtoxinA is what is known as Dysport, and rimabotulinumtoxinB is sold as Myobloc or NeuroBloc.

FORMULATIONS: DILUTION AND RECONSTITUTION

All three BoNT products have differing dosing, safety, and efficacy characteristics, and there are no established methodologies to calculate equivalent doses (Brin, 1997). Lyophilized BoNTA (Botox) is available in vials containing 100 units (U) of *Clostridium botulinum* type A neurotoxin complex; for migraine treatment, one vial is reconstituted with 3 ml, or more often with 4 ml, of preservative-free 0.9% sodium chloride (Blumenfeld et al., 2003; Samton and Mauskop, 2006). BoNTA (Dysport) is reconstituted with 1.0 ml sodium chloride (0.9%) to yield a solution containing 500 U/ml Dysport. BoNTB (Myobloc) is also available in the USA in vials containing either 2500 U/ml or 5000 U/ml in 0.05% human serum albumin. For the management of headaches and pain further dilution of BoNTB is often used. BoNTB solution has a highly acidic pH (5.6), which makes injections more painful.

INJECTION TECHNIQUE

While the injection technique varies somewhat among experienced injectors, most aspects are similar. The author provides his recommendations on the basis of over 7000 treatments administered to more than 2000 patients with headaches over 15 years. The use of a 30-gauge needle is recommended. Injection into the scalp areas can be done using a 0.5-inch (1.25-cm) needle, while in suboccipital, neck, and trapezii muscles a 1-inch (2.5-cm) needle is needed to deliver the toxin into the muscle rather than subcutaneous fat. Injections should be intramuscular rather than intradermal, avoiding the periosteum, eyelid region, and visible superficial blood vessels. Use of needles longer than 1 inch (2.5 cm) increases the risk of complications, such as pneumothorax, vascular injury, and spinal cord damage. Injections in the forehead should be bilateral and symmetrical in order to avoid facial asymmetry. To assure good compliance with continued treatment, it is important to achieve not only good headache relief, but also acceptable cosmetic outcome. There are no restrictions on postinjection activities. Application of an anesthetic cream to the forehead area for an hour prior to the procedure may reduce injection pain. However, most patients find that the injection pain, particularly with Botox, is minimal and very few choose to apply the cream.

A combination of fixed-site (FS) and follow-the-pain (FTP) methods is used for most headache conditions by most injectors. The sites injected depend on the distribution of headache pain and trigger points identified by palpation. It is not unusual for patients to report that headaches are confined to only one part of their head, but after treatment with Botox the location of the pain can shift to the opposite side or another area. Subsequent treatments are given to cover all of the involved areas. Recent studies of BoNTA in migraineurs with chronic daily headache (CDH) suggest that doses between 150 U and 225 U may provide best ratio of efficacy to adverse events (AEs) for chronic headache conditions (Mathew et al., 2005; Silberstein et al., 2005). In practice, the author and many injectors use 100 U for most headache patients. In rare cases when pain is strictly limited to one area, such as the forehead or temples, doses as low as 35 U have been found to be effective. In other patients with pain involving the entire head, neck, and shoulders as much as 300 U has been given by the author. In one large exploratory study in migraineurs with CDH ($n = 355$), the average total dose of BoNTA shown to be efficacious was 190 U (Mathew et al., 2005). In another large study ($n = 702$) in a similar population, BoNTA doses of 150 U and 225 U showed benefits over PBO (Silberstein et al., 2005). In one trial of BoNTA in episodic migraine, doses as low as 25 U were efficacious (Silberstein et al., 2000). BoNTA treatment is usually administered every 3 months, although the duration of effect can vary from 2 to 4 months.

Table 17.3

Published randomized controlled trials in episodic migraine for botulinum toxin type A (BoNTA)

Trial	*n*	Design/duration	Dose/method	Results
Elkind et al., 2006	418	Study I–III: 4 months each	Study I: 7.5, 25, or 50 U; FS Study II and III: 25 or 50 U; FS	BoNTA and PBO had similar decreases from baseline in frequency of migraines in all studies
Aurora, 2006	369	11 months	110–260 U; Varied sites	BoNTA patients with ≥12 HA days (but ≤15 HA days) at baseline had significant reductions in HA episodes at 6 months compared with PBO There were no significant between-group differences in the frequency of migraine episodes/month
Relja et al., 2006	495	11 months	75, 150, 255 U; FS	BoNTA and PBO showed improvement in frequency of migraine at 6 months with no significant between-group differences
Evers et al., 2004	60	3 months	16 U/100 U (frontal and neck); varied sites	Reductions from baseline in migraine frequency and number of days with migraine occurred in BoNTA and PBO with no significant between-group differences
Barrientos and Chana, 2003	30	3 months	50 U; FS	BoNTA showed significantly greater reductions in frequency of migraine at 2 and 3 months compared with PBO
Blumenfeld et al., 2008	59	Randomized, double-blind comparative (versus DVPX); 9 months	100 U Botox; FTP	Both treatments resulted in significant improvements in MIDAS scores and reductions in the number of HA days and in HA index from baseline Compared with BoNTA a significantly greater percentage of DVPX patients reported adverse events, Possibly related to treatment and discontinued due to adverse events
Silberstein et al., 2000	123	4 months	25 U or 75 U; FS	Pericranial injections of 25 U BoNTA significantly decreased migraine frequency and severity, and acute medication use compared with PBO Global assessments were significantly better in the 25 and 75 U groups versus PBO

FS: fixed-site; HA: headache; PBO: placebo.

all patients in each treatment group had a decrease from baseline of 50% or more migraine episodes per 30-day period.

A similar 11-month study ($n = 495$) by Relja et al. (2006) evaluated the safety and efficacy of multiple treatments of BoNTA (225, 150, or 75 U). The primary efficacy endpoint was the mean reduction from baseline in the frequency of migraine episodes at day 180 in the PNR group. However, all treatment groups showed improvement, with no significant differences favoring BoNTA.

Another study examined efficacy based on injection site over 3 months (Evers et al., 2004). In this study, 60 patients with migraine were randomly assigned to receive either PBO injections in the frontal and neck muscles; or 16 U BoNTA in the frontal muscles and PBO in the neck muscles; or a total of 100 U BoNTA in the frontal and neck muscles. In both BoNTA treatment groups, 30% of patients experienced a ≥50% reduction in migraine frequency at 3 months compared with baseline versus 25% of patients in the PBO group. There were no significant differences between the three study groups with respect to reduction of migraine frequency, number of days with migraine, and the number of total single doses to treat a migraine attack. In the *post hoc* analysis, the reduction of all accompanying symptoms was significantly greater in the 16-U treatment group compared with the PBO group. In the 100-U treatment group significantly more AEs occurred compared with the PBO group; all AEs were characterized as mild and transient (Evers et al., 2004).

In a double-blind, randomized, 90-day PBO-controlled study that enrolled 30 adult migraineurs (Barrientos and

Chana, 2003), 50 U BoNTA produced significantly greater reductions in the frequency of migraine attacks of any severity at day 90 and in the frequency of severe migraine attacks at days 60 and 90, compared with PBO.

A 4-month study by Silberstein et al. (2000) assessed the safety and efficacy of 25 U and 75 U BoNTA in 123 patients with a history of episodic migraine. Those in the 25-U group had significantly fewer migraine attacks per month, less severe migraines, fewer days when they needed acute migraine medication, and less migraine-associated vomiting versus PBO. Global assessment scores, indicating treatment response, were significantly better in the 25-U and 75-U groups than in the PBO group, but the 75-U group experienced more treatment-related AEs (Silberstein et al., 2000).

A number of open-label studies (Binder et al., 2000; Mauskop, 2002; Eross et al., 2005), a randomized, evaluator-masked comparator (Blumenfeld and Chippendale, 2006), and a randomized, double-blind comparator (Blumenfeld et al., 2007) trial have looked at the efficacy and safety of BoNTA in episodic migraine (Table 17.4). Significant reductions in migraine disability were observed in uncontrolled trials to last upwards of 15 months (Mauskop, 2002). In addition, treatment responses to acute attacks were seen in 1–2 h (Binder et al., 2000). In the randomized, evaluator-masked comparator trial with divalproex sodium (DVPX), a significantly greater percentage of BoNTA-treated patients had a ≥50% reduction from baseline in the mean number of headache days at 3 months, compared with DVPX (Blumenfeld and Chippendale, 2006). In the randomized, double-blind comparator trial, over 9 months, BoNTA and DVPX treatment resulted in significant improvements in disability, but without any between-group significance (Blumenfeld et al., 2007). In both comparator trials, significantly more patients receiving DVPX discontinued due to AEs than patients receiving BoNTA (Blumenfeld and Chippendale, 2006; Blumenfeld et al., 2007).

The evidence of efficacy of BoNTA in episodic migraine is still inconclusive (Mauskop and Mathew, 2008). Although several studies failed to meet primary endpoint or show substantial treatment effect over PBO, other studies suggested benefits. In some cases, the investigators speculated that the high PBO response that is common in studies of pain medications and other issues specific to some studies (e.g., high concomitant use of acute and prophylactic medications) may have confounded the results (Aurora et al., 2006; Elkind et al., 2006; Relja et al., 2006).

Tension-type headache and chronic tension-type headache

Three recent trials examining the efficacy and safety of BoNTA in CTTH (Table 17.5) have demonstrated conflicting results (Ondo et al., 2004; Padberg et al., 2004; Relja and Telarović, 2004; Silberstein et al., 2006). A double-blind, randomized, PBO-controlled, parallel-group study by Silberstein et al. (2006) evaluated the safety and efficacy of 0–150 U BoNTA for the prophylaxis of CTTH in 300 patients. While all treatment groups, including PBO, improved at day

Table 17.4

Other published trials in episodic migraine for botulinum toxin type A (BoNTA)

Trial	*n*	Design/duration	Dose/method	Results
Eross et al., 2005	61	Open-label; 6 months	25 U; FS and FTP	At 3-months, MIDAS scores, number of HA days, and HA intensity significantly decreased Duration of illness may be a predictor of treatment response
Binder et al., 2000	106	Open-label; 12 months	5–110 U; FS	Of 77 migraine patients treated prophylactically, 51% reported complete response with 2.6 months' duration of benefit Of 10 migraine patients treated for acute attack, 70% reported complete response and experienced improvement within 1–2 h
Mauskop, 2002 (abstract)	60	Retrospective, open-label; 17 months BoNTA tx (range 5–46 months)	25–200 U; varied sites	Sustained relief reported over periods of up to 46 months

FS: fixed-site; FTP: follow-the-pain; MIDAS: Migraine Disability Assessment Scale; HA: headache; DVPX: divalproex sodium; tx: treatment.

Table 17.5

Published randomized controlled trials in tension-type headache (TTH)/chronic tension-type headache (CTTH) for botulinum toxin type A (BoNTA)

Trial	*n*	Design/duration	Dose/method	Results
Ondo, et al., 2004	60 (46 CTTH, 14 CM)	Double-blind, PBO-controlled; 12 weeks, followed by an open label injection	200 U BoNTA, FTP	Primary outcome measure of headache-free days over 12 weeks was not met, but during weeks 8–12 the difference was statistically significant
Porta, 2000	20; TTH	Randomized, comparative versus methylprednisolone; 2 months	5–15 U BoNTA	Methylprednisolone decreased pain at day 30 BoNTA was associated with reduced pain at days 30 and 60, and improvements in the symptom profile up to day 60 BoNTA produced more prolonged pain relief than did methylprednisolone
Sebastian and de Bruijn, 2003 (abstract)	40; CTTH	Double-blind, PBO-controlled; 12 weeks	100 U	No significant between-group differences were observed in reduction in HA days and HA hours/day, or patient global assessments

60 in mean change from baseline in TTH-free days per month (primary endpoint), there were no significant differences between PBO and four of the five BoNTA treated groups; a statistically significant difference between PBO versus BoNTA 150-U group was observed at day 60 (favoring PBO). However, significantly greater percentages of patients in three BoNTA groups at day 90 and two BoNTA groups at day 120 had $\geq$50% decrease in TTH days compared with the PBO group (Silberstein et al., 2006).

Ondo et al. (2004) studied patients ($n = 60$) with primarily CTTH receiving 200 U BoNTA or PBO in a double-blind, PBO-controlled, parallel-design trial (weeks 0–12), with an open-label crossover for another 12 weeks (Ondo et al., 2004). Over a 12-week period after injections, headache-free days significantly improved in the BoNTA group from week 8 to 12 and tended to improve over the entire 12-week period, but did not meet the significance criterion. At week 24 (open-label), headache-free days were significantly higher in the twice-BoNTA-injected group compared with the once-injected group (Ondo et al., 2004). In another double-blind, PBO-controlled study in which 40 CTTH patients received lower dosage of BoNTA (maximum 100 U) or PBO, there was no significant difference between the two treatment groups in decrease of headache intensity, mean number of headache days, headache hours per day, days on which symptomatic treatment was taken, and number of analgesics taken per day (Padberg et al., 2004). There was also no significant difference in patients' assessment of improvement after weeks 4, 8, and 12 (Padberg et al., 2004).

In a relatively small ($n = 16$) prospective, randomized, double-blind, PBO-controlled crossover study of 8 weeks followed by a larger ($n = 30$) prospective, open-label study for 18 months (Relja and Telarović, 2004), patients received 40–95 U BoNTA. Compared with PBO, patients receiving BoNTA treatment demonstrated significantly reduced maximum severity of headache, reduced pericranial muscle tenderness, and increased headache-free days. Moreover, a constant and cumulative trend of improvement was present during the long-term study, suggesting better QoL during BoNTA treatment (Relja and Telarović, 2004).

Earlier studies also illustrate conflicting findings for prophylactic BoNTA treatment in CTTH (Smuts et al., 1999; Schmitt et al., 2001). A randomized, PBO-controlled study was conducted to examine the effect of 20 U BoNTA injected into frontal and temporal muscles in patients with CTTH (Schmitt et al., 2001). Patients were evaluated during the 4-week baseline period and the 8-week posttreatment period. Some improvement in affective variables were demonstrated in the BoNTA group, but other outcome variables, such as pain intensity, the number of pain-free days, and consumption of analgesics, were not statistically different between the groups. Reasons for these moderate effects may include the injection sites, dose of BoNTA, and duration of treatment (Schmitt et al.,

2001). Conversely, Smuts et al. (1999) assessed the efficacy of BoNTA (100 U) in the prophylaxis of CTTH ($n = 41$) over 3 months; 37 patients completed the study. The number of headache-free days improved significantly in the BoNTA group at month 3 compared with baseline, and patients randomized to BoNTA reported improvement in QoL after the injections (Smuts et al., 1999).

A number of smaller trials, including comparative (Porta, 2000), open-label (Freund and Schwartz, 2002), and pilot (Sebastian and De Bruijn, 2003) studies, have been conducted in TTH and CTTH patients. They also yielded some positive and some negative findings (Table 17.6).

Several published studies have also addressed headache prophylaxis in mixed populations of patients, with many patients displaying characteristics of both TTH and migraine, and in headache of other etiologies (e.g., cluster, cervicogenic, craniocervical dystonia) (Troost, 2002; McAllister, 2003; Miller and Denney, 2003; Troost et al., 2003). These were retrospective and open-label studies, which limits their value (Table 17.7).

Published trials for Dysport and Myobloc

Clinical experience with Dysport and Myobloc is far less extensive in the treatment of headache than that of BoNTA. Few preliminary studies have assessed the efficacy of Dysport and Myobloc in the prophylactic treatment of headache disorders (Table 17.8) (Rollnik et al., 2000; Fadeyi and Adams, 2002; Opida, 2002a, b; Gwynn et al., 2003; Lake and Saper, 2003; Schulte-Mattler et al., 2004).

In a double-blind, PBO-controlled study of 21 patients with TTH (Rollnik et al., 2000), patients received pericranial injection of (10 × 20 U: 200 U total) Dysport or PBO. After 4, 8, and 12 weeks, no significant differences between groups were observed in the Visual Analogue Scale (VAS) scores, frequency and duration of headache attacks, consumption of analgesics, pressure pain threshold, total tenderness score, and QoL parameters. Nevertheless, both groups showed improvement in the VAS scores. The investigators suggested that higher doses or other injection sites might be necessary to achieve therapeutic effects of Dysport in TTH (Rollnik et al., 2000).

In a prospective, randomized, double-blind, PBO-controlled trial, multiple pericranial muscles in 112 patients with CTTH were treated either with 500 U Dysport or with PBO (Schulte-Mattler et al., 2004). There were no significant differences between groups in any of the primary or secondary effect measures (the relative change of the area under the headache curve from baseline to the 6-week period beginning 5 weeks after the treatment (primary variable); number of days with headache, number of days with intake of analgesics, duration of nocturnal sleep, and Beck Depression Inventory score (secondary variables)).

Table 17.6

Other published trials in tension-type headache (TTH)/chronic tension-type headache (CTTH) for botulinum toxin type A (BoNTA)

Trial	*n*	Design/duration	Dose/method	Results
Freund and Schwartz, 2002	60	Open-label; 3 months	150 U; FS	63% of BoNTA patients reported a 50% improvement in facial pain Patients with TMD and CTTH reported ≥50% pain relief
Eross et al., 2005	61	Open-label; 6 months	25 U; FS and FTP	At 3-months, MIDAS scores, number of HA days, and HA intensity significantly decreased Duration of illness may be a predictor of treatment response
Binder et al., 2000	106	Open-label; 12 months	5–110 U; FS	Of 77 migraine patients treated prophylactically, 51% reported complete response with 2.6 months' duration of benefit Of 10 migraine patients treated for acute attack, 70% reported complete response and experienced improvement within 1–2 h
Mauskop, 2002 (abstract)	60	Retrospective, open-label; 17 months BoNTA tx (range 5–46 months)	25–200 U; Varied sites	Sustained relief reported over periods of up to 46 months

FS: fixed-site; HA: headache.

Table 17.7

Trials in mixed chronic populations for botulinum toxin type A (BoNTA)

Trial	*n*/population	Design/duration	Dose/method	Results
Blumenfeld et al., 2008	59; episodic and chronic	Randomized, double-blind comparative (versus DVPX); 9 months	100 U Botox; FTP	Both treatments resulted in significant improvements in MIDAS scores and reductions in the number of HA days and in HA index from baseline Compared with BoNTA a significantly greater percentage of DVPX patients reported adverse events, possibly related to treatment and discontinued due to adverse events
McAllister, 2003 (abstract)	116; migraine, TTH, and cervicogenic	Retrospective; 1–3 months postinjection tx response assessed	40–280 U; FS and FTP	While all patients reported some improvement, 76% reported a ≥75% improvement in HA 9% reported complete remission of HA
Miller and Denney, 2003 (abstract)	68; chronic, intractable HA with or without neck pain	Retrospective; 1 month postinjection tx response assessed	100 U; FTP	Significant reduction of pain was observed in 75% of patients Efficacy was similar in patients with and without neck pain
Troost et al., 2003 (abstract)	436; intractable HA: migraine/ETTH/CDH	Retrospective; 3-year open-label, assessment of 3-month tx periods	25–300 U; FS	91% of patients reported improvements in HA Improvements were cumulative through 3 cycles and sustained through 8 treatments
Troost, 2002 (abstract)	134; intractable HA: CDH, migraine with or without aura, ETTH	Open-label; patients assessed 2 months after tx; 1–4 tx cycles	30–200 U (CDH), 15–240 U (migraine); varied sites	Higher percentage of patients improved with multiple treatments: 77%, 94%, 90%, and 92% for treatments 1–4, respectively

TTH: tension-type headache; tx: treatment; FS: fixed-site; FTP: follow-the-pain; HA: headache; ETTH: episodic tension-type headache; CDH: chronic daily headache.

Seven patients in the Dysport group had transient weakness of the eyelids, the neck, or both, indicating that a higher dose than used in this study does not seem to be appropriate for the treatment of headache (Schulte-Mattler et al., 2004).

SAFETY AND TOLERABILITY

Two decades of clinical use have established BoNTA as a remarkably safe drug. Clinical AEs associated with BoNTs are typically of four types: (1) those due to expected effects on the target muscle (e.g., local muscle weakness); (2) those due to migration of the neurotoxin to nearby uninjected adjacent muscles; (3) those due to systemic spread to distant sites; and (4) temporary worsening of pain and muscle spasm due to the effect of needling. In addition, rash and flu-like symptoms can rarely occur as a result of an allergic reaction. However, serious allergic reactions have never been reported, which is surprising considering that BoNT is a protein. Injection of anterior neck muscles can cause dysphagia (swallowing difficulties) in a small number of patients; few cases have been reported where nasogastric tube feeding has been required. Dysphagia and dry mouth appear to be more common with injections of BoNTB because of its wider diffusion pattern (Titner et al., 2005). The most common side-effects when treating facial muscles are cosmetic and include ptosis or asymmetry of the position of the eyebrows, which usually resolves over a period of several weeks. In rare instances it may last for up to 2–3 months (Mauskop, 2004). Additional BoNT

Table 17.8

Published trials for botulinum toxin type A (BoNTA) (Dysport) and BoNTB (Myobloc)

Trial	*n*/population	Design/duration	Dose/method	Results
Dysport				
Rollnik et al., 2000	21; TTH	RCT, PBO-controlled; 12 weeks	200 U; FS	After 4, 8, and 12 weeks, both groups showed improvements in VAS scores, but no significant differences between PBO and Dysport were observed in VAS scores, frequency and duration of HAs, and analgesic consumption
Schulte-Mattler et al., 2004	112; CTTH	RCT, PBO-controlled; 12 weeks	500 U; FS	No significant differences between Dysport and PBO in HA curve of 6 weeks before and 12 weeks after tx, number of days with HA, or analgesic use
Myobloc				
Fadeyi and Adams, 2002	2 female patients; refractory HA	2 case studies: patient 1: follow-up 1 week after injection; second injection after 3 months	Patient 1: total 5000 U; FS Patient 2: total 2500 U; FS	Patient 1: reduction in HA severity and frequency at week 1; HA frequency declined from 7–10 episodes/week to 1/week Patient 2: at 2 weeks, patient reported a reduction in HA frequency but HA severity increased within 4 weeks of BoNTB injections
Lake and Saper, 2003 (abstract)	21; migraine	Open-label; 4 months	Total 5000 U	Significant reductions occurred in HA index, frequency, and average HA intensity following Myobloc treatment Significant improvements were seen in VAS and MIDAS scores and HA Impact Test
Opida, 2002a (abstract)	47; CM	Open-label; 4 weeks	Total 5000 U	64% of patients reported improvements in the severity of symptoms
Opida, 2002b (abstract)	31; chronic HA	Open-label; N/A	Total 5000 U	71% of patients reported improvements in neck motion and HA intensity and severity
Gwynn et al., 2003 (abstract)	39; CM, CTTH	RCT, PBO-controlled; N/A	5000 U to 7500 U	There was no significant difference between BoNTB and PBO in HA pain or dysfunction at 4, 8, and 12 weeks Reduction in HA severity was significantly greater than PBO at visit 4 (12 weeks)

TTH: tension-type headache; RCT: randomized, double-blind, controlled trial; FS: fixed-site; VAS: Visual Analogue Scale; PBO: placebo; HA: headache; tx: treatment; MIDAS: Migraine Disability Assessment Scale.

injections can correct asymmetry and even ptosis. Another possible, but rare, side-effect is difficulty in holding the head erect because of neck muscle weakness. This can be addressed by isometric neck exercises and, in more pronounced cases, by a soft cervical collar. Headache patients occasionally develop a headache following the injection procedure, although, in some, immediate relief of an acute attack can also occur.

The latter is most likely due to trigger point injection effect. Worsening of headaches and neck pain can occur for several days or, rarely, weeks after the injections because of the irritating effect of the needling and delay in the muscle-relaxing effect of BoNT (Mauskop, 2004).

As a non-human protein BoNT may evoke antibody formation. Once neutralizing antibodies are present in the body, the efficacy of the neurotoxin may be lost (Aoki, 2004). The antigenicity of a BoNT preparation depends on the amount of neurotoxin presented to the immune system, which is determined by biological activity of the preparation (Dressler and Hallett, 2006). For BoNTB this translates into an antibody-induced therapy failure rate of 44% in patients treated for cervical dystonia, whereas for BoNTA preparations this figure is approximately 5% and is likely associated with dose and frequency of treatment regimen (Mathew and Kaup, 2002; Dressler and Hallett, 2006). For the current formulation of Botox, the rate of antibody-induced therapy failure is $<1\%$ (Dressler and Hallett, 2006; Yablon et al., 2006). Factors that increase the risk for antibody formation include higher doses and short intervals between doses (Greene et al., 1994; Jankovic and Schwartz, 1995). Recommendations for minimizing immunoresistance include using the lowest effective dose at the longest possible intervals and avoiding booster injections (Greene et al., 1994).

CONCLUSIONS

Despite the number of available prophylactic treatments for primary headache disorders, many patients do not respond to therapy or cannot tolerate treatment. Many drugs have been studied for the prophylactic treatment of episodic migraine, with four being approved by the Food and Drug Administration, but far fewer treatments have been systematically studied for the treatment of CDH or CM.

Two recent large phase III double-blind PBO-controlled trials have established the efficacy of BoNTA (Botox, onabotulinumtoxinA) in the treatment of CM. Clinical experience also suggests efficacy, safety, and tolerability of BoNTA in the treatment of patients with episodic migraine; however, controlled trials are lacking. Clinical experience in the treatment of headaches with abobotulinumtoxinA (Dysport) and rimabotulinumtoxinB (Myobloc) is limited. Due to differences in formulation and actions, the various BoNTs are not interchangeable and both efficacy and safety profiles may differ. Thus, the current data set provides information on the efficacy and safety of onabotulinumtoxinA while further studies are warranted to establish the clinical profiles of other formulations in the treatment of headaches.

BoNTA (onabotulinumtoxinA, Botox) represents a unique and remarkably safe form of treatment for headache sufferers. BoNTA injections are usually given at 3-month intervals, thereby obviating the common problem of compliance with daily medications. It appears from current data that BoNTA is an effective prophylactic treatment for CM. Additional controlled trials may help define the most appropriate patient populations for successful treatment and the optimal doses and regimens.

Recent reports suggest that improved formulations of botulinum toxin with faster onset of action and longer duration of effect may become available in the future through protein engineering (Wang et al., 2008).

Disclosure

Dr. Mauskop has participated in clinical trials sponsored and paid for by Allergan. He had been a paid speaker for Allergan and had served on Allergan's advisory committees.

References

Aoki KR (2004). Botulinum toxin: a successful therapeutic protein. Curr Med Chem 11: 3085–3092.
Aoki KR (2005a). Pharmacology and immunology of botulinum neurotoxins. Int Ophthalmol Clin 45: 25–37.
Aoki KR (2005b). Review of a proposed mechanism for the antinociceptive action of botulinum toxin type A. Neurotoxicology 26: 785–793.
Aoki KR, Guyer B (2001). Botulinum toxin type A and other botulinum toxin serotypes: a comparative review of biochemical and pharmacological actions. Eur J Neurol 8 (Suppl. 5): 21–29.
Aurora S (2006). Botulinum toxin type A for the treatment of migraine. Exp Opin Pharmacother 7: 1085–1095.
Aurora SK, Gawel M, Brandes JL et al. (2006). Botulinum toxin type A prophylactic treatment of episodic migraine: a randomized, double-blind, placebo-controlled exploratory study. Headache 47: 486–499.
Aurora SK, Gawel M, Brandes JL et al. (2007). Botulinum toxin type A prophylactic treatment of episodic migraine: a randomized, double-blind, placebo-controlled exploratory study. Headache 47: 486–499.
Aurora SK, Schim JD, Cutrer FM et al. (2009a). Botulinum neurotoxin type A for treatment of chronic migraine: PREEMPT 1 trial double-blind phase. Cephalalgia 29 (Suppl. 1): 29.
Aurora SK, Winner P, Freeman MC et al. (2009b). Botulinum neurotoxin type A for treatment of chronic migraine: pooled analyses of the PREEMPT clinical program 32-week open-label phase. Cephalalgia 29 (Suppl. 1): 7.
Barrientos N, Chana P (2003). Botulinum toxin type A in prophylactic treatment of migraine headaches: a preliminary study. J Headache Pain 4: 146–151.
Binder WJ, Brin MF, Blitzer A et al. (2000). Botulinum toxin type A (Botox) for treatment of migraine headaches: an

open-label study. Otolaryngol Head Neck Surg 123: 669–676.

Blumenfeld A, Chippendale T (2006). Botulinum toxin type A compared with divalproex sodium for the prophylactic treatment of migraine: a randomized, evaluator-masked trial [poster]. Presented at: The 16th Migraine Trust International Symposium; September 19, 2006; London, UK.

Blumenfeld A, Binder W, Silberstein SD et al. (2003). Procedures for administering botulinum toxin type A for migraine and tension-type headache. Headache 43: 884–891.

Blumenfeld A, Schim J, Chippendale TJ (2008). Botulinum toxin type a and divalproex sodium for prophylactic treatment of episodic or chronic migraine. Headache 48: 210–220.

Brin MF (1997). Botulinum toxin: chemistry, pharmacology, toxicity, and immunology. Muscle Nerve 20 (Suppl. 6): S146–S168.

Conway S, Delplanche C, Crowder J et al. (2005). Botox therapy for refractory chronic migraine. Headache 45: 355–357.

Cui M, Khanijou S, Rubino J et al. (2004). Subcutaneous administration of botulinum toxin A reduces formalin-induced pain. Pain 107: 125–133.

de Paiva A, Meunier FA, Molgó J et al. (1999). Functional repair of motor endplates after botulinum neurotoxin type A poisoning: biphasic switch of synaptic activity between nerve sprouts and their parent terminals. Proc Natl Acad Sci U S A 96: 3200–3205.

Dodick DW, Mauskop A, Elkind AH et al. (2005). Botulinum toxin type A for the prophylaxis of chronic daily headache: subgroup analysis of patients not receiving other prophylactic medications: a randomized double-blind, placebo-controlled study. Headache 45: 315–324.

Dodick DW, Smith TR, Becker WJ et al. (2009a). Botulinum neurotoxin type A for treatment of chronic migraine: PREEMPT 2 trial double-blind phase. Cephalalgia 29 (Suppl. 1): 29.

Dodick DW, Aurora SK, Turkel CC et al. (2009b). Botulinum neurotoxin type A for treatment of chronic migraine: the double-blind phase of the PREEMPT clinical program. Cephalalgia 29 (Suppl. 1): 34.

Dolly O (2003). Synaptic transmission: inhibition of neurotransmitter release by botulinum toxins. Headache 43 (Suppl. 1): S16–S24.

Dressler D, Hallett M (2006). Immunological aspects of Botox®, Dysport® and Myobloc/neurobloc®. Eur J Urol 13 (Suppl. 1): 11–15.

Edwards KR, Dreyer MD (2002). Botulinum toxin type A (Botox) for chronic daily headaches. Presented at: The 44th Annual Scientific Meeting of the American Headache Society; June 21–23, 2002; Seattle, WA. Abstract S136.

Elkind AH, O'Carrol PO, Blumenfeld A et al. (2006). A series of three sequential, randomized, controlled studies of repeated treatments with botulinum toxin type A for migraine prophylaxis. J Pain 10: 688–696.

Eross EJ, Gladstone JP, Lewis S et al. (2005). Duration of migraine is a predictor for response to botulinum toxin type A. Headache 45: 308–314.

Evers S, Vollmer-Haase J, Schwaag S et al. (2004). Botulinum toxin A in the prophylactic treatment of migraine – a randomized, double-blind, placebo-controlled study. Cephalalgia 24: 838–843.

Fadeyi MO, Adams QM (2002). Use of botulinum toxin type B for migraine and tension headaches. Am J Health Syst Pharm 59: 1860–1862.

Freitag FG, McAllister P, Freund B et al. (2005). Botulinum toxin type A for the prophylaxis of chronic daily headache in migraineurs: effect on acute headache pain medication use [poster]. Presented at: The 47th Annual Scientific Meeting of the American Headache Society; June 25, 2005; Philadelphia, PA.

Freitag FG, Diamond S, Diamond M et al. (2008). Botulinum toxin type A in the treatment of chronic migraine without medication overuse. Headache 48: 201–209.

Freund BJ, Schwartz M (2002). Relief of tension-type headache symptoms in subjects with temporomandibular disorders treated with botulinum toxin-A. Headache 42: 1033–1037.

Greene P, Fahn S, Diamond B (1994). Development of resistance to botulinum toxin type A in patients with torticollis. Mov Disord 9: 213–217.

Gwynn MW, English JB, Baker TS (2003). Double-blind, placebo-controlled study of Myobloc (botulinum toxin type B) for the treatment of chronic headache (abstract). Headache 43: 577–578 (abstract S145).

Headache Classification Subcommittee of the International Headache Society (2004). The international classification of headache disorders, 2nd edn. Cephalalgia 24: 1–160.

Huang W, Foster JA, Rogachefsky AS (2000). Pharmacology of botulinum toxin. J Am Acad Dermatol 43: 249–259.

Jakubowski M, McAllister P, Bajwa Z et al. (2006). Exploding vs. imploding headache in migraine prophylaxis with botulinum toxin A. Pain 125: 286–295.

Jankovic J, Schwartz K (1995). Response and immunoresistance to botulinum toxin injections. Neurology 45: 1743–1746.

Klapper JA, Mathew NT, Klapper A et al. (2000). Botulinum toxin type A (BTX-A) for the prophylaxis of chronic daily headache. Cephalalgia 20: 291–295.

Lake AE, Saper JR (2003). Botulinum toxin type B for migraine prophylaxis: a 4-month open-label prospective outcome study. Headache 43: 578 (abstract S146).

Lipton RB, Varon S, Grosberg B et al. (2009). Botulinum neurotoxin type A treatment improves health-related quality of life and reduces the impact of chronic migraine: results from the double-blind phase of the PREEMPT clinical program. Cephalalgia 29 (Suppl. 1): 32–33.

Mathew NT, Kaup AO (2002). The use of botulinum toxin type A in headache treatment. Curr Treat Options Neurol 4: 365–373.

Mathew NT, Stubits E, Nigam MP (1982). Transformation of episodic migraine into daily headache: analysis of factors. Headache 22: 66–68.

Mathew NT, Frishberg BM, Gawel M et al. (2005). Botulinum toxin type A (Botox®) for the prophylactic treatment of chronic daily headache: a randomized, double-blind, placebo-controlled trial. Headache 45: 293–307.

Mauskop A (2002). Long-term use of botulinum toxin type A (Botox) in the treatment of episodic and chronic migraine headaches [abstract] Presented at: The 44th Annual Scientific Meeting of the American Headache Society; June 21–23, 2002; Seattle, WA.

Mauskop A (2004). The use of botulinum toxin in the treatment of headaches. Pain Physician 7: 377–387.

Mauskop A, Mathew N (2008). Letter to the editor. Assessment: Botulinum neurotoxin in the treatment of autonomic disorders and pain (an evidence-based review): Report of the Therapeutics and Technology Assessment Subcommittee of the American Academy of Neurology. Neurology Online, July 14, 2008.

McAllister P (2003). Patient-reported improvement in headache and change in headache medication usage in a cohort treated with botulinum toxin type A (Botox). Headache 43: 577 (abstract S143).

Meng J, Wang J, Lawrence G et al. (2007). Synaptobrevin I mediates exocytosis of CGRP from sensory neurons and inhibition by botulinum toxins reflects their anti-nociceptive potential. J Cell Sci 120: 2864–2874.

Miller T, Denney L (2003). Botulinum toxin A (Allergan) for chronic intractable headache; equally effective with or without concomitant neck pain. Headache 43: 579 (abstract S148).

Naumann M, So Y, Argoff CE et al. (2008). Assessment: Botulinum neurotoxin in the treatment of autonomic disorders and pain (an evidence-based review): Report of the Therapeutics and Technology Assessment Subcommittee of the American Academy of Neurology. Neurology 70: 1707–1714.

Ondo WG, Vuong KD, Derman HS (2004). Botulinum toxin A for chronic daily headache: a randomized, placebo-controlled, parallel design study. Cephalalgia 24: 60–65.

Opida CL (2002a). Open-label study of Myobloc (botulinum toxin type B) in the treatment of patients with transformed migraine headaches. Arch Pharmacol 365 (Suppl. 2): R33 (abstract 97).

Opida CL (2002b). Evaluation of Myobloc (botulinum toxin type B) in patients with post-whiplash headaches (abstract). Pain Med 3: 178–179.

Padberg M, De Bruijn SF, de Haan RJ et al. (2004). Treatment of chronic tension-type headache with botulinum toxin: a double-blind, placebo-controlled clinical trial. Cephalalgia 24: 675–680.

Porta M (2000). A comparative trial of botulinum toxin type A and methylprednisolone for the treatment of tension-type headache. Curr Rev Pain 4: 31–35.

Relja M, Telarović S (2004). Botulinum toxin in tension-type headache. J Neurol 251 (Suppl. 1): I/12–I/14.

Relja M, Poole AC, Schoenen J et al. (2006). A multicenter, double-blind, randomized, placebo-controlled, parallel group study of multiple treatments of botulinum toxin type A (BoNTA) for the prophylaxis of episodic migraine headaches. Cephalalgia 27: 492–503.

Rollnik JD, Tanneberger O, Schubert M et al. (2000). Treatment of tension-type headache with botulinum toxin type A: a double-blind, placebo-controlled study. Headache 40: 300–305.

Samton J, Mauskop A (2006). Treatment of headache with botulinum toxin. Exp Rev Neurother 6: 313–322.

Schmitt WJ, Slowey E, Fravi N et al. (2001). Effect of botulinum toxin A injections in the treatment of chronic tension-type headache: a double-blind, placebo-controlled trial. Headache 41: 658–664.

Schulte-Mattler WJ, Krack P; BoNTTH Study Group (2004). Treatment with chronic tension-type headache with botulinum toxin type A: a randomized, double-blind, placebo-controlled multicenter study. Pain 109: 110–114.

Sebastian FT, De Bruijn M (2003). Treatment of chronic tension-type headache with botulinum toxin: a double-blind placebo controlled clinical trial. Neurology 60: 148.

Shukla HD, Sharma SK (2005). *Clostridium botulinum*: a bug with beauty and weapon. Crit Rev Microbiol 31: 11–18.

Silberstein SD, Stark SR, Lucas SM et al. (2005). Botulinum toxin type a for the prophylactic treatment of chronic daily headache: a randomized, double-blind, placebo-controlled trial. Mayo Clin Proc 80: 1126–1137.

Silberstein SD, Gobel H, Jensen R et al. (2006). Botulinum toxin type A in the prophylactic treatment of chronic tension-type headache: a multicentre, double-blind, randomized, placebo-controlled, parallel-group study. Cephalalgia 26: 790–800.

Silberstein SD, Blumenfeld AM, Cady RK et al. (2009). Botulinum neurotoxin type A for the treatment of chronic migraine: analysis of the PREEMPT chronic migraine subgroup with baseline acute headache medication overuse. Cephalalgia 29 (Suppl. 1): 31.

Silberstein S, Mathew N, Saper J et al. (2000). Botulinum toxin type A as a migraine preventive treatment. Headache 40: 445–450.

Smuts JA, Baker MK, Smuts HM et al. (1999). Prophylactic treatment of chronic tension-type headache using botulinum toxin type A. Eur J Neurol 6 (Suppl. 4): S99–S102.

Tepper SJ, Bigal ME, Sheftell FD et al. (2004). Botulinum neurotoxin type A in the preventive treatment of refractory headache: a review of 100 consecutive cases. Headache 44: 794–800.

Titner R, Gross R, Winzer UF et al. (2005). Autonomic function after botulinum toxin type A or B: a double blind, randomized trial. Neurology 65: 765–767.

Troost B (2002). Botulinum toxin type A (Botox®) therapy for intractable headache. Presented at: The 44th Annual Scientific Meeting of the American Headache Society; June 21–23, 2002; Seattle, WA. Abstract S137.

Troost T, Rosenberg JR, Wiles R (2003). Improvement in intractable headache with repeated botulinum toxin type A treatment. Poster PO4.153. Neurology 60 (Suppl. 1): A323–A324.

Wang J, Meng J, Lawrence GW et al. (2008). Novel chimeras of botulinum neurotoxins A and E unveil contributions from the binding, translocation, and protease domains to their functional characteristics. J Biol Chem 283: 16993–17002.

Yablon SA, Daggett S, Lai F et al. (2006). The development of toxin neutralizing antibodies with botulinum toxin type A (BoNTA) treatment [poster]. Presented at: The 4th World Congress of NeuroRehabilitation; February 14, 2006; Hong Kong, China.

expectations and the therapeutic approach may need to be revised. In general, the goals of therapy shift from cure to care, with the principal focus on maximizing function and avoiding disability, iatrogenic harm from overly aggressive treatments that are unlikely to be effective, and monitoring patients for the development of depression.

It is increasingly common, however, to encounter patients for whom effective treatment of headaches might be possible but cannot be attempted because of external limits on treatment availability. These limits often take the form of payment denials or bureaucratic limitations that affect access to recommended drugs or treatments (Haas et al., 2005). Payment systems that do not adequately reimburse cognitive services are a serious barrier to the availability of specialist headache care in the USA. Physicians literally cannot afford to devote the necessary time to orchestrating and supervising complex treatment regimens that are most likely to help seriously ill headache patients (Wynia, 2006). This limits the ability of physicians to provide headache care, and the willingness of hospitals and clinics to develop systems of care for chronic headache patients. These systemic barriers to optimal headache care cannot be solved by individual physician or patient action. They point to a need to develop professional and consumer disease advocacy and political action campaigns such as those that have been successful for other chronic, difficult-to-treat medical problems.

References

Ashina S, Zeeberg P, Jensen RH et al. (2006). Medication overuse headache. [Medicinoverforbrugshovedpine]. Ugeskr Laeger 168: 1015–1019.

Bailer J, Witthoft M, Paul C et al. (2005). Evidence for overlap between idiopathic environmental intolerance and somatoform disorders. Psychosom Med 67: 921–929.

Bantick SJ, Wise RG, Ploghaus A et al. (2002). Imaging how attention modulates pain in humans using functional MRI. Brain J Neurol 125: 310–319.

Bolen J (2006). Getting informed consent and agreement for treatment right: a legal perspective on key obligations for practitioners who use controlled substances to treat chronic pain. J Opioid Manag 2: 193–200.

Breslau N, Merikangas K, Bowden CL (1994). Comorbidity of migraine and major affective disorders. Neurology 44 (Suppl. 7): S17–S22.

Breslau N, Lipton RB, Stewart WF et al. (2003). Comorbidity of migraine and depression: investigating potential etiology and prognosis. Neurology 60: 1308–1312.

Drahovzal DN, Stewart SH, Sullivan MJ (2006). Tendency to catastrophize somatic sensations: pain catastrophizing and anxiety sensitivity in predicting headache. Cogn Behav Ther 35: 226–235.

Elder N, Ricer R, Tobias B (2006). How respected family physicians manage difficult patient encounters. J Am Board Fam Med 19: 533–541.

Gigineishvili DA, Shakarishvili RR (2006). Unexplained somatic symptoms and underlying psychologic disorders in the neurology clinic. Georgian Med News 132: 50–53.

Goadsby PJ (2003). Medically unexplained symptoms. J R Soc Med 96: 368–369.

Grant BF, Compton WM, Crowley TJ et al. (2007). Errors in assessing DSM-IV substance use disorders. Arch Gen Psychiatry 64: 379–380; author reply 381–382.

Grilo CM, Sanislow CA, Skodol AE et al. (2007). Longitudinal diagnostic efficiency of DSM-IV criteria for borderline personality disorder: a 2-year prospective study. Can J Psychiatry 52: 357–362.

Haas LJ, Leiser JP, Magill MK et al. (2005). Management of the difficult patient. Am Fam Physician 72: 2063–2068.

Henningsen P, Zipfel S, Herzog W (2007). Management of functional somatic syndromes. Lancet 369: 946–955.

Jackson JL, Kroenke K (1999). Difficult patient encounters in the ambulatory clinic: clinical predictors and outcomes. Arch Intern Med 159: 1069–1075.

Karp JF, Scott J, Houck P et al. (2005). Pain predicts longer time to remission during treatment of recurrent depression. J Clin Psychiatry 66: 591–597.

Katz RC (1996). "Difficult patients" as family physicians perceive them. Psychol Rep 79: 539–544.

Krebs EE, Garrett JM, Konrad TR (2006). The difficult doctor? Characteristics of physicians who report frustration with patients: an analysis of survey data. BMC Health Serv Res 6: 128.

Lake AE, 3rd, Lipchik GL, Penzien DB et al. (2006). Psychiatric comorbidity with chronic headache: evidence-based clinical implications – introduction to the supplement. Headache 46 (Suppl. 3): S73–S75.

Loder E, Biondi D (2005). Headache attributed to psychiatric disorder: a case series. Psychosomatics 46: 326–333.

Maizels M, Burchette R (2004). Somatic symptoms in headache patients: the influence of headache diagnosis, frequency, and comorbidity. Headache 44: 983–993.

Mullen PE, Martin JL, Anderson JC et al. (1996). The long-term impact of the physical, emotional, and sexual abuse of children: a community study. Child Abuse Neglect 20: 7–21.

Nakao M, Barsky AJ (2007). Clinical application of somatosensory amplification in psychosomatic medicine. Biopsychosoc Med 1: 17.

Paemeleire K, Crevits L, Goadsby PJ et al. (2006). Practical management of medication-overuse headache. Acta Neurol Belg 106: 43–51.

Rief W, Barsky AJ (2005). Psychobiological perspectives on somatoform disorders. Psychoneuroendocrinology 30: 996–1002.

Romans SE (1997). Childhood sexual abuse: concerns and consequences. Med J Aust 166: 59–60.

Saper JR (2006). "Are you talking to me?" Confronting behavioral disturbances in patients with headache. Headache 46 (Suppl. 3): S151–S156.

Saper JR, Lake AE, 3rd (2002). Borderline personality disorder and the chronic headache patient: Review and management recommendations. Headache 42: 663–674.

Saper JR, Lake AE, 3rd (2006). Medication overuse headache: type I and type II. Cephalalgia 26: 1262.

Saper JR, Lake AE, 3rd, Hamel RL et al. (2004). Daily scheduled opioids for intractable head pain: long-term observations of a treatment program. Neurology 62: 1687–1694.

Tietjen GE, Brandes JL, Digre KB et al. (2007a). High prevalence of somatic symptoms and depression in women with disabling chronic headache. Neurology 68: 134–140.

Tietjen GE, Brandes JL, Digre KB et al. (2007b). History of childhood maltreatment is associated with comorbid depression in women with migraine. Neurology 69: 959–968.

Von Korff M, Lin EH, Fenton JJ et al. (2007). Frequency and priority of pain patients' health care use. Clin J Pain 23: 400–408.

Wynia MK (2006). Routine screening: informed consent, stigma and the waning of HIV exceptionalism. Am J Bioethics 6: 5–8.

Yucel B, Ozyalcin S, Sertel HO et al. (2002). Childhood traumatic events and dissociative experiences in patients with chronic headache and low back pain. Clin J Pain 18: 394–401.

Handbook of Clinical Neurology, Vol. 97 (3rd series)
Headache
G. Nappi and M.A. Moskowitz, Editors

Chapter 19

Ethical issues in headache management

TIMOTHY J. STEINER *
Division of Neuroscience and Mental Health, Imperial College London, London, UK

Practical ethics – those that are generally invoked as a guide to clinical practice today – are concerned much less with the idea that final solutions to ethical problems exist as truths than with the perception of tensions, to be resolved by applying generally accepted principles. Four key ethical principles established in medical practice – respect for autonomy (of patients), justice, non-maleficence, and beneficence (Beauchamp and Childress, 1989) – are complemented by the medical professional ethical principles of veracity (truth-telling), fidelity (the keeping of promises), and confidentiality (International Headache Society Ethics Subcommittee, 1998). An alternative, more general, approach seeks solutions to ethical dilemmas not through "principlism" but by recognizing – and attributing value to – the needs of patients, the responsibilities of doctors, the good of society as a whole, and desserts (International Headache Society Ethics Subcommittee, 1998).

Both approaches lead sometimes to philosophical conflict, and a realization that what appears ethical in one sense is less so in another. The Declaration of Helsinki, at least in its earlier versions (World Medical Association, 1964), provides a clear and often debated example, and shows that the term "needs of patients" is not the same as "needs of the patient." It enjoins physicians that "The health of my patient will be my first consideration," but it opens with: "It is the duty of the physician to safeguard the health of *the people*" (emphasis added). Although the tensions this illustrates arise most noticeably in proposals for research, which commonly "uses" – and may harm – present patients in the hope of benefiting future patients, they also are very much present in the sometimes challenging conflicts created by lack of resources, where one patient's treatment must be at the cost of another's because society cannot fund both. This is a scenario expressed worldwide in headache care – or rather the lack of it – because headache everywhere is given low (or no) priority in the health-care queue. It is a theme that will recur throughout this review.

In such situations, practical ethics become an expression of what a society thinks is right, and, in particular, of the weight a society gives to individual interests versus its own (i.e., society's) interests. Sometimes this leads to circular argument, since it is in the interests of individuals within a society that full protection be given to the interests of that same society. It also poses the question as to whether some things are absolutely right – or absolutely not right – such that no moral society could have a contrary view of them. This question is properly explored in moral philosophical texts, and no attempt at an answer will be put forward here; instead, it is assumed that we all share the view that alleviating suffering, whenever and to the greatest extent we reasonably can, is highly desirable.

This brief and somewhat selective review draws freely upon material published elsewhere (International Headache Society Ethics Subcommittee, 1998; Steiner and Riis, 2000) in order to consider a small number of ethical issues. They are those that appear most pertinent to headache management, and that are reflected worldwide.

LIMITED RESOURCES, IGNORANCE, DISTRIBUTIVE INJUSTICE

Limited access to care is foremost amongst these, in the sense of having the greatest practical impact. Everywhere, there are barriers preventing access to effective headache treatment (American Association for the Study of Headache and International Headache Society, 1998; Steiner, 2004). Some of these may be unavoidable, the inevitable consequence of non-existent means; some can at the very least be mitigated, by better use of available means; others are entirely artificial.

*Correspondence to: Dr Timothy J Steiner, Division of Neuroscience and Mental Health, Imperial College London, London W6 8RP, UK, E-mail: t.steiner@imperial.ac.uk

Competition for limited resources in most countries means that patients with some illnesses are less likely to receive treatment than those with other illnesses. Each society must make decisions that set and respect priorities, and what these are will vary. Although distributive justice calls for fair shares to all who need them, standing against it is an unsophisticated public perception of headache that regards it as not a disease at all, or as benign and therefore undeserving of health-care resources. "How," people ask, "can headache be considered alongside diseases that cause permanent severe disability or death?"

Reasonable and challenging though this question may seem, its answer is readily to hand. For, to dismiss headache altogether, or even to belittle it, rejects the clear evidence of its high cost: a burden of illness that comes not only from the suffering and disablement of large numbers of individual people (Stovner et al., 2007) but also from the scale of consequential lost work time and productivity (Steiner et al., 2003). Each of these pleads forcefully for a larger slice of the health-care cake than headache currently receives in most, if not all, countries (Steiner, 2004). Of course there may be other priorities; restricting treatment for headache lessens the demand upon resources needed for treatment of other important conditions (opportunity gain). But no one has reason to believe that the humanitarian burden of headache weighs less in populations that are, and because they are, beset by other illness.

There is a question of balance, which at present does not appear to be right, and if this is so it is because of ignorance. Ignorance about headache is widespread: in the general population as to nature, cause, treatment, and prognosis; amongst governments and captains of industry (who pay the cost of headache) as to prevalence, consequential disability, and the economic burden; amongst doctors at all levels (who receive little training in this field) as to mechanisms, diagnosis, and management. The last of these is a direct cause of under- or mistreatment, and it should not be insoluble; but the first two create apathy towards headache, and tolerance of the lack of political will that engenders and perpetuates the third, militating against any solution.

Whilst the right solution cannot be achieved quickly (Steiner, 2004), it is necessary to begin the process of finding it. This requires, first of all, acknowledgment that the problem exists. Importantly, the World Health Organization has formally made this acknowledgement on several separate occasions (World Health Organization, 2000, 2001, 2004, 2006). The need is for governments to follow.

Paradoxically, research – and the development of new treatments that open fresh opportunities for some – can make matters worse for many others. Premium pricing of a new treatment is likely to mean that many people have little real opportunity to benefit from it. At the same time, important relationships between cost and effect in medical management not only occur at the level of individual patients but also raise serious issues of distributive justice. It is self-evident that the appearance in the market of new, highly effective but very expensive treatments will cause serious perturbations in health-care budgets if the target population is large, as with headache. There is predictability about this. Failure to assess cost implications of this sort during a drug development program – through formal cost–utility evaluation – denies prescribers an ethical basis for rationing the treatment if simple economics dictate that it cannot be prescribed to everyone who might benefit. Yet such failure is the norm.

MARKETING, DRUG COMPANIES, COMMERCIAL SPONSORSHIP

Drug marketing, which might be based on economic analysis but very rarely is, generally seeks to raise awareness not only of a product but also of a need for treatment in which the product is a candidate for use. This can be good: heightened awareness of need is exactly what is necessary for headache to receive anything like its due priority. Unfortunately, it is sometimes made bad. A recent example of misdirected promotion (in the utilitarian sense of producing far less benefit to patients than might have been achieved at similar cost) is the huge expenditure aimed at increasing use of triptan *x* rather than triptan *y* when, in most populations, the much-needed message is that headache treatments generally, including triptans, are grossly underutilized.

Marketing sometimes targets health-care providers, sometimes consumers, and occasionally both. Direct-to-consumer advertising and the promotion of over-the-counter (OTC) products are especially relevant to headache because of its high general-population prevalence and the low levels of contact between doctors and affected people. Advertising to the general public of OTC painkillers for headache is particularly widespread and often intensive. Again this raises awareness, but not always in a wholly helpful way. Messages that product *z* is the "rapid and complete solution to headache," for example, may mislead by suggesting efficacy regardless of diagnosis. With its potential to generate uncontrolled demand, such advertising may and almost certainly does contribute to medication overuse headache – a major public health problem worldwide (Diener and Limmroth, 2004; Stovner et al., 2007) that places further, quite unnecessary, demands upon resources.

Marketing to health-care providers sometimes masquerades as education when this is commercially sponsored, particularly in primary care (Prosser et al., 2003; Watkins et al., 2003). This creates a dilemma: deficient education, at all levels, has already been identified as an issue in itself, with major ethical implications in its consequences. It has to be said that commercial sponsors support a great many educational initiatives that would otherwise not be possible, and that this is not of itself a bad thing. For example, education on some aspects of the therapeutic use of drugs is best given by people in industry who have most familiarity with them.

The problem is the perceived, if not actual, conflict between the commercial interests of pharmaceutical companies who sponsor education and the *prima facie* requirement that education be unaffected by considerations other than the needs of patients: balanced and non-promotional (Kessler, 1991). This concern arises not only from professional education, where influence may be wielded overtly or covertly upon content, but also in lay meetings. Even where there is no direct influence on content, speakers may be chosen by lay organizers from an industry-favored shortlist because their attendance and participation will be supported by industry.

A similar dilemma arises from sponsored clinical services. In certain countries – the UK is a prime example – some specialist headache clinics rely on direct commercial sponsorship. Often this is used to employ nurses. This is not unique to headache (Scott, 1993), but it is especially relevant to headache because of the lack of health service provision for it. When clinical services are otherwise inadequate, commercially supported services fill a vacuum, and this may be of major and direct benefit to patients. However, wherever such arrangements exist, there is possible influence over prescribing. It is not known what impact, if any, this has (Scott, 1993).

Of more concern, perhaps, are occasions when a service becomes established through commercial sponsorship that is then withdrawn, forcing the allocation to it of public health-care resources. Whilst this may be perceived as a good outcome, and even when it is so in reality, normal service development processes and priority determination are undermined. This is not generally desirable, nor is it likely to lead to best-planned services making best use of limited resources. The solution here again lies, primarily, at governmental level, requiring recognition by those responsible for health service policy of the unmet health-care needs of large numbers of people affected by headache. This, the fundamental prerequisite for optimal service provision, is not happening.

HEADACHE DIAGNOSIS: A PROBLEM, AND WRONG SOLUTIONS

Doctors, responsible at the front end for providing for these needs, also must recognize them. It is an unfortunate truth that, whereas headache is very common both in primary care and in neurological practice, interest in it is not. Whatever may be patients' "rights" to timely and correct diagnosis as a prelude to timely and correct treatment, and whatever protection those rights command as "inalienable human rights" (World Medical Association, 1981; Council of Europe, 1997a, b, 2003a, b), the reality is often a dismal shortfall (American Association for the Study of Headache and International Headache Society, 1998; Steiner, 2004).

It is another truth that the diagnosis of most headache disorders, certainly the common ones, is based on history and examination rather than on diagnostic tests, and a third truth that the set of clinical skills that history and examination require cannot be substituted by anything less. There is no suggestion here that headache diagnosis belongs or must be kept within the province of specialist physicians – far from it: primary-care physicians have all the requisite skills, and most need only a little more knowledge of the common headache disorders to diagnose perfectly competently the great majority of patients who present with headache as their main complaint. But, with all due respect to nurses and pharmacists – highly trained and skilled masters of their own professions – attempts to shift diagnosis of headache disorders to these practitioners aim to do exactly what should not be done: to replace doctors' clinical skills with something less.

This is not a good way forward. The underlying purpose where it is occurring may be to improve access, and it may sometimes achieve this. The concern is that it truly throws the baby out with the bath water, replacing one failing system – which is potentially remediable, given some support – with another that is not fit for purpose. Concern is much greater when this is happening simply as part of a drive to reduce costs, achieved through a general strategy of "demoting" a range of clinical services. Such health service reorganizations tend to seek and sometimes claim "better outcomes" framed as political objectives: greater patient throughput, shorter waiting lists. These might be laudable if there were any evidence that they would translate into better care, but the underpinning emphasis on quantity over quality hardly promises this.

But if this is not the way forward for headache diagnosis, nor is the *status quo* particularly desirable. The International Headache Society's classification of headache, in its second edition (ICHD-II) (International Headache Society Classification Subcommittee, 2004), has clarified the diagnostic criteria for many headache types. The hope is that headache diagnosis will improve through its widespread application (chapter 11), but the classification is a tool for the knowledgeable. The underlying problem leading to misdiagnosis, however, as has already been mentioned, is poor knowledge.

Are these ethical issues? They are, for two reasons. First, the consumption of health-care resources in pursuit of wrong objectives matters greatly to people with headache because headache is so low down in the queue for whatever is left. Second, shortcomings in headache diagnosis lead directly to failure to alleviate suffering when this can (or could if the correct diagnosis were made) often be easily achieved.

HEADACHE MANAGEMENT: EVIDENCE, GUIDELINES, EFFICIENCY

Of course, correct and timely diagnosis translates into alleviated suffering only when followed by effective treatment. It is nowadays axiomatic that therapeutic methods applied to headache patients should be based on reliable evidence of effect (Steiner, 1998), evaluated relative to side-effects and, as noted earlier, cost. Promotion of new treatments without such evidence is very obviously unethical. In the case of drugs, legally backed regulation in many countries prevents this. The same may not, unfortunately, apply to surgical techniques, to many complementary therapies, to devices marketed directly to the public, and to existing drugs used off-license. There has been limited scope in headache management for the first of these, although recent examples include closure of patent foramen ovale and implantation of occipital nerve stimulators, both of which, at present, belong firmly in the realms of research and have largely been kept there. Most readers will readily bring to mind multiple examples of the other three offered as treatments, usually in a commercial setting. If these involve ethical violations (and not all do), it is not only the general ethical principles of beneficence and non-maleficence (Beauchamp and Childress, 1989) but also the professional ethical principles of veracity and fidelity (International Headache Society Ethics Subcommittee, 1998) that are put aside.

On the other hand, the use in headache management of many standard treatments is based on so-called clinical experience rather than on more formally adduced evidence. This has to be acceptable: the alternative is "a state of paralysis until some piece of research is done" (Descartes, 1901), with little prospect (in the case of drugs long devoid of patent protection) of the research ever being done.

The question this raises is of management guidelines – perhaps the therapeutic equivalent of ICHD-II for diagnosis. Clinical experience is all very well when it exists, solidly founded on expert understanding of the disease(s) and of the treatments in use and on long-term specialist practice subjected to review by self- or peer-audit and careful and critical reflection upon outcomes. Yet – simply because of the numbers of people in need of it (coupled with people's preferences in relation to easy access to care) – the management of most headache belongs in primary care, where, with a few exceptions, skills are those of the non-specialist. There are, accordingly, ethical imperatives both for specialists to produce management guidelines in headache care for use within primary care and for primary-care physicians, unless they undertake additional training, to be directly guided by them. There is no other way for non-specialists to find the optimum balance between simple but effective remedies and newer, "proven," but usually much more expensive, treatments. Anything else is inefficient.

Efficiency is an ethical issue because whatever is expended on diagnostic or treatment methods that are ineffective is wasted, and, wherever costs are reimbursed by a health service, those resources are then not available for others (opportunity cost). That is, sub-optimal use of health-care resources deprives both the patient being treated of the best outcome, and other patients of whatever might have been used for their benefit had it not been wasted. To put this into one context, estimates of the prevalence of medication overuse headache are of the order of 1% in many adult populations (Stovner et al., 2007). This is a condition often involving prescription-only drugs, which are often reimbursed: wasted and causing ill health.

PLACEBO: THE TREATMENT OF CHOICE?

To conclude will be a change of tack, reproducing an argument published elsewhere (Steiner, 2005). It relates to a report of a 76-year-old man with a chronic daily headache syndrome refractory to all active medications but showing sustained response to and well controlled by placebo (Pascual-Lozano et al., 2005). This was a man whose quality of life had been horrible, and was now vastly improved.

Hyland (2003) described the placebo effect in clinical practice as useful but fickle. These two descriptors may seem somewhat incompatible, but probably all clinicians who manage patients with headache succeed sometimes – to their patients' benefit – not by their experienced and skillful selection of the right treatment but through the placebo effect of whatever they happen to choose. It is tempting in such cases to view placebo medications as the treatment of choice: "their undoubted effectiveness in ... some disorders, along with their obvious safety and lack of side-effects, makes them in some ways an ideal form of treatment" (Anonymous editorial, 2003). And placebo is happily inexpensive! But it is clear that not every patient will benefit from placebo.

Such cases as the one above defy explanation, since it would be illogical to postulate that active treatments do not also exert a placebo effect. They also raise an important ethical issue, because the administration of placebo with therapeutic intent necessitates the employment of deceit.

Analysis of this issue might invoke any or all of the four general ethical principles of respect for autonomy, beneficence, non-maleficence, and justice (Beauchamp and Childress, 1989). Gillon (2003) added consideration of scope to these, and the relevance of this will become apparent. As observed already, whilst the four principles themselves may not be contentious, they are found not uncommonly to be in conflict; the problem then is how to rank them in importance if one has to be favored over another.

In the case in question, the authors of the report were guided by beneficence, seeking the best clinical outcome for their patient. They achieved this at the expense of respect for his autonomy, and at the expense of veracity, since it was necessary to deceive the patient as to the nature of his medication. A utilitarian analysis might take the view that the benefit to the patient was clear, and therefore the action was (and presumably remains) entirely justified. On the surface this appears so. Some ethicists argue that being deceived is of itself harmful, and they would hold that non-maleficence was also sacrificed here. Even so, the utilitarian analysis might still lead to a conclusion that, on balance, the good outweighed the harm and that, with all other therapeutic options apparently exhausted, the action of using placebo was, and is, not merely justified but mandated by the doctors' overriding duty to help their patient.

Utilitarian arguments of this sort are highly seductive, but they are commonly flawed. Often standing against them – as it does here – is the principle that the consent of patients is required for whatever is done to them. This principle is stated explicitly or implicitly in virtually all codes of ethics and guidance on ethical practice since the Nuremberg trials (United States *vs* Karl Brandt, 1948-49). It upholds autonomy, or the right to self-determination, and the notion of respect for persons, against the paternalistic view that doctors know best. Not everyone may agree with Gillon (2003) that the ethical principle of respect for autonomy is first among equals, but few doctors nowadays will be comfortable to override autonomy without strong justification.

The utilitarian analysis, as outlined, argues that strong justification indeed exists in this case. However, this analysis not only discards the concept of need for consent but also restricts itself to the case and to the situation now, and so is incomplete. Further questions line up, and press to be answered. Is the deceit to be maintained for ever? Is the harm embedded in the deceit multiplied by the time duration of it, or by each instance of its execution? What, above all, might happen if the patient were to discover it? Going beyond the confines of the case, if this usage of placebo were to become accepted practice, what would patients more generally think of it? It is easy to imagine a future scenario in which patients were never sure that their treatment was not placebo. Every patient might be forced to have his or her medication analyzed. With trust in their physicians gone (Hill, 2003), so would be the placebo effect – the very thing from which are derived these benefits that we sometimes rely on.

This is how considerations of scope must come into the analysis: it is not only the immediate parties to a health-care transaction who may be affected by it. And when these wider considerations are included, even utilitarians must admit that it is much less clear where the balance between good and harm lies.

References

American Association for the Study of Headache and International Headache Society (1998). Consensus statement on improving migraine management. Headache 38: 736.

Anonymous editorial (2003). The placebo effect. Clin Med 3: 397–398.

Beauchamp TL, Childress JF (1989). Principles of Biomedical Ethics. 3rd edn. OUP, New York.

Council of Europe (1997a). Convention on human rights and biomedicine. Council of Europe, Oviedo, Spain.

Council of Europe (1997b). Explanatory report to the convention on human rights and biomedicine. Council of Europe, Strasbourg.

Council of Europe (2003a). Draft additional protocol to the convention on human rights and biomedicine, on biomedical research. Council of Europe, Strasbourg.

Council of Europe (2003b). Draft explanatory report to the draft additional protocol to the convention on human rights and biomedicine, on biomedical research. Council of Europe, Strasbourg.

Descartes R (1901). Principles of human knowledge. Translated by J Veitch. In: The Meditations and Selections from the Principles. Open Court, Illinois p. 130 (reprinted 1988).

Diener H-C, Limmroth V (2004). Medication-overuse headache: a worldwide problem. Lancet Neurol 3: 475–483.

Gillon R (2003). Ethics needs principles – four can encompass the rest – and respect for autonomy should be "first among equals". J Med Ethics 29: 307–312.

Hill J (2003). Placebos in clinical care: for whose pleasure? Lancet 362: 254.

Hyland ME (2003). Using the placebo response in clinical practice. Clin Med 3: 347–350.

International Headache Society Classification Subcommittee (2004). The international classification of headache disorders, 2nd edition. Cephalalgia 24 (Suppl. 1): 1–160.

International Headache Society Ethics Subcommittee (1998). Ethical issues in headache research and management: report and recommendations. Cephalalgia 18: 505–529.

Kessler DA (1991). Drug promotion and scientific exchange. The role of the clinical investigator. N Engl J Med 325: 201–203.

Pascual-Lozano AM, Chamarro-Lazáro R, Láinez MJA (2005). Placebo response in a patient with chronic migraine and ergotic overuse. Cephalalgia 25: 391–394.

Prosser H, Almond S, Walley T (2003). Influences on GPs' decision to prescribe new drugs – the importance of who says what. Fam Pract 20: 61–68.

Scott S (1993). Sponsorship of nurses. In: P Turner (Ed.), Commercial Sponsorship in the Provision of Healthcare. Royal Society of Medicine, London, pp. 28–36.

Steiner TJ (1998). Treating headache from an evidence base: the Cochrane Collaboration. Cephalalgia 18 (Suppl. 21): 63–65.

Steiner TJ (2004). Lifting the burden: the global campaign against headache. Lancet Neurol 3: 204–205.

Steiner TJ (2005). Using placebo in headache management [editorial]. Cephalalgia 25: 321–322.

Steiner TJ, Riis P (2000). Ethical issues in headache research and management. In: J Olesen, P Tfelt-Hansen, KMA Welch (Eds.), The Headaches. Lippincott-Raven, Philadelphia, pp. 49–54.

Steiner TJ, Scher AI, Stewart WF et al. (2003). The prevalence and disability burden of adult migraine in England and their relationships to age, gender and ethnicity. Cephalalgia 23: 519–527.

Stovner LJ, Hagen K, Jensen R et al. (2007). The global burden of headache: a documentation of headache prevalence and disability worldwide. Cephalalgia 27: 193–210.

United States vs Karl Brandt (1948). Trials of War Criminals Before the Nuremberg Military Tribunals Under Control Council Law No. 10, Vols 1 and 2: The Medical Case. Military Tribunal I, 1947. US Government Printing Office, Washington, DC.

Watkins C, Moore L, Harvey I et al. (2003). Characteristics of general practitioners who frequently see drug industry representatives: national cross sectional survey. BMJ 326: 1178–1179.

World Health Organization (2000). Headache disorders and public health. WHO, Geneva.

World Health Organization (2001). The World Health Report 2001. WHO, Geneva.

World Health Organization (2004). Atlas: Country Resources for Neurological Disorders 2004: Results of a Collaborative Study of the World Health Organization and the World Federation of Neurology. WHO, Geneva.

World Health Organization (2006). Neurological Disorders: Public Health Challenges. WHO, Geneva.

World Medical Association (1964). Declaration of Helsinki: Recommendations Guiding Medical Doctors in Biomedical Research Involving Human Subjects. 18th World Medical Assembly, Helsinki, Finland (revised 1975, Tokyo, Japan: 29th World Medical Assembly; revised 1983, Venice, Italy: 35th World Medical Assembly; revised 1989, Hong Kong: 41st World Medical Assembly; revised 1996, Somerset West, South Africa: 48th World Medical Assembly; revised 2000, Edinburgh: 52nd World Medical Assembly).

World Medical Association (1981). Declaration of Lisbon: The Rights of the Patient. 33rd World Medical Assembly, Lisbon.

Handbook of Clinical Neurology, Vol. 97 (3rd series)
Headache
G. Nappi and M.A. Moskowitz, Editors

Chapter 20

The role of lay associations

AUDREY CRAVEN*
European Headache Alliance and Migraine Association of Ireland, Dublin, Ireland

THE ROLE OF LAY ASSOCIATIONS

It took years of advocacy and argument to have migraine and other headache disorders acknowledged and recognized as a leading cause of disability. It is now generally accepted that migraine is the most common neurological condition in the world, affecting an estimated 600 million people worldwide. It is therefore more common than arthritis, asthma, and diabetes, but does not yet have the recognition or service provision that many less common disorders attract, despite being rated alongside dementia, quadriplegia, and psychosis as one of the most disabling chronic disorders. It is this huge area of need and suffering that has prompted the establishment of lay associations catering for people with migraine and other headache disorders.

Many doctors mistakenly believe that patients have unrealistic expectations of a magic bullet or miraculous cure when they seek treatment. In fact, they require a clear explanation and an empathetic approach to the management of this complex condition. Various studies have demonstrated that the typical severe headache patient usually explores numerous avenues in search of treatment. Recourse may be made to unlikely and unorthodox remedies in a desperate quest for relief: the author has vivid memories of ingesting a foul herbal decoction, formulated by a traditional healer, every day for 3 months with no beneficial effect whatsoever!

In reality what patients require most is reliable information and support on their journey to better management. Despite increasing recognition of migraine as a complex neurological disorder, it is apparent that many patients still feel that it is not being recognized as a debilitating condition and they can suffer stigmatization and discrimination as a result. This is especially evident in the case of workplace prejudice, where migraineurs have a fear of being seen as work-shy or lacking commitment if they take time off during migraine episodes. It has been proposed that the fact that migraine is predominantly a female disorder and that headache sufferers have a normal life expectancy may explain why these disorders have received considerably less attention and resources than they deserve. The reality of everyday life for most sufferers is that normal function is interrupted by migraine episodes at irregular and unpredictable intervals, and this can impose severe limitations on their daily lives, whether at school, at work, or during leisure time.

THE GENESIS OF A LAY ASSOCIATION

A lay association can be a valuable adjunct to the medical profession in the care and treatment of patients. Most lay associations have come into existence in response to an unmet need. In the case of the Migraine Association of Ireland (MAI: the example with which the author is most familiar), the MAI stemmed from an unmet and individual need. If information, support, and reassurance are needed for persons affected by headache disorders, then a lay association can supplement (not supplant) medical services. The reliable information and support that patients need on the way to developing management of their condition can be supplied by an effective and well-organized lay association: tailoring information to the individual is one of the most important functions of any lay association, especially when conveyed in an empathetic manner. The isolation and bewilderment that militate against a lone individual finding coping strategies for the disorder can be greatly assisted by the active involvement of a lay association in reducing that isolation and the accompanying feelings of inadequacy and loneliness by talking through the complexities of the condition.

*Correspondence to: Audrey Craven, President, European Headache Alliance and Migraine Association of Ireland, Unit 14, Block 5, Port Tunnel Business Park, Clonshaugh, Dublin 17, Ireland, Tel: 0035318510990, Fax: 0035318022044, E-mail: audreycraven@migraine.ie

The major functions that a well-organized lay association can perform will be user-focused, based on concern for people living with migraine and a belief that everyone has a right to accurate reliable information. What the lay associations can do for their members includes the following:

- Help the person to understand the condition by providing information on migraine
- Help the person to manage attacks by isolating trigger factors and identifying early-warning signs
- Provide a forum for sharing information and linking up with other migraineurs
- Provide information on treatments, both conventional and complementary
- Increase awareness of migraine and other headache disorders with the general public and health professionals
- Encourage research into the condition
- Advocate for better services.

As an example, practical help would include helpful hints and practical information on how to deal with migraine at work or at school. Allied to this would be promotional material to employers and school authorities to raise their levels of awareness, leading to better understanding and mutually beneficial strategies for dealing with problems or avoiding them entirely.

Google the word "migraine" on the internet and thousands of remedies are offered to the enquirer. Many are from quacks and charlatans ready to exploit those who are so desperate. One of the most valuable roles of the lay association lies in sifting and filtering these indiscriminate tranches of information, by working in tandem with the scientific community and other partners to ensure that all important information on conventional and complementary therapies is reliable, readily available, and up to date.

MEETING THE UNMET NEED

The role of the lay association is primarily to help the individual sufferer with information and support. Another, hugely important, function is to provide information to policy-makers and the public at large, by raising awareness of the condition and by encouraging research. These roles are probably best illustrated by reference to the development and operation of services provided by the MAI in recent times. MAI examples are quoted simply because they are the ones with which the author is most familiar.

It all began as an unexpected outcome to a personal quest for information. That quest led to research, travel abroad, media interest, rallying calls to fellow sufferers, followed by general interest and a group of like-minded people sitting at a kitchen table deciding to light a candle instead of railing against the darkness. From very basic beginnings the MAI has in 12 years become a properly organized and staffed center for sharing information and providing support, and an active advocate for better services. A brief description of the MAI's major successes to date follows.

Migraine clinics

MAI promoted and actively assisted in the establishment of clinics for headache/migraine sufferers in Dublin (1998) and Cork (2000). The clinics have yielded excellent outcomes from the close cooperation they facilitate between patients and health professionals. There is regular liaison between MAI, the consultants and staff of these clinics, with the clinical directors serving as medical advisors to the MAI, and MAI publications providing a two-way conduit to and from the clinics.

Information pack for medical professionals

This was developed by the MAI in collaboration with its medical advisors and consists of detailed advice and information on headache/migraine management, endorsed by the doctors' professional organization, the Irish College of General Practitioners. The information pack included patient leaflets and was distributed to all general practitioners in Ireland. (This project earned the Patient Association of the Year award for MAI in 2003.)

Health professional migraine website: www.migraine.ie

This was established in 2005 and marks another milestone in the cooperation between the lay association and the medical profession. It operates in parallel with the patient website.

An editorial board made up of health professionals and lay experts devised the site as a comprehensive medical resource for doctors and health workers. General practitioners can now consult this site from their surgeries, and are able to refer their clients to the patient section.

The site is regularly updated and doctors are encouraged to download leaflets for their patients. The website was launched in 2005 and won MAI the award for best use of information technology at the Irish Healthcare Pharmaceutical Awards in 2006. The site has grown in popularity and receives tens of thousands of hits each month.

Core information services

However, it is undoubtedly the telephone helpline which is the most direct and tangible benefit to patients taking the most vital first step to receiving information and support, although an increasing number will have already accessed the website as a background check on the organization. The helpline is supplemented by an advice line, which is staffed by a specialist nurse answering queries on specific medications and treatment regimens. This specialist nurse advice line is an extremely valuable outcome of the cooperation and liaison between the headache/migraine clinics, which allows the specialist nurse from the Dublin clinic to take calls referred from the MAI helpline. It is planned to expand this service further and a recent survey of members listed the advice line as the most beneficial service to the public.

Surprisingly, surveys of members' needs repeatedly demonstrate the overwhelming popularity of our newsletter (*Brainstorm*) as a source of information – perhaps its portability and ease of use compared to a laptop explain the preference!

The MAI also produces booklets for people with migraine on various aspects of the condition, including:

- *Managing Migraine*
- *Migraine in the Workplace*
- *Migraine Medications*
- *Migraine Triggers*
- *Migraine in Teenagers* resource pack.

Cooperative alliances

In addition to the cooperation between a lay association such as MAI and the relevant health professionals in the provision of services to patients, there is significant scope for joint endeavors in the area of advocacy and policy promotion with government departments and business interests. These joint endeavors tend to focus on budgetary matters, development of services, and research topics, where interests overlap and positive outcomes can be mutually advantageous. This mutuality prompted the establishment in Ireland of an alliance between the various lay associations representing neurological conditions. The Neurological Alliance of Ireland (NAI) is an umbrella organization for 23 voluntary groups. No government in the world wants to talk to 23 individual organizations, so by working together, delivering a unified message in partnership with the scientific community, some progress has been made. The group has already had an enormous impact and influence on government policies and funding programs and has produced policy papers that have been adopted by the Department of Health in Ireland and are now in the process of being implemented. Similar organizations have been and are being established in many countries.

The emerging role of lay associations

The role of lay associations can best be described as emerging, with patients becoming the new resource in neurology. Many headache associations are at different stages of development and several are newly established. In Spain the Asociación Española de Pacientes con Cefalea (AEPAC), founded in 2005, has not yet secured appropriate funding or staff, yet has already become actively involved in promoting awareness and generating interest in migraine. This was demonstrated at the European Headache Federation's Congress held in Valencia in April 2006, at which AEPAC conducted a very successful patient information forum, which attracted significant media coverage. This, in turn, greatly improves AEPAC's progress towards establishing itself on a better basis to serve the needs of Spanish migraine sufferers.

The Swedish Migraine Alliance has worked vigorously to put migraine and other headache disorders on their government's agenda. They are confident this will happen and should benefit many generations to come.

Alleanza Cefalalgici in Italy have a very popular interactive website. They collaborated with a sister lay association, Associazione Italiana per la lotta contro le Cefalee, to produce a grid for the quantification of headache-related disability that has recently been published as a regional decree (*Bollettino Regionale Lombardia* 2007; 3, pp. 198–203).

Partnership for progress

All successful lay associations have an impetus to develop their services; for example, five long-established headache organizations in the UK have become more effective in their advocacy work with government since forming an alliance to enable a joint approach. The three lay associations – Migraine Action Association, Migraine Trust, and the Organization for the Understanding of Cluster Headache – joined forces with the two groups representing health professionals, Migraine in Primary Care Advisors and the British Association for the Study of Headache, to form an alliance called Headache UK. This has led to the formation of an all-party parliamentary group for primary headache disorders which is actively promoting a parliamentary review of headache services. In March 2008 this group held an event championed by Shadow Health Minister Stephen O'Brien in the Houses of Parliament, London, and called for an early order motion requiring the signatures of 60 Members of Parliament.

Quite apart from the extensive cooperation that can exist within national boundaries, between the relevant lay associations and health professionals, there is an established and growing level of liaison and mutual international support between lay associations themselves, particularly between European countries. Some of the liaison is formalized on a Europe-wide basis, through the European Federation of Neurological Associations (EFNA), which combines European umbrella bodies of neurological patient advocacy groups. Its current involvements includes the foundation of the European Brain Council, which combines the European federations of neurologists, psychiatrists, pharmaceutical and health insurance industries, and has already actively promoted the establishment of Europe-wide federations of national patients' organizations in the neurological field, such as the Stroke Alliance for Europe in 2004 and the European Headache Alliance (EHA) in 2006.

European Headache Alliance partners

EHA was launched in 2006 and already represents patient associations from Austria, Finland, Germany, Iceland, Ireland, Italy, Luxembourg, the Netherlands, Norway, Serbia, Spain, Sweden, Switzerland, and the UK. A major benefit which is anticipated from international alliances (apart from increased lobbying potential) is the sharing of expertise and information, and the expansion of research opportunities beyond national patient groups. An example of the type of initiative which can be replicated on this international framework would be the specialist patient program pioneered by the Migraine Action Association in the UK; this has empowered sufferers to manage their condition more effectively and to become specialist patients, providing assistance to other migraine sufferers and raising awareness in their own local area.

EFNA has been successful in establishing a lobby group of Members of the European Parliament who are interested in brain disorders, to encourage informed debate, and to influence European Community policies on behalf of lay associations. EHA is involved in the dissemination of information on the latest headache research published in *Cephalalgia*. EHA and Blackwell, the publishers of the official journal of the International Headache Society, will collaborate on this project to translate scientific articles into lay language for wider distribution. These articles will appear in the articles digests section of Blackwell's website.

Lifting the burden of headache worldwide

These national and European alliances were preceded by the establishment of the World Headache Alliance (WHA) in 1997. WHA is a collaborative global alliance of lay associations from all over the world, representing 37 such organizations from 26 countries. It has an active liaison with the International Headache Society in developing services and support for people affected by headache disorders. Perhaps the most significant, ambitious, and far-reaching program devised by WHA is the campaign under way, entitled Lifting the Burden, which is a global campaign aimed >at reducing the burden of headache worldwide. Progress to date includes the Kyoto Declaration on Headache, which pledges a joint program of work to be undertaken as a first step between the relevant medical, scientific, and lay associations of Japan. The program includes raising awareness; educational programs for health-care providers; introduction of diagnostic aids; influencing health policy-makers and legislative bodies in Japan; and monitoring the effects of these initiatives in order to demonstrate beneficial change. The program is set against a background, in Japan, of 8 million sufferers and a cost to the Japanese economy in lost productivity of 288 billion yen every year.

Awareness-raising projects

An important innovation in raising awareness continues to be World Headache Awareness Month, which seeks a declaration from national governments encouraging migraine awareness activities each September. This initiative has been further enhanced by a European Migraine Day of Action on 12 September, spearheaded by the newly formed EHA. For this project, each member association highlights a particular theme chosen by EHA annually. For example, the theme for 2006 was to reduce the intolerance and prejudice against people living with migraine by promoting the message that "migraine is common, disabling, and treatable!"

Lay associations exist to assist all those affected directly and indirectly by headache disorders. The indirect concerns center on issues such as the need for research into obstacles to diagnosis and treatment of migraine and other headache disorders. It is important to direct publicity and awareness-raising programs towards delivering the message that headache/migraine disorders are real and treatable. This should in turn lead to greater awareness in the general public and improvements in medical training, leading to more accurate diagnosis and better treatment.

Encouraging research

There is huge potential in the field of headache/migraine for research and improvements in treatments and services to sufferers. The lay associations, of their nature and purpose, present an obvious and extremely cooperative resource for piloting research initiatives and trialing treatment and medical innovations. For health professionals anxious to promote improvements in facilities and care regimes to headache/migraine sufferers, the relevant national organizations and international federations and alliances of lay associations have a demonstrable value, and proven track record, in lobbying at national, European, and worldwide levels for policy and budgetary goals, in tandem with relevant health professional interests. Recent studies have demonstrated the importance of headache/migraine disorders from the health economic and public health perspectives. Such studies have gained fresh impetus and importance from the recognition of these disorders as seriously disabling by the World Health Organization. It should be stressed that this recognition is, in itself, a testament to the efficacy of sustained cooperative effort on the part of patient advocates and health professionals under the auspices of the WHA and the International Headache Society.

Advocacy

When lay associations combine with the scientific community in lobbying for improved services, or funding for research initiatives, they form a powerful and persuasive partnership. All politics are local and politicians understand the power of the electorate. Patient organizations have learned that political persuasion is most readily achieved by positive publicity and public relations; learning from the success of campaigns for cancer research and heart disease, and their methodologies can only yield better outcomes for headache and migraine sufferers. Evidence-based argument, repeated by patient associations and the relevant health professionals, is the most effective means of persuading key opinion leaders such as those formulating policies, devising budgets, and ordering priorities. Despite the growing body of research into headache and migraine disorders there is huge scope for further research. It is surprising that so much remains to be discovered about such a widespread and commonplace disorder. For example, it is well known that migraine is more prevalent amongst women and that it is affected by cyclical hormonal factors. However, sex differences in migraine rates persist well beyond menopause and the reasons for these differences have not been satisfactorily explained, thus yielding scope for further investigation.

Measuring the burden

Much valuable work has recently been undertaken in the area of health economics relating to the costs to society of headache and migraine. A recent calculation of the cost to the European Union economy each year in terms of work days lost and reduced productivity was €27 billion. This is the most compelling argument for the importance of these disorders in economic as well as social terms. Such studies have an obvious bearing on the importance that policy-makers attach to preventive therapies and services. It is important that comparative studies of treatment regimes using standard methodologies based on up-to-date statistical data be devised so that impact and burden can be properly evaluated.

Hope for the future

The growth in the development of well-organized, properly resourced, and interlinked lay associations should be viewed positively by the scientific community and can be regarded as a worthwhile and valuable resource in the shared goal of improving treatments, services, and beneficial research in the field of migraine and other headache disorders.

More information on the lay activities mentioned in the text can be found at the following websites:

AEPAC (Asociación Española Pacientes con Cefalea) – Spain: http://www.dolordecabeza.net/
Alleanza Cefalalgici – CIRNA Foundation – Italy: http://www.cefalea.it/interna.cfm?idmenu=2
Associazione Italiana per la lotta contro le Cefalee (AIC) – Italy: http://www.aicefalee.it/
Dutch Headache Patient Association – The Netherlands: http://www.hoofdpijnpatienten.nl/
European Federation of Neurological Associations (EFNA): http://www.efna.net/
European Headache Alliance (EHA): http://www.european-headache-alliance.eu/
Finnish Migraine Association – Finland: http://www.migreeni.org/
German Green Cross – Germany: http://www.dgk.de/
Migraine Action Association – UK: http://www.migraine.org.uk/
Migraine Association of Ireland – Ireland: http://www.migraine.ie/
Migraine Trust – UK: http://www.migrainetrust.org/
Norwegian Migraine Association – Norway: http://www.migrene.no/
Swedish Migraine Association – Sweden: http://www.migran.org
Swiss Migraine Action – Switzerland: http://www.migraine-action.ch/
Understanding Cluster Headache: http://www.ouchuk.org/html/
World Headache Alliance (WHA): http://www.w-h-a.org/

Section 4

Primary headache

Handbook of Clinical Neurology, Vol. 97 (3rd series)
Headache
G. Nappi and M.A. Moskowitz, Editors

Chapter 21

Migraine: general aspects

MICHAEL A. MOSKOWITZ[1]* AND M. GABRIELLA BUZZI[2]

[1]*Stroke and Neurovascular Regulation Laboratory, Departments of Radiology and Neurology, Massachusetts General Hospital, Harvard Medical School, Charlestown, MA, USA*
[2]*Headache Center, IRCCS Santa Lucia Foundation, Rome, Italy*

INTRODUCTION

Migraine is a complex group of disorders with several phenotypes and different clinical presentations. According to the latest international guidelines (Headache Classification Subcommittee of the International Headache Society, 2004), migraine phenotypes are grouped into 19 subtypes. Although the definition of the term "migraine" derives from the word hemicrania and refers to the unilateral localization of pain, bilateral pain is often present. In more typical subtypes, diagnostically important features include pain that is throbbing, the presence of focal neurological symptoms (the aura), photophobia, phonophobia, osmophobia, and aggravating factors such as cyclical hormones. With few exceptions, the neurological examination is normal during and between attacks. Proper diagnosis is essential in order to ensure adequate follow-up and to avoid drug misuse and abuse. Finally, careful attention should be given to family history because migraine headaches cluster in families (Russell, 2007).

This introductory chapter will briefly review the epidemiology, clinical and pathophysiological features of migraine, as well as pharmacological approaches to treatment. Many of these topics will be discussed in more detail in the sections that follow.

EPIDEMIOLOGY AND BURDEN OF DISEASE

Headache epidemiology is still a young discipline, although headaches are among the most common disorders of the nervous system. Most studies are descriptive and concern the demographics of migraine and related headaches in the general population. Other studies explore the economic and social impact of headache on patients and their families. More recent epidemiological approaches seek to identify potential causes of migraine and associations between candidate risk factors and headache.

Headache is a global problem that is underestimated in scope and scale, and underrecognized and undertreated worldwide. Because of its importance, the World Health Organization (WHO), in collaboration with non-governmental agencies, committed to the Lifting the Burden project, the global campaign to reduce the burden of headache worldwide (Steiner, 2004; Leonardi et al., 2005). One of the main goals of this campaign is to understand the scale and scope of the headache burden in order to assess disability with greater precision.

One of the most outstanding population-based epidemiological studies, the Head-HUNT study (Hagen et al., 2007), reported that migraine prevalence was 12% (16% in women and 8% in men), confirming other population-based studies in western countries. Among different age groups, the peak prevalence occurs during the fourth decade of life. The prevalence of headache is 47% in the general population based on epidemiological studies (Stovner et al., 2007) that consider migraine and tension-type headache according to their classification in the International Statistical Classification of Diseases and Related Health Problems, 10th revision (ICD-10; WHO, 2007) with code G43 and G44.2, respectively. Migraine and tension-type headaches have a prevalence of 10% and 38%, respectively. Migraine is most prevalent among adults, and is most common in Europe (15%) and reportedly lowest in Africa (5%). Migraine burden (headache days/year per person × intensity) is relatively evenly

*Correspondence to: Michael A. Moskowitz, MD, Stroke and Neurovascular Regulation Laboratory, Departments of Radiology and Neurology, Massachusetts General Hospital, Harvard Medical School, 149 13th Street, Room 6403, Charlestown, MA 02129, USA, E-mail: moskowitz@helix.mgh.harvard.edu

distributed across continents for which there is sufficient information. The contribution of migraine and tension-type headache to total headache burden accounts for 58% and 42%, respectively. The duration of attacks changes the burden in favor of tension-type headache (47% in migraine and 53% in tension-type headache). WHO favors using the disability-adjusted life year (DALY) as a compound measure, multiplying the sum of years of life lost (YLL) due to premature mortality with years lived with disability (YLD). YLD is defined as incidence × disability × disease weight. Migraine ranks in the highest tier of neurological disorders according to WHO criteria (i.e., ranging from 0.7 to 1.0, on a scale from 0 to 1). Migraine ranks 19th among all causes of disability, 12th in women, based on YLD.

PATHOPHYSIOLOGY AND TARGETED TREATMENTS

The most outstanding feature that distinguishes migraineurs from normal subjects is the susceptibility to recurrent activation of the trigeminovascular and upper cervical systems (Cutrer, 2006). Recurrence of attacks may be due to an enhanced susceptibility to activation, either because of relatively low activation thresholds or because of loss of inhibitory modulation (Cutrer, 2006). More likely, it is caused by upstream triggers such as cortical spreading depression (CSD) as well as others that await discovery.

Until the early 1980s, the vascular theory held sway and proposed that migraine was a manifestation of vascular dysregulation. In this view, the aura was caused by transient ischemia and the head pain was a result of rebound vasodilation. According to this view, vasodilation caused depolarization of primary nociceptive afferents within the adventitia of dilated intra- and extracerebral vessels due to distension (Wolff, 1963). The theory was supported by the vasoconstrictive actions of ergot alkaloids, the most effective compounds to abort migraine pain at that time. Although the importance of cephalic blood vessels to migraine pathophysiology remains unchallenged, the vasoconstrictor mechanism has been criticized by a number of investigators.

The trigeminovascular system

Since the early 1980s, researchers have studied the sensory innervation of cephalic blood vessels to elucidate mechanisms relevant to migraine pathophysiology, and, by so doing, to acquire knowledge about the anatomy, neurochemistry, physiology, and pharmacology of afferent neurotransmission (Mayberg et al., 1984; Moskowitz, 1984). Of particular importance to headache pathogenesis, nociceptive information is transmitted via perivascular unmyelinated C fibers projecting mainly from trigeminal and cervical primary sensory neurons. These axons are capsaicin-sensitive and express receptor populations and signaling mechanisms that are typical of unmyelinated C fibers innervating other tissues (with notable exceptions). Afferent fibers provide a final common pathway upon which numerous factors trigger or modulate pain. With depolarization, these axons transmit centrally to synapses within the trigeminal nuclear complex. They also release vasoactive neuropeptide transmitters from peripheral axons into the vessel wall. Released neuropeptides cause local plasma extravasation and vasodilation. Hence, neurogenic inflammation develops from peptide release and pain develops as a consequence of central processing of inputs into the trigeminal nucleus caudalis (TNC) (Moskowitz, 1984) (Figure 21.1). Headache pain is triggered by activation or modulation of the trigeminovascular system by biochemical, mechanical, immunological, ionic, and neuronal factors within the meninges. However, the contribution of neurogenic inflammation itself has not yet been established in humans.

The discovery of the trigeminovascular system and the consequences of its activation by electrical or chemical stimuli led to the hypothesis and demonstration that drugs used to treat migraine attack, such as ergot derivatives, bind to prejunctional receptors and inhibit the development of neurogenic inflammation in the rat (Markowitz et al., 1987; Saito et al., 1988). Sumatriptan, the first drug designed to target migraine treatment, was then found to be effective in the same model (Buzzi and Moskowitz, 1990). Sumatriptan also blocked c-fos expression in lamina I and II of the TNC in response to stimulation of trigeminal afferents (Nozaki et al., 1992). Because stimuli that evoke c-fos expression in TNC are noxious and C fiber-dependent, these findings support the notion that peripheral trigeminal branches and their central connections provide a final common pathway of importance to migraine headache. Specific serotonin (5-HT) binding sites for ergot alkaloids and triptans are expressed by such fibers and probably contribute to clinical efficacy (Moskowitz and Buzzi, 1991). Peptide release, as measured by calcitonin gene-related peptide (CGRP) levels in superior sagittal sinus blood, increased during intense stimulation of the trigeminal ganglion in the rat (Buzzi et al., 1991a). The antimigraine drugs ergot alkaloids and sumatriptan reduced CGRP release when given prior to stimulation (Buzzi et al., 1991a). Presumably triptans also inhibited neuropeptide release from the central terminations of trigeminovascular axons within the brainstem (Levy et al., 2004). Inhibition of this release by presynaptic receptors has been reported using electrophysiological criteria. Although these data are

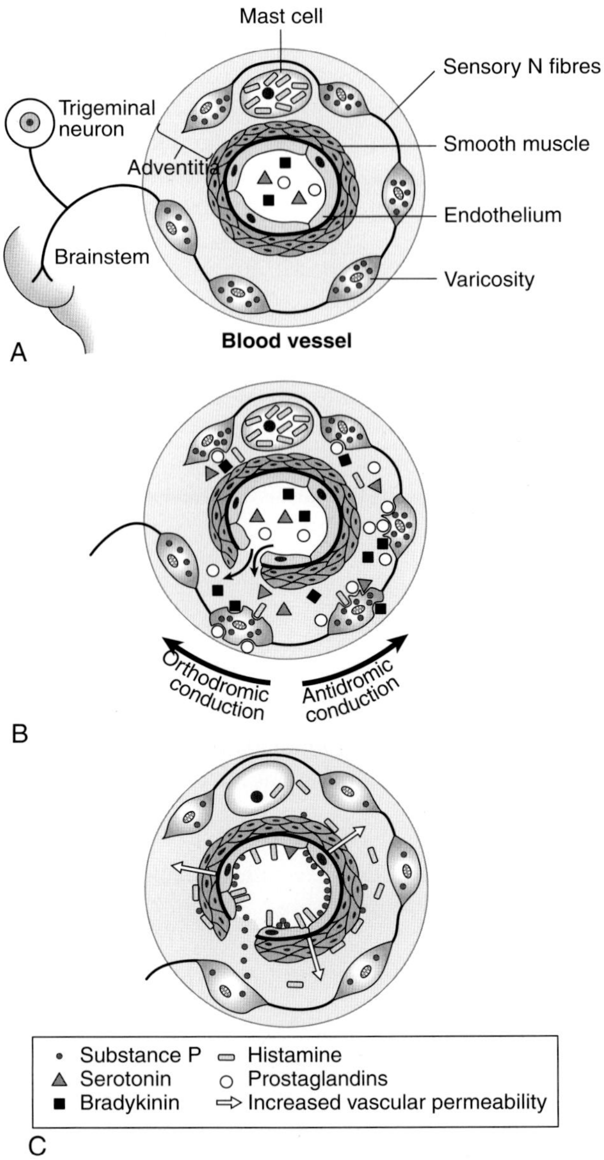

Fig. 21.1. (A–C) The activation of trigeminovascular system and neurogenic inflammation in tissues innervated by trigeminal fibers. (Reproduced from Moskowitz, 1984.)

compelling, it remains to be determined in humans whether sumatriptan penetrates the blood–brain barrier within the brainstem and specifically within the TNC. Despite limitations and expected species differences, the above findings support the notion that animal models may serve as useful screening tools to discover potential antimigraine compounds (Buzzi and Moskowitz, 1991).

Cortical spreading depression

The mechanisms that link migraine triggers to activation of the trigeminovascular system are complex. Leão's hypothesis that CSD could play a role in migraine has become very credible (Leão, 1944). Functional magnetic resonance imaging (fMRI) data from human visual cortex provides strong evidence that CSD underlies migraine visual aura (Hadjikhani et al., 2001), and similar findings may underlie migraine auras emanating from other brain regions. For example, experimental data show that CSD is noxious and can activate trigeminovascular afferents. Spreading depression provokes the expression of c-fos protein-like immunoreactivity within neurons of the TNC via trigeminovascular mechanisms (Moskowitz et al., 1993). Also CSD induces long-lasting blood flow enhancement within the middle meningeal artery, consistent with the consequences of a noxious stimulus within the trigeminal receptive field (Bolay et al., 2002). Vasodilation is caused by release of vasoactive agents from parasympathetic projections originating from parasympathetic nuclei of cranial nerve VII. Parasympathetic neurons are activated by monosynaptic connections to the TNC (see below). CSD also causes plasma protein leakage into the ipsilateral dura mater (Bolay et al., 2002). Protein extravasation is mediated via release of proinflammatory peptides from trigeminal axon collaterals innervating the meninges. Because meningeal inflammation persists after CSDs subside, it appears that intense and transient brain activity can cause sustained meningeal events and C fiber discharge. The precise mechanism awaits clarification.

The ability of five prophylactic drugs to suppress CSD in experimental animals further underscores the importance of CSD to migraine (see below). These data, combined with emerging findings showing that genetically engineered mice expressing "migraine" mutations (familial hemiplegic migraine: FHM) exhibit a CSD phenotype, emphasize the emerging importance of CSD to migraine pathophysiology (van den Maagdenberg et al., 2004).

CSD activates a class of enzymes called matrix metalloproteinases (MMPs) in brain blood vessels and parenchyma (Gursoy-Ozdemir et al., 2004). These enzymes are cleaved and activated within cortical vessels early after CSD. Levels remain elevated in brain for nearly 48 h. MMPs contribute to an inflammatory cascade triggered by the generation of oxygen species (e.g., nitric oxide) and provide indirect evidence for up regulation of a proinflammatory state in brain and its connective tissue coverings in migraine. Such changes may contribute to the delayed headache response to nitroglycerine and to disruption of the blood–brain barrier as seen during complicated or prolonged migraine attacks. These findings support the notion that inflammation may contribute to migraine pathophysiology (Bolay and Moskowitz, 2005).

It is not yet clear how CSD is triggered in human cortex to evoke migraine aura (Sanchez-del-Rio et al., 2006).

However, a number of stimuli trigger CSD in experimental animals, including direct cortical trauma, exposure to high concentrations of excitatory amino acids or K^+, direct electrical stimulation, inhibition of Na^+/K^+ ATPase, and energy failure. Genetic and environmental factors may modulate individual susceptibility by lowering the CSD threshold, and cortical excitation may cause sufficient elevation in extracellular K^+ and glutamate to initiate CSD (Moskowitz et al., 2004).

Recently identified genetic mutations in different forms of FHM (Table 21.1) provide some clues as to how genetic mutations may render the brain more susceptible to CSDs. Those include excessive synaptic glutamate release or decreased removal of glutamate and potassium from the synaptic cleft (Figure 21.2). Interestingly, a genetic pattern similar to FHM2 has been found in patients with basilar-type migraine, suggesting that a common genetic background may underlie diverse symptoms of migraine aura (Ambrosini et al., 2005). Mice carrying a human (FHM) type 1 mutation in P/Q-type Ca^{2+} channel were shown to express an abnormally low CSD threshold, and this phenotype was associated with enhanced glutamate release (van den Maagdenberg et al., 2004).

Other proteins (e.g., transporters or channels) relevant to CSD may also render the nervous system susceptible to CSD and migraine. For example, mutations in the sodium pump (Na/ATPase) cause FHM-2 (De Fusco et al., 2003) and may increase extracellular K^+ or decrease glutamate clearance to enhance susceptibility to CSD. FHM-2 is caused by mutations in the alpha 2 subunit of the sodium pump, and is encoded by a gene residing on chromosome 1. To date, 28 point mutations in this gene have been discovered within affected families. The mutations significantly inhibit or suppress the function of this key ion translocator.

The brainstem has been postulated as a key initiating site or migraine generator. Weiller and co-workers (1995) found an 11% increase in regional cerebral blood flow in the medial brainstem contralateral to the headache. Blockade of the head pain with subcutaneous sumatriptan did not reduce this flow change, although it did reverse flow increases in insula and anterior cingulate gyrus. It was posited that migraine attacks emanate from a brainstem generator either through direct activation or through failure of inhibition. The authors found that midbrain activation was not observed during a headache-free interval, nor was it observed in another study in which forehead pain was elicited by subcutaneous capsaicin injection (May et al., 1998). Although these results are of obvious importance, they should stimulate more detailed follow-up investigations to understand their particular relevance to migraine pathophysiology. For example, further experiments are needed to determine whether such findings may be due to aversive activity as shown previously for the periaqueductal gray, or reflect a true migraine generator.

Table 21.1

Migraine as a genetically determined disease

Chromosome locus	Gene/protein	Migraine type	Reference
19p13	CACNA1A	FHM1	Ophoff et al., 1996
1q23	ATP1	FHM2	De Fusco et al, 2003
2q24	SCN1A	FHM3	Dichgans et al, 2005

FHM: familial hemiplegic migraine.

Functional imaging

The development of non-invasive functional neuroimaging has become fundamental to the real-time study of brain events during migraine attacks in human patients. Over 20 years ago, Olesen, Lauritzen, and their co-workers utilized intra-arterial ^{133}Xe blood flow techniques to investigate whether changes in blood flow occurred during aura-like symptoms induced by carotid angiography (Olesen et al., 1981; Lauritzen et al., 1983). According to their findings, regional cerebral blood flow was reduced by 17–35% in the posterior parietal and occipital lobes after the onset of visual aura. Hypoperfusion was also observed occasionally in frontal cortex in combination with a decrease in blood flow within the posterior circulation. The decreases in regional cerebral blood flow persisted for up to 1 h but were not large enough to cause ischemia. Hence, the term "oligemia" was applied (Lauritzen and Olesen, 1984). The oligemia did spread anteriorly beyond individual vascular territories. Hence, the results tended to support a parenchymal rather than vascular origin for migraine aura.

Interestingly, Woods and co-workers (1994) fortuitously captured the onset of a spontaneous attack in a migraine patient undergoing blood flow measurements in an unrelated positron emission tomography (PET) study. They reported bilateral spreading oligemia that began in the visual association cortex within a few minutes of the onset of bilateral occipital throbbing headache (Brodman areas 18 and 19). The flow changes spread anteriorly across vascular and anatomical boundaries. The patient with known migraine without aura reported no visual symptoms other than transient

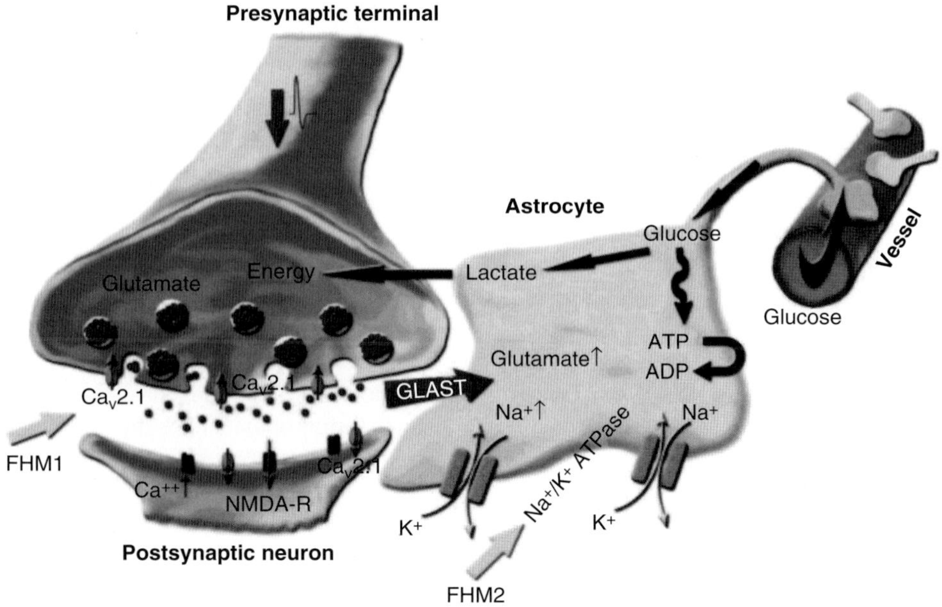

Fig. 21.2. Genetic modulation of glutamate activity in the synaptic cleft. Excessive synaptic glutamate release in familial hemiplegic migraine 1 (FHM1) or decreased removal of glutamate and potassium in the synaptic cleft may render the brain more susceptible to cortical spreading depression events. ATP: adenosine triphosphate; ADP: adenosine diphosphate; GLAST: astrocyte uptake of glutamate via transporters; NMDA-R: *N*-methyl-D-aspartate receptor. (Reproduced from Moskowitz et al., 2004.)

difficulty focusing on a target during the PET study. This case report is important because it illustrates that patients are often unable to experience significant changes in brain activity during migraine attacks (i.e., silent aura). Hence, as imaging methods become more sophisticated, the utility of classifying headaches based solely on clinical criteria may diminish.

fMRI techniques, diffusion-weighted imaging (DWI), including perfusion-weighted imaging (PWI) and blood oxygen level-dependent (BOLD) imaging, are also being applied to study migraine aura. The rapid acquisition times for many fMRI techniques allow the evaluation of metabolic as well as hemodynamic parameters within a single attack. One case series reported DWI findings during five spontaneous migraine visual auras in four patients (Cutrer et al., 1988). DWI has been applied to the study of spontaneous migraine visual aura in humans. Spreading depression evoked in animal models has been associated with waves of reduced apparent diffusion coefficient (ADC), moving at a rate of 3 mm/min. The decreased cortical ADC areas returned to normal levels after 30 s (Gardner-Medwin et al., 1994).

There is increasing evidence that metabolic and neurophysiological differences exist between the cortices of non-migraine subjects and patients with migraine with aura. Welch and colleagues (1989), using ^{31}P magnetic resonance spectroscopy, reported a decrease in the phosphocreatinine/inorganic phosphate ratio and normal pH during headache in migraine with aura but not in normal controls or migraine without aura. They concluded that migraine aura was characterized by defective aerobic metabolism. Low levels of brain magnesium possibly augmenting *N*-methyl-D-aspartate receptor activity (and thereby lowering the threshold for CSD) were also found in migraine patients (Welch et al., 1992). Lack of habituation is the most reproducible interictal abnormality in sensory processing of migraineurs. This may result from dysfunction within subcorticocortical aminergic pathways (Ambrosini et al., 2003). How it relates to the triggering of an attack remains to be determined.

Sensitization

Thus far, the aura is the best-characterized phase of a migraine attack. The prodromal period is well described clinically, but not understood. As noted in the introduction, symptoms vary considerably and the duration is uneven between patients. As a general rule, the aura persists for an hour or less and usually resolves before the headache is fully developed, according to International Headache Society (IHS) guidelines (Headache Classification Committee of the International Headache Society, 1988; Headache Classification Subcommittee of the International Headache

Society, 2004). If activation of the trigeminal system is transient and relatively brief, other mechanisms probably intervene to sustain the headache. Two processes may be important (Burstein, 2001): (1) peripheral sensitization of the primary afferent neuron; and (2) central sensitization of higher-order neurons within the spinal cord and brain.

Peripheral sensitization is characterized by increased excitability of primary afferents in response to triggers such as mechanical stimulation. This may be caused by excessive firing of primary afferents as well. The result is that second-order neurons are bombarded with high-frequency impulses from primary afferents innervating the meninges. Stimulation of the dural receptive fields by inflammatory mediators directly excites trigeminovascular axons and also enhances their mechanical sensitivity. After chemical stimulation, primary afferents became strongly activated by mechanical stimuli that are normally innocuous. These findings suggest that chemosensitivity and sensitization may contribute to the hypersensitivity of migraine patients to small changes in intracranial pressure and to the throbbing quality of a migraine headache.

Upon activation, trigeminal nociceptive fibers release proinflammatory vasoactive neuropeptides from their peripheral terminals in animal models (Buzzi et al., 1991a) and in humans during migraine pain (Goadsby et al., 1990). The resulting vasodilation, mast cell activation (Dimitriadou et al., 1991, 1992), and membrane disruption may contribute to the peripheral sensitization of the trigeminal primary afferent neurons.

Upon increased inputs from sensitized primary afferents, second-order neurons become sensitized within the TNC and now respond to weaker stimuli that were previously below threshold (Burstein et al., 1998). Because central neurons within the trigeminovascular system receive convergent inputs from both intracranial meningeal/vascular and cutaneous structures, changes in extracranial sensation (facial skin) develop following central sensitization during an attack. The existence of central sensitization was confirmed by a study in which 42 patients underwent repeated measurement of mechanical and thermal pain thresholds during and between attacks (Burstein et al., 2000a, b). Seventy-nine percent of subjects exhibited allodynia in periorbital and forearm skin during the acute migraine attack.

Despite the growing body of evidence regarding migraine pathophysiology, an attempt to identify a single unifying theory to explain susceptibility continues to be unsuccessful. The increasing evidence for genetic heterogeneity, combined with wide variations in migraine phenotype, argues for a syndrome approach to future study (Cutrer, 2006). A syndrome approach recognizes an acute migraine attack as a clinical "final common pathway" reflecting activation of the trigeminocervical pain system, which may arise from more than one initiating process. Research based on such a view may ultimately yield more useful information because it fosters the study of pathophysiology in clinically and perhaps genetically definable subgroups.

SELECTED CLINICAL FEATURES OF MIGRAINE AND THE ICHD-II DIAGNOSTIC CRITERIA

The complex mechanisms that underlie migraine (genetic, environment) are mirrored by the complexity of its phenotype and symptoms even within the same patient. In fact, the presentation of migraine varies from patient to patient, even though the diagnosis is based upon universally accepted criteria (Buzzi et al., 2005a). It is common in clinical practice to diagnose migraine in a patient with features that vary between attacks. Localization of pain may be unilateral or bilateral, and duration of attacks (if untreated) may vary depending on the phase of the menstrual cycle, being longer in those attacks temporarily related to menses. Among accompanying symptoms, vomiting may or may not be present from attack to attack and there might be other accompanying symptoms, such as osmophobia.

Attacks may be organized into five stages: the premonitory phase, the aura, the headache phase, resolution, and postdrome, although the IHS (Headache Classification Subcommittee of the International Headache Society, 2004) guidelines provide criteria only for stages related to aura and pain. However, these five phases do not necessarily occur in a single attack and there is usually no definable onset or termination for each phase, except the aura.

Patients should be questioned about premonitory symptoms as part of the routine visit (Giffin et al., 2003; Schoonman et al., 2006). Migraineurs often recognize the impending onset of a migraine attack hours or days before onset and the clinicians can suggest early treatment for the pain phase. Clinical signs of sensory hyperexcitability (Schoenen, 2006) often begin during the premonitory phase and include photophobia, phonophobia, hyperosmia, and cutaneous allodynia. Yawning, malaise, acute mood changes, food cravings, and nausea may also be experienced. In our view, understanding the pathophysiology of the premonitory phase may help to clarify the genesis of an acute attack and develop better treatments to prevent an attack (Buzzi et al., 2005b).

The aura may begin just before or simultaneously with the headache. The neurological symptoms that characterize the aura (visual, sensory, motor, language, or brainstem) vary in their complexity. Headaches during migraine with or without aura do not differ. Many patients who have frequent attacks with aura also have attacks without aura.

Pain often starts in the occipital/cervical regions, later becoming frontotemporal in location. It is throbbing and aggravated by physical activity. Although detailed, the description of the headache phase often lacks information about time-dependent changes (Linde, 2006), and no simple relationship exists between time and symptom intensity during untreated migraine attacks (Linde et al., 2006). When plotting time versus intensity, the curves are heterogeneous even in the same patient.

The latest International Classification of Headache Disorders (ICHD-II) provides a revised classification of cranial pain (Table 21.2). The ICHD-II emphasizes the need for additional clinical studies because some presentations may not satisfy the proposed criteria (see 1.6, probable migraine). Ophthalmoplegic migraine, previously coded as a subtype of migraine with aura, has been moved to a different ICHD-II chapter (secondary headaches), emphasizing the possibility that this form may be due to lesions in the central nervous system. Motor symptoms during migraine aura have become a mandatory criterion for hemiplegic migraine (whether familial, FHM, or sporadic), while basilar migraine has been renamed basilar-type migraine and kept distinct from hemiplegic migraine, although this form and hemiplegic migraine may share a common genetic susceptibility (Ambrosini et al., 2005).

Migraine patients exhibit comorbidity with other disorders or illnesses. The term "comorbidity" refers to the existence of two conditions within the same individual, and this coexistence implies that the two disorders may alter their respective clinical course (i.e., the time of presentation, the prognosis, the treatment, and the outcome). Comorbidity may be due to common risk factors, or causation, or random concurrence of the two. Comorbidity has been reported in clinical series, case–control studies, and epidemiological surveys. To summarize, the strongest associations with migraine include allergies, mitral valve prolapse, hypotension, hypertension, stroke, and depression and anxiety (Table 21.3) (Merikangas and Rasmussen, 2000). More recently, an association with patent foramen ovale has been linked to migraine with aura (Kimmelstiel et al., 2007; Slavin et al., 2007).

Finally, unilateral cranial autonomic symptoms (UAs), usually identifying trigeminal autonomic cephalalgias, may not be as rare in patients with migraine as thought. In one study (Barbanti et al., 2002), a prevalence of 45.8% was reported in migraine patients attending a tertiary referral center. UAs are spontaneously reported by migraine patients with more marked symptoms (i.e., pain severity or longer duration

Table 21.2

Migraine classification according to the International Classification of Headache Disorders, 2nd edition (ICHD-II) (Headache Classification Subcommittee of the International Headache Society, 2004)

1.	**Migraine**
1.1	Migraine without aura
1.2	Migraine with aura
1.2.1	Typical aura with migraine headache
1.2.2	Typical aura with non-migraine headache
1.2.3	Typical aura without headache
1.2.4	Familial hemiplegic migraine
1.2.5	Sporadic hemiplegic migraine
1.2.6	Basilar-type migraine
1.3	Childhood periodic syndromes that are commonly a precursor of migraine
1.3.1	Cyclical vomiting
1.3.2	Abdominal migraine
1.3.3	Benign paroxysmal vertigo of childhood
1.4	Retinal migraine
1.5	Complications of migraine
1.5.1	Chronic migraine
1.5.2	Status migrainosus
1.5.3	Persistent aura without infarction
1.5.4	Migrainous infarction
1.5.5	Migraine-triggered seizures
1.6	Probable migraine
1.6.1	Probable migraine without aura
1.6.2	Probable migraine with aura
1.6.3	Probable chronic migraine

Table 21.3

Medical disorders most strongly associated with migraine

Disorder	Evidence
Allergies	+++
Asthma	++
Mitral valve prolapse	++
Hypotension	++
Hypertension	++
Myocardial infarction	+
Patent foramen ovale	+
Depression/anxiety	+++
Colitis, irritable bowel, ulcers	++
Stroke	+++
Epilepsy	++

(Modified from Merikangas and Rasmussen, 2000.)

of the attack), and they may emerge following specific questioning in those patients with milder symptoms (Barbanti et al., 2002; Obermann et al., 2007). Interestingly, this feature may predict response to triptans (Barbanti et al., 2003).

Severe pain and/or intense activation of the TNC triggers the trigeminal autonomic reflex during a migraine attack (Goadsby and Lipton, 1997), a mechanism previously proposed for parasympathetic activation in cluster headache (Moskowitz, 1988). There is probably an activation threshold above which autonomic symptoms appear. The activation of the trigeminal afferent arm of this reflex, which is always present in patients with migraine, is presumably coupled with UAs with activation of the parasympathetic efferent arm (typically active in cluster headache), which provides secretomotor innervation to structures such as the lacrimal glands, nasal mucosa, and the meninges. As noted above, this monosynaptic reflex develops in experimental animals following CSD as well as other intense noxious stimuli (Hirata et al., 2000; Bolay et al., 2002). It has been proposed that overactivation of trigeminal afferents in migraineurs with UAs recruits peripheral neurovascular 5-$HT_{IB/ID}$ receptors to axonal membranes (Barbanti et al., 2003). Hence, this mechanism may explain the higher patient response rate to 5-$HT_{IB/ID}$ receptor agonists in trigeminal autonomic cephalalgias. Accordingly, increased trigeminal activation (as measured in patients with autonomic signs by CGRP and neurokinin A (NKA) levels in the external jugular vein blood) predicts a better response to rizatriptan (Sarchielli et al., 2006). In migraine patients responding to rizatriptan, pain was unilateral, severe, and pulsating. At least one sign suggestive of parasympathetic system activation was recorded. In non-responders, the pain tended to be bilateral and non-pulsating, but often severe. In non-responders, CGRP and NKA levels showed less significant variations at all time points compared with rizatriptan responders (Sarchielli et al., 2006).

MIGRAINE EVOLUTION AND PROGRESSION

Cyclical vomiting, abdominal migraine, and paroxysmal vertigo represent precursors of adulthood migraine according to IHS criteria, and their presentation supports the notion that migraine is present early in life, albeit with different manifestations than in adults. These manifestations represent non-specific and low-grade paroxysmal events, perhaps as a reflection of an immature brain (Buzzi et al., 2005a). There is reportedly evidence that the above-noted precursors of adult migraine are neurobiologically related to migraine (Li and Balint, 2000; Al-Twaijri and Shevell, 2002), and therefore the diagnosis of migraine should be considered in young children with these manifestations. Interestingly, the diagnosis in adolescents may not be as recognizable as in adults (Wang et al., 2005). In a 3-year follow-up, a large proportion convert to "probable migraine without aura" in the revised IHS (Headache Classification Subcommittee of the International Headache Society, 2004) criteria (formerly "migrainous disorder not fulfilling the criteria," Headache Classification Committee of the International Headache Society, 1988).

Longitudinal studies report that around 40% of patients with migraine either with or without aura stop having attacks (Cologno et al., 1998; Eriksen et al., 2004; Lyngberg et al., 2005), with the most significant changes occurring in the fifth and sixth decades of life. Migraine may, nevertheless, persist in patients over 60, although its characteristics may change with advancing age (Martins et al., 2006). Changes from episodic into chronic forms are possible in the elderly; drug overuse is one of the most frequent causes. With aging, migraine with aura may not be followed by headache (Fisher, 1980). The new onset of aura-like symptoms in an elderly person raises the possibility of an organic cause for the focal neurological symptom(s), and diagnostic procedures should be undertaken accordingly. Comorbid conditions, namely hypertension, should be considered in new-onset headache in elderly subjects, and investigated and treated accordingly (Haan et al., 2007).

Migraine attacks tend to disappear following severe traumatic brain injury and to recur after cognitive functioning significantly improves (Buzzi et al., 2003). Therefore, the more severe the brain damage, the later the recovery of a fully developed migraine attack. Neurodegenerative diseases presenting with focal brain damage in dopaminergic areas, such as substantia nigra, may shorten the lifetime clinical course of migraine (Barbanti et al., 2000).

PHARMACOLOGICAL TREATMENT

Preventive treatment

Prophylactic treatment is specifically intended to reduce frequency and intensity of headache attacks, improve the response to acute medications, and reduce migraine disability. The decision whether to prescribe preventive drugs is based upon the response to acute therapies and number of attacks. Also, patients should be alerted to external factors that are potentially avoidable. Identifying trigger factors can reduce the need for either acute or preventive medications.

None of the preventive treatments were specifically designed for prophylaxis. In large part, the effectiveness was observed serendipitously. First-line medication for migraine prevention presently consists of amitriptyline, flunarizine (where available on the market), beta-blockers (propranolol and timolol), and anticonvulsants (divalproex and topiramate) (Silberstein and Freitag, 2003). However, the choice of one or another has to consider the relative or absolute contraindications and comorbid conditions.

Most preventive medications are thought to act, at least in part, by normalizing neuronal firing and increasing the neuronal discharge threshold. Suppression of central hyperexcitability due to changes in voltage-gated channels may partly explain the basis for the effectiveness of calcium channel blockers or anticonvulsants, whereas modulation of neurotransmitter release may be the most relevant mechanism of action for serotonin reuptake inhibitors as well as beta-blockers. However, there is evidence for more complex mechanisms of action. For example, amitriptyline inhibits sodium channels, and beta-blockers and calcium antagonists exhibit inhibition of both sodium and calcium channels (Cohen, 2005). Among anticonvulsants (Table 21.4), topiramate shows the highest complexity of action, being able to modulate ion channels as well as gamma-aminobutyric acid, glutamate, and kainate receptors.

In animal models, chronic daily administration of migraine prophylactic drugs (topiramate, valproate, propranolol, amitriptyline, and methysergide) dose-dependently suppressed CSD frequency by 40–80% and increased the stimulation threshold, whereas acute treatment was ineffective (Ayata et al., 2006). Longer treatment durations produced stronger CSD suppression. Chronic treatment with D-propranolol (not effective in clinical practice) did not differ from saline control, whereas the racemate was effective. The treatment duration dependency of CSD inhibition is reminiscent of the gradual build-up of therapeutic efficacy observed in migraineurs. The above preclinical data also suggest that at least 3–4 weeks of treatment may be necessary to achieve therapeutic efficacy (Ayata et al., 2006), and that if treatment continues beyond 3–4 weeks the drugs may become even more effective. Interestingly, 1–3 months of valproate or topiramate treatment suppresses cortical hyperexcitability in migraineurs (Aurora et al., 2005a).

These data further support the hypothesis that CSD provides a common therapeutic target for widely prescribed migraine prophylactic drugs and suggest that assessing the CSD threshold may prove useful for developing new prophylactic drugs and improving existing ones (Ayata et al., 2006). Although CSD is considered a key factor for migraine aura, CSD or CSD-like events may also play a role in the pathophysiology of migraine without aura, perhaps after CSD is generated within clinically silent brain regions (see functional imaging section, above). After all, the five tested drugs are successfully used as prophylactic strategies in migraine without aura. Although the precise molecular mechanisms by which the above migraine prophylactic drugs suppress CSD remains to be elucidated, modulation of ion channels, pumps, neurotransmitter receptors, or transporter genes implicated in CSD deserves further scrutiny.

Table 21.4

Anticonvulsant drugs used in migraine prophylaxis and ion channels

Targets	Valproate	Lamotrigine	Gabapentin	Topiramate
Sodium channel	SCNA SCNB	SCN2A		SCNA SCNB
Calcium channel	CACNA CACNB	CACNA	CACN $\alpha 2\delta$	CACNA CACNB
Gamma-aminobutyric acid (GABA)	GABA degradation		GABA degradation	GABAR
Kainic acid (KA)/ α-amino-3-hydroxy-5-methyl-4-isoxazolepropionic acid (AMPA)				GluR1–4 GluR5–7 KA1 KA2
Binding proteins	Non-specific	Non-specific	Non-specific	Non-specific
Transporters	SLC02A (monocarboxylate)		GABA transporter	

Acute treatment

Sumatriptan was first synthesized in the mid-1980s (Humphrey et al., 1988), and subsequently evaluated in animal models (see above) and humans (Buzzi and Moskowitz, 1990; Buzzi et al., 1991b; Subcutaneous Sumatriptan International Study Group, 1991). The subcutaneous preparation has become the treatment of choice for cluster headache attack treatment (Ekbom et al., 1995).

As noted above, activation of the trigeminal nerve is a key component of the cascade that leads to, and perpetuates, a migraine attack (Buzzi and Moskowitz, 2005). Specific 5-HT receptor binding sites expressed by the trigeminovascular system include 5-HT_{1B}, 5-HT_{1D} and 5- HT_{1F} receptor subtypes (Bouchelet et al., 1996). Triptans are potent agonists of the 5-HT_{1B} and 5-HT_{1D} receptors, and some bind potently to 5-HT_{1F} receptors. Second-generation triptans, i.e., triptans that were synthesized after sumatriptan and are capable of crossing the blood–brain barrier at therapeutic doses, exhibit more favorable pharmacokinetic properties. Seven triptans are now available: almotriptan, eletriptan, frovatriptan, naratriptan, rizatriptan, sumatriptan, and zolmitriptan. They increase the choice of migraine attack-specific therapies, which translates into a more individually tailored treatment. Unfortunately, enhanced pharmacokinetic and preclinical pharmacodynamic profiles do not equate with substantial clinical improvement over sumatriptan, as measured by improving efficacy, reducing adverse events, or eliminating cardiovascular contraindications (Ferrari et al., 2001; Saxena and Tfelt-Hansen, 2006). Thus, alternative pharmacological treatments are still needed to expand the number of patients responding to acute treatment and to reduce the occurrence of adverse events. Gi proteins promote the antimigraine effects of triptans via 5-$HT_{1B/1D}$ receptors. Hence, agonists at Gi protein-coupled receptor types should be examined for their effects on the trigeminovascular system. They may provide a novel approach to the design of new antimigraine drugs (Humphrey, 2007).

Among migraine therapies, triptans are, so far, the most extensively evaluated. They have been investigated in preclinical studies and in well-designed trials based on universally adopted migraine diagnostic criteria (Headache Classification Committee of the International Headache Society, 1988; Headache Classification Subcommittee of the International Headache Society, 2004) and the IHS Guidelines for Clinical Trials (International Headache Society Committee on Clinical Trials in Migraine, 1991; International Headache Society Clinical Trials Subcommittee, 2000). There are patients who do not meet diagnostic IHS criteria for migraine but, nevertheless, respond to triptans. Other concomitant therapy, as well as attack frequency and susceptibility to drug abuse, deserves consideration when prescribing triptans.

Triptans are recommended for acute therapy in patients with moderate to severe migraine pain and in those with migraine pain of any severity whose mild to moderate headache does not respond sufficiently to non-specific agents (Silberstein, 2000). However, it has been estimated that up to 25% of all migraine sufferers and up to 40% of all migraine attacks do not respond to a triptan (Diener and Limmroth, 2001). Various hypotheses to explain non-response have been proposed, including differences in 5-HT receptor profile, inadequate absorption, overuse of analgesics, variant migraine, and use in tension-type headache with migraine features (Diener and Limmroth, 2001; Dodick, 2005). It may be that many non-responders are using triptans too late in the migraine attack (Burstein et al., 2004; Dodick, 2005). The recommendations for timing of triptan administration have been influenced by both clinical and economic factors. The placebo-controlled pivotal trials for efficacy and tolerability specified delaying triptan use until headache pain was moderate or severe (International Headache Society Committee on Clinical Trials in Migraine, 1991). Because of supply and reimbursement restrictions imposed by insurance companies and governmental or private health systems, patients may hesitate to use a triptan when headache pain is mild (i.e., "do not waste the dose") and instead wait until the attack is moderate or severe.

The efficacy of triptan use during the aura phase has been investigated. Several reports have indicated that treatment with almotriptan, eletriptan, sumatriptan, and naratriptan during aura or prodromes prevented or delayed the headache, or improved its outcome (Luciani et al., 2000; Aurora et al., 2005b). However, in several other studies treating during the aura, the proportion of patients who developed a moderate to severe headache was not significantly different from placebo, and the duration of aura was not shortened (Olesen et al., 2004). Migraine therapy may be more efficacious if initiated before the onset of cutaneous allodynia. In an open-label study, Burstein et al. (2004) evaluated the effect of time of triptan administration relative to the development of cutaneous allodynia in 31 patients who had a total of 27 non-allodynic attacks and 34 attacks with cutaneous allodynia. Prior to triptan administration, pain levels were not significantly different for non-allodynic and allodynic attacks. However, 2-h pain-free rates were 93% for non-allodynic attacks compared with 15% for allodynic attacks. Accumulating clinical trial data indicate that oral triptan treatment is more efficacious when migraine headache pain is mild. In addition, the proportion of patients reporting other migraine symptoms (nausea, vomiting, phonophobia, and photophobia) at 2 h after administration was lower in the early intervention group than after later intervention. As noted above, another distinguishing feature between responses to triptan may be the presence of local autonomic signs during headache.

Anecdotal experience teaches that patients with a poor response to one triptan can benefit from treatment with a different one. This should be considered when making therapeutic decisions after a single drug failure. Most probably the susceptibility to a given drug is determined by genetic differences, stages of drug metabolism, and differences in targets. However, very little is known about this subject. Polymorphisms in the 5-HT_{1B} receptor do not seem to predict the response to sumatriptan (Maassen Van DenBrink et al., 1996). Among triptans, sumatriptan and rizatriptan are metabolized by monoamine oxidase-A; eletriptan, naratriptan, and frovatriptan are metabolized by cytochrome P450 enzymes; whereas almotriptan can be metabolized by different metabolic pathways involving monoamine oxidase-A, cytochrome P450s, and flavin monooxygenase-3 (Armstrong and Cozza, 2002; Ferrari et al., 2003). Multiple routes for metabolism offer an advantage, so if one pathway is disrupted, others can take over to ensure the effectiveness of the drug and possibly to avoid drug accumulation. Drugs with single metabolic pathways may accumulate if metabolism is reduced. While this may prolong efficacy, it also increases the risk of adverse events (Buzzi, 2007) and altered interaction with other drugs metabolized by the same pathway, as seen, for example, in migraine patients receiving rizatriptan plus propranolol (Goldberg et al., 2001).

P-glycoprotein efflux transporter (belonging to the adenosine triphosphate-binding cassette) regulates the amount of drug entering the brain and reaching central sites of action. It represents another genetically determined system that may change the disposition of triptans (Evans et al., 2003). For example, there was a 40-fold difference in brain exposure to eletriptan between mice expressing the gene for the P-glycoprotein efflux pump and those lacking the pump (Evans et al., 2003). The activity of the P-glycoprotein efflux pump gene had a much smaller effect on brain exposure to other triptans, possibly due to their lower lipophilicity. It is noteworthy that, in clinical practice, a higher lipophilicity does not necessarily translate to improved migraine efficacy, whereas it is related to higher central nervous system adverse events and possibly to lower recurrence rates (Pascual and Munoz, 2005).

Pharmacogenomics offers the future option of tailoring a unique therapeutic approach to individual patients. Pharmacogenomics is the application of technology to analyze gene and protein expression to identify genetic polymorphisms and phenotypic traits that govern individual responses and adverse events to drug treatment (Ross et al., 2004), Genetic polymorphisms in drug-metabolizing enzymes, transporters, and other drug targets have been linked to interindividual differences in the efficacy and toxicity of many medications (Evans and Relling, 1999). Pharmacogenomics may become useful to help physicians to predict whether a patient will respond to a triptan or experience adverse events. It has the potential to match patients' genotypes to the most suitable drug for their metabolism and avoid drugs that may interfere with competing metabolic pathways. So far, association studies to assess polymorphisms of candidate genes encoding known metabolic pathways do not distinguish responders from non-responders (Asuni et al., 2007). Studies should be addressed to identify poor, normal, or fast drug metabolizers (Buzzi, 2007). The approach would also be useful to identify possible drug–drug interactions in patients receiving both preventive and attack treatments and to make the best choice to obtain the highest efficacy of both.

References

Al-Twaijri WA, Shevell MI (2002). Pediatric migraine equivalents: occurrence and clinical features in practice. Pediatr Neurol 6: 365–368.

Ambrosini A, de Noordhout AM, Sandor PS et al. (2003). Electrophysiological studies in migraine: a comprehensive review of their interest and limitations. Cephalalgia 23 (Suppl. 1): 13–31.

Ambrosini A, D'Onofrio M, Grieco GS et al. (2005). Familial basilar migraine associated with a new mutation in the ATP1A2 gene. Neurology 13: 1826–1828.

Armstrong SC, Cozza KL (2002). Med-psych drug–drug interactions update. Triptans. Psychosomatics 43: 502–504.

Asuni C, Cherchi A, Congiu D et al. (2007). Association study between clinical response to rizatriptan and some candidate genes. J Headache Pain 3: 185–189.

Aurora SK, Barrodale P, Chronicle EP et al. (2005a). Cortical inhibition is reduced in chronic and episodic migraine and demonstrates a spectrum of illness. Headache 45: 546–552.

Aurora SK, Barrodale PM, McDonald SM et al. (2005b). Preliminary evidence for improved efficacy when patients treat with sumatriptan 100 mg formulated with RT technology during visual aura in migraine. Cephalalgia 25: 928.

Ayata C, Jin H, Kudo C et al. (2006). Suppression of cortical spreading depression in migraine prophylaxis. Ann Neurol 59: 652–661.

Barbanti P, Fabbrini G, Vanacore N et al. (2000). Dopamine and migraine: does Parkinson's disease modify migraine course? Cephalalgia 20: 720–723.

Barbanti P, Fabbrini G, Pesare M et al. (2002). Unilateral cranial autonomic symptoms in migraine. Cephalalgia 22: 256–259.

Barbanti P, Fabbrini G, Vanacore N et al. (2003). Sumatriptan in migraine with unilateral cranial autonomic symptoms: an open study. Headache 43: 400–403.

Bolay H, Moskowitz MA (2005). The emerging importance of cortical spreading depression in migraine headache. Rev Neurol (Paris) 161: 655–657.

Bolay H, Reuter U, Dunn AK et al. (2002). Intrinsic brain activity triggers trigeminal meningeal afferents in a migraine model. Nat Med 8: 136–142.

Bouchelet I, Cohen Z, Case B et al. (1996). Differential expression of sumatriptan-sensitive 5-hydroxytryptamine receptors in human trigeminal ganglia and cerebral blood vessels. Mol Pharmacol 50: 219–223.

Burstein R (2001). Deconstructing migraine headache into peripheral and central sensitization. Pain 89: 107–110.

Burstein R, Yamamura H, Malick A et al. (1998). Chemical stimulation of the intracranial dura induces enhanced responses to facial stimulation in brain stem trigeminal neurons. J Neurophysiol 79: 964–982.

Burstein R, Yarnitsky D, Goor-Aryeh I et al. (2000a). An association between migraine and cutaneous allodynia. Ann Neurol 47: 614–624.

Burstein R, Cutrer MF, Yarnitsky D (2000b). The development of cutaneous allodynia during a migraine attack clinical evidence for the sequential recruitment of spinal and supraspinal nociceptive neurons in migraine. Brain 123: 1703–1709.

Burstein R, Collins B, Jakubowski M (2004). Defeating migraine pain with triptans: a race against the development of cutaneous allodynia. Ann Neurol 55: 19–26.

Buzzi MG (2007). Triptan efficacy in migraine attacks: from appropriate diagnosis to metabolic profiles and pharmacogenomics. Drug Dev Res 68: 335–340.

Buzzi MG, Moskowitz MA (1990). The antimigraine drug, sumatriptan (GR43175), selectively blocks neurogenic plasma extravasation from blood vessels in dura mater. Br J Pharmacol 99: 202–206.

Buzzi MG, Moskowitz MA (1991). Evidence for 5-HT1B/1D receptors mediating the antimigraine effect of sumatriptan and dihydroergotamine. Cephalalgia 11: 165–168.

Buzzi MG, Moskowitz MA (2005). The pathophysiology of migraine: year 2005. J Headache Pain 6: 105–111.

Buzzi MG, Carter WB, Shimizu T et al. (1991a). Dihydroergotamine and sumatriptan attenuate levels of CGRP in plasma in rat superior sagittal sinus during electrical stimulation of the trigeminal ganglion. Neuropharmacology 30: 1193–1200.

Buzzi MG, Moskowitz MA, Peroutka SJ et al. (1991b). Further characterization of the putative 5-HT receptor which mediates blockade of neurogenic plasma extravasation in rat dura mater. Br J Pharmacol 103: 1421–1428.

Buzzi MG, Bivona U, Matteis M et al. (2003). Cognitive and psychological patterns in post-traumatic headache following severe traumatic brain injury. Cephalalgia 23: 581.

Buzzi MG, Cologno D, Formisano R (2005a). Migraine disease: evolution and progression. J Headache Pain 6: 304–306.

Buzzi MG, Cologno D, Formisano R et al. (2005b). Prodromes and the early phase of the migraine attack: therapeutic relevance. Funct Neurol 20: 179–183.

Cohen GL (2005). Migraine prophylactic drugs work via ion channels. Med Hypotheses 65: 114–122.

Cologno D, Torelli P, Mazoni GC (1998). Migraine with aura. A review of 81 patients at 10-20 years follow-up. Cephalalgia 18: 690–696.

Cutrer FM (2006). Pathophysiology of migraine. Semin Neurol 26: 171–180.

Cutrer FM, Sorensen AG, Weisskoff RM et al. (1988). Perfusion weighted imaging defects during spontaneous migrainous aura. Ann Neurol 43: 25–31.

De Fusco M, Marconi R, Silvestri L et al. (2003). Haploinsufficiency of ATP1A2 encoding the Na^+/K^+ pump alpha2 subunit associated with familial hemiplegic migraine type 2. Nat Genet 33: 192–196.

Dichgans M, Freilinger T, Eckstein G et al. (2005). Mutation in the neuronal voltage-gated sodium channel SCN1A in familial hemiplegic migraine. Lancet 366: 371–377.

Diener HC, Limmroth V (2001). Advances in pharmacological treatment of migraine. Exp Opin Invest Drugs 10: 1831–1845.

Dimitriadou V, Buzzi MG, Moskowitz MA et al. (1991). Trigeminal sensory fiber stimulation induces morphological changes reflecting secretion in rat dura mater mast cells. Neuroscience 44: 97–112.

Dimitriadou V, Buzzi MG, Theoharides TC et al. (1992). Ultrastructural evidence for neurogenically mediated changes in blood vessels of the rat dura mater and tongue following antidromic trigeminal stimulation. Neuroscience 48: 187–203.

Dodick DW (2005). Triptan non-responder studies: implications for clinical practice. Headache 45: 156–162.

Ekbom K, Krabbe A, Micieli G et al. (1995). Cluster headache attacks treated for up to three months with sucutaneous sumatriptan (6 mg). Cephalalgia 15: 230–236.

Eriksen MK, Thomsen LL, Russell MB (2004). Prognosis of migraine with aura. Cephalalgia 24: 18–22.

Evans DC, O'Connor D, Lake BG et al. (2003). Eletriptan metabolism by human hepatic CYP450 enzymes and transport by human P-glycoprotein. Drug Metab Dispos 31: 861–869.

Evans WE, Relling MV (1999). Pharmacogenomics: translating functional genomics into rational therapeutics. Science 286: 487–491.

Ferrari A, Sternieri E, Ferraris E et al. (2003). Emerging problems in the pharmacology of migraine: interactions between triptans and drugs for prophylaxis. Pharmacol Res 48: 1–9.

Ferrari MD, Roon KI, Lipton RB et al. (2001). Oral triptans (serotonin 5-HT agonists) in acute migraine treatment. Lancet 358: 1668–1675.

Fisher CM (1980). Late-life migraine accompaniments as a cause of unexplained transient ischemic attacks. Can J Neurol Sci 7: 9–17.

Gardner-Medwin AR, van Bruggen N, Williams SR et al. (1994). Magnetic resonance imaging of propagating waves of spreading depression in the anaesthetised rat. J Cereb Blood Flow Metab 14: 7–11.

Giffin NJ, Ruggiero L, Lipton RB et al. (2003). Premonitory symptoms in migraine: an electronic diary study. Neurology 60: 935–940.

Goadsby PJ, Lipton RB (1997). A review of paroxysmal hemicranias, SUNCT syndrome and other shortlasting headaches with autonomic feature, including new cases. Brain 120: 193–209.

Goadsby PJ, Edvinsson L, Ekman R (1990). Vasoactive peptide release in the extracerebral circulation of humans during migraine headache. Ann Neurol 28: 183–187.

Goldberg MR, Sciberras D, De Smet M et al. (2001). Influence of beta-adrenoceptor antagonists on the pharmacokinetics of rizatriptan, a 5-HT1B/1D agonist: differential effects of propranolol, nadolol and metoprolol. Br J Clin Pharmacol 52: 69–76.

Gursoy-Ozdemir Y, Qiu J, Matsuoka N et al. (2004). Cortical spreading depression activates and upregulates MMP-9. J Clin Invest 113: 1447–1455.

Haan J, Hollander J, Ferrari MD (2007). Migraine in the elderly: a review. Cephalalgia 27: 97–106.

Hadjikhani N, Sanchez Del Rio M, Wu O et al. (2001). Mechanisms of migraine aura revealed by functional MRI in human visual cortex. Proc Natl Acad Sci U S A 98: 4687–4692.

Hagen K, Stovner LJ, Zwart J-A (2007). Potentials and pitfalls in analytical headache epidemiological studies – lessons to be learned by the Head-HUNT Study. Cephalalgia 27: 403–413.

Headache Classification Committee of the International Headache Society (1988). Classification and diagnostic criteria for headache disorders, cranial neuralgias and facial pain. Cephalalgia 8 (Suppl. 7): 1–96.

Headache Classification Subcommittee of the International Headache Society (2004). The International Classification of Headache Disorders, 2nd edn. Cephalalgia 24 (Suppl. 1): 1–160.

Hirata H, Takeshita S, Hu JW et al. (2000). Cornea-responsive medullary dorsal horn neurons: modulation by local opioids and projections to thalamus and brain stem. J Neurophysiol 84: 1050–1061.

Humphrey PA (2007). The discovery of a new drug class for the acute treatment of migraine. Headache 47 (Suppl. 1): S10–S19.

Humphrey PP, Feniuk W, Perren MJ et al. (1988). GR43175, a selective agonist for the 5-HT1-like receptor in dog isolated saphenous vein. Br J Pharmacol 94: 1123–1132.

International Headache Society Clinical Trials Subcommittee (2000). Guidelines for controlled trials of drugs in migraine: second edition. Cephalalgia 20: 765–786.

International Headache Society Committee on Clinical Trials in Migraine (1991). Guidelines for controlled trials of drugs in migraine: first edition. Cephalalgia 11: 1–12.

Kimmelstiel C, Gange C, Thaler D (2007). Is patent foramen ovale closure effective in reducing migraine symptoms? A controlled study. Catheter Cardiovasc Interv 69: 740–746.

Lauritzen M, Olesen J (1984). Regional cerebral blood flow during migraine attacks by xenon-133 inhalation and emission tomography. Brain 107: 447–461.

Lauritzen M, Skyhoj Olsen T, Lassen NA et al. (1983). Changes of regional cerebral blood flow during the course of classical migraine attacks. Ann Neurol 13: 633–641.

Leão AAP (1944). Spreading depression of activity in the cerebral cortex. J Neurophysiol 7: 359–390.

Leonardi M, Steiner TJ, Scher A et al. (2005). The global burden of migraine measuring disability in headache disorders with WHO's classification of functioning, disability and health (ICF). J Head Pain 6: 429–440.

Levy D, Jakubowski M, Burstein R (2004). Disruption of communication between peripheral and central trigeminovascular neurons mediates the antimigraine action of 5HT 1B/1D receptor agonists. Proc Natl Acad Sci USA 101: 4274–4279.

Li BU, Balint JP (2000). Cyclic vomiting syndrome: evolution in our understanding of a brain–gut disorder. Adv Pediatr 47: 117–160.

Linde M (2006). Migraine: a review and future directions for treatment. Acta Neurol Scand 114: 71–83.

Linde M, Mellberg A, Dahlof C (2006). The natural course of migraine attacks. A prospective analysis of untreated attacks compared to treated. Cephalalgia 26: 712–721.

Luciani R, Carter D, Mannix L et al. (2000). Prevention of migraine during prodrome with naratriptan. Cephalalgia 20: 122–126.

Lyngberg AC, Rasmussen BK, Jorgensen T et al. (2005). Prognosis of migraine and tension-type headache. A population-based follow-up study. Neurology 65: 580–585.

Maassen Van DenBrink A, Vergouwe MN, Ophoff RA et al. (1996). 5-HT1B receptor polymorphism and clinical response to sumatriptan. Headache 3: 268–291.

Markowitz S, Saito K, Moskowitz MA (1987). Neurogenically mediated leakage of plasma protein occurs from blood vessels in dura mater but not brain. J Neurosci 7: 4129–4136.

Martins KM, Bordini CA, Bigal ME et al. (2006). Migraine in the elderly: a comparison with migraine in young adults. Headache 46: 312–316.

May A, Kaube H, Buchel C et al. (1998). Experimental cranial pain elicited by capsaicin: a PET study. Pain 74: 61–66.

Mayberg MR, Zervas NT, Moskowitz MA (1984). Trigeminal projections to supratentorial pial and dural blood vessels in cats demonstrated by horseradish peroxidase histochemistry. J Comp Neurol 223: 46–56.

Merikangas KR, Rasmussen BK (2000). Migraine comorbidity. In: J Olesen, P Tfelt-Hansen, KMA Welch (Eds.), The Headaches, 2nd edn. Lippincott Williams & Wilkins, Philadelphia, pp. 235–240.

Moskowitz MA (1984). The neurobiology of vascular head pain. Ann Neurol 16: 157–168.

Moskowitz MA (1988). Cluster headache: evidence for a pathophysiologic focus in the superior pericarotid cavernous plexus. Headache 28: 584–586.

Moskowitz MA, Buzzi MG (1991). Neuroeffector functions of sensory fibres: implications for headache mechanisms and drug actions. J Neurol 238 (Suppl. 1): S18–S22.

Moskowitz MA, Nozaki K, Kraig RP (1993). Neocortical spreading depression provokes the expression of c-fos protein-like immunoreactivity within trigeminal nucleus caudalis via trigeminovascular mechanisms. J Neurosci 13: 1167–1177.

Moskowitz MA, Bolay H, Dalkara T (2004). Deciphering migraine mechanisms: clues from familial hemiplegic migraine genotypes. Ann Neurol 55: 276–280.

Nozaki K, Boccalini P, Moskowitz MA (1992). Expression of c-foslike immunoreactivity in brainstem after meningeal irritation by blood in the subarachnoid space. Neuroscience 49: 669–680.

Obermann M, Yoon M-S, Dommes P et al. (2007). Prevalence of trigeminal autonomic symptoms in migraine: a population-based study. Cephalalgia 27: 504–509.

Olesen J, Larsen B, Lauritzen M (1981). Focal hyperemia followed by spreading oligemia and impaired activation of rCBF in classic migraine. Ann Neurol 9: 344–352.

Olesen J, Diener HC, Schoenen J et al. (2004). No effect of eletriptan administration during the aura phase of migraine. Eur J Neurol 11: 671–677.

Ophoff RA, Terwindt GM, Vergouwe MN et al. (1996). Familial hemiplegic migraine and episodic ataxia type-2 are caused by mutations in the Ca^{2+} channel gene CACNL1A4. Cell 87: 543–552.

Pascual J, Munoz P (2005). Correlation between lipophilicity and triptan outcomes. Headache 45: 3–6.

Ross JS, Schenkein DP, Kashala O et al. (2004). Pharmacogenomics. Adv Anat Pathol 11: 211–220.

Russell MB (2007). Genetics in primary headaches. J Headache Pain 8: 190–195.

Saito K, Markowitz S, Moskowitz MA (1988). Ergot alkaloids block neurogenic extravasation in dura mater: proposed action in vascular headaches. Ann Neurol 24: 732–737.

Sanchez-del-Rio M, Reuter U, Moskowitz MA (2006). New insights into migraine pathophysiology. Curr Opin Neurol 19: 294–298.

Sarchielli P, Pini LA, Zanchin G et al. (2006). Clinical–biochemical correlates of migraine attacks to rizatriptan responders and non-responders. Cephalalgia 26: 257–265.

Saxena PR, Tfelt-Hansen P (2006). Triptans, 5-HT1B/1D receptor agonists in the acute treatment of migraines. In: J Olesen, PJ Goadsby, NM Ramadan et al. (Eds.), The Headaches, 3rd edn. Lippincott Williams and Wilkins, Philadelphia, pp. 469–503.

Schoenen J (2006). Neurophysiological features of the migrainous brain. Neurol Sci 27 (Suppl. 2): S77–S81.

Schoonman GG, Evers DJ, Terwindt GM et al. (2006). The prevalence of premonitory symptoms in migraine: a questionnaire study in 461 patients. Cephalalgia 26: 1209–1213.

Silberstein SD (2000). Practice parameter: evidence-based guidelines for migraine headache (an evidence-based review): report of the quality standards subcommittee of the American Academy of Neurology. Neurology 55: 754–762.

Silberstein SD, Freitag FG (2003). Preventive treatment of migraine. Neurology 60: S38–S44.

Slavin L, Tobis JM, Rangarajan K et al. (2007). Five-year experience with percutaneous closure of patent foramen ovale. Am J Cardiol 99: 1316–1320.

Steiner TJ (2004). Lifting the burden: the global campaign against headache. Lancet Neurol 3: 204–205.

Stovner LJ, Hagen K, Jensen R et al. (2007). The global burden of headache: a documentation of headache prevalence and disability worldwide. Cephalalgia 27: 193–210.

Subcutaneous Sumatriptan International Study Group (1991). Treatment of migraine attacks with sumatriptan. N Engl J Med 325: 316–321.

van den Maagdenberg AM, Pietrobon D, Pizzorusso T et al. (2004). A CACNA1A knockin migraine mouse model with increased susceptibility to cortical spreading depression. Neuron 41: 701–710.

Wang SJ, Fuh JL, Juang KD et al. (2005). Evolution of migraine diagnoses in adolescents: a 3-year annual survey. Cephalalgia 25: 333–338.

Weiller C, May A, Limmroth V et al. (1995). Brain stem activation in spontaneous human migraine attacks. Nat Med 1: 658–660.

Welch KMA, Levine SR, D'Andrea G et al. (1989). Preliminary observations on brain energy metabolites in migraine studied by in vivo 31-phosphorus NMR spectroscopy. Neurology 39: 538–541.

Welch KMA, Barkley GL, Ramadan NM et al. (1992). NMR spectroscopic and magnetoencephalographic studies in migraine with aura: support for the spreading depression hypothesis. Pathol Biol (Paris) 40: 349–354.

Wolff HG (1963). Headache and Other Head Pain. 2nd edn. Oxford University Press, New York.

Woods RP, Iacoboni M, Mazziotta JC (1994). Bilateral spreading cerebral hypoperfusion during spontaneous migraine headache. N Engl J Med 331: 1689–1692.

World Health Organization (2007). International Statistical Classification of Diseases and Related Health Problems (ICD-10). World Health Organization, Geneva.

Handbook of Clinical Neurology, Vol. 97 (3rd series)
Headache
G. Nappi and M.A. Moskowitz, Editors

Chapter 22

Pathophysiology of migraine

SHEENA K. AURORA[1]* AND VIJAYA NAGESH[2]
[1]*Swedish Headache Center, Seattle, WA, USA*
[2]*Department of Radiation Oncology, University of Michigan Medical School, Ann Arbor, MI, USA*

INTRODUCTION

Headache is one of the most common presenting symptoms to a physician's office. The majority of headaches are in the category known as primary headaches where there are no structural disturbances. Secondary headaches are uncommon and usually occur in less than 10% of patients. The mechanisms of secondary headaches are usually due to the underlying pathology. These are usually quite evident on neuroimaging or laboratory testing. This chapter will mainly focus on mechanisms of migraine.

There have been remarkable strides in the last few decades mainly brought about by advanced imaging techniques which have helped to unravel the underlying basis of primary headache disorders. The vascular theory has been superseded by the neurovascular phenomenon which seems to be the permissive triggering factor in migraine and cluster headache. This has been achieved through new imaging modalities such as positron emission tomography (PET) and functional magnetic resonance imaging (fMRI). Prior to these imaging techniques it was impossible to study the primary headache disorders since these headaches had no structural basis. There is now an increasing body of evidence that the neuronal structures are involved primarily in cluster and migraine headaches and that vessel dilation is an epiphenomenon.

The exact pathogenesis of migraine remains to be determined. The pendulum for concepts of migraine pathophysiology swung between primary vascular and primary neural mechanisms. Harold G. Wolff, a pioneer of the vascular theory of migraine, proposed that the neurological symptoms of the migraine aura were caused by cerebral vasoconstriction, and the headache by vasodilation (Wolff, 1963). Lashley's experience of his own visual aura led him to the concept that the cortical spreading depression (CSD) of Leão was the primary cause (Lashley, 1941), thus promulgating the neural theory of migraine (Leão, 1944; Teive et al., 2005). Newer imaging techniques have made it possible to study the very early events of migraine; thus both theories have been reconciled by contemporary proponents of a neurovascular mechanism of the migraine attack. There is evidence for an inherited disorder that occurs in susceptible individuals.

There is also an increasing body of evidence for the concept of central neuronal hyperexcitability as a pivotal physiological disturbance predisposing to migraine (Welch et al., 1990). The reasons for increased neuronal excitability may be multifactorial. Through genetic studies abnormality of calcium channels has been introduced as a potential mechanism of interictal neuronal excitability (Ophoff et al., 1996). Mutant voltage-gated P/Q-type calcium channel genes likely influence presynaptic neurotransmitter release, possibly of excitatory amino acid systems' lack of inhibitory control. Other genetic studies have demonstrated dysfunction in the *ATP1A2* gene which encodes an ion pump (De Fusco et al., 2003; Marconi et al., 2003). This mutation may make the migraine brain more vulnerable to events like CSD.

Recently data in episodic ataxia and hemiplegic migraine patients with no mutation in either *CACNA1A* or *ATP1A2* demonstrated a heterozygous mutation in *EAAT1* that can lead to decreased glutamate uptake, which can contribute to neuronal hyperexcitability to cause seizures, hemiplegia, and episodic ataxia (Jen et al., 2005). It could therefore be hypothesized that genetic abnormalities result in a lowered threshold of response to trigger factors, since migraine is an episodic disorder involving head pain and cortical

*Correspondence to: S.K. Aurora, MD, Swedish Headache Center, 1101 Madison, Suite 200, Seattle, WA 98104, USA, E-mail: Sheena.Aurora@swedish.org

phenomena without structural abnormalities (Haan et al., 2005). Therefore, investigations aimed at studying the function of the brain provide insight into migraine pathophysiology. In this chapter the mechanism of aura and head pain will be discussed followed by a discussion of interictal disturbances which lead to a propensity to developing migraine.

MECHANISMS OF AURA

The unpredictable and elusive nature of migraine has prevented many investigators from systematically studying migraine aura. Studies by Cao et al. (1999a), where migraine was reliably visually triggered in 50% of subjects, enabled the immediate early events of the migraine attack to be measured for the first time. A red and green checkerboard was used for visual stimulation since migraineurs are known to be sensitive to linear stimuli. Using the recently developed fMRI methods, based on the blood oxygen level-dependent (BOLD) technique, the authors were able to measure, with millimeter resolution, the second-to-second activation of the occipital cortex to visual stimulation. None of six normal controls developed a headache and displayed normal patterns of BOLD signals on visual activation. Six patients with migraine with aura and two patients with migraine without aura had experienced visually triggered headache; two also had accompanying visual change. Headache was preceded by suppression of brain activation that slowly propagated into contiguous occipital cortex at a rate ranging from 3 to 6 mm/min. This neuronal suppression was accompanied by an increase in baseline contrast intensity, indicative of vasodilation and tissue hyperoxygenation. The baseline contrast increases indicated that tissue hyperoxygenation was similar to those witnessed in experimental CSD (Gardner-Medwin et al., 1994). These spreading events accompanied visually triggered headache whether or not it was associated with visual change.

In this study patients were selected based on a history of visually triggered headache, so that generalizing these findings to all migraine patients must be done with caution. Nevertheless, previously hypothesized mechanisms of CSD in migraine were clarified by this study, and the previously controversial findings of ischemia accompanying migraine aura were not supported.

Spontaneous migraine with aura has been described by Hadjikhani et al. (2001) with similar changes on BOLD fMRI as described by Cao et al. (1999a). Although it was only a case report, a critical study demonstrated spreading events on PET during migraine without aura (Woods et al., 1994). These studies and one critical case report demonstrate spreading-like events of blood flow during migraine. These phenomena are reminiscent of CSD and convincing proof of this came from magnetoencephalography (MEG) studies discussed in this review later. Recently, propogating calcium channel waves have been reported to occur convincingly using models to trigger CSD. These waves seemed to occur in multiple areas and were not restricted to the area of application of potassium chloride. This preliminary work suggests that there may be a spreading event that accompanies migraine which seem akin but does not exactly match the animal events of CSD (Brennan et al., 2007).

In a different study using perfusion-weighted imaging (PWI), another novel functional neuroimaging technique particularly suited to study short-lived events such as migraine aura, 19 patients were studied during spontaneous migraine (Sanchez del Rio et al., 1999). Twenty-eight attacks were studied because some patients were imaged more than once. There was a relative reduction of cerebral blood flow in the occipital cortex contralateral to the visual defect during migraine with aura, but this was observed only in the occipital cortex and not other brain regions. One subject who experienced attacks of both migraine with aura and migraine without aura demonstrated these phenomena only during migraine with aura. No significant changes in blood flow were observed in migraine without aura. The hemodynamic changes were demonstrated only on PWI and not on diffusion-weighted imaging (DWI); DWI is sensitive to ischemia and thus further supports migraine with aura not being an ischemic event.

These imaging studies, although they favor the neural basis of migraine, are not able to demonstrate CSD as the putative mechanism of migraine aura. To date, CSD has been recorded successfully in animal models (Bowyer et al., 1999a, b). In animals, the CSD's band of hyperexcited neurons travels into sulci or fissures eliciting signals that can be detected on MEG. Using the seven channels of MEG, Barkley et al. (1990) reported direct-current (DC) shifts in spontaneous migraine.

A further study of a larger number of patients has not been possible because of the unpredictable nature of migraine and time of capture of these spontaneous events. Using the visual trigger modeled by Cao et al. (1999b), Bowyer et al. (2001) have now been able to detect DC shifts when headache or aura was precipitated. These studies were performed using a whole-head MEG (148 channels), which permits a precise localization of signals. In this study headache was triggered in 5 of 8 migraine patients and none of 6 controls. DC MEG shifts were observed in migraine subjects during visually triggered aura and in a patient studied during the first few minutes of spontaneous aura. No DC

MEG shifts were seen in control subjects. This is additional evidence supporting the primary neural basis of migraine and confirms MEG-recorded DC shifts typical of those found during CSD, reported previously in migraine attacks.

DC MEG waveforms arising during migraine aura were used to determine the effectiveness of prophylactic medication therapy valproate on neuronal hyperexcitability. Using visual stimulation, widespread regions of hyperexcitability were detected throughout the occipital cortex in migraine patients, explaining the susceptibility for triggering CSD and migraine aura. After 30 days of prophylactic treatment, reduced DC MEG shifts in the occipital cortex and reduced incidence of migraine attacks were observed. This study confirmed that MEG can non-invasively determine the status of neuronal excitability before and after therapy (Bowyer et al., 2005). Similar findings have been found with topiramate (unpublished Henry Ford Hospital MEG laboratory).

MECHANISM OF MIGRAINE PAIN

From recent experimental and clinical data the brainstem and specifically the trigeminovascular system have been implicated as playing a large role during a migraine attack (Raskin et al., 1987). It is hypothesized that a sterile inflammatory response occurs due to the release of neuropeptides, i.e., calcitonin gene-related peptide, neurokinin A, and substance P (Raskin et al., 1987). The development of novel antimigraine drugs for the treatment of migraine has been based predominantly on these animal models The importance of the trigeminovascular system is further strengthened by the discovery of binding sites for the serotonin (5-HT) 1B/1D agonists on central terminals of primary afferents within human brainstem (Moskowitz, 1984; Raskin et al., 1987; Goadsby and Gundlach, 1991; Longmore et al., 1997).

The first human study to show activation in the brainstem used PET performed in subjects during spontaneous migraine. Recently we have completed PET scans on 10 migraine subjects and demonstrated increased cerebral metabolism in areas of the brainstem compared to global flow (Aurora et al., 2007). There were also decreased areas of cerebral metabolism in the medial frontal and parietal as well as the somatosensory cortex. This would suggest perhaps that the normal inhibitory tone of the higher cortical centers is disturbed and therefore the brainstem may have increased activity in the pain pathways in chronic migraine. Because PET lacks sufficient resolution for exact anatomical localization, we hypothesized that the activation was in the regions of dorsal raphe nuclei, periaqueductal gray (PAG), and locus coeruleus (Weiller et al., 1995). An isolated case report found red nucleus (RN) and substantia nigra (SN) to be activated in a spontaneous migraine attack (Welch et al., 1998). The same authors also now report that RN and SN were activated in subjects with visually triggered migraine (Cao et al., 1999b). RN and SN are best known for their functional roles in motor control. RN, however, has also been associated with pain and/or nociception (Iadarola et al., 1998). Numerous animal studies have documented a response of RN neurons to a variety of sensory and noxious stimuli. In a PET study performed on normal volunteers during capsaicin-induced pain, ipsilateral activation of RN was documented. It remains to be clarified whether or not RN is involved in the pain pathways or in the motor response to pain.

The PAG has a large influence on the nociceptive pathways with extensive networks from thalamus, hypothalamus, and autonomic nervous system. The PAG was found to be dysfunctional in migraine with an increased non-heme content, which increased with the chronicity of migraine studied interictally (Welch et al., 2001). During migraine the PAG was shown to be hyperactive in PET studies (Bahra et al., 2001). The ventrolateral subdivision of the PAG is of particular importance to trigeminal nociceptive modulation (Knight and Goadsby, 2001). A genetic link to the predisposition of hyperactivity in the nociceptive system in migraine has been established (Knight et al., 2002). Using a microinjection of the P/Q channel blocker ω-agatoxin-IVA into the rat ventrolateral PAG, a facilitation of neuronal activity was noted in the trigeminal nociceptive pathway (Knight and Goadsby, 2001). This study demonstrated the influence of both the P/Q-type calcium channels and PAG in trigeminal pronociception.

The link between aura and pain

The mystery of how a brain event, i.e. CSD, starting in an insensate part of the brain evolves into a painful disorder has been elucidated. Bolay et al. (2002) demonstrated an increase in flow of the middle meningeal artery (MMA) after CSD, which was triggered by pinprick in experimental animals. To clarify the mechanisms underlying these events the trigeminal nerve was transected, resulting in a lack of the delayed phase of increased blood flow in MMA. Further, the expression of c-fos as a surrogate marker of pain was increased in lamina I and II in the nucleus caudalis. There was also plasma protein extravasation observed in the experiment, which was noted to be mediated by neurokinin I. This landmark study clearly demonstrated the link between the head pain of migraine and CSD as the putative mechanism of aura.

The exact neurotransmitters are unknown. One potential important mediator of plasma protein extravasation may be nitric oxide (NO). Migraine may be induced in patients by an infusion of nitroglycerine. This induction may be delayed by 4–6 h (Olesen et al., 1993). The underlying pathogenetic mechanism has been noted to be a delayed inflammatory response in the dura mater, increased expression of inducible NO synthase (iNOS), and upregulation of proinflammatory cytokines interleukin (IL)-1β and IL-6 (Reuter et al., 2001). Thus NO is intimately involved with the process of plasma protein extravasation. Interestingly, as patients after glyceryl trinitrate infusion never develop aura, one may therefore hypothesize that NO may be induced after CSD. During migraine NO metabolites, i.e., nitrites/nitrates and secondary messengers of NO, i.e., cyclic guanosine monophosphate, have been demonstrated to be increased in platelets (Read et al., 1997; Stepien and Chalimoniuk, 1998). One might hypothesize that fluctuation in NO may be an independent reason for plasma protein extravasation leading to activation of the trigeminal vascular system, resulting in migraine headache but without involvement of cortical structures.

Evidence of interictal disturbances

Electroencephalography (EEG) was one of the first techniques that was undertaken to discern physiological differences between migraine patients and controls. A thorough review suggests that EEG is not a valuable diagnostic tool for primary headache disorders (Gronseth and Greenberg, 1995). The enhanced photic drive response on the EEG, known as the H-response, was thought to be characteristic of migraine (Golla and Winter, 1982) and has been confirmed by spectral analysis (Golla and Winter, 1982; Simon et al., 1982). The specificity of the H-response, however, has been questioned since it may occur with other primary headache disorders (Pechadre and Gibert, 1987). Abnormal steady-state response evoked by a sine-wave visual stimulus was seen in migraineurs, and improved after administration of propranolol (Nyrke et al., 1984, 1989). Finally, following a repetitive pattern reversal stimulation, migraineurs, but not controls, displayed potentiation of visual evoked potential (VEP) amplitude, which reached its maximum in the second to fourth blocks (Schoenen et al., 1995). Similar results were seen using prolonged stimulation (Afra et al., 1998a). However, in agreement with VEP studies, strong interictal dependence of the auditory evoked potentials on stimulus intensity was demonstrated in migraine patients (Wang et al., 1996). Furthermore, the response was modulated by zolmitriptan (Cecchini et al., 1997).

Transcranial magnetic stimulation (TMS) has been developed to study cortical physiology non-invasively (Barker et al., 1985, 1987) and this technique is now increasingly being used to study migraine.

TMS OF MOTOR CORTEX IN MIGRAINE

Several studies have been performed investigating the motor cortex of migraineurs using TMS. Three studies have been performed on the motor cortex, two of which reported increased excitability in migraineurs and suggested that this neurophysiological correlate may have a role in migraine mechanisms (Bettucci et al., 1992; Maertens de Noordhout et al., 1992). The first study compared subjects with migraine with and without aura to controls and demonstrated an increased motor threshold in classic migraine (Maertens de Noordhout et al., 1992). The motor threshold was increased on the side corresponding to the aura. The threshold difference could not be attributed to attack frequency. The second study was performed on menstrual migraineurs during the cycle compared to controls (Bettucci et al., 1992). An increased threshold was demonstrated, similar to the first study, but in this study the patients had migraine without aura.

Following these studies two other studies were performed. In the first study there was a difference in amplitude of motor evoked potentials in migraine with aura compared to controls, but no differences were found in the motor threshold (van der Kamp et al., 1996). The differences in this study compared to previous reports of increased threshold were explained on the basis of attack frequency, which was higher in this group of patients.

In a second study performed in familial hemiplegic migraine, the threshold of motor cortex was higher on the side corresponding to the aura (van der Kamp et al., 1997). Using paired pulses a study demonstrated reduced motor cortical excitability after administration of zolmitriptan, a centrally acting 5-$HT_{IB/D}$ receptor agonist used in the treatment of migraine (Werhahn et al., 1998). This technique thus provides a new opportunity to study cortical physiology and the effects of drugs in migraine.

CORTICAL SILENT PERIOD IN MIGRAINE

Two studies have examined the cortical silent period (CSP), which is thought to be a marker of inhibitory function. Although the results were judged to be preliminary, both reported no differences in CSP at high levels of stimulus intensity (Afra et al., 1998b; Aurora et al., 1999a), but at low stimulus intensity a shorter

CSP was documented in migraine with aura compared to controls (Aurora et al., 1999a). Since the CSP, in part, is a measure of central inhibition of motor pathways, this shortening of the CSP suggests reduced central inhibition, inferring increased excitability.

TMS OF OCCIPITAL CORTEX IN MIGRAINE

Using TMS to study the occipital cortex is perhaps more relevant to migraine because enhanced excitability of the occipital cortex may underlie either spontaneous or visually triggered migraine aura (Teive et al., 2005). Occipital cortex excitability in migraine has been evaluated by the generation of phosphenes by TMS in the occipital cortex. The first study reported a low threshold for generation of phosphenes in subjects with migraine with aura, inferring hyperexcitability of the occipital cortex (Aurora et al., 1999b). In contrast, occipital cortex hypoexcitability was reported in migraine with aura based on a lower prevalence of phosphenes stimulated by TMS (Afra et al., 1998b). Important technical differences, such as the type of stimulator or coil size, might explain these conflicting findings (Aurora and Welch, 1999).

Since these early reports there have been two more studies performed on the occipital cortex using TMS, both confirming the initial reports of hyperexcitability (Aggugia et al., 1999; Aurora et al., 1999c). In one of these studies hyperexcitability of the occipital cortex was associated with a propensity to visually triggered headache in the same patients (Aurora et al., 1999c).

Battelli and colleagues (2002) investigated the extrastriate visual area V5, which is important for the perception of motion. Both migraine with and migraine without aura groups required significantly lower magnetic field strength for the induction of moving phosphenes, as compared to the control group; this difference was significant for V5 in both left and right hemispheres. In addition the phosphenes were better defined and had clearer presentation in migraine groups, whereas in controls they tended to be more transient and ill defined.

Most studies with TMS utilized the subjective sensation of phosphenes as a measure of excitability. Although these studies have shown important differences in migraine, the lack of objectivity makes data interpretation difficult. We have therefore developed objective physiological measures to assess differences in cortical excitability. To assess inhibitory function of the occipital cortex a visual suppression method was utilized. Timed TMS impulses, usually 10% above phosphene threshold or where suppression was noted, were delivered to the visual cortex. Subjects were asked to report letters projected at a fixed luminance on the screen. Visual suppression was calculated based on the number of errors the subjects made. Using an automated analysis our results confirmed that migraineurs had reduced errors, demonstrating a reduction in visual suppression (Aurora et al., 2005). We have recently completed a study demonstrating a spectrum of illness in chronic migraine. A cohort of these subjects demonstrated decreased metabolism in cerebral metabolism, thus correlating with the magnetic suppression of perceptual accuracy studies. Using this objective model we have some data on topiramate demonstrating dynamic changes in episodic and chronic migraine in two subjects. Topiramate seemed to balance the dysfunction in cortical inhibition seen in chronic migraine.

SUMMARY

We currently conceive of a migraine attack as originating in the brain. Triggers of an attack initiate a depolarizing neuroelectrical and metabolic event likened to the spreading depression of Leão. This event activates the headache and associated features of the attack by mechanisms that remain to be determined, but appear to involve either peripheral trigeminovascular or brainstem pathways, or both. Excitability of cell membranes, perhaps in part genetically determined, determines the brain's susceptibility to attacks. Factors that increase or decrease neuronal excitability constitute the threshold for triggering attacks.

Using a model of visual stress-induced migraine or by studying spontaneous attacks, and applying advanced imaging and neurophysiological methods, results have been obtained that support spreading neuronal inhibition as the basis of aura. This neuroelectrical event is accompanied by hyperoxia of the brain, possibly associated with vasodilation. Evidence has also been obtained that the spreading cortical event can activate subcortical centers possibly involved in nociception and associated symptoms of the migraine attack. Susceptibility to migraine attacks appears related to brain hyperexcitability. Newer techniques of functional neuroimaging have confirmed the primary neural basis of the migraine attack with secondary vascular changes, reconciling previous theories into a neurovascular mechanism.

References

Afra J, Cecchini AP, DePasqua V et al. (1998a). Visual evoked potentials during long periods of pattern-reversal stimualtion in migraine. Brain 121: 233–241.

Afra J, Mascia A, Gérard P et al. (1998b). Interictal cortical excitability in migraine: a study using transcranial magnetic stimulation of motor and visual cortices. Ann Neurol 44: 209–215.

Aggugia M, Zibetti M, Febbraro A et al. (1999). Transcranial magnetic stimulation in migraine with aura: further evidence of occipital cortex hyperexcitability. Cephalalgia 19: 465.

Aurora SK, Welch KMA (1999). Phosphene generation in migraine. Ann Neurol 45: 416.

Aurora SK, Al-Sayed F, Welch KMA (1999a). The cortical silent period is shortened in migraine with aura. Cephalalgia 19: 708–712.

Aurora SK, Al-Sayed F, Welch KMA (1999b). The threshold for magnetophoshenes is lower in migraine. Neurology 52: A472.

Aurora SK, Cao Y, Bowyer SM et al. (1999c). The occipital cortex is hyperexcitable in migraine; evidence from TMS, fmri and MEG studies (Wolff Award 1999). Headache 39: 469–476.

Aurora SK, Barrodale P, Chronicle EP et al. (2005). Cortical inhibition is reduced in chronic and episodic migraine and demonstrates a spectrum of illness. Headache 45: 546–552.

Aurora SK, Barrodale PM, Tipton RL et al. (2007). Brainstem dysfunction in chronic migraine as evidenced by neurophysiological and positron emission tomography studies. Headache 47(7): 996–1003.

Bahra A, Matharu MS, Buchel C et al. (2001). Brainstem activation specific to migraine headache. Lancet 357: 1016–1017.

Barker AT, Jalinous R, Freeston IL (1985). Non-invasive magnetic stimulation of human motor cortex. Lancet 1: 1106–1107.

Barker AT, Freeston IL, Jalinous R et al. (1987). Magnetic stimulation of the human brain and peripheral nervous system: an introduction and the results of an initial clinical evaluation. Neurosurgery 20: 100–109.

Barkley GL, Tepley N, Nagel-Leiby S et al. (1990). Magnetoencephalograhic studies of migraine. Headache 30: 428–434.

Battelli L, Black KR, Wray SH (2002). Transcranial magnetic stimulation of visual area V5 in migraine. Neurology 58: 1066–1069.

Bettucci D, Cantello R, Gianelli M et al. (1992). Menstrual migraine without aura: cortical excitability to magnetic stimulation. Headache 32: 345–347.

Bolay M, Reuter U, Dunn A et al. (2002). Intrinsic brain activity triggers trigeminal meningeal afferents in a migraine model. Nat Med 8: 136–142.

Bowyer SM, Okada YC, Papuashvili N et al. (1999a). Analysis of MEG signals of spreading cortical depression with propagation constrained to a rectangular cortical strip: I. Lissencephalic rabbit model. Brain Res 843: 79–86.

Bowyer SM, Tepley N, Papuashvili N et al. (1999b). Analysis of MEG signals of spreading cortical depression with propagation constrained to a rectangular cortical strip: II. Gyrencephalic swine model. Brain Res 843: 71–78.

Bowyer SM, Aurora SK, Moran JE et al. (2001). Magnetoencephalographic fields from patients with spontaneous and induced migraine aura. Ann Neurol 50: 582–587.

Bowyer SM, Moran JE, Tepley N et al. (2005). Cortical hyperexcitability in a migraine patient before and after sodium valproate treatment. J Clin Neurophysiol 22: 65–67.

Brennan KC, Beltrán-Parrazal L, López-Valdés HE et al. (2007). Distinct vascular conduction with cortical spreading depression. J Neurophysiol 97: 4143–4151.

Cao Y, Welch KMA, Aurora SK et al. (1999a). Functional MRI-BOLD of visually triggered headache and visual change in migraine sufferers. Arch Neurol 56: 548–554.

Cao Y, Aurora SK, Vikingstad EM et al. (1999b). Functional MRI of the red nucleus and occipital cortex during visual stimulation of subjects with migraine. Cepahalalgia 19: 462.

Cecchini AP, Afra J, Schoenen J (1997). Intensity dependence of the cortical auditory evoked potentials as a surrogate marer of CNS serotonin transmission in man: demonstration of a central effect for the 5-HT1B/1D agonist zomitriptan (311C90, Zomig). Cephalalgia 17: 1–18.

De Fusco M, Marconi R, Silvestri L et al. (2003). Haploinsufficiency of ATP1A2 encoding the Na^+/K^+ pump alpha2 subunit associated with familial hemiplegic migraine type 2. Nat Genet 33: 192–196.

Gardner-Medwin AR, Bruggen NV, Williams SR et al. (1994). Magnetic resonance imaging of propagating waves of spreading depression in the anaesthetised rat. J Cereb Blood Flow Metab 14: 7–11.

Goadsby PJ, Gundlach AL (1991). Localization of ^{3}H-dihydroergotamine-binding sites in cat central nervous system: relevance to migraine. Ann Neurol 29: 91–94.

Golla FL, Winter AL (1982). Analysis of cerebral responses to flicker in patients complaining of episodic headache. Electroencephalogr Clin Neurophysiol 53: 270–276.

Gronseth GS, Greenberg MK (1995). The utility of the electroencephalogram in the evaluation of patients presenting with headache: a review of the literature. Neurology 45: 1263–1267.

Haan J, Kors EE, Vanmolkot KR et al. (2005). Migraine genetics: an update. Curr Pain Headache Rep 9: 213–220.

Hadjikhani N, Sanchez Del Rio M, Wu O et al. (2001). Mechanisms of migraine aura revealed by functional MRI in human visual cortex. Proc Natl Acad Sci U S A 98: 4687–4692.

Iadarola MJ, Berman KF, Zeffiro TA et al. (1998). Neural activation during acute capsaicin-evoked pain and allodynia assessed with PET. Brain 121: 931–947.

Jen JC, Wan J, Palos TP et al. (2005). Mutation in the glutamate transporter EAAT1 causes episodic ataxia, hemiplegia, and seizures. Neurology 65: 529–534.

Knight YE, Goadsby PJ (2001). The periaqueductal grey matter modulates trigeminovascular input: a role in migraine? Neuroscience 106: 793–800.

Knight YE, Bartsch T, Kaube H et al. (2002). P/Q-type calcium-channel blockade in the periaqueductal gray facilitates trigeminal nociception: a functional genetic link for migraine. J Neurosci 22: 1–6.

Lashley KS (1941). Patterns of cerebral integration indicated by the scotomas of migraine. Arch Neurol Psychiatry 46: 331–339.

Leão AAP (1944). Spreading depression of activity in the cerebral cortex. J Neurophysiol 8: 379–390.

Longmore J, Shaw D, Smith D et al. (1997). Differential distribution of 5-HT 1D and 5-HT 1B immunoreactivity within the human trigemino-cerebrovascular system: implications for the discovery of new anti-migraine drugs. Cephalalgia 17: 835–842.

Maertens de Noordhout AL, Pepin JL, Schoenen J et al. (1992). Percutaneous magnetic stimulation of the motor cortex in migraine. Electroencephalogr Clin Neurophysiol 85: 110–115.

Marconi R, De Fusco M, Aridon P et al. (2003). Familial hemiplegic migraine type 2 is linked to 0.9Mb region on chromosome 1q23. Ann Neurol 53: 376–381.

Moskowitz MA (1984). The neurobiology of vascular head pain. Ann Neurol 15: 157–168.

Nyrke T, Kangasniemi P, Lang AH (1984). Steady-state visual evoked potentials during migraine prophylaxis by propranolol and femoxetine. Acta Neurol Scand 69: 9–14.

Nyrke T, Kangasniemi P, Lang AH (1989). Difference of steady-state visual evoked potential in classic and common migraine. Electroencephalopgr Clin Neurophysiol 73: 284–294.

Olesen J, Iversen HK, Thomsen LL (1993). Nitric oxide supersensitivity: a possible molecular mechanism of migraine pain. Neuroreport 4: 1027–1030.

Ophoff RA, Terwindt GM, Vergouwe MN et al. (1996). Familial hemiplegic migraine and episodic ataxia type-2 are caused by mutations in the Ca^{+2} channel gene CACNL1A4. Cell 87: 543–552.

Pechadre JC, Gibert J (1987). Demonstration, by the cartographic test, of an unusual reaction to intermittent light stimulation in patients with migraine. Encephale 13: 245–247.

Raskin NH, Hosobuchi Y, Lamb S (1987). Headache may arise from perturbation of the brain. Headache 27: 416–420.

Read SJ, Smith MI, Hunter AJ et al. (1997). Enhanced nitric oxide release during cortical spreading depression following infusion of glyceryl trinitrate in the anaesthetized cat. Cephalalgia 17: 159–165.

Reuter U, Bolay H, Jansen-Olsen I et al. (2001). Delayed inflammation in rat meinges: implications for migraine pathophysiology. Brain 124: 2490–2502.

Sanchez del Rio M, Bakker D, Wu O et al. (1999). Perfusion weighted imaging during migraine spontaneous visual aura and headache. Cephalalgia 19: 701–707.

Schoenen J, Wang W, Albert A et al. (1995). Potentiation instead of habituation characterizes visual evoked potentials in migraine patients between attacks. Eur J Neurol 2: 115–122.

Simon RH, Zimmerman AW, Tasman A et al. (1982). Spectral analysis of photic stimulation in migraine. Electroencephalogr Clin Neurophysiol 53: 270–276.

Stepien A, Chalimoniuk M (1998). Level of nitric oxide-dependent cgmp in patients with migraine. Cephalalgia 18: 631–634.

Teive HAG, Kowacs PA, Maranhão Filho P et al. (2005). Leão's cortical spreading depression:from experimental "artifact" to physiological principle. Neurology 65: 1455–1459.

van der Kamp W, Maassenvandenbrink A, Ferrari MD et al. (1996). Interictal cortical hyperexcitability in migraine patients demonstrated with transcranial magnetic stimulation. J Neurol Sci 139: 106–110.

van der Kamp W, Maassenvandenbrink A, Ferrari MD et al. (1997). Interictal cortical excitability to magnetic stimulation in familial hemiplegic migraine. Neurology 48: 1462–1464.

Wang W, Timsit-Berthier M, Schoenen J (1996). Intensity dependence of auditory evoked potentials is pronounced in migraine: An indication of cortical potentiation and low serotonergic neurotransmission? Neurology 46: 1404–1409.

Weiller C, May A, Limmroth V et al. (1995). Brainstem activation in spontaneous human migraine attacks. Nat Med 1: 658–660.

Welch KMA, Cao Y, Aurora SK et al. (1998). MRI of the occipital cortex, red nucleus, and substantia nigra during visual aura of migraine. Neurology 51: 1465–1469.

Welch KMA, D'Andrea G, Tepley N et al. (1990). The concept of migraine as a state of central neuronal hyperexcitabiliy. Neurol Clin 8: 817–828.

Welch KMA, Nagesh V, Aurora SK et al. (2001). Periaqueductal gray matter dysfunction in migraine: cause or the burden of illness. Headache 41: 629–637.

Werhahn KJ, Förderreuther S, Straube A (1998). Effects of serotonin 1B/1D receptor agonist zolmitriptan on motor cortical excitability in humans. Neurology 51: 896–898.

Wolff HG (1963). Headache and other head pain. 2nd edn. Oxford University Press, New York.

Woods RP, Iacoboni M, Mazziotta JC (1994). Bilateral spreading cerebral hypoperfusion during spontaneous migraine headache. N Engl J Med 22: 1689–1692.

Handbook of Clinical Neurology, Vol. 97 (3rd series)
Headache
G. Nappi and M.A. Moskowitz, Editors

Chapter 23

Migraine – clinical neurophysiology

ANNA AMBROSINI,[1] DELPHINE MAGIS,[2] AND JEAN SCHOENEN[2,3]*

[1]*Headache Clinic, INM Neuromed, IRCCS, Pozzilli (Isernia), Italy*

[2]*Headache Research Unit, Department of Neurology, University of Liège, Liège, Belgium*

[3]*Research Center for Cellular and Molecular Neurobiology, University of Liège, Liège, Belgium*

Migraine is an ictal neurological disorder in which no consistent structural disturbances are found, but a dysfunction of the central nervous system (CNS) is supposed to be the culprit. Several neuronal structures are probably involved in migraine pathophysiology, such as the cerebral cortex, the brainstem (periaqueductal gray matter, aminergic nuclei), and both peripheral and central components of the trigeminovascular system. Thus, clinical neurophysiology methods seem particularly suited to study migraine pathophysiology and the effects of pharmacological treatments (Sandrini et al., 2004). Because of a high interindividual variability, however, these methods have poor diagnostic utility.

In this chapter we will critically review the available data published for neurophysiological tests in headache. In particular we will summarize the studies performed in migraine patients on electroencephalogram (EEG), evoked and event-related potentials, transcranial magnetic stimulation (TMS), electromyographic techniques and cerebellar tests, and we will focus on those tests that have provided the most relevant information for the understanding of migraine pathophysiology.

ELECTROENCEPHALOGRAPHY

Electroencephalography was one of the first techniques used to explore cortical functions in migraine patients. Studies have addressed four EEG aspects in migraine: (1) background rhythm; (2) photic drive (or "H-response"); (3) mapping techniques using spectral analysis; and (4) magnetoencephalography (MEG).

Slowing of background rhythm, both generalized (Logar et al., 1986; Genco et al., 1994) and focal (Sand, 1991; Pothmann, 1993; Seri et al., 1993; Kramer et al., 1994), has been described during migraine attacks, but not in all studies (Lauritzen et al., 1981; Neurfeld et al., 1991; Lia et al., 1995). An enhanced photic drive response on the EEG, the so-called "H-response," was found in migraineurs (Golla and Winter, 1982; Simon et al., 1982; Pechadre and Gibert, 1987). However, its specificity is low, since it may occur in other primary headache disorders and in normal subjects (Schoenen et al., 1987).

Brain mapping using quantitative topographical EEG (qEEG) (Sauer et al., 1997) showed unilateral reduction of alpha activity during and within 3 days of an attack in migraine with visual aura (Schoenen et al., 1987; Cerquiglini et al., 1993), as well as in migraine without aura (MO) on the side of the headache, and in patients with menstrual migraine up to 24 h before the attack (Schoenen et al., 1987). In some studies an increase in alpha1 power was observed (Facchetti et al., 1990; Hughes and Robbins, 1990; Sauer et al., 1997) but in children there was no difference compared to controls (Valdizan et al., 1994). In one study, non-specific abnormalities on EEG were modified with flunarizine (Formisano et al., 1988). Multichannel EEG recorded during repetitive flash stimulation demonstrated hypersynchronization of the alpha rhythm in MO (De Tommaso et al., 2005d).

With non-linear multielectrode sleep EEG analysis preictally, a pronounced focus of maximum change in dimensional complexity was observed in the area of the scalp where subsequently the migraine pain would be perceived (Fritzer et al., 2004).

Seven-channel MEG studies revealed long-lasting suppressions in spectral power of all frequencies faster than 1 Hz, and prolonged direct-current (DC) shifts during attacks of MA or MO (Lauritzen et al., 1981;

*Correspondence to: Professor Dr. J Schoenen, Headache Research Unit, Department of Neurology and Research Center for Cellular and Molecular Neurobiology, University of Liège, CHR Citadelle, Bd du 12ème de Ligne 1, B-4000 Liège, Belgium, Tel: +32/4.223.86.63, Fax: +32/4.225.64.51, E-mail: jschoenen@ulg.ac.be

Barkley et al., 1990). These electromagnetic phenomena are similar to those described in experimental cortical spreading depression (CSD) (Okada et al., 1988). More recently, using whole-head MEG (Bowyer et al., 2001), DC shifts were observed during visually triggered aura and during the first few minutes of a spontaneous aura in migraine subjects, but not in control subjects. These findings add further support to the hypothesis that CSD is the likely culprit for the migrainous aura. MEG in a patient with aura without headache also showed alpha-band desynchronization in the left extrastriate and temporal cortex for the duration of the visual disturbance, and gamma-frequency desynchronization in the left temporal lobe persisting for 8–10 min after the aura (Hall et al., 2004).

EVOKED POTENTIALS

Visual evoked potentials (VEPs)

Visual evoked responses to stimuli repeated at low rates are defined as transient VEPs. VEPs can be elicited by either patterned or unpatterned stimuli. The most commonly used are pattern reversal, pattern onset–offset, and flash stimuli. Steady-state VEPs (SVEPs) are responses to visual stimuli at relatively high stimulation frequencies (above 3.5/s).

In early VEP studies in migraine patients single flashes were used to evoke visual potentials (flash-evoked visual potentials). In almost all of these pilot studies, the main evoked components showed higher amplitudes in migraineurs than in controls (Lehtonen, 1974; Connolly et al., 1982; Brinciotti et al., 1986), except one (Richey et al., 1966). Early VEP components were reduced on the side opposite to the aura (MacLean et al., 1975).

Subsequently, most VEP studies have used pattern reversal stimulation (PR-VEP). Their results were heterogeneous (Table 23.1). VEP amplitudes were found to be normal (Brinciotti et al., 1986; Mariani et al., 1988; Lai et al., 1989; Drake et al., 1990; Schoenen et al., 1995; Rossi et al., 1996; Sener et al., 1997; Áfra et al., 1998a, 2000b; Wang et al., 1999a; Sand and Vingen, 2000), increased between attacks (Kennard et al., 1978; Mariani et al., 1988; Aloisi et al., 1997; Lahat et al., 1997, 1999; Shibata et al., 1997a, b; Khalil et al., 2000) or in temporal proximity to an attack (Raudino, 1988), or decreased (Polich et al., 1986; Tagliati et al., 1995). In one study the PR-VEP amplitude decreased over time with the duration of the disease (Khalil et al., 2000), but this was not confirmed in another study (Yucesan et al., 2000). VEP amplitude or latency asymmetries were found in subgroups of patients (Benna et al., 1985; Tsounis et al., 1993; Tagliati et al., 1995; Shibata et al., 1997b, 1998; Logi et al., 2001). In migraine with aura (MA) patients, vector analysis of VEP showed alterations suggesting asymmetrical visual cortex activation (Coutin-Churchman and Padron de Freytez, 2003).

PR-VEP latencies were found to be increased in some studies (Kennard et al., 1978; Raudino, 1988; Diener et al., 1989; Mariani et al., 1990; Sener et al, 1997; Yilmaz et al., 2001; Kochar et al., 2002; Oelkers et al., 2005) and decreased in others (Tsounis et al., 1993; Aloisi et al., 1997). Oelkers et al. (1999) found increased N2 latency only with high spatial frequency of the stimulation pattern and suggested that this reflects dysfunction of the magnocellular pathway in migraine. High contrast and spatial frequency were also reported to induce increased VEP amplitudes (Shibata et al., 2005).

The results of VEP studies were globally similar in MO and MA (Brinciotti et al., 1986; Raudino, 1988; Diener et al., 1989; Lai et al., 1989; Rossi et al., 1996; Aloisi et al., 1997; Sener et al., 1997; Khalil et al., 2000; Sand and Vingen, 2000), with the exception of an abnormal P100 amplitude found on the side of the visual aura in migraineurs with aura (Tagliati et al., 1995, Shibata et al., 1997b).

The heterogeneity of these results can in part be explained by methodological differences, diagnostic bias (i.e., for studies performed before the first Headache Classification of the International Headache Society (1988), or the timing of recordings, as evoked cortical responses undergo profound modifications in the periictal, ictal, and immediate postictal periods, which was not adequately controlled for in most studies.

A considerable advance towards the understanding of the cortical dysfunction in migraine patients was obtained when, instead of considering the global PR-VEP amplitudes, the amplitude change in successive blocks of a lower number of averaged responses was analyzed during continuous stimulation. Normally, when an innocuous/irrelevant stimulus is delivered repetitively a gradual decrease in the amplitude of the cortical response is observed. This phenomenon is known as "habituation." It is supposed to protect against sensory overload and to save attentional and memory resources for meaningful novel stimuli. Studies of VEP habituation show that the amplitude of the N1–P1 and P1–N2 components decreases (i.e., habituates) during repetitive stimulation in healthy volunteers, but they remain unchanged or increase (i.e., potentiate) in migraineurs between attacks (Schoenen et al., 1995; Áfra et al., 1998a; Wang et al., 1999a). Interestingly, the habituation deficit normalizes just before and during the attack (Judit et al., 2000).

The interictal lack of habituation in migraine was not totally confirmed in two studies where different methodologies were used (Oelkers et al., 1999) or recordings were preictal in many patients (Sand and Vingen, 2000).

Table 23.1

Visual evoked potential recordings in migraine

		Material			Methods		
First author	Year	Number of patients plus controls	Mean age (SD/range) (years)	Timing of recordings	Stimulation rate	Number of trials	Main findings in migraineurs
Kennard	1978	28 MA 30 CTRL	39 (?)	? Days after attack	2 Hz	256	Increased amplitude and latency of P1
Benna	1985	10 MO No CTRL	36 (25–46)	8 days after attack	?	?	Aspecific amplitude and latency asymmetries
Brinciotti	1986	24 MO 19 MA ? CTRL	11.4 (7–16)	7 days after attack	1.6 Hz	100 × 2	No difference from CTRL
Polich	1986	20 MA 20 CTRL	32.8 (23–44)	Headache-free at test	3.9 Hz	200 × 2	Reduced P1 amplitude
Mariani	1988	22 MO 20 CTRL	39.4 (17–60)	2 days after attack	1 Hz	128 × 2	No difference from CTRL
Raudino	1988	34 MO 6 MA 20 CTRL	34.8 (14–78)	Headache-free at test	1.5 Hz	?	Increased P1 amplitude and latencies close to the attack
Diener	1989	54 MO 4 MA 87 CTRL	42.3 (?)	Baseline (?/attack), after 4 months' treatment and 3 months after washout period	1.56 Hz	64	At baseline, significantly increased latencies and higher amplitudes
Lai	1989	13 MO 25 MA No CTRL	29 (17–38)	During attacks precipitated by food and fasting	?	128	Latencies and amplitudes within normal limits
Drake	1990	50 MO 37 CTRL	? (16–67)	?	1.88 Hz	200 × 2	No difference from CTRL
Mariani	1990	20 MA 20 CTRL	34.2 (19–55)	2 days after attack	1 Hz	128 × 2	Increased latencies of P1
Tsounis	1993	22 MO 20 MA 37 CTRL	36.5 (15–56)	2 weeks after attack	1 Hz	128 × 2	P1 latencies shorter on the symptomatic side (hemifield stimulation)
Schoenen	1995	27 MO 9 MA 16 CTRL	32 (?)	At least 1 week after attack	3.1 Hz	50 × 5	No difference in amplitude or latencies. Potentiation of N1–P1 and P1–N2 amplitudes in migraineurs; habituation in CTRL

(Continued)

Table 23.1

Continued

		Material			Methods		
First author	Year	Number of patients plus controls	Mean age (SD/range) (years)	Timing of recordings	Stimulation rate	Number of trials	Main findings in migraineurs
Tagliati	1995	8 MO 7 MA 15 CTRL	31.7 (17–56)	7 days after attack	1 Hz	240	Reduced amplitudes ipsilateral to visual aura around Oz
Rossi	1996	71 MO, MA plus TTH 19 CTRL	? Children	2 days after attack	1.7 Hz	100 × 2	No difference from CTRL
Aloisi	1997	16 MO 4 MA ? CTRL	10.1 (6–13)	7 days after attack	1.1 Hz	256 × 2	Inverse correlation between P1 amplitude and serum magnesium levels
Lahat	1997	44 MO ? CTRL	? (3–17)	?	2 Hz	?	Increased P1–N2 amplitude
Sener	1997	23 MO 16 MA 17 CTRL	33.4 (7.2)	1 week after attack	2 Hz	200 × 2	No difference from CTRL
Shibata	1997a	14 MO 19 MA 43 CTRL	41.3 (20–70)	2–20 days after attack	2 Hz	100 × 2	Increased P1 amplitude
Shibata	1997b	14 MO 15 MA 23 CTRL	42.9 (22–65)	5 days after attack	2 Hz	100 × 2	Increased P1 amplitude in MA, higher on the contralateral side of visual aura
Áfra	1998a	25 MO 15 MA 25 CTRL	36 (?)	5 days after attack	3.1 Hz	100 × 15	Trend to lower first block N1–P1 amplitude Lack of habituation during long-lasting visual stimulation
Shibata	1998	20 MA 19 ME 34 CTRL	41, 48	1–30 days after attack	2 Hz	100 × 2	Increased N1–P1 amplitude soon after the attack. Amplitude asymmetry correlated to disease duration
Lahat	1999	53 "headache" No CTRL	Under 5 years	?	?	?	P1–N2 amplitude significantly larger
Oelkers	1999	13 MO 13 MA 28 CTRL	29.1 (5.9)	At least 3 days before and after attack	1 Hz	50 × 5	Prolonged N2 latency in MA when small checks presented

Sándor	1999a	40 MO (20 parents and their children) No CTRL	44.4 (7.5) 17 (6.1)	At least 3 days before and after attack	3.1 Hz	50 × 5	Similar lack of habituation patterns in related migrainous pairs
Wang	1999a	22 MO 13 ETTH 20 CTTH 26 CTRL	35.3 (9.6) 27.1 (10.9) 27.8 (8.4)	At least 1 week after attack	3 Hz	50 × 5	Elongated N2 latency in MA interictally Reduced habituation in migraine but not CTTH or ETTH
Khalil	2000	37 MO 47 MA 8 MO + MA 62 CTRL	40.2 (12)	Headache-free at test	2 Hz	240	P1 amplitude increased in migraineurs but decreased in MA with long disease duration
Sand	2000	15 MO 6 MA 22 CTRL	39.3 (9.2)	3 days after attack, 24 h within test or interictal	2 Hz	100 × 2	Significant habituation to small checks in CTRL but not in migraineurs (except preattack subgroup) Potentiation in CTRL for medium-sized checks
Yucesan	2000	22 MO <2 years disease 27 MO >10 years disease 17 CTRL	29 (8.1) 37 (6.9) 35.6 (8.5)	At least 1 week after attack	2 Hz	250 × 2	No correlation between amplitude of visual evoked potentials and duration of the disease
Áfra	2000a	12 MA 10 CTRL	34 (16)	At least 3 days before and after an attack	3.1 Hz	50 × 5	Increased amplitude and potentiation with red light in CTRL and not in MA
Áfra	2000b	37 MO 22 MA 23 CTRL	36 (11)	At least 3 days before and after an attack	3.1 Hz	50 × 5	Negative correlation between first block amplitude and potentiation of visual evoked potential in all subject groups
Judit	2000	69 MO 4 MA 4 MO + MA No CTRL	?	At least 3 days before and after, just before, during, 1 day or 2 days after attack	3.1 Hz	100 × 5	Normalization of evoked potential habituation just before and during the attack
Logi	2001	40 MO 19 MA 30 CTRL	35.8 (13.7) 38.3 (9.6)	Interictal (> 10 days)	1 Hz	Minimum 100 × 2 or 3	Asymmetry in right–left amplitude
Marrelli et al.	2001	20 MO 14 MA 14 TTH 10 CTRL	11.9 (1.8) 11.5 (2.3)	Attack-free for at least 1 week	1.1 Hz 8.1 Hz (SS)	256 at 1.1 Hz 100 at 8.1 Hz	No difference from CTRL

(Continued)

Table 23.1

Continued

		Material			Methods		
First author	Year	Number of patients plus controls	Mean age (SD/range) (years)	Timing of recordings	Stimulation rate	Number of trials	Main findings in migraineurs
Yilmaz	2001	16 MO 29 MA 22 CTRL	31.5 (11–64) 33.5 (15–60)	During and between attacks	2 Hz	200	Elongated N2 latency in MA interictally
Kochar	2002	25 "migraine" No CTRL	?	During and 7 days after attack	?	?	Prolonged P1 latency at the time of acute attack
Ozkul and Bozlar	2002	44 MO 35 MA 40 CTRL	33 (8)	At least 3 days before and after the attack	3.1 Hz	50 × 5	Significant lack of habituation in migraineurs corrected after fluoxetine prophylaxis
Coutin-Churchman	2003	23 MA 50 CTRL	? (18–53) ? (18–47)	Interictal period	2 Hz	100 × 2	No difference in latency or amplitude Significant alteration in vector orientation, laterality of deviation correlated with laterality of symptoms
Oelkers-Ax	2005	67 MO 32 MA 24 TTH 82 CTRL	? (6–18)	Headache-free at test	1 Hz	?	Decline of N2 latency with increasing age shifted to lower spatial frequencies in headache patients
Spreafico et al.	2004	53 "migraine" 20 CTRL	?	During migraine prophylactic treatment, or without prophylaxis	?	?	Lower P1 latencies
Oelkers-Ax	2005	123 "headache" 82 CTRL	? (6–18)	At least 72 h before and after an attack	1 Hz	50 × 5	Lack of N2 latency reduction with age No difference in habituation

MO: migraine without aura; MA: migraine with aura; TTH: tension-type headache; ME: migraine equivalent (aura without headache); CTRL: healthy controls; SS: steady-state; CTTH: chronic tension-type headache; ETTH: episodic tension-type headache.

VEP habituation is negatively correlated with amplitude in the first block of averaged responses (Áfra et al., 2000b). Red light, supposed to represent the most effective stimulus for the visual cortex, induces VEP potentiation in healthy subjects, but not in migraineurs (Áfra et al., 2000a), suggesting that the visual cortex is less responsive in migraine.

The degree of the VEP habituation deficit was very similar in related parent–child pairs of migraineurs, but not in unrelated pairs (Sándor et al., 1999a), which favors its familial, most probably genetic, character.

In migrainous children, some authors reported normal VEP (Brinciotti et al., 1986; Rossi et al., 1996), others increased amplitudes (Aloisi et al., 1997; Lahat et al., 1997, 1999); this was associated with decreased latencies in one study (Aloisi et al., 1997). Deficient habituation to PR-VEP was not found in one study of childhood migraine (Oelkers et al., 2005).

Drug treatments may influence VEPs in migraine patients. PR-VEP (Diener et al., 1989) and PR-VEP habituation (Sándor et al., 2000) tended to normalize during prophylactic treatment with beta-blockers. The latter normalizes also during prolonged treatment with the specific serotonin reuptake blocker fluoxetine (Ozkul and Bozlar, 2002). MEG signals evoked by visual stimulation are reduced in migraine patients during prophylactic treatment with sodium valproate (Bowyer et al., 2005).

High-frequency (10 Hz) repetitive TMS (rTMS) over the occipital region, supposed to activate the underlying cortex, was followed by a normalization of VEP habituation in migraineurs, while low-frequency (1 Hz) rTMS, which has an inhibitory effect, induced a deficit of VEP habituation in normal controls (Bohotin et al., 2002). After daily sessions of rTMS, these effects on habituation may last from hours to weeks in both controls and migraine patients (Fumal et al., 2006).

An analysis of high-frequency oscillations in the gamma range (GFOs: 20–60 Hz) embedded in broadband VEPs (Coppola et al., 2007b) showed that the late GFO components, which are supposed to represent postsynaptic cortical activities, present a significant habituation deficit in MO and MA patients. On the other hand, the early GFOs, which seem to be related to presynaptic mechanisms, have increased amplitudes in MA, which may account for the interictal visual discomfort more frequently reported in this migraine type.

Auditory evoked potentials (AEPs)

Studies of short latency, i.e., brainstem auditory evoked responses (BAERs), provide contrasting and heterogeneous results in migraine. Normal interictal latencies (Benna et al., 1985; Yamada et al., 1986; Podoshin et al., 1987; Battistella et al., 1988; Sand and Vingen, 2000), increased latencies (especially for wave V) (Bussone et al., 1985; Drake et al., 1990), in particular during the attack (Yamada et al., 1986; Podoshin et al., 1987), and interaural asymmetries (Bussone et al., 1985; Schlake et al., 1990) were reported. A negative correlation was described between discomfort to low-intensity stimulations (55 dB) and wave IV–V amplitude (Sand and Vingen, 2000).

The few studies of cortical long-latency AEPs did not show significant differences between migraineurs and controls with regard to N1, P2, and N2 latencies or amplitudes (Drake et al., 1989; Sand and Vingen, 2000).

Only a few studies have explored habituation of cortical AEPs. The first one reported potentiation of N1–P2 amplitude only at high stimulus intensities, contrasting with habituation in healthy volunteers (Wang et al., 1996). This was not confirmed in another report (Sand and Vingen, 2000), possibly because of methodological differences. In a subsequent study (Ambrosini et al., 2003b), the intensity dependence of auditory N1–P2 and habituation for each stimulation intensities were measured simultaneously and potentiation was found in migraineurs, greater for high- than for low-intensity stimulations, as opposed to habituation or absence of amplitude change for all stimulation intensities in controls.

"Gating" of sensory input is another characteristic of central processing of incoming information. A typical example of this phenomenon is the suppression of the cortical response to a test stimulus delivered after an identical preceding conditioning stimulus. The middle-latency P50 component of the auditory evoked cortical potential is very sensitive to gating. Gating of the auditory P50 response was markedly reduced in migraine patients compared to healthy volunteers (Ambrosini et al., 2001a), which was considered as an expression of reduced short-term habituation (Siniatchkin et al., 2003).

Intensity dependence of AEPs (IDAP), i.e., the amplitude increase of auditory evoked cortical responses with increasing stimulation intensities, was found to be enhanced in migraine patients (Wang et al., 1996). IDAP is supposed to be inversely related to central serotoninergic neurotransmission (Hegerl and Juckel, 1993). The increased IDAP normalizes during the migraine attack (Judit et al., 2000). IDAP abnormalities correlate with personality profiles thought to be associated with lower serotonergic transmission in migraine, but not in posttraumatic headache (Wang et al., 1999b).

Two independent studies (Sándor et al., 2000; Siniatchkin et al., 2000b) found evidence for a familial influence on IDAP in migraineurs, pointing towards a genetic background, though up to now no direct genetic link has been identified.

IDAP is not useful for diagnostic purposes because of its limited repeatability both in pathophysiological

(Sándor et al., 1999b) and in pharmacological (Roon et al., 1999) studies. This may be related to the fact that the major part of the IDAP increase in migraine could be due to the AEP habituation deficit at high intensity stimulations (Ambrosini et al., 2003b). Interestingly, IDAP amplitude–stimulus function slopes and PR-VEP habituation slopes were not significantly correlated when investigated together in the same migraine patients (Áfra et al., 2000b).

Somatosensory evoked potentials

Overall, no significant abnormalities of standard somatosensory evoked potentials (SSEP) after median nerve or index-finger stimulation were found in migraine patients (Montagna et al., 1985; Firenze et al., 1988; Chayasirisobhon, 1995; Marlowe, 1995), apart form some subtle changes such as prolonged N13 latency interictally (Montagna et al., 1985), reduced P22/N30 amplitude interictally (de Tommaso et al., 1997), prolonged N19 latency, and reduced amplitude during the aura (Chayasirisobhon, 1995).

Habituation of SSEPs was found to be replaced by potentiation in one study (Ozkul and Uckardes, 2002).

Recently, more sophisticated methods were used to analyze SSEPs. The shorter SSEP recovery cycle found in migrainous children was interpreted as reflecting a dysfunction of inhibitory interneurons (Valeriani et al., 2005). High-frequency oscillations (HFOs) embedded in SSEPs, which are supposed to reflect spike activity in thalamocortical cholinergic fibers (early HFOs) and in cortical inhibitory GABAergic interneurons (late HFOs), were found to be globally reduced in amplitude in one study (Sakuma et al., 2004), whereas in the other one (Coppola et al., 2005) early but not late HFOs were reduced in amplitude in migraineurs, suggesting reduced thalamocortical activation, but normal intracortical inhibition.

The response pattern of the somatosensory cortex in migraine has also been investigated with MEG (Lang et al., 2004); the equivalent current dipole of the first MEG cortical component, the N20m, was increased in migraine patients and positively related to their mean attack frequency. Curiously, in this study both migraine patients and controls did not habituate to repeated stimuli, which contrasts with all previous evoked potential studies in healthy subjects.

Laser-evoked nociceptive potentials

CO_2 laser-evoked potentials (LEPs) have been studied only recently in migraine. The main component of LEPs is the long-latency N2–P2 vertex complex. It mainly originates in the cingulate cortex (Bentley et al., 2003), which belongs to the limbic system and is involved in the emotional and unpleasant component of pain. The N2–P2 can thus be significantly affected by the subject's attentional and emotional state at the time of recording. During spontaneous migraine attacks, LEP N2–P2 amplitude – especially its P2 component – was increased when the symptomatic supraorbital zone and the dorsum of the ipsilateral hand were stimulated (de Tommaso et al., 2002, 2004a, 2005c). Efficient symptomatic treatment of the attack with lysine acetylsalicylate or almotriptan reduced the P2 amplitude (de Tommaso et al., 2005c). A P2 amplitude increase was also found in migraine patients when an attack was provoked by oral administration of nitroglycerine (de Tommaso et al., 2004b).

Interictally, migraineurs are characterized by a lack of habituation of the LEP N2–P2 amplitude compared with healthy volunteers (Valeriani et al., 2003; de Tommaso et al., 2005a) or tension-type headache patients (Valeriani et al., 2003). In one study (de Tommaso et al., 2005b) this lack of N2–P2 habituation persisted during the attack, in contrast with results from other stimulation modalities. This ictal lack of habituation was found to be correlated with frequency and duration of migraine (de Tommaso et al., 2005b). The authors explained their finding by an abnormal processing in the nociceptive system of migraineurs during the attack. Further support to this hypothesis comes from a recent study, in which a distractive painful stimulus (capsaicin application on the dorsum of the hand) failed to produce in migraineurs the LEP amplitude decrease found in normal subjects (de Tommaso et al., 2007a).

EVENT-RELATED POTENTIALS

Contingent negative variation

Contingent negative variation (CNV), a slow negative cortical potential appearing during a reaction time task between a warning and an imperative stimulus, has an early component modulated by noradrenergic systems and a late component thought to be related to motor readiness and to be under dopaminergic control (Rohrbaugh et al., 1986; Birbaumer et al., 1990).

Consistent results from different laboratories have shown that CNV amplitude is increased in migraineurs between attacks, mainly in those suffering from MO (Schoenen et al., 1985a, b; Maertens de Noordhout et al., 1986; Bocker et al., 1990; Kropp and Gerber, 1993). This increase was more pronounced for the early component (Kropp and Gerber, 1993), which may reflect an overweight of excitatory versus inhibitory processes, and seems to be enhanced by stress and the premenstrual phase of the ovarian cycle (Siniatchkin et al., 2006a, b). Modifications of early (Kropp et al., 1999) and late (Bender et al., 2002) CNV amplitude with aging were found in healthy volunteers but not in migraineurs, which

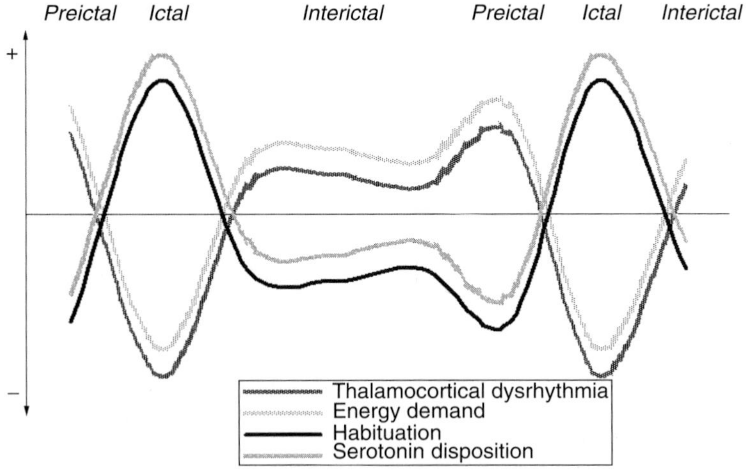

Fig. 23.1. Model for the chronobiology of the cerebral cortex in migraine.

system of the brain, the trigeminovascular system, and thus to the migraine attack. During the migraine attack, activation of the endogenous pain control systems would lead to increased central serotonergic transmission and normalization of cortical responsiveness, "by which this condition is dispersed and the equilibrium for the time restored" (Liveing, 1873).

References

Áfra J, Cecchini AP, De Pasqua V et al. (1998a). Visual evoked potentials during long periods of pattern-reversal stimulation in migraine. Brain 121: 233–241.

Áfra J, Mascia A, Gérard P et al. (1998b). Interictal cortical excitability in migraine: a study using transcranial magnetic stimulation of motor and visual cortices. Ann Neurol 44: 209–215.

Áfra J, Ambrosini A, Genicot R et al. (2000a). Influence of colors on habituation of visual evoked potentials in patients with migraine with aura and in healthy volunteers. Headache 40: 36–40.

Áfra J, Proietti Cecchini A, Sandor PS et al. (2000b). Comparison of visual and auditory evoked cortical potentials in migraine patients between attacks. Clin Neurophysiol 111: 1124–1129.

Aguggia M, Zibeti M, Febbraro A et al. (1999). Transcranial magnetic stimulation in migraine with aura: further evidence of occipital cortex hyperexcitability. Cephalalgia 19: 465.

Aktekin B, Yaltkaya K, Ozkaynak S et al. (2001). Recovery cycle of the blink reflex and exteroceptive suppression of temporalis muscle activity in migraine and tension-type headache. Headache 41: 142–149.

Aloisi P, Marrelli A, Porto C et al. (1997). Visual evoked potentials and serum magnesium levels in juvenile migraine patients. Headache 37: 383–385.

Ambrosini A, de Noordhout AM, Alagona G et al. (1999). Impairment of neuromuscular transmission in a subgroup of migraine patients. Neurosci Lett 276: 201–203.

Ambrosini A, De Pasqua V, Afra J et al. (2001a). Reduced gating of middle-latency auditory evoked potentials (P50) in migraine patients: another indication of abnormal sensory processing? Neurosci Lett 306: 132–134.

Ambrosini A, Maertens de Noordhout A, Schoenen J (2001b). Neuromuscular transmission in migraine: a single fiber EMG study in clinical subgroups. Neurology 56: 1038–1043.

Ambrosini A, Maertens de Noordhout A, Schoenen J (2001c). Neuromuscular transmission in migraine patients with prolonged aura. Another suggestion of the possible involvement of P/Q Ca^{2+}-channels in common forms of migraine. Acta Neurol Belg 101: 166–170.

Ambrosini A, Pierelli F, Schoenen J (2003a). Acetazolamide acts on neuromuscular transmission abnormalities found in some migraineurs. Cephalalgia 23: 75–78.

Ambrosini A, Rossi P, De Pasqua V et al. (2003b). Lack of habituation causes high intensity dependence of auditory evoked cortical potentials in migraine. Brain 126: 2009–2015.

Antal A, Arlt S, Nitsche MA et al. (2006). Higher variability of phosphene thresholds in migraineurs than in controls: a consecutive transcranial magnetic stimulation study. Cephalalgia 26: 865–870.

Aurora SK, Ahmad BK, Welch KMA et al. (1998). Transcranial magnetic stimulation confirms hyperexcitability of visual cortex in migraine. Neurology 50: 1105–1110.

Aurora SK, al-Sayeed F, Welch KM (1999a). The cortical silent period is shortened in migraine with aura. Cephalalgia 19: 708–712.

Aurora SK, Cao Y, Bowyer SM et al. (1999b). The occipital cortex is hyperexcitable in migraine: experimental evidence. Headache 39: 469–476.

Aurora SK, Welch KM, Al-Sayed F (2003). The threshold for phosphenes is lower in migraine. Cephalalgia 23: 258–263.

Bahra A, Matharu MS, Buchel C et al. (2001). Brainstem activation specific to migraine headache. Lancet 357: 1016–1017.

Bank J, Bense E, Kiraly C (1992). The blink reflex in migraine. Cephalalgia 12: 289–292.

Barbiroli B, Montagna P, Cortelli P et al. (1992). Abnormal brain and muscle energy metabolism shown by ^{31}P magnetic resonance spectroscopy in patients affected by migraine with aura. Neurology 42: 1209–1214.

Barkley GL, Tepley N, Nagel-Leiby S et al. (1990). Magnetoencephalographic studies of migraine. Headache 30: 428–434.

Baslo B, Coban A, Baykan B et al. (2007). Investigation of neuromuscular transmission in some rare types of migraine. Cephalalgia 27: 1201–1205.

Battelli L, Black KR, Wray SH (2002). Transcranial magnetic stimulation of visual area V5 in migraine. Neurology 58: 1066–1069.

Battistella PA, Suppiej A, Casara G et al. (1988). Brainstem auditory evoked potentials (BAEPs) in childhood migraine. Headache 28: 204–206.

Bender S, Weisbrod M, Just U et al. (2002). Lack of age-dependent development of the contingent negative variation (CNV) in migraine children? Cephalalgia 22: 132–136.

Benna P, Bianco C, Costa P et al. (1985). Visual evoked potentials and brainstem auditory evoked potentials in migraine and transient ischemic attacks. Cephalalgia 5 (Suppl. 2): 53–58.

Bentley DE, Derbyshire SW, Youell PD et al. (2003). Caudal cingulate cortex involvement in pain processing: an inter-individual laser evoked potential source localisation study using realistic head models. Pain 102: 265–271.

Bettucci D, Cantello M, Gianelli M et al. (1992). Menstrual migraine without aura: cortical excitability to magnetic stimulation. Headache 32: 345–347.

Birbaumer N, Elbert T, Canavan AG et al. (1990). Slow potentials of the cerebral cortex and behavior. Physiol Rev 70: 1–41.

Bocker KB, Timsit-Berthier M, Schoenen J et al. (1990). Contingent negative variation in migraine. Headache 30: 604–609.

Bohotin V, Fumal A, Vandenheede M et al. (2002). Effects of repetitive transcranial magnetic stimulation on visual evoked potentials in migraine. Brain 125: 1–11.

Bohotin V, Fumal A, Vandenheede M et al. (2003). Excitability of visual V1-V2 and motor cortices to single transcranial magnetic stimuli in migraine: a reappraisal using a figure-of-eight coil. Cephalalgia 23: 264–270.

Bowyer SM, Aurora SK, Moran JE et al. (2001). Magnetoencephalographic fields from patients with spontaneous and induced migraine aura. Ann Neurol 50: 582–587.

Bowyer SM, Mason KM, Moran JE et al. (2005). Cortical hyperexcitability in migraine patients before and after sodium valproate treatment. J Clin Neurophysiol 22: 65–67.

Brighina F, Piazza A, Daniele O et al. (2002). Modulation of visual cortical excitability in migraine with aura: effects of 1 Hz repetitive transcranial magnetic stimulation. Exp Brain Res 145: 177–181.

Brighina F, Giglia G, Scalia S et al. (2005). Facilitatory effects of 1 Hz rTMS in motor cortex of patients affected by migraine with aura. Exp Brain Res 161: 34–38.

Brinciotti M, Guidetti V, Matricardi M et al. (1986). Responsiveness of the visual system in childhood migraine studied by means of VEPs. Cephalalgia 6: 183–185.

Buodo G, Palomba D, Sarlo M et al. (2004). Auditory event-related potentials and reaction times in migraine children. Cephalalgia 24: 554–563.

Bussone G, Sinatra MG, Boiardi A et al. (1985). Brainstem auditory evoked potentials in migraine patients in basal conditions and after chronic flunarizine treatment. Cephalalgia 5 (Suppl. 2): 177–180.

Cerquiglini A, Guidetti V, Seri S (1993). Computerized EEG topography in childhood migraine between and during attacks. Cephalalgia 13: 53–56.

Chadaide Z, Arlt S, Antal A et al. (2007). Transcranial direct current stimulation reveals inhibitory deficiency in migraine. Cephalalgia 27: 833–839.

Chayasirisobhon S (1995). Somatosensory evoked potentials in acute migraine with sensory aura. Clin Electroencephalogr 26: 65–69.

Chen W, Shen X, Liu X et al. (2007). Passive paradigm single-tone elicited ERPs in tension-type headaches and migraine. Cephalalgia 27: 139–144.

Coban A, Baslo M, Baykan B et al. (2007). Subclinical neuromuscular transmission abnormality detected by single-fibre EMG is more pronounced in cluster headache than in migraine with aura. Cephalalgia 27: 788–792.

Connolly JF, Gawel M, Rose FC (1982). Migraine patients exhibit abnormalities in the visual evoked potential. J Neurol Neurosurg Psychiatry 45: 464–467.

Coppola G, Vandenheede M, Di Clemente L et al. (2005). Somatosensory evoked high-frequency oscillations reflecting thalamo-cortical activity are decreased in migraine patients between attacks. Brain 128: 98–103.

Coppola G, Di Clemente L, Fumal A et al. (2007a). Inhibition of the nociceptive R2 blink reflex after supraorbital or index finger stimulation is normal in migraine without aura between attacks. Cephalalgia 27: 803–808.

Coppola G, Ambrosini A, Di Clemente L et al. (2007b). Interictal abnormalities of gamma band activity in visual evoked responses in migraine: an indication of thalamocortical dysrhythmia? Cephalalgia 27: 1360–1367.

Coutin-Churchman P, Padron de Freytez A (2003). Vector analysis of visual evoked potentials in migraineurs with visual aura. Clin Neurophysiol 114: 2132–2137.

Currà A, Pierelli F, Coppola G et al. (2007). Shortened cortical silent period in facial muscles of patients with migraine. Pain 132: 124–131.

De Marinis M, Pujia A, Natale L et al. (2003). Decreased habituation of the R2 component of the blink reflex in migraine patients. Clin Neurophysiol 114: 889–893.

de Tommaso M, Sciruicchio V, Tota P et al. (1997). Somatosensory evoked potentials in migraine. Funct Neurol 12: 77–82.

de Tommaso M, Guido M, Libro G et al. (2000a). The three responses of the blink reflex in adult and juvenile migraine. Acta Neurol Belg 100: 96–102.

de Tommaso M, Guido M, Libro G et al. (2000b). Zolmitriptan reverses blink reflex changes induced during the migraine attack in humans. Neurosci Lett 289: 57–60.

de Tommaso M, Guido M, Libro G et al. (2002). Abnormal brain processing of cutaneous pain in migraine patients during the attack. Neurosci Lett 333: 29–32.

de Tommaso M, Guido M, Libro G et al. (2004a). Topographic and dipolar analysis of laser-evoked potentials during migraine attack. Headache 44: 947–960.

de Tommaso M, Libro G, Guido M et al. (2004b). Nitroglycerin induces migraine headache and central sensitization phenomena in patients with migraine without aura: a study of laser evoked potentials. Neurosci Lett 363: 272–275.

de Tommaso M, Libro G, Guido M et al. (2005a). Habituation of single CO_2 laser-evoked responses during interictal phase of migraine. J Headache Pain 6: 195–198.

de Tommaso M, Lo Sito L, Di Fruscolo O et al. (2005b). Lack of habituation of nociceptive evoked responses and pain sensitivity during migraine attack. Clin Neurophysiol 116: 1254–1264.

de Tommaso M, Losito L, Libro G et al. (2005c). Effects of symptomatic treatments on cutaneous hyperalgesia and laser evoked potentials during migraine attack. Cephalalgia 25: 359–368.

de Tommaso M, Marinazzo D, Guido M et al. (2005d). Visually evoked phase synchronization changes of alpha rhythm in migraine: correlations with clinical features. Int J Psychophysiol 57: 203–210.

de Tommaso M, Difruscolo O, Sardaro M et al. (2007a). Effects of remote cutaneous pain on trigeminal laser-evoked potentials in migraine patients. J Headache Pain 8: 167–174.

de Tommaso M, Difruscolo O, Sardaro M et al. (2007b). Influence of MTHFR genotype on contingent negative variation and MRI abnormalities in migraine. Headache 47: 253–265.

Di Clemente L, Coppola G, Magis D et al. (2005). Nociceptive blink reflex and visual evoked potential habituations are correlated in migraine. Headache 45: 1388–1393.

Di Clemente L, Coppola G, Magis D et al. (2007). Interictal habituation deficit of the nociceptive blink reflex: an endophenotypic marker for presymptomatic migraine? Brain 130: 765–770.

Diener HC, Scholz E, Dichgans J et al. (1989). Central effects of drugs used in migraine prophylaxis evaluated by visual evoked potentials. Ann Neurol 25: 125–130.

Domitrz I, Kostera-Pruszczy KA, Kwiecinski H (2005). A single-fiber EMG study of neuromuscular transmission in migraine patients. Cephalalgia 25: 817–821.

Drake ME, Pakalnis A, Padamadan H (1989). Long-latency auditory event related potentials in migraine. Headache 29: 239–241.

Drake ME, Pakalnis A, Hietter SA et al. (1990). Visual and auditory evoked potentials in migraine. Electromyogr Clin Neurophysiol 30: 77–81.

Evers S, Bauer B, Suhr B et al. (1997). Cognitive processing in primary headache: a study of event-related potentials. Neurology 48: 108–113.

Evers S, Bauer B, Grotemeyer KH et al. (1998). Event-related potentials (P300) in primary headache in childhood and adolescence. J Child Neurol 13: 322–326.

Evers S, Quibeldey F, Grotemeyer KH et al. (1999). Dynamic changes of cognitive habituation and serotonin metabolism during the migraine interval. Cephalalgia 19: 485–491.

Facchetti D, Marsile C, Faggi L et al. (1990). Cerebral mapping in subjects suffering from migraine with aura. Cephalalgia 10: 279–284.

Ferrari MD, Odink J, Tapparelli C et al. (1989). Serotonin metabolism in migraine. Neurology 39: 1239–1242.

Firenze C, Del Gatto F, Mazzotta G et al. (1988). Somatosensory-evoked potential study in headache patients. Cephalalgia 8: 157–162.

Formisano R, Martucci N, Fabbrini G et al. (1988). Spectral EEG analysis and flunarizine treatment in migraine patients. Cephalalgia 8 (Suppl. 8): 31–33.

Fritzer G, Strenge H, Gader R et al. (2004). Changes in cortical dynamics in the preictal stage of a migraine attack. J Clin Neurophysiol 21: 99–104.

Fumal A, Coppola G, Bohotin V et al. (2006). Induction of long-lasting changes of visual cortex excitability by five daily sessions of repetitive transcranial magnetic stimulation (rTMS) in healthy volunteers and migraine patients. Cephalalgia 26: 143–149.

Genco S, de Tommaso M, Prudenzano AM et al. (1994). EEG features in juvenile migraine: topographic analysis of spontaneous and visual evoked brain electrical activity: a comparison with adult migraine. Cephalalgia 14: 41–46.

Golla FL, Winter AL (1982). Analysis of cerebral responses to flicker in patients complaining of episodic headache. Electroencephalogr Clin Neurophysiol 53: 270–276.

Gunaydin S, Soysal A, Atay T et al. (2006). Motor and occipital cortex excitability in migraine patients. Can J Neurol Sci 33: 63–67.

Hall SD, Barnes GR, Hillebrand A et al. (2004). Spatiotemporal imaging of cortical desynchronization in migraine visual aura: a magnetoencephalography case study. Headache 44: 204–208.

Harno H, Hirvonen T, Kaunisto MA et al. (2003). Subclinical vestibulocerebellar dysfunction in migraine with and without aura. Neurology 61: 1748–1752.

Headache Classification Committee of the International Headache Society (1988). Classification and diagnostic criteria for headache disorders, cranial neuralgias and facial pain. Cephalalgia 8: 1–96.

Hegerl U, Juckel G (1993). Intensity dependence of auditory evoked potentials as an indicator of central serotonergic neurotransmission: a new hypothesis. Biol Psychiatry 33: 173–187.

Hughes JR, Robbins LD (1990). Brain mapping in migraine. Clin Electroencephalogr 21: 14–24.

Judit A, Sandor P, Schoenen J (2000). Habituation of visual and intensity dependence of auditory evoked cortical potentials tends to normalize just before and during the migraine attack. Cephalalgia 20: 714–719.

Katsarava Z, Lehnerdt G, Duda B et al. (2002). Sensitization of trigeminal nociception specific for migraine but not pain of sinusitis. Neurology 59: 1450–1453.

Katsarava Z, Giffin N, Diener H et al. (2003). Abnormal habituation of "nociceptive" blink reflex in migraine – evidence for increased excitability of trigeminal nociception. Cephalalgia 23: 814–819.

Kaube H, Katsarava Z, Kaufer T et al. (2000). A new method to increase nociception specificity of the human blink reflex. Clin Neurophysiol 111: 413–416.

Kaube H, Katsarava Z, Przywara S et al. (2002). Acute migraine headache: possible sensitization of neurons in the spinal trigeminal nucleus? Neurology 58: 1234–1238.

Kennard C, Gawel M, Rudolph ND et al. (1978). Visual evoked potentials in migraine subjects. Res Clin Stud Headache 6: 73–80.

Khalil NM, Legg NJ, Anderson DJ (2000). Long term decline of P100 amplitude in migraine with aura. J Neurol Neurosurg Psychiatry 69: 507–511.

Khedr EM, Ahmed MA, Mohamed KA (2006). Motor and visual cortical excitability in migraineurs patients with or without aura: transcranial magnetic stimulation. Neurophysiol Clin 36: 13–18.

Kochar K, Srivastava T, Maurya RK et al. (2002). Visual evoked potential & brainstem auditory evoked potentials in acute attack and after the attack of migraine. Electromyogr Clin Neurophysiol 42: 175–179.

Kramer U, Nevo Y, Neufeld MY et al. (1994). The value of EEG in children with chronic headaches. Brain Dev 16: 304–308.

Kropp P, Gerber WD (1993). Contingent negative variation – findings and perspectives in migraine. Cephalalgia 13: 33–36.

Kropp P, Gerber WD (1995). Contingent negative variation during migraine attack and interval: evidence for normalization of slow cortical potentials during the attack. Cephalalgia 15: 123–128.

Kropp P, Siniatchkin M, Stephani U et al. (1999). Migraine – evidence for a disturbance of cerebral maturation in man? Neurosci Lett 276: 181–184.

Kropp P, Siniatchkin M, Gerber WD (2000). Contingent negative variation as indicator of duration of migraine disease. Funct Neurol 15 (Suppl. 3): 78–81.

Lahat E, Nadir E, Barr J et al. (1997). Visual evoked potentials: a diagnostic test for migraine headache in children. Dev Med Child Neurol 39: 85–87.

Lahat E, Barr J, Barzilai A et al. (1999). Visual evoked potentials in the diagnosis of headache before 5 years of age. Eur J Pediatr 158: 892–895.

Lai CW, Dean P, Ziegler DK et al. (1989). Clinical and electrophysiological responses to dietary challenge in migraineurs. Headache 29: 180–186.

Lang E, Kaltenhauser M, Neundorfer B et al. (2004). Hyperexcitability of the primary somatosensory cortex in migraine – a magnetoencephalographic study. Brain 127: 2459–2469.

Lauritzen M, Trojaborg W, Olesen J (1981). EEG during attacks of common and classical migraine. Cephalalgia 1: 63–66.

Lehtonen JB (1974). Visual evoked cortical potentials for single flashes and flickering light in migraine. Headache 14: 1–12.

Lia C, Carenini L, Degioz C (1995). Computerized EEG analysis in migraine patients. Ital J Neurol Sci 16: 249–254.

Liveing E (1873). On Megrim, Sick Headache. Arts & Boeve, Nijmegen.

Logar C, Grabmair W, Lechner H (1986). [EEG in migraine.] EEG EMG Z Elektroenzephalogr Elektromyogr Verwandte Geb 17: 153–156.

Logi F, Bonfiglio L, Orlandi G et al. (2001). Asymmetric scalp distribution of pattern visual evoked potentials during interictal phases in migraine. Acta Neurol Scand 104: 301–307.

MacLean C, Appenzeller O, Cordaro JT et al. (1975). Flash evoked potentials in migraine. Headache 14: 193–198.

Maertens de Noordhout A, Timsit-Berthier M, Timsit M et al. (1986). Contingent negative variation in headache. Ann Neurol 19: 78–80.

Maertens de Noordhout A, Pepin JL, Schoenen J et al. (1992). Percutaneous magnetic stimulation of the motor cortex in migraine. Electroencephalogr Clin Neurophysiol 85: 110–115.

Magis D, Joiris T, Di Clemente L et al. (2007). Interictal cognition in migraineurs: a study correlating psychometric and neurophysiological tests. Cephalalgia 27: E080.

Mariani E, Moschini V, Pastorino G et al. (1988). Pattern-reversal visual evoked potentials and EEG correlations in common migraine patients. Headache 28: 269–271.

Mariani E, Moschini V, Pastorino GC et al. (1990). Pattern reversal visual evoked potentials (VEP-PR) in migraine subjects with visual aura. Headache 30: 435–438.

Marlowe N (1995). Somatosensory evoked potentials and headache: a further examination of the central theory. J Psychosom Res 39: 119–131.

Marrelli A, Tozzi E, Porto C et al. (2001). Spectral analysis of visual potentials evoked by pattern-reversal checkerboard in juvenile patients with headache. Headache 41: 792–797.

Mazzotta G, Alberti A, Santucci A et al. (1995). The event-related potential P300 during headache-free period and spontaneous attack in adult headache sufferers. Headache 35: 210–215.

Mesulam MM (1990). Large-scale neurocognitive networks and distributed processing for attention, language and memory. Ann Neurol 28: 597–613.

Montagna P, Zucconi M, Zappia M et al. (1985). Somatosensory evoked potentials in migraine and tension headache. Headache 25: 115.

Montagna P, Cortelli P, Barbiroli B (1994). Magnetic resonance spectroscopy studies in migraine. Cephalalgia 14: 184–193.

Mulleners WM, Chronicle EP, Palmer JE et al. (2001a). Visual cortex excitability in migraine with and without aura. Headache 41: 565–572.

Mulleners WM, Chronicle EP, Palmer JE et al. (2001b). Suppression of perception in migraine: evidence for reduced inhibition in the visual cortex. Neurology 56: 178–183.

Mulleners WM, Chronicle EP, Vredeveld JW et al. (2002). Visual cortex excitability in migraine before and after valproate prophylaxis: a pilot study using TMS. Eur J Neurol 9: 35–40.

Neurfeld MY, Treves TA, Orczyn AD (1991). EEG and topographic frequency analysis in common and classic migraine. Headache 31: 232–236.

Oelkers R, Grosser K, Lang E et al. (1999). Visual evoked potentials in migraine patients: alterations depend on pattern spatial frequency. Brain 122: 1147–1155.

Oelkers-Ax R, Parzer P, Resch F et al. (2005). Maturation of early visual processing investigated by a pattern-reversal habituation paradigm is altered in migraine. Cephalalgia 25: 280–289.

Okada YC, Lauritzen M, Nicholson C (1988). Magnetic field associated with spreading depression: a model for the detection of migraine. Brain 442: 185–190.

Ozkul Y, Bozlar S (2002). Effects of fluoxetine on habituation of pattern reversal visually evoked potentials in migraine prophylaxis. Headache 42: 582–587.

Ozkul Y, Uckardes A (2002). Median nerve somatosensory evoked potentials in migraine. Eur J Neurol 9: 227–232.

Pechadre JC, Gibert J (1987). Demonstration, by the cartographic test, of an unusual reaction to intermittent light stimulation in patients with migraine. Encephale 13: 245–247.

Podoshin L, Ben-David J, Pratt H et al. (1987). Auditory brainstem evoked potentials in patients with migraine. Headache 27: 27–29.

Polich J, Ehlers CL, Dalessio DJ (1986). Pattern-shift visual evoked responses and EEG in migraine. Headache 26: 451–456.

Pothmann R (1993). Topographic EEG mapping in childhood headaches. Cephalalgia 13: 57–58.

Raudino F (1988). Visual evoked potential in patients with migraine. Headache 28: 531–533.

Richey ET, Kooi KA, Waggoner RW (1966). Visually evoked responses in migraine. Electroencephalogr Clin Neurophysiol 21: 23–27.

Rohrbaugh JW, McCallum WC, Gaillard AW et al. (1986). ERPs associated with preparatory and movement-related processes. A review. Electroencephalogr Clin Neurophysiol (Suppl. 38): 189–229.

Roon KI, Sándor PS, Schoonman GG et al. (1999). The use of auditory evoked potentials in the assessment of central nervous system effects of antimigraine drugs. Cephalalgia 19: 880–886.

Rossi LN, Pastorino GC, Bellettini G et al. (1996). Pattern reversal visual evoked potentials in children with migraine or tension-type headache. Cephalalgia 16: 104–106.

Sakuma K, Takeshima T, Ishizaki K et al. (2004). Somatosensory evoked high-frequency oscillations in migraine patients. Clin Neurophysiol 115: 1857–1862.

Sand T (1991). EEG in migraine: a review of the literature. Funct Neurol 6: 7–22.

Sand T, Vingen JV (2000). Visual, long-latency auditory and brainstem auditory evoked potentials in migraine: relation to pattern size, stimulus intensity, sound and light discomfort thresholds and pre-attack state. Cephalalgia 20: 804–820.

Sand T, Zwart JA (2004). The blink reflex in chronic tension-type headache, migraine, and cervicogenic headache. Cephalalgia 14: 447–450.

Sándor PS, Afra J, Proietti-Cecchini A et al. (1999a). Familial influences on cortical evoked potentials in migraine. Neuroreport 10: 1235–1238.

Sándor PS, Roon KI, Ferrari MD et al. (1999b). The repeatability of the intensity dependence of cortical auditory evoked potentials (IDAP) in the assessment of cortical information processing. Cephalalgia 19: 873–880.

Sándor PS, Afra J, Ambrosini A et al. (2000). Prophylactic treatment of migraine with beta-blockers and riboflavin: differential effects on the intensity dependence of auditory evoked cortical potentials. Headache 40: 30–35.

Sándor PS, Mascia A, Seidel L et al. (2001). Subclinical cerebellar impairment in the common types of migraine: a three-dimensional analysis of reaching movements. Ann Neurol 49: 668–672.

Sandrini G, Proietti Cecchini A, Milanov I et al. (2002). Electrophysiological evidence for trigeminal neuron sensitization in patients with migraine. Neurosci Lett 317: 135–138.

Sandrini G, Friberg L, Janig W et al. (2004). Neurophysiological tests and neuroimaging procedures in non-acute headache: guidelines and recommendations. Eur J Neurol 11: 217–224.

Sauer S, Schellenberg R, Hofmann HC (1997). Functional imaging of headache – first steps in an objective quantitative classification of migraine. Eur J Med Res 2: 367–376.

Schlake HP, Grotemeyer KH, Hofferberth B et al. (1990). Brainstem auditory evoked potentials in migraine – evidence of increased side differences during the pain-free interval. Headache 30: 129–132.

Schoenen J (1996a). Deficient habituation of evoked cortical potentials in migraine: a link between brain biology, behavior and trigeminovascular activation? Biomed Pharmacother 50: 71–78.

Schoenen J (1996b). Abnormal cortical information processing between migraine attacks. In: M Sandler, M Ferrari, S Harnett (Eds.), Migraine: Pharmacology and Genetics. Altman, London, pp. 233–253.

Schoenen J, Timsit-Berthier M (1993). Contingent negative variation: methods and potential interest in headache. Cephalalgia 13: 28–32.

Schoenen J, Maertens A, Timsit-Berthier A et al. (1985a). Contingent negative variation (CNV) as a diagnostic and physiopathologic tool in headache patients. In: FC Rose (Ed.), Migraine. Clinical and Research Advances. Karger, Basel, pp. 17–25.

Schoenen J, Timsit-Berthier M, Timsit M (1985b). Correlations between contingent negative variation and plasma levels of catecholamines in headache patients. Cephalalgia 5 (S1): 480.

Schoenen J, Jamart B, Delwaide PJ (1987). Topographic EEG mapping in common and classic migraine during and between attacks. In: F Clifford Rose (Ed.), Advances in Headache Research. Smith Gordon, London, pp. 25–33.

Schoenen J, Wang W, Albert A et al. (1995). Potentiation instead of habituation characterizes visual evoked potentials in migraine patients between attacks. Eur J Neurol 2: 115–122.

Sener HO, Haktanir I, Demirci S (1997). Pattern-reversal visual evoked potentials in migraineurs with or without visual aura. Headache 37: 449–451.

Seri S, Cerquiglini A, Guidetti V (1993). Computerized EEG topography in childhood migraine between and during attacks. Cephalalgia 13: 53–56.

Shibata K, Osawa M, Iwata M (1997a). Pattern reversal visual evoked potentials in classic and common migraine. J Neurol Sci 145: 177–181.

Shibata K, Osawa M, Iwata M (1997b). Simultaneous recording of pattern reversal electroretinograms and visual evoked potentials in migraine. Cephalalgia 17: 742–747.

Shibata K, Osawa M, Iwata M (1998). Pattern reversal visual evoked potentials in migraine with aura and migraine aura without headache. Cephalalgia 18: 319–323.

Shibata K, Yamane K, Iwata M et al. (2005). Evaluating the effects of spatial frequency on migraines by using pattern-reversal visual evoked potentials. Clin Neurophysiol 116: 2220–2227.

Simon RH, Zimmerman AW, Tasman A et al. (1982). Spectral analysis of photic stimulation in migraine. Electroencephalogr Clin Neurophysiol 53: 270–276.

Siniatchkin M, Gerber WD, Kropp P et al. (2000a). Are the periodic changes of neurophysiological parameters during the pain-free interval in migraine related to abnormal orienting activity? Cephalalgia 20: 20–29.

Siniatchkin M, Kropp P, Neumann M et al. (2000b). Intensity dependence of auditory evoked potentials in migraine families. Pain 85: 247–254.

Siniatchkin M, Kirsch E, Kropp P et al. (2000c). Slow cortical potentials in migraine families. Cephalalgia 20: 881–892.

Siniatchkin M, Kropp P, Gerber WD (2003). What kind of habituation is impaired in migraine patients? Cephalalgia 23: 511–518.

Siniatchkin M, Averkina N, Gerber WD (2006a). Relationship between precipitating agents and neurophysiological abnormalities in migraine. Cephalalgia 26: 457–465.

Siniatchkin M, Averkina N, Andrasik F et al. (2006b). Neurophysiological reactivity before a migraine attack. Neurosci Lett 400: 121–124.

Siniatchkin M, Kraner-Herwig B, Kocabiyik E et al. (2007). Intracortical inhibition and facilitation in migraine – a transcranial magnetic stimulation study. Headache 47: 364–370.

Spreafico C, Frigerio R, Santoro P et al. (2004). Visual evoked potentials in migraine. Neurol Sci 25 (Suppl. 3): S288–S290.

Tagliati M, Sabbadini M, Bernardi G et al. (1995). Multichannel visual evoked potentials in migraine. Electroenceph Clin Neurophysiol 96: 1–5.

Terwindt GM, Kors EE, Vein AA et al. (2004). Single-fiber EMG in familial hemiplegic migraine. Neurology 63: 1942–1943.

Tsounis S, Milonas J, Gilliam F (1993). Hemi-field pattern reversal visual evoked potentials in migraine. Cephalalgia 13: 267–271.

Valdizan JR, Andreu C, Almarcegui C et al. (1994). Quantitative EEG in children with headache. Headache 34: 53–55.

Valeriani M, de Tommaso M, Restuccia D et al. (2003). Reduced habituation to experimental pain in migraine patients: a CO_2 laser evoked potential study. Pain 105: 57–64.

Valeriani M, Rinalduzzi S, Vigevano F (2005). Multilevel somatosensory system disinhibition in children with migraine. Pain 118: 137–144.

Valli G, Cappellari A, Zago S et al. (2002). Migraine is not associated with hyperexcitability of the occipital cortex. A transcranial magnetic stimulation controlled study. 10th World Congress of Pain. Proceedings. 1580-P128, IASP Press, Seattle, p. 525.

Van der Kamp W, Maassen van den Brink M, Ferrari M et al. (1996). Interictal cortical hyperexcitability in migraine patients demonstrated with transcranial magnetic stimulation. J Neurol Sci 139: 106–110.

Van der Kamp W, Maassen van den Brink A, Ferrari M et al. (1997). Interictal cortical excitability to magnetic stimulation in familial hemiplegic migraine. Neurology 48: 1462–1464.

Wang W, Schoenen J (1994). Reduction of temporalis exteroceptive suppression by peripheral electrical stimulation in migraine and tension-type headaches. Pain 59: 327–334.

Wang W, Schoenen J (1996). Suppression of voluntary temporalis muscle activity by peripheral limb stimulations in healthy volunteers, migraineurs and tension-type headache sufferers. Funct Neurol 11: 307–315.

Wang W, Schoenen J (1998). Interictal potentiation of passive "oddball" auditory event-related potentials in migraine. Cephalalgia 18: 261–265.

Wang W, Schoenen J, Timsit-Berthier M (1995). Cognitive functions in migraine without aura between attacks: a psychophysiological approach using the "oddball" paradigm. Neurophysiol Clin 25: 3–11.

Wang W, Timsit-Berthier M, Schoenen J (1996). Intensity dependence of auditory evoked potentials is pronounced in migraine: an indication of cortical potentiation and low serotonergic neurotransmission? Neurology 46: 1404–1409.

Wang W, Wang GP, Ding XL et al. (1999a). Personality and response to repeated visual stimulation in migraine and tension-type headaches. Cephalalgia 19: 718–724.

Wang W, Wang YH, Fu XM et al. (1999b). Auditory evoked potentials and multiple personality measures in migraine and post-traumatic headaches. Pain 79: 235–242.

Weiller C, May A, Limmroth V et al. (1995). Brain stem activation in spontaneous human migraine attacks. Nat Med 1: 658–660.

Welch KM, Levine SR, D'Andrea G et al. (1989). Preliminary observations on brain energy metabolism in migraine studied by in vivo phosphorus 31 NMR spectroscopy. Neurology 39: 538–541.

Werhahn KJ, Wiseman K, Herzog J et al. (2000). Motor cortex excitability in patients with migraine with aura and hemiplegic migraine. Cephalalgia 20: 45–50.

Yamada T, Dickins QS, Arensdorf K et al. (1986). Basilar migraine: polarity-dependent alteration of brainstem auditory evoked potential. Neurology 36: 1256–1260.

Yilmaz M, Bayazit YA, Erbagci I et al. (2001). Visual evoked potential changes in migraine. Influence of migraine attack and aura. J Neurol Sci 184: 139–141.

Young WB, Oshinsky ML, Shechter AL et al. (2004). Consecutive transcranial magnetic stimulation: phosphene thresholds in migraineurs and controls. Headache 44: 131–135.

Yucesan C, Sener O, Mutluer N (2000). Influence of disease duration on visual evoked potentials in migraineurs. Headache 40: 384–388.

Handbook of Clinical Neurology, Vol. 97 (3rd series)
Headache
G. Nappi and M.A. Moskowitz, Editors

Chapter 24

Migraine: clinical diagnostic criteria

F. MICHAEL CUTRER[1]* AND VINCENT T. MARTIN[2]
[1]*Department of Neurology, Mayo Clinic, Rochester, MN, USA*
[2]*Division of General Internal Medicine, University of Cincinnati College of Medicine, Cincinnati, OH, USA*

INTRODUCTION

The criteria formulated by the International Headache Society (IHS), first in 1988 (Headache Classification Committee of the International Headache Society, 1988) and then revised and published in a second edition in 2004 (Headache Classification Subcommittee of the International Headache Society, 2004), are widely accepted as the basis for accurate clinical diagnosis of headache disorders. Over the past 18 years the IHS criteria have been very helpful in defining homogeneous populations for clinical research and have gradually had an important beneficial effect on daily clinical practice. Both editions of the IHS diagnostic criteria have employed a hierarchical structure which divides all headaches into two broad categories: secondary headache disorders, in which the headache may be attributed to an identifiable underlying abnormality (etiological diagnosis), and primary headache disorders, in which such a causal abnormality cannot be identified (syndromic or symptomatic diagnosis). The primary and secondary headache disorders are then, in turn, divided into headache types, subtypes, and subforms. Such a hierarchical system allows physicians and scientists to employ the criteria to the level of precision required for their purposes.

In the case of migraine, the disorder as a whole is coded as 1 based on the characteristics of the acute headache attack. The two major subtypes of migraine are then divided into 1.1 migraine without aura and 1.2 migraine with aura, based on the presence or absence of transient focal neurological symptoms. Migraine with aura is then further subdivided into 1.2.1 typical aura with migraine headache, 1.2.2 typical aura with non-migraine headache, and 1.2.3 typical aura without headache, based on the co-occurrence of focal neurological symptoms with headache. Other subforms of aura include 1.2.4 familial hemiplegic migraine (formerly motor aura) and 1.2.5 sporadic hemiplegic migraine, derived from new information about the genetic underpinnings of motor symptoms that can accompany migraine headache, as well as 1.2.6 basilar-type migraine, based on the presumed brainstem (non-cortical) origin of the neurological symptoms. Other subtypes of migraine include: 1.3 childhood precursors of migraine; 1.4 retinal migraine, in which visual disturbance is monocular (prechiasmal) rather than homonymous (retrochiasmal); 1.5 complications of migraine; and 1.6 probable migraine, in which the headache fails to fulfill one of the criteria required for definite diagnosis.

Because the criteria for the primary headache disorders are based on the symptom characteristics of the acute attack, the criteria for migraine and the other primary headache disorders always include the final caveat: "not attributable to another disorder." The diagnostic criteria for migraine remained fairly stable from the first edition to the second edition, with the most prominent changes including the addition of criteria for the diagnosis of chronic migraine and the separate categorization of hemiplegic migraine. The criteria for migraine are dynamic and likely to show continuing change over the coming decades as our knowledge of migraine genetics and pathophysiology evolves.

1.1. MIGRAINE WITHOUT AURA

Migraine without aura is defined by the specific characteristics of the headache attack, its duration, and the associated symptoms that accompany it. IHS criteria (the second edition of the International Classification of Headache Disorders (ICHD-II): Headache Classification Subcommittee of the International

*Correspondence to: F. Michael Cutrer, MD, Department of Neurology, Mayo Clinic, 200 First St. SW, Rochester, MN 55902, USA, Tel: 507-538-1036, Fax: 507-266-4419, E-mail: cutrer.michael@mayo.edu

Headache Society, 2004) require that an individual have five past attacks that fulfill the following criteria:

- Duration of 4–72 h
- Two of more of the following headache characteristics: unilateral location, pulsating quality, moderate to severe intensity, aggravation by physical activity
- One or more associated symptoms occurring during the attack: nausea/vomiting or both photophobia and phonophobia
- Attacks must not be attributable to another disorder. That is, the history and physical examination must not suggest any of the disorders identified as causative of headache in the IHCD-II classification, or history and/or physical and/or neurological examinations do suggest that such disorder is present but it is ruled out by appropriate investigations, or such disorder is present but attacks do not occur for the first time in close temporal relation to the disorder.

The 2004 criteria for migraine without aura (Headache Classification Subcommittee of the International Headache Society, 2004) are identical to those established in 1988 by the IHS (Headache Classification Committee of the International Headache Society, 1988). The interobserver reliability of these criteria has been established in past studies (Granella et al., 1994; Leone et al., 1994). Field testing of these criteria has suggested that the presence of associated symptoms (e.g., photophobia, phonophobia, nausea and vomiting) provides the greatest discrimination between migraine without aura and other headache subtypes (Keck, 1994). It has been suggested that osmophobia be added to the diagnostic criteria for migraine without aura. Studies have reported that the presence of osmophobia is very specific for the diagnosis of migraine without aura (Kelman, 2004; Zanchin et al., 2005). In fact, alternate diagnostic criteria for migraine without aura, which include osmophobia as an associated symptom, have been proposed in the appendix of the 2004 criteria to encourage future research in this area.

Note that a diagnosis of migraine without aura requires a specific grouping of symptoms to establish a diagnosis and that no single symptom absolutely defines this disorder. Past studies have shown that migraine is unilateral in 52–63%, throbbing in 62–78%, and moderate to severe in 85–91% (Rasmussen et al., 1991; Martin et al., 2005). For example, if one only diagnoses migraine when the headaches are unilateral then 37–48% of all cases would be missed. Therefore, an accurate diagnosis of migraine headache requires use of several migraine-related symptoms, as specified in the IHS criteria.

Other investigators have attempted to simplify the diagnosis of migraine through development of abbreviated criteria for use within primary care. Lipton et al. (2003) developed abbreviated diagnostic criteria and later validated them in a primary care setting. They determined that the presence of nausea, photophobia, and disability (any two of the three) had a sensitivity of 81%, a specificity of 75%, and a positive predictive value of 93% in the diagnosis of migraine within primary care settings. These criteria could be used by physicians who may not know the IHS criteria to increase the probability of a migraine diagnosis.

1.2.1.–1.2.3. MIGRAINE WITH TYPICAL AURA

The IHS criteria define migraine with aura as a "recurrent disorder manifesting in attacks of reversible focal neurological symptoms that usually develop gradually over 5–20 minutes and last for less than 60 minutes." Headache with the features of migraine without aura usually follows the aura symptoms. Less commonly, headache lacks migrainous features or is completely absent (Headache Classification Subcommittee of the International Headache Society, 2004).

To fulfill the IHS diagnostic criteria for migraine with aura an individual must have had at least two attacks involving an aura consisting of at least one of the following, but not motor weakness:

- Fully reversible visual symptoms, including positive features (flickering lights, spots, or lines) and/or negative features (loss of vision)
- Fully reversible sensory symptoms, including positive features (pins and needles) and/or negative features (numbness)
- Fully reversible dysphasic speech disturbance.

And the attacks must have at least two of the following characteristics:

- They include homonymous visual symptoms and/or unilateral sensory symptoms
- At least one aura symptom develops gradually over $\geq$5 min and/or different aura symptoms occur in succession over $\geq$5 min
- Each symptom lasts $\geq$5 min and $\leq$60 min
- Attacks must not be attributable to another disorder.

The typical aura consists of fully reversible visual, sensory, or language symptoms that generally precede or accompany the appearance of migraine headache. In both visual and sensory auras, the symptoms follow a bimodal progression with positive symptoms (shimmering lights, zigzagging line, or prickling paresthesias) appearing first, only to be followed by negative symptoms (blind spot or numbness). In the language aura, a bimodal pattern is less apparent, although patients experiencing language aura report both paraphasic errors (deranged function) and word retrieval difficulties (loss of function). Typical visual and sensory aura symptoms also have a spreading or migratory quality in which the visual symptoms expand or move across the visual field and sensory symptoms migrate over an extremity or across the face.

In ICHD-I (Headache Classification Committee of the International Headache Society, 1988), motor symptoms were included as a typical aura subtype. New genetic information became available in the interval between the first and second editions of the classification, which allowed a more precise definition of hemiplegic migraine. As a result, motor symptoms are now considered as diagnostic of hemiplegic migraine, a distinct type of migraine aura. However, typical aura symptoms (visual, sensory, and language) very frequently occur in hemiplegic migraine and their presence does not exclude the diagnosis.

Three types of attack may occur in patients who experience typical aura symptoms:

1. Typical aura with migraine headache (1.2.1) in which the aura is accompanied or is followed within an hour by a headache that meets the diagnostic criteria for migraine without aura (1.1)
2. Typical aura with non-migraine headache (1.2.2) in which the aura is accompanied or followed by a headache that does not fulfill criteria for migraine without aura (1.1)
3. Typical aura without headache (1.2.3) in which the aura symptoms are not followed by headache.

The characteristics of aura are identical regardless of the attack type. When aura symptoms occur in the absence of headaches fulfilling the criteria for migraine without aura, it is important it exclude conditions which may mimic aura, especially when the symptoms are of very short (seconds to under 10 min) or very long (more than 1 h) duration, they are primarily negative (loss of function), or they begin after the age of 40. Many patients experience only a single type of aura-associated attack. However, other patients may experience more than one attack type over the course of their lives.

Clinical research studies of typical aura based on the IHS criteria

One of the major benefits of validated criteria for migraine diagnosis is the ability to conduct nosographic studies of migraine in clinically homogeneous populations. Over the past 15 years, several such studies have been published. In 1996, a general population-based analysis of migraine aura was published in which 163 cases were identified from a sample of 4000 Danish citizens (Russell and Olesen, 1996). In this study, 62 patients reported that some of their migraine auras occurred with headache and some occurred without headache, whereas 7 patients reported only auras without headache. In this case series, visual aura was overwhelmingly the most common aura symptom, occurring in 99% of patients, followed by sensory, language, and motor auras. Visual aura occurred without any other aura symptoms in 64% of cases, whereas other aura types usually occurred with another aura type (usually visual).

These findings are similar to those seen in another small prospective study published in 1994 in which 54 attacks of migraine with aura in 20 patients were described in detail (Russell et al., 1994). In this study, visual and sensory aura symptoms developed over 15–25 min and persisted for 20–55 min. When visual and sensory symptoms preceded a headache, the headache typically had features of migraine. However, if the headache preceded the aura symptoms, the headache lacked migrainous features and was of the tension type.

In a study employing IHS criteria, Eriksen and co-workers (2004a) compared the characteristics of migraine with aura in patients with familial typical (non-motor) migraine with aura to those seen in migraineurs with aura from the1996 Danish general population-based study. Patients with familial migraine with typical aura began to have attacks at an earlier age and continued to have attacks until later in life. They also had a higher co-occurrence of migraine without aura.

In another IHS criteria-based study, a diagnostic scale for migraine aura, known as the Visual Aura Rating Scale (VARS), was developed and tested in an effort to improve assessment of typical aura. The scale is based on a quantification of the cardinal characteristics of the visual aura, the most commonly occurring type (Russell and Olesen, 1996). The VARS score was derived from the weighted sum of the presence of five visual symptom characteristics, including: duration 5–60 min (3 points), develops gradually (2 points), scotoma (2 points), zigzag lines (2 points), and unilaterality (1 point) (Eriksen et al., 2005). A VARS score of 5 or more predicted migraine with aura with a sensitivity of 96% and a specificity of 98% (Eriksen et al., 2004c).

In another IHS criteria-based study, the prognosis of migraine with aura was examined. In this outcomes study of 53 patients initially seen for migraine with aura between 1977 and 1984 (Eriksen et al., 2004b), at the time of a follow-up telephone interview, attacks had ceased for 2 years in 36% of patients. Attacks had stopped in 41% of patients who experienced visual aura alone and in 25% of those with sensory or language aura in addition to their visual aura ($P = 0.36$). In those who continued to have migraine attacks, the frequency of attacks was improved in 44% and headache intensity was improved in 41% of patients.

1.2.4. AND 1.2.5. FAMILIAL AND SPORADIC HEMIPLEGIC MIGRAINE

The availability of new genetic data regarding patients with transient focal motor symptoms has allowed a more precise diagnosis of hemiplegic migraine than was available in the past. As a result hemiplegic migraine was separated as a distinct diagnostic category from the other typical forms of migraine with aura. Hemiplegic migraine has been further subdivided into two forms: familial hemiplegic migraine (FHM) (1.2.4), in which a patient has motor aura and a first- or second-degree relative also has motor aura (Headache Classification Subcommittee of the International Headache Society, 2004), and sporadic hemiplegic migraine (1.2.5), in which there is not a first- or second-degree relative with motor aura symptoms. Thus far, the specific genetic mutations for three forms of FHM have been identified: in FHM1, mutations are found in the *CACNA1A* gene on chromosome 19 (Ophoff et al., 1996); in FHM2, mutations occur in the *ATP1A1* gene on chromosome 1 (De Fusco et al., 2003); and in FHM3 mutations are present in the *SCN1A* gene on chromosome 2 (Dichgans et al., 2005).

To fulfill the IHS diagnostic criteria for migraine with aura an individual must have had at least two attacks of fully reversible motor weakness and at least one of the following:

- Fully reversible visual symptoms, including positive features (flickering lights, spots, or lines) and/or negative features (loss of vision)
- Fully reversible sensory symptoms, including positive features (pins and needles) and/or negative features (numbness)
- Fully reversible dysphasic speech disturbance.

And the attacks must have at least two of the following characteristics:

- They include homonymous visual symptoms and/or unilateral sensory symptoms
- At least one aura symptom develops gradually over $\geq$5 min and/or different aura symptoms occur in succession over $\geq$5 min
- Each symptom lasts $\geq$5 min and $\leq$60 min
- Attacks must not be attributable to another disorder.

Attacks of familial and sporadic hemiplegic migraine have the same clinical profile (Thomsen et al., 2003). When compared with population-based migraine with typical aura (non-hemiplegic migraine), patients with both familial and sporadic hemiplegic migraine were more likely to experience more than one aura symptom during a single attack, to have more prolonged aura symptoms, and to have symptoms of basilar-type migraine (Eriksen et al., 2006).

1.2.6. BASILAR-TYPE MIGRAINE

The IHS criteria recognize a distinct subtype of migraine aura in which the aura symptoms originate from brainstem and/or bilateral cerebral hemispheric sources and are not associated with motor symptoms. Basilar-type symptoms frequently occur in FHM1. So the presence of motor symptoms, even if other symptoms suggestive of basilar-type migraine are present, would require the diagnosis of hemiplegic migraine (1.2.4 or 1.2.5) rather than basilar-type migraine (1.2.6).

To fulfill the IHS diagnostic criteria for basilar-type migraine (1.2.6) an individual must have at least two attacks involving an aura consisting of at least two of the following, but not motor weakness:

- Dysarthria
- Vertigo
- Tinnitus
- Hypacusia
- Diplopia
- Visual symptoms simultaneously in both temporal and nasal fields of both eyes
- Ataxia
- Decreased level of consciousness
- Simultaneous bilateral paresthesias.

And the attacks must have at least one of the following characteristics:

- At least one aura symptom develops gradually over $\geq$5 min and/or different aura symptoms occurring in succession over $\geq$5 min
- Each symptom lasts $\geq$5 min and $\leq$60 min
- Headache which meets the criteria for migraine without aura begins during or within 60 min of the resolution of the aura symptoms
- Attacks must not be attributable to another disorder.

Although basilar-type migraine may occur in either sex at any age, it is more commonly seen in young females (Panayiotopoulos, 1991). Although the term "basilar-type migraine" is used because of presumed abnormality in the territory of the basilar artery, whether the symptoms are due to involvement of the basilar artery or rather are bihemispheric in origin is uncertain. Occipital headache is more common in basilar-type migraine than in migraine with typical aura (Sturzenegger and Meienberg, 1985), which might weakly suggest posterior circulation (basilar) involvement, especially if bilateral sensory symptoms predominate.

1.3. CHILDHOOD PERIODIC SYNDROMES

Three syndromes described in children are recognized in the IHS criteria as precursors to migraine. Small population-based studies suggest a relationship between migraine and these disorders (Abu-Arafeh and Russell 1995a, b, c).

Cyclical vomiting (1.3.1) is a self-limited condition of childhood consisting of episodes of severe nausea, pallor, and lethargy separated by symptom-free periods. During attacks the child may also experience photophobia, phonophobia, and exercise intolerance. To fulfill the IHS diagnostic criteria for cyclical vomiting, the patient must have experienced at least five stereotypical attacks of intense nausea and vomiting lasting from 1 h to 5 days in which vomiting occurs at least four times per hour for at least 1 h, and which are separated by symptom-free periods and which cannot be attributed to another disorder.

Abdominal migraine (1.3.2) consists of episodic dull, midline, moderate to severe, abdominal pain in children. The episodes last from 1 to 72 h and are separated by symptom-free periods. In some cases flushing or vasomotor symptoms can occur. To fulfill the IHS diagnostic criteria for abdominal migraine, the patient must have experienced at least five stereotypical attacks of abdominal pain lasting from 1 h to 72 h and associated with all of the following characteristics:

- Midline location, periumbilical or poorly localized
- Dull or "just sore" quality
- Moderate to severe intensity.

And two of the following in combination with the abdominal pain:

- Anorexia
- Nausea
- Vomiting
- Pallor.

And which cannot be attributed to another disorder.

Benign paroxysmal vertigo of childhood (1.3.3) is characterized by recurrent episodes of vertigo which occur without warning and resolve spontaneously after minutes to hours. The attacks may be accompanied by vomiting, nystagmus, and headache.

To fulfill the IHS diagnostic criteria for benign paroxysmal vertigo, the patient must have experienced at least five stereotypical attacks of episodic vertigo lasting from minutes to hours which resolved spontaneously to a baseline with normal neurological, vestibular, and audiometric function, and the patient must have a normal electroencephalogram.

1.4. RETINAL MIGRAINE

Retinal migraine refers to a monocular visual impairment that occurs in temporal association with a headache that meets diagnostic criteria for migraine without aura. The monocular visual impairment generally represents a visual loss, but scotomata, flashing lights, haloes, and zigzag lines have been reported. The symptoms can last for seconds, days, or even weeks and may recur repeatedly in the same patient. The pathophysiology is unknown, but may occur as a result of vasospasm of ciliary or retinal arteries, or could represent a spreading depression of retinal neurons (Grosberg et al., 2005).

The IHS criteria (Headache Classification Subcommittee of the International Headache Society, 2004) require the following:

- Fully reversible monocular positive and/or negative visual phenomena confirmed by physical examination during an attack or by the patient's drawing of a monocular field defect
- Headache meeting criteria for migraine without aura that begins during the visual symptoms or follows them within 60 min
- Normal ophthalmoscopic examination between attacks
- Not attributable to another disorder.

1.5.1. CHRONIC MIGRAINE

Chronic migraine was a new addition to the revised IHS criteria published in 2004. A diagnosis of chronic migraine requires (Headache Classification Subcommittee of the International Headache Society, 2004):

- $\geq$15 days of headache per month that fulfills criteria for migraine without aura for longer than 3 months
- Not attributable to another disorder.

These criteria have been controversial for several reasons. First, chronic migraine often evolves from a less frequent episodic pattern and, as the headaches chronify, they may lose some of their migraine-like features and resemble tension-type headaches. This has been referred to as "transformed migraine." Second, with the advent of migraine-specific therapies (e.g., triptans and ergots) some patients may treat migraine attacks so early in their course that migraine symptoms may not develop. Third, there is evidence that when migraine and tension-type headaches coexist in the same patient they may represent spectrums of migraine headache (Lipton et al., 2000). Therefore, several researchers have proposed that the number of days of migraine per month be reduced to $\geq$8 to meet diagnostic criteria for chronic migraine. These criteria for chronic migraine were revised in 2006 and are included in the appendix of the current classification (Headache Classification Committee, 2006). They require the following:

- Headaches on $\geq$15 days per month for at least 3 months
- $\geq$5 previous attacks fulfilling criteria for migraine without aura
- $\geq$8 days per month of headache for 3 months that has two of four headache characteristics (i.e., unilateral location, pulsating quality, moderate to severe intensity, and aggravation by physical activity), one of two groupings of associated symptoms (nausea and/or vomiting or both photophobia and phonophobia), and treated by an ergot or triptan before the development of migraine symptoms
- No medication overuse and not attributed to another causative disorder.

Note that the above criteria state that chronic migraine cannot be diagnosed in the setting of medication overuse. Only after the overused abortive medication has been withdrawn can a patient meet criteria for chronic migraine headache. Field testing of the above criteria has been performed in patients with transformed migraine. Bigal et al. (2006a) reported that the revised 2006 criteria for chronic migraine identified a greater proportion of patients with transformed migraine than the 2004 criteria.

1.5.2. STATUS MIGRAINOSUS

Status migrainosus refers to the persistence of an attack of migraine without aura beyond the 72 h typically encountered with episode attacks. The headache attack also has to be severe and unremitting over that time period and not attributed to another disorder. Less severe migraines that persist beyond 72 h would be classified as probable migraine (see below) (Headache Classification Subcommittee of the International Headache Society, 2004).

1.5.3. PERSISTENT AURA WITHOUT INFARCTION

If a patient experiences persistence of a typical previously transient aura symptom for greater than 60 min and neuroimaging demonstrates no cerebral infarction in the relevant brain area, then the patient is considered to have persistent aura without infarction (1.5.3). This is a rare condition with no known reliably effective treatment. It should be differentiated from migrainous infarction and posterior leukoencephalopathy (Headache Classification Subcommittee of the International Headache Society, 2004).

1.5.4. MIGRAINOUS INFARCTION

A migrainous infarction is diagnosed when a patient has an aura typical of a past attack that lasts longer than >60 min and a cerebral infarction is noted on neuroimaging in the relevant brain area (Headache Classification Subcommittee of the International Headache Society, 2004). This could account for 0.5–1.5% of all strokes or 10% of strokes in younger patients (Sacquegna et al., 1989; Arboix et al., 2003). The pathophysiology of migrainous infarction is unknown, but has been postulated to result from oligemia as a result of spreading cortical depression. Before making a diagnosis of migrainous infarction one must exclude disorders that have been associated with migraine, but could also lead to stroke, such as arterial dissection, intracranial aneurysm, and patent foramen ovale (Agostoni and Aliprandi, 2006).

1.5.5. MIGRAINE-TRIGGERED SEIZURES

A diagnosis of migraine-triggered seizures is established in a patient who meets IHS criteria for migraine with aura (1.2) and seizure occurs during or within 1 h after a migraine aura (Headache Classification Subcommittee of the International Headache Society, 2004). Marks and Ehrenberg (1993) identified 395 patients who experienced both migraine as well as a seizure disorder and reported that 3% of these patients experienced a seizure during or immediately after an aura. The pathophysiology of migraine-triggered seizures is unknown, but it is possible that regional oligemia as encountered in the cortical spreading depression of the aura could trigger a seizure (Agostoni and Aliprandi, 2006).

1.6. PROBABLE MIGRAINE

Probable migraine refers to attacks and/or headache that fulfill all but one of the diagnostic criteria for a subtype of migraine headache (Headache Classification Subcommittee of the International Headache Society, 2004). Probable migraine is categorized into three subtypes: probable migraine without aura (1.6.1), probable migraine with aura (1.6.2), and probable chronic migraine (1.6.5). Epidemiological studies from France have reported that 11.2% of the general population meet strict criteria for migraine while another 10.1% meet criteria for probable migraine (Lanteri-Minet et al., 2005). The most common reason for a patient to be classified as having probable migraine is short attack duration (<4 h) (Rains et al., 2001; Lanteri-Minet et al., 2005). Migraineurs are more likely to be diagnosed with probable migraine as they age because migraine-related symptoms tend to decrease with age (Bigal et al., 2006b).

CONCLUSION

Migraine headache represents a diverse group of disorders that includes migraine with and without aura, childhood periodic syndromes, retinal migraine, complications of migraine, and probable migraine. The criteria as proposed by the IHS have standardized the diagnosis of migraine headache for use within clinical and research settings. Controversy exists with some of the proposed criteria (particularly with migraine without aura and chronic migraine), which only serves to emphasize the fact that these diagnostic criteria are in constant evolution. Further research in the field will guide future revisions of the diagnostic criteria to provide more precise and accurate diagnoses of this complex disorder called "migraine headache."

References

Abu-Arafeh I, Russell G (1995a). Cyclical vomiting syndrome in children: a population-based study. J Pediatr Gastroenterol Nutr 21 (4): 454–458.

Abu-Arafeh I, Russell G (1995b). Prevalence and clinical features of abdominal migraine compared with those of migraine headache. Arch Dis Child 72 (5): 413–417.

Abu-Arafeh I, Russell G (1995c). Paroxysmal vertigo as a migraine equivalent in children: a population-based study. Cephalalgia 15 (1): 22–25.

Agostoni E, Aliprandi A (2006). The complications of migraine with aura. Neurol Sci 27 (Suppl. 2): S91–S95.

Arboix A, Massons J, Garcia-Eroles L et al. (2003). Migrainous cerebral infarction in the Sagrat Cor Hospital of Barcelona stroke registry. Cephalalgia 23: 389–394.

Bigal ME, Tepper SJ, Sheftell FD et al. (2006a). Field testing alternative criteria for chronic migraine. Cephalalgia 26: 477–482.

Bigal ME, Liberman JN, Lipton RB (2006b). Age-dependent prevalence and clinical features of migraine. Neurology 67: 246–251.

De Fusco M, Marconi R, Silvestri L et al. (2003). Haploinsufficiency of ATP1A2 encoding the Na^+/K^+ pump alpha2 subunit associated with familial hemiplegic migraine type 2. Nat Genet 33: 192–196.

Dichgans M, Freilinger T, Eckstein G et al. (2005). Mutation in the neuronal voltage-gated sodium channel SCN1A in familial hemiplegic migraine. Lancet 366: 371–377.

Eriksen MK, Thomsen LL, Andersen I et al. (2004a). Clinical characteristics of 362 patients with familial migraine with aura. Cephalalgia 24: 564–575.

Eriksen MK, Thomsen LL, Russell MB (2004b). Prognosis of migraine with aura. Cephalalgia 24: 18–22.

Eriksen MK, Thomsen LL, Olesen J (2004c). New international classification of migraine with aura (ICHD-2) applied to 362 migraine patients. Eur J Neurol 11 (9): 583–591.

Eriksen MK, Thomsen LL, Olesen J (2005). The Visual Aura Rating Scale (VARS) for migraine aura diagnosis. Cephalalgia 25 (10): 801–810.

Eriksen MK, Thomsen LL, Olesen J (2006). Implications of clinical subtypes of migraine with aura. Headache 46: 286–297.

Granella F, D'Alessandro R, Manzoni GC et al. (1994). International Headache Society classification: interobserver reliability in the diagnosis of primary headaches. Cephalalgia 14: 16–20.

Grosberg BM, Solomon S, Lipton RB (2005). Retinal migraine. Curr Pain Headache Rep 9: 268–271.

Headache Classification Committee of the International Headache Society (1988). Classification and diagnostic criteria for headache disorders, cranial neuralgias and facial pain. Cephalalgia 8 (Suppl. 7): 1–96.

Headache Classification Subcommittee of the International Headache Society (2004). The international classification of headache disorders, 2nd edition. Cephalalgia 24: 1–30.

Headache Classification Committee, Olesen J, Bousser MG, Diener HC et al. (2006). New appendix criteria open for a broader concept of chronic migraine. Cephalalgia 26 (6): 742–746.

Keck PE Jr, Merikangas KR, McElroy SL, Strakowski SM (1994). Diagnostic and treatment implications of psychiatric comorbidity with migraine. Ann Clin Psychiatry 6 (3): 165–171.

Kelman L (2004). The place of osmophobia and taste abnormalities in migraine classification: a tertiary care study of 1237 patients. Cephalalgia 24: 940–946.

Lanteri-Minet M, Valade D, Geraud G et al. (2005). Migraine and probable migraine – results of FRAMIG 3, a French nationwide survey carried out according to the 2004 IHS classification. Cephalalgia 25: 1146–1158.

Leone M, Filippini G, D'Amico D et al. (1994). Assessment of International Headache Society diagnostic criteria: a reliability study. Cephalalgia 14: 280–284.

Lipton RB, Stewart WF, Cady R et al. (2000). 2000 Wolfe Award. Sumatriptan for the range of headaches in migraine sufferers: results of the Spectrum Study. Headache 40: 783–791.

Lipton RB, Dodick D, Sadovsky R et al. (2003). A self-administered screener for migraine in primary care: the ID Migraine validation study. Neurology 61: 375–382.

Marks DA, Ehrenberg BL (1993). Migraine-related seizures in adults with epilepsy, with EEG correlation. Neurology 43: 2476–2483.

Martin VT, Penzien DB, Houle TT et al. (2005). The predictive value of abbreviated migraine diagnostic criteria. Headache 45: 1102–1112.

Olesen J, Bousser MG, Diener HC et al. (2006). New appendix criteria open for a broader concept of chronic migraine. Cephalalgia 26: 742–746.

Ophoff RA, Terwindt GM, Vergouwe MN et al. (1996). Familial hemiplegic migraine and episodic ataxia type-2 are caused by mutations in the Ca^{2+} channel gene CACNL1A4. Cell 87: 543–552.

Panayiotopoulos CP (1991). Basilar artery migraine. Neurology 41: 1707.

Rains JC, Penzien DB, Lipchik GL et al. (2001). Diagnosis of migraine: empirical analysis of a large clinical sample of atypical migraine (IHS 1.7) patients and proposed revision of the IHS criteria. Cephalalgia 21: 584–595.

Rasmussen BK, Jensen R, Olesen J (1991). A population-based analysis of the diagnostic criteria of the International Headache Society. Cephalalgia 11: 129–134.

Russell MB, Olesen J (1996). A nosographic analysis of the migraine aura in a general population. Brain 119: 335–361.

Russell MB, Iversen HK, Olesen J (1994). Improved description of the migraine aura by a diagnostic aura diary. Cephalalgia 14: 107–117.

Sacquegna T, Andreoli A, Baldrati A et al. (1989). Ischemic stroke in young adults: the relevance of migrainous infarction. Cephalalgia 9: 255–258.

Sturzenegger MH, Meienberg O (1985). Basilar artery migraine: a follow-up study of 82 cases. Headache 25: 408–415.

Thomsen LL, Ostergaard E, Olesen J et al. (2003). Evidence for a separate type of migraine with aura: sporadic hemiplegic migraine. Neurology 25: 595–601.

Zanchin G, Dainese F, Mainardi F et al. (2005). Osmophobia in primary headaches. J Headache Pain 6: 213–215.

Handbook of Clinical Neurology, Vol. 97 (3rd series)
Headache
G. Nappi and M.A. Moskowitz, Editors

Chapter 25

Migraine and reproductive life

ROSSELLA E. NAPPI [1]* AND SARAH L. BERGA [2]

[1]*Research Center of Reproductive Medicine and Unit of Gynecological Endocrinology and Menopause, Department of Internal Medicine and Endocrinology, IRCCS Maugeri Foundation, University of Pavia, Pavia, Italy*
[2]*Department of Gynecology and Obstetrics, Emory University School of Medicine, Atlanta, GA, USA*

INTRODUCTION

The goddess Athena was born from the skull of Zeus who was suffering from severe recurrent headaches. There is evidence that migraine has been considered a "female disease" since ancient times. Even Sigmund Freud, the famous Viennese founder of psychoanalysis, back in the 19th century made significant observations on the nature of migraine, "a disease less common in the healthy man, more present in the active phase of sexual life, occurring following a certain amount of internal and external stimuli, characterized by periodic attacks of severe pain and with a complex etiology" (Karwautz et al., 1996).

Medical literature has linked gender to migraine, not only because of its preponderance in women from puberty to menopause but also because both neuroendocrine events related to reproductive stages (menarche, pregnancy, and menopause) and menstrual cyclicity and the use of exogenous sex hormones, such as hormonal contraception and replacement therapy, may cause significant change in the clinical pattern of migraine itself (Silberstein, 1992).

Geographical differences in migraine prevalence are not marked. The more recent studies of the general adult population indicate lifetime prevalence rates between 6% and 10% for men and between 15% and 26% for women (Lipton and Bigal, 2005). In European studies 1-year prevalence of migraine ranges from 6% to 15% in adult men and from 14% to 35% in adult women (Stovner et al., 2006). The epidemiological profile of migraine has remained stable over the years in both sexes (Lipton and Stewart, 1993; Rasmussen, 1993; Lyngberg et al., 2005; Lipton et al., 2007). Migraine prevalence in women displays a striking increase between 10 and 12 years, around the time of puberty, with a female-to-male ratio of 3:1 during the fertile age, and a gradual, progressive decline following the age of 40 years, around the time of menopause (Mortimer et al., 1992a; Rasmussen, 1995). In spite of the concept that "the femaleness of the migraine condition is inescapable" (Welch et al., 1984), the role of ovarian function remains to be fully elucidated. Endogenous sex hormone fluctuations throughout the female life cycle significantly affect individual migraine history but it is likely that the endocrine milieu is only one of the multiple triggers of migraine in susceptible women (Silberstein, 2000). However, an association between estrogen "withdrawal" and attacks of migraine without aura, as well as evidence for an association between high estrogen states and attacks of migraine with aura, are strongly supported by several lines of research (MacGregor, 2005). These data are highly relevant for prevention and treatment of migraine in women and further studies are warranted.

MENARCHE

Neuroendocrine aspects of puberty

Puberty is the end-point of a complex series of developmental events, defined by the dynamic interaction between genetic factors and environmental cues, ultimately leading to the attainment of reproductive capacity (Somerville, 1975c). The neuroendocrine basis of puberty has been the subject of extensive investigation in recent decades but the mechanisms controlling the pubertal increase in gonadotropin-releasing hormone

*Correspondence to: Rossella E. Nappi, MD PhD, Research Center of Reproductive Medicine and Unit of Gynecological Endocrinology and Menopause, Department of Internal Medicine and Endocrinology, IRCCS Maugeri Foundation, University of Pavia, Via Ferrata 8, 27100 Pavia, Italy, Tel: 39 0382 592201, Fax: 39 0382 520070, E-mail: renappi@tin.it

(GnRH) release, the key driver of reproductive function, are still unclear. Briefly, the onset of puberty in humans is marked by an increase in the amplitude of luteinizing hormone (LH) pulses, an indirect indicator of the increase in amplitude of GnRH pulses. The hypothalamic GnRH–pituitary gonadotropin complex is functional by at least 0.3 gestation in the human fetus; the sex difference in the fetal and neonatal pattern of secretion is an apparent consequence of imprinting of the fetal hypothalamus–pituitary apparatus by fetal testosterone. The intrinsic central nervous system (CNS) mechanisms responsible for the inhibition of the GnRH pulse generator during childhood (the juvenile phase) involve the major role of an inhibitory neuronal system – the CNS-inhibitory neurotransmitter gamma-aminobutyric acid (GABA) and GABAergic neurons, as revealed by studies in the rhesus monkey (Terasawa and Fernandez, 2001). With the onset of puberty, disinhibition and reactivation of the GnRH pulse generator are associated with a fall in GABAergic neurotransmission and a concomitant increase in the input of excitatory amino acid neurotransmitters (including glutamate) and possibly astroglial-derived growth factors (Grumbach, 2002). Several mechanisms have been hypothesized in the control of the onset of puberty, including a critical level of leptin, the adipocyte hormone signaling the size of body energy store which is involved in the metabolic control of the hypothalamic KiSS-1 system (Tena-Sempere, 2006). However, leptin signal is only one of the several permissive factors which are under investigation in the onset of human puberty.

Nocturnal augmentation of gonadotropin release, especially wake-time LH pulses, marks the onset of sexual development. With the rise in both LH and follicle-stimulating hormone (FSH) there is an increase in ovarian steroid production (namely testosterone and estradiol) and the development of secondary sexual characteristics. In girls, pubertal maturation of the hypothalamic–pituitary–ovarian (HPO) axis results in the dynamic hormonal milieu of the menstrual cycle with the occurrence of the first mid-cycle gonadotropin (FSH and especially LH) surge induced by estradiol increased levels.

Migraine and menarche

Menarche refers to the onset of menstruation during puberty. Less than 10% of US girls start to menstruate before 11 years, and 90% of all US girls are menstruating by 13.75 years of age, with a median age of 12.43 years. Ethnic differences remained even after adjustment for current body mass index and several social and economic variables (Chumlea et al., 2003). Irregular menstrual cycles occur most frequently within the first 2–3 years after menarche and are often anovulatory. By the third gynecological year, 60–80% of cycles are 21–34 days long, as is typical of adults, and within the sixth gynecological year most of the cycles are ovulatory (Adams Hillard, 2002). Approximately 4–5% of children aged under 12 suffer from migraine, with little apparent difference between boys and girls until the time around puberty (Mortimer et al., 1992b). After menarche, the incidence diverges and amongst girls there is a rapid increase which continues throughout early adult life (Stewart et al., 1992). Age- and sex-specific incidence rates for the onset of migraine headache with and without visual aura have been clearly described. Among both males and females, the incidence rate for migraine with visual aura appears to have peaked as much as 3–5 years earlier than the age peak for migraine without aura. For males, the age-specific incidence for migraine with visual aura appears to have peaked on or before 5 years of age, while the highest incidence for migraine without aura occurred between 10 and 11 years of age. By contrast, in girls experiencing migraine with aura the peak incidence was 12–13 years of age, while in those experiencing migraine without aura it was 14–17 years of age (Stewart et al, 1991). Notwithstanding, it is likely that the erratic estrogen secretion occurring in postmenarcheal anovulatory cycles may have a role in the onset of migraine with aura, while the establishment of the ovulatory menstrual cycle is significantly relevant to the onset of migraine without aura.

MENSTRUAL CYCLE

Neuroendocrine aspects of menstrual cycle

The human menstrual cycle represents a complex interplay of dynamic neuroendocrine events driving the activity of the HPO axis in order to ensue reproductive capacity. The pulsatile activity of hypothalamic GnRH is highly regulated by the integration of central and peripheral signals and any changes at the various levels of the HPO may modify target organ sensitivity, alter hormone secretion, and produce anovulation and/or reproductive failure. Virtually the entire array of neurotransmitters, neuropeptides, and neuromodulators, including norepinephrine (NE), dopamine, serotonin (5-HT), GABA, endogenous opioid peptides, and many others, are involved in the control of GnRH release. The endometrium is the target organ of sex steroids (estradiol and progesterone) secreted from the ovary under the regulation of pituitary FSH and LH (Genazzani et al., 1997).

By definition, the ideal menstrual cycle lasts 28 ± 7 days, begins with the first day of bleeding (day 1), and ends just before the next menstrual period. It is conventionally divided into phases and the length of each phase varies from woman to woman and from cycle to cycle. Unpredictable or longer menstrual cycles are normal for teenagers and women in their 40s due to the high rate of anovulatory cycles. The initial portion of the cycle which includes menstruation is the follicular (proliferative) phase. It is characterized by a relatively high ratio of FSH to LH. This is likely the result of a slow GnRH pulse frequency, as evidenced by LH release with an approximately 90-min interpulse interval. This period of FSH drive is critical for the recruitment and maturation of ovarian follicles. FSH induces granulosa cell expression of both LH receptors and levels of the enzyme aromatase, needed for the synthesis of estradiol from androgen precursors. Development of the dominant follicle with increasing gonadotropin and estradiol secretion, culminating in the mid-cycle gonadotropin surge, broadly characterizes the follicular phase, together with the formation of a new layer of endometrium in the uterus (proliferative phase). Indeed, by the middle of the follicular phase, LH pulse frequency has increased to a nearly hourly pattern. With this, LH levels rise and ovarian release of estradiol increases significantly toward mid-cycle. The increase in estradiol and ovarian production of the inhibins (dimeric peptides that selectively inhibit FSH synthesis and secretion) reduce FSH levels, perhaps playing an important role in limiting the final maturation of the non-dominant follicles. At the end of the follicular phase, or mid-cycle, the increasing levels of estradiol result in an enhancement of LH responsiveness, thereby inducing the LH surge. Also, progesterone levels begin to increase and may further augment the LH responses to the ongoing GnRH stimulus. During the surge, LH levels remain increased for 36–48 h, during which time ovulation occurs, estradiol levels decline, and luteinization of the follicle results in increasing production of progesterone (luteal phase). This increase in progesterone plays a critical role in regulating GnRH release by decreasing GnRH pulse frequency (every 2–5 h). In addition to gonadal steroids, the corpus luteum releases higher levels of inhibin, resulting in further reductions in FSH release and preventing recruitment of new follicles. In the luteal phase, progesterone plays a vital role in converting the proliferative endometrium into a secretory lining receptive for implantation and supportive of the early pregnancy (secretory phase). In the absence of fertilization, the corpus luteum regresses and gonadal steroid and peptide production declines, causing menstruation. As the inhibitory actions of progesterone are removed, GnRH pulse frequency increases and LH pulsatility returns to a near hourly pattern. The fall in inhibin and estradiol results in a rise in FSH secretion. Thus, the beginning of follicular recruitment for the subsequent menstrual cycle actually begins during the later portion of the prior luteal phase/menstrual cycle. In the event that pregnancy occurs, a hormone analogous to LH, human chorionic gonadotropin, is released by the developing embryo into the maternal circulation to maintain the corpus luteum and consequently to prevent menstruation.

In general, the menstrual phase lasts for a few days (usually 3–5 days, but anywhere from 2 to 7 days is considered normal). Menstrual cycles with intervals of 21 days or fewer are indicated with the medical term polymenorrhea, while the term for cycles with intervals exceeding 35 days is oligomenorrhea (or amenorrhea if intervals exceed 180 days) (MacGregor, 1996). The average blood loss during menstruation is 35 ml, with 10–80 ml considered normal. Very little flow (less than 10 ml) is called hypomenorrhea, while heavy flow is defined as hypermenorrhea. Metrorrhagia or menometrorrhagia is used to indicate prolonged flows with unpredictable pattern, while dysfunctional uterine bleeding refers to hormonally caused flow abnormalities, typically anovulation (Speroff et al., 1994; Yen and Jaffe, 2004). Menstruation depends on endometrial shedding which is an endocrine and vascular phenomenon involving a complex cascade of paracrine/autocrine and intracrine mechanisms crucial for implantation and, in the absence thereof, normal menstruation (Jabbour et al., 2006).

Apart from reproductive function, ovarian hormone fluctuations throughout the menstrual cycle are relevant to several aspects of female health and display a high degree of inter- and intraindividual variability. Serum estradiol levels typically are low during the early to mid-follicular phases (25–50 pg/ml range), peak during the late follicular and early luteal phase (100–400 pg/ml range), plateau during the mid-luteal phase (200–300 pg/ml range), and fall precipitously to levels of 25–50 pg/ml just prior to menstrual bleeding. Serum progesterone levels are undetectable during the follicular phase (<1 ng/ml range), peak during the mid-luteal phase (from 6 to 10 ng/ml), and then fall precipitously (<2 ng/ml) during the late luteal phase. Two elegant back-to-back reviews (Martin and Behbehani, 2006a, b) have recently summarized the relevance of ovarian hormones changes on the CNS of female migraineurs during the reproductive lifespan.

Menstrual migraine

The second edition of the International Classification of Headache Disorders (ICHD-II: Headache Classification Subcommittee of the International Headache Society, 2004) included menstrual migraine (MM) in the appendix and defined two subcategories in the

Table 25.1

International Classification of Headache Disorders II criteria for menstrual migraine (Headache Classification Subcommittee of the International Headache Society, 2004)

"Pure" menstrual migraine (PMM)	Menstrually related migraine (MRM)
Attacks fulfilling criteria for migraine without aura	Attacks fulfilling criteria for migraine without aura
Attacks occur exclusively on day 1 ± 2 (i.e., days −2 to +3) of menstruation in at least two out of three menstrual cycles and at no other times of the cycle	Attacks occur on day 1 ± 2 (i.e., days −2 to +3) of menstruation in at least two out of three menstrual cycles and additionally at other times of the cycle

diagnostic criteria (Table 25.1). "Pure" menstrual migraine (PMM) occurs exclusively on day 1 ± 2 of menstruation in at least two out of three menstrual cycles and at no other time of the cycle. Menstrually related migraine (MRM) occurs on day 1 ± 2 of menstruation in at least two out of three menstrual cycles and additionally at other times of the cycle. The recognition of a 5-day window is based on clinical data and is in line with the hypothesis of estrogen withdrawal as proposed by Somerville (1972a, b) several years ago. After pharmacologically induced prolonged estradiol elevation, migraine attacks were correlated to declining estradiol levels, as occurs before the onset of menstruation. Migraine seems independent of progesterone concentration (Somerville, 1975a). Even though many years have passed, such an intriguing hypothesis is still elusive due to the complexity of the neuroendocrine events driving the menstrual cycle. Indeed, the finding that a period of several days of exposure to high estrogen levels is necessary before estrogen withdrawal can result in migraine (Somerville, 1975b) explains very well PMM, but does not shed light on why women are prone to developing migraine throughout the entire menstrual cycle, pre- and postmenstrually, and at the time of ovulation (G. Nappi et al., 1997). However, some studies have not convincingly shown an increased frequency of migraine headache during the mid-cycle or ovulatory time period of the menstrual cycle (MacGregor et al., 1990; Stewart et al., 2000) and there are data suggesting that the mid-luteal intervals of the menstrual cycle might represent times of less frequent, severe, and disabling migraine headache (Beckham et al., 1992; Martin et al., 2005). A recent study investigating the relationship between urinary ovarian hormone levels and migraine across the menstrual cycle of women with menstrual and MRM found a significantly higher number of migraine attacks during the late luteal/early follicular phase of falling estrogen and lower number of attacks during phases of rising estrogen (MacGregor et al., 2006a). On the other hand, Martin et al. (2005) found that higher urinary progesterone metabolites were associated with a worsening of headache during mid-luteal time periods; this is at variance with the literature which is, however, quite poor regarding progesterone/progestins, that a progesterone threshold can be hypothesized in the occurrence of migraine. In this context, the use of headache diaries, which make it possible to record prospectively the characteristics of every attack, is of paramount importance for evaluating the time pattern of headache and for identifying a clear link with menstrual cycle-related features (G. Nappi et al., 2006).

That being so, many authors throughout the years, in absence of strict criteria of definition of the timing, have referred to MM in a variable way, finding a wide range of prevalence (from 4% to 73%). By using more strict criteria, "true" MM is far less frequent, concerning 7–12% of women (MacGregor et al., 1990; Granella et al., 1993; Dzoljic et al., 2002).

Population-based studies of women with migraine demonstrate little difference between the attack characteristics of menstrual and non-menstrual migraine (Johannes et al., 1995; Stewart et al., 2000). However, many clinicians are under the impression that migraine attacks related to menses are more severe, long-lasting, and refractory to both acute and prophylactic treatment (Silberstein et al., 1998; Stewart et al., 2000; Couturier et al., 2003). Menstrually related attacks may have a typical duration (no more than 72 h), but in some cases head pain can last several days and may be extremely severe and poorly responsive to analgesics (status migrainosus). Moreover, migraine attacks of longer duration and less responsive to acute treatment cover the entire perimenstrual period, from day −2 to day +7 (Granella et al., 2004). Migraine at menstruation is different in terms of severity from non-menstrual attacks, even within individuals, and the highest severity is evident on days 1–3 when menstrual bleeding starts (MacGregor and Hackshaw, 2004).

Theoretically, menstrual and non-menstrual attacks could have different clinical features and/or a different response to abortive and prophylactic therapy due to a different pathogenesis. Circulating levels of estradiol and progesterone measured across the menstrual cycle seem to be similar between menstrual and non-menstrual migraineurs (Epstein et al., 1975). Estrogen variations are highly implicated in modulating the threshold to challenges by altering neuronal excitability, cerebral vasoactivity, pain sensitivity, neuroendocrine axes, throughout the menstrual cycle and not only at the time of menstruation (Brandes, 2006). On the other hand, estrogen withdrawal may constitute a triggering factor for migraine in women with peculiar characteristics of vulnerability. Indeed, R.E. Nappi et al. (2003) have recently found that ovulatory women with extremely severe migraine attacks triggered by menstruation display a blunted neuroendocrine response to a challenge with meta-chlorophenylpiperazine (*m*-CPP), a 5-HT agent with a high affinity for several subtypes of 5-HT receptor, especially 1 and 2, in comparison with women with MM with typical duration of attacks (4–72 h) and controls. More interestingly, women with a clear window of vulnerability to migraine due to the abrupt withdrawal of synthetic estrogens, as occurs during the free week of hormonal contraception, showed the same pattern of neuroendocrine response to *m*-CPP, peculiar to long-lasting, severe, and poorly responsive migraine to acute treatments. Estradiol supplementation during the 7 days was able to restore the neuroendocrine response to the same 5-HT challenge and the pattern was similar to that in women suffering from MM with typical duration and adequate response to analgesics (R.E. Nappi et al., 2005). These two studies, conducted on a small sample of women, suggest that estradiol drop has the ability cyclically to disrupt 5-HT-mediated adaptive capacities implicated in the inhibition of pain. Even in women with migraine undergoing *in vitro* fertilization and embryo transfer treatment, headache was more frequently reported, specifically during the downregulation stage induced by GnRH, when very low levels of estradiol were measured (Amir et al., 2005).

A very elegant explanation of the estrogen withdrawal theory was recently given by Welch and coworkers (2006), suggesting a "mismatch" between the timing of estrogen effects on gene regulation in the CNS and its effects on cell membrane. The hypothesis is based on the idea that under ordinary circumstances estrogen-mediated gene regulation "modulates inhibitory peptide function in the trigeminal nerve," an action which counterbalances estrogen-mediated increases in neuronal membrane excitability. When estrogen levels fall, their downregulating effect on inflammatory genes is removed and compensatory mechanisms cannot always be rapidly active to prevent headache in "the migraine-prone brain."

A large amount of data concerning the role of ovarian hormone variations in modulating several systems probably involved in the overrepresentation of migraine in women are available and may be summarized as follows (Fioroni et al., 1995; R.E. Nappi et al., 1999).

Opioid system

When injected into the luteal phase, naloxone, a μ-receptor antagonist, induces a maximal rise of circulating LH levels, while the lowest response is observed in the early follicular phase. This is due to the fact that hypothalamic opioidergic tone, apart from being involved in analgesia and in affective/behavioral disorders related to adaptive responses to environmental and internal stimuli, controls gonadotropin secretion and is under the influence of gonadal steroids, in particular estrogens during the menstrual cycle. Patients with MRM display a failure of the naloxone-induced LH release in close proximity to the attack, similarly to what can be found in patients with premenstrual syndrome (PMS), free of any headache.

Hypothalamic–pituitary–adrenal (HPA) system

The influence of the reproductive system upon the stress response guarantees the female body a better adaptation during emergency situations. Indeed, HPA function is dynamic over the ovarian cycle and estrogens inflect the HPA axis sensitivity to stress. In MM patients cortisol response to high doses of naloxone is inhibited in the luteal phase, while it is normal during the follicular phase of the menstrual cycle. On the other hand, women with PMS exhibit an exaggerated plasma cortisol response to a corticotropin-releasing hormone bolus compared to asymptomatic controls, which is independent of the comorbidity with MM.

Adrenergic system

Several lines of evidence support the theory that the basal tone of sympathetic activity and its receptor sensitivity are modulated by menstrual cyclicity. An excessive fluctuation of dopamine β-hydroxylase plasma levels, with lower values in the late luteal period, has been reported in patients suffering from MM. As mentioned above, MM patients are characterized by a transient, cyclic failure of endogenous opioid activity. The evidence that the inhibitory effect of the opioid system at the central level is prevented by α_2-adrenergic receptor blockers suggests a possible interaction between opioids and catecholamines in the naloxone-induced endocrine effect. In women suffering from MM, clonidine stimulates β-endorphin and growth hormone release during the follicular phase and reduces 3-methoxy-4-hydroxyphenylethylene glycol (MHPG) and NE plasma levels. Clonidine also reduces

MPHG and NE concentrations in the late luteal phase, but the release of β-endorphin and growth hormone in the same patients is lost, suggesting a postsynaptic α_2-adrenoreceptor hyposensitivity during the premenstrual period. The possible defective integration between gonadal steroids and catecolamines at the central level is also supported by the evidence that controls and non-menstrual migraineurs show a marked luteal increase in platelet NE, which is absent in menstrual migraineurs who also show a platelet epinephrine decrease in the luteal phase.

Serotonergic system

Platelet function and 5-HT have been extensively studied in migraine sufferers. In normal women intraplatelet 5-HT does not change during the menstrual cycle but shows an increase at menstruation. On the other hand, platelet 5-HT significantly increases during the premenstrual and menstrual phases of the cycle in menstrual migraineurs. Moreover, in patients with MM the mean values of platelet 5-HT drop significantly during the attack in comparison with those found in basal conditions. 5-HT and monoamine oxidase B (MAO-B) appear to be compartmentalized together in neurons and platelets, and several studies suggest that MAO-B platelet activity is a good indicator of central serotoninergic activity. In addition, the endocrine milieu may play some role in the non-genomic regulation of MAO-B activity. Recent data suggest that in MM patients there could be a hypersensitivity of the serotonergic system to hormonal modulation, since MAO-B activity is significantly increased in the luteal phase more than in asymptomatic control women.

Prostaglandins

There is a threefold increase in prostaglandin levels in the uterine endometrium from the follicular to the luteal phase with a further increase during menstruation, which stimulates uterine contractions. Endometrial prostaglandins are known to be increased in women with either dysmenorrhea or MM and it is also known that plasma levels of some prostaglandins vary according to the phase of the menstrual cycle and during the migraine attack. In addition, prostaglandins modulate descending NE pain control systems as well as the release of 5-HT by platelets or serotoninergic neurons in response to ischemic stimuli in the brain, a phenomenon under estrogenic control which probably contributes to the pathogenesis of MM. In addition to platelet prostaglandins and serotoninergic metabolism, which is altered during the luteal phase of the cycle in MM, a direct involvement of other aspects of platelet function, such as aggregation, may be postulated because a change in platelet homeostasis, mainly evident in the luteal phase, has also been found in MM.

Prolactin

Dopamine antagonists produce enhanced prolactin release throughout the luteal phase in all women, and during the entire menstrual cycle in women suffering from MM, even though basal plasma prolactin levels do remain in the normal range in MM during the menstrual cycle. In addition, thyroid-releasing hormone infusion enhances prolactin release, but not thyroid-stimulating hormone, during a migraine attack and a supersensitivity of dopaminergic system coupled to a serotoninergic hyperfunction has been postulated to explain this endocrine feature.

Melatonin

Nocturnal urinary melatonin excretion decreases in patients suffering from migraine in all phases of the menstrual cycle and the normal rise in urinary melatonin excretion during the luteal phase is less evident in migraine sufferers. The significance of such subtle changes is not fully established but it can be hypothesized that an impairment of melatonin function is related to nociceptive function controlling circadian fluctuation of pain threshold.

Nitric oxide

The pivotal role of nitric oxide in migraine pain and the outstanding observation that there is an estrogen-mediated enhancement of the activity and/or the expression of endothelial nitric oxide synthase open a new field of investigation in the pathogenesis of MM. Indeed, an overactivation in the platelet arginine–nitric oxide pathway has recently been demonstrated during the luteal phase of the cycle in females affected by MM. On the other hand, nitroglycerine, an organic nitrate that has been used in the treatment of cardiac disease for over a century, consistently induces a specific headache attack in patients suffering from migraine. Experimental data (Pardutz et al., 2002) showed that there is a sexual dimorphic neuronal activation induced by nitroglycerine systemic injection, supporting the idea that estrogens significantly affect the rat brain structures implicated in the pathophysiology of migraine.

Even magnesium deficiency could theoretically play a role in MM, given the evidence that estrogen and progesterone fluctuations modulate cerebral vascular smooth-muscle cells' normal concentrations of magnesium ions which are essential to a number of functions within the CNS (Li et al., 2001). Facchinetti et al.

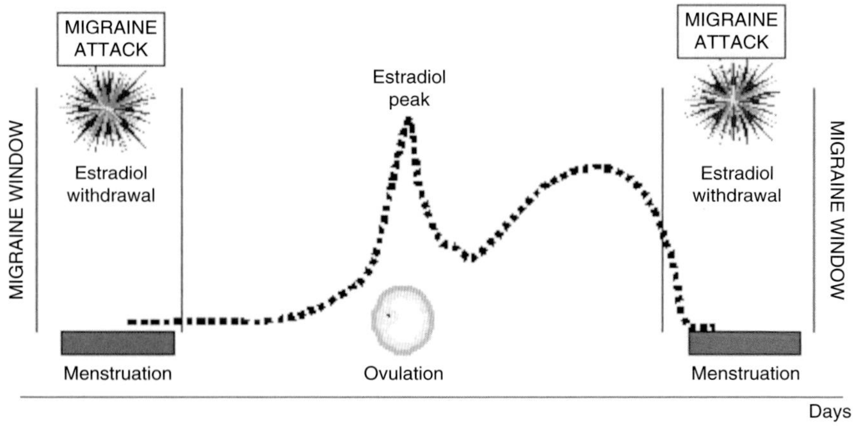

Fig. 25.1. Schematic representation of the concept of the "menstrual window" for menstrual migraine.

(1991) demonstrated that MM could be prevented by administration of oral magnesium during the last 15 days of the menstrual cycle.

Collectively, these data add a significant piece of information to the concept that "the menstrual window" may constitute a triggering factor for migraine in vulnerable women (Figure 25.1), but more research has to be done on the crucial role of estrogens in modulating the delicate balance of excitatory and inhibitory neurotransmission within the target systems during the luteal phase of the menstrual cycle. A very elegant study (Martin et al., 2003) investigated the threshold of sensitivity to estradiol variation in women with migraine with a clinical model of medical oophorectomy. The authors found an "overall" preventive effect with the transdermal estradiol patch compared with placebo, but even a small rise (11 pg/ml) in serum estradiol levels on the first 2 days of the patch might be provocative for migraine headache by increasing outcome measures by 45–50%. These results emphasize how exquisitely sensitive some women with migraine may be to small changes in serum estradiol levels and demonstrate that estrogen can be preventive in some situations and provocative in others. Strategies to prevent estradiol drop during the perimenstrual period have been tried with variable results (de Lignieres et al., 1986; Dennerstein et al., 1988; Pradalier et al., 1994). The dose of estrogens seems to be critical given the evidence that a clear benefit in preventing MM was documented only when a 100 μg patch or 1.5 mg estradiol gel was used with estradiol plasma levels above 45 pg/ml. However, in spite of reducing severity and duration of menstrual attacks, the timing and the duration of estradiol treatment across the "menstrual window" remain to be further established because of the evidence of a 40% increase in migraine in the 5 days after estradiol versus placebo was stopped (MacGregor et al., 2006b).

Data collected across the entire reproductive life (Stewart et al., 1991; Granella et al., 2000) indicate that migraine with and migraine without aura are triggered by different mechanisms. Stewart et al. (2000) reported that attacks of migraine without aura were 2.04 times more likely during the first 2 days of menstruation, while attacks of migraine with aura occurred with equal frequency throughout the menstrual cycle. Mattsson (2003) reported that 21% of patients experiencing migraine without aura reported >75% of attacks occurring during the perimenstrual time period as compared to only 4% of patients with migraine with aura. In a retrospective case–control study (Granella et al., 2000) carried out on 100 women affected by migraine with typical aura and 200 age-matched women with migraine without aura, menstrually triggered migraine was more frequently encountered among migraine without aura (53.5%) than among migraine with aura (15.0%) patients and PMS was found to be much more common among the patients with migraine with aura.

REPRODUCTIVE COMORBIDITIES OF MIGRAINE

A number of studies have estimated the prevalence of chronic pelvic pain to be similar to that reported for migraine, low back pain, and asthma (Zondervan et al., 1999). Dysmenorrhea and endometriosis are the two most common causes of pelvic pain. Primary dysmenorrhea is a very common gynecological problem in menstruating women and its prevalence is so high (up to 90%), especially during adolescence (Jamieson and Steege, 1996), that it is extremely difficult to draw a conclusion on the association with MM. The biological link between these two conditions should be the levels of prostaglandins and their metabolites, which are elevated in the systemic circulation during the first 48 h of menstruation in response to the withdrawal of estradiol and progesterone (Nattero et al., 1989). Endometriosis, a condition characterized by endometrial tissue growing outside the uterus, is seen in 5–10% of women in the general population and is thought to be more common in the mature woman, but it can also occur in adolescents, with a peak incidence between the ages of 25 and 30 years (US Department of Health and Human Services Public Health Service, 2006). Recent data corroborate early observations that women with endometriosis suffer headache significantly more often than those without endometriosis (Tervila and Marttila, 1975). Indeed, Ferrero et al. (2004) investigated the prevalence of migraine in a population of 133 women with histologically proven endometriosis and in 166 controls and found that the prevalence of migraine was significantly higher among women with endometriosis (38.3%) than in controls (15.1%). In addition, migraine with aura was observed in 18 women with endometriosis (13.5%) and in 2 controls (1.2%). The age at migraine onset was significantly lower in women with endometriosis than in controls, suggesting a common physiopathological background. However, the link between endometriosis and migraine remains elusive and several mechanisms can be proposed, including an excess of prostaglandin production and an impairment of nitric oxide synthesis. It is likely, as well, that the early use of hormonal preparations in women suffering from chronic pelvic pain may play a role in the overexpression of migraine in women with endometriosis.

Another recent study (Tietjen et al., 2007) examined the headache characteristics of women with migraine and endometriosis compared to female migraineurs without endometriosis, and the association of endometriosis with other comorbid conditions, such as irritable bowel syndrome, fibromyalgia, chronic fatigue syndrome (CFS), and interstitial cystitis (IC) among others, in women with migraine and in non-headache controls. The authors confirmed that endometriosis was reported more commonly in migraineurs than in controls (22% versus 9.6%). In addition, irritable bowel syndrome, fibromyalgia, CFS, and IC were more common in migraine with endometriosis than in controls, while IC and CFS were more common in migraine with endometriosis than in the cohort with migraine without endometriosis. These data suggest that such medical conditions may share a common neuroimmunoendocrine milieu involving mast cell activation and other mediators of inflammation.

A well-established comorbidity with migraine (Facchinetti, 1994; Kornstein and Parker, 1997) is PMS, which is characterized by a cluster of symptoms in the luteal phase, including physical, affective, behavioral, and cognitive symptoms, which resolve with the onset of menstruation. Women who have severe affective symptoms may also meet criteria for premenstrual dysphoric disorder (PMDD) which is diagnosed in 3–8% of cases. Up to 75% of women report some symptoms regularly during the luteal phase, including headache, but they deserve treatment in 20% of cases (Johnson, 2004). The premenstrual increase of each cluster of PMS symptoms is identical in MM and PMS subjects with the exception of negative affect (Facchinetti et al., 1993), confirming a common terrain of neuroendocrine vulnerability between these two conditions (Fioroni et al., 1995). More recently, Martin et al. (2006) determined the association between the severity of PMS symptoms and headache outcome measures during natural menstrual cycles and after medical oophorectomy, suggesting a moderate correlation between the severity of PMS symptoms and migraine and a possible modulation of PMS symptoms by the presence and severity of migraine.

PREGNANCY

Neuroendocrine aspects of pregnancy

Neuroendocrine adaptation to the pregnant state involves virtually every area of the female body, including the CNS, in order to achieve the normal course of gestation and parturition. The progressively increased level of progesterone, be it of either ovarian or placental origin, is critical for the establishment and maintenance of pregnancy, as well as high levels of estradiol. Indeed, during the third trimester, progesterone levels are 20 times higher and serum estradiol levels are 30–40 times higher than in the normal menstrual cycle. Other hormones, such as human chorionic gonadotropin, human placental lactogen, and prolactin, play a decisive role in the physiology of pregnancy (Speroff et al., 1994). The human placenta and its related membranes are also a neuroendocrine organ, since they are able to produce and release locally substances such as neurohormones, cytokines, and growth factors. These products act as endocrine, paracrine, and autocrine factors to control the secretion of other regulatory molecules, including the pituitary hormones of both mother and fetus and their placental counterparts. Furthermore, they may play a role in the regulation of maternal and fetal physiology during pregnancy, ranging from the control of placental anchoring to fetal growth and maturation, fine regulation of uterine blood flow, and/or initiation of labor (Petraglia et al., 1996). One of the most important actions of ovarian steroids is to modulate the central neural circuitries involved in the process of nociception, mainly the production of endogenous opioid peptides (Cogan and Spinnato, 1980; Genazzani et al., 1980; Dawson-Basoa and Gintzler, 1993). In addition, the placenta–CNS network is highly responsible for anxiolysis through the activity of neurosteroids, active metabolites of progesterone synthesized within the CNS by the same steroidogenic enzymes found in the gonads and the adrenals, that are able to influence neuronal exicitability, emotional states, and adaptive responses throughout pregnancy (Genazzani and Bernardi, 1999). That being so, physiological adaptations of pregnancy affect neurological function in health and disease (Lee, 2007). As far as migraine is concerned, the analgesic condition associated with gestation seems to be the most important factor capable of modulating the clinical expression of head pain.

Migraine and pregnancy

In western countries the age at first pregnancy and the number of children have changed considerably in recent years due to major psychosocial changes, with important consequences for reproductive health and behavior. Delayed motherhood is characterized by an increased probability of obstetric complications and/or fetal and perinatal problems (Tarin et al., 1998) and may have a significant impact on physical and mental well-being of women, including the natural history of migraine. Several studies have demonstrated that migraine improves or disappears, in most women, during pregnancy. *De novo* migraine during pregnancy is rare (<3%) and typically occurs during the first trimester (Somerville, 1972c). Migraine does not pose an increased risk for miscarriage, toxemia, congenital anomalies, or stillbirth. However, inadequately addressed and treated migraines can lead to poor nutritional intake, dehydration, sleep deprivation, increased stress, poor marital relations, and depression, with associated adverse sequelae on maternal and fetal well-being (Silberstein, 1997; Marcus, 2003). Thus, many pregnant or lactating migraineurs require intermittent use of medication for treatment and some also need preventive treatment aimed at decreasing the number or severity of migraine attacks (Loder, 2007). The majority of data available on the course of migraine during pregnancy are retrospective, the patients having been evaluated several years after pregnancy or, at best, in the postpartum period (Lance and Anthony, 1966; Callaghan, 1968; Somerville, 1972c; Epstein et al., 1975; Granella et al., 1993, 2000; Rasmussen, 1993; Cupini et al., 1995; Maggioni et al., 1997). In these studies, the percentage of migrainous women whose headache improved during pregnancy varies broadly, from 43% (Cupini et al., 1995) to 86% (Maggioni et al., 1997). These results could have been influenced by a number of factors: the geographical area in which a study was carried out, the type of population investigated (headache center, obstetrics department, general population), the diagnostic criteria of migraine employed (International Headache Society, Ad Hoc Committee), the type of migraine investigated (all types or only migraine without aura), and the definition of improvement. However, of all the possible factors, a major role was possibly played by the timing of the interview: the studies performed close to delivery showed percentages of improvement – ranging from 78% (Somerville, 1972c) to 86% (Maggioni et al., 1997) – that were higher than those found in studies carried out years after childbirth, in which the percentages ranged from 43% (Cupini et al., 1995) to 67% (Granella et al., 1993, 2000). It appears that the time elapsing since pregnancy biases recall, attenuating its positive effect.

By contrast, very few studies have investigated prospectively the course of migraine during pregnancy. Chen and Leviton (1994), studying 484 migraineurs drawn from a huge sample of pregnant women ($n = 40\,273$), found an improvement in 79% of cases, while 21% of the women reported no headaches during pregnancy. However, this study has several shortcomings. Even though the paper was published in 1994, it refers to data collected (as part of a study designed to identify the antecedents of neurological problems in children) way back in the years 1959–1966. Not only did it fail, obviously, to use the International Headache Society diagnostic criteria, but the very low prevalence of migraine (1.3%) suggests that it included only a small, and thus not representative, proportion of migrainous women. Moreover, the migraine course was assessed only very roughly: all that was established at each antenatal check-up was whether or not there had been a headache since the last antenatal check-up.

At variance with all the previous studies, Marcus et al. (1999), using a headache diary, prospectively monitored from the second trimester on a highly selected sample (women experiencing headache at least twice a month, recruited through advertisements placed in obstetricians' surgeries and local newspapers) of 49 primary headache sufferers, only 18 of whom were pure migraineurs, and found an improvement in only 41% of the women. The study also revealed a non-significant trend towards a greater improvement in migraineurs than in tension-type headache patients. Several factors reduce the validity of this study: the self-selection of the subject sample, the inclusion of subjects only from the second trimester (thus excluding women experiencing a first-trimester improvement), and the small number of migraineurs recruited.

Scharff et al. (1997) reported that migraine sufferers showed an increase in attacks during the third trimester of gestation. A prospective study conducted in pregnant women attending an obstetrics/gynecology clinic for a first routine antenatal check-up demonstrated a very favorable effect of pregnancy in the overwhelming majority of patients affected by migraine without aura, an effect that was more striking than that observed in almost all the retrospective studies. Indeed, migraine improved in 46.8% of sufferers during the first trimester, in 83.0% during the second, and in 87.2% during the third, with complete remission in 10.6%, 53.2%, and 78.7% of the women, respectively. Moreover, any residual attacks tended to be less severe, even though their duration did not alter. Furthermore, no women experienced a worsening of headache during pregnancy and around 10% of the women were attack-free throughout pregnancy (Sances et al., 2003).

These data, collected using a prospective headache diary, produce a percentage of improvement (87%) that is higher than the maximum values produced by retrospective studies performed close to the time of delivery, and very similar to that (86%) found by Maggioni et al. (1997) in their accurate survey. However, the positive effect of pregnancy was not exerted uniformly across the trimesters: having emerged in the first trimester, it increased substantially in the second with a further benefit in the third trimester, mainly in terms of a shift from improvement to complete remission. It is striking to observe that the amelioration of migraine without aura follows in some way the progressive rise of endogenous sex hormones throughout pregnancy. In line with the hypothesis that the "high estrogen milieu" of pregnancy could play a role in initiating attacks of migraine with aura, some studies (Wright and Patel, 1986; Chancellor et al., 1990) have reported "new-onset" visual, sensory, and motor aura during pregnancy with fewer women reporting improvement or remission (43.6%) in comparison to women with migraine without aura (76.8%) (Granella et al., 2000).

Among the factors possibly associated with lack of improvement of migraine without aura during pregnancy, very few attempts had been made in the literature. Somerville (1972b) failed to find differences between the plasma progesterone levels (measured during the 4 weeks before delivery) of improved and of non-improved women. Lance and Anthony (1966) reported greater relief in women who had had a menstrual periodicity (defined as the regular occurrence of migraine at the time of menses) prior to pregnancy, while the gender of the unborn child was not found to be correlated with the course of migraine. Most recent prospective data (Sances et al., 2003) indicate, quite surprisingly, that the occurrence of MRM prior to pregnancy constituted a risk factor for a lack of improvement in both the first and the third trimesters. An explanation of the phenomenon may lie in the definition of MRM used in the study, which included not only "true" MM, but also migraine occurring during and outside menses. Other major factors predicting lack of migraine improvement were evident during the second and third trimesters of pregnancy and consisted in the pathological course of pregnancy, and the persistence of hyperemesis after the first trimester. It is likely that physical problems arising during pregnancy, generating concern and anxiety over the health of both the mother and the fetus, or inducing the use of drugs, may cancel out the benefits normally accompanying pregnancy. Any significant differences between primiparous and multiparous women were observed, a finding that is in keeping with the conclusions of Maggioni et al. (1997).

A very interesting finding from the literature is the possible association between typical hypertensive disorders (gestational hypertension and pre-eclampsia) starting after the 20th week of pregnancy, in previously normotensive women, and migraine. However, studies available are retrospective and in most of them the diagnosis of migraine was not done according to the International Headache Society criteria for primary headaches and the criteria for the diagnosis of hypertensive disorders were not homogeneous (Moore and Redman, 1983; Marcoux et al., 1992; Scher et al., 2005). In the only retrospective case–control study in which rigorous criteria for both migraine and pre-eclampsia diagnosis were applied, a strong association was found between these two clinical conditions (Facchinetti et al., 2005), suggesting the need for further prospective studies to corroborate the hypothesis that a history of migraine may be considered a risk factor for hypertensive disorders in pregnancy.

LACTATION

Neuroendocrine aspects of lactation

The postpartum period is a unique condition characterized by a rapid ovarian hormone withdrawal which inevitably induces a wide range of neuroendocrine adaptive responses that have been associated with the occurrence or recurrence of neurological disorders (Lee, 2007). Lactation, which commonly inhibits ovulatory cycles during the puerperium with a mean time to ovulation after delivery of 6 months (Campbell and Gray, 1993), is characterized by increased levels of prolactin, hypoestrogenism, and elevated release of antinociceptive neuropeptides such as oxytocin and vasopressin (Buhimschi, 2004). In non-breast-feeding women the cyclic hormonal milieu is rapidly restored and the mean time to ovulation after delivery is 45 days (Campbell and Gray, 1993).

Migraine and lactation

There is very little in the literature on the course of migraine postpartum. Stein (1981) studied 71 women randomly selected from a postnatal ward during the first postpartum week. Postpartum headache developed in 37% of the subjects. This percentage rose to 61% among women with a family history of migraine and to 64% among previous migraineurs. In migraine patients, postpartum headache generally had some migrainous features, but was milder and less frequently unilateral than the patients' typical migraine. Sances et al. (2003) found a considerable rate of migraine recurrence in a prospective study: 34% within the first week and 55.3% within the first month following childbirth. Women reported that postnatal migraine attacks were indistinguishable from those experienced before pregnancy and more severe than those that had occurred during the third trimester. On the basis of the clinical characteristics of the headache attacks, postdural puncture headache in the women who had had epidural anesthesia for labor and cesarean section were excluded. Attacks that occurred early after delivery were probably triggered by the abrupt fall in the level of estrogens, while later headaches may have been favored by other factors, such as postpartum depression or the stress of adjusting to the new parental role and responsibilities.

The main risk factor for the postnatal recurrence of migraine, both early on (in the first week) and during the first month, was bottle-feeding, supporting the concept that a early return to menstrual cyclicity may have an unfavorable effect, while breast-feeding exerts a protective action which is possibly related to anovulation (Sances et al., 2003). Indeed, Marcus et al. (1999) found that the headache index during the first 3 postpartum months for women who breast-fed was similar to that obtained during the second trimester of pregnancy. No conclusive data are available on migraine with aura and lactation.

MENOPAUSE

Neuroendocrine aspects of menopause

The menopause, defined as the permanent cessation of menstruation resulting from the loss of ovarian follicular activity, marks the end of the natural female reproductive life. It is preceded by a period of menstrual cycle irregularity, the menopausal transition, which usually begins in the mid-40s and is conventionally divided into early and late phases. Briefly, the biology underlying the transition to menopause includes central neuroendocrine changes as well as changes within the ovary, the most striking of which is a profound decline in follicle numbers. Although traditionally it has been thought that both estradiol and progesterone levels decline with progression through the menopause transition, several studies suggest that prostaglandin E_2 levels can increase rather than decrease toward the final menstrual period in association with unpredictable ovulatory and anovulatory cycles. FSH is an established indirect marker of follicular activity. Serum FSH concentration begins to increase some years before there are any clinical indications of approaching menopause, particularly in the early follicular phase of the menstrual cycle. The rise in FSH is the result of declining levels of inhibin B, a dimeric protein that reflects the fall in ovarian follicle numbers, and plays a role in maintaining estradiol levels, which remain relatively unchanged or elevated throughout the transition.

The menopausal transition is a time of marked hormonal instability which affects central neuroendocrine circuitries, including a multitude of neurotransmitters, neuropeptides, and neuromodulators involved in thermoregulation, mood, cognition, and adaptation. Symptoms of the menopause (hot flushes, mood swings, sleep disturbances, fatigue, poor concentration, vaginal dryness, diminished libido) can be interpreted as resulting primarily from the profound fall in estradiol, occurring over a 3–4-year period around final menses. Plasma FSH levels higher than 40 IU/l and estradiol lower than 20 pg/ml are clear signs of menopause. Even concentrations of testosterone have been reported to fall by about 50% during reproductive life, between the ages of 20 and 40, as a result of ovarian aging. They change little during the transition and, after menopause, may even rise, while in surgical menopause testosterone is reduced by up to 75% in comparison with fertile age (Burger et al., 2007).

Migraine and menopause

Menopause is the last menstrual period; the mean age at menopause varies according to studies and is mostly between 48 and 52 years of age. More or less 90% of women have their menopause between 45 and 55 years of age and life expectancy after menopause is, therefore, longer than 30 years (Avis and McKinlay, 1991).

Migraine incidence generally decreases with advancing age and about two-thirds of patients no longer have migraines by age 65. The prevalence of migraine in the elderly population has been estimated to be around 5% and women continue to be affected twice as much as men (Solomon et al., 1990). Menopause has a variable effect on migraine depending on the neuroendocrine adjustment to the new hormonal environment and on the length of menopausal transition. Erratic estrogen secretion and unbalanced estrogen exposure due to anovulatory cycles and/or progesterone deficiency may worsen or even initiate migraine during the perimenopausal period and such endocrine aberrations often precede by several years the stable and low plasma levels of gonadal steroids typical of the postmenopausal period (MacGregor, 1997). In addition, the intensity of climacteric symptomatology such as hot flushes, palpitations, night sweats, disturbed sleep, and negative emotions may more or less contribute to triggering or aggravating migraine attacks (Fettes, 1999).

MacGregor (2000) has reported that the perimenopausal years are extremely critical for first consultations, meaning that migraine becomes a problem for women later in fertile life. On the other hand, a low prevalence of migraine at menopause emerged from a retrospective study, indicating that only about 12% of 1300 women suffering from migraine were referred to a headache center during the postmenopausal years (Granella et al., 1993).

The controversy over the real role played by menopause in the natural history of migraine may also be ascribed to the fact that neurologists and gynecologists have often carried out studies from different points of view. Indeed, migraine sufferers referring to headache centers are not representative of the general population and are probably the ones who worsen after menopause, while patients recruited in clinics for menopause are generally evaluated during menopausal transition and may lack accurate diagnostic criteria, since the "headache" symptom is commonly included in the majority of scales assessing menopausal wellbeing (MacGregor and Barnes, 1999).

The effect of menopausal transition on the frequency of migraine has been explored in a cross-sectional community-based survey conducted in Chinese women aged 40–54 years (Wang et al., 2003). The prevalence of migraine was similar in premenopausal and early perimenopausal women (16.7%) and much higher in the late perimenopausal group (31%). The spontaneous menopausal group had the lowest prevalence (7%), while women who had had a hysterectomy reported the highest migraine prevalence (27%), particularly in those with PMS (44%). The presence of low estradiol (<50 pg/ml) and high FSH (>30 mIU/ml) levels was associated with lower migraine prevalence, even in premenopausal and early perimenopausal women. Another study conducted in women aged 40–74 years attending a population-based mammography screening program indicated a decrease in risk for migraine without aura in postmenopausal women (Mattsson, 2003). Collectively, these data support the idea that migraine prevalence increases before menopause, when hormonal imbalance is present, particularly in women vulnerable to hormonal changes, and declines after menopause, when estradiol is definitively low.

In a menopause clinic the postmenopausal course of headache with a premenopausal onset differed according to the type of headache and the type of menopause. While migraine improved in almost two-thirds of cases, tension-type headache worsened or was unchanged in 70% of cases. On the other hand, women who had a physiological menopause experienced a more favorable course of migraine than women who had a surgical menopause with bilateral oophorectomy, suggesting abrupt estrogen withdrawal as a well-defined aggravating factor of migraine, probably coupled to the emotional impact of hysterectomy (Neri et al., 1993). Even in a sample of postmenopausal women collected in a tertiary headache center, surgical menopause was found to be significantly associated with a worsening of migraine (Granella et al., 1993), confirming the clinical impression that the severity of the climacteric syndrome related to the lack of both ovarian estrogen and androgen may have a role in aggravating migraine condition. Indeed, a cross-sectional population questionnaire survey conducted in the Netherlands in women aged 39–60 years has shown that hysterectomy with ovarian retention is significantly more present in women reporting moderate to severe migraine (15.1%) compared with non-hysterectomized women (8.8%) (Oldenhave et al., 1993).

MIGRAINE AND EXOGENOUS HORMONES

Hormonally associated migraine

Loder et al. (2007) very elegantly revised the issue of hormonally associated migraine and stated the difficulties of establishing a causal relationship between the use of exogenous hormones and migraine, especially in women already suffering from the disease. Indeed, even though it is of paramount importance for further research, the attempt to classify ICHD-II hormonally associated headaches in the group of secondary headaches, serious diagnostic inconsistencies and clinical variability are evident, as a consequence of not well-proven scientific findings. To fulfill the criteria for exogenous hormone-induced headache, criteria require that the headache begins or "markedly worsens" within 3 months of beginning exogenous hormones and "revolves or reverts to previous pattern" within 3 months of stopping exogenous hormones. On the other hand, to fulfill the criteria of estrogen withdrawal headache, headache should develop within at least 5 days of discontinuation of estrogen used for at least 21 days and should resolve within 3 days. Such a temporal association is, however, based on anecdotal and personal beliefs and it does not take into account many variables related to reproductive biology that may be relevant to a better understanding of the role of exogenous hormones in migraine. Indeed, the multitude of clinical gynecological conditions and the large variety of exogenous hormones available in terms of biochemical nature, route, scheme of treatment, and dose should be taken into account to produce scientific evidence. In addition, it is also possible that, by understanding the hormonal nature of some migraine attacks, hormonal compounds can be proposed as therapeutic options for migraine relief. Hormonally sensitive women may be recognized on the basis of their migraine history, i.e., onset of migraine during menarche, MM, PMS, and severe climacteric symptomatology at menopausal transition, and may be considered a special subgroup of patients.

Migraine and hormonal contraception

Contraceptive options available on the market allow women to select the best hormonal combination to control fertility by achieving several advantages for reproductive and general health. Hormonal contraception is primarily composed of a synthetic estrogen, ethinylestradiol, in combination with progestins of different generations. Throughout the decades, a significant reduction of the estrogenic content and the development of new progestins, with less androgenic properties, have substantially improved the risk/benefit profile of users. Apart from the oral route of administration on a daily basis, the transdermal combination to be taken once a week and the vaginal ring to be inserted once a month are recently offered alternatives for safe hormonal contraception. In addition, periodic injectable preparations and long-term subcutaneous implants containing progestogens are used worldwide to protect women from unwanted pregnancies. Finally, oral hormonal contraception may be delivered in monophasic, biphasic, and triphasic estro-progestin combinations, as well as preparations containing only progestins. Usually there is a week off, during which bleeding due to hormonal discontinuation occurs. Interestingly enough, extended regimens of hormonal contraception have been designed with the aim of reducing menstrually related symptoms (Benagiano et al., 2006). The variety of hormonal products and the significant changes over time of the types of molecules most commonly used by women are responsible for the conflicting results regarding hormonal contraception and the course of migraine. Even though headache is one of the most common side-effects reported in studies related to hormonal contraception, a clear impact of hormonal contraception on the course of migraine has only been reported in women referring to headache centers (Kudrow, 1975; Silberstein and Merriam, 1991). However, there is a paucity of prospective well-controlled studies with clear-cut endpoints (improvement, remission, worsening, no change) and a high degree of variability between the general population and clinical samples is also evident. A worsening of migraine in terms of frequency and severity has been documented in 18–50% of cases, an improvement in 3–35% of women, and no change in 39–65% of cases, demonstrating a lack of consensus. Ryan (1978) reported that headaches worsened in 70% and improved in 30% during treatment with oral hormonal contraception containing 50 μg ethinylestradiol/0.5 mg norgestrel in a randomized placebo-controlled crossover trial. Other case series (Whitty et al., 1966; Dalton, 1976) have reported that migraine headaches typically occur during the week of discontinuation in susceptible patients. Other studies confirmed the evidence of variable effects of different formulations of hormonal contraception but the paucity of information on the types of association that were used limits any definitive conclusion (Granella et al., 1993; Cupini et al., 1995; Mueller, 2000). The use of oral contraceptives worsened migraine in women with migraine with aura (56.4%) more frequently than in patients with migraine without aura (25.3%) (Granella et al., 2000).

Collectively, these studies suggest that exogenous hormones may contribute to the occurrence of neurological symptoms, such as aura; the use of oral contraceptives may coincide with the onset of migraine, more often in women with a family history of migraine, and such new onset may usually occur in the early cycles of use or rarely after prolonged use; sometimes no improvement may be observed following discontinuation of treatment and remission may take a long time; lowering the estrogen dose may be useful in limiting the occurrence of migraine, but sometimes fluctuations in endogenous plasma estrogen levels may not be prevented (R.E. Nappi et al., 1999; Loder et al., 2005).

A recent large cross-sectional population-based study in Norway regarding use of contraceptives and headache in premenopausal women demonstrated that headache, especially migraine, was more likely in women using hormonal contraception containing estrogens (Aegidius et al., 2006). In the absence of firm guidelines, Massiou and MacGregor (2000) concluded that the contraceptive choice should be based on clinical judgment and personal experience, and hormonal contraception should be discontinued or used with caution to avoid the increased risk of stroke (MacGregor, 2001; Curtis et al., 2002).

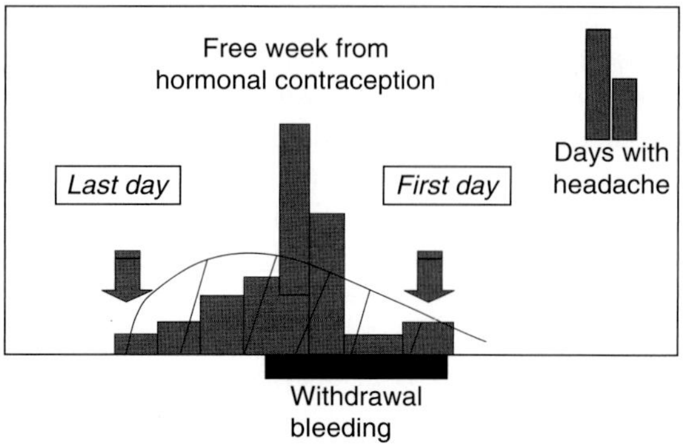

Fig. 25.2. Schematic representation of the concept of the "menstrual window" for hormonally related headaches.

The free interval is a good model to study the "menstrual window" vulnerability to severe migraine attacks because it is a well-defined period of abrupt exogenous estrogen withdrawal (MacGregor, 2004) that may eventually represent a major insult to neuroendocrine adaptive phenomena. Indeed, the onset of migraine triggered by oral contraception during the pill-free interval is very common in obstetric/gynecology practice (Sulak et al., 2000) and migraine may occur virtually every day during discontinuation (Figure 25.2). Menstrually related attacks may be evident during the pill-free interval in some women presenting with unrelenting headache lasting more than 72 h, nausea and vomiting, and showing a lack of responsiveness to conventional non-specific and specific therapy (R.E. Nappi et al., 2005). That being so, even though hormonal manipulations are not the first-line strategies for hormonal withdrawal headache, some hormonal tricks, such as tricycling the pill, altering the ratio of estrogens to progestins, inducing medical castration with GnRH analogues, interfering with the menstrual cycle by using danazol, an androgen derivative, tamoxifen, an antiestrogen, or bromocriptine, a dopamine receptor agonist which inhibits prolactin release, adding phytoestrogens, using estrogen supplementation during the pill-free week, have been proposed to relieve MRM (Murray and Muse, 1997; Massiou and MacGregor, 2000; Sulak et al., 2002; Loder, 2007). In order to stabilize endogenous hormonal fluctuation in some women with a history of intractable migraine, hormonal contraception may be proposed as an attempt to reduce the frequency of attacks.

It is, indeed, of great interest that a series of data has suggested that the use of an extended regimen of hormonal contraception may help to limit the frequency of migraine (Loder et al., 2005). Cachrimanidou et al. (1993) reported an incidence of headache complaints of 9.7% in participants receiving extended duration and 17.3% in those receiving standard oral contraception. Miller and Notter (2001) found that headache was less severe in women receiving a 49-day cycle regimen compared with those on a traditional cyclic regimen. Most recently, Sulak et al. (2007) compared a 21/7-day oral contraceptive regimen with a 168-day extended placebo-free regimen containing 30 μg ethinylestradiol and 3 mg of the novel progestin drospirenone, which showed a positive effect on headache severity along with improvement in work productivity and involvement in activities. In addition, Coffee et al. (2007) reported a significant improvement of mood, headaches, and pelvic pain scores throughout 1 year of use on the same extended regimen. Another randomized study compared an extended regimen (12 weeks) with the standard one (3 weeks) by using transdermal contraception with ethinylestradiol/norelgestromin and claimed a beneficial effect on headache which did not reach statistical significance (LaGuardia et al., 2005). That being so, even though it is reasonable proceed with more studies attempting to manipulate the time of hormonal withdrawal, it is critical to use accurate diagnostic criteria for migraine in order to reach any valuable conclusion. On the other hand, the notion that oral contraceptive use and migraine might interact in predisposing young women to ischemic stroke has to be kept in mind when prescribing the pill or any hormonal supplementations in order to choose the lowest effective dose of synthetic estrogens, and to stop treatment if migraine changes from without aura to migraine with aura (Bousser et al., 2000).

The evidence deriving from estrogen supplementation during the hormonal contraception-free interval is interesting and deserves further studies. Indeed, 100 μg of transdermal estradiol supplementation during the oral contraception-free interval was able to induce a significant improvement of severe migraine in terms of both duration and severity by modulating neuroendocrine responses following a 5-HT challenge. These data conducted against placebo in a small sample of women suggest that estradiol supplementation may modulate pain control mechanisms mediated by 5-HT_2 and 5-HT_1 receptors, which are relevant for analgesic responsiveness in hormonally associated migraine (R.E. Nappi et al., 2005).

Migraine and hormonal replacement therapy (HRT)

Many types of HRT are available on the market in order to personalize treatments according to women's need and risk/benefit profile. The estrogen preparations most commonly used for replacement contain natural estradiol or conjugated estrogens, which display a lower potency in comparison with synthetic estrogens contained in hormonal contraception. Progestins include natural progesterone as well as synthetic progestins (e.g., medroxyprogesterone) and should be co-administered with estrogens to prevent endometrial hyperplasia. According to their biochemical nature, estrogens and progestins can display different effects in target organs, especially at vascular and neuronal levels (Genazzani et al., 2000; Modena et al., 2005). The most common routes of delivery of HRT include pills, transdermal patches/gels, subcutaneous implants, and vaginal suppositories (Kaufman, 1997). To minimize systemic side-effects, an intrauterine system delivering a progestin may also be used (Hampton et al., 2005).

In clinical practice, it is very common to observe a benefit from HRT when women are in the menopausal transition because the treatment prevents erratic hormonal secretion, particularly when stable plasma estrogen levels are provided by the use of a continuous regimen, and this significantly improves quality of life (MacGregor, 2006). On the other hand, the cyclic administration of progestins, which is mandatory in non-hysterectomized women, may induce migraine attacks (de Lignieres and MacGregor, 2000). In these cases, on the basis of their clinical experience Silberstein and Merriam (1991) suggested the use of a progestin with low androgenic properties, natural progesterone, and even a combined estrogen–progestin continuous therapy. MacGregor, in a preliminary uncontrolled retrospective study, suggested that transdermal estradiol was associated with more improvement in migraine than oral conjugated estrogens (MacGregor, 1999b). In addition, a high dose of exogenous estrogens may induce migraine with aura, as happens during pregnancy and hormonal contraception (MacGregor, 2004). Aura may develop *de novo* or estrogens may increase the frequency of pre-existing attacks. Higher dosages of estrogen replacement therapy may be more capable of inducing aura symptoms, while lowering the dosage or changing to another type of estrogen replacement may lead to the amelioration of aura symptoms (MacGregor, 1999a).

Hodson et al. (2000) found that headache is a substantial problem at menopause and in HRT users, since 259 women out of 1000 reported a worsening of the number of attacks. In addition, by using logistic regression models the same authors showed reported history of migraine and more difficulty coping with stress to be strong predictors for worse headache at menopause and with HRT. A greater use of antimigraine preparations by estrogen users than by non-users was reported (Small et al., 2001) and a cross-sectional study found that current HRT use was associated with higher rates of migraine headache than non-use. Migraine was experienced by 11.2% in 1 year and was also significantly associated with a younger age, a younger age at menopause, and surgical menopause (Misakian et al., 2003).

A recent large cross-sectional population-based study in Norway regarding use of HRT and headache in postmenopausal women demonstrated that headache, especially migraine, was more likely in women using HRT (Aegidius et al., 2007). The Postmenopausal Estrogen/Progestin Interventions Trial showed an improvement in headache with oral conjugated estrogens when compared with placebo in women with a history of headache at baseline, whereas if there was no history of headache women were more likely to develop headache as a side-effect (Greendale et al., 1998). Having a history of premenopausal MRM predisposes to develop a migraine attack following estrogen deprivation in postmenopausal women (Lichten et al., 1996). These data imply that HRT worsen the clinical picture of migraine when menopause is already well established.

Some prospective studies based on the use of headache diaries have been conducted to investigate the impact of various HRT regimens on the course of postmenopausal headache. HRT significantly affects the course of migraine, but not of episodic tension-type headache, in postmenopausal women (R.E. Nappi et al., 2001). This observation fits with the common knowledge that migraine is more sensitive to hormones, in comparison with tension-type headache, which is likely more affected by psychological distress and coping strategies (Bono et al., 1995). Moreover, it was interesting to observe different effects exerted by the different routes of administration of HRT on the course of migraine. In particular, outcome measures worsened in women receiving an oral conjugated estrogen and medroxyprogesterone combination, while they did not change as compared to baseline in those receiving a 50-μg transdermal estradiol patch and medroxyprogesterone. These data could suggest that the best way to give hormonal replacement to a postmenopausal woman suffering from migraine is by using the transdermal route of estradiol administration because it maintains a more stable hormonal milieu (R.E. Nappi et al., 2001). Facchinetti et al. (2002) showed that the oral route of HRT administration progressive increase attack frequency, days with headache and analgesic consumption over 6 months. However, women receiving regimens of daily continuous combined HRT had lower outcome measures than those receiving HRT regimens with intermittent dosing regimens (continuous sequential oral cyclic sequential), generating the idea that giving the same dose of exogenous hormones on a daily basis is superior in the hormonal replacement in postmenopausal women with migraine. The dose of the progestin apparently does not make any difference on adverse events, including headache (Nand et al., 1998). Recent experience in a sample of postmenopausal women referred to a tertiary headache center with a longstanding history of disease proposed the use of tibolone, a tissue-selective steroid with estrogenic, progestogenic, and androgenic properties for alleviating climacteric symptoms, as a valid alternative to low-dose conventional HRT with estrogens and progestins. Indeed, such a unique version of HRT may offer some benefits in terms of analgesic responsiveness in long-term migraine sufferers reporting analgesic overuse (R.E. Nappi et al., 2006).

CONCLUSIONS

The field of research linking migraine to reproductive endocrinology needs to be further expanded to develop better preventive and acute treatment across the lifespan of women. The brain–gonad "liaison" is highly operational from prenatal life to the aging period and the enormous advances that basic scientists and clinicians will achieve should be based on the belief that the "female nature" makes a difference in neuroendocrine adaptive phenomena in order to fulfill reproductive goals.

References

Adams Hillard PJ (2002). Menstruation in young girls: a clinical perspective. Obstet Gynecol 99: 655–662.

Aegidius K, Zwart JA, Hagen K et al. (2006). Oral contraceptives and increased headache prevalence: the Head-HUNT Study. Neurology 66: 349–353.

Aegidius KL, Zwart JA, Hagen K et al. (2007). Hormone replacement therapy and headache prevalence in postmenopausal women. The Head-HUNT study. Eur J Neurol 14: 73–78.

Amir BY, Yaacov B, Guy B et al. (2005). Headaches in women undergoing in vitro fertilization and embryo-transfer treatment. Headache 45: 215–219.

Avis NE, McKinlay SM (1991). A longitudinal analysis of women's attitudes toward the menopause: results from the Massachusetts Women's Health Study. Maturitas 13: 65–79.

Beckham JC, Krug LM, Penzien DB et al. (1992). The relationship of ovarian steroids, headache activity and menstrual distress: a pilot study with female migraineurs. Headache 32: 292–297.

Benagiano G, Bastianelli C, Farris M (2006). Contraception today. Ann N Y Acad Sci 1092: 1–32.

Bono G, Neri I, Granella F et al. (1995). Factors associated with pain complaints in a clinical sample of postmenopausal women. J Psychosom Obstet Gynecol 16: 117–121.

Bousser MG, Conard J, Kittner S et al. (2000). Recommendations on the risk of ischaemic stroke associated with use of combined oral contraceptives and hormone replacement therapy in women with migraine. The International Headache Society Task Force on Combined Oral Contraceptives and Hormone Replacement Therapy. Cephalalgia 20: 155–156.

Brandes JL (2006). The influence of estrogen on migraine: a systematic review. JAMA 295: 1824–1830.

Buhimschi CS (2004). Endocrinology of lactation. Obstet Gynecol Clin North Am 31: 963–979, xii.

Burger HG, Hale GE, Robertson DM et al. (2007). A review of hormonal changes during the menopausal transition: focus on findings from the Melbourne Women's Midlife Health Project. Hum Reprod Update 13: 559–565.

Cachrimanidou AC, Hellberg D, Nilsson S et al. (1993). Long-interval treatment regimen with a desogestrel-containing oral contraceptive. Contraception 48: 205–216.

Callaghan N (1968). The migraine syndrome in pregnancy. Neurology 18: 197–201.

Campbell OM, Gray RH (1993). Characteristics and determinants of postpartum ovarian function in women in the United States. Am J Obstet Gynecol 169: 55–60.

Chancellor AM, Wroe SJ, Cull RE (1990). Migraine occurring for the first time in pregnancy. Headache 30: 224–227.

Chen T-C, Leviton A (1994). Headache recurrence in pregnant women with migraine. Headache 34: 107–110.

Chumlea WC, Schubert CM, Roche AF et al. (2003). Age at menarche and racial comparisons in US girls. Pediatrics 111: 110–113.

Coffee AL, Sulak PJ, Kuehl TJ (2007). Long-term assessment of symptomatology and satisfaction of an extended oral contraceptive regimen. Contraception 75: 444–449.

Cogan R, Spinnato JA (1980). Pain and discomfort thresholds in late pregnancy. Pain 27: 63–68.

Couturier EG, Bomhof MA, Neven AK et al. (2003). Menstrual migraine in a representative Dutch population sample: prevalence, disability and treatment. Cephalalgia 23: 302–308.

Cupini LM, Matteis M, Troisi E et al. (1995). Sex-hormone-related events in migrainous females. A clinical comparative study between migraine with aura and migraine without aura. Cephalalgia 15: 140–144.

Curtis KM, Chrisman CE, Peterson HB (2002). Contraception for women in selected circumstances. Obstet Gynecol 99: 1100–1102.

Dalton K (1976). Migraine and oral contraceptives. Headache 15: 247–251.

Dawson-Basoa MB, Gintzler AR (1993). 17-Beta-estradiol and progesterone modulate an intrinsic opioid analgesic system. Brain Res 601: 241–245.

de Lignieres B, MacGregor EA (2000). Risks and benefits of hormone replacement therapy. Cephalalgia 20: 164–169.

de Lignieres B, Vincens M, Mauvais-Jarvis P et al. (1986). Prevention of menstrual migraine by percutaneous oestradiol. BMJ 293: 1540.

Dennerstein L, Morse C, Burrows G et al. (1988). Menstrual migraine: a double-blind trial of percutaneous estradiol. Gynecol Endocrinol 2: 113–120.

Dzoljic E, Sipetic S, Vlajinac H et al. (2002). Prevalence of menstrually related migraine and nonmigraine primary headache in female students of Belgrade University. Headache 42: 185–193.

Epstein MT, Hockaday JM, Hockaday TDR (1975). Migraine and reproductive hormones throughout the menstrual cycle. Lancet 1: 543–547.

Facchinetti F (1994). The premenstrual syndrome belongs in the diagnostic criteria for menstrual migraine. Cephalalgia 14: 413–414.

Facchinetti F, Sances G, Borella P et al. (1991). Magnesium prophylaxis of menstrual migraine: effects on intracellular magnesium. Headache 31: 298–301.

Facchinetti F, Neri I, Martignoni E et al. (1993). The association of menstrual migraine with the premenstrual syndrome. Cephalalgia 13: 422–425.

Facchinetti F, Nappi RE, Tirelli A et al. (2002). Hormone supplementation differently affects migraine in postmenopausal women. Headache 42: 924–929.

Facchinetti F, Allais G, D'Amico R et al. (2005). The relationship between headache and preeclampsia: a case-control study. Eur J Obstet Gynecol Reprod Biol 121: 143–148.

Ferrero S, Pretta S, Bertoldi S et al. (2004). Increased frequency of migraine among women with endometriosis. Hum Reprod 19: 2927–2932.

Fettes I (1999). (1999). Migraine in the menopause. Neurology 53: S29–S33.

Fioroni L, Martignoni E, Facchinetti F (1995). Changes of neuroendocrine axes in patients with menstrual migraine. Cephalalgia 15: 297–300.

Genazzani AR, Bernardi F (1999). The brain as a new frontier for reproductive endocrinology. Curr Opin Obstet Gynecol 11: 237–240.

Genazzani AR, Facchinetti F, Parrini D (1980). β-Lipotrophin and β-endorphin plasma levels during pregnancy. Clin Endocrinol 14: 409–418.

Genazzani AR, Petraglia F, Gamba O et al. (1997). Neuroendocrinology of the menstrual cycle. Ann N Y Acad Sci 816: 143–150.

Genazzani AR, Stomati M, Morittu A et al. (2000). Progesterone, progestagens and the central nervous system. Hum Reprod 15: S14–S27.

Granella F, Sances G, Zanferrari C et al. (1993). Migraine without aura and reproductive life events: a clinical epidemiological study in 1300 women. Headache 33: 385–389.

Granella F, Sances G, Pucci E et al. (2000). Migraine with aura and reproductive life events: a case control study. Cephalalgia 20: 701–707.

Granella F, Sances G, Allais G et al. (2004). Characteristics of menstrual and non-menstrual attacks in women with menstrually-related migraine. Cephalagia 24: 707–716.

Greendale GA, Reboussin BA, Hogan P et al. (1998). Symptom relief and side effects of postmenopausal hormones: results from the Postmenopausal Estrogen/Progestin Interventions Trial. Obstet Gynecol 92: 982–988.

Grumbach MM (2002). The neuroendocrinology of human puberty revisited. Horm Res 57: S2–S14.

Hampton NR, Rees MC, Lowe DG et al. (2005). Levonorgestrel intrauterine system (LNG-IUS) with conjugated oral equine estrogen: a successful regimen for HRT in perimenopausal women. Hum Reprod 20: 2653–2660.

Headache Classification Subcommittee of the International Headache Society (2004). The international classification of headache disorders, 2nd edn. Cephalalgia 24: 1–160.

Hodson J, Thompson J, Al-Azzawi F (2000). (2000). Headache at menopause and in hormone replacement therapy users. Climacteric 3: 119–124.

Jabbour HN, Kelly RW, Fraser HM et al. (2006). Endocrine regulation of menstruation. Endocr Rev 27: 17–46.

Jamieson DJ, Steege JF (1996). The prevalence of dysmenorrhea, dyspareunia, pelvic pain, and irritable bowel syndrome in primary care practices. Obstet Gynecol 87: 55–58.

Johannes CB, Linet MS, Stewart WF et al. (1995). Relationship of headache to phase of the menstrual cycle among young women: a daily diary study. Neurology 45: 1076–1082.

Johnson SR (2004). Premenstrual syndrome, premenstrual dysphoric disorder, and beyond: a clinical primer for practitioners. Obstet Gynecol 104: 845–859.

Karwautz A, Wöber-Bingöl C, Wöber C (1996). Freud and migraine: the beginning of a psychodynamically oriented view of headache a hundred years ago. Cephalalgia 16: 22–26.

Kaufman JM (1997). Pharmacokinetics of estrogens and hormone replacement therapy. Eur Menopause J 4: 14–22.

Kornstein SG, Parker AJ (1997). Menstrual migraines: etiology, treatment, and relationship to premenstrual syndrome. Curr Opin Obstet Gynecol 9: 154–159.

Kudrow L (1975). The relationship of headache frequency to hormone use in migraine. Headache 15: 36–40.

LaGuardia KD, Fisher AC, Bainbridge JD et al. (2005). Suppression of estrogen-withdrawal headache with extended transdermal contraception. Fertil Steril 83: 1875–1877.

Lance JW, Anthony M (1966). Some clinical aspects of migraine. A prospective survey of 500 patients. Arch Neurol 15: 356–361.

Lee LK (2007). Physiological adaptations of pregnancy affecting the nervous system. Semin Neurol 27: 405–410.

Li W, Zheng T, Altura BM et al. (2001). Sex steroid hormones exert biphasic effects on cytosolic magnesium ions in cerebral vascular smooth muscle cells: possible relationships to migraine frequency in premenstrual syndromes and stroke incidence. Brain Res Bull 54: 83–89.

Lichten EM, Lichten JB, Whitty A et al. (1996). The confirmation of a biochemical marker for women's hormonal migraine: the depo-estradiol challenge test. Headache 36: 367–371.

Lipton RB, Bigal ME (2005). Migraine: epidemiology, impact, and risk factors for progression. Headache 45 (Suppl. 1): S3–S13.

Lipton RB, Stewart WF (1993). Migraine in the United States: a review of epidemiology and health care use. Neurology 43: S6–S10.

Lipton RB, Bigal ME, Diamond M et al. (2007). Migraine prevalence, disease burden, and the need for preventive therapy. Neurology 68: 343–349.

Loder E (2007). Migraine in pregnancy. Semin Neurol 27: 425–433.

Loder EW, Buse DC, Golub JR (2005). Headache and combination estrogen–progestin oral contraceptives: integrating evidence, guidelines, and clinical practice. Headache 45: 224–231.

Loder E, Rizzoli P, Golub J (2007). Hormonal management of migraine associated with menses and the menopause: a clinical review. Headache 47: 329–340.

Lyngberg AC, Rasmussen BK, Jorgensen T et al. (2005). Has the prevalence of migraine and tension-type headache changed over a 12-year period? A Danish population survey. Eur J Epidemiol 20: 243–249.

MacGregor A (2000). Gynecological aspects of migraine. Rev Contemp Pharmacother 11: 75–90.

MacGregor EA (1996). "Menstrual" migraine: towards a definition. Cephalalgia 16: 11–21.

MacGregor EA (1997). Menstruation, sex hormones, and migraine. Neurol Clin 15: 125–141.

MacGregor EA (1999a). Estrogen replacement and migraine aura. Headache 39: 674–678.

MacGregor EA (1999b). Effect of oral and transdermal estrogen replacement on migraine. Cephalalgia 19: 124–125.

MacGregor EA (2001). Hormonal contraception and migraine. J Fam Plann Reprod Health Care 27: 49–52.

MacGregor EA (2004). Oestrogen and attacks of migraine with and without aura. Lancet Neurol 3: 354–361.

MacGregor EA (2005). Female sex hormones and migraine. Rev Neurol (Paris) 161: 677–678.

MacGregor EA (2006). Migraine and the menopause. J Br Menopause Soc 12: 104–108.

MacGregor EA, Barnes D (1999). Migraine in a specialist menopause clinic. Climacteric 2: 218–223.

MacGregor EA, Hackshaw A (2004). Prevalence of migraine on each day of the natural menstrual cycle. Neurology 63: 351–353.

MacGregor EA, Chia H, Vohrah RC et al. (1990). Migraine and menstruation: a pilot study. Cephalalgia 10: 305–310.

MacGregor EA, Frith A, Ellis J et al. (2006a). Incidence of migraine relative to menstrual cycle phases of rising and falling estrogen. Neurology 67: 2154–2158.

MacGregor EA, Frith A, Ellis J et al. (2006b). Prevention of menstrual attacks of migraine: a double-blind placebo-controlled crossover study. Neurology 67: 2159–2163.

Maggioni F, Alessi C, Maggino T et al. (1997). Headache during pregnancy. Cephalalgia 17: 765–769.

Marcoux S, Berube S, Brisson J et al. (1992). History of migraine and risk of pregnancy-induced hypertension. Epidemiology 3: 53–56.

Marcus DA (2003). Headache in pregnancy. Curr Pain Headache Rep 7: 288–296.

Marcus DA, Scharff L, Turk D (1999). Longitudinal prospective study of headache during pregnancy and postpartum. Headache 39: 625–632.

Martin VT, Behbehani M (2006a). Ovarian hormones and migraine headache: understanding mechanisms and pathogenesis – part I. Headache 46: 3–23.

Martin VT, Behbehani M (2006b). Ovarian hormones and migraine headache: understanding mechanisms and pathogenesis – part 2. Headache 46: 365–386.

Martin V, Wernke S, Mandell K et al. (2003). Medical oophorectomy with and without estrogen add-back therapy in the prevention of migraine headache. Headache 43: 309–321.

Martin V, Wernke S, Mandell K et al. (2005). Defining the relationship between ovarian hormones and migraine headache. Headache 45: 1190–1201.

Martin VT, Wernke S, Mandell K et al. (2006). Symptoms of premenstrual syndrome and their association with migraine headache. Headache 46: 125–137.

Massiou H, MacGregor EA (2000). Evolution and treatment of migraine with oral contraceptives. Cephalalgia 20: 170–174.

Mattsson P (2003). Hormonal factors in migraine: A population-based study of women aged 40 to 74 years. Headache 43: 27–35.

Miller L, Notter KM (2001). Menstrual reduction with extended use of combination oral contraceptive pills: randomized controlled trial. Obstet Gynecol 98: 771–778.

Misakian AL, Langer RD, Bensenor IM et al. (2003). Postmenopausal hormone therapy and migraine headache. J Womens Health 12: 1027–1036.

Modena MG, Sismondi P, Mueck AO et al. (2005). New evidence regarding hormone replacement therapies is urgently required transdermal postmenopausal hormone therapy differs from oral hormone therapy in risks and benefits. Maturitas 52: 1–10.

Moore MP, Redman CWG (1983). Case-control study of severe pre-eclampsia of early onset. BMJ 287: 580–583.

Mortimer MJ, Kay J, Jaron A (1992a). Childhood migraine in general practice: clinical features and characteristics. Cephalalgia 12: 238–243.

Mortimer MJ, Kay J, Jaron A (1992b). Epidemiology of headache and childhood migraine in an urban general practice using Ad Hoc, Vahlquist and IHS criteria. Dev Med Child Neurol 34: 1095–1101.

Mueller L (2000). Predictability of exogenous hormone effect on subgroups of migraineurs. Headache 40: 189–193.

Murray SC, Muse KN (1997). Effective treatment of severe menstrual migraine headaches with gonadotropin-releasing hormone agonist and "add-back" therapy. Fertil Steril 67: 390–393.

Nand SL, Webster MA, Baber R et al. (1998). Menopausal symptom control and side-effects on continuous estrone sulfate and three doses of medroxyprogesterone acetate. Ogen/Provera Study Group. Climacteric 1: 211–218.

Nappi G, Facchinetti F, Rossi F (Eds.) (1997). Headache and menstrually related disorders: in search of a consensus. Cephalalgia 17 (Suppl. 20).

Nappi G, Jensen R, Nappi RE et al. (2006). Diaries and calendars for migraine. A review. Cephalalgia 26: 905–916.

Nappi RE, Veneroni F, Chiapparini I et al. (1999). Gonadal hormones and migraine: a tight bondage within the female brain. Semin Headache Manage 4: 11–15.

Nappi RE, Cagnacci A, Granella F et al. (2001). Course of primary headaches during hormone replacement therapy. Maturitas 38: 157–163.

Nappi RE, Sances G, Brundu B et al. (2003). Neuroendocrine response to the serotonin agonist m-chlorophenylpiperazine in women with menstrual status migrainosus. Neuroendocrinology 78: 52–60.

Nappi RE, Sances G, Brundu B et al. (2005). Estradiol supplementation modulates neuroendocrine response to M-chlorophenylpiperazine in menstrual status migrainosus triggered by oral contraception-free interval. Hum Reprod 20: 3423–3428.

Nappi RE, Sances G, Sommacal A et al. (2006). Different effects of tibolone and low-dose EPT in the management of postmenopausal women with primary headaches. Menopause 13: 818–825.

Nattero G, Allais G, De Lorenzo C et al. (1989). Relevance of prostaglandins in true menstrual migraine. Headache 29: 233–238.

Neri I, Granella F, Nappi R et al. (1993). Characteristics of headache at menopause: a clinico-epidemiologic study. Maturitas 17: 31–37.

Oldenhave A, Jaszmann LJ, Everaerd WT et al. (1993). Hysterectomized women with ovarian conservation report more severe climacteric complaints than do normal climacteric women of similar age. Am J Obstet Gynecol 168: 765–771.

Pardutz A, Multon S, Malgrange B et al. (2002). Effect of systemic nitroglycerin on CGRP and 5-HT afferents to rat caudal spinal trigeminal nucleus and its modulation by estrogen. Eur J Neurosi 15: 1803–1809.

Petraglia F, Florio P, Nappi C et al. (1996). Peptide signaling in human placenta and membranes: autocrine, paracrine, and endocrine mechanisms. Endocr Rev 17: 156–186.

Pradalier A, Vincent D, Beaulieu P et al. (1994). Correlation between oestradiol plasma level and therapeutic effect on menstrual migraine. In: C Rose (Ed.), New Advances in Headache Research, Vol. 4. Smith-Gordon, London, pp. 129–132.

Rasmussen BK (1993). Migraine and tension-type headache in a general population: precipitating factors, female hormones, sleep pattern and relation to lifestyle. Pain 53: 65–72.

Rasmussen BK (1995). Epidemiology of headache. Cephalalgia 15: 45–68.

Ryan RE (1978). A controlled study of the effect of oral contraceptives on migraine. Headache 17: 250–251.

Sances G, Granella F, Nappi RE et al. (2003). Course of migraine during pregnancy and postpartum: a prospective study. Cephalalgia 23: 197–205.

Scharff L, Marcus DA, Turk DC (1997). Headache during pregnancy and in the postpartum: a prospective study. Headache 37: 203–210.

Scher AI, Terwindt GM, Picavet HSJ et al. (2005). Cardiovascular risk factors and migraine: the GEM population-based study. Neurology 64: 614–620.

Silberstein SD (1992). The role of sex hormones in headache. Neurology 42: 37–42.

Silberstein SD (1997). Migraine and pregnancy. Neurol Clin 15: 209–231.

Silberstein SD, Lipton RB, Goadsby PJ (1998). Headache in clinical practice. Oxford: Isis Medical Media, 1998: 61–90.

Silberstein SD (2000). Sex hormones and headache. Rev Neurol (Paris) 156 (Suppl. 4):4S30–4S41.

Silberstein SD, Merriam GR (1991). Estrogens, progestins and headache. Neurology 41: 786–793.

Small R, Friedman GD, Ettinger B (2001). Concomitant medication use in postmenopausal women using estrogen therapy. Menopause 8: 120–126.

Solomon GD, Kunkel RS Jr, Frame J (1990). Demographics of headache in elderly patients. Headache 30: 273–276.

Somerville BW (1972a). Plasma estradiol level linked to migraine during menstrual period. JAMA 221: 845–846.

Somerville BW (1972b). The role of estradiol withdrawal in the etiology of menstrual migraine. Neurology 22: 355–365.

Somerville BW (1972c). A study of migraine in pregnancy. Neurology 22: 824–828.

Somerville BW (1975a). Estrogen-withdrawal migraine. Neurology 25: 239–244.

Somerville BW (1975b). Estrogen-withdrawal migraine. I. Duration of exposure required and attempted prophylaxis by premenstrual estrogen administration. Neurology 25: 239–244.

Somerville BW (1975c). Estrogen-withdrawal migraine. II. Attempted prophylaxis by continuous estradiol administration. Neurology 25: 245–250.

Speroff L, Glass RH, Kase NG (1994). Clinical Gynecologic Endocrinology and Infertility, 5th edn. Williams and Wilkins, Baltimore.

Stein GS (1981). Headaches in the first post partum week and their relationship to migraine. Headache 21: 201–205.

Stewart WF, Linet MS, Celentano DD et al. (1991). Age- and sex-specific incidence rates of migraine with and without visual aura. Am J Epidemiol 134: 1111–1120.

Stewart WF, Lipton RB, Celentano DD et al. (1992). Prevalence of migraine headache in the United States. Relation to age, income, race, and other sociodemographic factors. JAMA 267: 64–69.

Stewart WF, Lipton RB, Chee E et al. (2000). Menstrual cycle and headache in a population sample of migraineurs. Neurology 55: 1517–1523.

Stovner LJ, Zwart JA, Hagen K et al. (2006). Epidemiology of headache in Europe. Eur J Neurol 13: 333–345.

Sulak PJ, Scow RD, Preece C et al. (2000). Hormone withdrawal symptoms in oral contraceptive users. Obstet Gynecol 95: 261–266.

Sulak PJ, Kuehl TJ, Ortiz M et al. (2002). Acceptance of altering the standard 21-day/7-day oral contraceptive regimen to delay menses and reduce hormone withdrawal symptoms. Am J Obstet Gynecol 186: 1142–1149.

Sulak P, Willis S, Kuehl T et al. (2007). Headaches and oral contraceptives: impact of eliminating the standard 7-day placebo interval. Headache 47: 27–37.

Tarin JJ, Brines J, Cano A (1998). Long-term effects of delayed parenthood. Hum Reprod 13: 2371–2376.

Tena-Sempere M (2006). Kiss-1 and reproduction: focus on its role in the metabolic regulation of fertility. Neuroendocrinology 83: 275–281.

Terasawa E, Fernandez DL (2001). Neurobiological mechanisms of the onset of puberty in primates. Endocr Rev 22: 111–151.

Tervila L, Marttila P (1975). Headache as a symptom of endometriosis externa. Ann Chir Gynaecol Fenn 64: 239–241.

Tietjen GE, Bushnell CD, Herial NA et al. (2007). Endometriosis is associated with prevalence of comorbid conditions in migraine. Headache 47: 1069–1078.

US Department of Health and Human Services Public Health Service (2006). Fast Facts About Endometriosis. National Institute of Child Health and Human Development, New York.

Wang SJ, Fuh JL, Lu SR et al. (2003). Migraine prevalence during menopausal transition. Headache 43: 470–478.

Welch KM, Darnley D, Simkins RT (1984). The role of estrogen in migraine: a review and hypothesis. Cephalalgia 4: 227–236.

Welch KM, Brandes JL, Berman NE (2006). Mismatch in how oestrogen modulates molecular and neuronal function may explain menstrual migraine. Neurol Sci 27: S190–S192.

Whitty CW, Hockaday JM, Whitty MM (1966). The effect of oral contraceptives on migraine. Lancet 1: 856–859.

Wright GD, Patel MK (1986). Focal migraine and pregnancy. BMJ 293: 1557–1558.

Yen MK, Jaffe MK (2004). Reproductive Endocrinology. 5th edn. Elsevier Saunders, Philadelphia.

Zondervan KT, Yudkin PL, Vessey MP et al. (1999). Prevalence and incidence in primary care of chronic pelvic pain in women: evidence from a national general practice database. Br J Obstet Gynaecol 106: 1149–1155.

Handbook of Clinical Neurology, Vol. 97 (3rd series)
Headache
G. Nappi and M.A. Moskowitz, Editors

Chapter 26

Acute treatment of migraine

J.L. BRANDES, [1]* T.M. BUCHANAN, [2] AND K.M.A. WELCH [3]

[1]*Department of Neurology, Vanderbilt University Medical Center, Nashville Neuroscience Group, St Thomas Health Services, Department of Neurology, Vanderbilt University School of Medicine, Nashville, Tennessee, USA*

[2]*Department of Neurology, University of Utah, Salt Lake City, Utah, USA*

[3]*Department of Neurology, Chicago Medical School, Rosalind Franklin University of Medicine and Science, Chicago, Illinois, USA*

INTRODUCTION

Acute treatment of migraine has benefited first from major advances in pharmacological science followed in short order, sometimes preceded, by an improved understanding of pathogenesis, especially of headache. This chapter will briefly review mechanisms of migraine that provide understanding of the pharmacology and therapeutic use of acute migraine medications. General clinical approaches to acute therapy (e.g., stratified versus stepped care, early approaches) will be reviewed, and some indices of acceptable acute therapeutic outcomes will be discussed (e.g., 24-h relief from IHS). Currently the serotonin (5-HT) agonist group of drugs, triptans, forms the mainstay of acute therapeutic regimens and thus will be emphasized in this review, as we describe the basic pharmacology, clinical trials, and safety profile that have established therapeutic dominance for these drugs. Despite such dominance, another approach to acute treatment is often called for, so we will review some of the more longstanding therapies (simple analgesics, non-steroidal anti-inflammatory drugs (NSAIDs), ergots, and combination medications), and then alternative medications. We will conclude with notation of the newest acute treatments that are currently exploratory or under clinical investigation, and speculate on future targets culled from experimental observations.

MECHANISMS OF MIGRAINE

Knowledge of the pathogenesis of migraine is incomplete but understanding is evolving; multiple pathophysiological mechanisms seem to be involved in the peripheral and central nervous system. Interictal susceptibility, aura mechanisms, potential migraine generators, and especially cascading molecular events underlying migraine-associated pain and related symptoms must be contemplated in understanding the pharmacotherapeutics of an attack.

Prevailing concepts of susceptibility to attacks center on neuronal hyperexcitability (Welch, 2003). Hyperexcitability appears to be a common brain state due to one or more factors, such as genetically determined neuronal membrane channelopathies (Ophoff et al., 1996), or certain metabolic determinants such as low magnesium (Boska et al., 2002). Hyperexcitability may also be secondary to disruption in central inhibitory neuromodulation, of which the mechanism is less well known (Afra et al., 1998). Cortical spreading depression (CSD), a slowly spreading wave of neuronal depolarization (activation) that may be followed by a longer-lasting suppression of neuronal activity in the occipital cortex, is now generally accepted as the underlying mechanism of the stimulative followed by suppressive character of the clinical features of the migraine aura that mostly precedes the headache phase (Bowyer et al., 2001).

How aura activates headache remains to be established, however. Migraine without aura is thought to be associated either with CSD invading "silent" brain areas, or activation of subcortical centers. Migraine susceptibility and aura-triggering factors constitute the targets for preventive therapies. Few studies have exploited the potential of targeting the interface between aura and headache; it is hard to define whether preventive or acute

*Correspondence to: J.L. Brandes, Assistant Clinical Professor, Department of Neurology, Vanderbilt University Medical Center, Nashville Neuroscience Group, St Thomas Health Services, Assistant Clinical Professor, Department of Neurology, Vanderbilt University School of Medicine, Nashville, TN 37203, USA, Tel: 615-284-4680, Fax: 615-284-4681, E-mail: jbrandes@nashvilleneuroscience.com

medications also act at this intracerebral level during activation of trigeminovascular terminals by certain neuroactive substances. For example, CSD releases nitric oxide (NO) (Read et al., 1997), which couples neuronal activity with vascular tone by causing release of calcitonin gene-related peptide (CGRP) (Wei et al., 1992), vasodilation, and nociceptor activation.

Due to significant sensory innervation, meninges are a principal source of migraine headache (Feindel et al., 1960; Moskowitz, 1990; Goadsby and Hoskin, 1997). Trigeminovascular system activation involves a cascade of reactions likely initiated by release of inflammatory cytokines in trigeminal neurons, CGRP, substance P, and neurokinin A on to meningeal blood vessels (Liu-Chen et al., 1984; Uddman et al., 1985; Edvinsson et al., 1988). CGRP has been implicated most in the headache of migraine patients, having been detected in jugular venous blood during a migraine attack (Goadsby et al., 1988; Gallai et al., 1995). Further, infusion of CGRP to susceptible individuals elicited migraine-like headache (Lassen et al., 1998b). One consequence of release of these neuroactive substances is neurogenic inflammation accompanied by vasodilation, disruption of membrane barriers, and plasma protein extravasation, a point of controversy in understanding mechanisms of migraine headache, however (Roon et al., 2000).

Hypersensitization of trigeminal nerve endings may be the basis for peripheral sensitization and prolongation of migraine pain. Central sensitization of the trigeminal system may also account for the severe prolonged pain of migraine headache, also manifest as pain returning on head movement or scalp pressure after attacks have subsided, and allodynia of the head. Allodynia and pain of the upper trunk and limbs suggest supraspinal origins of sensitization in addition (Burstein et al., 2000; Kaube et al., 2002). Abnormal supraspinal pain modulation is in keeping with periaqueductal gray dysfunction and aberrance of its balanced nociceptive facilitatory or inhibitory functions (Welch et al., 2001). The critical importance of central sensitization has been underlined most recently by observations that triptans may be ineffective after allodynia is established (Burstein et al., 2004).

Based on a positron emission tomography (PET) study of acute migraine without aura, central brainstem structures were proposed as loci for a primary "generator" role for migraine headache (Weiller et al., 1995). Although the observations were seminal in first demonstrating convincing brainstem involvement in migraine attacks, the activated regions, periaqueductal gray matter, dorsal raphe nucleus, and the locus coeruleus were contralateral to the side of head pain, provoking an alternative explanation that these centers were not directly responsible for pain, but responsible instead for modulating the flow of pain impulses. It does seem likely, however, that a network of cortical and subcortical structures with modulatory nociceptive and antinociceptive function might become abnormally activated in a migraine attack, or even may be abnormal between attacks (Terr Host et al., 2001). Thus episodic dysfunction of certain brainstem centers may play a key role in migraine pain, through either aberrant activation or modulation of impulse flow in the trigeminal system.

In sum, migraine pathogenesis involves nociception, inflammation, and peripheral and central sensitization. Therefore, a rational approach to therapeutics of the acute attack might rationally combine pharmacotherapies that target nociception, inflammation, and sensitization.

THERAPEUTICS

Maximizing response to therapy

Population studies have probed the treatment attributes deemed important by patients with acute migraine attacks (Lipton and Stewart, 1997). Medications should bring about: (1) complete pain relief; (2) no headache recurrence; and (3) rapid relief. The International Headache Society used these requirements in deriving a testable endpoint for clinical trials of acute medication, namely sustained pain-free at 24 h. The US Headache Consortium has provided more general directions to clinical practitioners, which include: (1) treat attacks rapidly and consistently without recurrence; (2) restore the patient's ability to function; (3) minimize use of back-up (rescue) medications; (4) be cost-effective for overall management; and (5) minimal or no adverse events (Lipton and Silberstein, 2001).

Two broad management approaches have been introduced in recent years for acute treatment (Lipton et al., 2000). Stratified care entails matching treatment to illness severity, using the most powerful antimigraine drugs at the outset if called for. For example, patients disabled with frequent attacks of intense pain attaining high scores on disability scales may be managed best with triptans plus preventive therapies. Patients with few but severe and disabling attacks may require only acute triptan therapy. Infrequent attacks of mild intensity may respond to NSAIDs, combination analgesics, and simple modifications in lifestyle (e.g., caffeine regulation, sleep pattern adjustments).

In contrast, stepped care does not rely on severity indices but entails first using simple analgesics, escalating over time to more powerful drugs depending on response. With this approach, patients' satisfaction may not be achieved for weeks to months as several different treatment steps may be required. In a study of stratified versus stepped care, the former improved headache response and reduced disability measured as time missed from work, school, or leisure activities (Lipton et al., 2000). Overall costs associated with care were reduced over the long term, measured by fewer office visits, less use of rescue medication, and less time missed from work or school.

Drugs administered early in an acute attack can bring about a shortened time to pain-free response. Further, the earlier administered and effective, the less the opportunity for central sensitization of the trigeminal system. Unfortunately, many patients delay taking medication because of inconvenience, hoping for spontaneous resolution, waiting to establish the headache type, worrying about side-effects, or avoiding needless expense. Studies of early treatment when attacks are mild, versus delay until moderate or severe, first appeared in 1998 (The International 311C90 Long-term Study Group, 1998). For example, the proportion of patients reporting 2-h pain-free rates for mild, moderate, or severe attacks after oral zolmitriptan was 80%, 57%, and 35%, respectively; results were replicated with the nasal spray (Syrett et al., 2003). Cady et al. (2000) reported results from a placebo-controlled, retrospective analysis of patients who treated mild migraine attacks with sumatriptan 100 mg oral tablet in violation of the study protocol. Highest 2-h pain-free rates were observed for participants ($n = 40$) who treated mild attacks (52% versus placebo 0%), compared to those who treated moderate or severe attacks (29% versus placebo 8%, $n = 36$). Subsequently, similar findings were reported (Hu et al., 2002; Pascual and Cabarrocas, 2002). Studies cited above were unblended, used protocol violators, or were based on retrospective analyses. In a prospective study, patients who treated mild attacks had a 2-h pain-free response rate of 43% as compared to 18% in placebo recipients; the 2-h pain-free response rate rose to 57% of patients treating within the first 15 min after onset of pain. Treating earlier in a migraine attack while the pain is still mild therefore confers additional therapeutic benefit, emphasizing the early time factor since treating mild headache does not always mean early treatment.

Acute therapy

5-HT_1 agonists – Triptans

Activation of the trigeminal nerve is a key component of the cascade that leads to, and perpetuates, a migraine attack. Specific 5-HT receptor subtypes that are found on the trigeminovascular system include 5-HT_{1B}, 5-HT_{1D}, and 5-HT_{1F} receptor subtypes (Waeber and Moskowitz, 2005; Hamel and Saxena, 2006). Sumatriptan and the other triptans currently on the market (almotriptan, eletriptan, frovatriptan, naratriptan, rizatriptan, zolmitriptan) are potent agonists of the 5-HT_{1B} and 5-HT_{1D} receptors, and some are potent 5-HT_{1F} agonists (Table 26.1) (Saxena and Tfelt-Hansen, 2006).

Table 26.1

Affinity of marketed triptans to 5-HT_1 receptors. Data represent human binding affinity (pKi) values. Numbers in parentheses are standard errors

Compound	pKi (h 5-HT_{1B})	pKi (h 5-HT_{1D})	pKi (h 5-HT_{1F})
Almotriptan	8.15 (0.15)	7.80 (0.20)	7.49
Eletriptan	8.14 (0.24)	8.85 (0.04)	7.99
Frovatriptan	8.24 (0.20)	8.31 (0.16)	7.10 (0.08)
Naratriptan	8.64 (0.20)	8.55	8.31
Rizatriptan	7.70 (0.29)	8.18 (0.20)	6.74 (0.08)
Sumatriptan	7.77 (0.11)	8.13 (0.17)	7.81 (0.06)
Zolmitriptan	8.40 (0.23)	9.07 (0.18)	7.47 (0.09)

(Adapted from Ramadan et al., 2003, with permission.)

Sumatriptan succinate was the first of the triptan classes to be developed specifically for acute migraine. Initially, sumatriptan was advanced because of its potent vasoconstrictive properties in animal and human blood vessels (Humphrey and Feniuk, 1991). Sumatriptan was discovered later to inhibit neurogenic inflammation, which may or may not have relevance to migraine (Peroutka, 2005), and the release of pro-inflammatory and vasoactive substances (e.g., CGRP) that are implicated in migraine (Saxena and Tfelt-Hansen, 2006). Similarly, second-generation triptans constrict cranial blood vessels by a 5-HT_{1B} receptor-mediated agonist action and inhibit trigeminal nerve firing with reduced release of proinflammatory mediators in response to neural stimulation of the trigeminal nerve via 5-HT_{1D} and 5-HT_{1F} receptor agonist actions (Longmore et al., 1999; Waeber and Moskowitz, 2005; Saxena and Tfelt-Hansen, 2006).

It is unclear whether the benefit of the 5-HT agonists in relieving migraine headache is through a peripheral or central action, or both. Further it is unclear if any peripheral action is by vasoconstriction or inhibition of peptide release, or both. Sumatriptan does not cross the blood–brain barrier, but can inhibit the trigeminal nucleus activation when disrupted (Kaube et al., 1993). Since in theory the blood–brain barrier may be altered during migraine (Ferrari, 1998), a central action cannot be ruled out for sumatriptan (Nozaki et al., 1992). All second-generation triptans developed after sumatriptan readily penetrate the blood–brain barrier, binding to key structures in central nociceptive structures.

Sumatriptan dramatically changed acute migraine therapy, as it provided pain relief and improvement in the majority of patients and disappearance of the associated symptoms of nausea, photophobia, and phonophobia. The limitations of sumatriptan, however, became evident with accumulating clinical data. Oral administration did not provide full pain relief to more than 50% of patients, was associated with headache recurrence in over 30% of patients who initially responded, and sumatriptan could not be given to patients with cardiovascular disease or at risk for it (Saxena and Tfelt-Hansen, 2006). Subcutaneous sumatriptan was more effective but had the same contraindications and precautions as the oral form, exaggerated side-effects such as chest tightness (see below), and possessed the inherent disadvantages of a needle injection. Shortfalls of sumatriptan kept alive various research programs aimed at discovering an enhanced triptan through optimizing the compound's pharmacokinetic properties; increasing the potency at the desired receptors; reducing adverse events; or minimizing cardiovascular complications.

Second-generation drugs (almotriptan, eletriptan, frovatriptan, naratriptan, rizatriptan, zolmitriptan) resulted from these research efforts. Also, alternative routes of compound delivery (e.g., intranasal or rectal sumatriptan; intranasal zolmitriptan) and enhanced enteral formulations (e.g., rapidly disintegrating sumatriptan) were brought to market. Second-generation triptans, for the most part, kept to the promise of enhanced pharmacokinetic properties. Also, they increased the choice of migraine-specific therapies, which translates into a more individually tailored treatment. Unfortunately, enhanced pharmacokinetic and preclinical pharmacodynamic profiles did not equate with meaningful and substantial clinical improvement over sumatriptan, whether in maximizing efficacy, reducing adverse events, or eliminating the cardiovascular contraindications (Ferrari et al., 2001; Saxena and Tfelt-Hansen, 2006).

Sumatriptan was the first 5-HT_{1BD} receptor agonist proven to be effective in migraine (Welch, 1993). Subcutaneous administration of 6 mg sumatriptan reduced headache severity within 2 h in up to 86% of patients. Nausea and vomiting were effectively relieved in most patients. Unfortunately, headache can recur in up to 46% of patients within 24 h, probably because of the short half-life of the drug. Sumatriptan nasal spray is also available, the standard dose being 20 mg. Patients have to deliver the spray with the head bent forward because of unpleasant taste. This preparation is useful, however, when a more rapid action than can be obtained by the oral route of the drug is required, or for patients who find the injection unacceptable but require more rapid pain relief. When sumatriptan is given orally in a dose of up to 100 mg, headache and associated symptoms are relieved within 4 h in 75% of patients. The optimal oral dose is currently accepted to be 100 mg at the outset of the attack. As with subcutaneous administration, headache recurrence is a problem.

Zolmitriptan, the second triptan developed and the first to penetrate the blood–brain barrier, is available in intranasal and oral form (Ryan, 2001). Zolmitriptan has higher bioavailablity (42%) when compared to sumatriptan (14%). The number of patients who are pain-free 2 h after treatment is nearly identical for both drugs. Nausea, vomiting, and photophonophobia are also effectively treated. Zolmitriptan is most effective taken early during the headache, and has equal efficacy across headache types (migraine with aura, migraine without aura, menstrual migraine).

Naratriptan is available only in oral form; the recommended dose is 2.5 mg. Adverse events occur overall at a lower rate than sumatriptan, however, and the drug is well tolerated (Klassen et al., 1997). Headache recurrence after treatment with naratriptan may be lowest of all the triptan drugs, and its efficacy at 2 h is less than that of other triptans.

The recommended dose of rizatriptan is 10 mg (Wellington and Plosker, 2002). Bioavailablity (45%) is comparable to that of zolmitriptan (42%) but lower than for naratriptan (74% for women, 63% for men). Studies have shown that rizatriptan 10 mg provides fast pain relief and a high percentage of patients with an absence of pain and normal functional ability at 2 h. The rate of headache recurrence may be higher than for other triptans, but otherwise the drug is generally well tolerated.

Eletriptan is rapidly absorbed when administered orally, and has good bioavailability and good central nervous system penetration due to its lipophilicity. Compared with other serotonin agonists, eletriptan has a longer duration of action, which contributes to its ability to prevent recurrent headaches. Eletriptan is metabolized through the cytochrome P450 3A4 system; therefore, it does have the potential for clinically significant drug interactions (Takiya et al., 2006).

Frovatriptan is a 5-$HT_{(1B/1D)}$ receptor agonist with high 5-$HT_{(1B)}$ potency, and apparently cerebroselective. Oral bioavailability of frovatriptan is 22–30%; time to maximum concentration is typically 2–3 h, although 60–70% of maximum plasma concentration is achieved within 1 h of dosing. Frovatriptan has a long terminal elimination half-life of 26 h, making it well suited for patients with migraine of long duration and those with frequent recurrence. Like naratriptan, frovatriptan has lower efficacy than the other triptans at 2 h.

Good tolerability is an added feature of value (Buchan et al., 2002).

Almotriptan is an effective drug for the acute treatment of moderate or severe attacks of migraine in adults with rapid onset of action (significant headache relief is observed 0.5 h after administration of a 12.5-mg dose), with a good adverse event and tolerability profile, especially a low incidence of chest symptoms (Keam et al., 2002; Linder et al., 2008). It is the only triptan approved by the Food and Drug Agency for use in adolescents.

Side-effects are similar for all triptans, though of variable prominence depending on route of delivery (subcutaneous greater than oral), and drug preparation. Most are mild to moderate in intensity, are short-lived, resolve spontaneously, and do not change with repeated use of the drug. The most common side-effects, popularly known as "triptan effects," are sensations of flushing, heat, and tingling, and neck pain with stiffness. Some 3–5% of patients experience chest tightness, heaviness, pressure, tingling, and pain. The cause of the chest symptoms is unknown, but in rare instances coronary vasospasm has undoubtedly occurred. The vasoconstrictive action of the triptans extends to the coronary vasculature, although it only occurs at concentrations well above those attained for aborting acute migraine headache. Although rare, cardiovascular complications have occurred in treated patients (Welch et al., 2000). For patients who are likely to have unrecognized coronary artery disease (e.g., postmenopausal women, men older than 40 years, and patients with risk factors for coronary artery disease), the first dose of triptan is best given under medical supervision. The use of vasoconstrictors, such as ergotamines, dihydroergotamine, and other triptans, is contraindicated within 24 h. Restricting the patient population that can receive triptans to those without coronary or cerebrovascular diseases, or the risk thereof, is an undesirable element of clinical practice. Thus triptans are contraindicated in patients with a history of myocardial infarction, symptomatic ischemic heart disease, Prinzmetal angina, and hypertension. The serious adverse events are considered a drug class effect.

Although the effectiveness of the triptans is generally of high order, it is far from absolute and this, plus the adverse event profile, demands the continued search for new drug targets, new drugs, and new approaches to treatment.

On the basis of multiple pathogenic mechanisms being involved in generating the migraine symptom complex, multimechanism targeted therapy may have advantages over monotherapy. In a strategy to enhance the effectiveness of sumatriptan, a fixed-dose tablet containing sumatriptan succinate and the NSAID naproxen sodium was tested relative to efficacy and safety of each monotherapy and placebo for the acute treatment of moderate or severe migraine attacks in randomized, double-blind, single-attack, parallel-group studies. Sumatriptan/naproxen sodium produced more favorable clinical benefits than either monotherapy or placebo, with an acceptable and well-tolerated adverse effect profile (Brandes et al., 2007). The precise reasons for this added benefit are uncertain but may be related to differing pharmacokinetics of absorption plus pre-empting or overcoming trigeminal sensitization.

Other medications used for acute headache

Although increasingly uncommon, some patients may also respond only to other established acute medications, find such medications more tolerable, or may have contraindications to the use of triptans. Ergot preparations are also 5-HT_1 agonists but much less specific. Triptans have largely replaced the ergots but they were used for many years for treatment of moderate to severe acute migraine attacks. Ergotamine, however, is effective in only half of patients when given orally, sublingually, rectally, or nasally. The addition of caffeine enhances the absorption and possibly the vasoconstrictive activity of ergotamine. Ergotamine is best absorbed rectally. An antiemetic drug (best given by suppository) may be needed together with ergotamine. Dihydroergotamine, which has a relatively long half-life, and is available for nasal, subcutaneous, and intravenous administration in the USA, is also effective in migraine attacks, and now constitutes the preferred ergot-derived preparation as a triptan alternative. Like triptans, dihydroergotamine is a vasoconstrictor (particularly of the venous system) and should not be given to patients with vascular disease.

Simple analgesic drugs such as aspirin and acetaminophen or NSAIDs are the commonest medications used for treating acute headache and may be used for the treatment of mild or moderate migraine attacks (Welch, 1993). Contemporary trials of the longer-established medications are rare in the current literature, however. In one large multicenter, randomized, double-blind, single-dose study patients received either oral acetylsalicylic acid effervescent 1000 mg ($n = 169$) or effervescent placebo ($n = 174$) for treating acute migraine attack (Lange et al., 2000). Response rates (reduction of headache severity from severe or moderate to mild or no pain at 2 h after administration) were 55.0% for acetylsalicylic acid and 36.8% for placebo ($P < 0.001$). Twenty-nine percent of patients in the active treatment group were pain-free after 2 h compared with 16.7% in the placebo group. No headache recurred within 24 h postdose in 84.6% of patients in the active group and in 85.1% of patients in the placebo group. Effervescent placebo reduced nausea and vomiting to the same degree as the active drug. Adverse events of acetylsalicylic acid (8.3%) were generally mild or moderate and comparable to those of placebo (2.9%). Although aspirin clearly was effective compared with placebo, the 2-h pain-free effectiveness is unlikely to satisfy the majority of sufferers who expect complete pain freedom at 2 h as the optimal outcome goal of therapy.

NSAIDs, being relatively recent additions to the formulary, have been tested in randomized clinical trials, and have established efficacy for acute migraine treatment (McNeely and Goa, 1999). Their effectiveness fits well with the inflammatory basis of migraine headache, being also effective in settings where inflammation leads to sensitization of pain systems. Naproxen and ibuprofen are most commonly used in the USA. Side-effects and contraindications are similar to those of aspirin, with easy bleeding and gastric toxicity. NSAIDs may be the acute treatment of choice when triptans or ergot derivatives are contraindicated.

Because gastric stasis often accompanies migraine attacks, metoclopramide, a drug that increases gut motility and promotes gastric emptying, enhances the effectiveness of analgesic drugs. However, metoclopramide should be used sparingly in adults and should not be used at all in young patients, because it can cause dystonia. When nausea and vomiting are prominent, suppository preparations of analgesic and antiemetic drugs can be given. The most frequently used antiemetic drugs are perphenazine, prochlorperazine, and chlorpromazine.

Symptomatic treatment in the emergency department

Migraine attacks that are severe, prolonged, and unresponsive to self-administered medication may be treated in the clinic or emergency department. If patients with such attacks have not received them already, they should be treated with sumatriptan given subcutaneously or dihydroergotamine given intravenously or subcutaneously. If these drugs fail, the preferred regimens are metoclopramide (10 mg intravenously), prochlorperazine (10 mg intravenously), or chlorpromazine administered in three intravenous injections of 0.1 mg/kg given 15 min apart. In addition to dystonia and tardive dyskinesia, the side-effects of the three drugs are drowsiness, nausea, vomiting, dizziness, and hypotension, all of which are infrequent.

Major narcotic analgesic drugs, particularly meperidine, are used in the emergency treatment of migraine attacks. The use of meperidine should be limited to patients who have attacks that do not respond to antimigraine preparations and patients in whom antimigraine drugs are contraindicated (e.g., those with peripheral vascular or coronary artery disease and pregnant women). Acute attacks may be so frequent and the patient's pain so severe and continuous that hospitalization is needed. In these patients, it may be effective to administer dihydroergotamine intravenously for 3–4 days, discontinue all other drugs, and administer intravenous fluid (Raskin, 1986). Intravenous administration of corticosteroids may also be effective.

NOVEL PHARMACOTHERAPEUTIC APPROACHES

Non-triptan 5-HT$_1$ agonists

5-HT$_{1D}$ agonists (PNU-109291 and PNU-142633)

5HT$_{1D}$ receptor agonists are potent inhibitors of dural plasma protein extravasation (PPE) (an animal model with some relevance to migraine) (Cutrer et al., 1999) and possess no vasoactive properties. Also, peptidergic nociceptors express these receptors (Potrebic et al., 2003) in an activation-dependent manner (Ahn et al., 2004). Two non-vasoactive 5-HT$_{1D}$-selective agonists have shown some promise in animal models of migraine. In one human randomized controlled trial (RCT), PNU-142633 failed to achieve significance, and subjects reported cardiovascular symptoms such as chest pain (Gomez-Mancilla et al., 2001). The PNU-142633 program was abandoned, but it can be argued that this 5-HT$_{1D}$ agonist proof-of-concept experiment did not address fully the 5-HT$_{1D}$ in migraine hypothesis because PNU-142633 is a partial 5-HT$_{1D}$ agonist at the gorilla receptor (33% of 5-HT efficacy in the functional GTPγS assay), whereas sumatriptan is a full agonist (93% of 5-HT efficacy) (Pregenzer et al., 1999). Also, the non-vasoactive hypothesis of 5-HT$_{1D}$ agonism needs further elucidation with the complaints of chest symptoms on PNU-142633. One tantalizing hypothesis is that 5-HT$_{1D}$ agonists are cardioactive but not vasoactive, and the chest symptoms are valvular in origin since 5-HT$_{1D}$ receptors are found on cardiac valves (Roy et al., 2000). Another explanation is that the chest symptoms are of pulmonary origin (see Dodick, 2004, for review).

5-HT$_{1F}$ agonists

There are several lines of evidence that implicate the 5-HT$_{1F}$ receptor in migraine (Ramadan et al., 2003). Animal experiments indicate that 5-HT$_{1F}$ agonists are effective in preclinical models of migraine, and are not vasoconstrictive. Also, it is argued that the activity in the PPE model correlates with affinity at 5-HT_{1F}, but not at 5-HT_{1D} or 5-HT_{1B} receptors. Furthermore, LY334370, which is a selective 5-HT_{1F} agonist, inhibits single cell firing in the trigeminal nucleus caudalis (TNC) without any effect on cerebral vessel lumen as measured by intravital microscopy (Shepheard et al., 1999). Anatomically, 5-HT_{1F} mRNA is on the trigeminal ganglion (TG). Functionally, 5-HT_{1F}, and 5-HT_{1B} and 5-HT_{1D} agonists can presynaptically inhibit the release of glutamate, which may participate in the migraine cascade (Ramadan, 2003).

Clinically, LY334370 is the prototype and first selective 5-HT_{1F} agonist that reached phase II clinical development (Goldstein et al., 2001; Ramadan et al., 2003). In a phase II RCT, 99 patients received oral placebo or LY334370 20 mg, 60 mg, or 200 mg for the acute treatment of moderate to severe migraine (Goldstein et al., 2001). Sustained headache response rates (headache response at 2 h and no headache recurrence or use of rescue medication from 2 to 24 h after treatment) were significantly higher on 60 mg LY334370 (37%) and 200 mg LY334370 (52%) than on placebo (8%) ($P<0.001$ for dose response). Adverse events that were more common on oral LY334370 than on placebo were asthenia, somnolence, and dizziness. The development of LY334370 was halted because of animal toxicity.

GABA agonists

Oral divalproate is a broad-spectrum antiepileptic drug with well-demonstrated efficacy in migraine prevention. The recent introduction of intravenous valproate for epileptic seizures and the demonstration that valproate acts on mechanisms of acute migraine such as inhibition of neurogenic PPE and nociceptive transmission (Cutrer and Moskowitz, 1996) led to the exploration of its value in severe attacks of migraine. Several open-label studies suggested that intravenous valproate is beneficial in acute severe migraine and other primary severe headaches (Freitag, 2003). A non-placebo-controlled trial, however, failed to demonstrate benefit of intravenous valproate, while the comparator drug prochlorperazine was effective as an acute antimigraine drug (Tanen et al., 2003).

Dopamine antagonists

Migraineurs may be hypersensitive to dopaminergic stimulation (Cerbo et al., 1997), which suggests that dopaminergic blockade is a valuable therapeutic strategy (Peroutka, 1997; Del Zompo, 2000), but this hypothesis is controversial (Akerman and Goadsby, 2005). Various dopamine antagonists are used widely in acute migraine therapy. More recently, the therapeutic value of droperidol, an antagonist of dopamine actions *in vivo*, in acute migraine was tested. A large randomized clinical trial that included over 300 patients with acute migraine demonstrated that intramuscular droperidol provides significant relief of acute migraine pain and associated symptoms (Silberstein et al., 2003). Adverse effects are a concern, as akathisia occurred in over 30%, and somnolence or anxiety was also common.

Glutamate modulators

The glutamate hypothesis of migraine has been discussed in detail (Ramadan, 2003). Briefly, ionotropic *N*-methyl-D-aspartate (NMDA) and non-NMDA (α-amino-3-hydroxy-5-methyl-4-isoxazolepropionic acid (AMPA), kainic acid (KA)) glutamate receptor subtypes, and metabotropic glutamate receptors are distributed widely in the trigeminal system (Tallaksen-Green et al., 1992; Sahara et al., 1997; Quartu et al., 2002). Also, noxious stimulation of the trigeminal nerve increases extracellular glutamate, which in turn excites TNC neurons. Furthermore, neurons in the TG that are 5-HT_{1B}, 5-HT_{1D}, and 5-HT_{1F} receptor-positive are glutamate receptor-positive, which may indicate that 5-HT_1 autoreceptors may inhibit the release of glutamate presynaptically (Ma, 2001). Lastly, several preclinical pharmacological studies have implicated the glutamatergic system in trigeminovascular trafficking (Mitsikostas et al., 1998, 1999; Goadsby and Classey, 2000; Classey et al., 2001).

Clinically, a genetic observation (Jen et al., 2005), biomarker studies, and clinical trials have implicated the glutamatergic system in migraine (Ramadan, 2003). For example, two studies demonstrated elevated plasma levels of glutamate in migraineurs but not in controls, and more so in migraine with aura as compared to migraine without aura (Ferrari et al., 1990; Alam et al., 1998). However, these results were not replicated in other studies (Cananzi et al., 1995). Also, in a small open-label trial, intranasal ketamine prevented migraine aura in 5 of 11 patients with familial hemiplegic migraine but had no effect on the headache (Kaube et al., 2000a). Finally, in hemiplegic migraine, mutations reduce the glial cell's ability to clear glutamate from the synaptic cleft, which would contribute to postsynaptic hyperexcitation (De Fusco et al., 2003).

LY293558

LY293558 is a non-selective AMPA/KA antagonist that has demonstrated efficacy for pain relief in allodynia, hyperalgesia, and lumbar monoradiculopathy (Sang et al., 1998). The potential efficacy of LY293558 in migraine was also assessed in a RCT (Sang et al., 2004). In this multicenter RCT ($n = 45$), the efficacy and safety of intravenous LY293558 were compared to placebo, and subcutaneous sumatriptan was included as a positive control. The drug was significantly superior to placebo on all efficacy measures. Generally mild and reversible visual distortion is the most consistently reported adverse effect of LY293558 (Sang et al., 1998, 2004). Dizziness and sedation can occur.

Adenosine-1 receptor agonists

Adenosine modulates nociception through its A_1 receptor (Sawynok, 1998), and A_1 receptor protein is on human trigeminal ganglia (Schindler et al., 1998, 2001). Furthermore, prejunctional selective A1 agonists can inhibit trigeminovascular activation, both in the trigeminal nucleus and by inhibition of release of CGRP in the cranial circulation (Goadsby et al., 2002). Lastly, glutamate may modulate nociception, in part by releasing adenosine which inhibits prejunctional A1 receptors (Ramadan, 2003).

GR79236

The antinociceptive activity of the potent and selective A1 agonist, GR79236, has been studied in animal models of migraine. In the cat, GR79236 reduced venous concentration of CGRP and nociceptive transmission from the trigeminal nerve (Goadsby et al., 2002). In the rat, GR79236 inhibited nociception-induced activity of neurons in the TNC (Bland-Ward et al., 2000), and trigeminally evoked dural vasodilation (Honey et al., 2002). However, in the pig, capsaicin-induced CGRP release was not affected by GR79236 administration (Arulmani et al., 2005).

In humans, GR79236 was effective in suppressing the nociceptive blink reflex in an open-label study of 12 adult healthy female volunteers (Kaube et al., 2000b), at doses that are inhibitory of trigeminal neurons and without vascular effects in experimental animals. Conventional migraine trials in humans are anticipated, but there is concern that the A1 agonist target has an adverse event profile that may preclude further development.

Calcitonin gene-related peptide antagonists

Several lines of evidence support the involvement of CGRP in the migraine cascade (Edvinsson, 2003). First, CGRP is located on sensory terminals of the trigeminal nerve, and is released following stimulation of the nerve. Also, CGRP mediates dilation of cerebral vasculature and increases in cerebral blood flow (Edvinsson et al., 1998; Edvinsson, 2003; Jansen-Olesen et al., 2003), which is a component of the trigeminovascular reflex that leads to inhibition of excessive cerebrovascular contraction (McCulloch et al., 1986). Furthermore, CGRP-induced vasodilation can activate nociceptors on cerebral vessels. In humans, intravenous human CGRP administration induces migraine-like headache in susceptible migraineurs (Lassen et al., 2002). Lastly, data from a RCT confirmed CGRP antagonism as a potentially useful migraine target (see below) (Olesen et al., 2004).

BIBN4096BS is a potent CGRP antagonist that was tested recently in a phase II RCT which used an adaptive dose design method (Olesen et al., 2004). Migraine patients ($n = 126$) were randomized to receive intravenous BIBN4096BS 0.25 mg, 0.5 mg, 1 mg, 2.5 mg, 5 mg, 10 mg, or placebo. Significantly more patients (66%) reported relief of headache (improvement from moderate or severe pain to mild or none at 2 h) on the optimal dose (2.5 mg) of BIBN4096BS than those who received placebo (26.8%). Paresthesia was the most common adverse event linked to BIBN4096BS. The mechanism of action of BIBN4096BS is independent of changes in cerebral blood flow (Petersen et al., 2004).

Telcagepant (MK-0974), a novel CGRP receptor antagonist, was found effective in acute migraine treatment and was well tolerated (Ho et al., 2008). While in trial as a preventive medication, however, longer-term use was associated with hepatic enzyme elevation, engendering uncertainty as to whether the drug will receive approval for clinical practice.

Nitric oxide synthase inhibitors

NO is a membrane-permeable, lipophilic gas that is found in endothelial cells, platelets, neutrophils, and the brain, and it has vasodilatory activity. Preclinical and clinical experiments support the validity of NO inhibition as a target in migraine therapeutics. An intravenous infusion of nitroglycerine releases NO, causes migraine in more than 60% of migraineurs (Olesen et al., 1993), and activates trigeminal neurons in experimental animals (Tassorelli et al., 1999). Also, nitroglycerine infusion induces delayed PPE in the dura mater of rats (Reuter et al., 2001). In the cat, CSD releases NO (Read et al., 1997), which couples neuronal activity with vascular tone by causing release of CGRP (Wei et al., 1992), vasodilation, and nociceptor activation. Lastly, the NO synthase (NOS) inhibitor N^G-methyl-L-arginine hydrochloride (LNMAH; 546C88) was effective in the clinic (Lassen et al., 1998a).

In a small RCT, 546C88, a non-selective NOS inhibitor, was administered intravenously to migraineurs during an acute attack (Lassen et al., 1998a). The 2-h headache response rate was 67% (10/15) on 546C88 versus 14% (2/14) on placebo. Symptoms such as phono- and photophobia were significantly improved as well. The authors concluded that 546C88 may be beneficial in migraine and acknowledged the study limitations (e.g., small sample size; use of historical controls). The effects of 546C88 in humans are believed to be independent of vascular changes as cerebral blood flow velocities measured by transcranial Doppler ultrasound did not change in a RCT that tested the compound in healthy subjects (Hjorth-Lassen et al., 2003).

Vanilloid receptor modulators

Capsaicin is the best-known vanilloid, and is an extract of chilli pepper. Capsaicin activates afferents involved in nociceptive transmission and neurogenic inflammation. Such activation is rapidly followed by desensitization, with loss of sensitivity to heat and chemical stimulation, and inability to release substance P and CGRP.

Capsaicin effects are mediated by the vanilloid receptors, which are coupled to Na^+ and Ca^{2+} channels preferentially (Watling, 2001). Thus far, only the VR_1 ($TRPV_1$) receptor has been cloned. A single endogenous vanilloid ligand is still elusive but noxious heat, hydrogen ions, and anandamide (endogenous cannabinoid) all activate the receptor. Interestingly, anandamide presynaptically inhibits the release of CGRP (Akerman et al., 2004).

Civamide, the *cis*-monomer of capsaicin, is a vanilloid receptor agonist and a neuronal calcium channel blocker. A non-placebo-controlled study of 34 patients with moderate to severe migraine with or without aura showed that intranasal civamide provided headache relief in 55% of patients at 2 h (Diamond et al., 2000). Adverse effects associated with civamide administration were largely local as $\geq$90% of patients experienced nasal burning and over 40% experienced lacrimation, which would question the effectiveness of blinding the experiment.

Miscellaneous acute therapy

Magnesium

Magnesium plays a key role in many physiological functions that have relevance to migraine mechanisms, including gating of the NMDA receptors and increasing the efficiency of the Na/K ATPase pump. Magnesium has been included in intravenous cocktails for abortive migraine therapy and has been effective in aborting all symptoms of migraine with aura but not the pain of migraine without aura (Bigal et al., 2002). However, the results of a more recent RCT indicated that intravenous magnesium was no better than placebo in relieving acute migraine (Cete et al., 2005). It is of note that the study also did not demonstrate any benefit from metoclopramide, which is an established intravenous therapy for acute migraine. Thus, the validity of the study is questionable when the positive control fails to separate from placebo.

Somatostatin receptor agonists

The 14-amino-acid peptide somatostatin inhibits the release of CGRP and other vasoactive peptides (Helyes et al., 2001). Also, somatostatin-positive neurons are distributed in nervous system regions that participate in head and neck nociception, such as TNC and the periaqueductal gray (Schindler et al., 1998). Five somatostatin receptors (sst1–5) have been cloned (Hoyer et al., 1995), with octreotide acting predominantly on sst2 and sst5 (Patel and Srikant, 1994).

Early small trials of somatostatin in migraine suggested benefit (Sicuteri et al., 1984). More recently, the somatostatin analogue octreotide was tested in migraineurs using a cross-over randomized controlled design, and found not to be superior to placebo when given as a 100-μg subcutaneous dose (Levy et al., 2005). In contrast, the same subcutaneously administered dose was modestly superior to placebo in relieving the pain of cluster headache in another cross-over RCT (Matharu et al., 2004). These data cast doubt on somatostatin modulation as a target for acute migraine, but provide a positive signal for cluster headache.

Summation and practical considerations in acute treatment

The goals of acute migraine therapy are many, but the primary one is interruption of the migraine attack itself. Attacks of migraine may very considerably within the same individual and the history establishing the various patterns of migraine attacks is critical is designing an effective treatment plan. Triptans have become established as drugs of first choice. Table 26.2 shows drugs available for acute treatment.

Compliance with acute therapy in migraine treatment is often related to confidence in the diagnosis. Patients who have a clear understanding of their attacks and why specific acute medications are chosen for them are more likely to be compliant with treatment regimens. It is important to remember that most patients with migraine have self-treated with acute "off-the-shelf" medications available to them before seeking medical attention for their migraine attacks.

The history of an individual's migraine attacks should question the presence of prodrome, aura, the sequence of events in severe attacks, with specific questions about quality and intensity of the pain at

Table 26.2

Current acute migraine pharmacotherapy. List of non-parenteral (oral and nasal) therapies with at least one randomized controlled trial demonstrating efficacy of the active compound versus either placebo or another comparator. Doses are those that have demonstrated efficacy in clinical trials

Drug class/mechanism	Drug/compound	Daily dose range (mg)
Analgesic	Acetaminophen	1000
Simple	AAC*	600 + 400 + 200
Compound	Acetaminophen + codeine	(250–500) + 30
	Isometheptane + dichloralphenazone + acetaminophen	(65–130) + (100–200) + (325–650)
Ergots	DHE intranasal	2–4
	Ergotamine	1–6
NSAIDs	Aspirin	650–1000
	Diclofenac	50–100
	Flurbiprofen	100
	Ibuprofen	400–1200
	Ketoprofen	75–150
	Mefenamic acid	500
	Naproxen	750–825
	Rofecoxib	25–50
	Tolfenamic acid*	200
Triptans	Almotriptan	6.25–12.5
	Eletriptan	40–80
	Frovatriptan	2.5–5.0
	Naratriptan	1.0–2.5
	Rizatriptan	5–10
	Sumatriptan	25–100
	Zolmitriptan	2.5–5.0

*Not available in the USA.
NSAIDs: non-steroidal anti-inflammatory drugs; AAC: aspirin–acetaminophen–caffeine; DHE: dihydroergotamine.

onset along with escalation of pain and onset of nausea and vomiting. The history should establish differences between severity of attacks, including lack of awareness of escalation during sleep prompting severe early-morning attacks, or attacks worse under changes in hormonal status. The abortive or acute therapy should be chosen on the basis of these features. For example, early-onset vomiting would preclude oral acute medication, and intense early migraine symptoms argue for rapid-onset migraine-specific therapies.

Stratification of treatment for acute attacks should be aimed at achieving pain-free status within 2 h, and should optimally achieve migraine-free status when possible. Setting treatment goals for acute therapy should be done at the time of each patient visit, and headache calendars are essential in this process. Optimal acute treatment should be aimed at stopping the migraine attack as quickly as possible and for an individual patient more than one acute treatment regimen may be needed. Without specific goals and ways to measure acute treatment outcomes, patients may be at risk for prolonged attacks, simply on the basis of undertreatment, even with acute migraine-specific medication. Patients who wait to treat are known to be less likely to achieve pain freedom, even with the migraine-specific triptans, and may be more likely to suffer recurrence, prompting them to overuse acute medications in repeated attempts to abort the migraine attack. In patients with frequent attacks of migraine, this lack of a migraine-free response may lead to medication overuse headache. Asking the patient to describe the various patterns of attack also allows for the selection of specific formulations aimed at achieving a migraine-free state more quickly. If the escalation of headache pain is very rapid or if early onset of nausea or vomiting occurs, then injectable or nasal spray formulations are more appropriate than oral formulations. An important consideration in measuring any acute treatment should be disability from an attack.

References

Afra J, Mascia A, Gerard P et al. (1998). Interictal cortical excitability in migraine: a study using transcranial magnetic stimulation of motor and visual cortices. Ann Neurol 44: 209–215.

Ahn AH, Fields HL, Basbaum AI (2004). The triptan receptor 5HT1D is dynamically regulated in the central terminal of primary afferents in models of pain. Neurology 62: A440–444.

Akerman S, Goadsby PJ (2005). The role of dopamine in a model of trigeminovascular nociception. J Pharmacol Exp Ther 314: 162–169.

Akerman S, Kaube H, Goadsby PJ (2004). Anandamide is able to inhibit trigeminal neurons using an in vivo model of trigeminovascular-mediated nociception. J Pharmacol Exp Ther 309: 56–63.

Alam Z, Coombes N, Waring RH et al. (1998). Plasma levels of neuroexcitatory amino acids in patients with migraine or tension headache. J Neurol Sci 156: 102–106.

Arulmani U, Heiligers JP, Centurion D et al. (2005). Lack of effect of the adenosine A1 receptor agonist, GR79236, on capsaicin-induced CGRP release in anaesthetized pigs. Cephalalgia 25: 1082–1090.

Bigal ME, Bordini CA, Tepper SJ et al. (2002). Intravenous magnesium sulphate in the acute treatment of migraine without aura and migraine with aura. A randomized, double-blind, placebo-controlled study. Cephalalgia 22: 345–353.

Bland-Ward PA, Feniuk W, Humphrey PPA (2000). The adenosine A1 receptor agonist GR79236 inhibits evoked firing of trigeminal nucleus caudalis (TNC) neurons in the rat (Abstract). Cephalalgia 20: 271.

Boska MD, Welch KM, Barker PB et al. (2002). Contrasts in cortical magnesium, phospholipid and energy metabolism between migraine syndromes. Neurology 58 (8): 1227–1233.

Bowyer SM, Aurora SK, Moran JE et al. (2001). Magnetoencephalographic fields from patients with spontaneous and induced migraine aura. Ann Neurol 50 (5): 582–587.

Brandes JL, Kudrow D, Stark SR et al. (2007). Sumatriptan-naproxen for acute treatment of migraine: a randomized trial. JAMA 297 (13): 1443–1454.

Buchan P, Keywood C, Wade A et al. (2002). Clinical pharmacokinetics of frovatriptan. Headache 42 (Suppl. 2): S54–S62.

Buchanan TM, Ramadan NM (2006). Prophylactic pharmacotherapy for migraine headaches. Semin Neurol 26 (2): 188–198.

Burstein R, Yarnitsky D, Goor-Aryeh I et al. (2000). An association between migraine and cutaneous allodynia. Ann Neurol 47: 614–624.

Burstein R, Collins D, Yakubowski M (2004). Defeating migraine pain with triptan: a race against the development of cutaneous allodynia. Ann Neurol 55 (1): 19–26.

Cady RK, Lipton RB, Hall C et al. (2000). Treatment of mild headache in disabled migraine sufferers: results of the Spectrum Study. Headache 40 (10): 792–797.

Cananzi AR, D'Andrea G, Perini F et al. (1995). Platelet and plasma levels of glutamate and glutamine in migraine with and without aura. Cephalalgia 15: 132–135.

Cerbo R, Barbanti P, Buzzi MG et al. (1997). Dopamine hypersensitivity in migraine: role of the apomorphine test. Clin Neuropharmacol 20: 36–41.

Cete Y, Dora B, Ertan C et al. (2005). A randomized prospective placebo-controlled study of intravenous magnesium sulphate vs. Metoclopramide in the management of acute migraine attacks in the Emergency Department. Cephalalgia 25: 199–204.

Classey JD, Knight YE, Goadsby PJ (2001). The NMDA receptor antagonist MK-801 reduces Fos-like immunoreactivity within the trigeminocervical complex following superior sagittal sinus stimulation in the cat. Brain Res 907: 117–124.

Cutrer FM, Moskowitz MA (1996). The actions of valproate and neurosteroids in a model of trigeminal pain. Headache 36: 579–585.

Cutrer FM, Yu XJ, Ayata G et al. (1999). Effects of PNU-109,291, a selective 5-HT1D receptor agonist, on electrically induced dural plasma extravasation and capsaicin-evoked c-fos immunoreactivity within trigeminal nucleus caudalis. Neuropharmacology 38: 1043–1053.

De Fusco M, Marconi R, Silvestri L et al. (2003). Haploinsufficiency of ATP1A2 encoding the Na^+/K^+ pump alpha2 subunit associated with familial hemiplegic migraine type 2. Nat Genet 33 (2): 192–196.

Del Zompo M (2000). Dopaminergic hypersensitivity in migraine: clinical and genetic evidence. Funct Neurol 15 (Suppl. 3): 163–170.

Diamond S, Freitag F, Phillips S et al. (2000). Intranasal civamide for the acute treatment of migraine headache. Cephalalgia 20: 597–602.

Dodick DW (2004). Triptans and chest symptoms: the role of pulmonary vasoconstriction. Cephalalgia 24: 298–304.

Edvinsson L (2003). New therapeutic target in primary headaches – blocking the CGRP receptor. Expert Opin Ther Targets 7: 377–383.

Edvinsson L, Brodin E, Jansen I et al. (1988). Neurokinin A in cerebral vessels: characterization, localization and effects in vitro. Regul Pept 20: 181–197.

Edvinsson L, Mulder H, Goadsby PJ et al. (1998). Calcitonin gene-related peptide and nitric oxide in the trigeminal ganglion: cerebral vasodilatation from trigeminal nerve stimulation involves mainly calcitonin gene-related peptide. J Auton Nerv Syst 70: 15–22.

Feindel W, Penfield W, McNaughton F (1960). The tentorial nerves and localization of intracranial pain in man. Neurology 10: 555–563.

Ferrari MD (1998). Migraine. Lancet 351: 1043–1051.

Ferrari MD, Odink J, Bos KD et al. (1990). Neuroexcitatory plasma amino acids are elevated in migraine. Neurology 40: 1582–1586.

Ferrari MD, Roon KI, Lipton RB et al. (2001). Oral triptans (serotonin 5-HT agonists) in acute migraine treatment. Lancet 358: 1668–1675.

Freitag FG (2003). Divalproex in the treatment of migraine. Psychopharmacol Bull 37 (Suppl. 2): 98–115.

Gallai V, Sarchielli P, Floridi A et al. (1995). Vasoactive peptides levels in the plasma of young migraine patients with and without aura assessed both interictally and ictally. Cephalalgia 15: 384–390.

Goadsby PJ, Classey JD (2000). Glutamatergic transmission in the trigeminal nucleus assessed with local blood flow. Brain Res 875: 119–124.

Goadsby PJ, Hoskin KL (1997). The distribution of trigeminovascular afferents in the non-human primate brain *Macaca nemestrina*: a c-fos immunocytochemical study. J Anat 190: 367–375.

Goadsby PJ, Edvinsson L, Ekman R (1988). Release of vasoactive peptides in the extracerebral circulation of man and the cat during activation of the trigeminovascular system. Ann Neurol 23: 193–196.

Goadsby PJ, Hoskin KL, Storer RJ et al. (2002). Adenosine (A1) receptor agonists inhibit trigeminovascular nociceptive transmission. Brain 125: 1392–1401.

Goldstein DJ, Roon KI, Offen WW et al. (2001). Selective serotonin 1F (5HT(1F)) receptor agonist LY334370 for acute migraine: a randomized controlled trial. Lancet 358: 1230–1234.

Gomez-Mancilla B, Cutler NR, Leibowitz MT et al. (2001). Safety and efficacy of PNU-142633, a selective 5-HT_{1D} agonist, in patients with acute migraine. Cephalalgia 21: 727–732.

Hamel E, Saxena PR (2006). 5-Hydroxytryptamine involvement in migraine. In: J Olesen, PJ Goadsby, NM Ramadan et al. (Eds.), The Headaches. 3rd edn. Lippincott Williams & Wilkins, Philadelphia, pp. 275–280.

Helyes Z, Pinter E, Nemeth J et al. (2001). Anti-inflammatory effect of synthetic somatostatin analogues in the rat. Br J Pharmacol 134: 1571–1579.

Hjorth-Lassen L, Klingenberg Iversen H, Olesen J (2003). A dose–response study of nitric oxide synthase inhibition in different vascular beds in man. Eur J Clin Pharmacol 59: 499–505.

Ho TW, Mannix LK, Fan X et al. (2008). Randomized controlled trial of an oral CGRP receptor antaganist, MK-0974, in acute treatment of migraine. 70 (16): 1304–1312.

Hoyer D, Bell GI, Berelowitz M et al. (1995). Classification and nomenclature of somatostatin receptors. Trends Pharmacol Sci 16: 86–88.

Hu XH, Raskin NH, Cowan R et al. (2002). Treatment of migraine with rizatriptan: when to take the medication. Headache 42: 16–20.

Humphrey PP, Feniuk W (1991). Mode of action of the anti-migraine drug sumatriptan. Trends Pharmacol Sci 2: 444–446.

Jansen-Olesen I, Jorgensen L, Engel U et al. (2003). In-depth characterization of CGRP receptors in human intracranial arteries. Eur J Pharmacol 481: 207–216.

Jen JC, Wan J, Palos TP et al. (2005). Mutation in the glutamate transporter EAAT1 causes episodic ataxia, hemiplegia, and seizures. Neurology 65: 529–534.

Kaube H, Hoskin KL, Goadsby PJ (1993). Sumatriptan inhibits central trigeminal neurons only after blood–brain barrier disruption. Br J Pharmacol 109: 788–792.

Kaube H, Herzog J, Kaufer T et al. (2000a). Aura in some patients with familial hemiplegic migraine can be stopped by intranasal ketamine. Neurology 55: 139–141.

Kaube H, Katsarava Z, Kaufer T et al. (2000b). A new method to increase the nociception specificity of the human blink reflex. Clin Neurophysiol 111: 413–416.

Kaube H, Katsarava Z, Przywara S et al. (2002). Acute migraine headache: possible sensitization of neurons in the spinal trigeminal nucleus? Neurology 58 (8): 1234–1238.

Keam SJ, Goa KL, Figgitt DP (2002). Spotlight on almotriptan in migraine. CNS Drugs 16 (7): 501–507.

Klassen A, Elkind A, Asgharnejad M et al. (1997). Naratriptan is effective and well tolerated in the acute treatment of migraine. Results of a double-blind placebo-controlled, parallel group study. Naratriptan S2WA3001 study group. Headache 37 (10): 640–645.

Lange R, Schwarz JA, Hohn M (2000). Acetylsalicylic acid effervescent 1000 mg (aspirin) in acute migraine attacks; a multicentre, randomized, double-blind, single-dose, placebo-controlled parallel group study. Cephalalgia 20 (7): 663–667.

Lassen LH, Ashina M, Christiansen I et al. (1998a). Nitric oxide synthase inhibition: a new principle in the treatment of migraine attacks. Cephalalgia 18: 27–32.

Lassen LH, Jacobsen VB, Petersen P et al. (1998b). Human calcitonin gene-related peptide (hCGRP)-induced headache in migraineurs. Eur J Neurol 5 (Suppl. 3): S63, 28.

Lassen LH, Haderslev PA, Jacobsen VB et al. (2002). CGRP may play a causative role in migraine. Cephalalgia 22: 54–61.

Levy MJ, Matharu MS, Bhola R et al. (2005). Octreotide is not effective in the acute treatment of migraine. Cephalalgia 25: 48–55.

Linder SL, Mathew NT, Cady RK et al. (2008). Efficacy and tolerability of almotriptan in adolescents: a randomized, double-blind, placebo-controlled trial. Headache 48 (9): 1326–1336.

Lipton RB, Silberstein S (2001). The role of headache-related disability in migraine management: implications for headache treatment guidelines. Neurology 56 (Suppl. 1): S35–S42.

Lipton RB, Stewart WF (1997). Clinical application of zolmitriptan (311C90). Cephalalgia 17 (18): 53–59.

Lipton RB, Stewart WF, Stone AM et al. (2000). Disability in Strategies of Care Study Group. Stratified care vs. step care strategies for migraine: the Disability in Strategies of Care (DISC) Study: a randomized trial. JAMA 284: 2599–2605.

Liu-Chen L-Y, Gillespie SA, Norregaard TV et al. (1984). Co-localization of retrogradely transported wheat germ agglutinin and the putative neurotransmitter substance P within trigeminal ganglion cells projecting to cat middle cerebral. J Comp Neurol 225: 187–192.

Longmore J, Dowson AJ, Hill RG (1999). Advances in migraine therapy – 5-HT receptor subtype-specific agonist drugs. Curr Opin CPNS Invest Drug 1: 39–53.

Ma QP (2001). Co-localization of 5-HT (1B/1D/1F) receptors and glutamate in trigeminal ganglia in rats. Neuroreport 12: 1589–1591.

Matharu MS, Levy MJ, Meeran K et al. (2004). Subcutaneous octreotide in cluster headache-randomized placebo-controlled double-blind cross-over study. Ann Neurol 56: 488–494.

McCulloch J, Uddman R, Kingman TA et al. (1986). Calcitonin gene-related peptide: functional role in cerebro-vascular regulation. Proc Natl Acad Sci U S A 83: 5731–5735.

McNeely W, Goa KL (1999). Diclofenac-potassium in migraine: a review. Drugs 57 (6): 991–1003.

Mitsikostas DD, Sanchez del Rio M, Waeber C et al. (1998). The NMDA receptor antagonist MK-801 reduces capsaicin-induced *c-fos* expression within rat trigeminal nucleus caudalis. Pain 76: 239–248.

Mitsikostas DD, Sanchez del Rio M, Waeber C et al. (1999). Non-NMDA glutamate receptors modulate capsaicin induced c-fos expression within trigeminal nucleus caudalis. Br J Pharmacol 127: 623–630.

Moskowitz MA (1990). (1990). Basic mechanisms in vascular headache. Neurol Clin 8: 801–815.

Nozaki K, Moskowitz MA, Boccalini P (1992). CP-93, 129, sumatriptan, dihydroergotamine block c-fos expression within the rat trigeminal nucleus caudalis caused by chemical stimulation of the meninges. Br J Pharmacol 106: 409–415.

Olesen J, Iverson HK, Thomsen LL (1993). Nitric oxide supersensitivity. A possible molecular mechanism of migraine pain. Neuroreport 4: 1027–1030.

Olesen J, Diener HC, Husstedt IW et al. (2004). Calcitonin gene-related peptide receptor antagonist BIBN 4096 BS for the acute treatment of migraine. N Engl J Med 350: 1104–1110.

Ophoff RA, Terwindt GM, Vergouwe MN et al. (1996). Familial hemiplegic migraine and episodic ataxia type-2 are caused by mutations in the Ca^{2+} channel gene CACNLA4. Cell 87: 543–552.

Pascual J, Cabarrocas X (2002). Within-patient early versus delayed treatment of migraine attacks with almotriptan: the sooner the better. Headache 42 (1): 28–31.

Patel YC, Srikant CB (1994). Subtype selectivity of peptide analogs for all five cloned human somatostatin receptors (hsstr 1–5). Endocrinology 135: 2814–2817.

Peroutka SJ (1997). Dopamine and migraine. Neurology 49: 650–656.

Peroutka SJ (2005). Neurogenic inflammation and migraine: implications for the therapeutics. Mol Intervent 304–311.

Petersen KA, Birk S, Doods H et al. (2004). Inhibitory effect of BIBN4096BS on cephalic vasodilatation induced by CGRP or transcranial electrical stimulation in the rat. Br J Pharmacol 143: 697–704.

Potrebic S, Ahn AH, Skinner K et al. (2003). Peptidergic nociceptors of both trigeminal and dorsal root ganglia express serotonin 1D receptors: implications for the selective antimigraine action of triptans. J Neurosci 23: 10988–10997.

Pregenzer JF, Alberts GL, Im WB et al. (1999). Differential pharmacology between the guinea-pig and the gorilla 5-HT1D receptor as probed with isochromans (5-HT1D-selective ligands). Br J Pharmacol 127: 468–472.

Quartu M, Serra MP, Ambu R et al. (2002). AMPA-type glutamate receptor subunits 2/3 in the human trigeminal sensory ganglion and subnucleus caudalis from prenatal ages to adulthood. Mech Ageing Dev 123: 463–471.

Ramadan NM (2003). The link between glutamate and migraine. CNS Spectr 8: 446–449.

Ramadan NM, Skljarevski V, Phebus LA et al. (2003). 5-HT_{1F} receptor agonists in acute migraine treatment: a hypothesis. Cephalalgia 23: 776–785.

Raskin NH (1986). Repetitive intravenous dihydroergotamine as therapy for intractable migraine. Neurology 36 (7): 995–997.

Read SJ, Smith MI, Hunter AJ et al. (1997). Enhanced nitric oxide release during cortical spreading depression following infusion of glyceryl trinitrate in the anaesthetized cat. Cephalalgia 17: 159–165.

Reuter U, Bolay H, Jansen-Olesen I et al. (2001). Delayed inflammation in rat meninges: implications for migraine pathophysiology. Brain 124: 2490–2502.

Roon KI, Olesen J, Diener HC et al. (2000). No acute antimigraine efficcy of CP-122, 288, a highly potent inhibitor of neurogenic inflammation: results of two randomized double-blind placebo-controlled clinical trials. Ann Neurol 47: 238–241.

Roy A, Brand NJ, Yacoub MH (2000). Expression of 5-hydroxytryptamine receptor subtype messenger RNA in interstitial cells from human heart valves. J Heart Valve Dis 9: 256–260.

Ryan RE Jr (2001). Patient treatment preferences and the 5HT 1B/1D agonists. Arch Intern Med 161 (21): 2545–2553.

Sahara Y, Noro N, Iida Y et al. (1997). Glutamate receptor subunits GluR5 and KA-2 are coexpressed in rat trigeminal ganglion neurons. J Neurosci 17: 6611–6620.

Sang CN, Hostetter MP, Gracely RH et al. (1998). AMPA/kainate antagonist LY293558 reduces capsaicin-evoked hyperalgesia but not pain in normal skin in humans. Anesthesiology 89: 1060–1067.

Sang CN, Ramadan NM, Wallihan RG et al. (2004). LY293558, a novel AMPA/GluR5 antagonist, is efficacious and well-tolerated in acute migraine. Cephalalgia 24: 596–602.

Sawynok J (1998). Adenosine receptor activation and nociception. Eur J Pharmacol 17: 1–11.

Saxena PR, Tfelt-Hansen P (2006). Triptans, 5-HT1B/1D receptor agonists in the acute treatment of migraines. In: J Olesen, PJ Goadsby, NM Ramadan et al. (Eds.), The Headaches. 3rd edn. Lippincott Williams & Wilkins, Philadelphia, pp. 469–503.

Schindler M, Holloway S, Hathway G et al. (1998). Identification of somatostatin sst2(a) receptor expressing neurones in central regions involved in nociception. Brain Res 798: 25–35.

Schindler M, Harris CA, Hayes B et al. (2001). Immunohistochemical localization of adenosine A1 receptors in human brain regions. Neurosci Lett 297: 211–215.

Shepheard S, Edvinsson L, Cumberbatch M et al. (1999). Possible antimigraine mechanisms of action of the 5HT1F receptor agonist LY334370. Cephalalgia 19: 851–858.

Sicuteri F, Geppetti P, Marabini S et al. (1984). Pain relief by somatostatin in attacks of cluster headache. Pain 18: 359–365.

Silberstein SD, Young WB, Mendizabal JE et al. (2003). Acute migraine treatment with droperidol: a randomized, double-blind, placebo-controlled trial. Neurology 60: 315–321.

Syrett N, Abu-Shakra S, Yates R (2003). Zolmitriptan nasal spray: advances in migraine treatment. Neurology 61 (8 Suppl. 4): S27–S30.

Takiya L, Piccininni LC, Kamath V (2006). Safety and efficacy of eletriptan in the treatment of acute migraine. Pharmacotherapy 26 (1): 115–128.

Tallaksen-Greene SJ, Young AB, Penney JB et al. (1992). Excitatory amino acid binding sites in the trigeminal principal sensory and spinal trigeminal nuclei of the rat. Neurosci Lett 141: 79–83.

Tanen DA, Miller S, French T et al. (2003). Intravenous sodium valproate versus prochlorperazine for the emergency department treatment of acute migraine headaches: a prospective, randomized, double-blind trial. Ann Emerg Med 41: 847–853.

Tassorelli C, Joseph SA, Buzzi MG et al. (1999). The effects on central nervous system of nitroglycerin-putative mechanism and mediators. Prog Neurobiol 57: 607–624.

The International 311C90 Long-term Study Group (1998). The long-term tolerability and efficacy of oral zolmitriptan (Zomig, 311C90) in the acute treatment of migraine: an international study. Headache 38 (3): 173–183.

Uddman R, Edvinsson L, Ekman R et al. (1985). Innervation of the feline cerebral vasculature by nerve fibers containing calcitonin gene-related peptide: trigeminal origin and co-existence with substance P. Neurosci Lett 62: 131–136.

Waeber C, Moskowitz MA (2005). Migraine as an inflammatory disorder. Neurology 64 (10 Suppl. 2): S9–S15.

Watling KJ (2001). Vanilloid receptors. In: KJ Watling (Ed.), The Sigma-RBI Handbook of Receptor Classification and Signal Transduction. Sigma-RBI, Natick, MA, pp. 143–144.

Wei EP, Moskowitz MA, Baccalini P et al. (1992). Calcitonin gene related peptide mediates nitroglycerin and sodium nitroprusside induced vasodilation in feline cerebral arteries. Circ Res 70: 1313–1319.

Weiller C, May A, Limmroth V et al. (1995). Brain stem activation in spontaneous human migraine attacks. Nat Med 1: 658–660.

Welch KMA (1993). Drug therapy of migraine. N Engl J Med 329 (20): 1476–1483.

Welch KMA (2003). Contemporary concepts of migraine pathogenesis. Neurology 61 (8 Suppl 4): S2–S8.

Welch KMA, Mathew NT, Stone P et al. (2000). Tolerability of sumatriptan: clinical trials and post-marketing experience. Cephalalgia 20 (8): 687–695.

Welch KMA, Nagesh V, Aurora SK et al. (2001). Periaqueductal gray matter dysfunction in migraine: cause or the burden of illness? Headache 4 (1): 629–637.

Wellington K, Plosker GL (2002). Rizatriptan: an update of its use in the management of migraine. Drugs 62 (10): 1539–1574.

Handbook of Clinical Neurology, Vol. 97 (3rd series)
Headache
G. Nappi and M.A. Moskowitz, Editors

Chapter 27

Migraine: preventive treatment

STEPHEN D. SILBERSTEIN*
Jefferson Headache Center, Philadelphia, PA, USA

INTRODUCTION

Migraine is a chronic neurological disease characterized by episodic attacks of headache and associated symptoms (Headache Classification Committee, 2004). Effective migraine treatment begins with making an accurate diagnosis, ruling out alternate causes, ordering appropriate studies, and addressing the headache's impact on the patient. The pharmacological treatment of migraine may be acute (abortive) or preventive (prophylactic), and patients with frequent, severe headaches often require both approaches.

Comorbidity is the presence of two or more disorders, the association of which is more likely than chance. Conditions that occur in migraineurs with a higher prevalence than coincidence include stroke, epilepsy, mitral valve prolapse, Raynaud's syndrome, and certain psychological disorders, which include depression, mania, anxiety, and panic (Table 27.1).

Preventive therapy is given, even in the absence of a headache, in an attempt to reduce the frequency, duration, or severity of attacks. Additional benefits include improving responsiveness to acute attack treatment, improving function, and reducing disability. Preventive treatment may also prevent episodic migraine's progression to chronic migraine and result in health-care cost reductions (Silberstein et al., 2003). The changes in health-care utilization occur at a variety of levels, beginning with a decrease in triptan use (Etemad et al., 2005).

Silberstein et al. (2003) found that adding migraine-preventive drug therapy to therapy that consisted of only an acute medication was effective in reducing resource consumption. During the second 6 months after the initial preventive medication, as compared with the 6 months preceding preventive therapy, migraine diagnosis-related office and other outpatient visits decreased by 51.1%, emergency department visits with a migraine diagnosis decreased 81.8%, computed tomography (CT) scans decreased 75.0%, magnetic resonance imaging (MRI) decreased 88.2%, and other migraine medication dispensements decreased 14.1% (Silberstein et al., 2003).

In another study, Silberstein et al. (2007a) evaluated the medical resource utilization and overall cost of care among patients treated with topiramate for migraine prevention in a commercially insured population that included 2645 plan members. Topiramate utilization was associated with significantly less triptan utilization. In postindex period 1, there was a 46% decrease in emergency department visits, a 39% decrease in diagnostic procedures (e.g., CT and MRI scans), and a 33% decrease in hospital admissions; physician office visits were unchanged. In postindex period 2, there was a 46% decrease in emergency department visits, a 72% decrease in diagnostic procedures, a 61% decrease in hospital admissions, and a 35% decrease in physician office visits (Silberstein et al., 2007a).

Preventive treatment can be pre-emptive, short-term (miniprophylaxis), or chronic.

- Pre-emptive treatment is used when there is a known headache trigger, such as exercise or sexual activity. Patients can be instructed to pretreat prior to the exposure or activity.
- Short-term prevention is used when patients are undergoing a time-limited exposure to a provoking factor, such as ascent to a high altitude or menstruation. These patients can be treated with daily medication just before and during the exposure (Silberstein et al., 1998).

The Revised United States Evidence-Based Guidelines for Migraine (Silberstein and Rosenberg, 2000; Silberstein

*Correspondence to: Stephen D. Silberstein, MD, Jefferson Headache Center, 111 South 11th Street, Suite 8130, Philadelphia, PA 19107, USA, Tel: 215.955.2072, Fax: 215.955.6682, E-mail: Stephen.Silberstein@Jefferson.edu

Table 27.1

Migraine comorbid disease

Cardiovascular	Psychiatric	Neurological	Gastrointestinal	Other
Hyper-/hypotension	Depression	Epilepsy	Irritable bowel syndrome	Asthma
Raynaud's	Mania	Essential tremor		Allergies
Mitral valve prolapse	Panic disorder	Positional vertigo		
Angina/myocardial infarction	Anxiety disorder	Restless legs syndrome		
Stroke				
Patent foramen ovale (migraine with aura)				

2010) and the European Guidelines (Evers et al., 2006) have established the circumstances that might warrant preventive treatment:

- Recurring migraine attacks that, in the patient's opinion, significantly interfere with his or her daily routines, despite appropriate acute treatment
- Frequent headaches ($\geq$4 attacks/month)
- Contraindication to, failure of, overuse of, or intolerance to acute therapies
- Patient preference
- Frequent, very long, or uncomfortable auras
- Presence of uncommon migraine conditions, including hemiplegic migraine, basilar migraine, migraine with prolonged aura, or migrainous infarction (to attempt to reduce neurological damage).

Prevention is not being utilized to the extent it should be; only 13% of all migraineurs currently use medication that can be used as preventive therapy to control their attacks (Lipton et al., 2005). According to the American Migraine Prevalence and Prevention Study, 38.8% of patients with migraine should be considered for (13.1%) or offered (25.7%) migraine-preventive therapy based on migraine frequency and disability associated with the headaches (Silberstein et al., 2005).

The major medication groups for preventive migraine treatment (Table 27.2) include β-adrenergic blockers, antidepressants, calcium channel antagonists, serotonin antagonists, anticonvulsants, non-steroidal anti-inflammatory drugs, and others (including riboflavin, minerals, and herbs). If preventive medication is indicated, the agent should be preferentially chosen from one of the first-line categories, based on the drug's side-effect profile and the patient's coexistent and comorbid conditions (Tfelt-Hansen and Lipton, 1993). The following principles will help increase the chance of success:

- Start the chosen drug at a low dose and increase it slowly until therapeutic effects develop, the ceiling dose for the chosen drug is reached, or side-effects become intolerable.

Table 27.2

Preventive prescription drugs

ACE inhibitors/angiotensins receptor antagonists
Anticonvulsants
Valproate, gabapentin, topiramate
Antidepressants
TCAs, SSRIs, SNRIs
β-Adrenergic blockers
Propranolol/nadolol/metoprolol/atenolol
Calcium channel antagonists
Verapamil/flunarizine
Neurotoxins
Serotonin antagonists
Methysergide/methergine
Others: NSAIDs, riboflavin, magnesium, feverfew, butterroot, neuroleptics

ACE: angiotensin-converting enzyme; TCAs: tricyclic antidepressants; SSRIs: selective serotonin reuptake inhibitors; SNRIs; selective serotonin and norepinephrine reuptake inhibitors; NSAIDs: non-selective anti-inflammatory drugs.

- Give each treatment an adequate trial. A full therapeutic trial may take 2–6 months.
- Avoid interfering, overused, and contraindicated drugs.
- Re-evaluate therapy: migraine headaches may improve independently of treatment; if the headaches are well controlled, slowly taper and, if possible, discontinue the drug.
- Be sure that a woman of child-bearing potential is aware of any potential risks and pick the medication that will have the least adverse effect on the fetus (Silberstein, 1997).
- To maximize compliance, involve patients in their care. Discuss the rationale for a particular treatment, when and how to use it, and what side-effects are likely. Address patient expectations. Set realistic goals.

- Set realistic expectations regarding adverse events. Most adverse events are self-limited and dose-dependent, and patients should be encouraged to tolerate the early adverse events that may develop when a new medication is started.
- Consider comorbidity, which is the presence of two or more disorders whose association is more likely than chance (Table 27.1).

MECHANISM OF ACTION OF PREVENTIVE MEDICATIONS

The migraine aura is probably due to cortical spreading depression (CSD). Spreading depression (SD) is characterized by a slowly spreading wave (at a rate of 2–3 mm/min) of neuronal and glial depolarization that lasts about 1 min (Gold et al., 1998; Bradley et al., 2001). SD develops within brain areas, such as the cerebral cortex, cerebellum, or hippocampus, after electrical or chemical stimulation. SD is associated with a marked decrease in neuronal membrane resistance, a massive increase in extracellular K^+ and neurotransmitters, and an increase in intracellular Na^+ and Ca^{2+}. The threshold for SD is believed to be reduced in patients with migraine; this has been shown to be true for familial hemiplegic migraine-1. How CSD is triggered in the human cortex during a migraine attack is uncertain (Dichgans et al., 2005).

Headache probably results from activation of meningeal and blood vessel nociceptors combined with a change in central pain modulation. Headache and its associated neurovascular changes are subserved by the trigeminal system. Trigeminal sensory neurons contain substance P, calcitonin gene-related peptide, and neurokinin A. Stimulation results in the release of substance P and calcitonin gene-related peptide from sensory C-fiber terminals and neurogenic inflammation. The neuropeptides interact with the blood vessel wall, producing dilation, plasma protein extravasation, and platelet activation (Dimitriadou et al., 1992). Neurogenic inflammation sensitizes nerve fibers (peripheral sensitization), which now respond to previously innocuous stimuli, such as blood vessel pulsations, causing, in part, the pain of migraine. Central sensitization (CS) of trigeminal nucleus caudalis neurons can also occur. CS may play a key role in maintaining the headache. Brainstem activation also occurs in migraine without aura, in part due to increased activity of the endogenous antinociceptive system. The migraine aura can trigger headache: SD activates trigeminovascular afferents. How does a headache begin in the absence of aura? SD may occur in silent areas of the cortex or the cerebellum. In addition, direct activation of the trigeminal nerve can occur. Stress can also activate meningeal plasma cells via a parasympathetic mechanism, leading to nociceptor activation (Kandere-Grzybowska et al., 2003).

Migraine may be a result of a change in pain and sensory input processing. The aura is triggered in the hypersensitive cortex (CSD). Headache is generated by central pain facilitation and neurogenic inflammation. CS can occur, in part mediated by supraspinal facilitation. Decreased antinociceptive system activity and increased peripheral input may be present.

Most migraine-preventive drugs were designed to treat other disorders. Serotonin (5-HT) antagonists were developed based on the pathophysiological concept that migraine is due to excess 5-HT. Antidepressants down regulate 5-HT_2 and β-adrenergic receptors. Anticonvulsant medications decrease glutamate and enhance $GABA_A$. Potential mechanisms of migraine-preventive medications include: raising the threshold to migraine activation by stabilizing a more reactive nervous system; enhancing antinociception; inhibiting SD; inhibiting peripheral and CS; blocking neurogenic inflammation; and modulating sympathetic, parasympathetic, or serotonergic tone. Oshinsky and Luo (2006) have shown that descending control from the upper brainstem, through serotonergic and noradrenergic systems, modulates the trigeminal nucleus caudalis and prevents CS. Moskowitz has shown that preventive medications given chronically, but not acutely, block CSD (Silberstein, 2004). Chronic daily administration of migraine-preventive drugs (topiramate, valproate, propranolol, amitriptyline, and methysergide) dose-dependently suppressed CSD frequency by 40–80% and increased the cathodal stimulation threshold, whereas acute treatment was ineffective. Longer treatment durations produced stronger CSD suppression. Chronic D-propranolol (the inactive enantiomer of propranolol) treatment did not differ from saline control. Assessing the CSD threshold may prove useful for developing new preventive drugs and improving upon existing ones (Ayata et al., 2006).

ANTIDEPRESSANTS

Antidepressants consist of a number of different classes of drugs with different mechanisms of action:

1. Monoamine oxidase inhibitors (MAOIs)
   (a) Selective and reversible
   (b) Non-selective and irreversible
2. Monoamine reuptake inhibitors
   (a) Non-selective tricyclic antidepressants (TCAs)
   (b) Selective serotonin reuptake inhibitors (SSRIs)
   (c) Selective serotonin and norepinephrine reuptake inhibitors (SNRIs)

3. Monoamine receptor-targeted drugs
   (a) Serotonin (trazodone)
   (b) Norepinephrine α_2-antagonist (mirtazepine)
   (c) Dopamine (bupropion).

The mechanism by which antidepressants work to prevent headache is uncertain, but it does not result from treating masked depression. Antidepressants are useful in treating many chronic pain states, including headache, independent of the presence of depression, and the response occurs sooner than the expected antidepressant effect (Couch et al., 1976; Kishore-Kumar et al., 1990; Panerai et al., 1990). In animal pain models, antidepressants potentiate the effects of coadministered opioids (Feinmann, 1985). The clinically effective antidepressants in headache prophylaxis either inhibit 5-HT reuptake or are antagonists at the 5-HT_2 receptors (Richelson, 1990).

Amitriptyline is the only antidepressant with fairly consistent support for efficacy in migraine prevention (Gray et al., 1999). Recently, Dodick and colleagues (2007) compared the relative efficacy and tolerability profiles of topiramate (100 mg/day) and amitriptyline (100 mg/day) as preventive treatment for migraine in a large, randomized, double-blind, parallel-treatment trial. Both treatments were associated with a lower mean monthly attack frequency, although treatment with topiramate was associated with a significant improvement of daily activities in all three domains of the Migraine-Specific Quality-of-Life Questionnaire compared with amitriptyline (Dodick et al., 2007). These studies showed that amitriptyline is effective for migraine prevention (efficacious doses in clinical trials: 30–150 mg/day; Ramadan et al., 2000). Collectively, these studies confirm that amitriptyline is effective for migraine prevention.

Fluoxetine was significantly better than placebo in one (Adly et al., 1992) but not a second (Saper et al., 1994) migraine prevention trial. In a small, retrospective study, Adelman et al. (2000) reported that mean reduction in migraine fell from 16.1 to 11.1 headaches per month with venlafaxine treatment. Bulut and colleagues (2004) also assessed the relative efficacy of venlafaxine versus amitriptyline and found that the two agents were equally effective in reducing pain outcomes for migraine, but, based on study drop-out rates, venlafaxine may be better tolerated.

Anticholinergic symptoms were frequently reported with the TCAs studied (including amitriptyline). Adverse events were less common with SSRIs, with nausea and sexual dysfunction the most frequently observed symptoms (Gray et al., 1999).

The TCAs most commonly used for migraine (and tension-type) headache prevention include amitriptyline, nortriptyline, doxepin, and protriptyline. Imipramine and desipramine have been used at times. Most have not been vigorously evaluated; their use is based on anecdotal or uncontrolled reports.

Principles of antidepressant use

- The TCA dose range is wide and must be individualized.
- With the exception of protriptyline, TCAs are prone to causing sedation. Start with a low dose of the chosen TCA at bedtime, except when using protriptyline, which should be administered in the morning.
- If the TCA is too sedating, switch from a tertiary TCA (amitriptyline, doxepin) to a secondary TCA (nortriptyline, protriptyline). If a patient develops insomnia or nightmares, give the TCA in the morning.
- Bipolar patients who are depressed can become manic on antidepressants.

Adverse events are common with TCA use. The antimuscarinic adverse events are most common; they include dry mouth, a metallic taste, epigastric distress, constipation, dizziness, mental confusion, tachycardia, palpitations, blurred vision, and urinary retention. Antihistaminic activity may be responsible for carbohydrate cravings, which contribute to weight gain. Adrenergic activity is responsible for the orthostatic hypotension, reflex tachycardia, and palpitations that patients may experience. Any antidepressant treatment may change depression to hypomania or frank mania (particularly in bipolar patients). Ten percent of patients may develop tremors, and confusion or delirium may occur, particularly in older patients who are more vulnerable to the muscarinic adverse events. Antidepressant treatments may also reduce the seizure threshold, although this is not generally a problem in antimigraine treatment (Baldessarini, 1990). There are differences among the TCAs and properties that may be useful in selecting an agent and modifying drug regimens to reduce adverse effects.

Clinical use

See Table 27.3.

Tertiary amines

Amitriptyline (Elavil, Endep) is a tertiary amine tricyclic that is sedating. Patients with depression are more tolerant and require higher doses of amitriptyline than patients with migraine. Start at a dose of 10–25 mg at bedtime. The dose ranges from 10 to 400 mg a day.

Doxepin (Sinequan, Adapin) is a sedating tertiary amine TCA. Start at a dose of 10 mg at bedtime. The dose ranges from 10 to 300 mg a day.

Table 27.3

Antidepressants in the preventive treatment of migraine

Agent	Daily dose	Comment
Tertiary amines		
Amitriptyline	10–400 mg	Start at 10 mg at bedtime
Doxepin	10–300 mg	Start at 10 mg at bedtime
Secondary amines		
Nortriptyline	10–150 mg	Start at 10–25 mg at bedtime If insomnia, give early in the morning
Protriptyline	5–60 mg	Start at 10–25 mg in the morning
Selective serotonin reuptake inhibitors (SSRIs)		
Citalopram	10–80 mg	Evidence in the treatment of migraine is controversial
Escitalopram	10–20 mg	Some may worsen the migraine pattern
Fluoxetine tablets	10–80 mg	May be used as an adjuvant in the treatment of migraine and severe depression
Sertraline tablets	25–100 mg	
Paroxetine tablets	10–30 mg	
Selective serotonin and norepinephrine reuptake inhibitors (SNRIs)		
Venlafaxine tablets	37.5–300 mg	Some evidence in the treatment of migraine
Duloxetine	20–60 mg	
Other		
Mirtazapine tablets	15–45 mg	
Monoamine oxidase inhibitors		
Phenelzine	30–90 mg	Strict diet considerations

Secondary amines

Nortriptyline (Pamelor, Aventyl) is a secondary amine that is less sedating than amitriptyline. Nortriptyline is a major metabolite of amitriptyline. If insomnia develops, give the drug earlier in the day or in divided doses. Start at a dose of 10–25 mg at bedtime. The dose ranges from 10 to 150 mg a day.

Protriptyline (Vivactil) is a secondary amine similar to nortriptyline. Start at a dose of 5 mg a day in the morning. The dose ranges from 5 to 60 mg a day.

Selective serotonin reuptake inhibitors

Evidence for the use of SSRIs is poor. The combination of an SSRI and a TCA can be beneficial in treating refractory depression (Weilburg et al., 1989) and, in our experience, resistant cases of migraine. The combination may require dose adjustment of the TCA because levels may significantly increase.

Selective serotonin and norepinephrine reuptake inhibitors

Venlafaxine has been shown to be effective in a double-blind, placebo-controlled trial and a separate placebo and amitriptyline controlled trial (Bulut et al., 2004). The effective dose is 150 mg/day. Start with the extended-release tablet of 37.5 mg for 1 week, then 75 mg for 1 week, and then extended-release 150 mg in the morning. Side-effects include insomnia and nervousness, mydriasis, and seizures. As with the TCAs and SSRIs, weight gain may occur.

Duloxetine is available as 20-, 30-, or 60-mg capsules. The dose ranges from 20 to 60 mg/day. A 20-mg daily starting dose is begun and slowly titrated upwards.

Other antidepressants

Mirtazepine is an antagonist at central α_2-presynaptic norepinephrine receptor that results in increased norepinephrine and 5-HT action. In addition, it is a potent 5-HT_2 and 5-HT_3 receptor antagonist. The dose ranges from 15 to 45 mg at bedtime.

Other antidepressants can be tried in resistant cases, particularly those complicated by depression. Bupropion is useful for smoking cessation and neuropsychiatric comorbidity.

ANTIEPILEPTIC DRUGS

Antiepileptic drugs (Table 27.4) are increasingly recommended for migraine prevention because of placebo-controlled, double-blind trials that prove them effective. With the exception of valproic acid, phenobarbital, and topiramate (dose 200 mg/day), many anticonvulsants interfere with the efficacy of oral contraceptives (Coulam and Annagers, 1979; Hanston and Horn, 1985).

Table 27.4

Selected antiepileptic drugs in the preventive treatment of migraine

Agent	Daily dose	Comment
Carbamazepine	600–1200 mg	Three times daily
Gabapentin	600–2400 mg	Dose can be raised to 3000 mg
Lamotrigine	100–200 mg	Start at 25 mg Very slow titration May be effective in migraine with aura Discontinue if rash occurs
Topiramate	100–600 mg	Start at 15–25 mg at bedtime Increase by 15–25 mg/week Attempt to reach 50–100 mg Increase further if necessary Associated with weight loss
Valproate/ divalproex	500–1500 mg	Start at 250–500 mg/day Monitor levels if compliance is an issue Maximum dose is 60 mg/kg per day

Carbamazepine

There is insufficient evidence to demonstrate clearly carbamazepine is an effective migraine-preventive treatment (Gray et al., 1999).

In our experience, carbamazepine (Tegretol) 600–1200 mg/day (beginning at 100 mg twice a day) may be effective in the preventive treatment of migraine, particularly in patients who have coexisting mania or hypomania, especially if rapid cycling is present; however, monitoring of plasma levels and white blood cell count is essential.

Gabapentin

Gabapentin (600–1800 mg) was effective in episodic migraine and chronic migraine in a 12-week open-label study (Mathew, 1996). Gabapentin was not effective in one placebo-controlled, double-blind study (Wessely et al., 1987), but a more recent trial reported clinical efficacy for gabapentin in migraine prevention (Mathew et al., 1998). This randomized, placebo-controlled, double-blind trial showed that gabapentin 1800–2400 mg was superior to placebo in reducing the frequency of migraine attacks. The study involved 145 subjects (81% women) who experienced 3–8 migraine episodes a month and who had failed no more than two prophylactic antimigraine regimes. The responder rate was 36% for gabapentin and 14% for placebo ($P = 0.02$). The two treatment groups were comparable with respect to treatment-limiting adverse events. Limited data were reported on adverse events. The most common adverse events were dizziness or giddiness, and drowsiness. Relatively high patient withdrawal rates due to adverse events were reported in some trials (Gray et al., 1999).

Lamotrigine

Lamotrigine blocks voltage-sensitive sodium channels, leading to inhibition of neuronal release of glutamate, which is essential in the propagation of CSD. Lamotrigine was studied as combination therapy for headache prevention in one relatively large, prospective, open-label trial of 65 patients, most of whom had chronic migraine (Wheeler, 2001). Those who had migraine with aura had a better response rate (12/18 or 67%). Another open-label study assessed the impact of lamotrigine on aura itself, and found that the drug significantly reduced both the frequency and duration of aura (Wheeler, 2001). Chen et al. (2001) reported 2 patients with migraine with persistent, aura-like, visual phenomena for months to years. After 2 weeks of lamotrigine treatment, both patients had resolution of the visual symptoms.

Steiner et al. (1997) compared the safety and efficacy of lamotrigine (200 mg/day) and placebo in migraine prophylaxis in a double-blind, randomized, parallel-groups trial. Improvements were greater on placebo, and these changes, not statistically significant, indicate that lamotrigine was ineffective for migraine prophylaxis. There were more adverse events on lamotrigine than on placebo, most commonly rash. With slow dose escalation, their frequency was reduced and the rate of withdrawal for adverse events was similar in both treatment groups.

Despite lamotrigine's overall lack of efficacy in migraine headache prevention, it may have a special role in the treatment of migraine with aura.

Oxcarbazepine

Silberstein and colleagues (2008) evaluated the efficacy, safety, and tolerability of oxcarbazepine (1200 mg/day) versus placebo as preventive therapy for patients suffering from migraine headaches. Oxcarbazepine did not show efficacy in the prophylactic treatment of migraine headaches.

Topiramate

Topiramate is a derivative of the naturally occurring monosaccharide D-fructose and contains a sulfamate moiety. Topiramate was originally marketed for the treatment of epilepsy (Shank et al., 1994); it is now approved by the Food and Drug Administration (FDA) for migraine.

Storer and Goadsby (2003) studied the effect of topiramate on trigeminocervical activation in the anesthetized cat. Activation of neurons within the trigeminocervical complex is likely to be the biological substrate for pain in migraine and cluster headache. The superior sagittal sinus (SSS) was isolated and electrically stimulated. Units linked to SSS stimulation were recorded in the caudalmost part of the trigeminal nucleus. Topiramate reduced SSS-evoked firing of neurons in the trigeminocervical complex in a dose-dependent fashion. Its inhibition is a plausible mechanism of the action of migraine or cluster headache-preventive medicines.

Clinical profile

Two large, pivotal, multicenter, randomized, double-blind, placebo-controlled clinical trials assessed the efficacy and safety of topiramate (50, 100, and 200 mg/day) in migraine prevention. In the first pivotal placebo-controlled clinical trial of 487 patients, Silberstein et al. (2004) found that the responder rate (patients with $\geq$50% reduction in monthly migraine frequency) was 52% with topiramate 200 mg/day ($P < 0.001$), 54% with topiramate 100 mg ($P < 0.001$), 36% with topiramate 50 mg/day ($P = 0.039$), and 23% with placebo.

Topiramate treatment was also associated with reduced consumption of acute-treatment medications. The onset of efficacy was observed within the first week of treatment using the combined data from the primary efficacy trials (Freitag et al., 2007). The 200-mg dose was not significantly more effective than the 100-mg dose. However adverse events, including adverse events resulting in discontinuation from the study, were more common at the 200-mg dose. The most common adverse events were paresthesias, fatigue, nausea, anorexia, and abnormal taste. Body weight was reduced by an average of 3.8% in the 100- and 200-mg groups (Silberstein et al., 2004).

In the second (MIGR-002) pivotal trial (Brandes et al., 2004), significantly more patients exhibited at least a 50% reduction in mean monthly migraines in the groups treated with 50 mg/day of topiramate (39%, $P = 0.009$), 100 mg/day of topiramate (49%, $P = 0.001$), and 200 mg/day of topiramate (47%, $P = 0.001$).

A third (MIGR-003) randomized, double-blind, parallel-group, multicenter trial (Diener et al., 2004b) compared two doses of topiramate (100 or 200 mg/day) to placebo or propranolol (160 mg/day) in 575 subjects in 13 countries. Topiramate 100 mg/day was superior to placebo as measured by reduction in monthly migraine frequency, overall 50% responder rate (37%), reduction in monthly migraine days, and reduction in the rate of daily rescue medication use. Propranolol 160 mg/day and topiramate 100 mg/day were similar with respect to reductions in migraine frequency, responder rate (43%), migraine days, and daily rescue medication usage. Topiramate 100 mg and propranolol 160 mg had similar adverse events rates and both were better tolerated than topiramate 200 mg.

Safety and tolerability

Topiramate's most common adverse event is paresthesia, which, when bothersome, can be controlled with potassium supplementation (Silberstein, 2002). Other common adverse events were fatigue, decreased appetite, nausea, diarrhea, weight decrease, taste perversion, hypoesthesia, and abdominal pain. In the migraine trials, body weight was reduced by an average of 2.3% in the 50-mg group, 3.2% in the 100-mg group, and 3.8% in the 200-mg group. Patients on propranolol gained 2.3% of their baseline body weight.

The most common central nervous system (CNS) adverse events were somnolence, insomnia, difficulty with memory, language problems, difficulty with concentration, mood problems, and anxiety. Renal calculi can occur with topiramate use. The reported incidence is about 1.5%, representing a two- to fourfold increase over the estimated occurrence in the general population (Sachedo et al., 1997).

Patients receiving topiramate infrequently develop a syndrome consisting of acute myopia associated with secondary angle-closure glaucoma. Symptoms include the acute onset of decreased visual acuity and/or ocular pain. The primary treatment to reverse symptoms is to discontinue topiramate as rapidly as possible, according to the judgment of the treating physician. Other measures, in conjunction with discontinuation, may be helpful (Thomson Healthcare, 2003).

Oligohidrosis, infrequently resulting in hospitalization, has been reported in association with elevated body temperature. Some of the cases were reported after exposure to elevated environmental temperatures. Most of the reports have involved children.

Clinical usage

Topiramate is available as a 15-mg spansule and as 25-, 50-, 100-, and 200-mg tablets. Start at a dose of 15–25 mg at bedtime. Increase by 15–25 mg/week. Do not increase the dose if bothersome adverse events develop; wait until they resolve (they usually do). If they do not resolve, decrease the drug to the last tolerable dose, then increase by a lower dose more slowly. Attempt to reach a dose of 50 mg/day given twice a day. Patients who tolerate the lower doses with only partial improvement often have increased benefit with higher doses (600 mg/day or higher).

Valproic acid

Valproic acid possesses anticonvulsant activity in a wide variety of experimental epilepsy models. Valproate at high concentrations increases GABA levels in synaptosomes, perhaps by inhibiting its degradation; it enhances the postsynaptic response to GABA, and, at lower concentrations, it increases potassium conductance, producing neuronal hyperpolarization. Valproate turns off the firing of the 5-HT neurons of the dorsal raphe, which are implicated in controlling head pain.

Divalproex sodium and sodium valproate are effective for migraine prevention (Gray et al., 1999). Two placebo-controlled trials of each of these agents showed them to be significantly better than placebo at reducing headache frequency (Jensen et al., 1994; Mathew et al., 1995a; Klapper, 1997). One double-blind, randomized, controlled trial showed that extended-release divalproex sodium 500–1000 mg (once a day) significantly reduced the mean 4-week migraine headache rate versus placebo (Freitag et al., 2002).

Valproic acid is a simple 8-carbon, 2-chain fatty acid with 80% bioavailability after oral administration. It is highly protein-bound, with an elimination half-life of between 8 and 17 h.

Nausea, vomiting, and gastrointestinal distress are valproate's most common adverse events. These are generally self-limited and are slightly less common with divalproex sodium than with sodium valproate. When the therapy is continued, the incidence of gastrointestinal symptoms decreases, particularly after 6 months. Later, tremor and alopecia can occur. Valproate has little effect on cognitive function and it rarely causes sedation. On rare occasions, valproate administration is associated with severe adverse events, such as hepatitis or pancreatitis. The frequency varies with the number of concomitant medications used, the patient's age, the presence of genetic and metabolic disorders, and the patient's general state of health. These idiosyncratic reactions are unpredictable (Pellock and Willmore, 1991).

Valproate is potentially teratogenic and should not be used by pregnant women or women considering pregnancy (Silberstein, 1996). Hyperandrogenism, resulting from elevated testosterone levels, ovarian cysts, and obesity, is of particular concern in young women with epilepsy who use valproate (Vainionpaa et al., 1999).

Absolute contraindications to valproate are pregnancy and a history of pancreatitis or a hepatic disorder, such as chronic hepatitis or cirrhosis of the liver. Other important contraindications are hematological disorders, including thrombocytopenia, pancytopenia, and bleeding disorders.

Valproic acid is available as 250-mg capsules and as syrup (250 mg/5 ml). Divalproex sodium is a stable coordination complex comprising sodium valproate and valproic acid in a 1:1 molar ratio. An enteric-coated form of divalproex sodium is available as 125-, 250-, and 500-mg capsules and a sprinkle formulation. Start with 250–500 mg a day in divided doses and slowly increase the dose. The maximum recommended dose is 60 mg/kg/day. An extended-release form of divalproex sodium demonstrated comparable efficacy to the tablet formulation. The adverse events profile in the clinical trial, however, showed almost identical adverse events rates for the placebo and active treatment arms (Freitag et al., 2001).

BETA-ADRENERGIC BLOCKERS

Beta-blockers (Table 27.5) are approximately 50% effective in producing a >50% reduction in attack frequency. Rabkin et al. (1966) serendipitously discovered propranolol's effectiveness in headache treatment when patients being treated for angina experienced headache improvement (Weber and Reinmuth, 1972; Diamond and Medina, 1976).

Evidence consistently showed propranolol's efficacy in a daily dose of 120–240 mg for migraine prevention (Gray et al., 1999). The relative efficacy of the different beta-blockers has not been clearly established, and most studies show no significant difference between drugs.

Results from four trials comparing metoprolol with placebo reported mixed results (Gray et al., 1999). Direct comparisons of metoprolol with propranolol (Steardo et al., 1982; Andersson et al., 1983; Olsson et al., 1984;

Table 27.5

Beta-blockers in the preventive treatment of migraine

Agent	Daily dose	Comment
Atenolol	50–200 mg	Use four times daily Fewer side-effects than propranolol
Metoprolol	100–200 mg	Use the short-acting form twice daily Use the long-acting form four times daily
Nadolol	20–160 mg	Use four times daily Fewer side-effects than propranolol
Propranolol	40–400 mg	Use the short-acting form twice daily or three times daily Use the long-acting form four times daily or twice daily 1–2 mg/kg in children
Timolol	20–60 mg	Divide the dose Short half-life

Gerber et al., 1991), flunarizine (Grotemeyer et al., 1990; Sorensen et al., 1991), and pizotifen (Vilming et al., 1985) demonstrated few significant differences, suggesting that metoprolol is effective for migraine prevention. Timolol, atenolol, and nadolol are also likely to be beneficial based on comparisons with placebo or with propranolol (Gray et al., 1999). Beta-blockers with intrinsic sympathomimetic activity (acebutolol, alprenolol, oxprenolol, pindolol) have not been found to be effective for the prevention of migraine (Gray et al., 1999).

Three randomized, double-blind trials tested the efficacy of beta-blockers in migraine prevention (Rao et al., 2000; Diener et al., 2001, 2002). Diener and colleagues (2001) found that metoprolol (200 mg/day) was more effective than aspirin (300 mg/day) in achieving a 50% reduction in migraine frequency. Diener et al. (2002) reported that propranolol LA 120 mg/day was similar in efficacy to flunarizine 5 or 10 mg/day as measured by attack frequency and responder rates (reduction $\geq$50% in attack frequency from baseline). Rao and colleagues (2000) reported that propranolol (80 mg/day) was as effective as cyproheptadine (4 mg/day) in reducing migraine frequency and severity. The combination of cyproheptadine and propranolol was more effective than monotherapy.

The action of beta-blockers is most likely central and could be mediated by: (1) inhibition of central β-receptors that interfere with the vigilance-enhancing adrenergic pathway; (2) interaction with 5-HT receptors (but not all beta-blockers bind to the 5-HT receptors); and (3) cross-modulation of the serotonin system (Koella, 1985; Silberstein and Silberstein, 1990). Propranolol inhibits nitric oxide production by blocking inducible nitric oxide synthase (NOS). Propranolol also inhibits kainate-induced currents and is synergistic with *N*-methyl-D-aspartate blockers, which reduce neuronal activity and have membrane-stabilizing properties (Ramadan, 2004).

Beta-blockers that are clinically useful in the treatment of migraine consist of both the non-selective blocking agents (propranolol, nadolol, and timolol) and the selective β_1-blockers (metoprolol and atenolol).

All beta-blockers can produce behavioral adverse events, such as drowsiness, fatigue, lethargy, sleep disorders, nightmares, depression, memory disturbance, and hallucinations, indicating that they all affect the CNS. The central effect of beta-blockers is used to treat anxiety (Koella, 1985). Other common adverse events include nausea, dizziness, insomnia, and decreased exercise tolerance. These symptoms appear to be fairly well tolerated and were seldom the cause of premature withdrawal from trials (Gray et al., 1999). Common adverse events include gastrointestinal complaints. Less common are orthostatic hypotension, significant bradycardia, impotence, and aggravation of intrinsic muscle disease. Propranolol has been reported to have an adverse effect on the fetus (Featherstone, 1983). Severe congestive heart failure, asthma, and insulin-dependent diabetes are contraindications to the use of non-selective beta-blockers.

Treatment with beta-blockers must be individualized. It is best to taper beta-blockers slowly as stopping them abruptly can cause increased headache (Kangasniemi et al., 1987) and the withdrawal symptoms of tachycardia and tremulousness (Frishman, 1987).

Clinical use (Table 27.5)

Propranolol (Inderal; approved by the FDA for migraine) is a non-selective beta-blocker with a half-life of 4–6 hours, and is also available in an effective long-acting formulation (Inderal LA) (Diamond et al., 1987; Pradalier et al., 1989). The dose ranges from 40 to 400 mg a day, with no correlation between propranolol and 4-hydroxypropranolol plasma levels and headache relief (Cortelli et al., 1985). The short-acting form can be given three to four times a day, the long-acting form once or twice a day (we recommend twice a day). Start with 40 mg a day of propranolol (Inderal 60 LA) in divided doses and slowly increase to tolerance. An advantage of the regular propranolol is its greater dosing flexibility. The dose for children is 1–2 mg/kg a day.

Nadolol (Corgard) is a non-selective beta-blocker with a long half-life. It is less lipid-soluble than propranolol and has fewer CNS side-effects. The dose ranges from 20 to 160 mg a day given once daily or in split doses. Some authorities prefer it to propranolol since it has fewer side-effects (Sudilovsky et al., 1987).

Timolol (Blocadren; approved by the FDA for migraine) is a non-selective beta-blocker with a short half-life. The dose ranges from 20 to 60 mg a day in divided doses.

Atenolol (Tenormin) is a selective β_1-blocker with fewer side-effects than propranolol. The dose ranges from 50 to 200 mg a day once daily.

Metoprolol (Lopressor) is a selective β_1-blocker with a short half-life. The dose ranges from 100 to 200 mg a day in divided doses. The long-acting preparation may be given once a day.

CALCIUM CHANNEL ANTAGONISTS

The mechanism of action of the calcium channel antagonists (Table 27.6) in migraine prevention is uncertain. They were introduced into the treatment of migraine on the assumption that they prevent hypoxia of cerebral neurons, contraction of vascular smooth muscles, and inhibition of the Ca^{2+}-dependent enzymes

Table 27.6

Selected calcium channel blockers in the preventive treatment of migraine

Agent	Daily dose	Comment
Verapamil	120–640 mg	Start 80 mg twice daily or three times daily Sustained release can be given four times daily or twice daily
Flunarizine	5–10 mg	Give at bedtime Weight gain is the most common adverse effect

that are involved in prostaglandin formation. Perhaps it is their ability to block 5-HT release, interfere with neurovascular inflammation, or interfere with the initiation and propagation of spreading depression that is critical (Wauquier et al., 1985). The discovery that an abnormality in an α_{1A} subunit (P/Q channel) can produce familial hemiplegic migraine (Ophoff et al., 1996) has led to a search for more fundamental associations.

The Agency for Health Care Policy and Research (AHCPR) technical report identified 45 controlled trials of calcium antagonists, including flunarizine (25 trials), nimodipine (11 trials), nifedipine (five trials), verapamil (three trials), cyclandelate (three trials), and nicardipine (one trial) (Gray et al., 1999). A meta-analysis of these seven heterogeneous trials was statistically significant in favor of flunarizine (Gray et al., 1999).

Nimodipine had mixed results in placebo-controlled trials. Three placebo-controlled studies suggested no significant differences (Ansell et al., 1988; Migraine-Nimodipine European Study Group (MINES), 1989), while two reported relatively large and statistically significant differences in favor of nimodipine (Gelmers, 1983; Ansell et al., 1988).

The evidence for nifedipine was difficult to interpret. Two comparisons with placebo yielded similar effect sizes that were statistically insignificant, but the 95% confidence intervals associated with these estimates were large and did not exclude either a clinically important benefit or harm associated with nifedipine (McArthur et al., 1989; Shukla et al., 1995). Similarly ambiguous results were reported in one comparison with flunarizine (Lamsudin and Sadjimin, 1993) and in two comparisons with propranolol (Albers et al., 1989; Gerber et al., 1991). One trial found that metoprolol was significantly better than nifedipine at reducing headache frequency (Gerber et al., 1991).

Verapamil was more effective than placebo in two of three trials, but both positive trials had high dropout rates, rendering the findings uncertain (Markley et al., 1984; Solomon, 1986). The single negative placebo-controlled trial that included a propranolol treatment arm reported no significant difference between verapamil, propranolol, and placebo (Solomon, 1986). The efficacy of nicardipine is supported by a single comparison with placebo in 30 patients with migraine with aura (Leandri et al., 1990). Diltiazem (60–90 mg four times a day) was effective in two small open studies (Riopelle and McCans, 1982; Smith and Schwartz, 1984).

Adverse events of the Ca^{2+} antagonists depend on the drug, and include dizziness and headache (particularly with nifedipine), depression, vasomotor changes, tremor, gastrointestinal complaints (including constipation), peripheral edema, orthostatic hypotension, and bradycardia. Adverse events most commonly associated with flunarizine were sedation, weight gain, and abdominal pain. Symptoms reported with other calcium channel antagonists included dizziness, edema, flushing, and constipation. Adverse events associated with nifedipine use were frequent (54%) and included dizziness, edema, flushing, headache, and mental symptoms (McArthur et al., 1989).

Clinical use (Table 27.6)

Verapamil (Calan, Isoptin) is available as a 40-, 80-, or 120-mg tablet or as a 120-, 180-, or 240-mg sustained-release preparation. Start at a dose of 80 mg two to three times a day, increasing to 480 mg a day (or more) in divided doses. The sustained-release preparation of verapamil can be given once or twice a day, but unreliable absorption reduces reliability. The most common adverse event is constipation; dizziness, nausea, hypotension, headache, and edema are less common.

Diltiazem (Cardizem) is available in 30-, 60-, 90-, and 120-mg tablets. Start at a dose of 30 mg two to three times a day, with a maximal dose of 360 mg a day in divided doses. Adverse events are infrequent: hypotension, arteriovenous block, and headaches are occasionally seen. Bioavailability is 50%; the drug is tightly protein-bound.

Nifedipine (Procardia) is available in 10- or 20-mg capsules. Start at a dose of 10 mg a day. This can be increased to a maximum of 120 mg a day in divided doses. Adverse events are common and include hypotension, headache, nausea, and vomiting. Bioavailability is 50%; almost all the drug is protein-bound.

Nimodipine (Nimotop) is available in 30-mg capsules. The dose is 30–60 mg four times a day. Adverse events are infrequent. However, the cost of the drug may be prohibitive in the USA.

Flunarizine (Sibelium) is not available in the USA. The dose is 5–10 mg a day. The most prominent adverse events include weight gain, somnolence, dry mouth, dizziness, hypotension, and occasional extrapyramidal reactions. The elimination half-life of flunarizine is 19 days.

SEROTONIN ANTAGONISTS (TABLE 27.7)

Methysergide (Sansert)

Methysergide is a semisynthetic ergot alkaloid that is structurally related to methylergonovine. The AHCPR technical report identified 17 controlled trials of methysergide for migraine prevention (Gray et al., 1999). Four placebo-controlled trials suggested that methysergide was significantly better than placebo at reducing headache frequency (Lance et al., 1963; Shekelle and Ostfeld, 1964; Pedersen and Moller, 1966; Ryan, 1968).

Methysergide was associated with a higher incidence of adverse events than was placebo. Adverse events noted in trials and clinical practice included transient muscle aching, claudication, gastrointestinal complaints (nausea, vomiting, abdominal pain, and diarrhea), leg cramps, hair loss, weight gain, dizziness, giddiness, drowsiness, lassitude, paresthesia, and hallucinations. Frightening hallucinatory experiences after the first dose are not uncommon (Curran et al., 1967). Curran and Lance (1964) have treated leg claudication with vasodilators with some enhancement of methysergide's effectiveness, suggesting that its action on headache is not a result of vasoconstriction. The major complication of methysergide is the rare (1/5000) development of retroperitoneal, pulmonary, or endocardial fibrosis (Graham et al., 1966; Graham, 1967; Elkind et al., 1968; Bana et al., 1974).

Table 27.7

Miscellaneous medications in the preventive treatment of migraine

Agent	Daily dose	Comment
Serotonin antagonists		
Methysergide	2–8 mg	Higher doses given twice daily or three times daily Start at 1 mg and increase by 1 mg every 3 days Should not be taken continuously for long periods
Cyproheptadine	12–36 mg	Twice daily or three times daily Useful in children Weight gain in most patients
Pizotifen	1.5–3 mg	Three times daily Weight gain and drowsiness are common adverse events
Miscellaneous		
Feverfew	50–82 mg	Controversial evidence
Petasites	50–100 mg	75 and 100 mg better than placebo in independent trials
Riboflavin	400 mg	Positive small controlled trial
Coenzyme Q	150–300 mg	Two positive controlled trials
Magnesium	400–600 mg	Controversial evidence

Methysergide is indicated for the treatment of migraine and cluster headache. The dose ranges from 2 to 8 mg a day, with the higher doses being given two or three times a day. Some clinicians find they can use higher doses, up to 14 mg a day, without adverse events and with higher efficacy (Raskin, 1988a). Methysergide, in general, should not be taken continuously for long periods, since doing so may produce retroperitoneal fibrosis. Instead, the drug should be given for 6 months, stopped for 1 month, and then restarted. Some authorities use methysergide on a continuous basis with careful monitoring (Raskin, 1988a), which includes auscultation of the heart and annual echocardiography, chest X-ray, and abdominal MRI. The drug should be discontinued immediately if pulmonary or cardiac retroperitoneal fibrosis is suspected (Raskin, 1988a).

Contraindications to methysergide use include pregnancy, peripheral vascular disorders, severe arteriosclerosis, coronary artery disease, severe hypertension, thrombophlebitis or cellulitis of the legs, peptic ulcer disease, fibrotic disorders, lung diseases, collagen disease, liver or renal function impairment, valvular heart disease, debilitation, or serious infection. Patients who receive methysergide should remain under the supervision of the treating physician and be examined regularly for development of pulmonary, cardiac, or peritoneal fibrosis or vascular complications.

Cyproheptadine (Periactin)

Cyproheptadine (Periactin), an antagonist at the 5-HT_2, histamine H_1, L-calcium channels and muscarinic cholinergic receptors, is widely used in the preventive treatment of childhood migraine (Barlow, 1984; Forsythe and Hockaday, 1988; Raskin, 1988b). Curran and Lance (1964) found cyproheptadine to be more effective than placebo but less effective than methysergide. Cyproheptadine (Periactin) is available as 4-mg tablets. The total dose ranges from 12 to 36 mg a day (given twice to three times a day or at bedtime). Common adverse events are sedation and weight gain; dry mouth, nausea, lightheadedness, ankle edema, aching legs, and diarrhea are less common. Cyproheptadine may inhibit growth in children (Smyth and Lazarus, 1974) and reverse the effects of SSRIs. Rao and colleagues (2000) reported that cyproheptadine (4 mg/day) was as effective as propranolol (80 mg/day) in reducing migraine frequency and severity. The combination of cyproheptadine and propranolol was more effective than monotherapy.

Pizotifen

Pizotifen, a 5-HT_2 receptor antagonist structurally similar to cyproheptadine, is not available in the USA.

The evidence was inconsistent for its efficacy from 11 placebo-controlled trials (Gray et al., 1999) and 19 comparisons with other agents (Gray et al., 1999). Analysis of the placebo-controlled trials suggested a large clinical effect that was statistically significant. Pizotifen was generally poorly tolerated (Gray et al., 1999). Substantial weight gain, tiredness, and drowsiness were frequently reported. Pizotifen was associated with a high withdrawal rate due to adverse events. Controlled and uncontrolled studies in Europe (Peatfield, 1986) have shown this drug to benefit 40–79% of patients. The dose recommendation is 0.5–1 mg, three times daily by titration. Adverse events include drowsiness and weight gain (Capildeo and Rose, 1982).

MEDICINAL HERBS, VITAMINS, AND MINERALS (TABLE 27.7)

Feverfew

Feverfew (*Tanacetum parthenium*) is a medicinal herb used in self-treatment of migraine. Four trials were conducted, two in the AHCPR, and two after the report. One trial, conducted in a self-selected group of feverfew users, showed that withdrawing feverfew led to a statistically significant increase in headache frequency (Johnson et al., 1985). A pilot study of 17 migraineurs who ate fresh feverfew leaves daily was undertaken at the City of London Migraine Clinic. Patients were given capsules of freeze-dried feverfew or placebo. Those receiving placebo had a tripling in the frequency of migraine attacks. Patients on placebo reported increased nervousness, tension headaches, insomnia, or joint stiffness, constituting a "post-feverfew syndrome" (perhaps another example of rebound).

A second, more conventional, trial was conducted in a larger group of migraineurs, most of whom (71%) had never used feverfew (Murphy et al., 1988). This trial reported a smaller difference between feverfew and the control treatment than did the other trial, but still found the difference to be statistically significant in favor of feverfew. Another double-blind, randomized, crossover trial that tested the efficacy of feverfew compared with placebo reported that treatment with feverfew was associated with a significant reduction in pain intensity and non-headache symptoms (nausea, vomiting, photophobia, and phonophobia) (Palevitch et al., 1997). A fourth trial reported no significant differences between feverfew given as an alcoholic extract and placebo for reducing migraine frequency (Deweerdt et al., 1996).

Limited information indicates that adverse events were no more common with feverfew than with the control treatment (Gray et al., 1999). Feverfew has adverse events that include mouth ulceration and a more widespread oral inflammation associated with loss of taste. The mechanism of action of feverfew is uncertain. Feverfew is rich in sesquiterpene lactones, especially parthenolide, which may be a non-specific norepinephrine, 5-HT, bradykinin, prostaglandin, and acetylcholine antagonist. The biological variation in the sesquiterpene lactone content and the long-term safety and effectiveness of feverfew are of concern (Johnson et al., 1985).

The clinical effectiveness of feverfew for migraine prevention has not been established beyond reasonable doubt. More clinical trials are needed, both on a larger scale and with various feverfew extracts, including parthenolide-free sesquiterpene lactone chemotypes (Vogler et al., 1998).

MIG-99

MIG-99 is a stable extract of *Tanacetum parthenium* (feverfew). Three studies of MIG-99 for migraine prevention have been published. One dose-finding trial of MIG-99 (2.08 mg, 6.25 mg, 18.75 mg three times daily) reported the highest reduction in attack frequency with the 6.25-mg dose (Pfaffenrath et al., 2002). A second study confirmed that MIG-99 (6.25 mg three times daily) is effective in reducing the mean number of migraine attacks versus placebo (Diener et al., 2005).

Riboflavin

Schoenen et al. (1998) compared riboflavin (400 mg) with placebo in migraineurs in a randomized trial of 3 months' duration. Riboflavin was significantly superior to placebo in reducing the attack frequency ($P = 0.005$), headache days ($P = 0.012$), and migraine index ($P = 0.012$). The proportion of patients improved by at least 50% in headache days, i.e., "responders," was 15% for placebo, 59% for riboflavin ($P = 0.002$) and the number-needed-to-treat for effectiveness was 2.3. Only three adverse events occurred: two in the riboflavin group (diarrhea and polyuria) and one in the placebo group (abdominal cramps). None was serious. Because of its high efficiency, excellent tolerability, and low cost, riboflavin is an interesting option for prophylaxis and a candidate for a comparative trial with an established prophylactic drug.

Coenzyme Q

Rozen et al. (2002) assessed the efficacy of coenzyme Q10 as a preventive treatment for migraine headaches in an open-label trial. Thirty-two patients with a history of episodic migraine with or without aura were treated with coenzyme Q10 at a dose of 150 mg a day. Thirty-one of 32 patients completed the study; 61.3% of patients had a

>50% reduction in number of days with migraine headache. There were no side-effects noted with coenzyme Q10. From this open-label investigation, coenzyme Q10 appears to be a good migraine preventive. Sandor et al. (2003) performed a double-blind, placebo-controlled trial of coenzyme Q10 (100 mg three times daily) in 42 patients for 3 months. The 50% responder rate was 47.6% for coenzyme Q10 and 14.3% for placebo.

Petasites hybridus root

Petasites hybridus root (butterbur) is a perennial shrub whose extracts have been used for therapeutic purposes in traditional medicine for centuries. Lipton et al. (2004) conducted a randomized, double-blind, placebo-controlled trial of *Petasites*'s efficacy in migraine prophylaxis. Over 4 months of treatment, migraine attack frequency was reduced by 26% for placebo, 48% for *Petasites* extract 75 mg twice daily ($P = 0.0012$ versus placebo), and 36% for *Petasites* extract 50 mg twice daily ($P = 0.127$ versus placebo). The most frequently reported adverse event was burping.

Diener et al. (2004a) performed an independent reanalysis of a randomized, placebo-controlled, parallel-group study on the efficacy and tolerability of a special butterbur root extract (Petadolex) for the prophylaxis of migraine. The responder rate (improvement of migraine frequency >50%) was 45% in the active group (25-mg capsules of butterbur twice a day) and 15% in the placebo group. Butterbur was well tolerated and may be effective in the prophylaxis of migraine.

RECOMMENDATIONS

The goals of preventive treatment are to reduce the frequency, duration, or severity of attacks, improve responsiveness to acute attack treatment, improve function, and reduce disability. It may also prevent episodic migraine's progression to chronic migraine and result in health-care cost reductions. The medications used to treat migraine can be divided into five major categories: (1) drugs that have been proven effective (some beta-blockers, amitriptyline, topiramate, and divalproex); (2) drugs that are probably effective; (3) drugs that are possibly effective; (4) drugs for which evidence is inadequate or conflicting; and (5) drugs that are probably ineffective (Table 27.8).

- All drugs in group 1 should be used for the preventive treatment of migraine (level A).
- All drugs in group 2 should be considered for the preventive treatment of migraine (level B).
- All groups in group 3 may be considered for the preventive treatment of migraine (level C).
- All drugs in group 4 have no recommendation (level U).
- All drugs in group 5 should not be considered for migraine prevention (level B).

Choice of a preventive medication should be made based on a drug's proven efficacy, the patient's preferences and headache profile, the drug's adverse events, and the presence or absence of coexisting or comorbid disease (Table 27.1). The drug chosen should be the one that has the best risk-to-benefit ratio for the individual patient and takes advantage of the drug's adverse event profile.

Comorbid and coexistent diseases have important implications for treatment. The presence of a second illness provides therapeutic opportunities but also imposes certain therapeutic limitations. In some instances, two or more conditions can be treated with a single drug. However, there are limitations to using a single medication to treat two illnesses. Giving a single medication may not treat two different conditions optimally: although one of the two conditions may be adequately treated, the second illness may require a higher or lower dose, and therefore the patient is at risk of the second illness not being adequately treated. In an effort to use a single medication to treat two conditions, the physician may choose a second- or third-tier drug for treating either or both conditions, and this may not provide adequate efficacy for either illness. The risk is that one condition is managed appropriately, but the second condition requires a higher dose or additional therapy. Therapeutic independence may be needed should monotherapy fail. For example, a higher or lower dose of medication may be needed for migraine prevention than the dose commonly used for other indications. Usually, medicine is started with a minimally effective dose and then titrated over weeks or months. Avoiding drug interactions or increased adverse events is a primary concern when using polypharmacy. For example, when a patient is undergoing treatment for depression, adding a beta-blocker for migraine management may exacerbate the depression and put the patient at unnecessary risk.

For some patients, a single medication may adequately manage comorbid conditions. When migraine and hypertension and/or angina occur together, beta-blockers or calcium channel blockers may be effective for all conditions (Solomon, 1989). However, this is likely to be the exception rather than the rule. A beta-blocker may be poorly tolerated (or even contraindicated) in the presence of other conditions, such as depression or coexisting asthma. Co-pharmacy may enable therapeutic adjustments based on the status of each illness. TCAs are often recommended for patients with migraine and

Table 27.8

Preventive therapies for migraine

Group 1	Group 2	Group 3	Group 4	Group 5
Antiepileptic drugs	**ACE inhibitors**	**Alpha agonists**	**Anticoagulants**	**Antiepileptic drugs**
Divalproex sodium	Lisinopril	Clonidine	Acenocoumarol	Clonazepam
Sodium valproate	Candesartan	**Anticonvulsants**	Coumadin	Oxycarbamazepine
Topiramate	Antiepileptic drugs	Carbamazepine	Picotamide	Acetazolamide
Antidepressants	Gabapentin	**Ca^{2+} blockers**	**Antiepileptic drugs**	Lanepitant
Amitriptyline	Antidepressants/SSRI/SSNRI	Diltiazem	Lamotrigine	Montelukast
Beta-blockers	Fluoxetine	Nicardipine	Tiagabine	Omega-3
Metoprolol	Venlafaxine	Nifedipine	**Antidepressants**	Vitamin E
Propranolol	**Antihistamines/leukotriene antagonists**	Nimodipine	*TCAs*	
Timolol	Cyproheptadine	Verapamil	Doxepin	
Other	Histamine		Imipramine	
Petasites	**Beta-blockers**		Nortriptyline	
Serotonin agonists (MRM)	Atenolol		Protriptyline	
Frovatriptan*	Nadolol		*SSNRI/SSNRI*	
Serotonin antagonists	**NSAIDs**		Fluvoxamine	
Methysergide	Aspirin*		Paroxetine	
	Fenoprofen		Sertraline	
	Flurbiprofen		*Other*	
	Ibuprofen		Mirtazapine	
	Ketoprofen		Phenylzine	
	Mefenamic acid*		**Beta-blockers**	
	Naproxen		Acebutolol	
	Naproxen sodium		Bisoprolol	
	Other		Pindolol	
	Coenzyme Q10		**Serotonin antagonists**	
	MIG-99 (feverfew)		Methylergonovine	
	Vitamin B_2			
	Serotonin agonists (MRM)			
	Naratriptan*			
	Zolmitriptan*			

*For short-term prophylaxis.

MRM: menstrually related migraine; ACE: angiotensin-converting enzyme; SSRIs: selective serotonin reuptake inhibitors; SNRIs; selective serotonin and norepinephrine reuptake inhibitors; NSAIDs: non-selective anti-inflammatory drugs; TCAs: tricyclic antidepressants.

Group 1: Medications with proven high efficacy based on two class I trials; group 2: medications are probably effective based on one class I or two class II studies; group 3: medication use is possibly effective based on class II studies or two class III studies or conflicting studies; group 4: medication use cannot be recommended based on inadequate or conflicting data with no class I–III trials (class IV studies or no studies); group 5: medications probably ineffective (based on one class I or two case II studies).

depression (Silberstein et al., 1995). However, appropriate management of depression often requires higher doses of TCAs, which may be associated with more adverse events. A better approach might be to treat the depression with a SSRI or SNRI and the migraine with a cortical excitability stabilizer (antiepileptic drug, e.g., topiramate). For the patient with migraine and epilepsy (Mathew et al., 1995b), one may achieve control of both conditions with antiepileptic drugs, such as topiramate or divalproex sodium. Divalproex and topiramate are the drugs of choice for the patient with migraine and bipolar illness (Bowden et al., 1994; Silberstein, 1996). The pregnant migraineur who has a comorbid condition that needs treatment should be given a medication that is effective for both conditions and has the lowest potential for fetal adverse events. When individuals have more than one disease, certain categories of treatment may be relatively contraindicated. For example, beta-blockers should be used with caution in the depressed migraineur, while TCAs or neuroleptics may lower the seizure threshold and should be used with caution in the epileptic migraineur.

SUMMARY

Most migraine patients require acute headache treatment. Some require preventive treatment. Patients on preventive medication still require acute treatment for breakthrough attacks. Many patients find that their acute attacks are more manageable if they are on a preventive medication. The choice of preventive treatment depends on the individual drug's efficacy and adverse events, the patient's clinical features, frequency, and response to prior treatment, and the presence of any comorbid or coexistent disease.

References

Adelman LC, Adelman JU, Von Seggern R et al. (2000). Venlafaxine extended release (XR) for the prophylaxis of migraine and tension-type headache: a retrospective sutdy in a clinical setting. Headache 40: 572–580.

Adly C, Straumanis J, Chesson A (1992). Fluoxetine prophylaxis of migraine. Headache 32: 101–104.

Albers GW, Simon LT, Hamik A et al. (1989). Nifedipine versus propranolol for the initial prophylaxis of migraine. Headache 29: 215–218.

Andersson PG, Dahl S, Hansen JH et al. (1983). Prophylactic treatment of classical and nonclassical migraine with metoprolol: a comparison with placebo. Cephalalgia 3: 207–212.

Ansell E, Fazzone T, Festenstein R et al. (1988). Nimodipine in migraine prophylaxis. Cephalalgia 8: 269–272.

Ayata C, Jin H, Kudo C et al. (2006). Suppression of cortical spreading depression in migraine prophylaxis. Ann Neurol 59: 652–661.

Baldessarini RJ (1990). Drugs and the treatment of psychiatric disorders. In: AG Gilman, TW Rall, AS Nies et al. (Eds.), The Pharmacological Basis of Therapeutics. Pergamon, New York, pp. 383–435.

Bana DS, MacNeal PS, LeCompte PM et al. (1974). Cardiac murmurs and endocardial fibrosis associated with methysergide therapy. Am Heart J 88: 640–655.

Barlow CF (1984). Headaches and Migraine in Children. JB lippincott, Philadelphia, PA.

Bowden CL, Brugger AM, Swann AC (1994). Efficacy of divalproex vs lithium and placebo in the treatment of mania. JAMA 271: 918–924.

Bradley DP, Smith MI, Netsiri C et al. (2001). Diffusion-weighted MRI used to detect in vivo modulation of cortical spreading depression: comparison of sumatriptan and tonabersat. Exp Neurol 172: 342–353.

Brandes JL, Saper JR, Diamond M et al. (2004). Topiramate for migraine prevention: a randomized controlled trial. JAMA 291: 965–973.

Bulut S, Berilgen MS, Baran A et al. (2004). Venlafaxine versus amitriptyline in the prophylactic treatment of migraine: randomized, double-blind, crossover study. Clin Neurol Neurosurg 107: 44–48.

Capildeo R, Rose FC (1982). Single-dose pizotifen, 1.5mg nocte: a new approach in the prophylaxis of migraine. Headache 22: 272–275.

Chen WT, Fuh JL, Lu SR et al. (2001). Persistent migrainous visual phenomena might be responsive to lamotrigine. Headache 41: 823–825.

Cortelli P, Sacquegna T, Albani F et al. (1985). Propranolol plasma levels and relief of migraine. Arch Neurol 42: 46–48.

Couch JR, Ziegler D, Hassanein R (1976). Amitriptyline in the prophylaxis of migraine: effectiveness and relationship of antimigraine and antidepressant effects. Neurology 26: 121–127.

Coulam CB, Annagers JR (1979). New anticonvulsants reduce the efficacy of oral contraception. Epilepsia 20: 519–525.

Curran DA, Lance JW (1964). Clinical trial of methysergide and other preparations in the management of migraine. J Neurol Neurosurg Psychiatry 27: 463–469.

Curran DA, Hinterberger H, Lance JW (1967). Methysergide. Res Clin Stud Headache 1: 74–122.

Deweerdt CJ, Bootsma HP, Hendriks H (1996). Herbal medicines in migraine prevention: randomized double-blind placebo-controlled crossover trial of feverfew preparation. Phytomedicine 3: 225–230.

Diamond S, Medina JL (1976). Double-blind study of propranolol for migraine prophylaxis. Headache 16: 24–27.

Diamond S, Solomon GD, Freitag FG et al. (1987). Long-acting propranolol in the prophylaxis of migraine. Headache 27: 70–72.

Dichgans M, Freilinger T, Eckstein G et al. (2005). Mutation in the neuronal voltage-gated sodium channel SCN1A in familial hemiplegic migraine. Lancet 366: 371–377.

Diener HC, Hartung E, Chrubasik J et al. (2001). A comparative study of oral acetylsalicyclic acid and metoprolol for the prophylactic treatment of migraine. A randomized, controlled, double-blind, parallel group phase III study. Cephalalgia 21: 120–128.

Diener HC, Matias-Guiu J, Hartung E et al. (2002). Efficacy and tolerability in migraine prophylaxis of flunarizine in reduced doses: a comparison with propranolol 160 mg daily. Cephalalgia 22: 209–221.

Diener HC, Rahlfs VW, Danesch U (2004a). The first placebo-controlled trial of a special butterbur root extract for the prevention of migraine: reanalysis of efficacy criteria. Eur Neurol 51: 89–97.

Diener HC, Tfelt-Hansen P, Dahlof C et al. (2004b). Topiramate in migraine prophylaxis–results from a placebo-controlled trial with propranolol as an active control. J Neurol 251: 943–950.

Diener HC, Pfaffenrath V, Schnitker J et al. (2005). Efficacy and safety of 6.25 mg t.i.d. feverfew CO_2-extract (MIG-99) in migraine prevention–a randomized, double-blind, multicentre, placebo-controlled study. Cephalalgia 25: 1031–1041.

Dimitriadou V, Buzzi MG, Theoharides TC et al. (1992). Ultrastructural evidence for neurogenically mediated changes in blood vessels of the rat dura mater and tongue following antidromic trigeminal stimulation. Neuroscience 48: 187–203.

Dodick DW, Silberstein SD, Frietag F (2007). Topiramate versus amitriptyline for migraine prophylaxis: a multicenter randomized, double-blind, parallel treatment group trial. Cephalalgia 26: 1373 (Abstract).

Elkind AH, Friedman AP, Bachman A et al. (1968). Silent retroperitoneal fibrosis associated with methysergide therapy. JAMA 206: 1041–1044.

Etemad LR, Wang W, Globe D et al. (2005). Costs and utilization of triptan users who receive drug prophylaxis for migraine versus triptan users who do not receive drug prophylaxis. J Manag Care Pharm 11: 137–144.

Evers S, Afra J, Frese A et al. (2006). EFNS guideline on the drug treatment of migraine – report of an EFNS task force. Eur J Neurol 13: 560–572.

Featherstone HJ (1983). Low dose propranolol therapy for aborting acute migraine. West J Med 138: 416–417.

Feinmann C (1985). Pain relief by antidepressants: possible modes of action. Pain 23: 1–8.

Forsythe I, Hockaday JM (1988). Management of childhood migraine. In: JM Hockaday (Ed.), Migraine in Childhood. Butterworths, London, pp. 63–74.

Freitag FG, Diamond S, Diamond M et al. (2001). Divalproex in the long-term treatment of chronic daily headache. Headache 41: 271–278.

Freitag FG, Collins SD, Carlson HA et al. (2002). A randomized trial of divalproex sodium extended-release tablets in migraine prophylaxis. Neurology 58: 1652–1659.

Freitag FG, Forde G, Neto W et al. (2007). Topiramate effectively prevents migraine: analyzing pooled data from pivotal controlled trials. Analysis of pooled data from two pivotal controlled trials on the efficacy of topiramate in the prevention of migraine. J Am Osteopath Assoc 107: 251–258.

Frishman WH (1987). Beta adrenergic blocker withdrawal. Am J Cardiol 59: 32F.

Gelmers HJ (1983). Nimodipine, a new calcium antagonist, in the prophylactic treatment of migraine. Headache 23: 106–109.

Gerber WG, Diener H, Scholz E et al. (1991). Responders and nonresponders to metoprolol, propranolol and nifedipine treatment in migraine prophylaxis: a dose–range study based on time-series analysis. Cephalalgia 11: 37–45.

Gold L, Black T, Arnold G et al. (1998). Cortical spreading depression-associated hyperemia in rats: involvement of serotonin. Brain Res 783: 1983.

Graham J (1967). Cardiac and pulmonary fibrosis during methysergide therapy for headache. Am J Med Sci 254: 1–12.

Graham JR, Suby HI, LeCompte PR et al. (1966). Fibrotic disorders associated with methysergide therapy for headache. N Engl J Med 274: 360–368.

Gray RN, Goslin RE, McCrory DC et al. (1999). Drug treatments for the prevention of migraine headache. Prepared for the Agency for Health Care Policy and Research, Contract No. 290-94-2025. Available from the National Technical Information Service, Accession No. 127953.

Grotemeyer KH, Scharafinski HW, Schlake HP et al. (1990). Acetylsalicylic acid vs metoprolol in migraine prophylaxis: a double-blind crossover study. Headache 30: 639–641.

Hanston PP, Horn JR (1985). Drug interaction. Newsletter 5: 7–10.

Headache Classification Committee (2004). The international classification of headache disorders, 2nd edition. Cephalalgia 24: 1–160.

Jensen R, Brinck T, Olesen J (1994). Sodium valproate has a prophylactic effect in migraine without aura. Neurology 44: 647–651.

Johnson ES, Kadam NP, Hylands DM et al. (1985). Efficacy of feverfew as prophylactic treatment of migraine. BMJ 291: 569–573.

Kandere-Grzybowska K, Gheorghe D, Priller J et al. (2003). Stress-induced dura vascular permeability does not develop in mast cell-deficient and neurokinin-1 receptor knockout mice. Brain Res 980: 213–220.

Kangasniemi P, Andersen AR, Andersson PG et al. (1987). Classic migraine: effective prophylaxis with metoprolol. Cephalalgia 7: 231–238.

Kishore-Kumar R, Max MB, Schafer SC et al. (1990). Desipramine relieves post-herpetic neuralgia. Clin Pharmacol Ther 47: 305–312.

Klapper JA (1997). Divalproex sodium in migraine prophylaxis: a dose-controlled study. Cephalalgia 17: 103–108.

Koella WP (1985). CNS-related (side-)effects of β-blockers with special reference to mechanisms of action. Eur J Clin Pharmacol 28: 55–63.

Lamsudin R, Sadjimin T (1993). Comparison of the efficacy between flunarizine and nifedipine in the prophylaxis of migraine. Headache 33: 335–338.

Lance JW, Fine RD, Curran DA (1963). An evaluation of methysergide in the prevention of migraine and other vascular headaches. Med J Aust 1: 814–818.

Leandri M, Rigardo S, Schizzi R et al. (1990). Migraine treatment with nicardipine. Cephalalgia 10: 111–116.

Lipton RB, Gobel H, Einhaupl KM et al. (2004). *Petasites hybridus* root (butterbur) is an effective preventive treatment for migraine. Neurology 63: 2240–2244.

Lipton RB, Diamond M, Freitag F et al. (2005). Migraine prevention patterns in a community sample: results from the American Migraine Prevalence and Prevention (AMPP) study. Headache 45: 792–793 (Abstract).

Markley HG, Cleronis JCD, Piepko RW (1984). Verapamil prophylactic therapy of migraine. Neurology 34: 973–976.

Mathew NT (1996). Gabapentin in migraine prophylaxis. Cephalalgia 16: 367.

Mathew NT, Saper JR, Silberstein SD et al. (1995a). Migraine prophylaxis with divalproex. Arch Neurol 52: 281–286.

Mathew NT, Saper JR, Silberstein SD et al. (1995b). Prophylaxis of migraine headaches with divalproex sodium. Arch Neurol 52: 281–286.

Mathew N, Saper J, Magnus-Miller L (1998). Efficacy and safety of gabapentin (Neurontin®) in migraine prophylaxis. 17th Annual Meeting of the American Pain Society, San Diego, CA (Abstract).

McArthur JC, Marek K, Pestronk A et al. (1989). Nifedipine in the prophylaxis of classic migraine: a crossover, double-masked, placebo-controlled study of headache frequency and side-effects. Neurology 39: 284–286.

Migraine-Nimodipine European Study Group (MINES) (1989). European multicenter trial of nimodipine in the prophylaxis of common migraine (migraine without aura). Headache 29: 633–638.

Murphy JJ, Heptinstall S, Mitchell JR (1988). Randomized double-blind placebo controlled trial of feverfew in migraine prevention. Lancet 2: 189–192.

Olsson JE, Behring HC, Forssman B et al. (1984). Metoprolol and propranolol in migraine prophylaxis: a double-blind multicenter study. Acta Neurol Scand 70: 160–180.

Ophoff RA, Terwindt GM, Vergouwe MN (1996). Familial hemiplegic migraine and episodic ataxia type-2 are caused by mutations in the Ca^{2+} channel gene CACNLA4. Cell Tiss Res 87: 543–552.

Oshinsky ML, Luo J (2006). Neurochemistry of a rat migraine model. Headache 46 (Suppl. 1): S39–S44.

Palevitch D, Earon G, Carusso R (1997). Feverfew (*Tanacetum parthenium*) as a prophylactic treatment for migraine: a double-blind placebo-controlled study. Phytother Res 11: 508–511.

Panerai AE, Monza G, Movilia P et al. (1990). A randomized, within-patient, cross-over, placebo-controlled trial on the efficacy and tolerability of the tricyclic antidepressants chlorimipramine and nortriptyline in central pain. Acta Neurol Scand 82: 34–38.

Peatfield R (1986). Drugs acting by modification of serotonin function. Headache 26: 129–131.

Pedersen E, Moller CE (1966). Methysergide in migraine prophylaxis. Pharmacol Ther 7: 520–526.

Pellock JM, Willmore LJ (1991). A rational guide to routine blood monitoring in patients receiving antiepileptic drugs. Neurology 41: 961–964.

Pfaffenrath V, Diener HC, Fischer M et al. (2002). The efficacy and safety of *Tanacetum parthenium* (feverfew) in migraine prophylaxis: a double-blind, multicenter, randomized, placebo-controlled, dose–response study. Cephalalgia 22: 523–532.

Pradalier A, Serratrice G, Colard M et al. (1989). Long-acting propranolol on migraine prophylaxis: results of a double-blind, placebo-controlled study. Cephalalgia 9: 247–253.

Rabkin R, Stables DP, Levin NW et al. (1966). The prophylactic value of propranolol in angina pectoris. Am J Cardiol 370–383.

Ramadan NM (2004). Prophylactic migraine therapy: mechanisms and evidence. Curr Pain Headache Rep 8: 91–95.

Ramadan NM, Silberstein SD, Freitag FG et al. (2000). Evidence-based guidelines for migraine headache in the primary care setting: pharmacological management for prevention of migraine. Neurology. Available online at: http//www.neurology.org.

Rao BS, Das DG, Taraknath VR et al. (2000). A double blind controlled study of propranolol and cyproheptadine in migraine prophylaxis. Neurol India 48: 223–226.

Raskin NH (1988a). Headache. Churchill-Livingstone, New York.

Raskin NH (1988b). Migraine treatment. In: NH Raskin (Ed.), Headache. Churchill-Livingstone, New York.

Richelson E (1990). Antidepressants and brain neurochemistry. Mayo Clin Proc 65: 1227–1236.

Riopelle R, McCans JL (1982). A pilot study of the calcium channel antagonist diltiazem in migraine syndrome prophylaxis. Can J Neurol Sci 9: 269.

Rozen TD, Oshinsky ML, Gebeline CA et al. (2002). Open label trial of coenzyme Q10 as a migraine preventive. Cephalalgia 22: 137–141.

Ryan RE (1968). Double-blind crossover comparison of BC105, methysergide, and placebo in the prophylaxis of migraine headache. Headache 8: 118–126.

Sachedo RC, Reife RA, Lim P et al. (1997). Topiramate monotherapy for partial onset seizures. Epilepsia 38: 294–300.

Sandor PS, diClemente L, Coppola G et al. (2003). Coenzyme Q10 for migraine prophylaxis: a randomized controlled trial. Cephalalgia 23: 577 (Abstract).

Saper JR, Silberstein SD, Lake AE et al. (1994). Double-blind trial of fluoxetine: chronic daily headache and migraine. Headache 34: 497–502.

Schoenen J, Jacquy J, Lenaerts M (1998). Effectiveness of high-dose riboflavin in migraine prophylaxis. A randomized controlled trial. Neurology 50: 466–470.

Shank RP, Gardocki JF, Vaught JL et al. (1994). Topiramate: preclinical evaluation of structurally novel anticonvulsant. Epilepsia 35: 450–460.

Shekelle RB, Ostfeld AM (1964). Methysergide in the migraine syndrome. Clin Pharmacol Ther 5: 201–204.

Shukla R, Garg RK, Nag D et al. (1995). Nifedipine in migraine and tension headache: a randomized double-blind crossover study. J Assoc Phys India 43: 770–772.

Silberstein SD (1996). Divalproex sodium in headache – literature review and clinical guidelines. Headache 36: 547–555.

Silberstein SD (1997). Migraine and pregnancy. Neurol Clin 15: 209–231.

Silberstein SD (2002). Control of topiramate-induced paresthesias with supplemental potassium (letter). Headache 42: 85.

Silberstein SD (2004). Migraine pathophysiology and its clinical implications. Cephalalgia 24 (Suppl. 2): 2–7.

Silberstein SD on behalf of the Quality Standards Improvement Committee (2010). Practice parameter: evidence-based guidelines for treatment of migraine headache. Neurology (in press).

Silberstein SD, Rosenberg J (2000). Multispecialty consensus on diagnosis and treatment of headache. Neurology 54: 1553.

Silberstein SD, Silberstein MM (1990). New concepts in the pathogenesis of headache. Part II. Pain Mgt 3: 334–342.

Silberstein SD, Lipton RB, Breslau N (1995). Migraine: association with personality characteristics and psychopathology. Cephalalgia 15: 337–369.

Silberstein SD, Lipton RB, Goadsby PJ (1998). Migraine: diagnosis and treatment. In: SD Silberstein, RB Lipton, PJ Goadsby (Eds.), Headache in Clinical Practice. Isis Medical Media, Oxford, pp. 61–90.

Silberstein SD, Winner PK, Chmiel JJ (2003). Migraine preventive medication reduces resource utilization. Headache 43: 171–178.

Silberstein SD, Bhattacharaya S, Neto W et al. (2004). Topiramate in the prevention of migraine headache: a randomized, double-blind, placebo-controlled, multiple-dose study. For the MIGR-001 Study Group. Arch Neurol 61: 490–495.

Silberstein S, Diamond S, Loder E et al. (2005). Prevalence of migraine sufferers who are candidates for preventive therapy: results from the American Migraine Prevalence and Prevention (AMPP) Study. Headache 45: 770–771 (Abstract).

Silberstein SD, Feliu AL, Rupow MFT et al. (2007). Topiramate in migraine prophylaxis: long-term impact on resource utilization and cost. Headache 47: 500–510.

Silberstein S, Saper J, Berenson F et al. (2008). Oxcarbazepine in migraine headache: a double-blind, randomized, placebo-controlled study. Neurology 70: 548–555.

Smith R, Schwartz A (1984). Diltiazem prophylaxis in refractory migraine. N Engl J Med 310: 1327–1328.

Smyth GA, Lazarus L (1974). Suppression of growth hormone secretion by melatonin and cyproheptadine. J Clin Invest 54: 116–121.

Solomon GD (1986). Verapamil and propranolol in migraine prophylaxis: a double-blind crossover study. Headache 26: 325.

Solomon GD (1989). Management of the headache patient with medical illness. Clin J Pain 5: 95–99.

Sorensen PS, Larsen BH, Rasmussen MJ et al. (1991). Flunarizine versus metoprolol in migraine prophylaxis: a double-blind, randomized parallel group study of efficacy and tolerability. Headache 31 (10): 650–657.

Steardo L, Bonuso S, DiStasio E et al. (1982). Selective and nonselective beta-blockers: are both effective in prophylaxis of migraine? A clinical trial versus methysergide. Acta Neurol 4: 196–204.

Steiner TJ, Findley LJ, Yuen AW (1997). Lamotrigine versus placebo in the prophylaxis of migraine with and without aura. Cephalalgia 17: 109–112.

Storer RJ, Goadsby PJ (2003). Topiramate inhibits trigeminovascular traffic in the cat: a possible locus of action in the prevention of migraine. Neurology 60: A238 (Abstract).

Sudilovsky A, Elkind AH, Ryan RE et al. (1987). Comparative efficacy of nadolol and propranolol in the management of migraine. Headache 27: 421–426.

Tfelt-Hansen P, Lipton RB (1993). Prioritizing treatment. In: J Olesen, P Tfelt-Hansen, KMA Welch (Eds.), The Headaches. Raven Press, New York, pp. 359–362.

Thomson Healthcare (2003). Physicians' Desk Reference. Thomson PDR, Montvale, NJ.

Vainionpaa LK, Rattya J, Knip M et al. (1999). Valproate-induced hyperandrogenism during pubertal maturation in girls with epilepsy. Ann Neurol 45: 444–450.

Vilming S, Standnes B, Hedman C (1985). Metoprolol and pizotifen in the prophylactic treatment of classical and common migraine: a double-blind investigation. Cephalalgia 5: 17–23.

Vogler BK, Pittler MH, Ernst E (1998). Feverfew as a preventive treatment for migraine: a systematic review. Cephalalgia 18: 704–708.

Wauquier A, Ashton D, Marranes R (1985). The effects of flunarizine in experimental models related to the pathogenesis of migraine. Cephalalgia 5: 119–120.

Weber RB, Reinmuth OM (1972). The treatment of migraine with propranolol. Neurology 22: 366–369.

Weilburg JB, Rosenbaum JF, Biederman J et al. (1989). Fluoxetine added to nonMAOI antidepressants converts nonresponders to responders: a preliminary report. J Clin Psychiatry 50: 447–449.

Wessely P, Baumgartner C, Klinger D et al. (1987). Preliminary results of a double-blind study with the new migraine prophylactic drug gabapentin. Cephalalgia 7: 477–478.

Wheeler SD (2001). Lamotrigine efficacy in migraine prevention. Cephalalgia 21: 374 (Abstract).

Handbook of Clinical Neurology, Vol. 97 (3rd series)
Headache
G. Nappi and M.A. Moskowitz, Editors

Chapter 28

Tension-type headache: introduction and diagnostic criteria

PETER KROPP,[1]* GEORG EGLI,[2] AND PETER S. SÁNDOR[3]

[1]*Institute of Medical Psychology and Medical Sociology, Center of Nervous Diseases, Medical Faculty, University of Rostock, Rostock, Germany*

[2]*Kopfweh- & Schmerzabteilung, Neurologische Klinik/Unispital, Poliklinik, Zürich, Switzerland*

[3]*University of Zürich, Zürich, Switzerland; Headache and Pain Unit, Neurology Department, University Hospital, Zürich, Switzerland*

INTRODUCTION

Tension-type headache is regarded as the most common primary headache. In spite of this, it is considered, from a clinical point of view, less important than the other primary headaches, given the low intensity of the pain and, in a large section of the population, its low frequency (so-called infrequent tension-type headache).

Until 1988 there was no internationally accepted classification for primary headaches, including tension-type headache. The formerly used terms for tension-type headache were psychogenic headache, stress headache, psychomyogenic headache, idiopathic headache, and others. In 1988 the International Headache Classification was introduced, which also defined tension-type headache using clinical criteria (Headache Classification Committee of the International Headache Society, 1988). Until now one revision of these criteria has taken place (International Classification of Headache Disorders (ICHD-II), 2004) – the major changes were a division into subgroups of tension-type headache by means of their frequency. The diagnostic criteria for tension-type headache were not changed substantially in this revision, and the typical clinical profile of this headache was confirmed in the studies conducted in order to evaluate these criteria.

However, this chapter raises several issues that have been the focus of some debate.

Clinically, it seems difficult to distinguish tension-type headache from the early phase of a migraine attack in some patients. This is a particularly important issue, considering that the treatment of a migraine attack is clearly more effective if started when the pain is mild. Another controversial question is the role of pericranial muscle disorders. These do not appear to constitute a specific marker of tension-type headache, and there is no clear-cut difference between patients with and without muscular symptoms. The role of peripheral (muscular) factors is suggested on the basis of experimental models and aggravating factors in tension-type headache.

Prolonged muscular contraction and/or the activation of peripheral fibers could play an important role in the development of a typical central phenomenon: sensitization of the pain control system. Neurophysiological investigations confirm that central sensitization is a feature of tension-type headache, but it does not seem to be specific to this condition, since similar abnormalities are observed in migraine.

A fairly common pathogenetic mechanism could explain the frequent association between migraine and tension-type headache, the similarities between migraine and tension-type headache in the early phase of the migraine attack observed in some patients, as well as the effectiveness of some drugs which are able to prevent or to reduce pain in both these types of headache.

In particular, some drugs acting on the pain control system (e.g., amitriptyline) are effective in both migraine and in tension-type headache, while the effectiveness in tension-type headache of other drugs able to prevent migraine (i.e., antiepileptics) is unclear or unconfirmed. Similarly, the effectiveness of triptans, well known in migraine patients, is still debated in tension-type headache.

For all these reasons, both of the theories concerning migraine and tension-type headache (continuum spectrum versus two separate clinical entities) seem to be supported by contrasting clinical and experimental evidence.

*Correspondence to: Peter Kropp, Institute of Medical Psychology and Medical Sociology, Center of Nervous Diseases, Medical Faculty, University of Rostock, Gehlsheimer Strasse 20, D-18147 Rostock, Germany, Tel: +49-381-494-9530, Fax: +49-381-494-9532, E-mail: peter.kropp@med.uni-rostock.de

However, in clinical practice, it is fundamentally important to maintain a clear distinction between migraine and tension-type headache, since most patients present a typical clinical profile. Moreover, distinguishing migraine from tension-type headache helps research aimed at exploring the pathogenetic mechanisms of the two conditions.

The new concept of "probable" diagnosis, introduced in ICHD-II published in 2004, can provide information about the number of the patients who do not completely fulfill the diagnostic criteria for these two forms.

INTERNATIONAL HEADACHE SOCIETY (IHS) CLASSIFICATION OF TENSION-TYPE HEADACHE

The distinction between an episodic and a chronic type has been made in the first edition of the IHS classification. This distinction is important, as the chronic subtype causes a considerable impairment of quality of life and is comorbid with anxiety, mood disorders, and other pain syndromes.

Taking into account that almost everyone has experienced tension headache in their lives, in ICHD-II, episodic tension-type headache was subdivided into an infrequent and a frequent subtype. The infrequent subtype is defined as less than one headache episode per month on average (i.e., less than 12 headache days per year), and is considered part of normal life rather than a medical problem. The frequent subtype can lead to some disability, resulting in the need for treatment.

Episodic tension-type headache

Episodic tension-type headache is defined as lasting from 30 min to 7 days and is of pressing/tightening, non-pulsating quality. Intensity is mild or moderate, the pain occurs bilaterally, and is not aggravated by routine physical activity like walking or climbing stairs. Nausea or vomiting does not occur, but phonophobia or photophobia may be present during the pain period.

As mentioned above, there is a distinction within episodic tension-type headache: infrequent and frequent subtype has been introduced in the revised IHS classification (International Classification of Headache Disorders, 2004). The infrequent subtype occurs less than once per month, the frequent subtype between 1 and 15 episodes per month, but does not fit the criteria of the chronic tension-type headache. There is a further type of subdivision of each group using the criterion of presence of pericranial tenderness (Table 28.1, parts 2.1 and 2.2).

In clinical practice, frequent tension-type headache often coexists with migraine without aura and should be diagnosed separately. The distinction between the different headache types can probably best be identified by means of a diagnostic headache diary. This is important, as the treatment of migraine differs considerably from that of tension-type headache and it is important to educate patients to differentiate between these types of headache in order to select the right treatment and to prevent medication overuse headache.

Chronic tension-type headache

Chronic tension-type headache is to be diagnosed if headache occurs, on average, on more than 14 days per month for more than 3 months (Table 28.1, part 2.3). More than 60% of chronic tension-type headache patients report anxiety disorders, depression, sleep disturbances, and analgesic overuse (Juang et al., 2000).

Since the introduction of the category 1.5.1 chronic migraine (ICHD-II), the differential diagnosis from chronic tension-type headache can be difficult in clinical practice. Both diagnoses require headache (meeting the criteria for migraine or tension-type headache respectively) on at least 15 days a month. Therefore it is theoretically possible that a patient can be diagnosed with both chronic migraine and chronic tension-type headache. A very small group of patients has 15 or more headaches per month, fulfilling the diagnostic criteria for both 1.5.1 chronic migraine and 2.3 chronic tension-type headache. This is possible when two (and only two) of the four pain characteristics are present and headaches are associated with mild nausea. In these very rare cases, other clinical evidence that is not part of the explicit diagnostic criteria should be taken into account. The clinician should base thereon the best possible choice of diagnosis. Where there is some degree of uncertainty regarding how many of the attacks fulfill one or other set of criteria, a diagnostic headache diary which should be used prospectively can be of great help.

In many uncertain cases there is overuse of medication. The correct diagnostic procedure in these cases is rather complicated, as in the current version it is required that the headaches disappear after successful withdrawal. This is unsatisfactory and appears almost paradoxical in clinical practice as the majority of patients present while overusing acute headache medication. Further, after successful withdrawal, if the headaches disappear, they cannot be diagnosed any longer. To account for these practical problems, the International Headache Classification Committee has published appendix criteria that could prove very useful in clinical practice (Olesen et al., 2006). However, currently the criteria are not yet in the main text body of the classification, and need to be tested in studies before being recommended for use in clinical practice.

If the chronic headaches are daily and have become unremitting within 3 days of onset, they are classified as new daily persistent headache (category 4.8).

Table 28.1

Diagnostic criteria of tension-type headache (TTH)

2.1 Infrequent episodic TTH

A. At least 10 episodes occuring on <1 day/month (<12 day/year) and fulfilling criteria B–D
B. Headache lasting from 30 min to 7 days
C. Headache has ≥2 of the following characteristics:
   1. bilateral location
   2. pressing/tightening (non-pulsating) quality
   3. mild or moderate intensity
   4. not aggravated by routine physical activity
D. Both of the following:
   1. no nausea or vomiting (anorexia may occur)
   2. no more than one of photophobia or phonophobia
E. Not attributed to another disorder

2.2 Frequent episodic TTH

2.2.1 Frequent episodic tension-type headache associated with pericranial tenderness

A. Episodes fulfilling criteria A–E for 2.1 *Infrequent episodic tension-type headache*
B. Increased pericranial tenderness on manual palpation

2.2.2 Frequent episodic tension-type headache not associated with pericranial tenderness

A. Episodes fulfilling criteria A–E for 2.1 *Infrequent episodic tension-type headache*
B. No increased pericranial tenderness

***As 2.1 except*:**

A. At least 10 episodes occuring on ≥1 but <15 days/month for ≥3 months (≥12 and <180 days/year) and fulfilling criteria B–D

2.3 Chronic TTH

2.3.1 Chronic tension-type headache associated with pericranial tenderness

A. Headache fulfilling criteria A–E for 2.3 *Chronic tension-type headache*
B. Increased pericranial tenderness on manual palpation

2.3.2 Chronic tension-type headache not associated with pericranial tenderness

A. Episodes fulfilling criteria A–E for 2.3 *Chronic tension-type headache*
B. No increased pericranial tenderness

A. Headache occuring on ≥15 days/month (≥180 days/year) for >3 months and fulfilling criteria B–D
B. Headache lasts hours or may be continuous
C. Headache has ≥2 of the following characteristics:
   1. bilateral location
   2. pressing/tightening (non-pulsating) quality
   3. mild or moderate intensity
   4. not aggravated by routine physical activity
D. Both of the following:
   1. not >1 of photophobia, phonophobia, mild nausea
   2. neither moderate or serve nausea nor vomiting
E. Not attributed to another disorder

2.4 Probable TTH

2.4.1 Probable infrequent episodic TTH

A. Episodes fulfilling all but one of criteria A–D for 2.1 *Infrequent episodic tension-type headache*
B. Episodes do not fulfill criteria for 1.1 *Migraine without aura*
C. Not attributed to another disorder

2.4.2 Probable frequent episodic TTH

A. Episodes fulfilling all but one criteria for 2.2 *Frequent episodic tension-type headache*
B. Episodes do not fulfill criteria for 1.1 *Migraine without aura*

2.4.3 Probable chronic TTH

***As 2.3 except*:**

E. Not attributed to another disorder but there is, or has been within the last 2 months, medication overuse fulfilling criterion B for any of the subforms of 8.2 *Medication overuse headache*

(Reproduced from International Classification of Headache Disorders (ICHD-II), 2004.)

Probable tension-type headache

All patients meeting all but one criteria for episodic tension-type headache are listed here (Table 28.1, part 2.4). They are to be excluded from the condition of migraine without aura. Further patients with chronic tension-type headache and medication overuse are listed here until there is a significant improvement (or not) of headache after cessation of medication for 2 months (see above).

References

Headache Classification Committee of the International Headache Society (1988). Classification and diagnostic criteria for headache disorders, cranial neuralgias and facial pain, first edition. Cephalalgia 8 (Suppl. 7): 1–96.

International Classification of Headache Disorders (ICHD-II) (2004). Headache classification committee of the International Headache Society. Classification and diagnostic criteria for headache disorders, cranial neuralgias and facial pain, 2nd edition. Cephalalgia 24 (Suppl. 1): 1–160.

Juang K-D, Wang S-J, Fuh J-L et al. (2000). Comorbidity of depressive and anxiety disorders in chronic daily headache and its subtypes. Headache 40: 818–823.

Olesen J, Bousser M-G, Dienser H-C et al. (2006). New appendix criteria open for a broader concept of chronic migraine. Cephalalgia 26: 742–746.

Handbook of Clinical Neurology, Vol. 97 (3rd series)
Headache
G. Nappi and M.A. Moskowitz, Editors

Chapter 29

Tension-type headache: mechanisms

L. BENDTSEN[1]* A. FUMAL,[2] AND J. SCHOENEN[3]

[1]*Danish Headache Center, Department of Neurology, Glostrup Hospital, University of Copenhagen, Copenhagen, Denmark*
[2]*Headache Research Unit, Neurology and Neuroanatomy Departments, University of Liège, Liège, Belgium*
[3]*Headache Research Unit, Department of Neurology, and Research Center for Cellular and Molecular Neurobiology, University of Liège, Liège, Belgium*

INTRODUCTION

Tension-type headaches (TTHs) are very prevalent and responsible for substantial costs for both the individual and society (Schwartz et al., 1997). In contrast to migraine, no significant improvement in treatment possibilities has been seen in TTH within recent decades. This may partly be attributed to the fact that the understanding of TTH pathophysiology is less complete than that of migraine. Fortunately, we have gained much new knowledge on pathophysiological aspects of TTH within the last decade, and we are now beginning to understand some of the complex mechanisms leading to this prevalent disorder (Jensen, 1999; Bendtsen, 2000; Vandenheede and Schoenen, 2002; Ashina, 2004; Ashina et al., 2005; Bendtsen and Jensen, 2006; Mathew, 2006). This is the first step towards the development of more effective treatments. Previously, research into the mechanisms leading to TTH mainly focused on muscular factors. More recently it has become clear that central factors play a crucial role, in particular in the more severe forms of the disorder.

GENETIC PREDISPOSITION

Because of the enormous prevalence and variability in frequency and severity of TTH, any inheritance is almost certain to be polygenic. Sufferers of TTH must by chance have many affected first-degree relatives. The population relative risk in relatives compared with normal controls has been calculated in a single study. In chronic TTH, the risk was increased threefold, indicating a genetic predisposition (Østergaard et al., 1997). The transmission suggested complex inheritance (Russell et al., 1998). At present, we adopt the view that the great majority of the population, perhaps all, have the potential to develop TTH if exposed to sufficiently strong environmental factors.

ENVIRONMENTAL AND PSYCHOLOGICAL FACTORS

Headaches are generally reported to occur in relation to emotional conflict and psychosocial stress, but, as in migraine, the cause-and-effect relationship is not clear. Stress and mental tension are the most frequently reported precipitating factors but they occur with similar frequency in TTH and migraine (Jensen and Becker, 2005). A recent review (Heckman and Holroyd, 2006) concluded that there is no increase in anxiety or depression in patients with infrequent TTH, while frequent TTH is associated with higher rates of anxiety and depression. As in other chronic pain disorders, psychological abnormalities in TTH may be viewed as secondary rather than primary. However, maladaptive coping strategies, e.g., catastrophizing and avoidance, seem to be common in TTH (Heckman and Holroyd, 2006). In addition, it was recently demonstrated that depression increases vulnerability to TTH in patients with frequent headaches during and following a laboratory stress test and that the induced headache was associated with elevated pericranial muscle tenderness (Janke et al., 2004). The authors suggested that depression may aggravate existing central sensitization (see below) in patients with frequent headaches (Janke et al., 2004). Thus, there may be a bidirectional relationship between depression and frequent TTH.

It has been demonstrated that the 1-year prevalence of TTH increased significantly from 1989 to 2001 (Lyngberg

*Correspondence to: Lars Bendtsen, Danish Headache Centre, Department of Neurology, Glostrup Hospital, University of Copenhagen, DK-2600 Glostrup, Copenhagen, Denmark, Tel: +45 43232062, E-mail: larben01@glo.regionh.dk

et al., 2005a). Risk factors for the development of TTH were poor self-rated health, an inability to relax after work, and sleep disturbances (Lyngberg et al., 2005b). These findings are interesting, because they may lead to new ways of preventing or treating TTH.

PERIPHERAL FACTORS

Peripheral factors have traditionally been considered of major importance in TTH and numerous studies have reported increased tenderness and hardness of pericranial myofascial tissues in these patients (Jensen, 1999; Ashina et al., 2005; Bendtsen and Treede, 2005). The tenderness is uniformly increased throughout the pericranial region both in patients with episodic and in patients with chronic TTH (Langemark and Olesen, 1987; Jensen et al., 1998; Buchgreitz et al., 2006). Tenderness and hardness have been found to be increased both on days with and without headache (Ashina et al., 1999b; Jensen, 1999; Lipchik et al., 2000), indicating that these findings are not simply a consequence of the headache. In addition, it has been demonstrated that pericranial tenderness is positively associated with both the intensity and the frequency of TTH (Jensen et al., 1993; Buchgreitz et al., 2006) and with muscle hardness (Ashina et al., 1999b).

It was recently demonstrated that infusion of hypertonic saline into various pericranial muscles elicits referred pain that is perceived as head pain in healthy subjects (Schmidt-Hansen et al., 2006b). The existence and importance of trigger points (tenderness in a hypersensible spot within a palpable taut band, local twitch response elicited by snapping palpation, and elicited referred pain with palpation) (Fernandez-de-Las-Penas et al., 2006b) in myofascial pain disorders has long been debated. A recent series of pilot studies performed in a blinded fashion reported an increased number of active trigger points both in patients with frequent episodic TTH and in patients with chronic TTH (Fernandez-de-Las-Penas et al., 2006a, b, 2007). In chronic, but not in episodic, TTH the trigger points were positively correlated to headache severity.

What could be the pathophysiological basis for the possible pain originating in the myofascial tissues? Under normal conditions, myofascial pain is mediated by thin myelinated (Aδ) fibers and unmyelinated (C) fibers, while the thick myelinated (Aα and Aβ) fibers normally mediate innocuous sensations (Newham et al., 1994). Various noxious and innocuous events such as mechanical stimuli, ischemia, and chemical mediators could excite and sensitize Aδ and C fibers (Mense, 1993) and thereby play a role in the increased tenderness in TTH.

The role of the first two events, mechanical strain and ischemia, has been extensively studied in TTH. Sustained experimental tooth clenching induced headache in more patients than healthy controls (Jensen and Olesen, 1996), and it was demonstrated that TTH patients are more liable to develop shoulder and neck pain in response to static exercise than healthy controls (Christensen et al., 2005). Numerous electromyographic (EMG) studies using surface electrodes have demonstrated that muscle activity is only slightly increased in TTH (Jensen, 1999). However, it has been reported that EMG activity is significantly increased in myofascial trigger points (Hubbard and Berkoff, 1993). Continuous activity in a few motor units over a long period of time could be sufficient for excitation or sensitization of peripheral nociceptors (Bendtsen, 2000), but the findings by Hubbard and Berkoff (1993) have not yet been reproduced by other groups.

Muscle tenderness and hardness at tender muscle sites could also result from a local contracture (i.e., shortening of the contractile apparatus without action potentials in the muscle fibers) rather than normal contraction of motor units (Simons and Mense, 1998). This mechanism would explain the lack of EMG abnormalities in TTH, but the mechanisms of peripheral nociceptor activation by a contracture have not yet been studied in enough detail (Mense et al., 2003). Using a microdialysis technique, Ashina et al. (2002) demonstrated that lactate levels in a tender site in the trapezius muscle did not differ between patients and healthy subjects during rest and static exercise, ruling out muscle ischemia in these patients. However, the increase in muscle blood flow during exercise was lower in patients than in controls. The authors suggested that altered blood flow was caused by altered sympathetic outflow to blood vessels in striated muscle due to plastic changes in the central nervous system (central sensitization) (Ashina et al., 2002). Thus, it can be concluded that muscle pain in TTH is not caused by generalized excessive muscle contraction and muscle ischemia. However, it cannot be excluded that a locally increased muscle tone without EMG activity (contracture) may result in microtrauma of muscle fibers and tendon insertions, or that excessive activity in a few motor units may excite or sensitize peripheral nociceptors.

Peripheral muscle afferents could be activated and sensitized by endogenous substances such as serotonin and bradykinin (Mense, 1993). Mork et al. (2004) demonstrated that, when a combination of the endogenous substances bradykinin, serotonin, histamine, and prostaglandin E_2 was slowly infused into the trapezius muscle, patients with frequent episodic TTH developed more pain and tenderness (Mork et al., 2003) than healthy controls. Concomitant psychophysical measures indicated that peripheral sensitization of myofascial sensory afferents was responsible for the muscular hypersensitivity in these patients (Mork et al., 2003). However, Ashina et al. (2003) demonstrated that the *in vivo* interstitial concentrations of adenosine 5′-triphosphate, glutamate, glucose, pyruvate, urea, and prostaglandin E_2 in tender muscles during rest and static exercise did not differ between patients with chronic TTH and healthy controls. The authors concluded that tender muscle sites in these patients are not sites of ongoing inflammation.

To summarize, pericranial myofascial tenderness and muscle hardness are frequently observed in TTH. These findings are similar to trigger points in other myofascial diseases (Treede et al., 2002). Some studies indicate that the increased myofascial pain sensitivity in TTH may be caused by activation or sensitization of peripheral nociceptors. However, firm evidence for peripheral abnormalities as a cause of myofascial tenderness is still lacking.

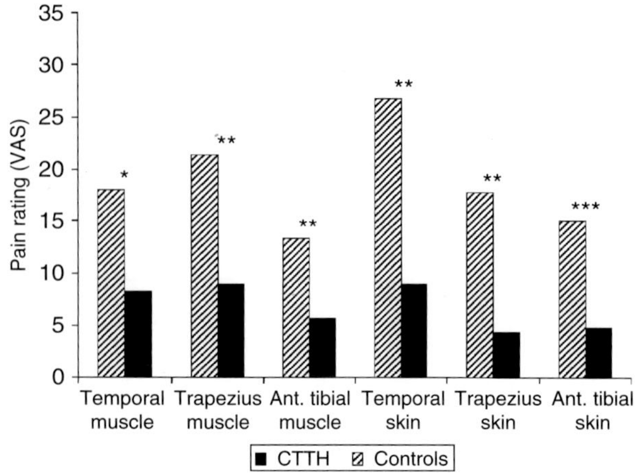

Fig. 29.1. Pain perception study demonstrating pronounced generalized hyperalgesia in patients with chronic tension-type headache (CTTH). Pain ratings to suprathreshold single electrical stimulation (Visual Analogue Scale: VAS) of skin and muscle in patients with CTTH and healthy controls. $*P < 0.05$, $**P < 0.01$, $***P < 0.001$. Data from Ashina et al. (2006).

CENTRAL FACTORS

The increased myofascial pain sensitivity in TTH could also be caused by central factors such as: (1) sensitization of second-order neurons at the level of the spinal dorsal horn/trigeminal nucleus; (2) sensitization of supraspinal neurons; and (3) decreased antinociceptive activity from supraspinal structures. The measurement of pain sensitivity to various types of stimulus applied to various parts of the body has provided important information about the nociceptive system in TTH. Pain detection thresholds have been reported normal in patients with episodic TTH in studies performed before the separation between the infrequent and frequent form was made (Bovim, 1992; Göbel et al., 1992; Jensen et al., 1993; Jensen, 1996). In contrast, pain detection thresholds have been reported to be decreased in patients with frequent episodic TTH (Mork et al., 2003; Schmidt-Hansen et al., 2006a), and both pain detection and tolerance thresholds have been found to be decreased in patients with chronic TTH in all studies performed with sufficient sample size (Langemark et al., 1989; Schoenen et al., 1991; Langemark et al., 1993; Bendtsen et al., 1996a; Ashina et al., 2006; Sandrini et al., 2006; Schmidt-Hansen et al., 2006a). Ashina et al. (2006) recently demonstrated that the difference in pain sensitivity is even more pronounced when recording pain sensitivity to clinically relevant stimuli, namely suprathreshold stimuli (Figure 29.1). Most importantly, the findings of abnormal pain modulation in patients with frequent headaches reported from clinical studies were recently confirmed in a population-based study demonstrating a close relation between altered pain perception and chronification of headache (Buchgreitz et al., 2006). In addition, it was demonstrated that a previously reported increase in TTH prevalence over a 12-year period was related to increased pain sensitivity (Buchgreitz et al., 2007).

Patients with chronic TTH have been found to be hypersensitive to each of the different stimulus modalities examined, namely, pressure (Langemark et al., 1989; Schoenen et al., 1991; Bendtsen et al., 1996a), thermal (Langemark et al., 1989) and electrical (Langemark et al., 1993; Bendtsen et al., 1996a; Ashina et al., 2006; Sandrini et al., 2006) stimuli as well as intramuscular infusions of painful substances (Schmidt-Hansen et al., 2006a). Sensitivity to the various stimulus modalities is increased at both cephalic and extracephalic locations (Langemark et al., 1989, 1993; Schoenen et al., 1991; Bendtsen et al., 1996a; Ashina et al., 2006), to stimulation of various tissues, i.e., muscle, skin, tendons, and peripheral nerves (Langemark et al., 1989, 1993; Schoenen et al., 1991; Bendtsen et al., 1996a; Ashina et al., 2006; Schmidt-Hansen et al., 2006a), and both during and outside headache (Schmidt-Hansen et al., 2006a). The fact that chronic TTH patients are hypersensitive to stimuli applied both at cephalic and at extracephalic, non-symptomatic locations strongly indicates that synaptic transmission of nociceptive input within the central nervous system is increased in this group of patients, because peripheral sensitization would have more localized effects (Treede et al., 1992; Milanov and Bogdanova, 2004). The expansion of hypersensitivity to other tissues such as skin is consistent with referred hyperalgesia, which may be explained by convergence of multiple peripheral sensory afferents on to sensitized spinal cord neurons. The widespread and non-specific nature of the hypersensitivity, however, suggests that the central sensitization involves supraspinal neurons as well. Decreased activity of the endogenous antinociceptive systems would have similar effects (disinhibition) (Sandrini et al., 2006). Thus, it can be concluded that nociceptive processing in the central nervous system is increased in patients with chronic TTH, while central nociceptive processing seems to be relatively normal in patients with infrequent episodic TTH.

The increase in myofascial tenderness is more pronounced than the increase in general pain sensitivity (Bendtsen, 2000). Moreover, a significant but not very high correlation between general pain hypersensitivity and pericranial tenderness has been demonstrated (Bendtsen et al., 1996a; Jensen et al., 1998). Thus, general hypersensitivity can explain only a part of the increased pericranial tenderness in patients with chronic TTH. It has been demonstrated that the stimulus–response function for pressure versus pain in pericranial muscles is not only quantitatively but also qualitatively altered in patients with chronic TTH (Bendtsen et al., 1996b). On the basis of results from animal studies this is most likely explained by central sensitization at the level of the spinal dorsal horn/trigeminal nucleus. Thus, the increased tenderness in patients with chronic TTH is probably partly caused by segmental central sensitization.

The hyperalgesia could be caused by prolonged nociceptive input from tender pericranial myofascial tissues resulting in segmental central sensitization at the level of the upper cervical spinal dorsal horn/trigeminal nucleus with secondary sensitization of supraspinal neurons, e.g., in the thalamus or somatosensory cortex (Bendtsen and Schoenen, 2005). This hypothesis was further supported by a study demonstrating decrease in volume of gray-matter brain structures involved in pain processing in patients with chronic TTH (Schmidt-Wilcke et al., 2005). This decrease was positively correlated with duration of headache and most likely a consequence of central sensitization generated by prolonged input from pericranial myofascial structures (Schmidt-Wilcke et al., 2005; Bendtsen and Jensen, 2006; Mathew, 2006). Decreased antinociceptive activity from supraspinal structures, i.e., deficient descending inhibition, may also contribute to the increased pain sensitivity in chronic TTH (Langemark et al., 1993; Pielsticker et al., 2005; Sandrini et al., 2006).

In an important recent study, Sandrini et al. (2006) demonstrated deficient diffuse noxious inhibitory control in chronic TTH. Impaired descending inhibition could be the primary abnormality or it could contribute to, or be a consequence of, central sensitization (Bendtsen, 2000). Longitudinal studies are needed to clarify this. Thus, present knowledge strongly suggests that the central nervous system is sensitized both at the level of the spinal dorsal horn/trigeminal nucleus and supraspinally in patients with chronic TTH, while the central pain processing seems to be normal in patients with infrequent episodic TTH. An animal model of TTH has been developed (Makowska et al., 2005a). This model allows investigation of the important interactions between peripheral myofascial factors and central sensitization and may prove to be of major importance for the investigations of pathophysiology (Makowska et al., 2005b) and drug development (Makowska et al., 2006; Panfil et al., 2006) in TTH.

The hypothesis of central sensitization in TTH is further supported by clinical pharmacological studies (Bendtsen, 2002). It has been demonstrated that the increased tenderness in patients with chronic TTH can be reduced by treatment with amitriptyline (Bendtsen and Jensen, 2000). Interestingly, the reduction in tenderness could be ascribed solely to the group of patients who responded to amitriptyline treatment while the smaller group of non-responders had unchanged levels of pericranial myofascial tenderness. The reduction of myofascial tenderness during treatment with amitriptyline may be caused by a segmental reduction of central sensitization in combination with an enhanced efficacy of noradrenergic or serotonergic descending inhibition (Bendtsen and Jensen, 2000).

Animal studies have shown that sensitization of pain pathways may be caused by or associated with activation of nitric oxide synthase (NOS) and the generation of nitric oxide (NO) and that NOS inhibitors reduce central sensitization in animal models of persistent pain (Meller and Gebhart, 1993). On the basis of these findings and the hypothesis of central sensitization in chronic TTH, Ashina et al. (2000) demonstrated that infusion of the NO donor, glyceryl trinitrate, induces TTH in these patients. In addition, the same group investigated the analgesic effect of the NOS inhibitor N^{G}-monomethyl-L-arginine hydrochloride (L-NMMA). This drug significantly reduced headache (Ashina et al., 1999c) as well as pericranial myofascial tenderness and hardness (Ashina et al., 1999a) in patients with chronic TTH. Sarchielli et al. (2002) reported increased platelet NOS activity in patients with chronic TTH, possibly reflecting central upregulation of NOS. These pharmacological data support that central sensitization is involved in the pathophysiology of chronic TTH. Moreover, these findings suggest that inhibition of NO and thereby central sensitization may become a novel means of future treatment of chronic TTH.

To summarize, a large number of pain perception studies and pharmacological studies consistently demonstrate that central pain modulation is abnormal in chronic TTH. It is most likely that central sensitization plays a pivotal role for the chronification of TTH.

A MODEL OF TENSION-TYPE HEADACHE

Individual episode

In healthy subjects, the processing of pain from myofascial tissues is finely regulated, such that the degree of perceived pain is appropriate for the actual situation. The nociceptive system allows the detection of potential harmful events and enables the individual to react appropriately to these, e.g., to avoid unphysiological working positions that cause painful pericranial muscles and headache. The painful stimulus from the periphery is usually eliminated by actions from the individual and, if necessary, by local reparative mechanisms in the myofascial tissues, and the properties of the nociceptive system will normally not be altered after a short-lasting painful episode. This may be representative for the nociceptive system in subjects with rare episodes of TTH.

Under some conditions, the painful stimulus from the pericranial myofascial tissues may be more prolonged or more intense than normal. The mechanisms behind this are not known but may include increased muscle activity or the release of various chemical mediators secondary to local pathological conditions. Increased muscle activity secondary to psychogenic stress is likely to be of relevance in this respect, because the psychogenic stress condition may cause a prolonged increase of muscle tone via the limbic system and at the same time potentiate pain facilitation from the brainstem to the spinal dorsal horn (Merskey, 1994). In most subjects these conditions will be self-limiting due to central pain modulatory mechanisms and local reparative processes, and will be experienced as frequent headache episodes for a limited period of time.

How chronicity may develop

In predisposed individuals, the prolonged nociceptive input from the pericranial myofascial tissues may lead to sensitization of nociceptive second-order neurons at the level of the spinal dorsal/trigeminal nucleus (Figure 29.2). The pathophysiological basis for the increased susceptibility to central sensitization is unknown. Possible mechanisms include an impaired

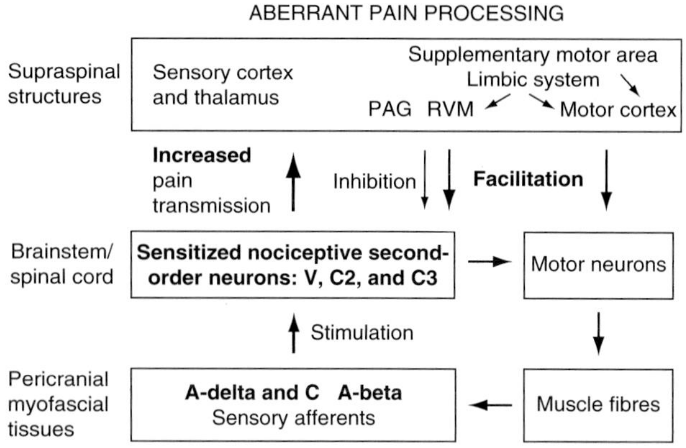

Fig. 29.2. A model of chronic tension-type headache. The model states that the main problem in chronic tension-type headache is sensitization of dorsal horn neurons due to increased nociceptive inputs from pericranial myofascial tissues. Important alterations from the normal pain state are presented in bold. The nociceptive input from myofascial A-delta and C fibers is increased for unknown reasons, resulting in plastic changes in the spinal dorsal horn/trigeminal nucleus. The increased nociceptive stimulation of supraspinal structures may result in increased facilitation and decreased inhibition of pain transmission at the level of the spinal dorsal horn/trigeminal nucleus and in increased pericranial muscle activity. Together these mechanisms may induce and maintain the chronic pain condition. V: Trigeminal nerve; C2 and C3: second and third cervical segment of the spinal cord; PAG: periaqueductal gray; RVM: rostral ventromedial medulla. (Modified from Bendtsen, 2000.)

supraspinal inhibition of nociceptive transmission in the spinal dorsal horn. In the sensitized state, the afferent Aβ fibers that normally inhibit Aδ and C fibers by presynaptic mechanisms in the dorsal horn will on the contrary stimulate the nociceptive second-order neurons. In addition, the effect of Aδ and C fiber stimulation of the nociceptive dorsal horn neurons will be potentiated, and the receptive fields of the dorsal horn neurons will be expanded (Coderre et al., 1993). The nociceptive input to supraspinal structures will therefore be considerably increased, which may result in increased excitability of supraspinal neurons as well as decreased inhibition or increased facilitation of nociceptive transmission in the spinal dorsal horn, i.e., in generalized pain hypersensitivity. The central neuroplastic changes may also increase the drive to motor neurons both at the supraspinal and at the segmental level, resulting in slightly increased muscle activity and in increased muscle hardness. It is possible that low-grade tension that normally does not result in pain does so in the presence of central sensitization. By these mechanisms the central sensitization may be maintained even after the initial eliciting factors have

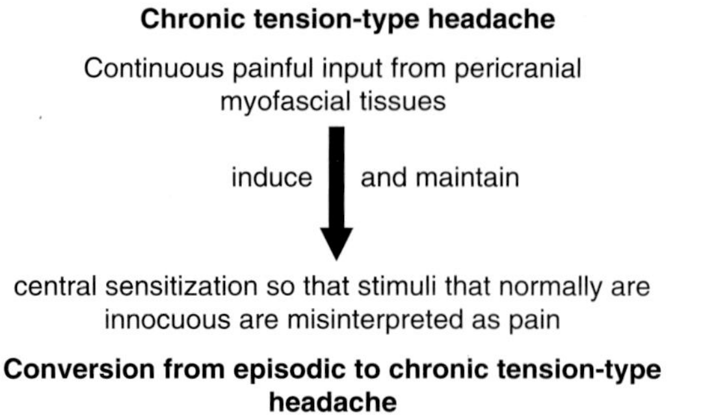

Fig. 29.3. The proposed pathophysiological model of chronic tension-type headache delineates two major aims for future research: (1) to identify the source of peripheral nociception in order to prevent the development of central sensitization in patients with episodic tension-type headache; and (2) to reduce established central sensitization in patients with chronic tension-type headache. (Modified from Bendtsen, 2000.)

been normalized, and the individual will experience daily headaches. This hypothesis (Bendtsen, 2000) may account for most, but not all, cases of chronic TTH. In some patients the central dysfunction, e.g., deficient supraspinal descending inhibition, may be the primary abnormality making the individual more susceptible to a normal level of nociceptive input, and in other patients the disorder may be purely central with no interaction with the periphery.

To summarize, pericranial myofascial mechanisms are probably of importance in episodic TTH whereas sensitization of pain pathways in the central nervous system due to prolonged nociceptive stimuli from pericranial myofascial tissues seems to be responsible for the conversion of episodic to chronic TTH (Figure 29.3). This hypothesis delineates two major targets for future treatment strategies: (1) to identify the source of peripheral nociception in order to prevent the development of central sensitization and thereby the conversion of episodic into chronic TTH; and (2) to reduce established central sensitization (Jensen, 1999; Bendtsen, 2000; Ashina, 2004; Milanov and Bogdanova, 2004).

References

Ashina M (2004). Neurobiology of chronic tension-type headache. Cephalalgia 24: 161–172.

Ashina M, Bendtsen L, Jensen R et al. (1999a). Possible mechanisms of action of nitric oxide synthase inhibitors in chronic tension-type headache. Brain 122: 1629–1635.

Ashina M, Bendtsen L, Jensen R et al. (1999b). Muscle hardness in patients with chronic tension-type headache: relation to actual headache state. Pain 79: 201–205.

Ashina M, Lassen LH, Bendtsen L et al. (1999c). Effect of inhibition of nitric oxide synthase on chronic tension-type headache: a randomised crossover trial. Lancet 353: 287–289.

Ashina M, Bendtsen L, Jensen R et al. (2000). Nitric oxide-induced headache in patients with chronic tension-type headache. Brain 123: 1830–1837.

Ashina M, Stallknecht B, Bendtsen L et al. (2002). In vivo evidence of altered skeletal muscle blood flow in chronic tension-type headache. Brain 125: 320–326.

Ashina M, Stallknecht B, Bendtsen L et al. (2003). Tender points are not sites of ongoing inflammation – in vivo evidence in patients with chronic tension-type headache. Cephalalgia 23: 109–116.

Ashina S, Bendtsen L, Ashina M (2005). Pathophysiology of tension-type headache. Curr Pain Headache Rep 9: 415–422.

Ashina S, Bendtsen L, Ashina M et al. (2006). Generalized hyperalgesia in patients with chronic tension-type headache. Cephalalgia 26: 940–948.

Bendtsen L (2000). Central sensitization in tension-type headache – possible pathophysiological mechanisms. Cephalalgia 20: 486–508.

Bendtsen L (2002). Sensitization: its role in primary headache. Curr Opin Invest Drugs 3: 449–453.

Bendtsen L, Jensen R (2000). Amitriptyline reduces myofascial tenderness in patients with chronic tension-type headache. Cephalalgia 20: 603–610.

Bendtsen L, Jensen R (2006). Tension-type headache: the most common, but also the most neglected, headache disorder. Curr Opin Neurol 19: 305–309.

Bendtsen L, Schoenen J (2005). Synthesis of tension-type headache mechanisms. In: J Olesen, PJ Goadsby, N Ramadan et al. (Eds.), The Headaches. Lippincott Williams & Wilkins, Philadelphia, pp. 677–681.

Bendtsen L, Treede RD (2005). Sensitization of myofascial pain pathways in tension-type headaches. In: J Olesen, PJ Goadsby, N Ramadan et al. (Eds.), The Headaches. Lippincott Williams & Wilkins, Philadelphia, pp. 635–639.

Bendtsen L, Jensen R, Olesen J (1996a). Decreased pain detection and tolerance thresholds in chronic tension-type headache. Arch Neurol 53: 373–376.

Bendtsen L, Jensen R, Olesen J (1996b). Qualitatively altered nociception in chronic myofascial pain. Pain 65: 259–264.

Bovim G (1992). Cervicogenic headache, migraine, and tension-type headache. Pressure–pain threshold measurements. Pain 51: 169–173.

Buchgreitz L, Lyngberg AC, Bendtsen L et al. (2006). Frequency of headache is related to sensitization: a population study. Pain 123: 19–27.

Buchgreitz L, Lyngberg A, Bendtsen L et al. (2007). Increased prevalence of tension-type headache over a 12-year period is related to increased pain sensitivity. A population study. Cephalalgia 27: 145–152.

Christensen M, Bendtsen L, Ashina M et al. (2005). Experimental induction of muscle tenderness and headache in tension-type headache patients. Cephalalgia 25: 1061–1067.

Coderre TJ, Katz J, Vaccarino AL et al. (1993). Contribution of central neuroplasticity to pathological pain: review of clinical and experimental evidence. Pain 52: 259–285.

Fernandez-de-Las-Penas C, Alonso-Blanco C, Cuadrado ML et al. (2006a). Myofascial trigger points and their relationship to headache clinical parameters in chronic tension-type headache. Headache 46: 1264–1272.

Fernandez-de-Las-Penas C, Alonso-Blanco C, Cuadrado ML et al. (2006b). Trigger points in the suboccipital muscles and forward head posture in tension-type headache. Headache 46: 454–460.

Fernandez-de-Las-Penas C, Cuadrado ML, Pareja JA (2007). Myofascial trigger points, neck mobility, and forward head posture in episodic tension-type headache. Headache 47: 662–672.

Göbel H, Weigle L, Kropp P et al. (1992). Pain sensitivity and pain reactivity of pericranial muscles in migraine and tension-type headache. Cephalalgia 12: 142–151.

Heckman BD, Holroyd KA (2006). Tension-type headache and psychiatric comorbidity. Curr Pain Headache Rep 10: 439–447.

Hubbard DR, Berkoff GM (1993). Myofascial trigger points show spontaneous needle EMG activity. Spine 18: 1803–1807.

Janke EA, Holroyd KA, Romanek K (2004). Depression increases onset of tension-type headache following laboratory stress. Pain 111: 230–238.

Jensen R (1996). Mechanisms of spontaneous tension-type headaches: an analysis of tenderness, pain thresholds and EMG. Pain 64: 251–256.

Jensen R (1999). Pathophysiological mechanisms of tension-type headache: a review of epidemiological and experimental studies. Cephalalgia 19: 602–621.

Jensen R, Becker WJ (2005). Symptomatology of episodic tension-type headaches. In: J Olesen, PJ Goadsby, N Ramadan et al. (Eds.), The Headaches. Lippincott Williams Wilkins, Philadelphia, pp. 685–692.

Jensen R, Olesen J (1996). Initiating mechanisms of experimentally induced tension-type headache. Cephalalgia 16: 175–182.

Jensen R, Rasmussen BK, Pedersen B et al. (1993). Muscle tenderness and pressure pain thresholds in headache. A population study. Pain 52: 193–199.

Jensen R, Bendtsen L, Olesen J (1998). Muscular factors are of importance in tension-type headache. Headache 38: 10–17.

Langemark M, Olesen J (1987). Pericranial tenderness in tension headache. A blind, controlled study. Cephalalgia 7: 249–255.

Langemark M, Jensen K, Jensen TS et al. (1989). Pressure pain thresholds and thermal nociceptive thresholds in chronic tension-type headache. Pain 38: 203–210.

Langemark M, Bach FW, Jensen TS et al. (1993). Decreased nociceptive flexion reflex threshold in chronic tension-type headache. Arch Neurol 50: 1061–1064.

Lipchik GL, Holroyd KA, O'Donnell FJ et al. (2000). Exteroceptive suppression periods and pericranial muscle tenderness in chronic tension-type headache: effects of psychopathology, chronicity and disability. Cephalalgia 20: 638–646.

Lyngberg AC, Rasmussen BK, Jorgensen T et al. (2005a). Has the prevalence of migraine and tension-type headache changed over a 12-year period? A Danish population survey. Eur J Epidemiol 20: 243–249.

Lyngberg AC, Rasmussen BK, Jorgensen T et al. (2005b). Incidence of primary headache: a Danish epidemiologic follow-up study. Am J Epidemiol 161: 1066–1073.

Makowska A, Panfil C, Ellrich J (2005a). Long-term potentiation of orofacial sensorimotor processing by noxious input from the semispinal neck muscle in mice. Cephalalgia 25: 109–116.

Makowska A, Panfil C, Ellrich J (2005b). Nerve growth factor injection into semispinal neck muscle evokes sustained facilitation of the jaw-opening reflex in anesthetized mice – possible implications for tension-type headache. Exp Neurol 191: 301–309.

Makowska A, Panfil C, Ellrich J (2006). ATP induces sustained facilitation of craniofacial nociception through P2X receptors on neck muscle nociceptors in mice. Cephalalgia 26: 697–706.

Mathew NT (2006). Tension-type headache. Curr Neurol Neurosci Rep 6: 100–105.

Meller ST, Gebhart GF (1993). Nitric oxide (NO) and nociceptive processing in the spinal cord. Pain 52: 127–136.

Mense S (1993). Nociception from skeletal muscle in relation to clinical muscle pain. Pain 54: 241–289.

Mense S, Simons DG, Hoheisel U et al. (2003). Lesions of rat skeletal muscle after local block of acetylcholinesterase and neuromuscular stimulation. J Appl Physiol 94: 2494–2501.

Merskey H (1994). Pain and psychological medicine. In: PD Wall, R Melzack (Eds.), Textbook of Pain. Churchill Livingstone, Edinburgh, pp. 903–920.

Milanov I, Bogdanova D (2004). Pain and tension-type headache: a review of the possible pathophysiological mechanisms. J Headache Pain 5: 4–11.

Mork H, Ashina M, Bendtsen L et al. (2003). Induction of prolonged tenderness in patients with tension-type headache by means of a new experimental model of myofascial pain. Eur J Neurol 10: 249–256.

Mork H, Ashina M, Bendtsen L et al. (2004). Possible mechanisms of pain perception in patients with episodic tension-type headache. A new experimental model of myofascial pain. Cephalalgia 24: 466–475.

Newham DJ, Edwards RHT, Mills KR (1994). Skeletal muscle pain. In: PD Wall, R Melzack (Eds.), Textbook of Pain. Churchill Livingstone, Edinburgh, pp. 423–440.

Østergaard S, Russell MB, Bendtsen L et al. (1997). Comparison of first degree relatives and spouses of people with chronic tension headache. BMJ 12: 1092–1093.

Panfil C, Makowska A, Ellrich J (2006). Brainstem and cervical spinal cord Fos immunoreactivity evoked by nerve growth factor injection into neck muscles in mice. Cephalalgia 26: 128–135.

Pielsticker A, Haag G, Zaudig M et al. (2005). Impairment of pain inhibition in chronic tension-type headache. Pain 118: 215–223.

Russell MB, Iselius L, Olesen J (1998). Inheritance of chronic tension-type headache investigated by complex segregation analysis. Hum Genet 102: 138–140.

Sandrini G, Rossi P, Milanov I et al. (2006). Abnormal modulatory influence of diffuse noxious inhibitory controls in migraine and chronic tension-type headache patients. Cephalalgia 26: 782–789.

Sarchielli P, Alberti A, Floridi A et al. (2002). L-Arginine/nitric oxide pathway in chronic tension-type headache: relation with serotonin content and secretion and glutamate content. J Neurol Sci 198: 9–15.

Schmidt-Hansen PT, Svensson P, Bendtsen L et al. (2006a). Increased muscle pain sensitivity in patients with tension-type headache. Pain 129: 113–121.

Schmidt-Hansen PT, Svensson P, Jensen TS et al. (2006b). Patterns of experimentally induced pain in pericranial muscles. Cephalalgia 26: 568–577.

Schmidt-Wilcke T, Leinisch E, Straube A et al. (2005). Gray matter decrease in patients with chronic tension type headache. Neurology 65: 1483–1486.

Schoenen J, Bottin D, Hardy F et al. (1991). Cephalic and extracephalic pressure pain thresholds in chronic tension-type headache. Pain 47: 145–149.

Schwartz BS, Stewart WF, Lipton RB (1997). Lost workdays and decreased work effectiveness associated with headache in the workplace. J Occup Environ Med 39: 320–327.

Simons DG, Mense S (1998). Understanding and measurement of muscle tone as related to clinical muscle pain. Pain 75: 1–17.

Treede RD, Meyer RA, Raja SN et al. (1992). Peripheral and central mechanisms of cutaneous hyperalgesia. Prog Neurobiol 38: 397–421.

Treede RD, Rolke R, Andrews K et al. (2002). Pain elicited by blunt pressure: neurobiological basis and clinical relevance. Pain 98: 235–240.

Vandenheede M, Schoenen J (2002). Central mechanisms in tension-type headaches. Curr Pain Headache Rep 6: 392–400.

Handbook of Clinical Neurology, Vol. 97 (3rd series)
Headache
G. Nappi and M.A. Moskowitz, Editors

Chapter 30

The clinical neurophysiology of tension-type headache

GIORGIO SANDRINI [1]* AND PAOLO ROSSI [1, 2]

[1] *University Center for Adaptive Disorders and Headache (UCADH) and Department of Neurological Sciences, IRCCS "C. Mondino Institute of Neurology" Foundation, Pavia, Italy*

[2] *University Center for Adaptive Disorders and Headache (UCADH), Pavia and Headache Clinic, INI, Grottaferrata (Rome), Italy*

INTRODUCTION

Despite being widely investigated, the pathogenesis of tension-type headache (TTH) continues to be debated. Among the different approaches used to explore the mechanisms underlying TTH, clinical neurophysiology plays an important role.

Studies to date have focused mainly on two areas: (1) evaluation of peripheral factors (i.e., by electromyography (EMG)); and (2) exploration of the role of the pain control system.

In the second of these areas, a large number of studies have explored trigeminal pathways, in particular using reflexes (e.g., the trigeminofacial reflex, trigemino-trigeminal reflexes).

More recently, the descending inhibitory system, known to modulate both the trigeminal and the spinal system, has also been investigated.

In addition, several studies have sought to establish whether there are neurophysiological parameters that could be markers of this condition, but the results of these were inconclusive, since some abnormalities could frequently be observed in migraine too.

ELECTROMYOGRAPHY

Chronic tension or contraction of the pericranial musculature has long been thought to be the primary cause of TTH. Thus, it is not surprising that many researchers turned to EMG in their bid to explore the possibility of a relationship between pericranial muscle activity and TTH. EMG studies in TTH include evaluation of baseline EMG activity and dynamic assessment of EMG changes induced by different experimental conditions or experimental stressors.

EMG surface recording of pericranial muscle activity has yielded contradictory results (for a review, see Pikoff, 1984, and Schoenen and Bendtsen, 2006). As reviewed by Pikoff, about half of the studies published before 1983 gave normal findings, whereas the other half reported increased EMG activity. More recent studies have come out more strongly in favor of increased EMG activity in TTH patients compared with controls under variable experimental conditions (Schoenen and Bendtsen, 2006). However, the differences that emerged related to average values, whereas in single cases EMG activity was of little help when seeking to assign individual subjects to diagnostic groups (Schoenen et al., 1991).

Contrasting results were also obtained when considering pericranial EMG activity in response to stressful laboratory situations (Schoenen and Bendtsen, 2006). In naturalistic studies conducted with portable EMG recorders, TTH patients and controls showed no significant differences in EMG activity variations in response to stressful events (Rugh et al., 1990; Hatch et al., 1991).

Discrepancies emerged in studies investigating EMG activity in patients with and without pericranial muscular disorders (Schoenen et al., 1987; Jensen and Olesen, 1998) and in a few studies using needle EMG to quantify EMG activity in trigger points in chronic TTH (CTTH) patients (McNulty et al., 1994; Schoenen and Bendtsen, 2006). More consistent evidence was found to suggest that pericranial EMG activity was not quantitatively or chronologically related to head pain (Schoenen et al., 1987, Jensen, 1996; Jensen and Olesen, 1996; Schoenen and Bendtsen, 2006). A tooth-clenching challenge used to induce headache in an experimental setting caused a similar decrease

*Correspondence to: Giorgio Sandrini, MD, University Center for Adaptive Disorders and Headache (UCADH) and Department of Neurological Sciences, IRCCS "C. Mondino Institute of Neurology" Foundation, Via Mondino 2, 27100, Pavia, Italy, Tel: 003 903 823 80279, Fax: 003 903 823 80244, E-mail: giorgio.sandrini@unipv.it

in EMG levels both in controls and patients, and in those who developed headache as well as in those who did not (Jensen, 1996). Heterotopic noxious stimulation (in the form of an ischemic pain task) produced dissociated effects on pain sensation and EMG signals (Lehrer and Murphy, 1991). Stress-induced pain was generalized and prolonged in TTH versus headache-free controls, but pain was not associated with increased EMG activity (Leistad et al., 2006). No consistent relationship has been found between a reduction of EMG activity and headache improvement after biofeedback (Schoenen et al., 1987; Rokicki et al., 2003). These data suggest that the increased EMG activity observed at rest was a secondary characteristic rather than a primary cause of pain.

In summary, the main findings of EMG recordings in TTH patients are the following: EMG has no diagnostic usefulness but it is helpful in the exploration of the pathophysiology of TTH. Data on EMG activity of pericranial and neck muscles are discrepant. This variability is partially explained by the use of different methodological conditions and sampling strategies and non-standardized techniques, and by the high intrinsic variability of EMG signals that allows only large effects to be detected. A small majority of the studies argue in favor of slightly increased EMG activity, suggesting insufficient muscle relaxation in TTH. However, experimental data did not show any relation between EMG levels and headache status, thus indicating that muscle activity has no causal role, and is possibly a secondary protective mechanism.

BRAINSTEM REFLEXES

Brainstem structures play a crucial role not only in conveying, but also in modulating nociceptive impulses. Descending modulation of sensory transmission occurs largely in the brainstem. Thus, the study of trigeminofacial and trigeminocervical reflexes (TCRs) may provide valuable insights into central pain control mechanisms.

Exteroceptive suppression of the temporalis muscle

Electrical stimulation of the infraorbital and mental nerves evokes a reflex inhibition of the jaw-closing muscles (the temporalis or masseter inhibitory reflex). On surface EMG recordings from contracted jaw-closers, this reflex appears as two suppression periods, an early one and a late one (SP1 and SP2), both of which are mediated by Aβ fibers. The SP1 response (or ES1, 10–12 ms latency) is mediated by an oligosynaptic pontine pathway. The SP2 response (or ES2, 40–50 ms latency) is mediated by a polysynaptic chain of interneurons probably belonging to the medullary lateral reticular formation. This area is modulated via peripheral and central afferents (the periacqueductal gray, nucleus raphe magnus, limbic cortex, orbitofrontal cortex). Thus, ES2 measurements constitute a neurophysiological correlate of the level of excitability and of the suprasegmental control of these brainstem inhibitory interneurons (Schoenen, 1992).

The duration of the ES2 in TTH at rest has been investigated by many authors, with contradictory results. In episodic TTH (ETTH) and in migraine, the ES2 has been found to be largely normal. In CTTH, the ES2 has been found to be shortened in some studies but not in others (Schoenen and Bendtsen, 2006). These differences between studies may be explained partially by considering the following factors. The analysis is the most critical part of the methodology and the use of manual and unblinded scoring procedures may, in some cases, have yielded spurious and unreliable findings. Methodological differences in the elicitation of the ES2 – up to the year 2000, no two studies used the same procedure and few were conducted according to published recommendations (Lipchik et al., 2000) – might be another important source of these discrepant findings, as might heterogeneous subject samples (with regard to age, sample size, comorbidities, and headache severity and frequency). It is noteworthy that blinded studies including a large number of patients and conducted according to rigorous methodologies have yielded negative findings, as has study of the recovery cycle of the ES2, which is considered more sensitive than baseline recording in measuring the excitability of the reflex (Bendtsen et al., 1996; Lipchik et al., 2000; Aktektin et al., 2001).

Most studies have not documented significant correlations between the ES2, headache severity, headache status, comorbid disorders, and other pain parameters, such as pain thresholds and pericranial muscle tenderness. Studies investigating the effect of conditioning stimuli on the ES2 have demonstrated a differential effect of experimental stressors in TTH patients and controls (Wang and Schoenen, 1994; Bendtsen et al., 1996; Neufeld et al., 2000). It has been documented that TTH patients are more aroused in the experimental situation than healthy controls (Bendtsen et al., 1996), suggesting that the ES2 may reflect the degree of arousal in the examined subject rather than endogenous supraspinal pain control system activity. Wang and Schoenen (1994) found that, when a prior electrical stimulus is applied peripherally, the ES2 is reduced and that this reduction is more pronounced in TTH patients than in controls, possibly on account of brainstem circuit hyperexcitability. Following a jaw-clenching challenge and appropriate placebo procedure, the ES2 area was found to be significantly increased in control subjects whereas it remained unchanged in young TTH patients. These findings have been interpreted as an early sign of central antinociceptive system dysfunction in TTH (Neufeld et al., 2000).

In short, static measurement of the ES2 in CTTH has yielded conflicting results. The majority of high-quality studies failed to find any difference between TTH patients and controls. Several studies suggest that dynamic evaluation of ES2 responses, such as those measuring ES2 reactivity to experimental stressors, might be more sensitive than baseline measures in detecting dysfunction of brain excitability and its supraspinal control.

Blink reflex

The blink reflex (BR) is the surface electromyographic recording (from the orbicularis oculi) of the reflex evoked by a stimulus applied in the area innervated by the trigeminal nerve or directly on a branch of the trigeminal nerve. The BR is commonly evoked by electrical stimulation of the supraorbital nerve and consists of three components: (1) an ipsilateral early component (R1) that is conducted by large afferent myelinated fibers (Aβ fibers) and follows an oligosynaptic pontine pathway passing through the principal trigeminal nucleus; (2) a bilateral late component (R2) that is mainly mediated by Aβ fibers but is relayed to the facial motoneurons through a multisynaptic chain of interneurons belonging to the reticular formation in the lower medulla (the R2 component receives a nociceptive contribution from Aδ afferents converging with Aβ fibers on wide dynamic range neurons in the trigeminal nucleus caudalis and is strongly modulated by suprasegmental influences); and (3) a bilateral ultralate component (R3) that is mainly mediated by activation of Aβ fibers and probably follows the same central pathways as the R2.

Although suggested to be a specific nociceptive component of the BR, the R3 may be part of an aspecific startle reflex and is not considered in clinical neurophysiology studies investigating brainstem function. To focus on the nociceptive component of the R2, Kaube et al. (2000) developed a novel stimulation technique, the nociceptive-specific BR (nBR). Until now, the BR has only been investigated by means of the standard technique. Sand et al. conducted two studies. In the first of these, published in 1994, the authors found no significant difference in the R1 and R2 latencies between 11 CTTH patients and 9 controls (Sand and Zwart, 1994). In a more recent study, the same authors evaluated R2 amplitude as an electrophysiological marker of brainstem excitability (Sand et al., 2006). The R2 integrated amplitude was not significantly affected in 12 CTTH patients compared with 17 controls.

Normal R2 amplitude and area were also reported by Avramidis et al. (1998) (10 ETTH patients examined during a headache phase and 30 controls) and Aktekin et al. (2001) (20 patients with CTTH, 12 patients with ETTH, 20 controls). In the latter study the authors evaluated the recovery cycle of the BR as a more sensitive index of brainstem excitability. They found a slowed recovery cycle of the R2 in both the ETTH and the CTTH patients compared with controls and migraineurs, in the presence of a normal recovery curve of the ES2. These findings were interpreted as an effect of a reduction of excitability of the brainstem interneurons rather than as an effect of excessive inhibition.

In summary, BR studies indicate that brainstem excitability, as explored by the standard, static evaluation of the reflex, is largely normal in TTH patients. As with other brainstem reflexes, a dynamic assessment of the BR (e.g., performed in a recovery cycle paradigm) revealed specific brainstem hypoexcitability in TTH. However this finding needs to be replicated in further blinded studies, also investigating larger samples, before definite conclusions can be drawn.

Trigeminocervical reflexes

The evaluation of trigeminal reflexes may be extended to the extracranial neck muscles by measuring cervical muscle responses after electrical stimulation of the supraorbital or infraorbital nerve. TCRs can be obtained by recording from several neck muscles (sternocleidomastoid muscle (SCM), semispinalis capiti muscle) at different levels of activity. They comprise early and late responses that probably have different functional significance. Whereas the early responses are mediated by non-nociceptive afferents and functionally resemble the R1 component of the BR, the late responses have been related to head retraction movements (protective responses to nociceptive stimuli applied to the face). An oligosynaptic pathway confined to the lower brainstem seems to mediate the early responses whereas a polysynaptic pathway involving the pontomedullary reticular formation seems to mediate the late responses.

The TCR may offer several potential advantages over the BR: (1) the TCR may make it possible to explore directly the anatomofunctional connection between the trigeminal afferents and the upper cervical spinal cord neurons and its modulation by supraspinal inhibitory pathways; (2) its early response is much easier to measure than the BR response, seems to be more sensitive in disclosing brainstem abnormality, and is less influenced by supratentorial abnormalities;

and (3) its late response has a clear nociceptive function and may be used as a clinical tool for pain evaluation.

Different patterns of abnormal findings have been found in two recent studies investigating the TCR in TTH patients using different methods and electrophysiological parameters. Milanov and Bogdanova (2003) investigated the late responses recorded in the resting SCM after stimulation of the supraorbital nerve in 15 CTTH patients and 15 migraineurs, suffering from predominantly unilateral headache, and 32 controls. In both the CTTH patients and the migraineurs the TCR on the painful side showed a shortened latency when compared with the non-painful side and with healthy individuals. The authors interpreted these findings as the effect of reduced inhibitory activity of brainstem interneurons reflecting abnormal endogenous pain mechanisms operating both in migraine and in TTH. Nardone and Tezzon (2003) investigated the early TCR recorded in the active SCM in 15 ETTH patients, 15 CTTH patients (outside the pain attack), and 15 controls. In the CTTH patients the TCR amplitude was significantly decreased bilaterally, whereas the TCR latency was significantly increased when compared with the controls. No significant difference was found in the ETTH patients. In the CTTH patients the occurrence of TCR abnormalities correlated with abnormal pericranial tenderness. The authors hypothesized the presence of disturbed brainstem interneuronal activity controlling the pericranial muscles, specific to CTTH patients, but the functional significance of these findings, which argue in favor of a hypoactive status, are unclear and difficult to fit into the current pathophysiological model of TTH.

NOCICEPTIVE FLEXION REFLEX

The nociceptive flexion reflex (NFR) recorded in the lower limbs is a polysynaptic, multisegmental spinal response inducing a complex, protective flexion synergy of the stimulated limb. It is mediated by a complex circuitry modulated at spinal and supraspinal levels (Sandrini et al., 2005). At rest, the flexion reflex appears as a double burst composed of an early, inconstantly present component, called the RII reflex, and a late, larger, and more stable component, called the RIII reflex. Due to its neurophysiological properties (namely, a strong correlation between the pain intensity stimulus–response curve and the reflex size stimulus–response curve, and good standardization and reproducibility), several researchers have used the RIII component of the NFR as an objective and quantitative measure of experimental pain in clinical research in order to investigate pain pathways at spinal and supraspinal level, and to study the pathophysiology of chronic painful disorders (Sandrini et al., 2005).

Studies using the NFR have been conducted only in patients with CTTH and have yielded conflicting data. A significant reduction of the pain threshold/reflex threshold (Tp/Tr) ratio, related to a significant reduction in the subjective pain threshold with normal Tr, has been suggested to be a distinctive feature of CTTH (Sandrini et al., 1991). In contrast, patients with chronic migraine, defined as "migraine with interparoxysmal headaches," presented a significant reduction of the RIII threshold but a normal Tp/Tr ratio (Sandrini et al., 1986, 1991). A significant correlation between Tp/Tr ratio and Hamilton Rating Scales for Anxiety was found in both groups. Taken together, these data indicate the existence of an impairment of psychological and neural mechanisms of pain in chronic headaches.

Amplification of subjective nociceptive perception seems to be a typical feature of the CTTH biotype while a reduced inhibitory tone of pain might characterize chronic migraineurs (Sandrini et al., 1993). Such findings have not been completely replicated in other studies. Boureau et al. (1991) found no difference in RIII threshold between patients with chronic pain (9 with headaches and 9 with myofascial syndromes) and controls, but these patients were on treatment, including antidepressants, which may explain the absence of reflex changes. These earliest studies are flawed by serious methodological biases, such as the failure to take medication overuse into consideration, the use of old diagnostic criteria, and the inclusion of a low number of patients under treatment.

In agreement with data obtained from pain sensitivity studies, the most recent research assessing the NFR in CTTH patients revealed a significantly lower reflex threshold than in the control group (Langemark et al., 1993; Sandrini et al., 2006). In the study by Langemark et al., a high degree of correlation was found between NFR threshold and tolerated stimulus strength, and the stimulus intensity/visual analogue scale pain rating response curves were steeper in patients with CTTH than in control subjects. In the paper by Sandrini et al. (2006), the NFR threshold and subjective pain threshold were significantly lower in CTTH patients (with no overt psychiatric comorbidity) than in controls, whereas no difference was found in episodic migraineurs. In this study the authors evaluated the function of supraspinal pain modulating systems subserving "diffuse noxious inhibitory controls" (DNICs) by studying the effects of heterotopic noxious conditioning stimulation, in the form of the cold pressor test, on the NFR.

A dysfunction of DNIC mechanisms has been found in patients with different chronic painful disorder (Kosek and Ordeberg, 2000; Desmeules et al., 2003), suggesting that defective DNIC activity may induce facilitation of central sensitization leading to chronic pain syndromes. As expected, Sandrini et al. (2006) observed a significant inhibition of the RIII reflex during the cold pressor test in controls (–30%, $P < 0.05$). Conversely, migraine and CTTH patients showed facilitation (+31%, $P < 0.05$ and +40%, $P < 0.01$, respectively) of the RIII reflex during the heterotopic noxious conditioning stimulation that persisted for a significantly prolonged time in the CTTH patients. No significant correlation was found between clinical parameters and neurophysiological findings. In CTTH, a deficient DNIC-like inhibitory mechanism with normal pain thresholds has been found by other authors using subjective methods (electrical threshold and pain threshold at cranial and extracranial sites: Pielsticker et al., 2005). These findings suggest that an impairment of endogenous supraspinal pain modulation systems, such as the descending inhibitory pathways subserving DNICs, may be an important common denominator in the pain mechanism of both CTTH and migraine.

In summary, if we consider only high-quality NFR studies on CTTH patients, the results confirm the presence of spinal cord hyperexcitability to peripheral noxious stimuli applied at extracephalic healthy sites, that is, central sensitization of nociceptive pathways. When considered in the context of available literature data (mainly data from pain sensitivity studies that show, in CTTH, a non-specific and widespread hypersensitivity to pain stimuli), and given the steeper pain intensity stimulus–response curve, and the defective DNIC-like mechanisms, these findings may be interpreted as evidence of a dysfunction of descending inhibitory pathways.

Interestingly, a very similar pattern of neurophysiological abnormalities (i.e., lowered NFR threshold, DNIC dysfunction, and qualitatively altered pain pressure function) has been found in fibromyalgia, another chronic musculoskeletal pain state. These similarities in the neurophysiological findings observed in a generalized and a regional pain syndrome raise several questions that future research must seek to answer. Are the neurophysiological findings specific to musculoskeletal chronic pain conditions or common to chronic pain states? Do the NFR abnormalities reflect common pathophysiological mechanisms, such as a prolonged input from muscle nociceptors, or are they the final effects of different dynamic pathogenic mechanisms? Do the neurophysiological findings precede or are they the consequence of the manifestations of the disease? What mechanisms account for pain location?

ELECTROENCEPHALOGRAPHY

Only a few studies have investigated electroencephalography (EEG) data in TTH patients and, as is to be expected when using a highly subjective and heterogeneously applied neurophysiological method (de Tommaso et al., 1999), the findings they have given have been inconclusive and contrasting. It is commonly held that EEG is not useful for discriminating primary headaches from secondary headaches and is not helpful in distinguishing TTH from migraine (Sandrini et al., 2004). In a pathophysiological setting, the study of sensory and cognitive evoked responses has proved to be much more useful than EEG recordings.

EVOKED POTENTIALS

Visual evoked potentials (VEPs)

VEPs are electrical potential differences recorded from the scalp in response to visual stimuli. VEPs to stimuli repeated at low rates are defined as transient VEPs. Steady-state visual evoked potentials (SVEPs) are responses to visual stimuli at relatively high frequencies (above 3.5/s). In normal subjects low-frequency VEPs are widely distributed over the scalp whereas SVEPs are restricted to a region lateral and anterior to the striate cortex. In migraine the majority of VEP studies demonstrate interictally increased amplitude of grand averages or lack of habituation in sequential blocks of averagings (Ambrosini et al., 2003). The habituation pattern may have a familial character. This indicates that information processing in the visual cortex is abnormal in migraineurs between attacks and that it could represent an endophenotypic marker for the disorder.

Only two studies have investigated VEPs in adult TTH. In an attempt to assess the possibility of discriminating between migraine and TTH using objective neurophysiological measures, de Tommaso et al. (1999) investigated SVEPs in 120 patients with migraine, 64 patients with TTH (33 ETTH, 31 CTTH), and 51 controls. The F1M was significantly increased in both migraine and TTH patients on multiple electrode sites. The TTH patients could not be distinguished from the migraineurs by SVEP measures and discriminative analysis could correctly distinguish only control subjects. These findings led the authors to hypothesize the presence of a common neural dysfunction in the two headache types consisting of exaggerated brain responses to visual stimuli, possibly secondary to abnormal cortical inhibition of subcortical origin.

Wang et al. (1999) investigated the habituation of low-frequency VEPs and arousal-related personality trait in 22 migraineurs, 13 ETTH patients, 20 CTTH patients, and 26 controls. In contrast with the migraineurs, the TTH patients had normal habituation slopes of the N1–P1 and P1–N2 components and no significant correlation between neurophysiological and neuropsycological measures. These findings suggest that a defective habituation response to repeated stimuli is specific to migraine, as confirmed by other studies using different sensory stimuli (Valeriani et al., 2003; Flor et al., 2004).

Laser evoked potentials (LEPs)

Over the past 25 years, several research groups have adopted LEPs for the objective and quantitative assessment of nociception and nociceptive pathways in both clinical and pathopysiological settings. Brief radiant heat pulses, such as those delivered by carbon dioxide laser beams, selectively activate the peripheral thermonociceptors without eliciting responses from Aβ mechanoceptors. The ascending signals following laser stimulation are conducted through Aδ fibers (and C fibers) and the spinothalamic tract. Unlike the standard electrical method, or (e)SEP, the LEP method does not detect the peripheral, spinal, or brainstem components of the LEP response and only identifies the "late" component. The Aδ nociceptors evoke two main late components: (1) an initial negativity which appears at least 150 ms after the onset of the stimulus and is referred to as N1 (-P1), or the middle-latency component, representing the first stage of sufficient neural synchronization; this component is thought to be specific to the secondary somatosensory cortex (SII); (2) a negative/positive biphasic deflection referred to as the vertex potential or N2a–P2 component. This is the most conspicuous response to laser stimulation and is thought to be an aspecific vertex response generated from a source in the cingulate cortex whose activity, after laser stimulation, is linked to the attention and orienting reaction triggered by pain and represents the physiological correlate of the integrated central nervous system processing that underlies the perception of pain.

LEP activity in CTTH patients was investigated by de Tommaso et al. and Valeriani et al., in three papers that gave partially contrasting findings. In a multicenter study, LEPs were studied in 19 CTTH patients, 24 migraineurs (pain-free phase), and 28 controls (Valeriani et al., 2003). No significant difference was found for the latency or amplitude value of any LEP component after either hand or face stimulation (supraorbital area). In addition, the CTTH patients and controls presented normal habituation of the LEP, whereas the migraineurs showed significantly reduced habituation. A normal pattern of habituation to painful electrical stimuli has been confirmed in another study using psychophysiological measures (Flor et al., 2004). These findings argue in favor of normal trigeminal nociceptive function and cortical pain processing in CTTH. In another study (de Tommaso et al., 2003), the authors evaluated the heat–pain threshold and LEP amplitude in 12 patients and 11 controls during a pain-free phase. The heat–pain threshold did not differ between patients and controls at the level of either the hand or of the pericranial skin, whereas the amplitude of the N2–P2 complex was significantly increased in the CTTH patients after stimulation of the skin over the pericranial muscles. LEP amplitude was significantly correlated with the total tenderness score but not with headache duration and frequency.

These findings were partly confirmed in a second study (de Tommaso et al., 2006), where a topographic analysis of LEPs was performed in 18 patients and 12 controls to examine simultaneously the discriminative and attentive components of pain. Pain ratings and the N1 component did not differ between patients and controls, whereas N2 and P2 amplitude was increased after stimulation of pericranial skin and the P2 amplitude was correlated with total tenderness score levels and anxiety scores. Topographic analysis showed a peculiar increase of N2 and especially P2 measured at the vertex region; a significant increase of LEP amplitude after stimulation of the hand was found as well. The authors interpreted these findings as evidence of an increased cortical pain-specific hypervigilance to pericranial stimuli facilitating the development of pericranial muscle tenderness.

Further studies conducted by different research groups and including larger samples and ETTH patients are necessary to establish the pathophysiological value of these findings.

Event-related potentials (ERPs)

ERPs are brain responses that are time-locked to some event, such as a sensory stimulus, a mental event, or the omission of a stimulus. Depending on the experimental paradigm used to evoke the brain responses, several ERPs may be investigated exploring different aspects of cognitive functioning.

Contingent negative variation (CNV) is an ERP recorded over the frontal area in a reaction time paradigm with a warning and an imperative stimulus. CNV is thought to reflect certain aspects of cortical information processing and to characterize the cortical activation level (Kropp and Berger, 1993). The early component seems to be modulated by the noradrenergic system and measures the level of expectation, whereas the late component is under the influence of the dopaminergic system and indicates motor readiness. In contrast to the findings of an increased CNV amplitude with reduced habituation (more pronounced for the early component) obtained in migraineurs (Ambrosini et al., 2003), patients with ETTH and CTTH had a normal CNV amplitude (Maertens de Noordhout et al., 1986).

The P300 component obtained by the classical active "oddball paradigm" (P3b) is a brain potential reflecting the neural activity elicited by mental work during evaluation and categorization of cognitive tests and depends on aminergic and cholinergic brain mediators. In conformity with CNV data, no abnormality of the P300 parameters was found in ETTH patients in the interictal phase (Mazzotta et al., 1995; Demirci and Savas, 2002) or during the headache attack (Mazzotta et al., 1995). ETTH patients presented a normal degree of habituation of the P300 when compared to chronic low-back pain patients, suggesting the presence of disturbed attentional processing in chronic pain sufferers (Demirci and Savas, 2002). The active P300 is a measure of active attentional processes. Passive attentional resources may be investigated by an ERP technique, the passive paradigm single-tone elicited ERP. This technique was used in a recent study by Chen et al. (2007) to investigate 32 patients suffering from CTTH, 17 with frequent ETTH, and 32 with interictal migraine without aura, as well as 28 healthy subjects. No significant differences were found among the groups in the latency and amplitude of the N1, P2, and N2 components or the P3 latency. By contrast, the P300 amplitude was significantly reduced in patients when compared to healthy subjects, but there was no difference between patient groups. These findings suggest the presence of a deficiency of passive attention that is common to TTH and migraine, unrelated to the headache frequency but possibly due to the experience of head pain *per se*.

In summary, the few studies investigating ERPs in ETTH and CTTH patients give largely normal findings. The finding of a deficiency of passive attention needs to be replicated in other studies using more extensive scalp recording and considering the potential influence of psychiatric comorbidity and headache status (Table 30.1).

CLINICAL NEUROPHYSIOLOGY OF TTH IN CHILDREN AND ADOLESCENTS

TTH is a common and disabling problem in children and adolescents. However, neurophysiological studies of TTH are rare in this age group, since researchers' attention has been focused more on migraine. As with adults, neurophysiological studies, in children, are of little value for the differential diagnosis of primary versus secondary headache and for the diagnosis of primary headache subtypes. Nevertheless, they are particularly interesting from a pathophysiological point of view for at least two reasons. First, they allow the disease to be investigated in its early stages, when it is little influenced by environmental factors and drug use. Second, they can be used to look for the presence of impaired maturation of sensory information processing in the brain. For ethical and practical reasons only non-painful techniques have been used.

No study investigating EMG, brainstem or spinal reflexes has been carried out in children with TTH. Few studies have evaluated the EEG (quantitative and qualitative analysis), VEPs and brainstem auditory EPs in TTH children. In contrast to young migraineurs, children with TTH did not show significant abnormalities when compared with healthy controls (Puca and de Tommaso, 1999; Ramirez-Segura et al., 1999).

CNV studies reported differences in CNV amplitudes between migraine children and children with TTH. Like affected adults, children with migraine had an increased amplitude of CNV and an increased motor postimperative negative variation, especially on and around the vertex (Besken et al., 1993; Cherniak et al., 2001). Instead, children with TTH, in contrast to findings obtained in adulthood, showed a tendency to suppression of CNV possibly secondary to an inhibitory effect of chronic pain or to the associated psychopathological status (Besken et al., 1993). However these differences have not been completely replicated in more recent studies (Bender et al., 2006). Bender et al. investigated the age-dependent development of ERPs in headache children (Bender et al., 2002, 2006, 2007). They found evidence of impaired maturation of information processing in migraine, mainly the lack of CNV age-dependent development around the vertex with no difference regarding the maturation of frontal and temporal contributions to N1b. The authors speculated that this neurophysiological pattern is underlain by an unspecific subcortical activation of the brainstem during all attention-demanding CNV tasks. Strong maturational abnormalities were not found in TTH but the sample size was too small to reveal significant age-dependent correlations and further studies are needed to provide definitive conclusions. In summary, neurophysiological studies of TTH in children and adolescents are rare. Preliminary findings seem to support the view that migraine and TTH are different disorders with regard to the information-processing activity.

Table 30.1

Clinical neurophysiology of tension-type headache (TTH)

Technique	Number of studies	Main findings	Comment
EMG activity	>20	A small majority of the studies are in favor of slightly increased EMG activity, indicating insufficient muscle relaxation in TTH. Experimental data did not show any relation between EMG levels and headache status, suggesting that muscle activity plays no causal role and is possibly a secondary protective mechanism.	Methodological differences have contributed to the variability of the results.
Exteroceptive suppression of temporalis muscle	>10	Static measurements of the ES2 in ETTH have been found to be largely normal. In CTTH the results are contradictory but high-quality studies gave negative findings.	Dynamic evaluation of ES2 responses, such as those measuring ES2 reactivity to experimental stressors, might be more sensitive than baseline measures in detecting dysfunction of brain excitability and its supraspinal control.
Blink reflex	4	The blink reflex is normal in both ETTH and CTTH. A single report indicates a slowed R2 recovery cycle, suggesting that TTH patients are characterized by reduced excitability of brainstem interneurons.	Further blinded studies including larger samples are needed to confirm these interesting blink reflex findings.
Trigeminocervical reflex	2	Late response: reduced latency on the painful side, in CTTH and migraine, suggests reduced inhibitory activity of brainstem interneurons in both disorders. Early response: abnormally increased latency and reduced amplitude in CTTH but not in ETTH suggest a brainstem impairment.	Further studies including larger samples, and using more correct sampling strategies and statistical methods, are needed to confirm these interesting trigeminocervical reflex findings.
Nociceptive flexion reflex	6	High-quality studies of CTTH reported a significantly reduced nociceptive flexion reflex threshold, suggesting central sensitization of nociceptive pathways. A DNIC dysfunction has been found in both CTTH and migraine, suggesting a dysfunction of descending inhibitory pathways.	Results need to be replicated by other research groups. Future studies, including larger samples, ETTH patients, and clinical controls (chronic pain subjects), will help to clarify the role, direction, and temporal pattern of the relationship between DNIC impairment and chronic pain.
EEG	<5	Inconsistent and contrasting findings.	It is commonly held that EEG is not helpful in either diagnostic or pathophysiological investigations.
Visual evoked potentials	2	One study suggests that TTH and migraine share an exaggerated brain response to visual stimuli, another that abnormal visual information processing is specific to migraine.	In contrast with findings obtained in migraineurs, the majority of the studies conducted on TTH suggest that cortical information processing of different sensory stimuli is normal.
Laser evoked potentials	3	Habituation to painful stimuli is normal in CTTH and controls but not in migraine. CTTH patients present neurophysiological signs of cortical pain-specific hypervigilance.	Further studies conducted by other research groups and including larger samples are necessary before any definitive conclusions can be drawn.
Event-related potentials	4	In contrast with migraine, event-related potential studies of ETTH and CTTH are largely normal. A deficiency in passive attention, common to TTH and migraine, has recently been described.	

EMG: electromyogram; EEG: electroencephalography; ES2: SP2 response; ETTH: episodic tension-type headache; CTTH: chronic tension-type headache; DNIC: diffuse noxious inhibitory controls.

CONCLUSIONS

As illustrated in the various sections of this chapter, clinical neurophysiological studies have helped to further understanding of several aspects of the pathophysiology of TTH. Regrettably, the majority of neurophysiological studies on TTH present serious methodological flaws. Most have been conducted on small samples of patients that preclude correct statistical analysis (statistical type 2 error, not enough statistical power). Second, the majority of the studies have been conducted only in highly selected patients drawn from headache clinics, who may present specific pathophysiological mechanisms. Different studies/centers have used different methods for eliciting the same neurophysiological responses, in spite of the existence of specific recommendations calling for improved standardization of research protocols. Little effort has been made to understand the role of potential confounding factors on neurophysiological parameters, factors such as the pain intensity, the onset of a new attack, and psychiatric comorbidity. Most studies have been conducted on CTTH whereas little has been done to explore differences in frequency-related subtypes or in patients presenting with or without pericranial tenderness. Several neurophysiological techniques have been applied only by single research groups and need to be replicated in further studies conducted by different researchers. Few researchers have used conditioning procedures, even though these have proved to be more helpful than baseline recording in testing pathophysiological hypotheses. Finally all the available studies have used a cross-sectional design that provides only limited information about the highly dynamic pain mechanisms underlying TTH. Future studies will have to overcome these limitations in order to further understanding of the mechanisms of TTH.

References

Aktekin B, Yaltkaya K, Ozkaynak S et al. (2001). Recovery cycle of the blink reflex and the exteroceptive suppression of temporalis muscle activity in migraine and tension-type headache. Headache 41: 142–149.

Ambrosini A, Maertens de Noordhout A, Sandor PS et al. (2003). Electrophysiological studies in migraine: a comprehensive review of their interest and limitations. Cephalalgia 23 (Suppl. 1): 13–31.

Avramidis TG, Podikoglu DG, Anastasopoulos IE et al. (1998). Blink reflex in migraine and tension-type headache. Headache 38: 691–696.

Bender S, Weisbrod M, Just U et al. (2002). Lack of age-dependent development of the contingent negative variation (CNV) in migraine children? Cephalalgia 22: 132–136.

Bender S, Oelkers-Ax R, Resch F et al. (2006). Frontal lobe involvement in the processing of meaningful auditory stimuli develops during childhood and adolescence. Neuroimage 33: 759–773.

Bender S, Weisbrod M, Resch F et al. (2007). Stereotyped topography of different elevated contingent variation components in children with migraine without aura points towards a subcortical dysfunction. Pain 127: 221–233.

Bendtsen L, Jensen R, Brennum J et al. (1996). Exteroceptive suppression of temporal muscle activity is normal in chronic tension-type headache and not related to actual headache state. Cephalalgia 16: 251–256.

Besken E, Pothmann R, Sartory G (1993). Contingent negative variation in childood migraine. Cephalalgia 13: 42–43.

Boureau F, Lou M, Doubrere JF (1991). Study of experimental pain measures in chronic pain patients and normal subjects. Pain 44: 131–138.

Chen W, Shen X, Liu X et al. (2007). Passive paradigm single-tone elicited ERPs in tension-type headaches and migraine. Cephalalgia 27: 139–144.

Cherniak ZV, Zenkov LR, Iakhno NN (2001). [Contingent negative deviation in children with headache.]. Zh Nevrol Psikhiatr Im S S Korsakova 103: 19–24.

de Tommaso M, Sciruicchio V, Guido M et al. (1999). Steady-state visual evoked-potentials in headache. Diagnostic value in migraine and tension-type headache. Cephalalgia 19: 23–26.

de Tommaso M, Libro G, Guido M et al. (2003). Heat–pain thresholds and cerebral event-related potentials following painful CO_2 laser stimulation in chronic tension-type headache. Pain 104: 111–119.

de Tommaso M, Shevel E, Pecoraro C et al. (2006). Topographic analysis of laser evoked potentials in chronic tension-type headache: correlations with clinical features. Int J Psychophysiol 62: 38–45.

Demirci S, Savas S (2002). The auditory event related potentials in episodic and chronic pain sufferers. Eur J Pain 6: 239–244.

Desmeules JA, Cedraschi C, Rapiti E et al. (2003). Neurophysiologic evidence for a central sensitization in patients with fibromyalgia. Arthritis Rheum 48: 1420–1429.

Flor H, Diers M, Bierbaumer N (2004). Peripheral and electrocortical responses to painful and non-painful stimulation in chronic pain patients, tension headache patients and healthy controls. Neurosci Lett 361: 147–150.

Hatch JP, Prihoda TJ, Moore PJ et al. (1991). A naturalistic study of the relationships among electromyographic activity, psychological stress, and pain in ambulatory tension-type headache patients and headache-free controls. Psychosom Med 53: 576–584.

Jensen R (1996). Mechanisms of spontaneous tension-type headaches; an analysis of tenderness, pain thresholds and EMG. Pain 64: 251–256.

Jensen R, Olesen J (1996). Initiating mechanisms of experimentally induced tension-type headache. Cephalalgia 16: 175–182.

Jensen R, Olesen J (1998). Muscular factors are of importance in tension-type headache. Headache 38: 10–17.

Kaube H, Katsarava Z, Käufer T et al. (2000). A new method to increase nociception specificity of the human blink reflex. Clin Neurophysiol 111: 413–416.

Kosek E, Ordeberg G (2000). Lack of pressure pain modulation by heterotopic noxious conditioning stimulation in patients with painful osteoarthritis before, but not following surgical pain relief. Pain 88: 69–78.

Kropp P, Berger WD (1993). Contingent negative variation – findings and perspectives in migraine. Cephalalgia 13: 33–36.

Langemark M, Bach FW, Jensen TS et al. (1993). Decreased nociceptive flexion reflex threshold in chronic tension-type headache. Arch Neurol 50: 1061–1064.

Lehrer PM, Murphy AI (1991). Stress reactivity and perception of pain among tension headache sufferers. Behav Res Ther 29: 61–69.

Leistad RB, Sand T, Westgaard RH et al. (2006). Stress induced pain and muscle activity in patients with migraine and tension-type headache. Cephalalgia 26: 64–73.

Lipchik GL, Holroyd KA, O'Donnel FJ et al. (2000). Exteroceptive suppression periods and pericranial muscle tenderness in chronic tension-type headache: effects of psychopathology, chronicity and disability. Cephalalgia 20: 638–646.

Maertens de Noordhout A, Timsit-Berthier M, Timsit M et al. (1986). Contingent negative variation in headache. Ann Neurol 86: 78–80.

Mazzotta G, Alberti A, Santucci A et al. (1995). The event-related potential P300 during headache-free period and spontaneous attack in adult headache sufferers. Headache 35: 210–215.

McNulty WH, Gevirtz RN, Hubbard DL et al. (1994). Needle electromyography evaluation of trigger point response to a psychological stressor. Psychophysiology 31: 313–316.

Milanov I, Bogdanova D (2003). Trigemino-cervical reflex in patients with headache. Cephalalgia 23: 35–38.

Nardone R, Tezzon F (2003). The trigemino-cervical reflex in tension-type headache. Eur J Neurol 10: 307–312.

Neufeld JD, Holroyd KA, Lipchik GL (2000). Dynamic assessment of abnormalities in central pain transmission and modulation in tension-type headache sufferers. Headache 40: 142–151.

Pielsticker A, Haag G, Zaudig M et al. (2005). Impairment of pain inhibition in chronic tension-type headache. Pain 118: 215–223.

Pikoff H (1984). Is the muscular model of headache still viable? A review of conflicting data. Headache 24: 186–198.

Puca F, de Tommaso M (1999). Clinical neurophysiology in childhood headache. Cephalalgia 19: 137–146.

Ramirez-Segura R, Campos-Castello J, Gonzalez-Mateos MJ et al. (1999). [Visual evoked potentials in children with tension headaches and migraine.] Rev Neurol 29: 1017–1019.

Rokicki LA, Houle TT, Dhingra LK et al. (2003). A preliminary analysis of EMG variance as an index of change in EMG biofeedback treatment of tension-type headache. Appl Psychophysiol Biofeedback 28: 205–215.

Rugh JD, Hatch JP, Moore PJ et al. (1990). The effect of psychological stress on electromyographic activity and negative affect in ambulatory tension-type headache patients. Headache 30: 216–219.

Sand T, Zwart JA (1994). The blink reflex in chronic tension-type headache, migraine and cervicogenic headache. Cephalalgia 14: 447–450.

Sand T, Møll-Nilsen B, Zwart JA (2006). Blink reflex R2 amplitudes in cervicogenic headache, chronic tension-type headache and migraine. Cephalalgia 26: 1186–1191.

Sandrini G, Martignoni E, Micieli G et al. (1986). Pain reflexes in the clinical assessment of migraine syndromes. Funct Neurol 1: 423–429.

Sandrini G, Ruiz L, Alfonsi E et al. (1991). Antinociceptive systems in primary headache disorders: a neurophysiological approach. In: G Nappi, G Bono, G Sandrini et al. (Eds.), Headache and Depression: Pathways as a Common Clue. Raven Press, New York, pp. 67–68.

Sandrini G, Arrigo A, Bono G et al. (1993). The nociceptive flexion reflex as a tool for exploring pain control systems in headache and other pain syndromes. Cephalalgia 13: 21–27.

Sandrini G, Friberg L, Janig W et al. (2004). Neurophysiological tests and neuroimaging procedures in non-acute headache. Guidelines and recommendations. Eur J Neurol 11: 217–224.

Sandrini G, Serrao M, Rossi P et al. (2005). The lower limb flexion reflex in humans. Progr Neurobiol 77: 353–395.

Sandrini G, Rossi P, Milanov I et al. (2006). Abnormal modulatory influence of diffuse noxious inhibitory controls in migraine and chronic tension-type headache patients. Cephalalgia 26: 782–789.

Schoenen J (1992). Clinical neurophysiology studies in headache: a review of data and pathophysiological limits. Funct Neurol 7: 191–204.

Schoenen J, Bendtsen L (2006). Neurophysiology of tension-type headache. In: J Olesen, PJ Goadsby, NR Ramadan et al. (Eds.), The Headaches. 3rd edn.. Lippincott Williams and Wilkins, Philadelphia, pp. 644–647.

Schoenen J, Jamart B, Gerard P et al. (1987). Exteroceptive suppression of temporalis muscle activity in chronic headache. Neurology 137: 1834–1836.

Schoenen J, Gerarrd P, De Pasqua V et al. (1991). Multiple clinical and paraclinical analyses of chronic tension-type headache associated or unassociated with disorder of pericranial muscles. Cephalalgia 11: 135–139.

Valeriani M, de Tommaso M, Restuccia D et al. (2003). Reduced habituation to experimental pain in migraine patients: a CO_2 laser evoked potentials study. Pain 105: 57–64.

Wang W, Schoenen J (1994). Reduction of temporalis exteroceptive suppression by peripheral electrical stimulation in migraine and tension-type headaches. Pain 59: 327–334.

Wang W, Wang GP, Ding XL et al. (1999). Personality and response to repeated visual stimulation in migraine and tension-type headache patients. Cephalalgia 19: 719–724.

Handbook of Clinical Neurology, Vol. 97 (3rd series)
Headache
G. Nappi and M.A. Moskowitz, Editors

Chapter 31

Treatment of tension-type headache

RIGMOR JENSEN[1]* AND PAOLA TORELLI[2]

[1]*The Danish Headache Center, Department of Neurology, University of Copenhagen, Glostrup Hospital, Glostrup, Denmark*
[2]*Headache Center, Department of Neuroscience, University of Parma and University Centre for Adaptive Disorders and Headache, Parma, Italy*

INTRODUCTION

Is tension-type headache (TTH) just a trivial, normal headache? Most patients and clinicians in specialized headache clinics tend to focus on the most severe headache, usually migraine, cluster headache, or the non-specific chronic daily headache (CDH) which may be a mixture of migraine, medication overuse headache (MOH), and TTH, and TTHs are therefore frequently overlooked as a specific entity. In contrast, epidemiological studies report TTH as the most prevalent and costly headache (Rasmussen et al., 1991, 1992a; Schwartz et al., 1998; Stovner et al., 2007). Recognition of TTH in the diagnostic process may therefore be essential for a correct individual evaluation and for a positive long-lasting treatment outcome.

PLANNING OF TENSION-TYPE HEADACHE TREATMENT

Patients usually expect a specific, simple treatment program at the first consultation and may be disappointed if they are just introduced to a diagnostic diary and prospective recordings instead of a specific treatment. In the following the most frequently asked questions from patients and professionals are discussed:

- Why is it important to keep a diary and have a specific diagnosis?
- Is the treatment strategy different if there is an underlying migraine or a TTH?
- Can headache triggers be identified and avoided in TTH?
- Which strategy should the doctor choose for the acute episode?
- Which strategy should the doctor choose to prevent TTH?

DIAGNOSIS OF TENSION-TYPE HEADACHE

A diagnosis of TTH is based on a diffuse, bilateral, mild to moderate headache without or with very mild accompanying symptoms and requires exclusion of other disorders (Headache Classification Committee of the International Headache Society, 1988; Headache Classification Subcommittee of the International Headache Society, 2004). The mild intensity and the absence of specific and distinguishing features may lead to the frequently used term "normal" headache and may explain why physicians, and subsequently patients, question the diagnosis, whereas migraine symptoms are more characteristic (Table 31.1).

The featureless headache may also mimic a secondary headache and explain why supplementary investigations are so frequently applied. The prospective use of a diagnostic headache diary with registration of all consumed drugs and a very careful history as well as a general and neurological examination are therefore of utmost importance to reach a precise diagnosis (Russell et al., 1992).

TTH was clearly defined in an episodic and a chronic form in the first international headache classification from 1988 (Headache Classification Committee of the International Headache Society, 1988), and this definition led to several epidemiological investigations illustrating the very high frequency of TTH affecting 45–87% of the general population (Rasmussen et al., 1991; Schwartz et al., 1998; Lyngberg et al., 2005a).

The classification of frequent headaches including TTH is also the part of the International Classification of Headache Disorders (ICHD-I) that has been most discussed and upon which much effort has been spent, with

*Correspondence to: Rigmor Jensen, The Danish Headache Center, Department of Neurology, University of Copenhagen, Glostrup Hospital, DK-2600 Glostrup, Denmark, Tel: 45-43233059, Fax: 45-43233839, E-mail: rigj@glo.regionh.dk

Table 31.1

Tension-type headache: International Headache Society diagnostic criteria (Headache Classification Subcommittee of the International Headache Society, 2004)

2.1 Infrequent episodic tension-type headache (TTH)
2.2 Frequent episodic TTH
2.3 Chronic TTH
- A. At least 10 episodes occurring on less than 1 day/month (2.1 = infrequent TTH)
  ≥12 and <180 days per year (2.2 = frequent episodic TTH)
  ≥180 days per year (2. 3= chronic TTH: CTTH) and fulfilling criteria B–E
- B. Headache lasting from 30 min to 7 days
- C. Headache has at least two of the following characteristics:
  1. Bilateral location
  2. Pressing/tightening (non-pulsating) quality
  3. Mild or moderate intensity
  4. Not aggravated by routine physical activity such as walking or climbing stairs
- D. Both of the following:
  1. No nausea or vomiting (anorexia may occur)
  2. No more than one of photophobia or phonophobia
- E. Not attributed to another disorder

various attempts to improve the diagnostic criteria of frequent headaches (Headache Classification Committee of the International Headache Society, 1988; Silberstein et al., 1996; Bigal et al., 2002). In the revised version of the headache classification (IHCD-II: Headache Classification Subcommittee of the International Headache Society, 2004), a further subgrouping of TTH was introduced, namely an infrequent form with fewer than 12 headache days per year, a frequent episodic form with 12–179 headache days per year, whereas the chronic form was kept unchanged with 180 headache days or more per year. This subdivision was created on the basis of epidemiological studies where infrequent episodic TTH (ETTH) is fairly "frequent" and probably a normal, protective reaction to lack of sleep, and mental stress. Thus, infrequent ETTH accounts for 40–50% of TTH cases in the general population (Rasmussen et al., 1991; Schwartz et al., 1998; Lyngberg et al., 2005a). The prevalence of frequent ETTH is rather stable at 37–39% and of chronic TTH (CTTH) 2–4% in several studies (Rasmussen et al., 1991; Schwartz et al., 1998; Lyngberg et al., 2005a).

The infrequent TTH is not regarded as a burden for either the individual or for society, whereas the frequent episodic and chronic subforms require further attention due to very high socioeconomic and personal costs (Rasmussen et al., 1991, 1992b; Schwartz et al., 1998; Lyngberg et al., 2005a).

In the general population, as many as 94% of migraineurs are bothered by coexisting TTH (Rasmussen et al., 1991; Lyngberg et al., 2005a) and, as coexisting migraine and TTH are important risk factors for a poor long-term prognosis and high use of health-care services, TTH certainly needs increased focus by specialists (Lyngberg et al., 2005b). Patients also usually seek medical attention for their most bothersome headache and a study revealed that ETTH was underestimated by 50% at the clinical interview compared to a prospective diagnostic diary (Russell et al., 1992). On the other hand, when a detailed headache history is taken, and a diary is used for a period of time, most patients are aware of their different headaches and can clearly describe them separately.

In clinical studies the prevalence of migraine is thus 70–80%, CDH with or without MOH accounts for 30–40%, and CTTH for 10–20% (Silberstein et al., 1996; Bigal et al., 2002; Zeeberg et al., 2005). Unfortunately, most clinical and some epidemiological publications do not report the coexisting TTH, only the migraines or the common denominator CDH.

As the treatment strategy and prognosis of MOH and migraine are completely different, recognition of the coexisting headache disorders is therefore of utmost importance and a diagnostic diary for at least a 4-week period is now regarded as mandatory in the diagnosis of headache.

IS THE TREATMENT STRATEGY DIFFERENT WHETHER THERE IS AN UNDERLYING MIGRAINE OR A TENSION-TYPE HEADACHE?

For the acute episode, simple analgesics and non-steroidal inflammatory drugs (NSAIDs) are generally accepted painkillers and are reported to have a significant effect in both migraine and TTH. The high pain intensity and accompanying symptoms in migraine indicate a fairly poor outcome with simple analgesics, whereas the milder pain intensity and lack of gastrointestinal symptoms in TTH predict a better treatment outcome, but comparative studies in properly classified patients have to our knowledge not yet been reported.

TRIPTANS

The triptans, serotonin (5-HT) agonists, are migraine-specific agents. While triptans are highly effective in the treatment of migraine, the efficacy of triptans in TTH is unclear. In one study, Brennum and colleagues (1992) reported that subcutaneous administration of sumatriptan 2 and 4 mg induced modest but significantly greater headache relief than placebo in patients with CTTH. It has also been reported that subcutaneous

injections of 6 mg sumatriptan in patients with TTH and coexisting migraine had an effect equal to response in migraine in subjects with coexisting migraine and TTH whereas there was no effect above placebo in subjects with pure TTH. These results indicate that, in patients with coexisting migraine and TTH, some mild headaches mimicking TTH may rather represent mild migraines (Cady et al., 1997). However, the oral formulation of sumatriptan 100 mg was not effective in the treatment of ETTH (Brennum et al., 1996). The possible mechanism responsible for the modest effect of subcutaneous sumatriptan in CTTH could be reduction of the increased excitability of neurons in the central nervous system (CNS). In support of this, animal studies have shown that 5-HT agonists can inhibit excitability of neurons in the CNS (Goadsby et al., 2002), and experimental studies in patients with CTTH suggested increased excitability of the CNS (Bendtsen, 2000). Using triptans for mild headaches includes a significant risk for developing MOH and should be avoided. Thus, until further convincing evidence is available, triptans play no role in the treatment of TTH.

Concerning prevention, the most frequently used headache prophylactics are migraine prophylactics such as beta-blockers, antiepileptics, antidepressants, or calcium channel blockers. All of them have been developed for disorders other than headache and have not been systematically tested in the prophylaxis of TTH. In one controlled study of the prophylactic effect of sodium valproate in migraine without aura there was absolutely no effect on coexisting TTH despite a marked effect on migraine frequency (Jensen et al., 1994). Only antidepressants such as tricyclic antidepressants and mirtazapine have a documented effect in TTH and a very modest, if any, effect in pure migraine (Bendtsen, 2004).

HEADACHE TRIGGERS

Triggers are very similar and quite non-specific in both TTH and migraine (Rasmussen et al., 1992b; Ulrich et al., 1996). Nevertheless, avoidance of triggers may have a very long-lasting and positive preventive effect, and a detailed analysis of possible triggers may therefore be very fruitful in each individual patient. The diagnostic diary can also be useful to identify triggers and advise the patient to eliminate the suspected trigger in a systematic way if possible. The most frequently reported triggers for TTH are: stress (mental or physical), irregular or inappropriate meals, high intake of coffee and other caffeine-containing drinks, dehydration, sleep disorders, too much or too little sleep, reduced or inappropriate physical exercise, psychological problems, as well as variations during the female menstrual cycle and hormonal substitution (Rasmussen et al., 1992b; Ulrich et al., 1996). Most triggers are self-reported and so far none of the triggers has been systematically tested.

COMBINATIONS OF TREATMENT

Most of the non-pharmacological and behavioral prophylactic treatments are non-specific and widely used in complex headache patients. Non-pharmacological treatment is widely used for TTH but the evidence for the various treatment modalities is, at best, sparse. Physical therapy is the most common of these therapies, but three independent reviews concluded that further studies of improved quality are needed either to support or to refute the effectiveness of physical modalities in TTH (Biondi, 2005; Lenssinck et al., 2004; Vernon et al., 1999). A controlled study reported a modest but significant effect of active physical therapy in both ETTH and CTTH patients (Torelli et al., 2004). Another study reported no effect of greater occipital nerve block in CTTH (Leinisch-Dahlke et al., 2005), while a large trial found acupuncture better than no treatment but not superior to minimal acupuncture (Melchart et al., 2005). It is therefore reassuring that the first study that has evaluated the efficacy of a multidisciplinary headache clinic reports positive results (Zeeberg et al., 2005). Treatment results for all patients discharged within 1 year were evaluated. Patients suffering from frequent ETTH, CTTH, migraine, cluster headache, MOH, and other headaches all had a significant positive treatment outcome by means of reduced headache frequency; only patients with posttraumatic headache had no effect. Patients with ETTH demonstrated a 50% reduction in frequency, 75% reduction in intensity, and 33% reduction in absence rate, whereas CTTH patients responded with 32%, 30%, and 40% reductions respectively (Zeeberg et al., 2005).

Psychological treatment strategies including biofeedback have also been used extensively, with promising results (Penzien et al., 2004). Future studies should also examine the relative efficacy of the various treatment modalities, e.g., physical, psychological, and pharmacological, and clarify how treatment programs should be optimized to suit the individual TTH patient best.

PLANNING THE PHARMACOLOGICAL TREATMENT OF THE ACUTE EPISODE OF TTH

Acute pharmacotherapy implies treatment of acute episode of TTH, i.e., frequent ETTH according to ICHD-II (Headache Classification Subcommittee of the International Headache Society, 2004). Non-opioids are widely used as an acute therapy. Unfortunately, there

is no selective or specific therapy and we will, therefore, focus on non-opioids in the treatment of ETTH. In contrast, acute therapy should be avoided in CTTH due to the risk of medication-induced headache (Zeeberg et al., 2006).

Simple analgesics

Aspirin and acetaminophen are the most commonly used analgesics in the treatment of acute episodes of TTH. Several randomized controlled trials have shown that aspirin (Ryan, 1977; Diamond, 1983; Peters et al., 1983; Langemark and Olesen, 1987; Nebe et al., 1995; Martinez-Martin et al., 2001; Steiner et al., 2003) and acetaminophen (Friedman and DiSerio, 1987; Miller et al., 1987; Schachtel et al., 1991, 1996; Migliardi et al., 1994; Dahlof and Jacobs, 1996; Steiner and Lange, 1998; Packman et al., 2000; Prior et al., 2002; Steiner et al., 2003) are effective in acute therapy of TTH. In one of the first placebo-controlled trials, 648 mg solid aspirin and 648 mg effervescent aspirin were more effective than placebo (Langemark and Olesen, 1987). However, the authors found no difference between solid and effervescent aspirin (Langemark and Olesen, 1987). In another randomized, parallel, double-blind study a subgroup of patients with TTH were treated with 1000 mg acetaminophen, 650 mg aspirin, and placebo (Peters et al., 1983). Both drugs were effective compared with placebo, but no difference was found when drugs were compared with each other. Steiner and colleagues (2003) reported that two different doses of aspirin (500 or 1000 mg) and acetaminophen 1000 mg were more effective than placebo. Two studies reported no difference between acetaminophen and placebo (Dahlof and Jacobs, 1996; Mehlisch et al., 1998). In the study by Dahlof and Jacobs (1996) there was no difference between 500 and 1000 mg acetaminophen and placebo. Authors suggested that severity at baseline of the treated headache episodes and the low number of evaluated patients might explain the lack of efficacy. In another study acetaminophen 1000 mg proved to be numerically, but not statistically, more favorable than placebo in most variables (Mehlisch et al., 1998). Martinez-Martin and colleagues (2001) reported that a non-opioid analgesic and antipyretic, dipyrone (not approved by Food and Drug Administration), at doses of 500 and 1000 mg, was more effective than placebo in treatment of patients with moderate ETTH. In another placebo-controlled trial intravenous dypirone 1000 mg was also shown to be more effective in treatment of patients with ETTH than placebo (Bigal et al., 2001).

In summary, most randomized controlled trials demonstrated that both acetaminophen and aspirin are effective in the treatment of an acute episode of TTH and should be included in the treatment of mild or moderate episodes. Acetaminophen may be recommended as the first choice because of a better gastric side-effect profile. Recommended doses are shown in Table 31.2.

Non-steroidal inflammatory drugs

NSAIDs comprise another group of drugs used as a non-specific acute pharmacotherapy of TTH. Efficacy of NSAIDs has been reported in several randomized controlled trials (Ryan, 1977; Diamond, 1983; Miller et al., 1987; Nebe et al., 1995; Dahlof and Jacobs, 1996; Schachtel et al., 1996; Van Gerven et al., 1996; Harden et al., 1998; Mehlisch et al., 1998; Diamond et al., 2000;

Table 31.2

Acute treatment of tension-type headache

Drug	Clinical efficacy	Scientific proof for efficacy	Side-effect	Examples of side-effects
Acetylsalicylic acid (ASA)	++++	++++	+++	Dyspepsia, gastric ulcers
Acetaminophen	+++	++++	++	Liver enzymes ↑, intoxication
NSAIDs				
Ibuprofen	+++	+++	++	Dyspepsia; gastric ulcers
Ketoprofene	+++	+++	++	Dyspepsia; gastric ulcers
Diclofenac	++	++	++	Dyspepsia; gastric ulcers
Combinations				
Paracetamol + codeine	++	+	++	As above, obstipation, MOH
ASA + caffeine	++	+	++	As above, MOH

NSAIDs: non-steroidal anti-inflammatory drugs; MOH: medication overuse headache.
Clinical efficacy, scientific proof of efficacy, and potential side-effects are rated on a scale from + to ++++ for drugs used in the acute treatment of tension-type headache.

Packman et al., 2000; Prior et al., 2002; Kubitzek et al., 2003). In one of the first randomized trials, Ryan (1977) reported that ibuprofen 400 mg was as effective as aspirin 650 mg in relieving pain in patients with muscle contraction headache (published before the International Headache Society classification). In another early double-blind randomized placebo-controlled trial, ibuprofen 400 and 800 mg and aspirin 650 mg were also more effective than placebo in patients with muscle contraction headache (Diamond, 1983). Onset of action after a single dose of 400 mg ibuprofen in treatment of TTH was determined in a double-blind randomized placebo-controlled trial (Schachtel and Thoden, 1988). The effect was detected within 15 min on a pain intensity scale, indicating that ibuprofen had an early onset of action.

Comparative studies have demonstrated that ibuprofen 400 mg was more effective than acetaminophen 1000 mg or placebo (Schachtel et al., 1996), and 200 mg ibuprofen was more effective than aspirin 500 mg or placebo (Nebe et al., 1995). A new solubilized formulation of ibuprofen 400 mg has been reported to be more effective than acetaminophen 1000 mg and placebo in the treatment of ETTH (Prior et al., 2002). Steiner and Lange (1998) evaluated efficacy of ketoprofen, another important drug in treatment of ETTH, in a multicenter placebo-controlled randomized parallel-group study. Ketoprofen 25 mg and acetaminophen 1000 mg were equally effective in pain relief and superior to placebo. Two doses of ketoprofen (25 and 50 mg) were reported to be more effective than ibuprofen 200 mg and placebo in the treatment of ETTH (Van Gerven et al., 1996). Mehlisch and colleagues demonstrated that low doses of ketoprofen 12.5 and 25 mg were also more effective than placebo (1998). In one comparative study Dahlof and Jacobs (1996) reported that ketoprofen 50 mg was more effective than acetaminophen 500 and 1000 mg or placebo. In the same study pain relief with ketoprofen 25 mg was intermediate between that with ketoprofen 50 mg and that with placebo, and not statistically significantly different (Dahlof and Jacobs, 1996). This outcome is probably due to a small number of patients.

Naproxen is another widely used NSAID in the treatment of TTH. The efficacy of naproxen was evaluated in comparative randomized controlled trials (Schachtel et al., 1991, Packman et al., 2000, Prior et al., 2002). Thus, naproxen 375 mg was reported to be more effective than placebo, but not better than acetaminophen 1000 mg (Schachtel et al., 1991). In a multicenter, randomized, double-blind, three-way parallel study, naproxen sodium 550 mg (rapidly absorbed formulation) was more effective than acetaminophen 650 mg and placebo (Packman et al., 2000). In a comparative study (not placebo-controlled) Lange and Lentz (1995) found no difference between naproxen 250 mg, ibuprofen 200 mg, and ketoprofen 12.5 or 25 mg. In addition, naproxen sodium 220 mg was reported to be as effective as ibuprofen 200 mg in the treatment of TTH (Autret et al., 1997).

Diclofenac potassium, known to be effective in migraine at doses of 50 or 100 mg (McNeely and Goa, 1999), was shown to be effective in the treatment of ETTH at low doses (12.5 and 25 mg) (Kubitzek et al., 2003). In addition, diclofenac potassium was found to be comparable to ibuprofen 400 mg.

Intramuscular injection of ketorolac 60 mg, an injectable NSAID approved for the management of acute pain, was found to be superior to placebo in relieving pain in patients with TTH compared with placebo (Harden et al., 1998).

Taking these data together demonstrates that NSAIDs are effective and should be included in the treatment of moderate or severe episodes of TTH. However, physicians should be aware of the risk of developing drug-induced headache due to frequent and excessive use of analgesics. Recommended doses are shown in Table 31.2.

Combination analgesics

Although there are only few randomized controlled trials, the combinations of simple analgesics with caffeine or codeine are widely used by physicians in the treatment of acute episodes of TTH. In a double-blind placebo-controlled trial Schachtel and co-workers (1996) showed that combination of aspirin 1000 mg with caffeine 64 mg was more effective than acetaminophen 1000 mg in the treatment of muscle contraction headache. In a randomized, double-blind, parallel, multicenter, single-dose, placebo- and active-controlled study Diamond and colleagues (2000) reported that more subjects obtained headache relief with combination of ibuprofen 400 mg and caffeine 200 mg than with ibuprofen 400 mg, caffeine 200 mg, or placebo. Another comparative study reported that a combination of acetaminophen 500 mg, aspirin 500 mg, and caffeine 130 mg and a combination of acetaminophen 1000 mg and 130 mg caffeine were more effective than acetaminophen 1000 mg alone or placebo (Migliardi et al., 1994).

Codeine, an opioid analgesic, is another compound which is combined in formulations containing aspirin or acetaminophen. One study reported that combination of acetaminophen and codeine (doses not reported) was better than placebo in relieving pain in patients with tension headache with an average of six attacks per month (Friedman and Di Serio, 1987).

In summary, data on combinations of simple analgesics demonstrate that more randomized controlled and comparative studies are needed to evaluate the efficacy and safety of combination analgesics in treatment of ETTH.

Muscle relaxants

Muscle relaxants are not considered to be effective in acute episodes of TTH, because of insufficient studies and the risk of habituation (Mathew and Schoenen, 2000; Jensen, 2001). Therefore, these drugs are generally not recommended.

PREVENTIVE THERAPY

Preventive treatment is generally considered if the patient has headache on more than 15 days per month, i.e., CTTH. For many years physicians have been prescribing tricyclic antidepressants and selective serotonin reuptake inhibitors (SSRIs) for the treatment of CTTH but they are far from effective or tolerated in all patients and improved treatment modalities are needed. In recent years there has been an increasing focus on other possible treatment strategies but unfortunately without significant success.

Amitriptyline

The tricyclic antidepressant amitriptyline is the most frequently prescribed drug for the treatment of CTTH (Mathew and Bendtsen, 2000). Controlled randomized trials have demonstrated that amitriptyline has a statistically significant and clinically relevant effect in the prophylactic treatment of CTTH (Lance and Curran, 1964; Diamond and Baltes, 1971; Göbel et al., 1994; Pfaffenrath et al., 1994; Bendtsen et al., 1996; Holroyd et al., 2001). In 1964, Lance and Curran conducted the first controlled crossover trial and demonstrated the superiority of amitriptyline compared to placebo. Later, Diamond and Baltes (1971) compared the efficacy of different doses and found that the lower dose range of between 10 and 60 mg/day was more effective than placebo. Interestingly there was no significant effect of higher dose range (25–150 mg/day). Göbel and colleagues (1994) demonstrated that amitriptyline 75 mg/day significantly reduced headache duration compared to placebo in the last week of a 6-week study. A large multicenter, parallel-group trial by Pfaffenrath and colleagues (1994) reported no difference between amitriptyline 50–75 mg/day, amitriptylinoxide 60–90 mg/day and placebo in all recorded endpoints of the study. The reason for these results is obscure. Amitriptyline has marked side-effects, but in the study by Pfaffenrath and colleagues there was no difference in side-effect report between amitriptyline and the placebo group. Therefore, inability to detect side-effects may suggest insensitivity of this study.

Bendtsen and colleagues (1996) conducted a three-way crossover trial of amitriptyline 75 mg per day, SSRI citalopram 20 mg/day, and placebo in CTTH. Amitriptyline reduced the area under the headache curve (calculated as headache duration multiplied by headache intensity) by 30% compared to placebo. In addition, amitriptyline reduced secondary efficacy parameters, such as headache duration and frequency, intake of analgesics, and myofascial tenderness (Bendtsen and Jensen, 2000). This latter finding suggests that amitriptyline elicits its analgesic effect by reducing transmission of painful stimuli from myofascial tissues and reduction of increased excitability in the CNS in patients with CTTH (Bendtsen and Jensen 2000). However, the exact mechanism of action of amitriptyline in TTH is far from clarified. Possible mechanisms may include a combination of 5-HT and norepinephrine reuptake in the CNS, potentiation of endogenous opioids, *N*-methyl-D-aspartate receptor antagonism, and blockade of ion channels (Watanabe et al., 1993; Eschalier et al., 1997; Sawynok et al., 2001). In a comparative study by Holroyd and colleagues (2001), amitriptyline and the tricyclic antidepressant nortriptyline were compared with stress management therapy and a combination of stress management and antidepressants in CTTH. All three treatments significantly reduced the headache index by 30% more than placebo. Moreover, this study demonstrated a long-lasting effect of amitriptyline in CTTH.

Collectively, randomized controlled studies demonstrated that amitriptyline is effective and should be considered as the first drug of choice in the preventive treatment of CTTH (Table 31.3).

Selective serotonin reuptake inhibitors

The efficacy of SSRIs has been shown in various chronic pain conditions (Jung et al., 1997). Two placebo-controlled studies investigated the efficacy of SSRIs in preventive therapy of CTTH. Bendtsen and colleagues (1996) compared citalopram (20 mg/day) with amitriptyline (25–75 mg/day) and placebo in a three-way crossover study. Amitriptyline reduced the area under the curve while citalopram had no significant effect in patients with CTTH. In a double-blind, placebo-controlled, randomized trial Singh and Misra (2002) investigated the efficacy of sertraline in patients with CTTH. Although the mean analgesic intake was significantly decreased in the sertraline group compared with placebo, headache index, which combined severity, duration, and frequency of headache, did not differ between groups.

Table 31.3

Prophylactic treatment of tension-type headache

Drug	Clinical efficacy	Scientific proof of efficacy	Side-effect potential	Examples of side-effects
Amitriptyline	+++	+++	++++	Weight gain, dry mouth, sedation
Nortriptyline	++	+	+++	Weight gain, dry mouth, sedation
Antiepileptics				
Sodium valproate	+	(+)	++++	Weight gain, tremor, hair loss wih divalproex, thrombocytopenia, liver enzymes ↑
NSAIDs				
Naproxen	++	+	++	Dyspepsia, peptic ulcer
Tolfenamic acid	++	+	++	Dyspepsia, peptic ulcer

NSAIDs: non-steroidal ant-inflammatory drugs.
Clinical efficacy, scientific proof of efficacy, and potential for side-effects rated on a scale from + to ++++ for drugs used in prophylaxis of tension-type headache.

In a randomized double-blind trial Manna and colleagues (1994) compared fluvoxamine (50–100 mg/day) with the tetracyclic antidepressant mianserine 30–60 mg/day and found a significant effect for both drugs. In another comparative randomized, double-blind, crossover study paroxetine (20–30 mg/day) was compared with sulpiride (200–400 mg/day), a D_2 antagonist, in 50 patients with CTTH (Langemark and Olesen, 1994). Both treatments resulted in a modest improvement in headache scores and decreased analgesic intake. However, sulpiride showed significantly better relief than paroxetine. Two placebo-controlled studies are clearly not enough to reach a conclusion on efficacy of SSRIs. More placebo-controlled trials are needed to demonstrate the efficacy of SSRIs in the preventive treatment of CTTH.

It has been demonstrated that the analgesic effect of amitriptyline in CTTH is not solely due to serotonin reuptake inhibition and that other mechanisms must be involved. In agreement with this the noradrenergic and specific serotonergic antidepressant mirtazapine was reported to be equally effective and better tolerated than amitriptyline (Bendtsen and Jensen, 2004). A recent study where very low-dose mirtazapine (4.5 mg) alone or in combination with ibuprofen was tested against placebo was, however, unable to demonstrate any positive effect (Bendtsen et al., 2007), In contrast, those subjects who received ibuprofen alone reported increased headache compared to placebo, indicating a possible early onset of MOH (Bendtsen et al., 2007). In conclusion, amitriptyline and mirtazapine are far from effective or tolerated in all patients and improved treatment modalities are greatly needed.

Muscle relaxants

The efficacy of muscle relaxants in the prevention of TTH has been investigated in three studies. Shimomura and colleagues (1991) suggested clinical usefulness of tizanidine for TTH in a controlled clinical trial. In a randomized double-blind placebo-controlled crossover study, Fogelholm and Murros (1992) investigated the efficacy of tizanidine in women with CTTH. Increasing dose from 6 to 18 mg/day was more effective than placebo. The authors suggested that tizanidine was effective in the treatment of CTTH in women (Fogelholm and Murros, 1992). In another study, modified-release formulations of tizanidine in doses up to 12 mg did not differ from placebo (Murros et al., 2000). The results from these two trials clearly demonstrate the need for more trials on effect and safety of muscle relaxants before they can be recommended in the preventive treatment of CTTH.

Botulinum toxin

Botulinum toxin is used in the treatment of dystonia and myofascial pain syndrome. The rationale for the use of botulinum toxin in pain conditions, and especially in TTH, is the combination of muscle relaxant and antinociceptive action in the peripheral nervous system and the CNS (Guyer, 1999). The efficacy of botulinum toxin in TTH was first evaluated in open-label studies (Relja, 1997) and indicated positive results. Unfortunately, randomized placebo-controlled trials produced conflicting, mostly negative, results (Göbel et al., 1999; Smuts et al., 1999; Rollnik et al., 2000) and the most recent large multicenter study in CTTH was also unable to demonstrate a positive effect (Silberstein et al., 2006).

In summary, data on efficacy of botulinum toxin in the treatment of TTH are based on a limited number of studies with several methodological reservations and, as large-scale randomized controlled trials are negative, botulinum toxin cannot be recommended in the preventive therapy of CTTH.

Future drug therapies should primarily focus on prevention of the frequent ETTH and CTTH, and both third-generation antidepressants, nitric oxide inhibitors, Na^+ and/or Ca^{2+} channel modulators, and new anticonvulsants are promising candidates. Developments in animal models of chronic pain and in more specific preventive compounds are also very promising and will undoubtedly require further investigation in randomized controlled trials.

FUTURE STRATEGY

Along with the substantial burden of TTH, the exciting evolution and enormous progress in genetic and molecular science call for a more systematic clinical and scientific approach to TTH. So, in conclusion, it should be mandatory to use a diagnostic headache diary and to characterize patients in as much detail as possible on the basis of the clinical diversity with several different diagnoses. It is also important to apply a dynamic and an academic approach to the difficult headache patient in the clinic and avoid the use of the nonspecific denominator, CDH, although this may be time-consuming at first glance. Headache patients deserve just as careful a scientific and systematic approach as other neurological patients and, until a precise diagnostic or genetic test for the various headaches has been developed, we have to rely on their history and develop further instruments to characterize our headache patients on a clinical basis. Specific diagnostic groupings of migraine have been used for more than a decade and it is now time that clinicians also recognized TTH. The effort usually proves to be cost-effective as patients may be withdrawn from their frequent medication overuse, receive a more focused therapy, and demonstrate a better treatment outcome. A compound developed and registered for the prophylaxis of TTH alone would be of major significance and a prominent step forward in the acceptance and recognition of TTH. We are only now beginning to understand the complex mechanisms leading to CTTH and other chronic pain conditions, and hopefully these results will lead to new treatment modalities in TTH. An increased focus on TTH in clinical, pathophysiological, and pharmaceutical research may thus lead us to the most important step forward since the triptan era in the 1990s.

REFERENCES

Autret A, Unger P, EURAXI group et al. (1997). Naproxen sodium versus ibuprofen in episodic tension headache (abstract). Cephalalgia 17: 446.

Bendtsen L (2000). Central sensitization in tension-type headache – possible pathophysiological mechanisms. Cephalalgia 20: 486–508.

Bendtsen L (2003). Amitriptyline in the treatment of primary headaches. Exp Rev Neurother 3: 165–173.

Bendtsen L, Jensen R (2000). Amitriptyline reduces myofascial tenderness in patients with chronic tension-type headache. Cephalalgia 20: 603–610.

Bendtsen L, Jensen R (2004). Mirtazapine is effective in the prophylactic treatment of chronic tension-type headache. Neurology 62: 1706–1711.

Bendtsen L, Jensen R, Olesen J (1996). A non-selective (amitriptyline), but not a selective (citalopram), serotonin reuptake inhibitor is effective in the prophylactic treatment of chronic tension-type headache. J Neurol Neurosurg Psychiatry 61: 285–290.

Bendtsen L, Buchgreitz L, Ashina S et al. (2007). Combination of low-dose mirtazapine and ibuprofen for profylaxis of chronic tension-type headache. Eur J Neurol 14: 187–193.

Bigal ME, Bordini CA, Speciali JG (2001). Intravenous metamizol (dipyrone) in acute migraine treatment and in episodic tension-type headache – a placebo-controlled study. Cephalalgia 21: 90–95.

Bigal ME, Sheftell FD, Rapaport AM et al. (2002). Chronic daily headache in a tertiary care population: correlation between the International Headache Society diagnostic criteria and proposed revisions of criteria for chronic daily headache. Cephalalgia 22: 432–438.

Biondi DM (2005). Physical treatments for headache: a structured review. Headache 45: 738–746.

Brennum J, Kjeldsen M, Olesen J (1992). The 5-HT1-like agonist sumatriptan has a significant effect in chronic tension-type headache. Cephalalgia 12: 375–379.

Brennum J, Brinck T, Schriver L et al. (1996). Sumatriptan has no clinically relevant effect in the treatment of episodic tension-type headache. Eur J Neurol 3: 23–28.

Cady RK, Gutterman D, Saiers JA et al. (1997). Responsiveness of non-IHS migraine and tension-type headache to sumatriptan. Cephalalgia 17: 588–590.

Dahlof CG, Jacobs LD (1996). Ketoprofen, paracetamol and placebo in the treatment of episodic tension-type headache. Cephalalgia 16: 117–123.

Diamond S (1983). Ibuprofen versus aspirin and placebo in the treatment of muscle contraction headache. Headache 23: 206–210.

Diamond S, Baltes BJ (1971). Chronic tension headache – treated with amitriptyline – a double-blind study. Headache 11: 110–116.

Diamond S, Balm TK, Freitag FG (2000). Ibuprofen plus caffeine in the treatment of tension-type headache. Clin Pharmacol Ther 68: 312–319.

Eschalier A, Ardid D, Dubray C (1997). Tricyclic and other antidepressants as analgesics. In: JCA Sawynok (Ed.),

Novel Aspects of Pain Management: Opioids and Beyond. John Wiley, New York, pp. 301–319.

Fogelholm R, Murros K (1992). Tizanidine in chronic tension-type headache: a placebo controlled double-blind cross-over study. Headache 32: 509–513.

Friedman AP, DiSerio FJ (1987). Symptomatic treatment of chronically recurring tension headache: a placebo-controlled, multicenter investigation of Fioricet and acetaminophen with codeine. Clin Ther 10: 69–81.

Goadsby PJ, Lipton RB, Ferrari MD (2002). Migraine – current understanding and treatment. N Engl J Med 346: 257–270.

Göbel H, Hamouz V, Hansen C et al. (1994). Chronic tension-type headache: amitriptyline reduces clinical headache-duration and experimental pain sensitivity but does not alter pericranial muscle activity readings. Pain 59: 241–249.

Göbel H, Lindner V, Krack PK et al. (1999). Treatment of chronic tension-type headache with botulinum toxin (abstract). Cephalalgia 19: 455.

Guyer BM (1999). Mechanism of botulinum toxin in the relief of chronic pain. Curr Rev Pain 3: 427–431.

Harden RN, Rogers D, Fink K et al. (1998). Controlled trial of ketorolac in tension-type headache. Neurology 50: 507–509.

Headache Classification Committee of the International Headache Society (1988). Classification and diagnostic criteria for headache disorders, cranial neuralgias and facial pain. Cephalalgia 8 (Suppl. 7): 1–96.

Headache Classification Subcommittee of the International Headache Society (2004). The international classification of headache disorders, 2nd edn. Cephalalgia 24: 1–160.

Holroyd KA, O'Donnell FJ, Stensland M et al. (2001). Management of chronic tension-type headache with tricyclic antidepressant medication, stress management therapy, and their combination: a randomized controlled trial. JAMA 285: 2208–2215.

Jensen R (2001). Tension-type headache. Curr Treat Options Neurol 3: 169–180.

Jensen R, Brinck T, Olesen J (1994). Sodium valproate has a prophylactic effect in migraine without aura: a triple-blind, placebo-controlled crossover study. Neurology 44: 647–651.

Jung AC, Staiger T, Sullivan M (1997). The efficacy of selective serotonin reuptake inhibitors for the management of chronic pain. J Gen Intern Med 12: 384–389.

Kubitzek F, Ziegler G, Gold MS et al. (2003). Low-dose diclofenac potassium in the treatment of episodic tension-type headache. Eur J Pain 7: 155–162.

Lance JW, Curran DA (1964). Treatment of chronic tension headache. Lancet 1: 1236–1239.

Lange R, Lentz R (1995). Comparison ketoprofen, ibuprofen and naproxen sodium in the treatment of tension-type headache. Drugs Exp Clin Res 21: 89–96.

Langemark M, Olesen J (1987). Effervescent ASA versus solid ASA in the treatment of tension headache. A double-blind, placebo controlled study. Headache 27: 90–95.

Langemark M, Olesen J (1994). Sulpiride and paroxetine in the treatment of chronic tension-type headache. An explanatory double-blind trial. Headache 34: 20–24.

Leinisch-Dahlke E, Jurgens T, Bogdahn U et al. (2005). Greater occipital nerve block is ineffective in chronic tension type headache. Cephalalgia 25: 704–708.

Lenssinck ML, Damen L, Verhagen AP et al. (2004). The effectiveness of physiotherapy and manipulation in patients with tension-type headache: a systematic review. Pain 112: 381–388.

Lyngberg AC, Rasmussen BK, Jørgensen T et al. (2005a). Has the prevalence of migraine and tension-type headache changed over a 12-year period? A Danish population survey. Eur J Epidemiol 20: 243–249.

Lyngberg AC, Rasmussen BK, Jørgensen T et al. (2005b). Prognosis of migraine and tension-type headache. Neurology 65: 580–585.

Manna V, Bolino F, Di Cicco L (1994). Chronic tension-type headache, mood depression and serotonin: therapeutic effects of fluvoxamine and mianserine. Headache 34: 44–49.

Martinez-Martin P, Raffaelli E Jr, Freimer ML et al. (2001). Efficacy and safety of metamizol vs. acetylsalicylic acid in patients with moderate episodic tension-type headache: a randomized, double-blind, placebo- and active-controlled multicentre study. Cephalalgia 21: 604–610.

Mathew NT, Bendtsen L (2000). Prophylactic pharmacotherapy of tension-type headache. In: J Olesen, P Tfelt-Hansen, KM Welch (Eds.), The Headaches. Lippincott-Raven, Philadelphia, pp. 667–673.

Mathew NT, Schoenen J (2000). Acute pharmacotherapy of tension-type headache. In: J Olesen, P Tfelt-Hansen, KM Welch (Eds.), The Headaches. Lippincott-Raven, Philadelphia, pp. 661–666.

McNeely W, Goa KL (1999). Diclofenac-potassium in migraine: a review. Drugs 57: 991–1003.

Mehlisch DR, Weaver M, Fladung B (1998). Ketoprofen, acetaminophen, and placebo in the treatment of tension headache. Headache 38: 579–589.

Melchart D, Streng A, Hoppe A et al. (2005). Acupuncture in patients with tension-type headache: randomised controlled trial. BMJ 331: 376–382.

Migliardi JR, Armellino JJ, Friedman M et al. (1994). Caffeine as an analgesic adjuvant in tension headache. Clin Pharmacol Ther 56: 576–586.

Miller DS, Talbot CA, Simpson W et al. (1987). A comparison of naproxen sodium, acetaminophen and placebo in the treatment of muscle contraction headache. Headache 27: 392–396.

Murros K, Kataja M, Hedman C et al. (2000). Modified-release formulation of tizanidine in chronic tension-type headache. Headache 40: 633–637.

Nebe J, Heier M, Diener HC (1995). Low-dose ibuprofen in self-medication of mild to moderate headache: a comparison with acetylsalicylic acid and placebo. Cephalalgia 15: 531–535.

Packman B, Packman E, Doyle G et al. (2000). Solubilized ibuprofen: evaluation of onset, relief, and safety of a novel formulation in the treatment of episodic tension-type headache. Headache 40: 561–567.

Penzien DB, Rains JC, Lipchik GL et al. (2004). Behavioral interventions for tension-type headache: overview of current therapies and recommendation for a self-management model for chronic headache. Curr Pain Headache Ther 8: 489–499.

Peters BH, Fraim CJ, Masel BE (1983). Comparison of 650 mg aspirin and 1000 mg acetaminophen with each other, and with placebo in moderately severe headache. Am J Med 74: 36–42.

Pfaffenrath V, Diener HC, Isler H et al. (1994). Efficacy and tolerability of amitriptylinoxide in the treatment of chronic tension-type headache: a multi-centre controlled study. Cephalalgia 14: 149–155.

Prior MJ, Cooper KM, May LG et al. (2002). Efficacy and safety of acetaminophen and naproxen in the treatment of tension-type headache. A randomized, double-blind, placebo-controlled trial. Cephalalgia 22: 740–748.

Rasmussen BK, Jensen R, Schroll M et al. (1991). Epidemiology of headache in a general population – a prevalence study. J Clin Epidemiol 44: 1147–1157.

Rasmussen BK, Jensen R, Olesen J (1992a). Impact of headache on sickness absence and utilisation of medical services: a Danish population study. J Epidemiol Community Health 46: 443–446.

Rasmussen BK, Jensen R, Schroll M et al. (1992b). Interrelations between migraine and tension-type headache in the general population. Arch Neurol 49: 914–918.

Relja M (1997). Treatment of tension-type headache by local injection of botulinum toxin. Eur J Neurol 4: S71–S73.

Rollnik JD, Tanneberger O, Schubert M et al. (2000). Treatment of tension-type headache with botulinum toxin type A: a double-blind, placebo-controlled study. Headache 40: 300–305.

Russell M, Rasmussen BK, Brennum J et al. (1992). Presentation of a new instrument. The diagnostic headache diary. Cephalalgia 12: 369–374.

Ryan RE (1977). Motrin – a new agent for the symptomatic treatment of muscle contraction headache. Headache 16: 280–283.

Sawynok J, Esser MJ, Reid AR (2001). Antidepressants as analgesics: an overview of central and peripheral mechanisms of action. J Psychiatry Neurosci 26: 21–29.

Schachtel BP, Thoden WR (1988). Onset of action of ibuprofen in the treatment of muscle-contraction headache. Headache 28: 471–474.

Schachtel BP, Thoden WR, Konerman JP et al. (1991). Headache pain model for assessing and comparing the efficacy of over-the-counter analgesic agents. Clin Pharmacol Ther 50: 322–329.

Schachtel BP, Furey SA, Thoden WR (1996). Nonprescription ibuprofen and acetaminophen in the treatment of tension-type headache. J Clin Pharmacol 36: 1120–1125.

Schwartz BS, Stewart WF, Simon D et al. (1998). Epidemiology of tension-type headache. JAMA 279: 381–383.

Shimomura T, Awaki E, Kowa H et al. (1991). Treatment of tension-type headache with tizanidine hydrochloride: its efficacy and relationship to the plasma MHPG concentration. Headache 31: 601–604.

Silberstein SD, Lipton RD, Solomon S et al. (1996). Classification of daily headaches or near daily headaches: field trial of revised IHS criteria. Neurology 47: 871–875.

Silberstein SD, Gobel H, Jensen R et al. (2006). Botulinum toxin type A in the prophylactic treatment of chronic tension-type headache: a multicentre, double-blind, randomized, placebo-controlled, parallel-group study. Cephalalgia 26: 790–800.

Singh NN, Misra S (2002). Sertraline in chronic tension-type headache. J Assoc Physicians India 50: 873–878.

Smuts J, Baker MK, Smuts HM (1999). Prophylactic treatment of chronic tension-type headache using botulinum toxin type A. Eur J Neurol 6 (Suppl. 4): S99–S102.

Steiner TJ, Lange R (1998). Ketoprofen (25 mg) in the symptomatic treatment of episodic tension-type headache: double-blind placebo-controlled comparison with acetaminophen (1000 mg). Cephalalgia 18: 38–43.

Steiner TJ, Lange R, Voelker M (2003). Aspirin in episodic tension-type headache: placebo-controlled dose-ranging comparison with paracetamol. Cephalalgia 23: 59–66.

Stovner LJ, Hagen K, Jensen R et al. (2007). The global burden of headache: a documentation of headache prevalence and disability world-wide. Cephalalgia 27: 193–210.

Torelli P, Jensen R, Olesen J (2004). Physiotherapy for tension-type headache: a controlled study. Cephalalgia 24: 29–36.

Ulrich V, Russell MB, Jensen R et al. (1996). A comparison of tension-type headache in migraineurs and in non-migraineurs: a population-based study. Pain 67: 501–506.

Van Gerven JMA, Schoemaker RC, Jacobs LD et al. (1996). Self-medication of single headache episode with ketoprofen, ibuprofen or placebo, home-monitored with an electronic patient diary. Br J Clin Pharmacol 42: 475–481.

Vernon H, McDermaid CS, Hagino C (1999). Systematic review of randomized clinical trials of complementary/alternative therapies in the treatment of tension-type and cervicogenic headache. Complement Ther Med 7: 142–155.

Watanabe Y, Saito H, Abe K (1993). Tricyclic antidepressants block NMDA receptor-mediated synaptic responses and induction of long-term potentiation in rat hippocampal slices. Neuropharmacology 32: 479–486.

Zeeberg P, Olesen J, Jensen R (2005). Effect of multidisciplinary treatment in a tertiary referral headache centre. Cephalalgia 25: 1159–1167.

Zeeberg P, Olesen J, Jensen R (2006). Probable medication-overuse headache: the effect of a 2-month drug-free period. Neurology 66: 1894–1898.

Handbook of Clinical Neurology, Vol. 97 (3rd series)
Headache
G. Nappi and M.A. Moskowitz, Editors

Chapter 32

Cluster headache and trigeminal autonomic cephalalgias: general aspects

GIUSEPPE NAPPI [1]* AND MICHAEL A. MOSKOWITZ [2]

[1]*Chair of Neurology, "Sapienza" University of Rome and IRCSS "C. Mondino Institute of Neurology" Foundation, Pavia, Italy*

[2]*Stroke and Neurovascular Regulation Laboratory, Departments of Radiology and Neurology, Massachusetts General Hospital, Harvard Medical School, Charlestown, MA, USA*

In the second edition of the International Classification of Headache Disorders (ICHD-II), the term trigeminal autonomic cephalalgias (TACs) was introduced to delineate a group of primary headache syndromes characterized by short-lasting pain with unilateral trigeminal distribution, associated with ipsilateral cranial autonomic symptoms. These forms include cluster headache (CH), paroxysmal hemicrania, short-lasting unilateral neuralgiform headache attacks with conjunctival injection and tearing (SUNCT), and probable TAC.

The etiology of these syndromes is largely unknown, notwithstanding the quite high number of investigations performed, at least in the case of CH. The lack of specific animal models for TACs and their rarity have probably contributed to hampering the process of understanding their underlying mechanisms.

The availability of more and more sophisticated neuroimaging techniques has recently allowed the identification of the central nervous system structures primarily involved. Functional neuroimaging findings, together with neurophysiological data on the functional modulation of nociceptive pathways, and in association with the first information from genetic studies on the possible existence of constitutional factors, will hopefully provide relevant information in the near future.

For now, it can be stated that CH is likely a disorder of the central nervous system, in particular the hypothalamus, possibly associated with the involvement of peripheral components, e.g., the inflammation of the cavernous sinus causing neurovascular dysfunction and pain.

If pathophysiological knowledge of TACs is far from satisfactory, the treatment of these conditions emerges as even more challenging. In the case of CH, only a few options are available for prophylactic treatment, with a rate of success which varies between and within subjects. With regard to symptomatic treatment, subcutaneous sumatriptan is very effective, but it has limitations in the daily frequency of intake and it is contraindicated when hypertension or other cardiovascular disorders are present. Unfortunately, sumatriptan – which was marketed more than 15 years ago – represents the last real breakthrough in the field of symptomatic treatment of CH.

The limited availability of therapeutic tools becomes particularly frustrating in the – fortunately rare – cases of intractable TACs, CH in particular. In recent years, various neurostimulation approaches have been tested for intractable chronic CH: deep brain stimulation (DBS) of the hypothalamus, occipital nerve stimulation, and vagal nerve stimulation. So far, studies on the DBS are limited to relatively small numbers of patients, placebo-controlled trials are not available, and the procedure has proved to be potentially at high risk of severe complications, which suggests the need to await further larger studies before delivering recommendations on its use. Occipital nerve stimulation is a safer procedure, but it is associated with a lower efficacy. Even lower – and

*Correspondence to: Professor Giuseppe Nappi, Chair of Neurology, "Sapienza" University of Rome and IRCSS "C. Mondino Institute of Neurology" Foundation, Pavia, Italy, E-mail: giuseppe.nappi@mondino.it

at present reported only in isolated patients – is the efficacy of neurostimulation of the vagus nerve.

In the case of paroxysmal hemicrania and SUNCT, the therapeutic armamentarium is even more limited, relying, in the case of paroxysmal hemicrania, mostly on indomethacin – as though the clock had stopped 30 years ago – and, in the case of SUNCT, on an empirical try-and-change approach, as shown in isolated case reports.

In conclusion, although considerable advances have been made in diagnostic and therapeutic approaches to TACs, much research is still needed to understand fully and manage better these challenging primary headache forms.

Handbook of Clinical Neurology, Vol. 97 (3rd series)
Headache
G. Nappi and M.A. Moskowitz, Editors

Chapter 33

Pathophysiology of cluster headache and other trigeminal autonomic cephalalgias

ELISABET WALDENLIND* AND CHRISTINA SJÖSTRAND
Department of Neurology, Karolinska University Hospital/Karolinska Institutet, Stockholm, Sweden

INTRODUCTION

In the second edition of the International Classification of Headache Disorders (ICDH-II) (Headache Classification Subcommittee of the International Headache Society, 2004), the term "trigeminal autonomic cephalalgias" (TACs) was introduced to delineate a group of primary headache syndromes with short-lasting headaches, unilateral trigeminal distribution of pain, and prominent ipsilateral cranial autonomic symptoms (Goadsby and Lipton, 1997). Experimental, clinical, and laboratory research has indicated important shared pathophysiology, i.e., excessive cranial parasympathetic autonomic reflex activation to nociceptive input in the ophthalmic division of the trigeminal nerve.

Cluster headache (CH) has been recognized for many years, whereas short-lasting unilateral neuralgiform pain with conjunctival injection and tearing (SUNCT) and the paroxysmal hemicranias (PH) are rare headache syndromes that have been described during recent decades. Consequently, there are far more studies regarding CH than SUNCT and PH, and thus this chapter will focus mainly on pathophysiological mechanisms in CH.

Still, the etiology of these syndromes is unknown. Since there is no animal model for the TACs, hypotheses about physiological mechanisms have to be tested in clinical studies or experimental human headache models. This is a slow procedure hampered by the relative rareness of CH and its episodic nature.

Challenging clinical features of CH (Headache Classification Subcommittee of the International Headache Society, 2004) have not yet been explained or are only partly understood. For instance, the unilaterality of pain, the self-limited headache attacks recurring with "clockwise regularity" (Ekbom, 1968) clustered in periods (Ekbom, 1947) or in some cases a chronic pattern (Ekbom and Olivarius, 1971); the male preponderance (although during recent years this is less pronounced Manzoni, 1998; Ekbom et al., 2002); and why substances like alcohol, histamine (Horton, 1941), and nitroglycerine (Ekbom, 1968) can provoke typical CH attacks only during cluster periods and not during remission. The main lines of research during recent decades have focused on whether CH is a disorder of the central nervous system, in particular the hypothalamus, or of a peripheral origin such as inflammation of the cavernous sinus, causing neurovascular dysfunction and pain. Further, epidemiological and genetic research has aimed at clarifying whether constitutional factors may predispose for CH.

UNILATERALITY

Typically CH attacks are strictly unilateral, with the maximal pain localized deep behind one eye or the temple, and associated with ipsilateral facial autonomic symptoms. This might indicate involvement of structures in the retro-orbital or cavernous sinus area. It has been speculated whether prior head trauma (Turkewitz et al., 1992) or constitutional anatomical variants like narrowness of the cavernous sinus or the hypophyseal fossa (Afra et al., 1998) would represent predisposing factors for CH, but there are hitherto no convincing data to prove this. In contrast, there are a number of reports where CH-like attacks have evolved secondary to various pathological processes, all located near the midline in proximity to the cavernous sinus, pituitary gland, and hypothalamus (Carter, 2004). Epidemiological data show that the risk for an individual to develop

*Correspondence to: Elisabet Waldenlind, Department of Neurology, Karolinska University Hospital/Karolinska Institutet, S-141 86 Stockholm, Sweden, Tel: 00-46-73-699 4530, 00-46-8-5858 7278, Fax: 00-46-8-774 4822, E-mail: elisabet.waldenlind@karolinska.se

CH on the contralateral side is 200 times higher than to develop CH at all (Sjaastad et al., 1985); this has been interpreted to indicate that midline structures would be affected.

The trigeminovascular system and the trigeminoautonomic reflex

Mapping of the trigeminovascular system and the trigeminoautonomic reflex has provided a new basis for the understanding of the TACs. The trigeminovascular system provides sensory innervation of the cerebral and dural vessels and it also has an efferent potential (May and Goadsby, 1999). The trigeminovascular system consists of neurons (Cushing, 1904; Penfield and McNaughton, 1940; Feindel et al., 1960; McNaughton and Feindl, 1977; May and Goadsby, 1999) with bipolar cell bodies in the trigeminal ganglion. Their peripheral fibers connect with vessels and other cranial structures and their central fibers project centrally to form synapses in the caudal brainstem and the upper cervical cord (Kaube et al., 1993; Goadsby and Hoskin, 1997; Hoskin et al., 1999). Several potent vasodilator peptides like calcitonin gene-related peptide (CGRP), substance P, and neurokinin A are co-localized with transmitters in various combinations within the cell bodies (Edvinsson et al., 1993). When the trigeminal ganglion was activated experimentally in humans, cerebral blood flow increased and there was facial flushing and increased concentrations of substance P and CGRP in the external jugular vein as markers of trigeminovascular activation (Goadsby et al., 1988).

The trigeminal autonomic brainstem reflex (Lambert et al., 1984; Goadsby et al., 1986) consists of an afferent limb, the trigeminal nerve, and an efferent limb, which is the facial/greater superficial petrosal nerve (parasympathetic) dilator pathway. It stems from the superior salivatory nucleus in the pons and supplies lacrimal glands and blood vessels in the upper part of the face. CGRP is a marker of trigeminal activation and vasoactive intestinal peptide (VIP) is a marker of parasympathetic activation. Sufficient painful stimulation of the ophthalmic trigeminal division produces reflex activation of the cranial parasympathetic outflow, with associated vasodilation of the internal carotid artery and watering and redness of the eye or nasal congestion (May et al., 2001).

There is now convincing evidence that the trigeminovascular system and the trigeminoautonomic reflex are activated in CH. An important step forward was a report showing increased concentrations of CGRP and VIP in jugular venous blood during spontaneous CH attacks (Goadsby and Edvinsson, 1994). Furthermore, there was a decrease of CGRP concomitant with pain relief after treatment with vasoconstrictors like oxygen and sumatriptan but not after injection of pethidine. It was also shown that CGRP increased after nitroglycerine provocation but only if an attack was induced (Fanciullacci et al., 1995, 1997). CGRP in external jugular venous blood remained higher than normal between attacks of CH (Fanciullacci et al., 1997), as an indication of abnormal cyclical activation of the trigeminovascular system (Mathiau et al., 1994; Fanciullacci et al., 1997). According to one hypothesis, nitroglycerine triggers a cluster attack by stimulating trigeminal nociceptive fibers to release CGRP (Fanciullacci et al., 1995), but this view seems unlikely since the CGRP levels do not increase until the attack is well established (Fanciullacci et al., 1997).

Local vasodilation is an essential aspect of CH pathophysiology. Firstly, there is dilation of the ophthalmic and middle cerebral arteries during attacks of CH (Ekbom and Greitz, 1970; Dahl et al., 1990; Waldenlind et al., 1993). Secondly, attacks can be induced by specific vasodilators as a sign of increased neurovascular reactivity (Ekbom, 1968), and thirdly, sumatriptan, a potent vasoconstrictor, gives prompt relief of pain (Ekbom et al., 1993). A prominent opinion is that the vasodilation is mainly a secondary phenomenon due to pain and activation of the trigeminoautonomic reflex, since a similar distribution of vasodilation is seen in experimental studies of induced pain (May and Goadsby, 1999; May et al., 2001). Notably, vasodilation *per se* is not painful, but if there is concomitant sensitization of vascular pain receptors caused by local processes or centrally induced mechanisms it may contribute to pain.

The role of the vasodilator nitric oxide (NO) in CH is not clear. Basal levels of nitrite, a metabolite and marker of NO, have been reported to be higher in CH patients (either in remission or in the active period) than in controls as a possible sign of a hyperactive L-arginine NO pathway (D'Amico et al., 2002) or to be normal (in the active period between attacks) (Martelletti et al., 1999; Costa et al., 2003). The increase of nitrite after nitroglycerine provocation did not differ between healthy controls and patients who suffered an induced CH attack (Costa et al., 2003). Other factors, at present not clarified, may render the CH patient hypersensitive to NO and other vasodilators but not all the time, since a few hours immediately after a spontaneous attack patients appear to be refractory to nitroglycerine provocation (Ekbom, 1968). A most challenging issue is to clarify how CH pain is induced by nitroglycerine and to clarify why this occurs only during the active cluster period (Fanciullacci et al., 1997).

AUTONOMIC FEATURES

Local

The ipsilateral facial autonomic symptoms associated with the cluster attack suggest both sympathetic deficit and parasympathetic hyperactivity. Several sources of the autonomic symptoms are presently under consideration at central as well as peripheral levels. As examples, the autonomic dysregulation may originate within the central nervous system in association with a hypothalamic disturbance. Sympathetic nerve fibers to the upper part of the face may be compromised due to vasodilation or perivascular edema within the carotid canal. Finally, autonomic symptoms may be secondary to trigeminal discharge as part of the trigeminal autonomic reflex.

About 3% of patients have no clinical autonomic symptoms (Nappi et al., 1992) and patients with and without autonomic symptoms have been described in the same families (Russell and Andersson, 1995; Leone et al., 2002). In some patients the ocular sympathetic deficit (miosis and ptosis) persists into remission and intensifies during attacks. Pain generally precedes autonomic disturbances and escalates within a few minutes to maximum (Drummond and Lance, 1984), and recruitment of secondary autonomic disturbances may cause pain to build up in a positive way (Drummond, 2006). Cyclical parasympathetic disturbances with or without headaches occasionally persist after trigeminal surgery (Matharu and Goadsby, 2002), suggesting that parasympathetic disturbances may be triggered centrally during attacks of CH and not necessarily by trigeminal activity. Besides, cyclical autonomic dysfunction without headache sometimes precedes (Salvesen, 2000) or follows typical cluster periods (Ashkenazi and Silberstein, 2004). These observations suggest that a central generator, for instance in the hypothalamus, may trigger pain and autonomic symptoms.

Activation of trigeminal autonomic parasympathetic reflexes probably mediates lacrimation, nasal congestion and secretion, forehead sweating, conjunctival injection, and vasodilation during CH attacks secondary to pain (Goadsby and Lipton, 1997). Thermoregulatory flushing and sweating are impaired on the symptomatic side of the forehead in CH patients with persistent signs of ocular sympathetic deficit (Drummond, 1992). During CH attacks, paradoxical sweating and increased blood flow often occur in this region (Sjaastad et al., 1981; Drummond and Lance, 1984). It was suggested that this paradoxical response may be explained by collateral sprouting of parasympathetic lacrimal fibers into sympathetically denervated blood vessels and sweat glands making functional connections with VIP receptors (Drummond and Lance, 1992; Drummond, 2006).

Miosis and ptosis are characteristic signs of a sympathetic deficit. Most evidence indicates a peripheral source of the sympathetic deficit in CH. Vasodilation or edema within the carotid canal (Ekbom and Greitz, 1970) or a proposed inflammation within the cavernous sinus (Hardebo, 1994) may injure sympathetic fibers on their way to the skull. Pain or anticipation of pain may also alter central sympathetic discharge (Drummond and Alessandro, 2005).

Peptide markers of sympathetic activity are not altered during CH attacks (Goadsby and Edvinsson, 1994). In the morning and at night when CH attacks frequently occur, however, lowered plasma norepinephrine levels as well as lowered spinal fluid levels of norepinephrine and catecholamine metabolites have been observed compared with healthy controls (Strittmatter et al., 1996). In contrast, muscular sympathetic nerve fibers show normal activation to vasodilation after nitroglycerine administration and during CH pain, and there are normal blood pressure responses (Nordin et al., 1997).

Other mechanisms may influence pupillary responses in CH, such as depletion of neuropeptide trigeminal stores after repeated attacks (Fanciullacci et al., 1989), or altered opioid control of pupillary activity (Tassorelli et al., 1998). Fanciullacci et al. (1989) found that brief electrical stimulation of the infratrochlear nerve induced a slowly developing noncholinergic miosis in healthy subjects. In CH the miotic response was attenuated on the symptomatic side during bouts and this was hypothesized to be due to depleted CGRP and VIP stores. Tassorelli et al. (1998) studied the miotic response after several minutes of hand immersion into painful cold water with or without naloxone as pretreatment. In controls the miotic response could be blocked by naloxone, while in CH at any phase of the disorder there was no miotic response except in individuals who were given naloxone. The persistence of this opioid disturbance during remission may indicate a vulnerability to CH.

Systemic autonomic function

Systemic autonomic disturbances during the cluster period, such as cardiac arrhythmias, bradycardia during attacks, and altered 24-h patterns of heart rate variability during cluster periods, have been recorded (Bruyn et al., 1976; Russell and Storstein, 1983; Micieli et al., 1993) and may be secondary to pain or disrupted sleep, but a primary generalized autonomic dysfunction may also be involved. In a study performed both during clinical remission and the active period (Meyer et al.,

2003), an apparently permanent metabolic disturbance of lipolysis was observed and hypothesized to be a result of sympathetic dysregulation, possibly at the hypothalamic level. Nocturnal adipose tissue lipolysis was lowered with an altered temporal profile in CH patients compared to controls. β-Receptor function in adipose tissue was found not to be deficient but rather to be upregulated in support of the hypothesis of a systemic decreased sympathetic tone (Meyer et al., 2006).

CIRCADIAN RHYTHMS, NEUROENDOCRINOLOGY, AND THE HYPOTHALAMUS

Due to its central role in rhythm regulation and autonomic control, the hypothalamus has been hypothesized to be involved in CH pathogenesis (Medina et al., 1979). The relapsing–remitting course of CH, the seasonal variation, and the "clockwise regularity" of attacks together with altered neuroendocrine, vascular, and pain control indicate that circadian and circannual rhythm regulation is affected. The timing of CH attacks also appears to be governed by the dark–light and sleep–activity cycles. Accordingly, there is an afternoon peak of CH attacks in Italy (Manzoni et al., 1983), which is not observed in Scandinavia (Russell, 1981), where there is no siesta during the work day.

A report of lowered basal testosterone levels in men with CH (Kudrow, 1976) was the first in a series of neuroendocrine studies that have provided ample indirect evidence that the hypothalamus is involved in CH pathophysiology. These studies have shown altered 24-h secretory patterns with phase shifts for hormones regulated via hypothalamus and the pituitary gland, like melatonin, cortisol, prolactin, testosterone, and growth hormone, during active periods but also during remission, as well as altered responses to various neuroendocrine tests (Leone and Bussone, 1993). Of particular interest is the pineal hormone melatonin which has been considered as a marker of the circadian system. Its endogenous circadian rhythm is driven by an oscillator in the hypothalamic suprachiasmatic nuclei which is entrained to external temporal variations of illumination via a retinohypothalamic norepinephric pathway. In humans plasma levels are high at night and low during the day. Reduced 24-h plasma levels of melatonin, as well as phase shifts (advanced or delayed) of the nocturnal peak, are observed during the cluster period (Chazot et al., 1984; Waldenlind et al., 1984a). It is unlikely that lowered melatonin levels are due to pain, since stress would rather increase secretion (Vaughan et al., 1978). Furthermore, in a longitudinal study (Waldenlind et al., 1994), the nocturnal excretion of melatonin was examined in urine monthly for a period of 14 months in patients with episodic CH. The 12-month mean levels were lower in patients than in controls, with no difference between cluster and remission periods. Similarly, nocturnal urinary excretion of 6-sulfatoxymelatonin, the chief metabolite of melatonin, was reduced in both phases of CH (Leone et al., 1998). Oral medication with melatonin has shown some efficacy as CH prophylaxis (Leone et al., 1994). Lowered melatonin production in CH may be considered as a marker for a vulnerability of the circadian regulation in CH rather than a causative agent.

The hypothalamic–pituitary–adrenal (HPA) axis is affected during both active disease and remission. During active cluster period and in chronic CH there is increased 24-h production of cortisol (Ferrari et al., 1983; Leone and Bussone, 1993) and a delayed nocturnal trough (Waldenlind et al., 1987), whereas during remission the circadian rhythm appears to be normal compared to healthy controls, with the exception of occasional reports of increased morning levels (Leone et al., 1994). The altered temporal pattern may be related to a disturbance of rhythm regulation, but long-term effects on sleep during cluster periods as well as stress-related responses also have to be considered. Normal dexamethasone suppression responses during both phases of CH indicate that the feedback mechanisms regulating plasma cortisol are normal (Devoize et al., 1986), while decreased responses to CRH (Leone et al., 1991), insulin (Leone et al., 1991), and the serotoninergic agonist *m*-chlorophenylpiperazine (Leone et al., 1997) indicate reduced responsiveness of the HPA axis during remission and active periods. The pro-opiomelanocortin-related peptides β-endorphin and β-lipotropin have also shown anomalies of their circadian production (Nappi et al., 1985; Franceschini et al., 1996).

The diurnal rhythm of prolactin has been reported to be normal (Ferrari et al., 1983; Chazot et al., 1984) or altered during the active period (Ferrari et al., 1979; Polleri et al., 1982). In patients not having cluster attacks although in an active period, the nocturnal peak appeared blunted (Polleri et al., 1982), and in remission the diurnal rhythm was flattened and lowered in men compared to controls and the same men during active periods (Waldenlind and Gustafsson, 1987a).

The 24-h data for blood pressure, body temperature, and pain sensitivity (Nappi et al., 1987) have shown that more patients than controls lack a significant circadian rhythm when the data are analyzed by cosinor rhythmometry (Halberg et al., 1977). Thus, there are several indications of circadian dysregulation in CH.

NEUROIMAGING

Functional and structural patterns

Functional neuroimaging with positron emission tomography (PET) and anatomical imaging with voxel-based magnetic resonance imaging (MRI) morphometry have made it possible to show directly that the posterior hypothalamic gray matter is indeed a key area in CH and other TACs.

The very first PET study in CH with ^{15}O-buthanol as a marker for regional cerebral blood flow was published in 1996 (Hsieh et al., 1996). Four patients were examined during nitroglycerine-provoked attacks of CH. There was a preferential activation of the non-dominant hemisphere in a similar pattern as seen in peripheral neuropathic pain. In particular the anterior cingulate cortex showed activation, an area involved in affective/cognitive processing of pain and willed attention. There was no specific mention of the hypothalamic region. In a later PET study with $H_2{}^{15}O$ in a larger patient series, significant activation during nitroglycerine-provoked attacks was observed in the ipsilateral hypothalamic gray matter when compared with the headache-free state (May et al., 1998a). This activation pattern could not be produced in patients in remission when compared to patients having acute attacks (May et al., 2000), in healthy volunteers exposed to experimental pain after injection of capsaicin into forehead skin (May et al., 1998b), or during migraine attacks. The hypothalamic activation appeared to be unique for CH pain, while in migraine there was activation in the brainstem suggesting different pathogenesis of the two syndromes. Hypothalamic activation has been reported in a patient during a spontaneous attack of CH (Sprenger et al., 2004). With functional MRI a similar pattern of hypothalamic activation during pain has been shown in SUNCT (May et al., 1999a) and hemicrania continua (Matharu et al., 2004). In hemicrania continua there was also activation in the brainstem. Thus, with functional neuroimaging methods it has been possible to visualize specific activation patterns during pain in CH, SUNCT, and hemicrania continua, and involvement of the hypothalamus as an indication of shared pathophysiological mechanisms.

With voxel-based morphometric analysis of the structural T_1-weighted MRI scans it has been possible to identify significant structural differences in gray-matter density in CH patients both during a cluster period and in remission (May et al., 1999b). An increase in volume was observed bilaterally in hypothalamus at virtually the same area in which activation was seen with PET during attacks. When mirror images were used to normalize for pain side, the structural change seemed slightly lateralized to the pain side. The nature of this structural change is not yet known. Thus, for the first time there is direct evidence showing structural pathology in CH, challenging the present definition of primary and secondary headaches.

With PET (Hsieh et al., 1996; May et al., 1998a, b), activation corresponding to the intracranial arteries and the cavernous sinus bilaterally has been observed and may indicate vasodilation and perhaps an increased venous inflow draining the dilated ophthalmic artery. According to May et al. (2001) this may be an epiphenomenon of trigeminovascular activation and not specific for CH. The prompt pain relief of sumatriptan injection has been claimed to be due to vasoconstriction, but decreased trigeminal release of vasoactive peptides has to be considered as well other non-vascular effects, for instance at the hypothalamic level.

Deep-brain stimulation

The activation of the inferior posterior hypothalamus and corresponding structural changes have inspired a completely new approach to treatment of intractable CH (Franzini et al., 2003). Deep-brain stimulation of posterior hypothalamus ipsilateral to the side of attacks has been shown to improve otherwise drug-resistant chronic CH (Leone et al., 2003; Schoenen et al., 2005). Pain disappearance was never immediate, but occurred from a few hours up to 4 weeks after starting stimulation, and the insertion of the electrode as such appeared not to affect pain attacks. Since there was no immediate cessation of attacks by deep-brain stimulation, a more complex mechanism involving several brain structures rather than simple inhibition or stimulation of hypothalamic nuclei was suggested. This would be consistent with PET studies showing that hypothalamic stimulation activates certain brain areas and deactivates others (May et al., 2003).

INFLAMMATION

CH has been attributed to a remittent inflammatory process within the cavernous sinus as the cause of unilateral pain (Moskowitz, 1988; Hannerz, 1991; Hardebo, 1994), obstruction of venous outflow, and damage to traversing sympathetic fibers based on pathological orbital phlebograms (Hannerz et al., 1987; Hannerz, 1991). However, there was no consistent correspondence between phlebopathic signs and symptoms, and similar phlebographic findings have been shown in healthy controls (Bovim et al., 1992). Further, with MRI (Sjaastad and Rinck, 1990) no definite abnormality was seen. With gallium single-photon emission computed tomography (SPECT), one study reported abnormal findings in the cavernous sinus during the active period in 3 out of 6 patients, suggesting inflammation (Gawel et al., 1990), which could not be confirmed in a later study showing no difference in labeling of the cavernous sinus between the CH period and remission, nor between cluster patients and migraineurs (Sianard-Gainko et al., 1994). Nor is there any abnormal labeling during nitroglycerine-induced cluster attacks (Schuh-Hofer et al., 2006). In conclusion, with available radiographic techniques there are hitherto no consistent findings supporting inflammation or any other type of structural pathology in the cavernous sinus region.

Inflammatory signs in blood (Hannerz, 1991) and in cerebrospinal fluid (CSF) (Hardebo and Ryberg, 1989) have been reported in some patients during the cluster period, but not by others in blood (Remahl et al., 2000; Empl and Straube, 2001). A number of studies have aimed at exploring the function of the immune system (Martelletti and Giacovazzo, 1996; Empl and Straube, 2001). With respect to the complex interaction between the hypothalamus and the immune system, inflammatory mechanisms in CH cannot be excluded. However, with the data available there is no consistent view as to the role of the immune system in CH pathophysiology, whether involved in the etiology or reflecting secondary phenomena due to pain or stress.

GENETIC ASPECTS

Heredity was previously regarded as being of minor importance for the etiology of CH. During recent decades this impression has changed since several studies have reported a positive family history. At the start of genetic research in CH other prevalence figures were used, i.e., CH was supposed to be less common. However, in more recent years investigations indicate a higher CH lifetime prevalence than previously thought. A study from Vågå (Norway) yielded a prevalence of CH of 0.38% (Sjaastad and Baaketeig, 2003). An Italian survey (Torelli et al., 2005) and a Swedish population-based twin study (Ekbom et al., 2006) showed the prevalence to be 0.2%. Thus, it is likely that the true prevalence of CH is about 1 per 500 rather than 1 per 1500, in many ways corresponding to the old extrapolated figures from Ekbom et al. (1978) and Kudrow (1980), although a later investigation might point to a lower prevalence (Black et al., 2005).

Genetic epidemiology

Four genetic epidemiological surveys have provided more complete information about CH patients and their relatives (Kudrow and Kudrow, 1994; Russell et al., 1995a; Leone et al., 2001; El Amrani et al., 2002). The following figures for familial risk are calculated (Russell, 2004) according to today's prevalence figures of about 1 in 500 inhabitants. Based on these studies the first-degree relatives had a 5–18-fold greater increased risk for CH than the general population. Second-degree relatives had a one to three times higher risk for CH. A complex segregation analysis of Danish families suggested an autosomal-dominant mode of inheritance in these families (Russell et al., 1995b). However, no common clear mode of inheritance was seen in all the reported families, although CH seems to be an autosomal-dominant inherited disorder in some families, but probably with incomplete penetrance. CH has been reported in seven concordant monozygotic twin pairs (Eadie, 1966; Sjaastad and Salvesen, 1986; Couturier et al., 1991; Roberge et al., 1992; Sjaastad et al., 1993; Lampl, 2002), although publication itself might introduce selection bias (Motulsky, 1978).The latter is emphasized in a twin survey based on the Swedish Twin Registry and the Swedish Inpatient Registry (Svensson et al., 2003). In this study two monozygotic and nine dizygotic twin pairs were all discordant for CH, and had been discordant for between 10 and 31 years. Nevertheless, the results from these genetic epidemiological studies indicate a genetic influence of the disease.

As for SUNCT and PH, there are case reports of single families with more than one member affected. In one family two patients with PH were identified, one of whom also had migraine with aura (Cohen et al., 2006). There were also other members with migraine in this family. Otherwise there are no other reports of PH families. However, in a series of 74 patients with PH, 80% did not have a family history of headache, while 15% had a family history of migraine and 5% a family history of CH, trigeminal neuralgia, or other headache (Boes and Dodick, 2002). As for SUNCT, a family with two affected family members has been reported, but one of them was diseased and thus the history was taken from the family members (Gantenbein and Goadsby, 2005).

Clinical picture of familial CH

Although there are several reports on familial CH there is little detailed information about the clinical characteristics of these families. Some studies have indicated that some familial CH cases might differ from the clinical pattern of sporadic CH. A lower age at onset has been seen in children than in parents, different clinical pattern in separate affected family members, worsening of symptoms in each successive generation, and a high frequency of attacks (1–8 attacks/day) respectively was found in a few separate families (Russell and Andersson, 1995). Females with familial CH had a lower age at onset than females with sporadic CH (Torelli and Manzoni, 2003). As described above, two patients who experienced attacks of autonomic symptoms without headache belonged to the same family (Leone et al., 2002). A higher frequency of females in familial CH than among sporadic cases has been observed (El Amrani et al., 2002). In an Italian survey several affected relatives had CH with undetermined periodicity (Leone et al., 2001) and about 1 in 5 of the affected had CH-like disorders not fulfilling International Headache Society criteria (Headache Classification Committee of the International Headache Society, 1988). Another family study also described CH cases not fulfilling criteria, mainly because of long duration of attacks (van Vliet et al., 2003). Furthermore, atypical cases not fulfilling criteria (Headache Classification Committee of the International Headache Society, 2004) have been observed in family members in a Swedish family material (Sjostrand et al., 2005). They all had clinical CH characteristics, but the attacks had a tendency to occur in a sporadic way, a tendency towards "mini-bouts"; they described milder pain and longer duration of attacks. However, attacks were strictly unilateral and the pain was orbital/periorbital. All but one had autonomic features during attacks. Thus, atypical cases are seen within families as well as in sporadic cases (Sjaastad et al., 1988; Martins et al., 2005) and these might represent an expanded spectrum of the TAC group. One might speculate whether these cases represent clinically different forms of the same disorder with activation of the trigeminoparasympathetic reflex as a common pathophysiological mechanism.

Molecular genetic studies of CH

The molecular genetic background of CH has until recently been an uninvestigated field, probably mostly due to the fact that CH was long regarded as a sporadic disorder. However, there are a few studies, or rather reports, including very small numbers of patients.

Some studies have reported human leukocyte antigen (HLA) frequencies in CH, mainly two studies of Italian material. An increased frequency of HLA-DR5 as well as a decreased frequency of HLA-B14 was shown (Martelletti et al., 1984). In patients responding well to lithium treatment, HLA-B18 was reported to be increased (Giacovazzo et al., 1985). However, the studied material was small and the finding in clear need of confirmation.

In a Japanese man with sporadic CH and no family history of mitochondrial encephalopathy, lactic acidosis, and stroke-like episodes (MELAS), a point mutation was reported in mitochondrial transfer RNA(Leu (UUR)) gene at nucleotide pair 3243 (Shimomura et al., 1994). This mutation could not be detected in either an Italian or a German study of CH patients (Cortelli et al., 1995; Seibel et al., 1996). Another report described multiple deletions of mitochondrial DNA in a Japanese man with CH and chronic progressive external ophthalmoplegia (Odawara et al., 1997). However, this patient did not fulfill the International Headache Society criteria for CH because his attacks were too long.

Calcium channel gene *CACNA1A*

At the end of the 1990s mutations in the *CACNA1A* gene were found to be responsible for several episodic neurological disorders and its importance especially in familial hemiplagic migraine was recognized in headache genetics (Ophoff et al., 1996). Consequently, several studies were performed to search for a plausible relevance of this gene in the more common forms of migraine. The *CACNA1A* gene has also been studied in CH. An association study of sporadic CH patients and controls did not reveal any significant differences as regards phenotype and allele frequencies (Sjostrand et al., 2001). A linkage study has been performed in an extended Dutch CH pedigree (Haan et al., 2001). Haplotype analysis did not reveal any obvious disease haplotype, and single-strand conformation polymorphism analysis of all 47 exons of the *CACNA1A* gene did not reveal a causative mutation in this family.

NOS

Polymorphic markers of the three NOS genes have also been studied in CH. However, an association study of CH patients and controls did not reveal any significant differences in this population (Sjostrand et al., 2002). A genetic study of trace amine receptors and CH has been published; this was a negative study (Aridon et al., 2004). However, these genes have not been studied in other populations.

Hypocretin

Hypocretin-1 and -2 (also called orexin-A and -B) are neuropeptides located exclusively in the lateral hypothalamus. They act on G-protein receptors, named HCRTR1 and HCRTR2, respectively. Hypocretins are important in regulating the sleep–wake cycle and a mutation in hypocretin has been reported to cause narcolepsy (Peyron et al., 2000). In 2004 a positive allelic association study on CH was published (Rainero et al., 2004). Several polymorphisms of the hypocretin/orexin system genes were evaluated in 109 CH patients and 211 controls. The 1246 G→A polymorphism of the gene was significantly different between cases and controls. Homozygosity for the G allele was associated with an increased disease risk for CH (odds ratio: 6.79, 95% confidence interval: 2.25–22.99). Furthermore, an allelic association study on the *HCRTR2* gene was performed in a Swedish, Danish, and British cohort comprising 257 patients and 272 controls, and in this cohort the former *HCRTR2* association could not be confirmed (Baumber et al., 2006). After stratification of single nucleotide polymorphism data into different populations it was still not confirmed. However, the *HCRTR2* gene has been further investigated in a German population consisting of 226 patients with CH and 266 controls (Schurks et al., 2006). The genotype and allele distribution varied significantly between patients and controls and in this cohort the homozygous carriers of the G allele had a twofold increase in risk for CH. It is evident that further studies are needed to clarify whether the *HCRTR2* gene is of importance in CH pathophysiology.

Linkage

A linkage study was performed on CH families from several countries (Baumber et al., 2006). First, a genome scan with almost 400 microsatellite markers covering the whole genome at 9-cM intervals was performed on five large Danish pedigrees. Four loci showed logarithm of odds of linkage (LOD) scores of potential significance, but when additional markers in additional individuals of Danish and Italian origin were added, the LOD scores were deflated and a single disease locus for CH was not identified. In summary, genetic predisposition for CH is likely to be complex and compounded by locus heterogeneity and variation in genes conferring only a small effect size.

BIOCHEMICAL BACKGROUND

A large number of biochemical studies have been performed more or less systematically in the search for disease-specific markers or markers indicating an increased vulnerability to CH. Many of the findings are at present fragmentary and not possible to fit into one single model of CH pathophysiology. Also, confirmatory studies are needed. Future molecular genetic studies might be able to re-evaluate the significance of these findings.

Most of the biochemical studies are presented in Table 33.1.

Histamine, mast cells, prostaglandins

Horton (1956) observed that CH was associated with an unusual histamine sensitivity since in more than 60% of his cases attacks could be induced with this drug. Histamine and mast cells have thereafter been subject to several studies. Histamine in blood has been reported to be higher during attacks (Anthony and Lance, 1971) and in urine (Sjaastad and Sjaastad, 1977) and increased numbers of mast cells have been found in skin biopsy from the temporal region (Appenzeller et al., 1981b; Liberski and Prusinski, 1982) both during and between cluster periods but also from the pain-free side compared to controls. Treatment with histamine H_1 (Friedman and Mikropoulos, 1958) and H_2 receptor blockers (Veger et al., 1976), or both (Anthony et al., 1978), as well as desensitization introduced by Horton (Symonds, 1956; Friedman and Mikropoulos, 1958), did not show any efficacy. Whether histamine release during attacks is secondary to trigeminal activation or whether it has a role in the induction of spontaneous CH attacks is not known.

Prostaglandins (PG) and leukotrienes (LT) have been proposed as mediators of neurovascular headache due to their vasoactive and hyperalgesic properties. They are not considered to be of primary pathogenetic importance in CH and non-steroidal anti-inflammatory drugs generally have no therapeutic effect (Waldenlind and Bussone, 2006).

Metencephalin and β-endorphin

Central mechanisms of pain control have been claimed to be disturbed in CH. In line with this, metencephalin-like activities (MET) in cerebrospinal fluid (CSF) were lower during (Anselmi et al., 1980; Hardebo and Ekman, 1985; Hardebo et al., 1985) and between (Hardebo et al., 1985) attacks of CH or did not differ (Vecchiet et al., 1987) compared with control patients. Low levels of CSF MET appear not to be caused by increased degradation since encephalinase and angiotensin-converting enzyme activities in CSF were not altered compared with controls (Spillanti et al., 1987). In plasma MET levels in chronic CH were lower during and after attacks than before the attack (Mosnaim et al., 1987), whereas in episodic CH higher levels have been reported during attacks (Hardebo and Ekman, 1987; Figuerola et al., 1990), and normal levels between attacks and during remission (Figuerola et al., 1990). The increase in plasma MET during pain may be secondary to sympathetic activation because MET in circulation is mainly derived from the adrenals, where it is stored with catecholamines. It may also be derived from neutrophils, in which a decrease of MET was observed parallel to the increase in plasma (Figuerola et al., 1991).

As regards β-endorphin (βEP) in CSF, there were no alterations during or between attacks of CH (Hardebo and Ekman, 1987). Plasma βEP has been reported to be increased (Appenzeller et al., 1981a) or normal

Table 33.1

Cluster headache pathophysiology: biochemical studies

Study	Reference	Specimen	*n*	Main findings	Cluster headache phase/ comparisons
Histamine	Anthony and Lance, 1971	Whole blood	22 CH	↑ histamine during versus before attacks	Before, during, and after attacks
	Sjaastad and Sjaastad, 1977	Urine	22 CH	↑ histamine in 7/22 patients during attack days	
Mast cells	Appenzeller et al., 1981b	Temporal skin biopsy	6 CH, 3 C	↑ number of mast cells in both phases perivascularly and near cutaneous nerves. No definitive change in degranulation	Period and remission
	Prusinski and Liberski, 1979	Temporal skin biopsy	13 CH, 6 C	↑ number of mast cells	Pain side versus C
	Liberski and Prusinski, 1982	Temporal skin biopsy	23 CH, 6 C	↑ number of mast cells versus C, but no difference between pain side versus pain-free side in CH	
	Joseph et al., 1985	Temporal skin biopsy	13 CH, 3 MA	↑ number of mast cells cluster period versus remission and versus MA, ↑ SP and ↑ 5-HT versus remission and MA	4 CH within 10 h of attack, 6 CH remission
	Dimitriadou et al., 1990	Temporal artery biopsy	19 CH, 10 C	↑ degranulation	Biopsy from pain side, between attacks
	Cuypers et al., 1980	Temporal skin biopsy	6 CH, 6 C	No difference in number, distribution, or morphology	3 in period and 3 in remission versus C
	Krabbe and Rank, 1985	Temporal artery biopsy	8 CCH, 7 ECH, 5 C	Number of mast cells and histology normal	14/15 in period or chronic
Opioid studies					
Encephalinase	Spillantini et al., 1987	CSF	5 CH, 5 C, 5 M	Similar range as M and C	Controls with non-painful neurological disorders
	Sicuteri et al., 1985	CSF	3 CH, 9 C	No sign difference versus C	Attack-free period
	Sicuteri et al., 1985	Plasma	18 CH, 20 C	↑ during (14) and between (18) spontaneous attacks versus C No significant difference before and during histamine-induced attacks versus C	During and between spontaneous and histamine-induced attacks
Angiotensin-converting enzyme (ACE)	Spillantini et al., 1987	CSF	5 CH, 5 C, 5 M	↓ ACE in CH and M versus C	Controls with non-painful neurological disorders

↑: increased; ↓: decreased; HVA: homovanillic acid; VMA: vanillyl mandelic acid; 5-HIAA: 5-hydroxyindole acetic acid; 5-HT: serotonin; BDNF, brain-derived nerve growth factor; NGF: nerve growth factor; PC/C: phosphatidylcholine/cholesterol ratio; NAA/Cr: *N*-acetyl aspartate/creatine ratio; Ch/Cr: choline/creatine ratio; β-TBG: β-thromboglobulin; PF4: platelet factor 4; CSF: cerebrospinal fluid; MRS: magnetic resonance spectroscopy; CH: cluster headache; C: controls; MA: migraine with aura; ECH: episodic cluster headache; M: migraine; MO: migraine without aura; TTH: tension-type headache; SP: substance P; NTG; nitroglycerine; CBF: cerebral blood flow; Li: lithium; PG: prostaglandin; ATP: adenosine triphosphate; PAF: platelet-activating factor; LP: lumbar puncture.

(Continued)

Table 33.1
Cluster headache pathophysiology: biochemical studies—Continued

Study	Reference	Specimen	*n*	Main findings	Cluster headache phase/ comparisons
Met-encephalin (MET)	Anselmi et al., 1980	CSF	5 CH, 5 C	MET below detection limit	Phase of disease not reported
	Hardebo et al., 1989	CSF	7 CH, 5 C	↓ MET in CH versus C ↑ MET after acupuncture	Period before and after acupuncture
	Vecchiet et al., 1987	CSF	5 CH, 34 C	No significant differences	Controls (LP for other reasons)
	Mosnaim et al., 1987	Plasma	8 CH, 18 C	↑ MET in plasma in 6/8 before attacks compared with attacks, remission, and C	During and after attacks
	Mosnaim et al., 1987	Platelets	8 CH, 18 C	↑ MET in platelets before versus after attack	During and after attacks
	Figuerola et al., 1990	Plasma	27 CH, 5 C	↑ during attacks compared to controls and remission	24 in period, 3 in remission, 2 longitudinal
	Figuerola et al., 1991	Neutrophils	27 CH, 9 C	↓ MET during (6) compared with after attack and remission ↑ MET after pain and remission versus C	
	Figuerola et al., 1994	Plasma	10 CH	No differences of MET after verapamil ↑ MET after prednisone	During period and 10 days after treatment
β-Endorphin (βEP)	Hardebo et al., 1989	CSF	7 CH, 7 C	No difference between CH and C No difference before and after acupuncture	Period before and after acupuncture
	Appenzeller et al., 1981a	Serum	6 CH, 4 MO	↑ in CH at height of attack	Onset, height, end, after attack
	Nappi et al., 1985	Plasma	7 CH, 55 C	No difference at 9 a.m. in CH versus C	CH period and controls
	Nappi et al., 1985	Plasma	7 CH, 7 C	No significant circadian rhythm in CH No attack-related changes	Blood samples over 24-h period
	Leone et al., 1993	Mononuclear leukocytes	65 CH, 50 C	↓ βEP during both phases of CH	33 cluster period, 32 remission
	Franceschini et al., 1996	Plasma	12 CH, 6 C	No significant circadian rhythm in CH period Delayed acrophase in CH period No attack-related changes	Blood samples over 24-h; period, attacks, remission versus controls
Nociceptin	Ertsey et al., 2004	Plasma	14 CH, 22 C	↓ during period but not in remission versus C May result in defective regulation of trigeminal activity	Period and remission versus controls

↑: increased; ↓: decreased; HVA: homovanillic acid; VMA: vanillyl mandelic acid; 5-HIAA: 5-hydroxyindole acetic acid; 5-HT: serotonin; BDNF, brain-derived nerve growth factor; NGF: nerve growth factor; PC/C: phosphatidylcholine/cholesterol ratio; NAA/Cr: *N*-acetyl aspartate/creatine ratio; Ch/Cr: choline/creatine ratio; β-TBG: β-thromboglobulin; PF4: platelet factor 4; CSF: cerebrospinal fluid; MRS: magnetic resonance spectroscopy; CH: cluster headache; C: controls; MA: migraine with aura; ECH: episodic cluster headache; M: migraine; MO: migraine without aura; TTH: tension-type headache; SP: substance P; NTG; nitroglycerine; CBF: cerebral blood flow; Li: lithium; PG: prostaglandin; ATP: adenosine triphosphate; PAF: platelet-activating factor; LP: lumbar puncture.

Other neuropeptides					
Calcitonin gene-related peptide	Goadsby and Edvinsson, 1994	Ext. jugular vein blood	13 CH, C	↑ during attacks	Spontaneous attacks versus controls
	Fanciullacci et al., 1995	Plasma	30 CH	↑ basal level in active period, ↑ during peak of attacks No increase after NTG in remission	18 in period, 12 in remission, NTG-induced CH attacks
	Fanciullacci et al., 1997	Plasma	19 CH	↑ basal level in active period ↑ during peak of pain if attack was provoked ↑ interpreted as activation of the trigeminovascular system	NTG-induced CH attacks; 11 in period, 19 in remission
	Nicolodi and Del Bianco, 1990	Saliva	15 CH, 18 C	↑ during versus between attacks ↑ during and between attacks versus C	10 in period, 5 in remission
Endothelin-1	Franceschini et al., 2002	Plasma	10 CH	↑ during attacks (in the absence of variations of mean arterial pressure)	During period, spontaneous attacks and remission
Neuropeptide Y	Goadsby and Edvinsson, 1994	Ext. jugular vein blood	13 CH, C (number not specified)	No significant changes	Spontaneous attacks versus age and sex-matched controls
Somatostatin	Sicuteri et al., 1985	Plasma	18 CH, 35 C	No change in CH versus C	Active period during and between attacks
	Caleri et al., 1987	Plasma	12 CH, 35 C	↓ during period and remission	Period and remission
	Vecchiet et al., 1987	CSF	5 CH, 10 M, 24 other	Comparable levels with other headache patients	CH versus controls (LP for other reasons)
Substance P	Sicuteri et al., 1985	Plasma	18 CH, 35 C	↓ during attack periods and remission versus C	During and between attacks
	Sicuteri et al., 1985	CSF	7 CH	No change before versus during mild attack	Histamine-induced headache
	Vecchiet et al., 1987	CSF	5 CH, 10 M, 24 other	No change versus C	CH versus controls (LP for other reasons)
	Hardebo and Ekman, 1985	CSF	8 CH, 15 C	No change during and between attacks versus C	Controls with minor neurological disorder
	Geppetti et al., 1987	CSF	7 CH, 32 C	No change versus C	Controls with minor neurological disorder
	Goadsby and Edvinsson, 1994	Ext. jugular vein blood	13 CH, C (number not specified)	No change versus C	CH attacks versus age and sex-matched controls

↑: increased; ↓: decreased; HVA: homovanillic acid; VMA: vanillyl mandelic acid; 5-HIAA: 5-hydroxyindole acetic acid; 5-HT: serotonin; BDNF, brain-derived nerve growth factor; NGF: nerve growth factor; PC/C: phosphatidylcholine/cholesterol ratio; NAA/Cr: *N*-acetyl aspartate/creatine ratio; Ch/Cr: choline/creatine ratio; β-TBG: β-thromboglobulin; PF4: platelet factor 4; CSF: cerebrospinal fluid; MRS: magnetic resonance spectroscopy; CH: cluster headache; C: controls; MA: migraine with aura; ECH: episodic cluster headache; M: migraine; MO: migraine without aura; TTH: tension-type headache; SP: substance P; NTG; nitroglycerine; CBF: cerebral blood flow; Li: lithium; PG: prostaglandin; ATP: adenosine triphosphate; PAF: platelet-activating factor; LP: lumbar puncture.

(Continued)

Table 33.1
Cluster headache pathophysiology: biochemical studies—Continued

Study	Reference	Specimen	*n*	Main findings	Cluster headache phase/ comparisons
	Fanciullacci et al., 1995	Plasma	30 CH	No change in period (12) versus remission (12) No change during attacks	NTG-induced CH attacks
	Nicolodi and Del Bianco, 1990	Saliva	15 CH, 18 C	↑ during versus between attacks No change during and between attacks versus C	10 in period, 5 in remission
Vasopressin	Franceschini et al., 1995	Plasma	12 CH	↑ during attacks versus between attacks and remission Similar variations of mean arterial pressure and osmolality	Spontaneous attacks, all studied in period and remission
Vasoactive intestinal peptide	Goadsby and Edvinsson, 1994	Ext. jugular vein blood	13 CH, C (number not specified)	↑ during attacks	Spontaneous attacks versus age and sex-matched controls
	Nicolodi and Del Bianco, 1990	Saliva	15 CH, 18 C	↑ during attacks versus between attacks ↑ during and between attacks versus C	10 in period, 5 in remission
Monoamine metabolism					
Dopamine	D'Andrea et al., 2006	Platelets, plasma	40 CH, 50 M, 36 C	↑ dopamine in platelets in period (20) and remission (20) versus C and M Dopamine not detectable in plasma	CH period and remission, M, and controls
Norepinephrine, epinephrine	Igarashi et al., 1985	Plasma	20 CH, 26 M, 33 C	No difference of norepinephrine in remission versus C or M ↑ norepinephrine and ↑ epinephrine during spontaneous attacks ↑ norepinephrine preceded NTG-induced attacks	NTG-induced and spontaneous attacks
Norepinephrine	Igarashi et al., 1987	Plasma	9 CH	↑ norepinephrine during beginning of attacks	5 NTG-induced, 1 alcohol-induced, 3 spontaneous, 6 during remission
Norepinephrine, epinephrine	Leston et al., 1987	Plasma	10 CH, 6 C	↑ conjugated norepinephrine and epinephrine in CH versus C	Period versus controls

↑: increased; ↓: decreased; HVA: homovanillic acid; VMA: vanillyl mandelic acid; 5-HIAA: 5-hydroxyindole acetic acid; 5-HT: serotonin; BDNF, brain-derived nerve growth factor; NGF: nerve growth factor; PC/C: phosphatidylcholine/cholesterol ratio; NAA/Cr: *N*-acetyl aspartate/creatine ratio; Ch/Cr: choline/creatine ratio; β-TBG: β-thromboglobulin; PF4: platelet factor 4; CSF: cerebrospinal fluid; MRS: magnetic resonance spectroscopy; CH: cluster headache; C: controls; MA: migraine with aura; ECH: episodic cluster headache; M: migraine; MO: migraine without aura; TTH: tension-type headache; SP: substance P; NTG; nitroglycerine; CBF: cerebral blood flow; Li: lithium; PG: prostaglandin; ATP: adenosine triphosphate; PAF: platelet-activating factor; LP: lumbar puncture.

Norepinephrine, epinephrine	Figuerola et al., 1990	Plasma	27 CH, 5 C	No difference in free norepinephrine and epinephrine in CH versus C	24 in period, 3 in remission, 2 longitudinal
Norepinephrine	Strittmatter et al., 1996	Plasma	12 CH, 15 C	↓ norepinephrine in the morning and at night, no difference in epinephrine in CH versus C	Period versus controls
Norepinephrine, epinephrine, HVA, VMA, 5-HIAA	Strittmatter et al., 1996	CSF	12 CH, 15 C	↓ norepinephrine, ↓ VMA, ↓ HVA, and ↓ 5-HIAA in CH versus C No difference in epinephrine or dopamine	Period versus controls
Monoamine oxidase (MAO)	Bussone et al., 1977	Platelets	7 CH, 8 M, 15 C	↓ MAO activity versus M and C; temporal pattern different in CH	Phase of CH not reported; 4 samples over 24h
	Bussone et al., 1979	Platelets	10 CH, 10 M, 20 C	Basal MAO levels lower in CH	Period
	Glover et al., 1981	Platelets	25 CH, 30 C (all men)	↓ MAO activity in men but not in women	Period and remission versus controls
	Summers et al., 1982	Platelets	15 CH, 16 C	Normal turnover number suggested that ↓ MAO activity was due to fewer molecules	CH headache-free (12 period, 3 remission), versus controls
	Littlewood et al., 1984	Platelets	41 CH, 48 M, 30 C (all men)	↓ MAO activity in M and CH versus controls	CH versus controls
	Waldenlind et al., 1984b	Platelets	33 CH (6 in period), 34 M, 128 C	↓ V_{max} , no change in K_m, indicating fewer MAO molecules in CH and migraine ↑ thermostable MAO in CH	CH versus controls and migraine
	Mosnaim et al., 1991	Platelets	8 chronic CH, 14 C	No sign difference before, during, and after attacks No sign change versus C	Before, during, and after attacks
Succinate dehydrogenase (SDH)	Littlewood et al., 1984	Platelets	41 CH, 48 M, 30 C	↓ in CH and M versus C No correlation in SDH versus MAO in the same platelets pointing against a generalized platelet deficit	Headache free, phase of CH not reported
Phenylsulpho-transferase (PST)	Littlewood et al., 1984	Platelets	41 CH, 48 M, 30 C	PST M similar in all groups	Headache free, phase of CH not reported
5-HT, 5-HIAA	Anthony and Lance, 1971	Plasma	26 CH, 10 M, 5 C	No sign difference CH versus C	Before, during, and after attacks
	Waldenlind et al., 1985	Platelets	33 CH, 34 M, 50 C	↓ 5-HT in CH and M; no difference between CH and M	30 CH in remission, 3 CH in period
	Strittmatter et al., 1996	CSF	12 CH, 15 C	↓ 5-HIAA in CH versus C	Period versus controls
	Blandini et al., 2006	Platelets	14 CH, 60 M, 57 C	↑ 5-HT and ↑ 5-HIAA in CH and M versus C	CH in interictal phase

↑: increased; ↓: decreased; HVA: homovanillic acid; VMA: vanillyl mandelic acid; 5-HIAA: 5-hydroxyindole acetic acid; 5-HT: serotonin; BDNF, brain-derived nerve growth factor; NGF: nerve growth factor; PC/C: phosphatidylcholine/cholesterol ratio; NAA/Cr: *N*-acetyl aspartate/creatine ratio; Ch/Cr: choline/creatine ratio; β-TBG: β-thromboglobulin; PF4: platelet factor 4; CSF: cerebrospinal fluid; MRS: magnetic resonance spectroscopy; CH: cluster headache; C: controls; MA: migraine with aura; ECH: episodic cluster headache; M: migraine; MO: migraine without aura; TTH: tension-type headache; SP: substance P; NTG; nitroglycerine; CBF: cerebral blood flow; Li: lithium; PG: prostaglandin; ATP: adenosine triphosphate; PAF: platelet-activating factor; LP: lumbar puncture.

(Continued)

Table 33.1
Cluster headache pathophysiology: biochemical studies—Continued

Study	Reference	Specimen	*n*	Main findings	Cluster headache phase/ comparisons
5-HT uptake	Swade et al., 1981	Platelets	10 CH, 31 C	↓ V_{max} versus controls	Phase of CH not reported
	Waldenlind et al., 1985	Platelets	33 CH, 34 M, 50 C	↓ V_{max} and ↓ K_m in CH and M versus C, no difference CH versus M	30 CH in remission, 3 CH in period
	Hannah et al., 1991	Platelets	12 CH, 75 M, 21 TTH, 29 C	K_m and V_{max} no different in CH versus C	Attack-free CH versus controls
β-Receptor response	Meyer et al., 2006	Adipose tissue	10 CH, 10 C	↑ β-receptor response to norepinephrine versus C	CH in remission
Trace amines					
Tyramine, octopamine, synephrine	D'Andrea et al., 2004	Plasma, platelets	44 CH, 50 M, 36 C	↑ tyramine, ↑ octopamine, and ↑ synephrine in period and remission in plasma versus C and M and in platelets versus C	24 CH in period, 20 in remission
Neurotropins					
BDNF, NGF	Blandini et al., 2006	Platelets, plasma	14 CH, 60 M, 57 C	↓ BDNF in plasma but not in platelets in CH versus C NGF no different in platelets or plasma in CH versus C	Period versus controls
Nitric oxide metabolism					
	D'Amico et al., 2002	Plasma	69 CH, 100 M, 112 C	↑ nitrite in CH period and remission, MA and MO versus C	32 in period and 37 in remission versus controls
	Costa et al., 2003	Plasma	18 CH, 12 C	Basal nitrite and L-citrulline did not differ in CH versus C ↑ nitrite after NTG in both CH and C	NTG-induced attacks versus controls
Membranes and phospholipids					
Choline	de Belleroche et al., 1984	Erythrocyte membrane	27 CH, 14 C	↓ choline in cluster period and remission; ↑↑ choline after Li treatment	Period, remission, and Li-treated versus controls
PC/C, cholesterol	de Belleroche et al., 1986	Erythrocyte membrane	12 CH, 10 C	↑ ratio PC/cholesterol untreated, ↑↑ PC/cholesterol after Li-treatment normal cholesterol level	8 in remission, and 4 Li treated versus controls
Arachidonic metabolism	Fragoso et al., 1989	Polymorphic leukocytes	12 CH, 24 C	↑ incorporation of 1-^{14}C-arachidonic acid into phosphatidyl-serine and phosphatidyl-etanolamine in CH; ↓ incorp. into phospatidylcholine	Period and remission mixed

↑: increased; ↓: decreased; HVA: homovanillic acid; VMA: vanillyl mandelic acid; 5-HIAA: 5-hydroxyindole acetic acid; 5-HT: serotonin; BDNF, brain-derived nerve growth factor; NGF: nerve growth factor; PC/C: phosphatidylcholine/cholesterol ratio; NAA/Cr: *N*-acetyl aspartate/creatine ratio; Ch/Cr: choline/creatine ratio; β-TBG: β-thromboglobulin; PF4: platelet factor 4; CSF: cerebrospinal fluid; MRS: magnetic resonance spectroscopy; CH: cluster headache; C: controls; MA: migraine with aura; ECH: episodic cluster headache; M: migraine; MO: migraine without aura; TTH: tension-type headache; SP: substance P; NTG; nitroglycerine; CBF: cerebral blood flow; Li: lithium; PG: prostaglandin; ATP: adenosine triphosphate; PAF: platelet-activating factor; LP: lumbar puncture.

Cell signaling function					
Adenylate cyclase	de Belleroche et al., 1986	Lymphocytes	12 CH, 10 C	↓ PG stimulation of adenylate cyclase, altered transduction function, ↓maximum response	Period, remission, and Li-treatment versus controls
Polyphosphoinositidol	de Belleroche et al., 1991	Platelets	7 CH, 27 M, 5 C	↑ activity in untreated, normalized in Li treated CH	CH before and after Li-treatment versus controls
G-proteins	Gardiner et al., 1998	Lymphocytes	12 CH, 20 MA, 8 C	↓ Giα in CH without medication versus C; Gqα and Gsα no different versus C	
	Galeotti et al., 2001	Lymphocytes	6 CH, 15 M, 18 C	↓ capability to inhibit forskolin-stimulated adenylate cyclase activity in headache patients versus C	Remission versus controls
Energy metabolism					
	Lodi et al., 1997	^{31}P MRS skeletal muscle	14 CH, 49 C	↓ max. mitochondrial ATP production versus C P-creatine and pH after work versus C	Isokinetic work, attack-free
	Lodi et al., 2001	^{31}P MRS brain	13 CH, 36 C, 78 M	↓ free energy release and ↓ free Mg^{2+} in occipital lobe in CH and M	Remission
NAA/Cr, Ch/Cr	Wang et al., 2006	^{1}H MRS brain/ hypothalamus	37 CH, 21 C	↓ NAA/Cr and ↓ Ch/Cr in CH versus C Similar in period versus remission	35 in period and 12 in remission
	Lodi et al., 2006	^{1}H-MRS brain/ hypothalamus	26 CH, 12 C	↓ NAA/Cr in CH versus C ↓ metabolism in remission, period, and chronic CH	Outside attacks
Excitatory amino acids					
Glycine	D'Andrea et al., 1991	Platelets	27 CH, 64 M, 17 C	↓ in CH attacks (12) and headache-free (27) versus C	CH versus controls, no info regarding phase
Aspartate	D'Andrea et al., 1991	Platelets	27 CH, 64 M, 17 C	no change in CH attacks (12) and headache-free (27) versus C	CH versus controls, no info regarding phase
Glutamate	D'Andrea et al., 1991	Platelets	37 CH, 17 C	no change in CH attacks (12) and headache-free (27) versus C	CH versus controls, no info regarding phase
Platelet aggregation	D'Andrea et al., 2003	Platelets	26 CH, 24 C	↓ aggregation to collagen and ADP ↑ aggregation to PAF	Period versus controls
β-TBG, PF4	D'Andrea et al., 1986	Plasma	17 CH, 10 C	↑ β-TBG and ↑ PF4 in remission (9) and cluster period (8) versus C); ↓ to normal during attacks	Period, attacks, remission

↑: increased; ↓: decreased; HVA: homovanillic acid; VMA: vanillyl mandelic acid; 5-HIAA: 5-hydroxyindole acetic acid; 5-HT: serotonin; BDNF, brain-derived nerve growth factor; NGF: nerve growth factor; PC/C: phosphatidylcholine/cholesterol ratio; NAA/Cr: *N*-acetyl aspartate/creatine ratio; Ch/Cr: choline/creatine ratio; β-TBG: β-thromboglobulin; PF4: platelet factor 4; CSF: cerebrospinal fluid; MRS: magnetic resonance spectroscopy; CH: cluster headache; C: controls; MA: migraine with aura; ECH: episodic cluster headache; M: migraine; MO: migraine without aura; TTH: tension-type headache; SP: substance P; NTG; nitroglycerine; CBF: cerebral blood flow; Li: lithium; PG: prostaglandin; ATP: adenosine triphosphate; PAF: platelet-activating factor; LP: lumbar puncture.

(Hardebo and Ekman, 1987) during attacks but without a normal circadian rhythmicity in several subjects (Nappi et al., 1985; Franceschini et al., 1996). Most likely, this finding is related to hypothalamic dysfunction since βEP in plasma is mainly released from the pituitary and synthesized from the same precursor as adrenocorticotropin and β-lipotropin. Lowered circulating levels of the opioid nociceptin during cluster periods compared to healthy controls was speculated to result in defective regulation of the trigeminal ganglion and insufficient protection against attacks (Ertsey et al., 2004).

Various other peptides

Endothelin-1 in plasma has been reported to increase during attacks compared to between attacks but with no significant changes in arterial blood pressure (Franceschini et al., 2002). Somatostatin is an inhibitory transmitter peptide found in sympathetic ganglia and in some primary afferent neurons, where it may inhibit substance P release from the C fibers. Somatostatin concentrations in plasma have been shown to be lower during (Sicuteri et al., 1985) and between (Sicuteri et al., 1985; Caleri et al., 1987) cluster attacks as well as during remission (Caleri et al., 1987) compared with controls. An injection of somatostatin appeared to relieve CH pain (Sicuteri et al., 1985), perhaps related to its venoconstrictive properties (Caleri et al., 1987). Due to rapid tachyphylaxis, somatostatin is not likely to become a choice for CH treatment. Vasopressin has been shown to increase during CH attacks without any concomitant variation of plasma osmolality or altered blood pressure variation (Franceschini et al., 1995). As a potent vasoconstrictor, the increase in vasopressin was suggested to counteract the vasodilation associated with the attack (Franceschini et al., 1995).

Involvement of Gi proteins in the modulation of pain is widely established and Gi inactivation may produce hyperalgesia and insensitivity to analgesic treatment. Gi proteins inhibit adenylate cyclase and modulate several K^+ and Ca^{2+} channels. As an example, in lymphocytes from CH and migraine patients but not in other pain syndromes, a hypofunctionality of Gi proteins has been shown (Galeotti et al., 2001).

Monoamines

Physical exercise and norepinephrine infusion reduce the pain of induced attacks (Ekbom and Lindahl, 1970), while spontaneous attacks often occur during relaxation and sleep. Attacks induced by nitroglycerine seemed to start after an initial increase of plasma norepinephrine had reversed to basal values (Igarashi et al., 1985). Norepinephrine increased during both spontaneous and induced attacks (Igarashi et al., 1985), maybe as a response to vasodilation, but evaluation during attacks may be difficult because posture affects norepinephrine levels. When examined before and after 5 min of standing, plasma concentrations of norepinephrine and epinephrine did not differ between patients in remission and controls, indicating normal postural responses (Igarashi et al., 1985). During the cluster period there are conflicting results. One study showed increased plasma concentrations of conjugated norepinephrine and epinephrine (Leston et al., 1987), and another showed decreased concentrations of norepinephrine in the morning and at night in comparison with healthy controls (Strittmatter et al., 1996). Further, CSF concentrations of norepinephrine and the metabolites vanillomandelic acid, homovanillic acid, and 5-hydroxyindoleacetic acid were all lowered in the active period (Strittmatter et al., 1996).

Monoamine metabolism has been studied in platelets due to similarities with monoaminergic synaptosomes in the brain. Monoamine oxidase (MAO) activity in platelets has been documented in several studies to be lowered during and between cluster periods, in both men and women and with respect to smoking habits, but with no further decrease during attacks (Mosnaim et al., 1991). The lowered MAO activity was explained by fewer enzyme molecules (Bussone et al., 1977) and lower V_{max} (capacity) but no change in K_m (affinity) (Summers et al., 1982; Waldenlind et al, 1984b). The enzyme was more thermostable than in controls (Waldenlind et al., 1984b). Since platelet MAO is of the B type, it does not metabolize norepinephrine, epinephrine, or serotonin, but it may affect these amines indirectly by its decreased ability to catabolize dopamine, tyramine, and other trace amines. Succinate dehydrogenase (SDH) and phenolsulfotransferase M (PST M) are other enzymes regulating amine metabolism. In one study SDH activity was lowered in CH, whereas PST M activity did not differ between patients and healthy controls (Littlewood et al., 1984). In the lowest range of MAO there was an inverse correlation between MAO and PST M, which was interpreted as a possible alternative route for metabolism of substrates like dopamine and tyramine.

As regards serotonin uptake into platelets, lowered V_{max} and lowered K_m (Waldenlind et al., 1985) or no difference (Hannah et al., 1991) in the kinetic parameters were reported in patients compared with controls. Circannual variation (Waldenlind et al., 1985; Malmgren, 1990) and medication may explain some of these differences.

With a sensitive high-performance liquid chromatography method for assessment of trace amines in human plasma and platelets (D'Andrea et al., 2004), increased levels of tyramine, octopamine, and synephrine were reported during remission and cluster periods in comparison with healthy controls. This finding was suggested to reflect sympathetic or hypothalamic dysfunction.

Membranes and phospholipids

Membrane composition and transduction properties have been studied in CH. Erythrocyte choline concentrations were found to be depressed both during and between cluster periods to values about 50% of those found in controls (de Belleroche et al., 1984), probably reflecting an abnormality in phospholipid metabolism. Also, the phosphatidylcholine content of erythrocyte membranes, from which choline is derived, was increased, suggesting decreased phosphatidylcholine turnover (de Belleroche et al., 1984). Lithium treatment is known to increase the choline content of erythrocytes. Accordingly, after lithium treatment of CH patients the erythrocyte choline content was normalized (de Belleroche et al., 1984). Other altered receptor-mediated membrane transduction functions in CH involve the adenylate cyclase and polyphosphoinositide systems. Adenylate cyclase is dependent on phospholipid constituents of membranes for its activity. Thus, a lower increase in the second-messenger cyclic adenosine monophosphate (cAMP) has been shown in lymphocytes from CH patients than from controls after *in vitro* stimulation of high-affinity prostaglandin receptors, and a similar trend was shown after stimulation of β-adrenoceptors (de Belleroche et al., 1986). In platelets stimulated with thrombin, the polyphosphoinositide system showed enhanced activity in untreated patients and normal activity in lithium-treated patients as compared with controls (de Belleroche et al., 1991). The prophylactic effect of lithium may therefore be related to dampening of an activated polyphosphoinositide system.

Energy metabolism

Phosphorus magnetic resonance spectroscopy (^{31}P-MRS) is a noninvasive method by which it is possible to measure high-energy phosphates and the efficacy of adenosine triphosphate production. Defective mitochondrial respiration in the brain was shown both during and after a CH period compared with matched healthy volunteers and it was associated with low free magnesium in the occipital lobes (Lodi et al., 2001). With ^{1}H-MRS, metabolism in the hypothalamus has been demonstrated to be lowered both in the cluster period and in remission (Lodi et al., 2006; Wang et al., 2006). This altered energy metabolism might render patients more susceptible to metabolic demands during stressful conditions.

Excitatory amino acids

Platelets take up glutamate and aspartate by an energy-dependent mechanism similar to that occurring in neurons. Glycine levels in platelets were similar during and between CH attacks but they were significantly lower in CH patients than in healthy controls, whereas the levels of aspartate and glutamate did not differ. This is in contrast to migraine with aura, where the concentrations of all three amino acids were increased (D'Andrea et al., 1991).

CONCLUSION

In conclusion, there is evidence for central as well as peripheral mechanisms in CH pathophysiology. The hypothalamus is definitely shown to be involved. The nature of the hypothalamic structural change is not known, whether acquired or constitutional, whether permissive or necessary for CH development. The episodic nature of CH, in particular the timing of single attacks and periods, circadian neurendocrine disturbances and systemic effects such as altered lipolysis, is likely to be related to hypothalamic dysfunction. Recurrent activation of the trigeminovascular system with parasympathetic recruitment and vasodilation explains many of the clinical features of CH but the trigger of this activation is unknown. Possibly attacks may be initiated by hypothalamic discharge (Goadsby, 2002). The local sympathoplegia, overt or subclinical, most probably is of peripheral origin and not a cause of the pain, but once the attack begins these autonomic disturbances may contribute to the rapid escalation of pain (Drummond, 2006).

References

Afra J, Cecchini AP, Schoenen J (1998). Craniometric measures in cluster headache patients. Cephalalgia 18: 143–145.

Anselmi B, Baldi E, Casacci F et al. (1980). Endogenous opioids in cerebrospinal fluid and blood in idiopathic headache sufferers. Headache 20: 294–299.

Anthony M, Lance JW (1971). Histamine and serotonin in cluster headache. Arch Neurol 25: 225–231.

Anthony M, Lord GD, Lance JW (1978). Controlled trials of cimetidine in migraine and cluster headache. Headache 18: 261–264.

Appenzeller O, Atkinson RA, Standefer JC (1981a). Serum betaendorphin in cluster headache and common migraine. In: FC Rose (Ed.), Progress in migraine. Pitman, London, pp. 106–109.

Appenzeller O, Becker WJ, Ragaz A (1981b). Cluster headache. Ultrastructural aspects and pathogenetic mechanisms. Arch Neurol 38: 302–306.

Aridon P, D'Andrea G, Rigamonti A et al. (2004). Elusive amines and cluster headache: mutational analysis of trace amine receptor cluster on chromosome 6q23. Neurol Sci 25 (Suppl. 3): S279–S280.

Ashkenazi A, Silberstein SD (2004). Periodic autonomic dysfunction without pain in a patient with cluster headache. Cephalalgia 24: 1005–1006.

Baumber L, Sjostrand C, Leone M et al. (2006). A genomewide scan and HCRTR2 candidate gene analysis in a European cluster headache cohort. Neurology 66: 1888–1893.

Black DF, Swanson JW, Stang PE (2005). Decreasing incidence of cluster headache: a population-based study in Olmsted County, Minnesota. Headache 45: 220–223.

Blandini F, Rinaldi L, Tassorelli C et al. (2006). Peripheral levels of BDNF and NGF in primary headaches. Cephalalgia 26: 136–142.

Boes CJ, Dodick DW (2002). Refining the clinical spectrum of chronic paroxysmal hemicrania: a review of 74 patients. Headache 42: 699–708.

Bovim G, Jenssen G, Ericson K (1992). Orbital phlebography: a comparison between cluster headache and other headaches. Headache 32: 408–412.

Bruyn GW, Bootsma BK, Klawans HL (1976). Cluster headache and bradycardia. Headache 16: 11–15.

Bussone G, Giovannini P, Boiardi A et al. (1977). A study of the activity of platelet monoamine oxidase in patients with migraine headaches or with 'cluster headaches'. Eur Neurol 15: 157–162.

Bussone G, Boiardi A, Cerrati A et al. (1979). Monoamine oxidase activities in patients with migraine or with cluster headache during the acute phases and after treatment with L-5-hydroxytryptophan. Riv Patol Nerv Ment 100: 269–274.

Caleri D, Marabini S, Panconesi A et al. (1987). A pharmacological approach to the analgesizing mechanism of somatostatin in cluster headache. Ric Clin Lab 17: 155–162.

Carter DM (2004). Cluster headache mimics. Curr Pain Headache Rep 8: 133–139.

Chazot G, Claustrat B, Brun J et al. (1984). A chronobiological study of melatonin, cortisol growth hormone and prolactin secretion in cluster headache. Cephalalgia 4: 213–220.

Cohen AS, Matharu MS, Goadsby PJ (2006). Paroxysmal hemicrania in a family. Cephalalgia 26: 486–488.

Cortelli P, Zacchini A, Barboni P et al. (1995). Lack of association between mitochondrial tRNA(Leu(UUR)) point mutation and cluster headache. Lancet 345: 1120–1121.

Costa A, Ravaglia S, Sances G et al. (2003). Nitric oxide pathway and response to nitroglycerin in cluster headache patients: plasma nitrite and citrulline levels. Cephalalgia 23: 407–413.

Couturier EG, Hering R, Steiner TJ (1991). The first report of cluster headache in identical twins. Neurology 41: 761.

Cushing H (1904). The sensory distribution of the fifth cranial nerve. Bull Johns Hopkins Hosp 15: 213–232.

Cuypers J, Westphal K, Bunge S (1980). Mast cells in cluster headache. Acta Neurol Scand 61: 327–329.

Dahl A, Russell D, Nyberg-Hansen R et al. (1990). Cluster headache: transcranial Doppler ultrasound and rCBF studies. Cephalalgia 10: 87–94.

D'Amico D, Ferraris A, Leone M et al. (2002). Increased plasma nitrites in migraine and cluster headache patients in interictal period: basal hyperactivity of L-arginine-NO pathway? Cephalalgia 22: 33–36.

D'Andrea G, Cananzi AR, Toldo M et al. (1986). Platelet activity in cluster headache. Cephalalgia 6: 163–167.

D'Andrea G, Cananzi AR, Joseph R et al. (1991). Platelet glycine, glutamate and aspartate in primary headache. Cephalalgia 11: 197–200.

D'Andrea G, Granella F, Cadaldini M (2003). Platelet aggregation profiles in cluster headache. Headache 43: 272–275.

D'Andrea G, Terrazzino S, Leon A et al. (2004). Elevated levels of circulating trace amines in primary headaches. Neurology 62: 1701–1705.

D'Andrea G, Granella F, Perini F et al. (2006). Platelet levels of dopamine are increased in migraine and cluster headache. Headache 46: 585–591.

de Belleroche J, Clifford Rose F, Das I et al. (1984). Metabolic abnormality in cluster headache. Headache 24: 310–312.

de Belleroche J, Kilfeather S, Das I et al. (1986). Abnormal membrane composition and membrane-dependent transduction mechanisms in cluster headache. Cephalalgia 6: 147–153.

de Belleroche J, Gardiner JM, Howley P et al. (1991). Membrane transduction in migraine and cluster headache: studies of G-proteins activation. In: FC Rose (Ed.), New Advances in Headache Research 2. Smith-Gordon, London, pp. 171–173.

Devoize JL, Rigal F, Eschalier A et al. (1986). Dexamethasone suppression test in cluster headache. Headache 26: 126–127.

Dimitriadou V, Henry P, Brochet B et al. (1990). Cluster headache: ultrastructural evidence for mast cell degranulation and interaction with nerve fibres in the human temporal artery. Cephalalgia 10: 221–228.

Drummond P (1992). The mechanism of facial sweating and cutaneous vascular reponses to painful stimulation of the eye. Brain 115: 1417–1428.

Drummond PD (2006). Mechanisms of autonomic disturbance in the face during and between attacks of cluster headache. Cephalalgia 26: 633–641.

Drummond PD, Alessandro M (2005). Neurophysiology and autonomic dysfunction in cluster headaches. In: J Olesen, PJ Goadsby, NM Ramadan et al. (Eds.), The Headaches. 3rd edn. Lippincott Willams & Wilkins, Philadelphia, pp. 767–773.

Drummond PD, Lance JW (1984). Thermographic changes in cluster headache. Neurology 34: 1292–1298.

Drummond PD, Lance JW (1992). Pathological sweating and flushing accompanying the trigeminal lacrimal reflex in patients with cluster headache and in patients with a confirmed site of cervical sympathetic deficit. Evidence for parasympathetic cross-innervation. Brain 115 (Pt 5): 1429–1445.

Eadie MJ (1966). Migrainous neuralgia. Med J Aust 1: 1053–1057.

Edvinsson L, McKenzie ET, McCulloch J (1993). Cerebral Blood Flow and Metabolism. Raven Press, New York.

Ekbom K (1947). Ergotamine tartrate orally in Horton's "histaminic cephalalgia" (also called Harris' "ciliary neuralgia"). Acta Psychiatr Scand 46: 106–113.

Ekbom K (1968). Nitrolglycerin as a provocative agent in cluster headache. Arch Neurol 19: 487–493.

Ekbom K, Greitz T (1970). Carotid angiography in cluster headache. Acta Radiol Diagn (Stockh) 10: 177–186.

Ekbom K, Lindahl J (1970). Effect of induced rise of blood pressure on pain in cluster headache. Acta Neurol Scand 46: 585–600.

Ekbom K, de Fine Olivarius B. (1971). Chronic migrainous neuralgia. A diagnostic and therapeutic aspects. Headache 11: 97–101.

Ekbom K, Ahlborg B, Schele R (1978). Prevalence of migraine and cluster headache in Swedish men of 18. Headache 18: 9–19.

Ekbom K, Monstad I, Prusinski A et al. (1993). Subcutaneous sumatriptan in the acute treatment of cluster headache: a dose comparison study. The Sumatriptan Cluster Headache Study Group. Acta Neurol Scand 88: 63–69.

Ekbom K, Svensson DA, Traff H et al. (2002). Age at onset and sex ratio in cluster headache: observations over three decades. Cephalalgia 22: 94–100.

Ekbom K, Svensson DA, Pedersen NL et al. (2006). Lifetime prevalence and concordance risk of cluster headache in the Swedish twin population. Neurology 67: 798–803.

El Amrani M, Ducros A, Boulan P et al. (2002). Familial cluster headache: a series of 186 index patients. Headache 42: 974–977.

Empl M, Straube A (2001). [The immune system and primary headache syndromes.]. Anaesthesist 50: 783–791.

Ertsey C, Hantos M, Bozsik G et al. (2004). Circulating nociceptin levels during the cluster headache period. Cephalalgia 24: 280–283.

Fanciullacci M, Fusco BM, Alessandri M et al. (1989). Unilateral impairment of pupillary response to trigeminal nerve stimulation in cluster headache. Pain 36: 185–191.

Fanciullacci M, Alessandri M, Figini M et al. (1995). Increase in plasma calcitonin gene-related peptide from the extracerebral circulation during nitroglycerin-induced cluster headache attack. Pain 60: 119–123.

Fanciullacci M, Alessandri M, Sicuteri R et al. (1997). Responsiveness of the trigeminovascular system to nitroglycerine in cluster headache patients. Brain 120: 283–288.

Feindel W, Penfield W, McNaughton FL (1960). The tentorial nerves and localization of intracranial pain. Neurology 10: 555–563.

Ferrari E, Nappi G, Vailati A et al. (1979). Circadian periodicity of plasma prolactin in some neurological diseases. Int J Chronobiol 6: 231–242.

Ferrari E, Canepari C, Bossolo PA et al. (1983). Changes of biological rhythms in primary headache syndromes. Cephalalgia 3 (Suppl. 1): 58–68.

Figuerola ML, Vindrola O, Barontini MB et al. (1990). Increase in plasma methionine-enkephalin levels during the pain attack in episodic cluster headache. Cephalalgia 10: 251–257.

Figuerola ML, Vindrola O, Barontini MB et al. (1991). Changes in neutrophil met-enkephalin containing peptides in episodic cluster headache. Headache 31: 406–408.

Figuerola ML, Levin G, Leston J et al. (1994). Opioid and sympathetic nervous system activity in cluster headache under verapamil or prednisone treatment. Headache 34: 257–260.

Fragoso YD, Seim A, Stovner LJ et al. (1989). Cluster headache: increased incorporation of (1-14C)arachidonic acid into phosphatidylserine in polymorphonuclear cells. Cephalalgia 9: 213–220.

Franceschini R, Leandri M, Cataldi A et al. (1995). Raised plasma arginine vasopressin concentrations during cluster headache attacks. J Neurol Neurosurg Psychiatry 59: 381–383.

Franceschini R, Leandri M, Gianelli MV et al. (1996). Evaluation of beta-endorphin secretion in patients suffering from episodic cluster headache. Headache 36: 603–607.

Franceschini R, Tenconi GL, Leandri M et al. (2002). Endothelin-1 plasma levels in cluster headache. Headache 42: 120–124.

Franzini A, Ferroli P, Leone M et al. (2003). Stimulation of the posterior hypothalamus for treatment of chronic intractable cluster headaches: first reported series. Neurosurgery 52: 1095–1099: discussion 1099–1101.

Friedman AP, Mikropoulos HE (1958). Cluster headaches. Neurology 8: 653–663.

Galeotti N, Ghelardini C, Zoppi M et al. (2001). Hypofunctionality of Gi proteins as aetiopathogenic mechanism for migraine and cluster headache. Cephalalgia 21: 38–45.

Gantenbein AR, Goadsby PJ (2005). Familial SUNCT. Cephalalgia 25: 457–459.

Gardiner IM, Ahmed F, Steiner TJ et al. (1998). A study of adaptive responses in cell signaling in migraine and cluster headache: correlations between headache type and changes in gene expression. Cephalalgia 18: 192–196.

Gawel MJ, Krajewski A, Luo YM et al. (1990). The cluster diathesis. Headache 30: 652–655.

Geppetti P, Frilli S, Spillanti MG et al. (1987). Evaluation of CSF neuropeptides and peptidase activities in primary headaches. Cephalalgia 7 (Suppl. 6): 43–45.

Giacovazzo M, Martelletti P, Romiti A et al. (1985). Relationship between HLA system in cluster headache and clinical response to lithium therapy. Headache 25: 268–270.

Glover V, Peatfield R, Zammit-Pace R et al. (1981). Platelet monoamine oxidase activity and headache. J Neurol Neurosurg Psychiatry 44: 786–790.

Goadsby PJ (2002). Pathophysiology of cluster headache: a trigeminal autonomic cephalgia. Lancet Neurol 1: 251–257.

Goadsby PJ, Edvinsson L (1994). Human in vivo evidence for trigeminovascular activation in cluster headache. Neuropeptide changes and effects of acute attacks therapies. Brain 117: 427–434.

Goadsby PJ, Hoskin KL (1997). The distribution of trigeminovascular afferents in the non-human primate brain *Macaca nemestrina*: a c-Fos immunocytochemical study. J Anat 190: 367–375.

Goadsby PJ, Lipton RB (1997). A review of paroxysmal hemicranias, SUNCT syndrome and other short-lasting headaches with autonomic feature, including new cases. Brain 120: 193–209.

Goadsby PJ, Lambert GA, Lance JW (1986). Stimulation of the trigeminal ganglion increases flow in the extracerebral but not the cerebral circulation of the monkey. Brain Res 38: 63–67.

Goadsby PJ, Edvinsson L, Ekman R (1988). Release of vasoactive peptides in the extracerebral circulation of man and the cat during activation of the trigeminovascular system. Ann Neurol 23: 193–196.

Haan J, van Vliet JA, Kors EE et al. (2001). No involvement of the calcium channel gene (CACNA1A) in a family with cluster headache. Cephalalgia 21: 959–962.

Halberg F, Carendente F, Cornelissen G (1977). Glossary of chronobiology. Chronobiologia IV: 3–199.

Hannah P, Jarman J, Glover V et al. (1991). Kinetics of platelet 5-hydroxytryptamine uptake in headache patients. Cephalalgia 11: 141–145.

Hannerz J (1991). Orbital phlebography and signs of inflammation in episodic and chronic cluster headache. Headache 31: 540–542.

Hannerz J, Ericson K, Bergstrand G (1987). Orbital phlebography in patients with cluster headache. Cephalalgia 7: 207–211.

Hardebo JE (1994). How cluster headache is explained as an intracavernous inflammatory process lesioning sympathetic fibers. Headache 34: 125–131.

Hardebo JE, Ekman R (1985). Substance P and opioids in cluster headache. In: F Sicuteri, L Vecchiet, M Fanciullacci (Eds.), Trends in Cluster Headache. Excerpta Medica, Amsterdam, pp. 145–157.

Hardebo JE, Ekman R (1987). Substance P and opioids in cluster headache. In: F Sicuteri, L Vecchiet, M Fanciullacci (Eds.), Trends in Cluster Headache. Elsevier Science, Amsterdam, pp. 145–157.

Hardebo JE, Ryberg B (1989). Cerebrospinal fluid shanges indicative of inflammatory recation or disease. Cephalalgia 9: 301–302.

Hardebo JE, Ekman R, Eriksson M et al. (1985). CSF opioid levels in cluster headache. In: F Clifford Rose (Ed.), Migraine: Proceedings of the 5th International Migraine Symposium. Karger, London, pp. 79–85.

Hardebo JE, Ekman R, Eriksson M (1989). Low CSF met-enkephalin levels in cluster headache are elevated by acupuncture. Headache 29: 494–497.

Headache Classification Committee of the International Headache Society (1988). Classification and diagnostic criteria for headache disorders, cranial neuralgias and facial pain. Cephalalgia 8 (Suppl. 7): 1–96.

Headache Classification Subcommittee of the International Headache Society (2004). (2004). International classification of headache disorders, 2nd edn. Cephalalgia 24 (Suppl. 1).

Horton BT (1941). The use of histamine in the treatment of specific types of headaches. JAMA 116: 377–383.

Horton BT (1956). Histaminic cephalalgia: Differential diagnosis and treatment. Mayo Clin Proc 31: 325–333.

Hoskin KL, Zagami A, Goadsby PJ (1999). Stimulation of the middle meningeal artery leads to bilateral Fos expression in the trigeminocervical nucleus: a comparative study of monkey and cat. J Anat 194: 579–588.

Hsieh JC, Hannerz J, Ingvar M (1996). Right-lateralised central processing for pain of nitroglycerin-induced cluster headache. Pain 67: 59–68.

Igarashi H, Sakai F, Tazaki Y et al. (1985). The role of the sympathetic nervous system in the pathogenesis of cluster headache. Cephalalgia 5: 362–363.

Igarashi H, Sakai F, Suzuki S et al. (1987). Cerebrovascular sympathetic nervous activity during cluster headaches. Cephalalgia 7 (Suppl. 6): 87–93.

Joseph R, Dhital K, Adams J et al. (1985). Cluster headache: a new approach using fluorescent histochemistry of nerves in temple skin. In: F Clifford Rose (Ed.), Migraine: Proceedings of the 5th International Migraine Symposium. Karger, Basel, pp. 162–165.

Kaube H, Keay K, Hoskin K et al. (1993). Expression of c-Fos-like immunoreactivity in the caudal medulla and upper cervical cord following stimulation of the superior sagittal sinus in the cat. Brain Res 629: 95–102.

Krabbe AA, Rank F (1985). Histological examinations of the superficial temporal artery in patients suffering from cluster headache. Cephalalgia 5 (Suppl. 3): 282–283.

Kudrow L (1976). [Changes of testosterone levels in the cluster headache syndrome. Preliminary study]. Minerva Med 67: 1850–1853.

Kudrow L (1980). Incidence, age at onset, sex and ethnic distribution. In: Kudrow L. Cluster Headache: Mechanisms and Managements. Oxford University Press, New York,, pp. 10–20.

Kudrow L, Kudrow DB (1994). Inheritance of cluster headache and its possible link to migraine. Headache 34: 400–407.

Lambert GA, Bogduk N, Goadsby PJ et al. (1984). Decreased carotid arterial resistence in cats in responsive to trigeminal stimulation. J Neurosurg 61: 307–315.

Lampl C (2002). Left-sided migraine headache interrupted by periods of right-sided cluster headaches in identical twins – another puzzle for modular headache theory. Cephalalgia 22: 583.

Leone M, Bussone GA (1993). Review of hormonal findings in cluster headache. Evidence for hypothalamic involvement. Cephalalgia 13: 309–317.

Leone M, Zappacosta BM, Valentini S et al. (1991). The insulin tolerance test and the ovine corticotrophin-releasing hormone test in episodic cluster headache. Cephalalgia 11: 269–274.

Leone M, Sacerdote P, D'Amico D et al. (1993). Beta-endorphin levels are reduced in peripheral blood mononuclear cells of cluster headache patients. Cephalalgia 13: 413–416.

Leone M, Maltempo C, Gritti A et al. (1994). The insulin tolerance test and ovine corticotrophin-releasing-hormone test in episodic cluster headache. II: Comparison with low back pain patients. Cephalalgia 14: 357–364; discussion 318–359.

Leone M, Attanasio A, Croci D et al. (1997). The m-chlorophenylpiperazine test in cluster headache: a study on central serotoninergic activity. Cephalalgia 17: 666–672.

Leone M, Lucini V, D'Amico D et al. (1998). Abnormal 24-hour urinary excretory pattern of 6-sulphatoxymelatonin in both phases of cluster headache. Cephalalgia 18: 664–667.

Leone M, Russell MB, Rigamonti A et al. (2001). Increased familial risk of cluster headache. Neurology 56: 1233–1236.

Leone M, Rigamonti A, Bussone G (2002). Cluster headache sine headache: two new cases in one family. Cephalalgia 22: 12–14.

Leone M, Franzini A, Broggi G et al. (2003). Hypothalamic deep brain stimulation for intractable chronic cluster headache: a 3-year follow-up. Neurol Sci 24 (Suppl. 2): S143–S145.

Leston J, Barontini M, Mancini A et al. (1987). Free and conjugated plasma catecholamines in cluster headache. Cephalalgia 7 (Suppl. 6):331.

Liberski PP, Prusinski A (1982). Further observations on the mast cells over the painful region in cluster headache patients. Headache 22: 115–117.

Littlewood J, Glover V, Sandler M et al. (1984). Low platelet monoamine oxidase activity in headache: no correlation with phenolsulphotransferase, succinate dehydrogenase, platelet preparation method or smoking. J Neurol Neurosurg Psychiatry 47: 338–343.

Lodi R, Kemp GJ, Montagna P et al. (1997). Quantitative analysis of skeletal muscle bioenergetics and proton efflux in migraine and cluster headache. J Neurol Sci 146: 73–80.

Lodi R, Iotti S, Cortelli P et al. (2001). Deficient energy metabolism is associated with low free magnesium in the brains of patients with migraine and cluster headache. Brain Res Bull 54: 437–441.

Lodi R, Pierangeli G, Tonon C et al. (2006). Study of hypothalamic metabolism in cluster headache by proton MR spectroscopy. Neurology 66: 1264–1266.

Malmgren R (1990). The central serotoninergic system. Cephalalgia 10: 199–204.

Manzoni GC (1998). Gender ratio of cluster headache over the years: a possible role of changes in lifestyle. Cephalalgia 18: 138–142.

Manzoni GC, Terzano MG, Bono G et al. (1983). Cluster headache – clinical findings in 180 patients. Cephalalgia 3: 21–30.

Martelletti P, Giacovazzo M (1996). Putative neuroimmunological mechanisms in cluster headache. An integrated hypothesis. Headache 36: 312–315.

Martelletti P, Romiti A, Gallo MF et al. (1984). HLA-B14 antigen in cluster headache. Headache 24: 152–154.

Martelletti P, Stirparo G, Giacovazzo M (1999). Nitric oxide (NO) as a coevolution factor in cluster headache pathophysiology: the NO pathway in both natural and NO-donor cluster attacks. EOS Riv Immunol Immunifarmacol XIX: 19–22.

Martins IP, Gouveia RG, Parreira E (2005). Cluster headache without autonomic symptoms: why is it different? Headache 45: 190–195.

Matharu MS, Goadsby PJ (2002). Persistence of attacks of cluster headache after trigeminal nerve root section. Brain 125: 976–984.

Matharu M, Cohen AS, McGonigle DJ et al. (2004). Posterior hypothalamic and brainstem activation in hemicrania continua. Headache 44: 747–761.

Mathiau P, Brochet B, Boulan P et al. (1994). Spontaneous and 5HT-induced cyclic contractions in superficial temporal arteries from chronic and episodic cluster headache patients. Cephalalgia 14: 419–429; discussion 393.

May A, Goadsby PJ (1999). The trigeminovascular system in humans: pathophysiologic implications for primary headache syndromes of the neural influences on the cerebral circulation. J Cereb Blood Flow Metab 19: 115–127.

May A, Bahra A, Buchel C et al. (1998a). Hypothalamic activation in cluster headache attacks. Lancet 352: 275–278.

May A, Kaube H, Buchel C et al. (1998b). Experimental cranial pain elicited by capsaicin: a PET study. Pain 74: 61–66.

May A, Bahra A, Buchel C et al. (1999a). Functional magnetic resonance imaging in spontaneous attacks of SUNCT: short-lasting neuralgiform headache with comjuntival injection and tearing. Ann Neurol 46: 791–794.

May A, Ashburner J, Buchel C et al. (1999b). Correlation between structural and functional changes in brain in an idiopathic headache syndrome. Nat Med 5: 836–838.

May A, Bahra A, Buchel C et al. (2000). PET and MRA findings in cluster headache and MRA in experimental pain. Neurology 55: 1328–1335.

May A, Buchel C, Turner R et al. (2001). Magnetic resonance angiography in facial and other pain: neurovascular mechanisms of trigeminal sensation. J Cereb Blood Flow Metab 21: 1171–1176.

May A, Leone M, Boecker H et al. (2003). Deep brain stimulation in cluster headache: preventing intractable pain by activating the pain network. Cephalalgia 22: 656.

McNaughton FL, Feindl WH (1977). Innervation of Intracranial Structures: A Reappraisal. Blackwell Scientific Publications, Oxford.

Medina JL, Diamond S, Fareed J (1979). The nature of cluster headache. Headache 19: 309–322.

Meyer EL, Waldenlind E, Marcus C (2003). Diminished nocturnal lipolysis in cluster headache: a sign of central sympathetic dysregulation? Neurology 61: 1250–1254.

Meyer EL, Waldenlind E, Marcus C (2006). Beta-receptor response to noradrenaline in cluster headache. A study of adipose tissue lipolysis. Cephalalgia 26: 831–836.

Micieli G, Cavallini A, Bosone D et al. (1993). Imbalance of heart rate regulation in cluster headache as based on continuous 24-h recordings. Clin Auton Res 3: 291–298.

Moskowitz MA (1988). Cluster headache: evidence for a pathophysiologic focus in the superior pericarotid cavernous sinus plexus. Headache 28: 584–586.

Mosnaim AD, Diamond S, Freitag F et al. (1987). Plasma and platelet methionine-enkephalin levels in chronic cluster patients during an acute headache episode. Headache 27: 325–328.

Mosnaim AD, Huprikar S, Wolff M et al. (1991). Studies of platelet monoamineoxidase activity during an acute cluster headache attack. Cephalalgia 11: 254–255.

Motulsky AG (1978). Biased ascertainment and the natural history of diseases. N Engl J Med 298: 1196–1197.

Nappi G, Facchinetti F, Martignoni E et al. (1985). Endorphin patterns within the headache spectrum disorders. Cephalalgia 5 (Suppl. 2): 201–210.

Nappi G, Micieli G, Facchinetti F et al. (1987). Changes in rhythmic temporal structures in cluster headache. In: F Sicuteri, I Vecciet, M Fanciullacci (Eds.), Trends in Cluster Headache. Elsevier Science, Amsterdam, pp. 351–359.

Nappi G, Micieli G, Cavallini A et al. (1992). Accompanying symptoms of cluster attacks: their relevance to the diagnostic criteria. Cephalalgia 12: 165–168.

Nicolodi M, Del Bianco E (1990). Sensory neuropeptides (substance P, calcitonin gene-related peptide) and vasoactive intestinal polypeptide in human saliva: their pattern in migraine and cluster headache. Cephalalgia 10: 39–50.

Nordin M, Fagius J, Waldenlind E (1997). Sympathetic vasoconstrictor outflow to extremity muscles in cluster headache. Recordings during spontaneous and nitroglycerin-induced attacks. Headache 37: 358–367.

Odawara M, Tamaoka A, Mizusawa H et al. (1997). A case of cluster headache associated with mitochondrial DNA deletions. Muscle Nerve 20: 394–395.

Ophoff RA, Terwindt GM, Vergouwe MN et al. (1996). Familial hemiplegic migraine and episodic ataxia type-2 are caused by mutations in the Casup^{2+}/sup channel gene CACNL1A4. Cell 87: 543–552.

Penfield W, McNaughton FL (1940). Dural headache and the innervation of the dura mater. Arch Neurol Psychiatry 44: 43–75.

Peyron C, Faraco J, Rogers W et al. (2000). A mutation in a case of early onset narcolepsy and a generalized absence of hypocretin peptides in human narcoleptic brains. Nat Med 6: 991–997.

Polleri A, Nappi G, Murialdo G et al. (1982). Changes in the 24-hour prolactin pattern in cluster headache. Cephalalgia 2: 1–7.

Prusinski A, Liberski PO (1979). Is the cluster headache local mastocytic diaethesis? Headache 19: 102.

Rainero I, Gallone S, Valfre W et al. (2004). A polymorphism of the hypocretin receptor 2 gene is associated with cluster headache. Neurology 63: 1286–1288.

Remahl IN, Waldenlind E, Bratt J et al. (2000). Cluster headache is not associated with signs of a systemic inflammation. Headache 40: 276–282.

Roberge C, Bouchard JP, Simard D et al. (1992). Cluster headache in twins [letter; comment]. Neurology 42: 1255–1256.

Russell D (1981). Cluster headache: severity and temporal profiles of attacks and patient activity prior to and during attacks. Cephalalgia 1: 209–216.

Russell D, Storstein L (1983). Cluster headache: a computerized analysis of 24 h Holter ECG recordings and description of ECG rhythm disturbances. Cephalalgia 3: 83–107.

Russell MB (2004). Epidemiology and genetics of cluster headache. Lancet Neurol 3: 279–283.

Russell MB, Andersson PG (1995). Clinical intra- and interfamilial variability of cluster headache. Eur J Neurol 1: 253–257.

Russell MB, Andersson PG, Thomsen LL (1995a). Familial occurrence of cluster headache. J Neurol Neurosurg Psychiatry 58: 341–343.

Russell MB, Andersson PG, Thomsen LL et al. (1995b). Cluster headache is an autosomal dominantly inherited disorder in some families: a complex segregation analysis. J Med Genet 32: 954–956.

Salvesen R (2000). Cluster headache sine headache: case report. Neurology 55: 451.

Schoenen J, Di Clemente L, Vandenheede M et al. (2005). Hypothalamic stimulation in chronic cluster headache: a pilot study of efficacy and mode of action. Brain 128: 940–947.

Schuh-Hofer S, Richter M, Israel H et al. (2006). The use of radiolabelled human serum albumin and SPECT/MRI co-registration to study inflammation in the cavernous sinus of cluster headache patients. Cephalalgia 26: 1115–1122.

Schurks M, Kurth T, Geissler I et al. (2006). Cluster headache is associated with the G1246A polymorphism in the hypocretin receptor 2 gene. Neurology 66: 1917–1919.

Seibel P, Grunewald T, Gundolla A et al. (1996). Investigation on the mitochondrial transfer RNA(Leu)(UUR) in blood cells from patients with cluster headache. J Neurol 243: 305–307.

Shimomura T, Kitano A, Marukawa H et al. (1994). Point mutation in platelet mitochondrial tRNA(Leu(UUR)) in patient with cluster headache. Lancet 344: 625.

Sianard-Gainko J, Milet J, Ghuysen V et al. (1994). Increased parasellar activity on gallium SPECT is not specific for active cluster headache. Cephalalgia 14: 132–133.

Sicuteri F, Fanciullacci M, Geppetti P et al. (1985). Substance P mechanism in cluster headache: evaluation in plasma and cerebrospinal fluid. Cephalalgia 5: 143–149.

Sjaastad O, Bakketeig LS (2003). Cluster headache prevalence. Vaga study of headache epidemiology. Cephalalgia 23: 528–533.

Sjaastad O, Rinck P (1990). Cluster headache: MRI studies of the cavernous sinus and the base of the brain. Headache 30: 350–351.

Sjaastad O, Salvesen R (1986). Cluster headache: are we only seeing the tip of the iceberg? Cephalalgia 6: 127–129.

Sjaastad O, Sjaastad OV (1977). Urinary histamine excretion in migraine and cluster headache. Further observations. J Neurol 216: 91–104.

Sjaastad O, Saunte C, Russell D et al. (1981). Cluster headache. The sweating pattern during spontaneous attacks. Cephalalgia 1: 233–244.

Sjaastad O, Saunte C, Fredriksen TA (1985). Bilaterality of cluster headache. An hypothesis. Cephalalgia 5: 55–58.

Sjaastad O, de Souza Carvalho D, Zhao JM (1988). "Mild" cluster headache(?). Cephalalgia 8: 121–126.

Sjaastad O, Shen JM, Stovner LJ et al. (1993). Cluster headache in identical twins. Headache 33: 214–217.

Sjostrand C, Giedratis V, Ekbom K, Waldenlind E et al. (2001). CACNA1A gene polymorphisms in cluster headache. Cephalalgia 21: 953–958.

Sjostrand C, Modin H, Masterman T et al. (2002). Analysis of nitric oxide synthase genes in cluster headache. Cephalalgia 22: 758–764.

Sjostrand C, Russell MB, Ekbom K et al. (2005). Familial cluster headache. Is atypical cluster headache in family members part of the clinical spectrum? Cephalalgia 25: 1068–1077.

Spillantini MC, Geppetti P, Marchionni A et al. (1987). "Enkephalinase" and converting enzyme activities in human CSF: their relation to pain an various pathology. In: F Sicuteri, L Vecchiet, M Fanciullacci (Eds.), Trends in Cluster Headache. Elsevier Science, Amsterdam, pp. 159–165.

Sprenger T, Boecker H, Tolle TR et al. (2004). Specific hypothalamic activation during a spontaneous cluster headache attack. Neurology 62: 516–517.

Strittmatter M, Hamann GF, Grauer M et al. (1996). Altered activity of the sympathetic nervous system and changes in the balance of hypophyseal, pituitary and adrenal hormones in patients with cluster headache. Neuroreport 7: 1229–1234.

Summers KM, Brown GK, Craig IW et al. (1982). Platelet monoamine oxidase: specific activity and turnover numbers. Clin Chim Acta 121: 134–146.

Svensson D, Ekbom K, Pedersen NL et al. (2003). A note on cluster headache in a population-based twin register. Cephalalgia 23: 376–380.

Swade CC, Carroll JD, Coppen A (1981). Platelet 5-hydroxytryptamine accumulation in migrainous neuralgia. In: FC Rose, KJ Zilkha (Eds.), Progress in Migraine Research. Pitman, London, pp. 89–92.

Symonds C (1956). A particular variety of headache. Brain 79: 217–232.

Tassorelli C, Micieli G, Osipova V et al. (1998). Combined evaluation of pupillary and cardiovascular responses to cold pressor test in cluster headache patients. Cephalalgia 18: 668–674.

Torelli P, Manzoni GC (2003). Clinical observations on familial cluster headache. Neurol Sci 24: 61–64.

Torelli P, Beghi E, Manzoni GC (2005). Cluster headache prevalence in the Italian general population. Neurology 64: 469–474.

Turkewitz LJ, Wirth O, Dawson GA et al. (1992). Cluster headache following head injury: a case report and review of the literature. Headache 32: 504–506.

van Vliet JA, Ferrari MD, Haan J (2003). Genetic factors in cluster headache. Exp Rev Neurother 3: 301–306.

Vaughan GM, McDonald SD, Jordan RM et al. (1978). Melatonin concentration in human blood and cereborspinal fluid: relationship to stress. J Clin Endocrinol Metab 47: 220–223.

Vecchiet L, Geppetti P, Marchionni A et al. (1987). Cerebrospinal fluid (methionin 5)-enkephalin, substance P, and somatostatin-like immunoreactivities in painful and painless human diseases. In: F Sicuteri, L Vecchiet, M Fanciullacci (Eds.), Trends in Cluster Headache. Elsevier Science, Amsterdam, pp. 135–143.

Veger T, Russell D, Sjaastad O (1976). Histamine H2 antagonists and cluster headache. BMJ 2: 585.

Waldenlind E, Bussone G (2006). Biochemistry, circannual and circadian rhythms, endocrinology and immunology of cluster headaches. In: J Olesen, PJ Goadsby, NM Ramadan et al. (Eds.), The Headaches. 3rd edn. Lippincott Williams & Wilkins, Philadelphia, pp. 755–773.

Waldenlind E, Gustafsson SA (1987). Prolactin in cluster headache: diurnal secretion, response to thyrotropin-releasing hormone, and relation to sex steroids and gonadotropins. Cephalalgia 7: 43–54.

Waldenlind E, Ekbom K, Friberg Y et al. (1984a). Decreased nocturnal serum melatonin levels during active cluster headache periods. Opusc Med 29: 207–213.

Waldenlind E, Saaf J, Ekbom K et al. (1984b). Kinetics and thermolability of platelet monoamine oxidase in cluster headache and migraine. Cephalalgia 4: 125–134.

Waldenlind E, Ross SB, Saaf J et al. (1985). Concentration and uptake of 5-hydroxytryptamine in platelets from cluster headache and migraine patients. Cephalalgia 5: 45–54.

Waldenlind E, Gustafsson SA, Ekbom K et al. (1987). Circadian secretion of cortisol and melatonin in cluster headache during active cluster periods and remission. J Neurol Neurosurg Psychiatry 50: 207–213.

Waldenlind E, Ekbom K, Torhall J (1993). MR-angiography during spontaneous attacks of cluster headache: a case report. Headache 33: 291–295.

Waldenlind E, Ekbom K, Wetterberg L et al. (1994). Lowered circannual urinary melatonin concentrations in episodic cluster headache. Cephalalgia 14: 199–204.

Wang SJ, Lirng JF, Fuh JL et al. (2006). Reduction in hypothalamic 1H-MRS metabolite ratios in patients with cluster headache. J Neurol Neurosurg Psychiatry 77: 622–626.

Handbook of Clinical Neurology, Vol. 97 (3rd series)
Headache
G. Nappi and M.A. Moskowitz, Editors

Chapter 34

Neuroimaging and clinical neurophysiology in cluster headache and trigeminal autonomic cephalalgias

LARS FRIBERG,[1] GIORGIO SANDRINI,[2]* AND ARMANDO PERROTTA[2,3]

[1]*Department of Clinical Physiology and Nuclear Medicine, Bispebjerb Hospital, Copenhagen, Denmark*
[2]*University Center for Adaptive Disorders and Headache (UCADH) and Department of Neurological Sciences, IRCCS "C. Mondino Institute of Neurology" Foundation, Pavia, Italy*
[3]*Headache Clinic, IRCCS "Neuromed" Institute, Pozzilli (Isernia) and University "Sapienza", Rome, Italy*

INTRODUCTION

Clinical neurophysiology and neuroimaging are two non-invasive approaches used to investigate the pathophysiological basis of primary headaches, including cluster headache (CH) and other trigeminal autonomic cephalalgias (TACs). The periodicity of the episodic form of CH and of other TACs makes it possible to study differences in neurophysiological responses or imaging across both active and remission periods. Furthermore, since it is possible to trigger CH attacks with alcohol (Horton, 1956), nitroglycerine (Ekbom, 1968), and by head-down tilt or breathing carbon dioxide (Hannerz and Jogestrand, 1995a, b), this entity lends itself well to the conducting of studies before, during, and after attacks.

In the past 10 years, modern neuroimaging has revolutionized understanding of the pathophysiology of primary headaches, and of TACs in particular, focusing from cerebrovascular dysfunction hypothesis toward a central triggering cause. The introduction of single-photon emission computed tomography (SPECT), positron emission tomography (PET), and voxel-based morphometry has allowed us new insights into mechanisms underlying TACs (both spontaneous and induced) and occurring during peripheral and/or central neuromodulation. The specific activation of neural structures that is observed exclusively in migraine and in TACs supports the hypothesis that primary headaches are driven predominantly by central nervous system dysfunction, and this has important implications from a therapeutic perspective.

While neurophysiological examinations are often of little or no value in the clinical setting, most of these tools offer vast potential for exploring further the pathophysiology of headaches and the effects of pharmacological treatments (Sandrini et al., 2004). Trigeminofacial reflexes, the nociceptive flexion reflex, and evoked potentials, in particular, have been used in TACs to explore the functional state of brainstem and spinal structures involved in pain processing, contributing to our understanding of the pathophysiology of these primary headaches.

NEUROIMAGING STUDIES IN CLUSTER HEADACHE AND OTHER TACS

Cluster headache

ANGIOGRAPHY

One of the first neuroimaging studies conducted in CH was an arteriographic evaluation of the internal carotid artery on the pain side in a single patient suffering from recurrent, strictly unilateral headache, but without a clear diagnosis of CH (Ekbom and Greitz, 1970). The authors described narrowing of the internal carotid artery just above the carotid canal during the attack; this narrowing progressed caudally into the upper part of the carotid canal as the attack continued.

The diameters of the carotid and basilar arteries were also evaluated before and after nitroglycerine administration in a magnetic resonance angiography study performed in 8 episodic CH patients, 5 during the active phase and 3 during the remission phase. In patients

*Correspondence to: Professor Giorgio Sandrini, University Center for Adaptive Disorders and Headache (UCADH) and Department of Neurological Sciences, IRCCS "C. Mondino Institute of Neurology" Foundation, Via Mondino 2, 27100 Pavia, Italy. Tel: +39 0382 380279, Fax: +39 0382 380448, E-mail: giorgio.sandrini@unipv.it

who developed a CH attack the vessels dilated before the onset of the attack but returned to baseline diameter at maximal pain intensity, within about 50 min of the nitroglycerine administration. Patients who did not develop a CH attack showed arterial dilation lasting only about 60 min (Hannerz and Greitz, 1992).

In addition, there are very few investigations of possible venous changes in CH. Orbital phlebography was carried out in CH patients in two studies (Hannerz, 1991; Bovim et al., 1992), but neither was able to confirm the presence of venous changes associated with CH.

Thus, these sparse and conflicting results fail to provide definitive evidence either for or against the vascular hypothesis, which postulates inflammation of the walls of the cavernous sinus (the only peripheral anatomical location where both trigeminal C fibers and sympathetic fibers could be involved in a single pathology) (Hardebo, 1991).

Regional cerebral blood flow and SPECT

Early functional neuroimaging studies of CH were cerebral blood flow (CBF) studies based on the direct intracarotid ^{133}Xe injection method with stationary detectors over one hemisphere. They showed a moderate, diffuse increase in CBF in 1 patient during a spontaneous CH attack (Norris et al., 1976) and unchanged regional CBF (rCBF) in 3 patients (Henry et al., 1978). Sakai et al. (1977), using a non-traumatic ^{133}Xe inhalation method with a battery of stationary detectors, measured a bilateral, global CBF increase during spontaneous CH attacks in 3 patients. Conversely, Nelson et al. (1980), using a similar detector system and intravenous injection of ^{133}Xe, failed to detect any consistent rCBF changes in 26 CH patients examined during spontaneous and/or nitroglycerine- or alcohol-induced attacks.

Subsequently, following the introduction of the SPECT technique, Krabbe et al. (1984), using ^{133}Xe inhalation, examined 8 CH patients during nitroglycerine- or alcohol-induced CH attacks but did not find any global or regional changes in CBF. Meanwhile, the absence of rCBF pattern changes in 5 CH patients studied during headache-free periods seemed to rule out permanent gross functional cerebral deficits.

Brain SPECT has also been used to explore the hypothesis that CH could be associated with inflammation in the cavernous sinus. However, no evidence of inflammation in the cavernous sinus was found either by studying ^{67}Ga accumulation in CH patients interictally (Sianard-Gainko et al., 1994), or by measuring accumulation of ^{99m}Tc-labeled human serum albumin (Schuh-Hofer et al., 2006).

In short, rCBF, considered both interictally and during CH attacks, does not seem to show systematic alterations, outside normal levels, that might help to explain the pathophysiology of CH. Neither has the SPECT technique offered any evidence to support the inflamed cavernous sinus theory.

Positron emission tomography and functional magnetic resonance imaging

PET allows functional imaging of the brain not only by studying rCBF as a surrogate marker of changes in local neuronal activation patterns, but also by recording local metabolic changes and the density of neuroreceptor-specific radiolabeled ligands. In functional magnetic resonance imaging (fMRI), it is possible to use an internal tracer as a marker of regional cortical blood supply: the blood oxygen level-dependent (BOLD) signal. Changes in the BOLD signal can be taken as a surrogate marker of changes in regional neuronal activity. However, in spite of the vast potential for application of both PET and fMRI in functional neuroimaging, surprisingly few studies have been published on the use of these techniques in CH, and those that have concern very small numbers of patients.

In a PET rCBF study, Hsieh et al. (1996) investigated 7 patients with right-handed, episodic CH, 4 during the active phase, and 3 during the remission period. Images were obtained before and 5 min after administration of 1 mg nitroglycerine, as well as at maximal pain and at remission after 6 mg sumatriptan injection. The main finding of this study was the activation of the anterior cingulate cortex (ACC) on the right, non-dominant hemisphere during maximal pain intensity. The authors speculate on the possibility of hemispheric specialization, involving the ACC in particular, in the affective processing of chronic ongoing pain syndromes (Hsieh et al., 1996). This study failed to show activation in the hypothalamic areas.

In a similar study set-up (PET rCBF), May et al. (1998) examined 9 right-handed patients with active chronic CH (study group) and 8 episodic CH patients during the remission phase (control group). All the patients in the study group and none in the control group developed a CH attack. During the acute attack, significant activations were found in the ipsilateral hypothalamic gray area, bilaterally in the ACC, in the contralateral posterior thalamus, in the ipsilateral basal ganglia, bilaterally in the insulae, and in the cerebellar hemispheres, when compared to the headache-free state. The specific activation of the ipsilateral hypothalamic gray area was only detected in the study group patients during the CH attack and not in the control group patients evaluated during the remission phase (May et al., 2000) (Figure 34.1A). This is worthy of note, because in migraine without aura attacks, Weiller

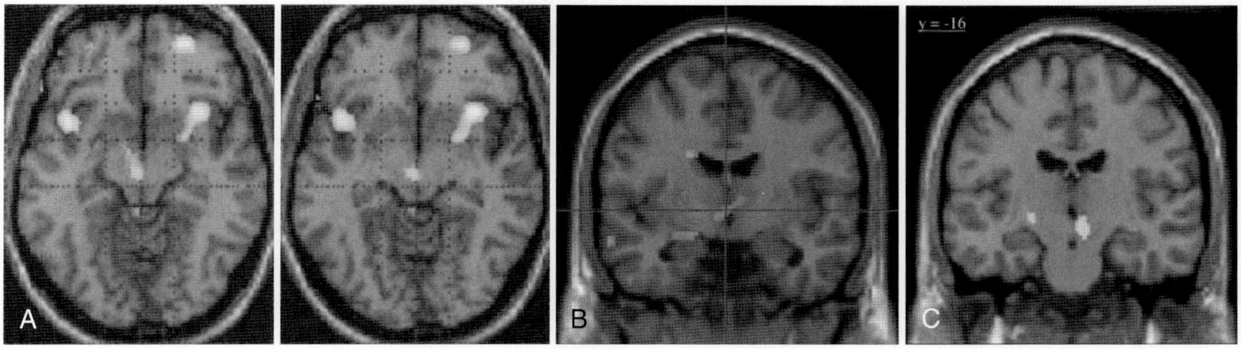

Fig. 34.1. (A) Activation in the posterior inferior hypothalamic gray area only on the pain side during an acute cluster headache attack. Significant activations are also seen in contralateral frontal cortex and bilateral insulae. $n = 9$; positron emission tomography (PET). (Reproduced from May et al., 2000.) (B) Bilateral positive hypothalamic activation during attacks of short-lasting unilateral neuralgiform headache attacks with conjunctival injection and tearing (SUNCT). $n = 1$; functional magnetic resonance imaging. (Reproduced from Cohen, 2007.) (C) Increased regional cerebral blood flow (rCBF) in the posterior hypothalamus during paroxysmal hemicrania headache $n = 7$; PET. (Reproduced from Matharu et al., 2006.)

et al. (1995) found brainstem but not hypothalamic activity, suggesting that different primary headaches could be underlain by different pathophysiological mechanisms, even though some of these syndromes may share common neuronatomical pathways.

The data from these functional mapping studies could support the hypothesis that the specific neural activation observed in CH plays a role in the pain process, exerting a permissive or trigger effect rather than simply constituting a response to ophthalmic division (nociceptive) activation. However, as activations in the hypothalamic region have also been demonstrated after nociceptive stimulation of the face (Kupers et al., 2004) and peripheral limbs (Petrovic et al., 2004), further investigations are needed in order to establish whether the hypothalamus acts as the primary generator of CH, via direct modulation of the activity of neural circuits involved in pain transmission, including the trigeminal nucleus caudalis, or whether it is a pain modulatory structure activated by primary nociceptive trigeminal inputs (Schoenen, 1998).

The findings of PET activation studies clearly show that deep-brain stimulation (DBS) of the posterior hypothalamus could be an effective treatment in patients suffering from intractable chronic CH (Schoenen et al., 2005; Leone et al., 2006).

In one PET study, 10 patients suffering from chronic intractable CH were submitted to DBS (8 were completely pain-free and 2 had sporadic attacks) and evaluated with the hypothalamic stimulator switched on and off alternately (May et al., 2006). The scans were taken immediately after turning the stimulator on or off. The stimulation induced activation in the ipsilateral hypothalamic gray (the site of the stimulator tip), the ipsilateral thalamus, somatosensory cortex and precuneus, the ACC, and the ipsilateral trigeminal nucleus and ganglion; and deactivation in the middle temporal gyrus, posterior cingulate cortex, and contralateral anterior insula. The authors hypothesized that a functional modulation of the pain-processing network, representing the mode of action of hypothalamic DBS in CH, might be responsible for the activation.

Morphometric studies

In addition to functional changes at hypothalamic level, May et al. (1999a) also demonstrated, on T_1-weighted MRI scans significantly increased density in an area corresponding to the posterior inferior hypothalamic gray matter in CH patients compared to healthy controls.

SUNCT, SUNA, paroxysmal hemicrania, and hemicrania continua

Given that CH and other TACs, including short-lasting unilateral neuralgiform headache attacks with conjunctival injection and tearing (SUNCT), short-lasting unilateral neuralgiform headache attacks with cranial autonomic symptoms (SUNA), and paroxysmal hemicrania, show a number of similarities (episodicity, unilaterality and autonomic symptoms) with other primary headaches with trigeminal autonomic features, including hemicrania continua, it has been suggested that these headaches share a common pathophysiological substrate. Data derived from functional neuroimaging studies using BOLD contrast MRI seem to support this hypothesis.

A BOLD fMRI study of six consecutive spontaneous pain attacks in a 71-year-old woman with a diagnosis of SUNCT revealed significant activation in the region of the ipsilateral hypothalamic gray, compared to the pain-free state (May et al., 1999b). The region of activation in this patient was the same as has been reported in acute attacks of CH. Similar findings were described in a second SUNCT case report where fMRI detected bilateral hypothalamic activation during the pain attacks, in addition to activation of several brain structures known to be involved in pain processing generally (Sprenger et al., 2005).

More recently, 9 patients with SUNCT and 2 with SUNA, drawn from a large series of patients with these conditions (respectively, 43 and 9 patients), were investigated using fMRI (Cohen, 2007). Hypothalamic activation was found in 7 patients with SUNCT: bilateral in 5 and contralateral in 2 (Figure 34.1B). The other 2 patients with SUNCT had ipsilateral negative activation. The SUNA patients showed negative activation bilaterally. No hypothalamic activation was found in a patient with SUNCT secondary to a brainstem lesion.

Activation in the hypothalamus was also seen in 7 patients with paroxysmal hemicrania studied using PET (Matharu et al., 2006) (Figure 34.1C). In untreated paroxysmal hemicrania, significant activation of the contralateral posterior hypothalamus and contralateral ventral midbrain, extending over the red nucleus and the substantia nigra, was demonstrated. In addition, persistent activation of the pain neuromatrix was observed during acute paroxysmal hemicrania attacks and during interictal pain-free states after the administration of indomethacin.

In 7 patients with hemicrania continua, significant activation of the contralateral posterior hypothalamus and ipsilateral dorsal rostral pons in association with the headache was described (Matharu et al., 2004). This primary headache shows both trigeminal autonomic and migraine features, whose neuroimaging markers seem to coexist.

CLINICAL NEUROPHYSIOLOGY IN CLUSTER HEADACHE AND TACS

Trigeminofacial reflexes

Studies of the blink reflex in CH have produced conflicting results, probably because of their great methodological variability and the small size of the samples investigated. During attacks, increased amplitude and duration as well as reduced habituation of the R2 responses were found on the affected side with respect to both the unaffected side and the pain-free period (Formisano et al., 1987). A reduced R2 response amplitude was found on the affected side when this was stimulated at the intensity able to elicit maximal R2 responses on the unaffected side during the active phase (Raudino, 1990). Furthermore, chronic CH patients have been found to show increased duration and area of the blink reflex R2 response on the painful side during the pain-free interval (de Tommaso et al., 2000).

Reduced inhibition of the R2 recovery curve on the headache side has been shown in patients with CH after segmental conditioning stimulation, and on both sides after extrasegmental conditioning stimulation (Lozza et al., 1997). The authors took these results to indicate hyperexcitability of the spinal trigeminal complex neurons (possibly caused by segmental sensitization of the trigeminal nucleus caudalis) and defective inhibitory control of reticular nuclei on medullary R2 interneurons.

Recently, baseline parameters (reflex threshold, latency, and area) and habituation of the R2 and R3 components of the blink reflex were evaluated in 27 patients with episodic CH (during the cluster period but outside the bout) and the results were compared with those of 22 patients with episodic migraine and 20 healthy subjects. No differences in the baseline parameters of the reflex components emerged among the groups. On the contrary, the habituation test showed significant differences. Patients with CH displayed significantly reduced habituation of the painful side R2 and R3 responses at all stimulation frequencies (0.2, 0.3, 0.5, 0.7, and 1 Hz for R2; 0.066 and 0.033 Hz for R3) when compared to healthy subjects (Figure 34.2). Interestingly, a marked habituation deficit in a large series of stimulation frequencies (0.2, 0.7, and 1 Hz for R2; 0.066 and 0.033 Hz for R3) was also found in patients with CH compared to patients with migraine. These data support the hypothesis of structural integrity of the trigeminofacial reflex arch and point to abnormal suprasegmental modulation of trigeminofacial reflex excitability in CH during the cluster period, even more pronounced than that seen in patients with migraine (Perrotta et al., 2008).

In summary, abnormal excitability of the blink reflex responses on the symptomatic side during the cluster period seems to be a recurrent finding in patients with CH.

The corneal reflex was evaluated in patients with CH during both active (15 subjects) and remission (6 patients) periods (Sandrini et al., 1991). Basic neurophysiological parameters, including latency, amplitude, and duration of the corneal reflex, as well as tactile sensation, were normal in both phases. A significant reduction of the pain threshold, more evident on the affected side, was found during the active period and followed by normalization of the values during the remission phase (Figure 34.3).

Nociceptive flexion reflex

The nociceptive flexion reflex of the lower limb is an objective tool for exploring the segmental processing of pain at spinal level as well as the supraspinal control

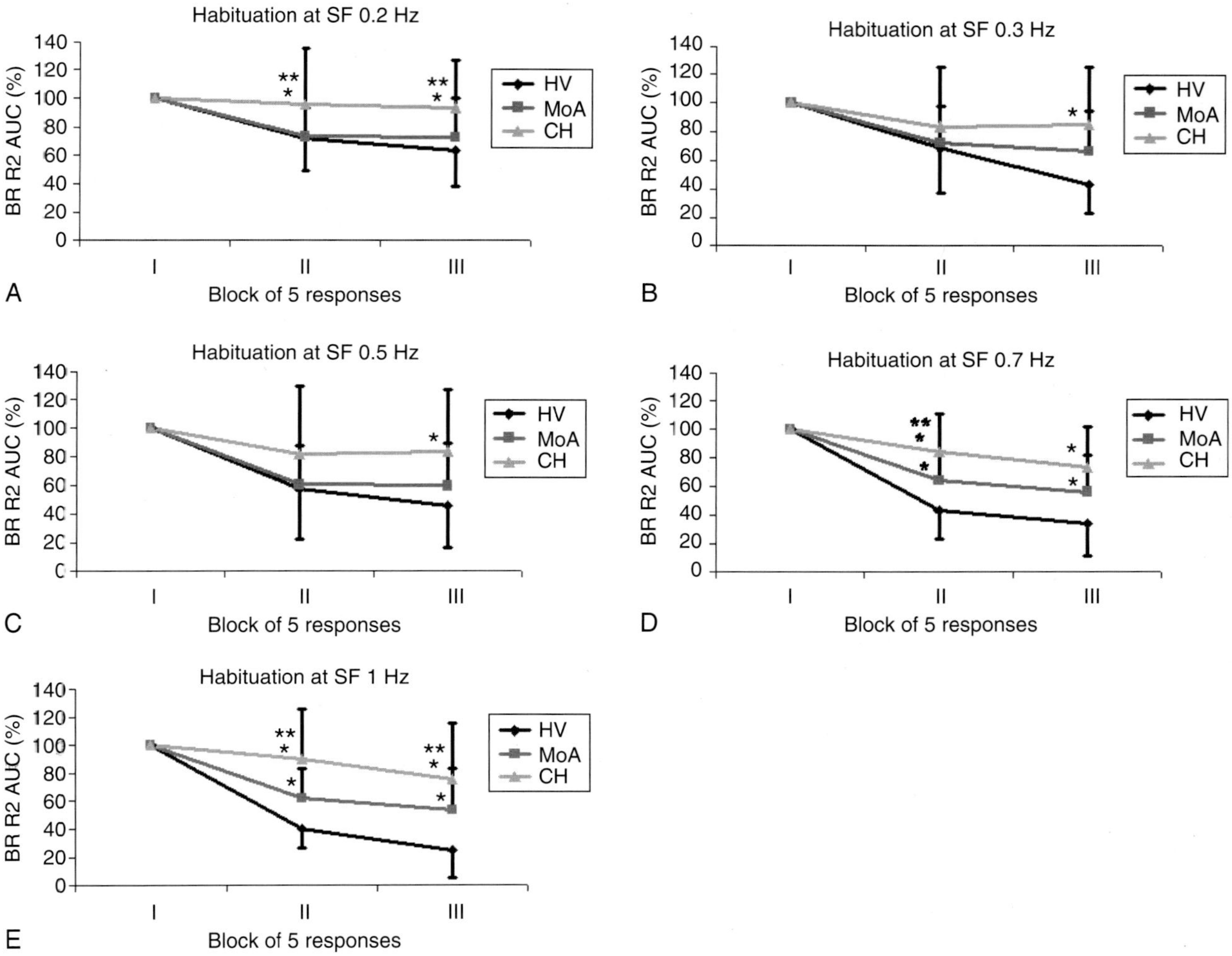

Fig. 34.2. Habituation of the ipsilateral R2 area under the curve (AUC) in three blocks of five averagings at increasing stimulation frequencies (SF) (A: 0.2 Hz; B: 0.3 Hz; C: 0.5 Hz; D: 0.7 Hz; E: 1 Hz) expressed as a percentage of the first block. Data are shown as mean values with standard deviations. BR: blink reflex; CH: cluster headache patients; MoA: migraine without aura patients; HVs: healthy volunteers. Bonferroni test *$P < 0.05$ versus HVs; **$P < 0.05$ versus MoA. (Reproduced from Perrotta et al., 2008.)

of pain (see Sandrini et al., 2005, for a review). The nociceptive flexion reflex was examined bilaterally in episodic (in both remission and active periods) and chronic CH (Sandrini et al., 2000). The results showed a significant reduction of the reflex threshold on the symptomatic side in patients with episodic CH during the active phase, and an inverse correlation emerged between the severity of CH and the pain threshold, suggesting a possible role for secondary central sensitization in pain pathways.

In view of the rythmicity of CH, the nociceptive flexion reflex has been used to explore the possibility of circadian failure of the pain control system in patients with episodic and chronic CH (Nappi et al., 2002). In episodic CH, the 24-h rhythm was conserved during both the active and the remission period, but a shift of the phase was observed during the active phase when compared with the remission period. In contrast, the patients with chronic CH showed a lack of circadian nociceptive flexion reflex threshold rhythmicity (Figure 34.4). In short, these data support the hypothesis of impaired central pain control and periodic failure of the mechanisms involved in the organization of biological rhythms in CH.

Evoked potentials

Different types of stimulation have been studied in CH, including somatosensory evoked, visual evoked, auditory evoked, and event-related potentials.

Somatosensory evoked potentials after median nerve stimulation were studied in patients with CH, before and after histamine administration (Firenze et al., 1988). Somatosensory evoked potential amplitudes did

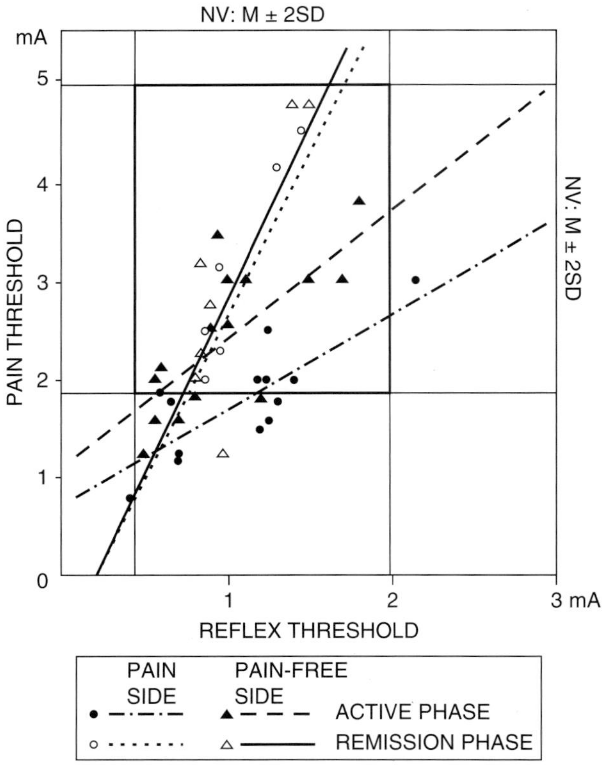

Fig. 34.3. Corneal pain threshold and reflex threshold on pain and pain-free side in cluster headache during active and remission phases. NV: Normal Values (Reproduced from Sandrini et al., 1991.)

not show any abnormalities, whereas the N1–P2 amplitude decreased after histamine stimulation.

Increased latencies of trigeminal somatosensory evoked potentials have been found in CH on the symptomatic side (Frese et al., 1999) and during attacks (Leandri et al., 2000), although it is difficult to compare these two studies. More recently, 28 patients with CH, compared with healthy controls, showed trigeminal somatosensory evoked potential latencies that were increased during the cluster period and more pronounced on the symptomatic side (van Vliet et al., 2003). On the basis of normal blink reflex latencies, the authors hypothesized permanent central dysregulation within higher cerebral regions rather than peripheral or pontine changes.

Decreased ipsilateral P100 amplitudes of visual evoked potentials were found when stimulating the pain side (Boiardi et al., 1986). However, this finding could not be reproduced (Polich et al., 1987).

In studies using auditory evoked potentials, patients with CH have been found to display a marked interaural asymmetry of responses (greater than that occurring in normal subjects) during both attacks and pain-free periods (Bussone et al., 1986), as well as mean amplitude–stimulus intensity function slopes that are significantly steeper than those found in controls both during the active period and interictally (Afra et al., 2005).

Event-related potentials are increased during the cluster period without medication, but normal during the cluster interval, showing a normal cognitive potential habituation pattern (Evers et al., 1997). These data on event-related potential latencies and the normal pattern of habituation in CH were confirmed in a subsequent study involving a larger series of patients with CH (episodic and chronic) and chronic paroxysmal hemicrania (Evers et al., 1999). Medication with prophylactic drugs normalized the event-related potential latencies in episodic CH, while,

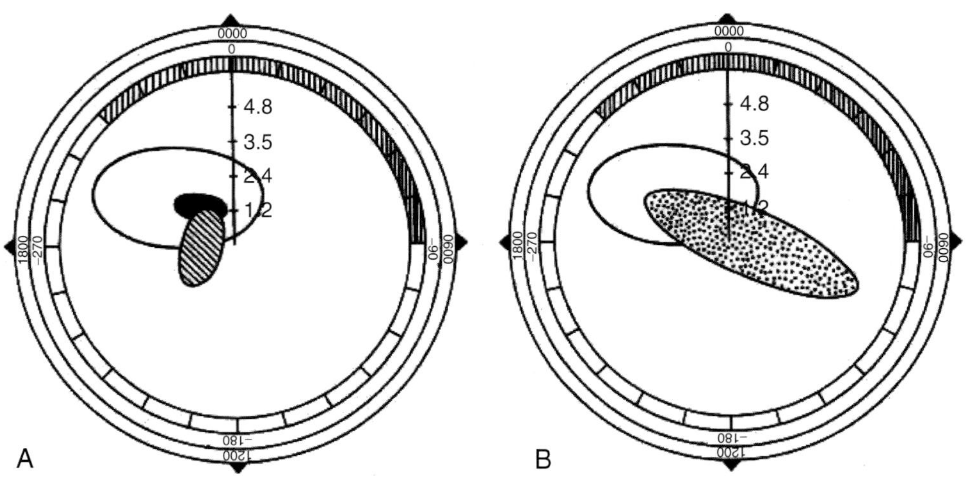

Fig. 34.4. Mean cosinor display of the circadian rhythm of nociceptive flexion reflex threshold in 10 healthy subjects versus 25 episodic cluster headache (ECH) (A) and 6 chronic cluster headache (CCH) subjects (B). The 360° circle represents 24-h clock time in the outer band; the hatched inner band, 6-h sleep time; 0° = midnight (00.00); open ellipse, healthy subjects; dotted ellipse, patients with CCH; hatched elipse, patients with ECH in active period; filled ellipse, patients with ECH in remission. (Reproduced from Nappi et al., 2002.)

in the chronic form, these latencies were decreased but not completely normalized. No event-related potential latency or amplitude changes were observed in chronic paroxysmal hemicrania.

These data suggest that central structures generating event-related potentials are involved in the pathophysiology of CH during but not outside the cluster period.

References

Afra J, Ertsey C, Bozsik G et al. (2005). Cluster headache patients show marked intensity dependence of cortical auditory evoked potentials during and outside the bout. Cephalalgia 25: 36–40.

Boiardi A, Carenini L, Frediani F et al. (1986). Visual evoked potentials in cluster headache: central structures involvement. Headache 26: 70–73.

Bovim G, Jenssen G, Ericson K (1992). Orbital phlebography: a comparison between cluster headache and other headaches. Headache 32: 408–412.

Bussone G, Sinatra MG, Boiardi A et al. (1986). Brainstem auditory evoked potential (baeps) in cluster headache (CH): new aspects for a central theory. Headache 26: 67–69.

Cohen AS (2007). Short-lasting unilateral neuralgiform headache attacks with conjunctival injection and tearing. Cephalalgia 27: 824–832.

de Tommaso MD, Guido M, Libro G et al. (2000). The blink reflex in chronic cluster headache: a comparison with migraine patients suffering from unilateral pain. J Headache Pain 2: 97–104.

Ekbom K (1968). Nitroglycerin as provocative agent in cluster headache. Arch Neurol 19: 487–493.

Ekbom K, Greitz T (1970). Carotid angiography in cluster headache. Acta Radiol Diagn (Stockh) 10: 177–186.

Evers S, Bauer B, Suhr B et al. (1997). Cognitive processing in primary headache: a study on event-related potentials. Neurology 48: 108–113.

Evers S, Bauer B, Suhr B et al. (1999). Cognitive processing is involved in cluster headache, but not in chronic paroxysmal hemicrania. Neurology 53: 357–363.

Firenze C, Del Gatto F, Mazzotta G et al. (1988). Somatosensory-evoked potential study in headache patients. Cephalalgia 8: 157–162.

Formisano R, Cerbo R, Ricci M et al. (1987). Blink reflex in cluster headache. Cephalalgia 7 (Suppl. 6): 353–354.

Frese A, Junker J, Suhr B et al. (1999). Somatosensory trigeminal evoked potentials and blink reflex in cluster headache. Cephalalgia 19: 387.

Hannerz J (1991). Orbital phlebography and signs of inflammation in episodic and chronic cluster headache. Headache 31: 540–542.

Hannerz J, Greitz D (1992). MRI of intracranial arteries in nitroglycerin induced cluster headache attacks. Headache 32: 485–488.

Hannerz J, Jogestrand T (1995a). Effects of increasing the intracranial blood volume in cluster headache patients and controls. Cephalalgia 15: 499–503.

Hannerz J, Jogestrand T (1995b). Provocation of unilateral pain in cluster headache patients by breathing CO_2. Headache 35: 38–43.

Hardebo JE (1991). Activation of pain fibers to the internal carotid artery intracranially may cause the pain and local signs of reduced sympathetic and enhanced parasympathetic activity in cluster headache. Headache 31: 314–320.

Henry PY, Vernhiet J, Orgogozo JM et al. (1978). Cerebral blood flow in migraine and cluster headache. Compartmental analysis and reactivity to anaesthetic depression. Res Clin Stud Headache 6: 81–88.

Horton BT (1956). Histaminic cephalagia. JAMA 160: 468–469.

Hsieh JC, Hannerz J, Ingvar M (1996). Right-lateralised central processing for pain of nitroglycerin induced cluster headache. Pain 67: 59–68.

Krabbe AA, Henriksen L, Olesen J (1984). Tomographic determination of cerebral blood flow during attacks of cluster headache. Cephalalgia 4: 17–23.

Kupers RC, Svensson P, Jensen TS (2004). Central representation of muscle pain and mechanical hyperesthesia in the orofacial region: a positron emission tomography study. Pain 108: 284–293.

Leandri M, Luzzani M, Gottlieb A (2000). Trigeminal evoked potentials in cluster headache. J Headache Pain 1: 43–46.

Leone M, Franzini A, Broggi G et al. (2006). Hypothalamic stimulation for intractable cluster headache: long-term experience. Neurology 67: 150–152.

Lozza A, Schoenen J, Delwaide PJ (1997). Inhibition of the blink reflex R2 component after supraorbital and index finger stimulations is reduced in cluster headache: an indication for both segmental and suprasegmental dysfunction? Pain 71: 81–88.

Matharu MS, Cohen AS, McGonigle DJ et al. (2004). Posterior hypothalamic and brainstem activation in hemicrania continua. Headache 44: 747–761.

Matharu MS, Cohen AS, Frackowiak RS et al. (2006). Posterior hypothalamic activation in paroxysmal hemicrania. Ann Neurol 59: 535–545.

May A, Bahra A, Büchel C et al. (1998). Hypothalamic activation in cluster headache attacks. Lancet 352: 275–278.

May A, Ashburner J, Büchel C et al. (1999a). Correlation between structural and functional changes in brain in an idiopathic headache syndrome. Nat Med 5: 836–838.

May A, Bahra A, Büchel C et al. (1999b). Functional magnetic resonance imaging in spontaneous attacks of SUNCT: short-lasting neuralgiform headache with conjunctival injection and tearing. Ann Neurol 46: 791–794.

May A, Bahra A, Büchel C et al. (2000). PET and MRA findings in cluster headache and MRA in experimental pain. Neurology 55: 1328–1335.

May A, Leone M, Boecker H et al. (2006). Hypothalamic deep brain stimulation in positron emission tomography. J Neurosci 26: 3589–3593.

Nappi G, Sandrini G, Alfonsi E et al. (2002). Impaired circadian rhythmicity of nociceptive reflex threshold in cluster headache. Headache 42: 125–131.

Nelson RF, du Boulay GH, Marshall J et al. (1980). Cerebral blood flow studies in patients with cluster headache. Headache 20: 184–189.

Norris JW, Hachinski VC, Cooper PW (1976). Cerebral blood flow changes in cluster headache. Acta Neurol Scand 54: 371–374.

Perrotta A, Serrao M, Sandrini G et al. (2008). Reduced habituation of trigeminal reflexes in patients with episodic cluster headache during cluster period. Cephalalgia 28 (9): 950–959.

Petrovic P, Petersson KM, Hansson P et al. (2004). Brainstem involvement in the initial response to pain. Neuroimage 22: 995–1005.

Polich J, Aung M, Dalessio DJ (1987). Pattern-shift visual evoked responses in cluster headache. Headache 27: 446–451.

Raudino F (1990). The blink reflex in cluster headache. Headache 30: 584–585.

Sakai F, Meyer JS, Ishihara N et al. (1977). Noninvasive 133Xe inhalation measurements of regional cerebral blood flow in migraine and related headaches. Acta Neurol Scand 64 (Suppl.): 196–197.

Sandrini G, Alfonsi E, Ruiz L et al. (1991). Impairment of corneal pain perception in cluster headache. Pain 47: 299–304.

Sandrini G, Antonaci F, Lanfranchi S et al. (2000). Asymmetrical reduction of the nociceptive flexion reflex threshold in cluster headache. Cephalalgia 20: 647–652.

Sandrini G, Friberg L, Jänig W et al. (2004). Neurophysiological tests and neuroimaging procedures in non-acute headache: guidelines and recommendations. Eur J Neurol 11: 217–224.

Sandrini G, Serrao M, Rossi P et al. (2005). The lower limb flexion reflex in humans. Prog Neurobiol 77: 353–395.

Schoenen J (1998). Cluster headaches – central or peripheral in origin? Lancet 352: 253–255.

Schoenen J, Di Clemente L, Vandenheede M et al. (2005). Hypothalamic stimulation in chronic cluster headache: a pilot study of efficacy and mode of action. Brain 128: 940–947.

Schuh-Hofer S, Richter M, Israel H et al. (2006). The use of radiolabelled human serum albumin and SPECT/MRI co-registration to study inflammation in the cavernous sinus of cluster headache patients. Cephalalgia 26: 1115–1122.

Sianard-Gainko J, Milet J, Ghuysen V et al. (1994). Increased parasellar activity on gallium SPECT is not specific for active cluster headache. Cephalalgia 14: 132–133.

Sprenger T, Valet M, Platzer S et al. (2005). SUNCT: bilateral hypothalamic activation during headache attacks and resolving of symptoms after trigeminal decompression. Pain 113: 422–426.

van Vliet JA, Vein AA, Le Cessie S et al. (2003). Impairment of trigeminal sensory pathways in cluster headache. Cephalalgia 23: 414–419.

Weiller C, May A, Limmroth V et al. (1995). Brain stem activation in spontaneous human migraine attacks. Nat Med 1: 658–660.

Handbook of Clinical Neurology, Vol. 97 (3rd series)
Headache
G. Nappi and M.A. Moskowitz, Editors

Chapter 35

Cluster headache and other trigeminal autonomic cephalalgias: diagnostic criteria

NINAN T. MATHEW*
Houston Headache Clinic, Houston, TX, USA

Trigeminal autonomic cephalalgias share clinical features of paroxysmal, usually short-lived, headaches and prominent cranial parasympathetic autonomic features. Experimental and human functional imaging suggests that these syndromes activate a normal human trigeminal parasympathetic reflex with clinical signs of cranial sympathetic dysfunction being secondary.

Cluster headache, one of the most severe forms of head pain, is a typical example of a periodic disease and is distinct from other forms of headache. The term "cluster headache" recognizes periodicity as a major clinical feature of the disorder (Ekbom, 1947; Kunkle et al., 1952).

CLASSIFICATION AND CLINICAL TERMS

The International Headache Society (IHS) recognizes various forms of trigeminal autonomic cephalalgia (Headache Classification Subcommittee of the International Headache Society, 2004). Table 35.1 gives the classification of cluster headache and other autonomic cephalalgias.

In the past, many terms have been used for cluster headache (Silberstein et al., 2002). These include erythroprosopalgia of Bing, ciliary neuralgia, migrainous neuralgia (Harris), erythromelalgia of the head, Horton's headache, histaminic cephalalgia, petrosal neuralgia (Gardner) or sphenopalatine neuralgia, vidian neuralgia, Sluder's neuralgia, and hemicrania angioparalytica.

CLUSTER HEADACHE

The terms used in describing cluster headache include "attack," meaning individual attacks of cluster headache pain; "cluster period," meaning periods during which patients have repeated attacks; "remission," a period of freedom from attacks; and "mini-bouts," periods of attacks lasting less than 7 days.

Description of cluster headache

The IHS diagnostic criteria are given in Table 35.2.

Cluster headache consists of attacks of severe, strictly unilateral pain, which is orbital, supraorbital, temporal, or in any combination of these sites, lasting 15–180 min and occurring from once every other day to eight times a day. The attacks are associated with one or more of the following, all of which are ipsilateral: conjunctival injection, lacrimation, nasal congestion, rhinorrhea, forehead and facial sweating, miosis, ptosis, and eyelid edema. Most patients are restless or agitated during an attack.

Diagnostic criteria

During a particular cluster period, some of the attacks may be very severe, whereas others may be less severe. The duration of the attack may also vary. Some are short and some are longer. The attacks may be less frequent at certain times during the cluster period, particularly at the beginning and towards the end.

Episodic cluster headache is characterized by cluster periods of 7 days to 1 year with periods of remission lasting 1 month or longer and occasional mini-bouts. Chronic cluster headache is characterized by absence of remission for 1 year or short remission of less than 1 month, increased frequency of attacks, and relative resistance to pharmacotherapy. Some patients may switch from chronic headache to episodic cluster headache. In a large series with good

*Correspondence to: Ninan T. Mathew, MD, FRCP(C), Director, Houston Headache Clinic, 1213 Hermann Drive, Suite 350, Houston, Texas 77004, USA, Tel: (713) 528–1916, Fax: (713) 526–6369, E-mail: ntmathew@houstonheadacheclinic.com

Table 35.1

International Headache Society classification (Headache Classification Subcommittee of the International Headache Society, 2004)

3. Cluster headache and other trigeminal autonomic cephalalgias
3.1 Cluster headache
  3.1.1 Episodic cluster headache
  3.1.2 Chronic cluster headache
3.2 Paroxysmal hemicrania
  3.2.1 Episodic paroxysmal hemicrania
  3.2.2 Chronic paroxysmal hemicrania
3.3 Short-lasting unilateral neuralgiform headache attacks with conjunctival injection and tearing (SUNCT)
3.4 Probable trigeminal autonomic cephalalgia
  3.4.1 Probable cluster headache
  3.4.2 Probable paroxysmal hemicrania
  3.4.3 Probable SUNCT

Table 35.2

International Headache Society diagnostic criteria for cluster headache (Headache Classification Subcommittee of the International Headache Society, 2004)

A. At least five attacks fulfilling criteria B–D
B. Severe or very severe unilateral orbital, supraorbital, and/or temporal pain lasting 15–180 min if untreated
C. Headache is accompanied by at least one of the following:
  1. Ipsilateral conjunctival injection and/or lacrimation
  2. Ipsilateral nasal congestion and/or rhinorrhea
  3. Ipsilateral eyelid edema
  4. Ipsilateral forehead and facial sweating
  5. Ipsilateral miosis and/or ptosis
  6. A sense of restlessness or agitation
D. Attacks have a frequency from one every other day to eight per day
E. Not attributed to another disorder

follow-up, 27% of patients had only a single cluster period (Sjostrand et al., 2000). These should be coded as 3.1 cluster headache.

Clinical manifestations

Cluster headache, predominantly a disease of males (the male-to-female ratio is approximately 9:1), has an approximate prevalence of 0.1–0.4% in the general population (Kudrow, 1980). Cluster headache may be inherited (autosomal dominant) in about 5% of cases (Russell et al., 1995). It usually begins between the ages of 20 and 40, although there are well-documented cases outside that range.

The unique head pain profile, periodicity, and autonomic features distinguish cluster headache from other headache disorders.

The headache pain profile

The headache pain profile consists of rapid onset of headache reaching a peak in intensity in 10–15 min, lasting generally 30–45 min. As indicated in the IHS diagnostic criteria, the range of pain duration could be 15–180 min. The pain may remain severe for an hour or more and then, after a period of fluctuating peaks of pain, rapidly subsides, leaving the sufferer exhausted. The headache is almost always unilateral, the most common site of pain being orbital, retro-orbital, temporal, supraorbital, and infraorbital in order of decreasing frequency. Rarer cases occur outside the trigeminal territory (Sanin et al., 1993). A few to several attacks usually occur with a frequency of range of one a week to eight or more per day.

In any cluster period, pain remains on the same side and may affect the same side year after year. Occasionally, pain may be contralateral in a subsequent cluster period; most rarely it alternates from side to side, from headache to headache. Pain is of terrible intensity and is usually described as boring or tearing, like a "hot poker in the eye" or as if "the eye is being pushed out." This is distinctly different from the dull, throbbing pain of migraine.

Periodicity

There is a clock-like regularity in the timing of attacks, a phenomenon thought to be due to a dysfunction of the hypothalamic biological clock mechanism. Acute attacks involve activation of posterior hypothalamic gray matter, as detected in imaging studies (May et al., 1998). Onset shortly after falling asleep is common and, at least in some subjects, corresponds to the onset of rapid eye movement (REM) sleep (Kudrow et al., 1984). Nocturnal attacks also occur during non-REM periods (Kudrow et al., 1984). Sleep apnea and resultant oxygen desaturation could act as a trigger for cluster headache attacks (Mathew et al., 1985). At times, three or four attacks per night rapidly lead to sleep deprivation, which in turn can result in frequent daytime naps, often with further painful attacks. Circumannual periodicity also occurs.

Autonomic symptoms

Parasympathetic overactivity resulting in ipsilateral lacrimation, injection of the conjunctiva, and nasal stuffiness or rhinorrhea are regular features. Partial sympathetic paresis resulting in ptosis and miosis also occurs. Facial flushing or pallor, scalp and facial tenderness, tenderness of the ipsilateral carotid artery, and bradycardia are other common associated symptoms. Some of these features also occur in patients with chronic paroxysmal hemicrania (CPH) or other conditions such as dissection of the carotid artery, but the temporal profile for cluster headache is virtually specific.

Behavior during attacks

During a cluster headache attack, patients have a sense of restlessness or agitation. Some patients pace the floor or sit in a position that gives them maximum relief (Kudrow, 1980). Patients find it difficult to lie down as this aggravates pain, distinct from migraine, during which the patient retreats into a dark, quiet room. Cluster headache patients may behave in irrational and bizarre ways, moaning, crying, or screaming, and may threaten suicide. Some patients find their relief by physical exercise such as jogging in place. They may press on the eye or temples with the hand or with an ice pack or a hot wash cloth. Many prefer to be alone or go outside, even in colder weather. After attacks, the patient may be exhausted. Fear of further attacks with the onset of sleep may lead to prolonged attempts to remain awake. This futile behavior results in rapid onset of REM activity when sleep eventually overcomes the subject and a further attack often occurs within minutes of falling asleep.

Provocation of attacks

Alcohol frequently triggers an attack while the patient is in an active cluster phase. In patients with periods of remission, alcohol rarely precipitates an attack during a pain-free period. Most subjects give up the use of alcohol as soon as they realize a cluster headache has begun. Some patients who are receiving prophylactic treatment can consume alcohol without developing an attack. Some can imbibe without any effect on the attacks, regardless of the phase of the disorder, and a very small percentage actually use excess quantities of alcohol to try to get to sleep without causing an attack to develop. Unlike migraine, cluster headache may be precipitated by any type of alcoholic beverage: beer, spirits, and wine have the same effect. Whether alcohol acts simply as a vasodilator is uncertain.

Other vasodilators such as nitroglycerine tablets (Ekbom, 1968) and histamine also induce attacks of cluster headache in susceptible patients. A transient, mild hypoxemia occurs following the administration of nitroglycerine (Hales and Westphal, 1978). Kudrow and Kudrow (1990) reported that cluster headache in patients in remission and non-headache controls had no headache following nitroglycerine despite transient oxygen desaturation. In the active cluster group, low-grade oxygen desaturation persisted, never returning to baseline, and this resulted in cluster attacks. Altitude hypoxemia and sleep apnea-induced hypoxemia can also induce cluster headache attacks during a cluster period. Kudrow and Kudrow (1993) offered the hypothesis, based on observations, that the carotid body chemoreceptors are involved in cluster headache pathogenesis.

Food items and food additives do not appear to be triggers for cluster headache attacks. Frequency of smoking is greatly increased among cluster headache patients and some achieve remission after abstinence.

For patients in the episodic phase, the factors that determine the beginning and end of a cluster period or period of remission are unknown. Stress, depression, and psychological factors seem to have less importance in the pathogenesis of cluster headache than other headache types. The behavior of some patients during the attack that resembles a manic episode, periodicity of the cluster headache, and the beneficial effects of lithium in some patients suggest some resemblance to manic depressive illness.

Course

Both the episodic form and the chronic form of cluster headache continue to occur for years. In the episodic form, remissions may last many years, but the subject remains at risk for recurrence until old age. In a large series of patients followed by Krabbe (1991), only a small minority appeared to have lost the propensity to attacks with age. The chronic form may revert to episodic form (Manzoni et al., 1983).

EXAMINATION

The only abnormal physical sign that may be seen between attacks of cluster headache, either permanently or for a few hours, is an ipsilateral partial Horner's syndrome with a minor degree of upper-lid ptosis and miosis. Pharmacological testing of the pupillary response suggests the Horner's syndrome is a third-order neuron disorder (Watson and Vijayan, 1982).

During an attack, an ipsilateral Horner's syndrome, conjunctival injection, tearing, and nasal obstruction are common. Flushing and ipsilateral facial sweating are relatively rare. An occasional patient will complain of swelling of the temple, cheek, palate, or gums ipsilateral to the pain. In most instances, swelling cannot be detected by an examiner, although occasionally there is apparent edema and soft-tissue swelling in the region described by the sufferer.

Results of neuroimaging studies, including computed tomography (CT) and magnetic resonance imaging (MRI) scans of the head and neck, are normal, and cerebral angiography, performed between attacks, is unremarkable. Arteriography or magnetic resonance angiography (MRA) during the attack has been performed only a few times (Ekbom and Greitz, 1970; Waldenlind et al., 1993). In the best-documented cases, the carotid artery appeared to be in spasm or to be irregularly compressed in the region of the siphon, with dilated ophthalmic artery (Ekbom and Greitz, 1970; Waldenlind et al., 1993).

Using positron emission tomography (PET), significant activation ascribable to the acute cluster headache was observed in the ipsilateral posterior hypothalamic gray matter when compared to the headache-free state (May et al., 1998) and in patients outside the cluster periods (Sprenger et al., 2004). In contrast to migraine (Weiller et al., 1995; Matharu et al., 2004), there was no brainstem activation during acute cluster headache attacks.

Using the voxel-based morphometric analysis of the structural T_1-weighted MRI scans, a significant structural difference in gray-matter density was found in patients with cluster headache when compared to healthy volunteers (May et al., 1999). This difference consists of an increase in volume and was present for the entire cohort. The difference was also present when patients in and outside a bout were compared with the control group. This structural difference is bilaterally situated in the diencephalon, adjacent to the third ventricle and rostral to the aqueduct, coinciding with the interior posterior hypothalamus. In terms of the stereotaxic coordinates, it is virtually the identical area in which activation during an acute cluster headache attack is demonstrated in the PET study.

Colocalization of morphometric and functional changes in cluster headache means that two different imaging techniques separately identify a highly specific brain area previously considered on clinical and biological grounds to be involved in the genesis of the cluster headache syndrome. The structural data relate to a morphometric change of the neuronal density in this region while the functional imaging data are related to the neuronal activity in this area. Together they demonstrate for the first time the precise anatomic location for the central nervous system lesion of cluster headache.

DIAGNOSIS

The diagnosis of cluster headache, which is primarily clinical, is based on the history of the attacks, a careful description of the pain, the temporal profile, the trigger factors, and the associated autonomic manifestations. The rapid escalation of the pain, the predominance of nocturnal attacks, and the limited duration of each headache are important details of the history. Despite the rarity of associated structural abnormalities, it is appropriate to obtain a MRI scan of the brain or a contrast-enhanced CT scan. PET and voxel-based morphomatic analysis of T_1-weighted MRI scans are only possible in specialized centers.

Differential diagnosis

Cluster headache is distinguished from migraine by the male predominance, strict unilaterality of pain, short-lived attacks (45 min to 1 h), multiple attacks per day, associated autonomic features, restlessness and inability to lie down during the attack, and the periodicity (clustering) of attacks. Migraines tend to occur primarily in females. Attacks may be associated with prodrome or aura and last a number of hours to days. Nausea, vomiting, and photophobia are prominent features in migraine; they may occur, but less frequently, in cluster headache (Table 35.3).

SYMPTOMATIC CLUSTER HEADACHE

Symptomatic cluster headaches (Mathew, 1993) are cluster headache-like attacks that occur as a result of an underlying intracranial lesion. Parasellar meningioma, adenoma of the pituitary, calcified lesion in the region of the third ventricle, anterior carotid artery aneurysm, epidermoid tumor of the clivus expanding into the suprasellar cistern, vertebral artery aneurysms, nasopharyngeal carcinoma, ipsilateral large hemispheric arteriovenous malformation, and upper cervical meningioma have been reported to produce

Table 35.3

Comparison of cluster headache and migraine

Clinical feature	Cluster headache	Migraine
Gender ratio (M:F)	90:10	25:75
Unilateral pain	100%	68%
Duration	15–180 min	4–72 h
Associated with:		
Nausea	+	+++
Photophobia, phonophobia	+	+++
Exacerbation by movement	−	+++
Family history	+	+++
Aura	±	++
Autonomic features, such as lacrimation, rhinorrhea, and ptosis	+++	±

symptomatic cluster headache, which should be suspected when clinical features are atypical. Atypical features include the following:

- Absence of typical periodicity seen in episodic cluster headache – in other words, the headaches behave more like chronic cluster headache
- A certain degree of background headache which does not subside between attacks
- Inadequate or unsatisfactory response to treatments that are effective in idiopathic cluster headache, such as oxygen inhalation, triptans, or dihydroergotamine
- Presence of neurological signs other than miosis and ptosis.

A careful neurological examination is essential. Diminished corneal reflex and other signs of involvement of the fifth nerve and signs of involvement of other cranial nerves have to be looked for. Most cases of symptomatic cluster headache reported have had some parasellar abnormality, especially around the distal portions of the carotid artery in the cavernous sinus area, where nociceptive fibers of the trigeminal nerve and sympathetic and parasympathetic nerves come together.

Cluster-like headaches have been reported following head and facial trauma involving the trigeminal nerve territory (Reik, 1987; Mathew and Rueveni, 1988).

Other short-lasting head pains, which should be differentiated from cluster headache, include primary stabbing headache, benign cough headache, hypnic headache, and trigeminal neuralgia.

CLUSTER HEADACHE WITH COEXISTENT TRIGEMINAL NEURALGIA (CLUSTER TIC SYNDROME)

Some patients have been reported who have both cluster headache and trigeminal neuralgia. They should receive both diagnoses, as both conditions must be treated simultaneously for effective control of head pain.

Trigeminal neuralgia is a short-lived lancinating pain confined to the second and third divisions of the trigeminal nerve. The most common areas of pain are perioral, around the angle of the mouth, or periorbital, in the distribution of the second division of the trigeminal nerve. Presence of trigger zones of the face, stimulation of which brings on severe attacks, is characteristic of trigeminal neuralgia. The patient prefers not to touch the face, unlike the patient with cluster headache, who may press on the areas to obtain some relief. Trigeminal neuralgia is more common above 50 years of age. Each attack lasts for only a few seconds.

PAROXYSMAL HEMICRANIAS

The paroxysmal hemicranias (PH) are a group of rare, benign headache disorders that clinically resemble cluster headache, but fail to remit with standard anticluster therapy. Attacks of PH have similar characteristics of pain and associated symptoms and signs to those of cluster headache, but are short-lasting, more frequent, occur more commonly in females, and exhibit an absolute responsiveness to indomethacin. CPH (Sjaastad and Dale, 1974, 1976) with an unremitting course was the first entity described in this group; later, an episodic variety (with remissions) was reported and the term "episodic paroxysmal hemicrania" (EPH) was given (Kudrow et al., 1987). CPH can evolve from EPH.

Sometimes, the responsiveness to indomethacin may be incomplete because of poor dosing. In general, a dose of 150 mg or more orally or rectally, or 100 mg by injection, may be required initially, with a lower maintenance dose later.

One of the major differences between cluster headache and paroxysmal hemicrania is the lack of male predominance. In fact, the female-to-male ratio is 3:1. Onset is usually in adulthood, although childhood cases have been reported. Table 35.4 shows the IHS diagnostic criteria for PH, including EPH and CPH.

In PH, the chronic form dominates the presentation, in contrast to cluster headache, in which the episodic form prevails.

A family history of CPH or EPH is uncommon. In 21% of reported cases, there was a documented family history of migraine. Only 1 patient reported a positive family history for PH (Antonaci and Sjaastad, 1989).

The pain is strictly unilateral and without side-shift in the vast majority of patients. Maximal pain is experienced in the ocular, temporal, maxillary, and frontal regions: nuchal, occipital, and retro-orbital pain has less often been described. The pain may occasionally radiate into the ipsilateral shoulder and arm. The pain is described as a throbbing, boring, pulsatile, or stabbing sensation that ranges in severity from moderate to excruciating headache and has an abrupt onset and cessation. In 28 previous reports, mild discomfort was noted interictally at the usual sites of pain in up to 60% (Cittadini and Goadsby, 2006). Restlessness or agitation may occur in up to 85% (Cittadini and Goadsby, 2006). The attacks occur regularly throughout the 24-h period without a preponderance of nocturnal attacks, as in cluster headache.

In CPH, attacks recur 1–40 times daily. However, there is a marked variability in attack frequency; the frequency of mild attacks ranges from 2 to 14 daily, and severe attacks recur 6–40 times daily. Most patients report 15 or more attacks per day. Headaches usually last between 2 and 25 min each (range 2–120 min).

Table 35.4

International Headache Society diagnostic criteria for paroxysmal hemicrania (Headache Classification Subcommittee of the International Headache Society, 2004)

A. At least 20 attacks fulfilling criteria B–D
B. Attacks of severe unilateral, orbital, supraorbital temporal pain lasting 2–30 min
C. Headache is accompanied by at least one of the following:
   1. Ipsilateral conjunctival injection and/or lacrimation
   2. Ipsilateral nasal congestion and/or rhinorrhea
   3. Ipsilateral eyelid edema
   4. Ipsilateral forehead and facial sweating
   5. Ipsilateral miosis and/or ptosis
D. Attacks are at frequency above five per day for more than half the time, although periods with lower frequency may occur
E. Attacks are completely prevented by therapeutic doses of indomethacin
F. Not attributed to another disorder

3.2.1 Episodic paroxysmal hemicrania

Description

Attacks of paroxysmal hemicrania occurring in periods lasting 7 days to 1 year separated by pain-free periods lasting 1 month or longer

Diagnostic criteria

A. Attacks fulfilling criteria A–F for 3.2 paroxysmal hemicrania
B. At least two attack periods lasting 7–365 days and separated by pain-free remission periods of $\geq$1 month

3.2.2 Chronic paroxysmal hemicrania

Description

Attacks of paroxysmal hemicrania occurring for more than 1 year without remission or with remissions lasting less than 1 month

Diagnostic criteria

A. Attacks fulfilling criteria A–F for 3.2 paroxysmal hemicrania
B. Attacks recur over $>$1 year without remission periods or with remission periods lasting $<$1 month

In EPH, the daily attack frequency ranges from 2 to 30, with attacks lasting 3–30 min each. The headache phase lasts from 2 weeks to 4.5 months, whereas remission periods range from 1 to 36 months.

Both EPH and CPH are characterized by excruciatingly severe throbbing or piercing headaches localized in the temple and orbital regions and accompanied by the ipsilateral autonomic features typical of cluster headache. Both EPH and CPH have clinically similar features: multiple short-duration daily headaches, nocturnal attacks, and absolute response to treatment with indomethacin.

Triggers

While the majority of attacks are spontaneous, approximately 10% of attacks may be precipitated mechanically, either by bending or by rotating the head. Attacks may also be provoked by external pressure against the transverse processes of C4–5, C2 root, or the greater occipital nerve. Alcohol ingestion triggers headaches in only 7% of patients (Antonaci and Sjaastad, 1989).

Diagnostic work-up

The differential diagnosis of PH is summarized in Table 35.5.

It is important to examine the patient carefully just like in any other headache disorder and rule out any organic condition.

Every patient with possible paroxysmal hemicrania must have diagnostic neuroimaging to exclude an underlying secondary cause. Structural mimics of CPH have included a parasellar pituitary adenoma, maxillary cyst, occipital infarction, gangliocytoma growing from the sella turcica, ophthalmic herpes zoster infection, arteriovenous malformation, cavernous sinus meningioma, frontal lobe tumor, and Pancoast tumor (Mathew, 2004). MRI is suggested as the neuroimaging procedure of choice because of its higher sensitivity than CT for visualizing tumors and vascular malformations. Contralateral posterior hypothalamic activation has been demonstrated in patients with PH, by PET imaging (Matharu et al., 2006).

PAROXYSMAL HEMICRANIA WITH COEXISTENT TRIGEMINAL NEURALGIA (CPH–TIC SYNDROME)

Patients who fulfill criteria for both paroxysmal hemicrania and trigeminal neuralgia may be seen occasionally. They should receive both diagnoses and should be treated for both conditions concomitantly.

Table 35.5

Differential diagnosis of paroxysmal hemicranias

Feature	Cluster headache	Chronic paroxysmal hemicrania	Episodic paroxysmal hemicrania	SUNCT	Primary stabbing headache	Trigeminal neuralgia
Gender (M:F)	9:1	1:3	1:1	8:1	F>M	F>M
Pain type	Boring	Throbbing/ boring	Throbbing	Stabbing	Stabbing	Stabbing
Severity	Very severe	Very severe	Very severe	More severe	Severe	Very severe
Location	Orbital Temporal	Orbital Temporal	Orbital Temporal	Orbital Temporal	Any part	V2/V3
Attack duration	15–180 min	2–45 min	1–30 min	5–240 s	<1 s	<1 s
Attack frequency	1–8/day	1–40/day	3–30/day	1/day to 30/h	Few to many/day	Few to many/day
Migraine features	+	+	+	–	–	–
Autonomic features	+++	++	++	+++	–	–
Alcohol trigger	++	+	+	–	–	–
Cutaneous trigger	–	–	–	++	–	–
Indomethacin	–	+++	+++	–	+	–

(Modified from Silberstein et al., 1998, with permission.)

SUNCT: short-lasting unilateral neuralgiform headache attacks with conjunctival injection and tearing; F: female; M: male; V1: ophthalmic; V2: maxillary; V3: mandibular divisions of the trigeminal innervation; +: precipitates headaches; ±: effect not consistent; –: no effect on headache.

SHORT-LASTING UNILATERAL NEURALGIFORM HEADACHE ATTACKS WITH CONJUNCTIVAL INJECTION AND TEARING (SUNCT)

SUNCT is a rare primary headache syndrome, characterized by unilateral orbital or temporal pain, which is stabbing or throbbing in quality and is severe. There should be at least 20 attacks, lasting for 5–240 s, and ipsilateral conjunctival injection and lacrimation should be present (Headache Classification Subcommittee of the International Headache Society, 2004). In recognition of the possibility that all patients with generically the same condition might not have both conjunctival injection and tearing, the classification committee considered that SUNCT syndrome may be a subset of short-lasting unilateral neuralgiform headache attacks with cranial autonomic features (SUNA), including the latter in the appendix. In SUNA there may be cranial autonomic symptoms other than conjunctival injection and lacrimation, or indeed only one of those symptoms may be present.

Diagnosis

Table 35.6 shows the IHS diagnostic criteria for SUNCT. The IHS describes the site of pain in SUNCT as unilateral orbital, supraorbital, or temporal pain (Headache Classification Subcommittee of the International Headache Society, 2004), although it is clear from a large series that the pain may be experienced anywhere in the head (Cohen et al., 2006). Clinical experience demonstrates that attacks may take on different characters: single stabs, which are usually short-lived, groups of stabs, or a longer attack comprising many stabs, between which the pain does not resolve to normal, thus giving a "saw-tooth" phenomenon with attacks lasting many minutes (Cohen et al., 2006).

Important clinical characteristics that lead to the suspicion of a diagnosis of SUNCT are the fact that the attacks can be triggered cutaneously (or otherwise), a lack of refractory period to triggering between attacks, and the lack of a response to indomethacin. Oxygen is unhelpful and the indomethacin test shows no distinction between indomethacin and saline placebo (Cohen et al., 2005). Apart from trigeminal sensory disturbance, the neurological examination is normal in primary SUNCT.

SECONDARY (SYMPTOMATIC) SUNCT

Secondary SUNCT is mainly seen with either posterior fossa or pituitary gland lesions, although other sites have been documented. It is a recommendation that a brain MRI with pituitary views and pituitary function tests should be a minimal work-up for SUNCT/SUNA. The diagnosis of SUNCT is often confused with trigeminal neuralgia, particularly in first-division trigeminal

Table 35.6

International Headache Society diagnostic criteria for SUNCT (Headache Classification Subcommittee of the International Headache Society, 2004)

3.3 Short-lasting unilateral neuralgiform headache attacks with conjunctival injection and tearing (SUNCT)
Description
This syndrome is characterized by short-lasting attacks of unilateral pain that are much briefer than those seen in any other trigeminal autonomic cephalalgia and very often accompanied by prominent lacrimation and redness of the ipsilateral eye
Diagnostic criteria
A. At least 20 attacks fulfilling criteria B–D
B. Attacks of unilateral orbital, supraorbital, or temporal stabbing or pulsating pain lasting 5–240 s
C. Pain is accompanied by ipsilateral conjunctival injection and lacrimation
D. Attacks occur with a frequency from 3 to 200 per day
E. Not attributed to another disorder (Ekbom, 1947)

neuralgia. Minimal or no cranial autonomic symptoms and a clear refractory period to triggering are useful pointers to a diagnosis of trigeminal neuralgia compared to SUNCT/SUNA.

Differential diagnosis

Hemicrania continua is another rare unilateral continuous headache disorder with some autonomic symptoms that responds to indomethacin (Sjaastad and Spierings, 1984). Remitting and unremitting forms have been described (Newman et al., 1994). Since the symptoms of hemicrania continua partly overlap with those of other trigeminal autonomic cephalgias, including cluster headache, it comes in the differential diagnosis (classification 4.7: Headache Classification Subcommittee of the International Headache Society, 2004).

Strictly unilateral headache without side-shift, and daily and continuous head pain without pain-free periods are characteristic. There is a background moderate-intensity headache most of the time with exacerbations of severe pain, during which conjunctival injections and lacrimation, nasal congestion and rhinorrhea, ptosis, and/or miosis may occur. The severity of autonomic symptoms in hemicrania continua is less than that of cluster headache. Complete or absolute responsiveness to indomethacin is diagnostic.

Hemicrania continua remains a rare disorder, with fewer than 120 reported cases found in the literature. Recent clinical experience suggests that the disorder may be more common than previously recognized. Hemicrania continua is one of the causes of refractory, unilateral, chronic daily headaches. This disorder demonstrates a marked female preponderance, unlike cluster headache, with a female-to-male ratio of 1.9:1. Age of onset of the disorder ranges from 11 to 58 years (mean 44 years). Table 35.7 lists indomethacin-responsive headache syndromes.

Table 35.7

Indomethacin-responsive headache syndromes (Mathew, 1980)

A. Absolute responsiveness
  1. Paroxysmal hemicranias
     Chronic paroxysmal hemicrania
     Episodic paroxysmal hemicrania
  2. Hemicrania continua
B. Relative or partial responsiveness
  1. Primary stabbing headache or idiopathic stabbing headache
  2. Benign cough headache
  3. Benign exertional headache

References

Antonaci F, Sjaastad O (1989). Chronic paroxysmal hemicrania (CPH): a review of the clinical manifestations. Headache 29: 648–656.

Cittadini F, Goadsby PJ (2006). Revisiting the International Headache Society criteria for paroxysmal hemicrania–series of 21 patients. Cephalalgia 26: 1401–1402.

Cohen AS, Matharu MS, Goadsby PJ (2005). Suggested guidelines for treating SUNCT and SUNA. Cephalalgia 25: 1200.

Cohen AS, Matharu MS, Goadsby PJ (2006). Short-lasting unilateral neuralgiform headache attacks with conjunctival injection and tearing (SUNCT) or cranial autonomic features (SUNA) – a prospective clinical study of SUNCT and SUNA. Brain 129: 2746–2760.

Ekbom KA (1947). Ergotamine tartrate orally in Horten's "histaminic cephalgia" (also called Harris's "ciliary neuralgia"). Acta Psychiatr Scand 46: 106–113.

Ekbom K (1968). Nitroglycerin as a provocative agent in cluster headache. Arch Neurol 19: 487–493.

Ekbom K, Greitz T (1970). Carotid angiography in cluster headaches. Acta Radiol Diagn 10: 177–183.

Hales CA, Westphal D (1978). Hypoxemia following the administration of sublingual nitroglycerin. Am J Med 65: 911–917.

Headache Classification Subcommittee of the International Headache Society (2004). The international classification of headache disorders, 2nd edn. Cephalalgia 24: 1–160.

Krabbe A (1991). The prognosis of cluster headache: a long-term observation of 226 cluster headache patients. Cephalalgia 11 (Suppl. 11): 250–251.

Kudrow L (1980). Cluster Headache. Mechanisms and Management. Oxford University Press, Oxford.

Kudrow L, Kudrow DB (1990). Association of sustained oxyhemoglobin desaturation and arrest of cluster headache attacks. Headache 30: 474–480.

Kudrow L, Kudrow DB (1993). The role of chemoreceptor activity and oxyhemoglobin desaturation in cluster headache. Headache 33: 483–484.

Kudrow L, McGinty DJ, Philips ER et al. (1984). Sleep apnea in cluster headache. Cephalalgia 4: 33–38.

Kudrow L, Esperanz AP, Vijaya NN (1987). Episodic paroxysmal hemicrania? Headache 7: 197–201.

Kunkle EC, Pfeiffer JB Jr, Wilhoit WM et al. (1952). Recurrent brief headache in cluster pattern. Trans Am Neurol Assoc 77: 240–243.

Manzoni GC, Terzano MG, Bono G et al. (1983). Cluster headache: clinical findings in 180 patients. Cephalalgia 3: 21–30.

Matharu MS, Bartsuch T, Ward N et al. (2004). Central neuromodulation in chronic migraine patients with suboccipital stimulations. A PET study. Brain 127: 220–230.

Matharu MS, Cohen AS, Frackowiak RS et al. (2006). Posterior hypothalamic activation in paroxysmal hemicrania. Ann Neurol 59: 535–545.

Mathew NT (1980). Indomethacin responsive headache syndrome. Headache 21: 147–150.

Mathew NT (1993). Symptomatic cluster. Neurology 43: 1270.

Mathew NT (2004). Cluster headache and other trigeminal autonomic cephalalgias. In: RW Evans, NT Mathew (Eds.), Handbook of Headache. 2nd edn. Lippincott, Williams & Wilkins, Philadelphia, PA, p. 168.

Mathew NT, Rueveni U (1988). Cluster-like headache following head trauma. Headache 28: 297.

Mathew NT, Glaze D, Frost JR (1985). Sleep apnea and other sleep abnormalities in primary headache disorders. In: F Clifford Rose (Ed.), Migraine Clinical and Research Advances. Karger, London, pp. 40–49.

May A, Bahara A, Buchel C et al. (1998). Hypothalamic activation in cluster headache. Lancet 352: 275–278.

May A, Ashburner J, Buchel C et al. (1999). Correlation between structural and functional changes in brain in an idiopathic headache syndrome. Nat Med 5: 836–838.

Newman LC, Lipton RB, Solomon S (1994). Hemicrania continua: ten new cases and a review of the literature. Neurology 44: 2111–2114.

Reik L (1987). Cluster headache after head injury. Headache 27: 509–511.

Russell MB, Anderson PG, Thompson LL et al. (1995). Cluster headache is an autosomal dominantly inherited disorder in some families: a complex segregation analysis. J Med Genet 32: 954–956.

Sanin LC, Mathew NT, Ali S (1993). Extratrigeminal cluster headache. Headache 33: 369–371.

Silberstein SD, Lipton RB, Goadsby PJ (1998). Headache in Clinical Practice. Isis Medical Media, Oxford.

Silberstein SD, Lipton RB, Goadsby PJ (2002). Headache in Clinical Practice. 2nd edn. Martin Dunitz, London.

Sjaastad O, Dale I (1974). Evidence for a new (?) Treatable headache entity. Headache 14: 105–108.

Sjaastad O, Dale I (1976). A new (?) clinical headache entity "chronic paroxysmal hemicrania" 2. Acta Neurol Scand 54: 140–159.

Sjaastad O, Spierings ELH (1984). "Hemicrania continua": another headache absolutely responsive to indomethacin. Cephalalgia 4: 65–70.

Sjostrand C, Waldelind E, Ekbom K (2000). A follow up study of 60 patients after an assumed first period of cluster headache. Cephalalgia 20: 653–657.

Sprenger T, Boecker H, Tollie TR et al. (2004). Specific hypothalamic activation during a spontaneous cluster headache attack. Neurology 62: 516–517.

Waldenlind E, Ekbom K, Torhall J (1993). MR angiography during spontaneous attacks of cluster headache. A case report. Headache 33: 291–295.

Watson C, Vijayan N (1982). Evaluation of oculocephalic sympathetic function in vascular headache syndromes. Part 1. Methods of evaluation. Headache 22: 192–199.

Weiller C, May A, Limmroth V et al. (1995). Brain stem activation in spontaneous human migraine attacks. Nat Med 1: 658–660.

Handbook of Clinical Neurology, Vol. 97 (3rd series)
Headache
G. Nappi and M.A. Moskowitz, Editors

Chapter 36

Acute and preventive treatment of cluster headache and other trigeminal autonomic cephalgias

GENNARO BUSSONE[1] AND ALAN RAPOPORT[2]*
[1]*Clinical Neurosciences Department, C. Besta National Neurological Institute, Milan, Italy*
[2]*Department of Neurology, The David Geffen School of Medicine at UCLA, Los Angeles, CA, USA*

ACUTE TREATMENT OF CLUSTER HEADACHE AND OTHER TACS

INTRODUCTION

Cluster headache (CH), without doubt the most excruciating form of head pain known, is a prime example of a periodic disorder that probably involves a biological pacemaker. The realisation that periodicity was an important clinical characteristic led to the affirmation of the now universal term "cluster headache" over other names for the condition used at various times in the past (Kunkle et al., 1952). But the suggestion that the periodicity was caused by a dysfunction in the hypothalamus was put forth by Lee Kudrow in the late 1970s. The intense, unilateral, orbital, periorbital or temporal pain attacks last 15-180 minutes and recur with a frequency ranging from once every two days to eight times a day (Headache Classification Committee of the International Headache Society, 1988). The individual headaches often begin at fixed times of the day or night. One or more of the following ipsilateral autonomic manifestations accompany the attack: lacrimation, conjunctival injection, nasal obstruction, rhinorrhea, miosis, palpebral ptosis, facial sweating, and palpebral edema (Headache Classification Committee of the International Headache Society, 1988). The cluster periods during which these headaches occur may last a few weeks or several months, and are usually separated by spontaneous remission phases that may endure for a few months or many years.

In about 10-20% of CH patients the condition is chronic; that is, there are no significant remission periods in the course of a year. The prevalence is around 0.1%-0.4% (D'Alessandro et al., 1986) and males are more commonly affected than females, in the ratio of about 3-4 to 1. Age at onset is generally between 18 and 40 years but can be as early as childhood or as late as the 8th decade. The cluster periods often begin in spring or autumn when the amount of available light from the sun is becoming either very low or high (Kudrow, 1987).

Treatment of cluster headache

The principles of treating cluster headache are no different from those of other primary headaches and may be summarized as follows: (a) educate the patient about the nature of the condition; (b) identify, and encourage the patient to avoid, conditions and factors that may trigger an attack; (c) identify the most appropriate acute care therapy; and (4) assess the need for prevention and determine the most appropriate preventive medication considering age, the clinical characteristics of the headache, and potential side effects from and contraindications to the available medications.

Educating the patient

The patient must be informed of and educated about his condition at an early stage. Because of the severity of the violent and intense pain, the new patient presenting with CH is often extremely concerned and agitated, and generally worries that he has a fatal or life-threatening condition. Later, patients may be terrified by and anxious about the spectre of a return of their attacks. Reassurance is all important. Full information should be given as to the nature of the disease, emphasizing its benign nature (Kudrow, 1990).

*Correspondence to: Alan M. Rapoport, M.D., Department of Neurology, The David Geffen School of Medicine at UCLA, 239 South Orange Drive, Los Angeles, CA 90036, USA, Tel: +1 323 939-9756, Fax: +1 323 939-9736, E-mail: alanrapoport@gmail.com

Although it may persist for years, around one third of cluster patients achieve complete remission, in another third the intensity of the attacks diminishes with time so that eventually medication is not required, and in the remaining third the pattern of attacks persists unchanged (Kudrow, 1982).

The patient should also be fully informed about available therapeutic options (acute care and preventive). Patients must be strongly encouraged to keep a headache diary, recording the time of onset, duration, intensity and therapeutic response of the attacks, in order to help the treating physician to more precisely tailor the therapy in successive cluster periods.

Triggering factors

Little is known about factors that can trigger the onset of a cluster period, although avoiding shift changes at work and long flights across multiple time zones is recommended. One can, however, hope to avoid individual attacks within a cluster period or at least attenuate their intensity. Moderate alcohol consumption may trigger an attack during the cluster period but not in remission phase (Kudrow, 1980). Paradoxically massive alcohol consumption not only fails to trigger an attack but may act preventively (Ekbom, 1987) with the length of remission being related to the quantity of ethanol imbibed (Klimek, 1978). The habit of drinking with meals may in part explain why attacks commonly begin around mealtimes. One should, therefore, advise the patient to completely abstain from drinking alcohol during a cluster period, even if preventive drugs such as verapamil or lithium have been prescribed. These medications may not prevent alcohol-triggered attacks, even though they are otherwise efficacious. The patient should also be advised to avoid exposure to vasodilating substances, as well as solvent vapors (in particular gasoline). High altitudes (above 5-7,000 feet above sea level), including flying in planes pressurized to 7-8,000 feet above sea level and especially aircraft with non-pressurized cabins, may also trigger an attack (Kudrow, 1982). Drastic changes in sleep-wake cycles including shift changes at work can start a cluster period or worsen attacks. For these reasons the habits of the CH patient should be extensively explored during history-taking.

Acute Therapy

Pharmacological treatment for cluster headache (CH) can be abortive (acute care), prophylactic (preventive), or a combination of the two. Bridge therapy means starting a patient on quicker acting treatments while you start preventive treatment which may take longer to take effect. Preventive treatment aims to shorten the cluster period and control the frequency of attacks in both the episodic and chronic forms. Acute care treatment aims to manage individual attacks by stopping them quickly. Individual attacks are extremely violent but usually of short duration; they often occur during sleep (waking the patient about 90 minutes after falling asleep) and reach full intensity with alarming rapidity. Drugs for acute relief must therefore be rapidly-acting. Subcutaneously, nasally or intramuscularly administered medications are indicated, as the oral or rectal route is generally too slow.

The first drug reported to be effective was ergotamine tartrate (Harris, 1936) Thereafter, dihydroergotamine mesylate and inhalation of 100% oxygen were also used successfully. (Horton, 1952; Friedman and Mikropoulos, 1958).

Application of intranasal cocaine hydrochloride or lidocaine to anaesthetize the sphenopalatine (pterygopalatine) ganglion on the symptomatic side has also proven effective in aborting cluster pain (Barrè, 1982; Kitrelle et al., 1985; Bussone et al., 1987).

The most effective treatments currently available for the acute care of a CH attack are subcutaneous sumatriptan and pure oxygen inhalation.

Sumatriptan

Sumatriptan has been in use since 1991 in Europe and 1993 in the USA (The Sumatriptan Cluster headache Study Group, 1991) and has effectively replaced ergotamine compounds which were the drugs of choice for acute CH attacks. Following subcutaneous injection of 6 mg sumatriptan, benefit is typically felt after about 5 min (Ekbom et al., 1993). Recent studies show that the drug is effective in relieving up to 88% of treated attacks: the pain disappears in about 15 min, with no reduction of efficacy when successive headaches are treated (Gobel et al., 1998). The tolerability of sumatriptan is also good (Gobel et al., 1998). Higher dose sumatriptan is not more effective and produces more side effects (McGeeney, 2005).

However, sumatriptan does not appear to be effective when used preventively, before an attack has commenced (Montsad et al., 1995). Ergotamine works better preventively.

Sumatriptan nasal spray is less effective but better tolerated than the injectable formulation (Hardebo and Dahlof, 1998). A double-blind, randomized, placebo-controlled trial of sumatriptan 20 mg nasal spray found that 56% of attacks responded within 30 minutes compared with a placebo response in 26% of attacks (vanVilet et al., 2001). An open label comparison study of sumatriptan 20 mg nasal spray with 6 mg of subcutaneous sumatriptan found that only 2 of the 26 enrolled patients preferred nasal spray to injectable sumatriptan (Hardebo and Dahlof, 1998).

Sumatriptan has a number of disadvantages:

(a) The high cost of the medication is an important drawback particularly for patients refractory to preventive therapy, those suffering very frequent attacks, and those with long cluster periods.
(b) In a recent study, 62% of treated patients reported adverse events from sumatriptan (Gobel et al., 1998). These were for the most part unpleasant local and general sensations occurring immediately after injection which, however, disappeared rapidly and were rarely severe enough to require changing therapy.
(c) Nevertheless sumatriptan can sometimes induce intolerable adverse events and caution must be exercised above all when treating middle-aged male CH patients who are tobacco abusers and often present risk factors for cardiovascular disease (Matharu et al., 2003). Sumatriptan (and all other triptans) are contraindicated in patients with ischemic heart and brain disease, peripheral vascular disease and uncontrolled hypertension. Other triptans will be discussed below.

Oxygen therapy

Oxygen inhalation, now a standard acute care treatment for CH, was first used by Horton in 1952 (Horton, 1952).

Oxygen inhalation can be dramatic in relieving the symptoms of an attack. Kudrow, who was first to popularize this safe and effective treatment for cluster headache, (Kudrow, 1981) has given the classic account of oxygen use: loose fitting facial mask over the nose and mouth attached at the onset of an attack; flow rate 7-10 L/min for up to 15 min with the patient sitting and bending forwards. This regimen is effective in approximately 70% of patients, usually within 5 minutes. Oxygen is well tolerated. Side effects are almost absent and the treatment can be repeated several times during the day. A recent report by Rozen suggested that high-flow oxygen therapy (15L/min) may be effective in those unresponsive to lower flow rates (Rozen, 2002). Oxygen's effectiveness may also depend on the timing of administration: it may be most effective when given at maximum pain intensity rather that at CH onset as suggested by Kudrow (Kudrow, 1981). In some patients, oxygen administration may delay rather than abort the attack, and pain may return. This rebound effect, which usually does not occur after ergot or sumatriptan treatment, may manifest 30-120 minutes later, and occur even after spontaneous resolution of an attack (Cerbo et al., 1999).

Oxygen therapy has several advantages. It has no contraindications and can be used in elderly patients and those with a heart condition or uncontrolled hypertension, in whom ergot derivatives and triptans are contraindicated. Oxygen can also be used during pregnancy. The speed of action is greater than that of ergots or subcutaneously administered sumatriptan. A major disadvantage of oxygen inhalation is lack of a truly practical administration device, especially when the patient is not at home or in the office. The apparatus is typically heavy and cumbersome, ruling it out for some patients. However, small portable devices are now available although tank capacity is insufficient for a single attack in some patients. The preferred method of prescribing oxygen at The New England Center for Headache in Stamford, Connecticut is to have the patient rent a large D cylinder which is placed in their bedroom and can only be used there. Many patients have the bulk of their attacks after work or in the middle of the night and are therefore at home. Caution should be exercised in the use of home oxygen with smokers and those with chronic obstructive pulmonary disease.

After the initial report by Weiss et al. (Weiss et al., 1989), other studies have confirmed that hyperbaric oxygen (2 atmospheres) is an effective and safe treatment of CH attacks. However the high cost, lack of readily available hyperbaric chambers, and time required to perform the treatment severely restrict the therapeutic utility of this modality, rendering it of theoretical interest only.

Little is known about the mechanism of action of oxygen in pain relief. Sakai and Meyer suggested that an hyper-reactivity of cerebral blood vessels to oxygen may be due to its potentiation of catecholamines, serotonin and other vasoconstricting substances at the receptor level (Sakai and Meyer, 1978, 1979). Kudrow first proposed that the carotid body was dysfunctional in CH and Mong's Disease, also called Chronic Mountain Sickness. The carotid glomus is sensitive to reduction in oxygen levels and increase in CO_2. Indeed hypercapnia has been suggested as a cause of CH (Rozen, 2002).

Ergotamine derivatives

Until fairly recently, ergotamine tartrate preparations were widely accepted as treatments of choice for the prevention and acute treatment of CH attacks, notwithstanding ergotamine's potential for serious side effects. Because ergotamine is poorly and erratically absorbed after oral administration, other routes are preferred, including inhalation, intramuscular, intravenous and rectal. (Dihydroergotamine has been also used intranasally). While peak plasma levels are obtained after only 5 min following inhalation, ergotamine bioavailability is greatest with the intramuscular and rectal routes of administration (Graham et al., 1984) and these routes are well suited for acute CH attacks as absorption is rapid (Bigal and Tepper, 2003). Ergotamine has a rather short half-life (2 h) but its biological action on the arteries lasts 24 h (Bigal and Tepper, 2003). This is because active metabolites persist and the drug dissociates slowly from vascular receptors. The latter phenomenon may be responsible for the drug-induced headaches that occur in chronic users, and also the two-step elimination kinetics: the first lasts about 90 min, and the second lasting about 20 h.

The side-effects of ergotamine and other ergot derivatives are well known and may limit their utility in CH. They are potent and long-acting vasoconstrictors and should be avoided in patients with coronary artery disease, vasospastic angina and other vascular diseases. They are also contraindicated in uncontrolled hypertension and pregnancy. Concomitant use with other vasoconstrictors, in particular triptans, should be avoided.

Ergotamine dosing should be limited to a maximum of 6 mg/day and 10 mg/week to avoid chronic peripheral vasoconstriction that may give rise to ergotism. Similar restrictions apply to DHE (not more than 2 mg/day) although this drug may be better tolerated Both of these medications have been given in higher doses and longer times to the severely ill chronic cluster patients without problem. But this should be done only by doctors very familiar with cluster headache and after informed consent of the patient. The nausea that occurs in about 10% of patients can be treated with anti-emetics, the leg cramps respond to dose reduction.

Ergotamine has central activity in addition to its peripheral vasoconstrictive effect mainly attributable to α-adrenergic blockade. It is a partial agonist of α-adrenergic receptors in the walls of cerebral arteries and blocks serotoninergic receptors in the brain (Aghjanin and Wang, 1978) and in the basilar and superficial temporal arteries (Ostergaard et al., 1981; Muller-Schweinitzer, 1983).

The drug also has a well-known dopaminergic effect which accounts for vomiting and dizziness. However, the most prominent mechanism of action of ergot derivatives in aborting CH attacks is a direct effect on post-junctional receptors located on vascular smooth muscle or on endothelial cells preventing neurogenic inflammation of the vessels (Buzzi and Moskowitz, 1991).

Unlike patients with migraine, those with CH do not commonly develop ergot dependence or rebound headache due to temporary reduction in ergot dosage. In episodic CH with short-lasting cluster periods characterized by attacks presenting at regular and predictable times, ergotamine may be usefully given 1-2 h before predicted onset. For nocturnal CH attacks, DHE may be given orally or intramuscularly at bedtime. These approaches – a mixture of the preventive and abortive treatments – are feasible when attack frequency is low (1-2/day).

The pharmacology of DHE is similar to that of ergotamine. Administered subcutaneously DHE is effective in relieving CH attacks in 15 minutes in 70% of patients (Klapper and Stanton, 1992). DHE 1 mg is injected at attack onset for not more than two injections per day or six injections per week. Usually 2-4 mg/24 h is well tolerated for several weeks. Anderson and Jasperson (Andersson and Jespersen, 1986) used a nasal spray to deliver 1 mg of DHE in a double blind trial versus placebo in 25 CH patients. The treatment reduced the intensity of the attack but not the duration. This poor result may have been due to the low dose employed. They suggested that the trial should be repeated using a larger dosage of DHE.

The principal side effects of intranasal DHE are local reactions (rhinorrhea, congestion and irritation).

Other triptans

The development and marketing of triptans with enhanced lipophilicity and hence with potentially more rapid oral absorption and greater penetration into the central nervous system (Goadsby, 1998; Millson, 1999) offer the possibility of more effective oral treatment of CH attacks.

Zolmitriptan, a triptan with enhanced lipophilicity, was the first orally administered triptan (sumatriptan is used subcutaneously) shown to be effective in the acute treatment of episodic CH, although at doses higher (5-10 mg) than those normally used for migraine (2.5 or 5 mg). In a trial of zolmitriptan tablet versus placebo, mild or no pain at 30 minutes was reported by 60%, 57% and 42% episodic CH patients treated with zolmitriptan 10 mg, zolmitriptan 5 mg and placebo respectively. For both zolmitriptan doses the differences compared to placebo were significant ($p \leq 0.01$). However, for patients with chronic CH, response rates following zolmitriptan 5 mg and 10 mg did not differ significantly from placebo for any endpoint. Both doses of zolmitriptan were well tolerated (Bahra et al., 2000). The lack of efficacy of zolmitriptan in patients with chronic CH is consistent with the finding that subcutaneous sumatriptan is less effective in chronic than acute CH patients and suggests that the pathophysiology of the chronic and episodic forms differs.

A recent double-blind, placebo-controlled, three way cross-over European study of nasal spray zolmitriptan 10 mg versus placebo explored the effectiveness of zolmitriptan in the acute treatment of CH in 69 patients. Headache relief at 30 minutes was reported by 62%, 40% and 21% patients treated with zolmitriptan 10 mg, zolmitriptan 5 mg and placebo. A pain free-state at 30 minutes was reported by 50%, 28% and 10% of patients treated with zolmitriptan 10 mg, zolmitriptan 5 mg and placebo. No serious adverse events were reported in either the placebo or zolmitriptan group.Similar results were found in an almost identical American study, which also found 10-15 minute post dose efficacy.

These findings indicate that zolmitriptan 10 mg nasal spray is effective at 30 min in 50% or more of cases and is well tolerated. It should therefore be considered for treatment of acute attacks in patients who do not respond well to subcutaneous sumatriptan or would prefer the nasal route to injection.

Nevertheless further randomized trials are required to investigate the efficacy of enhanced lipophilicity triptans and establish the optimal formulations for use in each of the CH variants (Cittadini et al., 2006).

Topical anaesthetics

Sympathetic, parasympathetic and nociceptive pathways from the craniofacial territory pass through the sphenopalatine ganglion (SPG) and application of local anaesthetic to the region of the SPG is often a useful block to abort various types of headaches and atypical facial pain. The SPG is easily accessed through the nasal passages, being located posterior to the middle nasal turbinate and covered by a thin layer of mucous membrane.

Sluder in 1913, Vail in 1929 and more recently Barrè in 1982 (Barrè, 1982) investigated the application of cocaine to the SPG during CH attacks. All found that the method aborted the attacks, however legal problems and those related to cocaine abuse severely limit the use of the method in clinical practice.

Intranasal application of 4% lidocaine has been proposed as an alternative to cocaine. Lidocaine nasal spray (4%) was studied in 30 male patients with CH (Robbins, 1995). Four ipsilateral sprays were applied with a further two if necessary. Only 27% of patients reported moderate relief, 27% mild relief, and 46% no relief.

Bussone et al. (Bussone et al., 1987) applied lidocaine 4% to the SPG region in 25 patients with spontaneous CH crises. In 16 the pain resolved completely within a minute, five patients obtained some relief, and four obtained no benefit. In the 16 responders the sympathetic symptoms disappeared some time after pain relief; more importantly the responders remained pain free for 1-30 days – longer than after treatment with subcutaneous sumatriptan. The three groups (responders, partial responders, and non-responders) did not differ significantly in terms of age, illness duration, annual cluster frequency, attack duration, or other clinical variables.

Application of local anesthetic nasal spray to the SPG region requires the patient supine with the head extended over the edge of the bed at an angle of about 35 degrees, with the pain side turned toward the side of the pain. After application the position is maintained for about 5 minutes. Other open label trials have explored the effectiveness of intranasal lidocaine (Kitrelle et al., 1985; Hardebo and Elner, 1987). Overall results suggest that intranasal lidocaine is useful as an adjuvant to other abortive treatments in selected cases.

Other medications

Give the limitations of the standard acute care agents discussed above, they are not acceptable or not effective in all CH patients. The literature contains reports on various other agents that may by useful for treating CH attacks, but are not usually in wide use.

Olanzapine was given to four chronic and one episodic CH patients in an open label trial. The initial dose was 5 mg, decreased to 2.5 mg if the 5 mg dose was effective but caused adverse effects. Each patient had to treat at least two attacks. Olanzapine reduced cluster pain by at least 80% within 20 minutes in the episodic patient and three of the chronic CH patients. The only adverse event was sleepiness (Rozen, 2001). This limited evidence therefore suggests that olanzapine appears effective in both episodic and chronic cluster headache.

Intravenous verapamil (5-7 mg) administered (after a check for contraindications such as bradycardia and atrioventricular conduction abnormalities) was administered to 15 chronic CH patients at peak pain after nitroglycerine-induced attacks. Pain decreased by more than 50% after about 30 minutes in 13 of the patients. The remaining two patients obtained no relief. No significant side effects were noted (Boiardi et al., 1986).

Two small randomized, double-blind trials using intravenous (Sicuteri et al., 1984) or subcutaneous somatostatin (Geppetti et al., 1985) in CH indicated that this substance could be better than placebo in blocking attacks with an efficacy comparable to that of intramuscular ergotamine, although it appears less effective than ergotamine in reducing pain duration.

Recently, octeotride, a somatostatin analogue with a half-life of approximately 1.5 hours, was used at the dose of 100 μg in a randomized, placebo-controlled, double-blind, crossover study for the treatment of CH attacks in patients with episodic and chronic form of the disease (Matharu et al., 2004). The primary endpoint was headache response at 30 minutes when initial pain was very severe, severe or moderate. Fifty-seven patients were recruited, 46 of whom provided efficacy data on attacks treated with octreotide and 45 on attacks treated with placebo. The headache response rate at 30 minutes was 52% in octeotride-treated attacks compared to 36% in placebo-treated attacks. The data suggest that subcutaneous octreotide 100 μg is effective in the acute treatment of CH when the attacks normally last longer than 45 minutes. However although octreotide was generally well-tolerated, eight of the patients (17%) treated with octreotide reported diarrhoea, abdominal bloating or nausea, compared with four patients (9%) treated with placebo. All adverse effects resolved spontaneously and were generally short-lived and mild in nature.

The rationale for using somatostatin and somatostatin analogues is that they are neuromodulators and neurotransmitters. Somatostatin-containing neurons are found in regions of the central and peripheral nervous system involved in nociception including peripheral sensory fibres, dorsal horn, trigeminal nucleus caudalis, periaqueductal grey matter and hypothalamus. Functional imaging with positron emission tomography (May et al., 1998), structural imaging with voxel-based morphometry (May et al., 1999) and results with deep brain stimulation (Leone et al., 2001; Leone et al., 2005) identify the posterior hypothalamic grey matter as involved CH pathophysiology and strongly suggest it is as the location as the basic defect in CH.

It is interesting that both verapamil and octreotide, which have no vasoconstrictor effect, offer a novel therapeutic approach to the treatment of acute cluster headache. This may suggest insights into understanding the more fundamental aspects of the pathophysiology of this most disabling form of primary headache.

Paroxysmal hemicranias

The treatment of both episodic and chronic paroxysmal hemicrania is entirely preventive as attacks are too short and intense for any acute oral treatment to be effective. Indomethacin is the drug of choice and it must have controlled the symptoms in order to confirm the diagnosis (according to IHS criteria, and not universally agreed upon) (Sjaastad, 1987). The dose should be increased to at least 150 mg per 24 hours or more for 3 to 4 days if there is no response. The beneficial effect is seen within 48 hours (range: a few hours to 5 days) (Pareja and Sjaastad, 1996).

In about 10% of cases indomethacin side-effects occur; the most serious are dyspepsia and gastrointestinal bleeding. Sumatriptan is not effective in chronic paroxysmal hemicrania probably because of the very short duration of the headache (Dahlof, 1993).

Short-lasting, unilateral, neuralgiform headache attacks with conjunctival injection and tearing (SUNCT)

SUNCT is an ultra-short head pain which is remarkably refractory to treatment. Most drugs, including indomethacin, fail to relive the pain. No studies on the acute treatment of SUNCT attacks have been published, again because, like paroxysmal hemicrania, the attacks are too short (15-240 seconds; frequency 3-200 per day).

Recent data suggest that lamotrigine is often effective in preventing or decreasing the attacks and in the absence of more effective treatments, may be considered the current first choice drug (Matharu et al., 2003; D'Andrea and D'Amico, 2005). Matharu et al., reported on four patients with SUNCT in whom intravenous lidocaine (1.3-3.3 mg/kg/h completely suppressed the headaches for the duration of the infusion. However the headaches returned after the cessation of treatment. This treatment is only feasible in the hospital setting in patients with intractable SUNCT, severely distressed by the frequency and severity of their attacks, while appropriate preventive strategies are being implemented (Matharu et al., 2004).

CONCLUSIONS

Cluster and the other TACs are severe, frequent short lived pains that can be treated in diverse ways, from oral and parenteral therapy to surgery and deep brain stimulation. One day there may be even better therapies for the more difficult to treat forms of TACs.

INTRODUCTION TO PREVENTIVE THERAPY FOR CLUSTER AND THE OTHER TACs

Before initiating any preventive treatment in a patient with cluster headache, a number of factors must be evaluated, including the frequency, duration, intensity, the patient's age, lifestyle, and the presence of other medical conditions. Moreover, when dealing with preventive treatment of episodic cluster headache, one must also consider the duration of the ongoing cluster period and whether it may be close to resolving spontaneously, so as not to subject the patient to powerful pharmacological treatment unnecessarily.

Patients with cluster headache are good candidates for preventive therapy when: (1) the attacks are frequent, severe, of rapid onset, or of too short a duration for acute treatment to be effective; (2) acute treatment postpones an attack, but has no effect on the course of the cluster period; (3) acute treatments are likely to be overused; and (4) the cluster period is likely to last for several months.

The aim of prevention is to bring about rapid cessation of the attacks and to maintain an attack-free state with minimal adverse events until the end of the cluster period. The principles of preventive pharmacotherapy are: (1) initiate the treatment as soon as possible after the onset of the cluster period; (2) continue treatment until the patient is attack-free for at least 2 weeks; (3) reduce the dose gradually without stopping the treatment abruptly; and (4) restart the medication at the beginning of the next cluster period. If a severe attack occurs while prevention is ongoing, acute attack treatments such as oxygen, injectable sumatriptan, or other effective triptans, such as zolmitriptan nasal spray, should be used (Rapoport et al., 2007).

The choice of preventive measures may depend on: (1) previous response; (2) previous adverse events and their severity; (3) the presence of contraindications; (4) whether the cluster headache is episodic or chronic; (5) the length of the cluster period by history. In difficult-to-treat cases, a combination of two or more preventive medications may sometimes be necessary.

VERAPAMIL

In recent years, new preventive treatments for cluster headache have been introduced. Verapamil is now considered the first-choice preventive therapy for cluster headache throughout the world; however, it has three important adverse effects: constipation, fluid retention, and sometimes hypotension. Before starting treatment, the patient should have an electrocardiogram to exclude major conduction defects. The first verapamil clinical trial compared the drug at 120 mg three times a day with the established preventive medication, lithium carbonate at 900 mg/day, in chronic cluster headache patients. It was found to have a greater than 75% efficacy in 80% of patients. Verapamil was also more rapidly effective than lithium: 50% of patients on verapamil improved in the first week of treatment compared to 37% on lithium (Bussone et al., 1990). In a clinical trial, verapamil was compared to placebo in 20 patients with episodic cluster headache. Attack frequency and analgesic consumption were significantly reduced after a week of treatment in the verapamil group and further reduced after 2 weeks, while in the placebo group there were no improvements. Adverse events in the verapamil arm were never sufficiently severe to warrant stopping the treatment (Leone et al., 2000). Based on these findings alone, verapamil should be considered the medication of choice in the prevention of both episodic and chronic cluster headache.

LITHIUM

Lithium is a valid alternative to verapamil, particularly for the prevention of chronic cluster headache. Considered the first-choice drug before the advent of verapamil, it is usually prescribed at a dose of 600–900 mg/day. Kidney and thyroid function, as well as lithium blood levels, should be checked when administering lithium so as to avoid polyuria, tremor, vomiting, diarrhea, edema, and the somnolence that appear when lithium blood levels rise above 1.2 mEq/l. The therapeutic effect of lithium in cluster headache is relatively independent of blood levels (Bussone et al., 1979).

PREDNISONE

Prednisone has proven efficacy, particularly in chronic cluster headache, and is useful in selected patients refractory to other treatments (May et al., 2006). Prednisone may also be given along with lithium or verapamil. Prednisone's adverse effects make it contraindicated for prolonged treatment, and it is best used as "bridge therapy" for a 2-week period at the start of a cluster cycle. It can also be given for a short time when chronic cluster attacks become intolerable. A typical starting dose is 50–80 mg/day with the dose tapering over a 2–3-week period.

Intravenous steroids should only be used for cluster headaches that are completely resistant to the medications described above, in patients with multiple daily attacks. Such patients should be hospitalized and carefully monitored during treatment (May et al., 2006). Long-term cortisone may be the only effective therapy in highly drug-resistant forms of chronic cluster headache; in such patients, long-term adverse events may be severe.

In general, chronic cluster headache should be treated with verapamil or lithium, either alone or in combination. Patients resistant to these drugs may benefit from add-on oral prednisone (50–80 mg/day) for 2–3 weeks followed by dose tapering. Another possibility is dexamethasone (8 mg/day for 1 week tapered to 4 mg/day the next week).

METHYSERGIDE

Methysergide is currently not available in US pharmacies after being withdrawn by the manufacturer, Novartis, which took over the company that previously made it, Sandoz. At a dose of 4–6 mg/day, it had been approved for migraine prevention in the US since 1962 but was also effective against episodic cluster headache. In the US, methylergonovine (an active metabolite of methysergide) is used at a dose of 0.6–1.2 mg/day as a substitute for methysergide. It is important to advise patients that this ergot alkaloid (which is not an ergotamine derivative) is structurally related to D-lysergic acid diethylamide (LSD) and should not be administered with other vasoconstrictive agents such as a triptan or other ergot alkaloids.

Rare yet serious complications of long-term use of both methysergide and methylergonovine – as well as other ergot alkaloids – are fibrotic reactions in pleural, pulmonary, retroperitoneal, valvular, aortic, and other tissues. Accordingly, some physicians recommend a monitoring scheme for patients on methysergide or methylergonovine, which includes renal function testing, abdominal ultrasound, chest X-ray, and electrocardiography after the first 4–6 months of treatment (Graham et al., 1966). It has been suggested that a 1-month drug holiday every 6 months on long-term methysergide or methylergonovine could mitigate the potential fibrotic reactions of these drugs.

CLONIDINE

Transdermal clonidine may be useful against chronic cluster headache (D'Andrea et al., 1995). However one study showed that this substance was scarcely effective as prophylaxis for episodic cluster headache (May et al., 2006).

MELATONIN

In a double-blind study melatonin was effective in 5 of 10 episodic cluster headache patients. The rationale for melatonin in cluster headache derives from the observation that nocturnal levels of melatonin are reduced in cluster periods. However, it is unclear whether melatonin acts directly on headache or is effective simply because it improves the quality of sleep; it is currently used almost exclusively as an add-on therapy (Leone et al., 1996).

ANTIEPILEPTICS

Valproate

Valproate has not been extensively investigated as a cluster headache preventive medication, although one study found it is effective in chronic cluster headache (Hering and Kuritzky, 1989). Interestingly, on the basis of this study, valproate was investigated for prevention of migraine in the US, and found to be effective and rapidly approved for this indication by the Food and Drug Administration. New interest in valproate for cluster headache prevention was generated by the observation that, in animal studies, it prevented plasma protein extravasation from the trigeminovascular system - an effect also exerted by sumatriptan and other triptans (May et al., 2006).

Topiramate

A study of 10 patients indicated that topiramate might be useful in cluster headache prevention. To investigate this possibility further a clinical trial was performed on 36 patients with episodic or chronic cluster headache. Results in this ample series did not support the early indications, and in fact the drug was effective in only 33% of patients (Leone et al., 2003). It was concluded that this drug should not be considered a first-choice medication for cluster headache prevention, but that it is useful in some patients.

SURGICAL TREATMENT OF CHRONIC, DRUG-RESISTANT CLUSTER HEADACHE

About 10% of patients with chronic cluster headache do not respond, or have major contraindications, to the preventive treatments mentioned above. Such patients may be candidates for surgical approaches. It is important, however, that any proposed surgery should have demonstrated efficacy in ample numbers of patients. Furthermore, surgery is only indicated in patients who have been shown to be totally unresponsive to all appropriate pharmaceutical treatments. Patient selection for surgical procedures is a difficult task. The physician should have extensive knowledge of and experience with refractory chronic cluster headache, a close professional relationship with the patient, and be prepared to dedicate time to test all possible medications and ascertain they are ineffective. The following criteria for selecting patients for surgery should be adhered to:

- Complete lack of efficacy of, and/or major contraindications to, all appropriate preventive medications for cluster headache
- Chronic headache for some time (at least a year)
- Frequent attacks (daily or almost daily)
- Strictly unilateral headache (no history of side-switch)
- Normal psychological profile
- No medical conditions contraindicating surgery.

Numerous surgical procedures have been used in the past; those involving the trigeminal nerve have generally provided the best results, although corneal damage and anesthesia dolorosa are severe – and not rare – side-effects. Pain is reduced or disappears in about 50% of cases; however, a significant proportion of patients experience a recurrence of pain attacks within a year of the operation. The persistence of the typical ocular pain of cluster headache has been noted even after total eye enucleation, while the onset of the cluster headache condition has been reported in patients who have had an eye removed. These data are further clear indications of the central origin of the pain of cluster headache, and may explain the limited efficacy of surgery directed to peripheral structures.

HYPOTHALAMIC STIMULATION

The discovery, by positron emission tomography (PET), that the hypothalamus is activated during cluster headache provided crucial support for the findings of numerous neuroendocrinological studies and the hypothesis put forth by Lee Kudrow (personal communication) in the 1970s that the hypothalamus is altered in cluster headache. Subsequently voxel-based morphometric analysis of magnetic resonance images showed significantly greater gray-matter density in the inferior posterior hypothalamus in cluster headache patients compared to controls, irrespective of whether or not the patients were in a cluster period. Thus, for the first time, a lesion associated with a primary headache had been identified, and the lesion site immediately suggested itself as a possible target for therapeutic intervention.

The Bussone/Leone group in Milan was the first to propose the use of electrode implant and stimulation to the inferior posterior hypothalamus in patients with severe, intractable chronic cluster headache (Leone et al., 2001). The rationale was that stimulation to this area might inhibit the activation revealed by PET. The technique of deep-brain stimulation is now widely employed to control intractable movement disorders, and experience accumulated over a decade or more has shown it to be safe and associated with few adverse events in cluster headache (Leone et al., 2006). It has the additional advantage of being completely reversible.

This new stereotactic neurosurgical approach was first attempted in a patient with severe daily cluster headache attacks and no significant remission, who had not obtained benefit from any medication for 5 years (Leone et al., 2001). The intervention proved successful in controlling the attacks, and 4 years after bilateral implants there were no significant side-effects. A total of twenty-two hypothalamic implants have now been performed by the Bussone/Leone group on patients with chronic cluster headache, with extremely encouraging results. A smaller number of similar operations have been tried in several countries.

These outcomes show hypothalamic stimulation to be a major new treatment for drug-resistant forms of chronic cluster headache; they also provide insight into the mechanism of the condition, confirming that the central nervous system in general, and the hypothalamus in particular, play a central role in the pathophysiology of cluster headache (Leone et al., 2006). The old term "vasomotor headache"– still unfortunately in use to refer to cluster headaches - should therefore be abandoned.

OCCIPITAL NERVE STIMULATION

Occipital nerve stimulation (ONS) has also shown a certain efficacy in treating drug-resistant, daily, chronic headaches, suggesting a putative therapeutic role also in cluster headaches as well as other primary headaches, through a non-specific mechanism (Popeney and Alo, 2003; Goadsby et al., 2008). In one trial, 5 of 8 operated cluster patients became pain-free or had headache frequency reduced by over 90% (Magis et al., 2007). Overall headache attack frequency in this study was much lower than usually reported in other surgical series, making efficacy comparisons difficult. Only 4 patients in this study had a sufficiently long follow-up (over 1 year) to provide a useful indication as to eventual outcome. It is still up for discussion as to which patients with just one to two attacks per week should undergo invasive surgical procedures (Leone et al., 2007).

In another study on greater occipital nerve stimulation in chronic cluster headache (Burns et al., 2007), only 3 of 8 operated patients improved. Surprisingly, when asked, all patients said they would recommend the operation to others with cluster headache. Factors other than pain relief *per se* might lead patients to express such positive judgments; the discrepancy between their opinions and established headache severity measures suggest the former might not be the most complete way to report on the efficacy of a surgical procedure in primary headaches (Leone et al., 2007).

NOTES ON THE TREATMENT OF OTHER TRIGEMINAL AUTONOMIC CEPHALALGIAS

Cluster headache is a form of trigeminal autonomic cephalalgia (TAC), with short, unilateral head pains associated with cranial autonomic signs. Short-lasting unilateral neuralgiform headache attacks with conjunctival injection and tearing (SUNCT) is another TAC syndrome at one time considered totally resistant to pharmaceutical treatment. However, studies have shown that lamotrigine is effective in some SUNCT patients (D'Andrea et al., 2001).

Functional magnetic resonance imaging studies have revealed that the posterior hypothalamus is activated during SUNCT attacks, just as seen in cluster headache. This finding, together with the close clinical similarities between SUNCT and cluster headache, suggest that hypothalamic stimulation might be useful in some SUNCT cases. The Bussone/Leone group proposed hypothalamic implant and stimulation for a patient with severe intractable SUNCT. The outcome was excellent: after 3 years of follow-up, stimulation remains effective in markedly reducing attacks and is very well tolerated. This clinical response reinforces the hypothesis of crucial hypothalamic involvement in TAC pathophysiology (Leone et al., 2005). Recently 2 other patients suffering from SUNCT were treated with deep-brain stimulation with good results.

CHRONIC PAROXYSMAL HEMICRANIA AND HEMICRANIA CONTINUA

The preventive treatment for paroxysmal hemicrania is indomethacin at a dose of about 150 mg/day, although lower doses may sometimes be effective; higher doses are rarely necessary (May et al., 2006). Hemicrania continua is a somewhat similar condition to paroxysmal hemicrania, although the pain is less severe and more constant on up to half of the head. Therefore it is not technically considered a TAC, although autonomic signs do occur during exacerbations. It, too, is highly responsive to indomethacin therapy.

CLUSTER–TIC SYNDROME

In this syndrome attacks of cluster headache and of trigeminal neuralgia occur in the same patient. Usually the attacks occur at different times but sometimes they occur together. Treatment needs to be specific for each condition (cluster headache and trigeminal neuralgia), even when both occur together (Klimek, 1987).

References

Aghjanin GK, Wang RY (1978). Physiology and pharmacology of central serotoninergic neurons. In: MA Lipton, A Di Mascio, KF Killman (Eds.), Psychopharmacology: A Generation of Progress. Raven, New York, pp. 171–183.

Andersson PG, Jespersen LT (1986). Dihydroergotamine nasal spray in the treatment of attacks of cluster headache. Cephalalgia 6: 51–54.

Bahra A, Gawel MJ, Hardebo JE et al. (2000). Oral Zolmitriptan is effective in the acute treatment of cluster headache. Neurology 54 (5):1832–1839.

Barrè F (1982). Cocaine a san abortive agent in cluster headache. Headache 22: 69–73.

Bigal ME, Tepper SJ (2003). Ergotamine and dihydroergotamine: a review. Curr Pain Headache Rep 7: 55–62.

Boiardi A, Gemma M, Porta E et al. (1986). Calcium entry blocker: treatment in acute pain in Cluster Headache patients. Ital J Neurol Sci 7: 531–534.

Burns B, Watkins L, Goadsby PJ (2007). Treatment of medically intractable cluster headache by occipital nerve stimulation: long-term follow-up of eight patients. Lancet 369: 1099–1106.

Bussone G, Boiardi A, Merati B et al. (1979). Chronic cluster headache: response to lithium treatment. J Neurol 221: 181–185.

Bussone G, Lamperti E, Grazzi L et al. (1987). Uso della Lidocaina nell'attacco acuto di Cluster Headache. Algos 4 (4):52–57.

Bussone G, Leone M, Peccarisi C et al. (1990). Double blind comparison of lithium and verapamil in cluster headache prophylaxis. Headache 30: 411–417.

Buzzi MG, Moskowitz MA (1991). Evidence for 5-HT1B/D receptors mediating the antimigraine effect of sumatriptan and dihydroergotamine. Cephalalgia 11: 165–168.

Cerbo R, Pascali MP, Barbanti P et al. (1999). Cluster headache: management of acute attacks before triptans. Ital J Neurol Sci 20: S63–S65.

Cittadini E, May A, Straube A et al. (2006). Effectiveness of Intranasal Zolmitriptan in Acute Cluster Headache: A Randomized, Placebo-Controlled, Double-blind Crossover Study. Arch Neurol 63 (11): 1537–1542.

D'Alessandro R, Gamberini G, Benassi G et al. (1986). Cluster headache in the Republic of San Marino. Cephalalgia 6: 159–162.

D'Andrea G, D'Amico D (2005). The women with orbital pain and tearing. In: A Purdy, A Rapoport, F Sheftell, SJ Tepper (Eds.), Advanced Therapy of Headache II Edition. BC Decker Inc, pp. 285–289.

Dahlof C (1993). Subcutaneous sumatriptan does not abort attacks of chronic paroxysmal hemicrania (CPH). Headache 33: 201–202.

D'Andrea G, Granella F, Ghiotto N et al. (2001). Lamotrigine in the treatment of SUNCT syndrome. Neurology 57: 1723–1725.

D'Andrea G, Perini F, Granella F et al. (1995). Efficacy of transdermal clonidine in short-term treatment of cluster headache: a pilot study. Cephalalgia 15: 430–433.

Ekbom K (1987). Pathogenesis of cluster headache. In: JN Blau (Ed.), Migraine. Clinical, Therapeutic, Conceptual and Research Aspects. Chapman and Hall, London, pp. 433–448.

Ekbom K, Mastad I, Prusinski A et al. (1993). Subcutaneous sumatriptan in the acute treatment of cluster headache. A dose comparison study. Acta Neurol Scand 88: 63–69.

Friedman AP, Mikropoulos HE (1958). Cluster headache. Neurology 8: 653–663.

Geppetti P, Brocchi A, Caleri D et al. (1985). Somatostatin for cluster headache attack. In: V Pfaffenrath, PO Lundberg, O Sjaastad (Eds.), Updating in Headache. Springer Verlag, Berlin, pp. 302–305.

Goadsby P (1998). A triptan too far? J Neurol Neurosurg Psychiatry 64: 143–147.

Table 37.1

Available neurostimulation studies in intractable chronic cluster headache

Reference	Neurostimulation therapy and site	Mean duration of chronic phase (years)	Mean number of attacks/day presurgery	Mean follow-up (months)	Outcome	Mean effect latency	Recurrence with stimulator off	Adverse effects
Broggi et al., 2007* Leone et al., 2006*	DBS ($n = 16$) Unilateral: 14 Bilateral: 2	3	5–8	23 (range 1–52)	10 patients pain-free 4 patients with sporadic attacks 4 patients requiring prophylaxis	42 days	9 patients switched off: 4: sporadic attacks 5: full-blown attacks after a mean of 2 months	Lead infection Arterial hypotension Diplopia (with voltage increase) Weight loss Electrode replacement Electrode migration Asymptomatic third-ventricle hemorrhage
Schoenen et al., 2005	DBS ($n = 6$) Unilateral	4.5	1–7	14.5 (range 12–17) at present: 34–40)	2 patients pain-free 1 patient with sporadic attacks (<3/month) 1 patient with transient remissions No patient requiring prophylaxis	Within 2 months	In 1 patient, switching off the stimulator followed by attack recurrence after 3 months	Diplopia with voltage increase Dizziness with voltage increase Panic attack in 1 patient: procedure interrupted Massive, fatal intracerebral hemorrhage in 1 patient
Rasche et al., 2008	DBS ($n = 1$) Unilateral	1.17	4–8	–	Marked reduction in attack frequency and intensity; attack stopped when stimulator switched on	Days	Not tested	Diplopia Tachycardia Panic attack
Starr et al., 2007	DBS ($n = 4$) Unilateral	? 19.7	3.64	12	1 patient >50% attack frequency reduction; 1 patient >50% attack intensity reduction All patients with drug prophylaxis	?	Not tested	Peroperative transient ischemic attack Oculomotor disturbances (diplopia, ophthalmoplegia, and skew deviation) Dizziness
Schwedt et al., 2006	ONS ($n = 1$) Unilateral	5	Up to 3/day	?	70% reduction in attack frequency and intensity	?	Not tested	?

(Continued)

Table 37.1

Continued

Reference	Neurostimulation therapy and site	Mean duration of chronic phase (years)	Mean number of attacks/day presurgery	Mean follow-up (months)	Outcome	Mean effect latency	Recurrence with stimulator off	Adverse effects
Schwedt et al., 2007	ONS (n = 3) Unilateral or bilateral	?	?	19 (range 5–42)	30% reduction in headache days 20% reduction in headache intensity	?	Not tested	Lead migration Battery replacement Neck stiffness Pain at battery site Contact dermatitis Pain at lead site Pain at myofascial incision site Lead revision
Magis et al., 2007	ONS (n = 8) Unilateral	5.1	1.91	15.1 (range 3–22)	Mean 79.9% frequency reduction 2 patients pain-free 3 patients ± 90% frequency reduction Mean intensity reduction of 50% Reduction, but no interruption, of preventive drug treatment	Several months; range 2–22	Yes	1 drop-out due to intolerance to stimulation 2 transient attack side-shifts Neck stiffness Battery replacements Pain at battery site Stimulator switch off by external magnetic field
Burns et al., 2007	ONS (n = 8) Bilateral	6	Range 1–8/day	Median: 20 (range 8–27)	2 patients: estimated improvement of 90% and 95% 4 with 25, 40, 60, 20–80% improvement	Several weeks/ months	Yes	First patient with attack side-shift Battery replacements Electrode migrations Scar pain Neck stiffness Muscle recruitment
Narouze and Kapural, 2007	SNS (n = 1) Unilateral	2	2–3	16	Complete remission	2 months	Yes	?
Mauskop, 2005	VNS (n = 2) Left	10	1–10	5–12	Patient 1: marked improvement, MIDAS decrease, but ongoing antidepressant abuse Patient 2: MIDAS decrease, but fentanyl dependence and poor functional level	2 months (patient 1)	Not tested	Neck pain

*The study of the first 2 patients of this cohort was published by Leone et al. in 2001; further patients were included and their follow-up is described in Franzini et al., 2003, Leone et al., 2003, 2004, 2006.

We chose to include the most recent available data in this table.

DBS: deep brain stimulation; ONS: occipital nerve stimulation; SNS: supraorbital nerve stimulation; VNS: vagal nerve stimulation; MIDAS: Migraine Disability Assessment Scale.

Although there is no placebo-controlled trial for DBS, two studies (Schoenen et al., 2005; Leone et al., 2006) reported attack recurrence at varying delays when the stimulator was switched off, suggesting that the clinical effect was probably not due to the natural history of the disorder. This does not rule out, however, a placebo effect which, contrary to common beliefs, may be as important in cluster headache as in migraine (Nilsson Remahl et al., 2003).

The mechanisms of action underpinning the effect of hDBS in iCCH remain obscure. May et al. (2006) performed $H_2^{15}O$ PET in 10 implanted patients from the Italian cohort (Franzini et al., 2003), at a time when 8 were pain-free and 2 had only sporadic attacks. They showed that DBS activated several areas of the pain neuromatrix in addition to the implanted hypothalamic area. In our study, algometric and electrophysiological measurements showed that hDBS decreased pain perception in peripheral limbs, but that it had no lasting effect on pain thresholds or nociceptive reflexes in the trigeminal territory. This suggests that the efficacy of hDBS in iCCH is not due to a simple generalized analgesic effect (Schoenen et al., 2005). We also showed that, after 1 month of hDBS, nitroglycerine, a classical trigger, was unable to provoke an attack in patients who were pain-free. There is also no explanation for the variability in effect latency and time to recurrence after switching off the stimulator; whether this could be related, as suggested (May et al., 2006), to a change in the hypothalamic clock-like function remains to be proven.

OCCIPITAL NERVE STIMULATION

Rationale and first results

Peripheral neurostimulation is a well-known non-destructive and minimally invasive way of controlling drug-resistant pain. Experimental studies have demonstrated that trigeminal and cervical afferents converge on second-order nociceptors in the spinal trigeminal nucleus (Bartsch and Goadsby, 2003). Suboccipital injections of steroids and/or local anesthetics in the region of the greater occipital nerve have shown efficacy in cluster headache (Anthony, 1985; Ambrosini et al., 2005). Finally, there were anecdotal reports of clinical benefit with ONS in various types of intractable headache, including some cluster patients (Matharu et al., 2004; Oh et al., 2004; Schwedt et al., 2007). Against this background systematic studies of ONS in iCCH were undertaken.

Available efficacy studies

Two open-label trials (Burns et al., 2007; Magis et al., 2007) and three case reports (Schwedt et al., 2007) with encouraging results have been published up to now (Table 37.1). In the Burns et al. study (2007), 8 iCCH patients were implanted and efficacy on attack frequency and intensity was assessed according to an estimate of percentage change and subjective satisfaction made by the patients. An improvement was reported by 6 patients, ranging from 20% to 95%. One patient had no change in attack frequency or intensity, but was nonetheless satisfied and willing to recommend the treatment to others. The first patient was implanted unilaterally and improved, after which the attacks shifted side; hence all subsequent patients were implanted bilaterally.

We performed the other large study (Magis et al., 2007) and published findings on 8 iCCH patients prospectively followed at baseline and after implantation using headache diaries. We found a mean 79.9% reduction of attack frequency and 50% of intensity; 2 patients became pain-free and 3 had an improvement of around 90%. Since publication, we have a useful follow-up for another patient and a maximal follow-up of 32 months. The therapeutic score is slightly lower with a mean attack frequency reduction of 54% and intensity decrease of 47%. Our patients were implanted unilaterally on the cluster side and up to now only a transient side-shift of attacks occurred in 2 patients. All of our patients were treated with several preventive medications at high doses before ONS. After ONS all of them were able to reduce preventive medication, but not to interrupt it completely. In the Burns et al. study, only 3 patients were taking prophylactic drugs before ONS; 2 of them continued with implantation of these drugs while 1 stopped because of side-effects. In both studies, the time latency to obtain a significant effect ranged from several weeks to several months.

A few ONS-treated iCCH patients were also reported by Schwedt et al. (2006, 2007). In 1 patient there was a 70% reduction of attack frequency and intensity, with persisting autonomic attacks, whereas in 3 others there was a 33% improvement in headache days and 20% in intensity.

Adverse events

Only mild and reversible side-effects have been reported with ONS. Batteries run flat rather rapidly because of the high stimulations used (range 2.4–10 V in our study). Local discomfort, such as neck stiffness, pain at the myofascial incision or the stimulator sites, was a common adverse effect. ONS-induced paresthesias in the territory of the greater occipital nerve are felt by all patients and may vary in intensity with head and neck position. They are used to assess lead positioning preoperatively if local anesthesia is used

(Burns et al., 2007), and to select or adjust the stimulation parameters. Their disappearance is often the first sign of a flat battery. In our study, 1 patient who had no beneficial effect found the stimulation-induced paresthesias unbearable and decided to switch his stimulator off after 4 months (Magis et al., 2007). If general anesthesia is required for technical reasons, or for the patient's comfort, the surgeon has to rely on anatomical landmarks (Oh et al., 2004; Magis et al., 2007). Hence, close contact of the lead with the greater occipital nerve may be lacking, which probably explains why high stimulation intensities are needed in several patients.

As for hDBS, there are no known prognostic factors for ONS efficacy. In particular, the response to greater occipital nerve blocks with steroids and local anesthetics seems not to be predictive of the therapeutic effect of ONS (Oh et al., 2004; Magis et al., 2007; Schwedt et al., 2007). There is at present no placebo-controlled trial of ONS because blinding of the patients is difficult to achieve due to the paresthesias. An alternative might be to use low voltage stimulations, barely producing paresthesias, as a control. However, the lowest effective stimulation intensity able to produce an effect of ONS has not yet been determined. It is nonetheless unlikely that the clinical improvements of iCCH found with ONS are due to a placebo effect or to the natural evolution of the disease, since in all patients responding to the neurostimulation severe attacks resumed rapidly after cessation of the stimulation due to an empty battery (Oh et al., 2004; Magis et al., 2007).

Mode of action

The neurobiological mechanisms by which ONS can improve iCCH are not known. We found no change in pain thresholds after ONS (Magis et al., 2007), which argues against a direct non-specific analgesic effect. As mentioned above, one rationale for ONS in headaches was the experimental evidence of convergence of cervical and trigeminal nociceptive afferents on second-order nociceptors in trigeminal nucleus caudalis (Bartsch and Goadsby, 2003). The nociception-specific blink reflex, mediated by a polysynaptic network in the medulla, increased with duration of ONS in our study (Magis et al., 2007), which could be due to sensitization in trigeminal nucleus caudalis and is probably not related to the clinical effect of ONS. A more likely explanation for the therapeutic effect of ONS in iCCH is the induction of slow neuromodulatory changes in centers belonging to the pain matrix or playing a pathogenic role in the disorder. For instance, in a functional imaging study of ONS in chronic migraine, activity of an area in the dorsal rostral pons, known to be activated during migraine attacks, was modulated proportionally to the pain, whereas activity in the left pulvinar was correlated with ONS-induced paresthesias (Matharu et al., 2004). Such slow plastic changes might explain why the therapeutic effect after ONS takes some time to appear.

We have undertaken a study of cerebral metabolism with fluorodeoxyglucose PET scanning in iCCH patients before and after implantation, which may disclose in the near future which brain areas are relevant for clinical improvement.

OTHER NEUROSTIMULATION METHODS

Supraorbital nerve stimulation

Narouze and Kapural (2007) recently published the case of a iCCH patient successfully treated with supraorbital nerve stimulation (SNS). After a convincing 7-day trial with a percutaneous quadripolar electrode, the subject received a permanent implant of the lead and attacks fully disappeared after 2 months of continuous stimulation. The patient was still pain-free 12 months later and was able to stop all preventive treatment. Switching off the stimulator led to attack recurrence within 24 h. SNS was also useful for aborting attacks. As for ONS, one hypothesis to explain the effect of SNS is the induction of slow neuromodulatory processes at the level of spinal trigeminal nucleus (Narouze and Kapural, 2007).

Vagus nerve stimulation

Lastly, neurostimulation of the vagus nerve (VNS) with a device similar to the one used to treat refractory epileptic patients may be an interesting option in iCCH. A few case reports presented at meetings suggest that, in epileptics who are also migraineurs, VNS may markedly improve both the epilepsy and the migraine. Mauskop (2005) reported modest improvement in 2 iCCH patients with VNS. In the first patient, who also had major depression, VNS reduced cluster headache attack frequency but he remained depressive and in need of various antidepressant drugs. The second subject had a significant decrease in MIDAS score after VNS, but was dependent on fentanyl patches, with a poor general functional level due to comorbidity with anxiety, fatigue, low-back pain, and depression. The time to obtain an effect in patient 1 was 2 months and neck pain was the only reported side-effect.

In the same study, excellent results were reported in 2 out of 4 chronic migraine patients.

CONCLUSIONS

Various neurostimulation methods offer new hope for distressed patients suffering from intractable chronic headaches and in particular from cluster headache. At present studies are limited to relatively small numbers of patients and placebo-controlled trials are not available, so that the precise positioning of neurostimulation therapy in the armamentarium for intractable chronic headaches has to await further, larger studies.

The most convincing studies performed up to now concern hDBS. Its effect can be spectacular (62.5% painfree rate in Broggi et al.'s (2007) series, 50% in Schoenen et al.'s (2005) trial) and rapid in onset. Minor and manageable adverse effects are due to the stimulation of the hypothalamus and neighboring areas (oculomotor disturbances, dizziness, panic attacks) or to the local tissue irritation at the site of stimulator implantation. Regrettably, as with the implantation of stimulation electrodes in other sites, hemorrhage may occur. Taking into account the 26 published patients treated with hDBS, intracerebral hemorrhage may be more prevalent than for other sites of stimulation, but this remains to be confirmed in larger series. DBS-induced hemorrhage may be minor and paucisymptomatic in most patients. Unfortunately, it was massive and fatal in 1 CCH patient.

By contrast, ONS is a risk-free procedure, but it should be preferred over hDBS only if it has similar or almost similar efficacy. Recent trials of a total of 16 patients show that ONS is an effective treatment for iCCH, but its efficacy seems slightly inferior to that of hDBS. With ONS only 18% of patients became painfree, but overall, 56% had a $\geq$50% reduction in attack frequency. Considering the severe disability of those patients before the implantation, it is of little surprise that 80% of them were satisfied with ONS, even those who had, percentagewise, a more modest improvement. Only minor local adverse effects were reported after ONS. At the present time, ONS could therefore be recommended for iCCH patients before hDBS (Schwedt et al., 2006, 2007; Burns et al., 2007; Magis et al., 2007).

Clearly more studies are needed to evaluate the usefulness of SNS and of VNS.

References

Ambrosini A, Vandenheede M, Rossi P et al. (2005). Suboccipital injection with a mixture of rapid- and long-acting steroids in cluster headache: a double-blind placebo-controlled study. Pain 118: 92–96.

Anthony M (1985). Arrest of attacks of cluster headache by local steroid injection of the occipital nerve. In: F Clifford Rose (Ed.), Migraine: Clinical and Research Advances. Karger, London, pp. 169–173.

Bartsch T, Goadsby PJ (2003). Increased responses in trigeminocervical nociceptive neurons to cervical input after stimulation of the dura mater. Brain 126: 1801–1813.

Broggi G, Franzini A, Leone M et al. (2007). Update on neurosurgical treatment of chronic trigeminal autonomic cephalalgias and atypical facial pain with deep brain stimulation of posterior hypothalamus: results and comments. Neurol Sci 28 (Suppl. 2): S138–S145.

Burns B, Watkins L, Goadsby PJ (2007). Treatment of medically intractable cluster headache by occipital nerve stimulation: long-term follow-up of eight patients. Lancet 369: 1099–1106.

Cruccu G, Aziz TZ, Garcia-Larrea L et al. (2007). EFNS guidelines on neurostimulation therapy for neuropathic pain. Eur J Neurol 14: 952–970.

Franzini A, Ferroli P, Leone M et al. (2003). Stimulation of the posterior hypothalamus for treatment of chronic intractable cluster headaches: first reported series. Neurosurgery 52: 1095–1099.

Goadsby PJ, Schoenen J, Ferrari MD et al. (2006). Towards a definition of intractable headache for use in clinical practice and trials. Cephalalgia 26: 1168–1170.

Headache Classification Subcommittee of the International Headache Society (2004). The international classification of headache disorders, 2nd edition. Cephalalgia 24 (Suppl. 1).

Kupers RC, Svensson P, Jensen TS (2004). Central representation of muscle pain and mechanical hyperesthesia in the orofacial region: a positron emission tomography study. Pain 108: 284–293.

Leone M, Franzini A, Bussone G (2001). Stereotactic stimulation of posterior hypothalamic gray matter in a patient with intractable cluster headache. N Engl J Med 345: 1428–1429.

Leone M, Franzini A, Broggi G et al. (2004). Long-term follow-up of bilateral hypothalamic stimulation for intractable cluster headache. Brain 127: 2259–2264.

Leone M, Franzini A, Broggi G et al. (2006). Hypothalamic stimulation for intractable cluster headache: long-term experience. Neurology 67: 150–152.

Lyons KE, Wilkinson SB, Overman J et al. (2004). Surgical and hardware complications of subthalamic stimulation: a series of 160 procedures. Neurology 63: 612–616.

Magis D, Allena M, Bolla M et al. (2007). Occipital nerve stimulation for drug-resistant chronic cluster headache: a prospective pilot study. Lancet Neurol 6: 314–321.

Matharu MS, Boes CJ, Goadsby PJ (2003). Management of trigeminal autonomic cephalgias and hemicrania continua. Drugs 63: 1637–1677.

Matharu MS, Bartsch T, Ward N et al. (2004). Central neuromodulation in chronic migraine patients with suboccipital stimulators: a PET study. Brain 127: 220–230.

Mauskop A (2005). Vagus nerve stimulation relieves chronic refractory migraine and cluster headaches. Cephalalgia 25: 82–86.

May A (2005). Cluster headache: pathogenesis, diagnosis, and management. Lancet 366: 843–855.

May A, Bahra A, Buchel C et al. (1998). Hypothalamic activation in cluster headache attacks. Lancet 352: 275–278.

May A, Ashburner J, Buchel C et al. (1999). Correlation between structural and functional changes in brain in an idiopathic headache syndrome. Nat Med 5: 836–838.

May A, Leone M, Boecker H et al. (2006). Hypothalamic deep brain stimulation in positron emission tomography. J Neurosci 26: 3589–3593.

Narouze SN, Kapural L (2007). Supraorbital nerve electric stimulation for the treatment of intractable chronic cluster headache: a case report. Headache 47: 1100–1102.

Nilsson Remahl AI, Laudon ME, Cordonnier C et al. (2003). Placebo response in cluster headache trials: a review. Cephalalgia 23: 504–510.

Oh MY, Ortega J, Bellotte JB et al. (2004). Peripheral nerve stimulation for the treatment of occipital neuralgia and transformed migraine using a C1-2-3 subcutaneous paddle style electrode: a technical report. Neuromodulation 7: 103–112.

Petrovic P, Petersson KM, Hansson P et al. (2004). Brainstem involvement in the initial response to pain. Neuroimage 22: 995–1005.

Rasche D, Foethke D, Gliemroth J et al. (2008). [Deep brain stimulation in the posterior hypothalamus for chronic cluster headache Case report and review of the literature.] Schmerz 22 (Suppl. 1): 37–40.

Schoenen J, Di Clemente L, Vandenheede M et al. (2005). Hypothalamic stimulation in chronic cluster headache: a pilot study of efficacy and mode of action. Brain 128: 940–947.

Schwedt TJ, Dodick DW, Trentman TL et al. (2006). Occipital nerve stimulation for chronic cluster headache and hemicrania continua: pain relief and persistence of autonomic features. Cephalalgia 26: 1025–1027.

Schwedt T, Dodick D, Hentz J et al. (2007). Occipital nerve stimulation for chronic headache-long-term safety and efficacy. Cephalalgia 27: 153–157.

Sjaastad O, Bakketeig LS (2003). Cluster headache prevalence. Vaga study of headache epidemiology. Cephalalgia 23: 528–533.

Sprenger T, Boecker H, Tolle TR et al. (2004). Specific hypothalamic activation during a spontaneous cluster headache attack. Neurology 62: 516–517.

Starr PA, Barbaro NM, Raskin NH et al. (2007). Chronic stimulation of the posterior hypothalamic region for cluster headache: technique and 1-year results in four patients. J Neurosurg 106: 999–1005.

Handbook of Clinical Neurology, Vol. 97 (3rd series)
Headache
G. Nappi and M.A. Moskowitz, Editors

Chapter 38

Other primary headaches – general aspects

GIUSEPPE NAPPI [1]* AND GIORGIO SANDRINI [2]

[1] *Chair of Neurology, "Sapienza" University of Rome and IRCSS "C. Mondino Institute of Neurology" Foundation, Pavia, Italy*
[2] *University Center for Adaptive Disorders and Headache (UCADH) and Department of Neurological Sciences, IRCCS "C. Mondino Institute of Neurology" Foundation, Pavia, Italy*

In the second edition of the International Headache Society Classification of Headache Disorders (ICHD-II), Chapter 4 emerges as one of the chapters to have undergone the most profound revision, as indicated by its title, which has been changed from "Primary Miscellaneous Headaches Unassociated with Structural Lesion" to "Other Primary Headaches".

This new chapter has been enriched by the addition of newly identified entities, whose clinical features have been adequately documented in the literature. On the other hand, other forms included in the original "Miscellaneous Primary Headaches" chapter, such as "external compression headache" and "cold stimulus headache", have, in view of their specific pathogenetic mechanisms, been moved to Chapter 13 of the ICHD-II.

The revised Chapter 4 thus includes eight primary headache forms: 4.1 Primary stabbing headache; 4.2 Primary cough headache; 4.3 Primary exertional headache; 4.4 Primary headache associated with sexual activity; 4.5 Primary hypnic headache; 4.6 Primary thunderclap headache; 4.7 Hemicrania continua; 4.8 New daily-persistent headache. The last four of these are the newly identified entities.

The headaches listed in Chapter 4 have, to date, received much less attention than the other three groups of primary headaches (i.e., migraine, tension-type headache, and cluster headache and other trigeminal-autonomic cephalalgias) mainly because, with the exception of primary stabbing headache, they show a low prevalence. However, it is now becoming clear, given the increase in the number of reports that have appeared in the literature in recent years, that these "other primary headaches" are a major issue in neurological practice.

Indeed, severe forms of headache can mimic, especially at their onset, serious forms of symptomatic headache due to organic disease of underlying structures. Intracranial structural lesions or ocular conditions, structural cranial disease at the level of the foramen magnum, subarachnoid haemorrhage, any kind of intracranial space-occupying lesion, arterial dissection, low cerebrospinal fluid pressure or increased intracranial pressure, arterial hypertension, and sleep apnoea must all be ruled out by brain neuroimaging findings and by careful evaluation of the results of other appropriate tests. Differential diagnosis versus secondary headaches is a crucial concern and the ICHD-II subcommittee has been at pains to emphasise and stress this particular aspect, starting with this chapter.

Clearly, since these headaches are clinically heterogeneous, their pathogenesis is still poorly understood; consequently their treatment continues to be guided by anecdotal reports and the results of uncontrolled trials. Most of them seem to be responsive to indomethacin administered preventively in patients in whom certain manoeuvres or actions give rise to the typical pain, although it is only in hemicrania continua that this response can be considered a reliable diagnostic tool.

Finally, some of these "other primary headaches" may occur more frequently in patients suffering from migraine, but the reason for this association is, as yet, unclear.

*Correspondence to: Professor Giuseppe Nappi, Chair of Neurology, "Sapienza" University of Rome and IRCSS "C. Mondino Institute of Neurology" Foundation, Pavia, Italy, E-mail: giuseppe.nappi@mondino.it

grunt, mild expletive, or stereotyped swearing, was an integral part of paroxysms, in about 5% of cases (Sjaastad et al., 2002).

The association between stabs/jabs and migraine may need a special comment. There may be three types of association (Sjaastad et al., 2005):

1. Regular jabs may appear outside or mainly inside a migraine attack, haphazardly, without any particular impact on it.
2. Paroxysms – of regular duration or "prolonged" ones – have been observed regularly to appear in front of migraine ± aura attacks (Raskin and Schwartz, 1980; Dangond and Spierings, 1993; Sjaastad et al., 2005); they may possibly play an "igniting" role.
3. Extremely severe and markedly prolonged paroxysms may appear towards the culmination of severe migraine/migraine-like attacks. These latter attacks are bizarre, with anopsia/autokinesis/undulation ($n = 2$: Sjaastad et al., 2005). The nature of such long-lasting paroxysms (10–120 s) has not been fully clarified.

Precipitating mechanisms

The paroxysms generally occur spontaneously and haphazardly. In exceptional cases (3.4% of cases), paroxysms could be provoked by neck movements, cough, abdominal strain, and touching the hair (Sjaastad et al., 2002). Occasionally, bright light, emotional stress, and postural changes have been reported to trigger attacks (Pareja et al., 1996a).

PSH may concur, synchronously or independently, with other primary headaches, such as migraine (Lansche, 1964; Raskin and Schwartz, 1980; Dangond and Spierings, 1993; Pareja et al., 1996a; Piovesan et al., 2001; Sjaastad et al., 2005; Sjaastad and Bakketeig, 2006) (see above), tension-type headache (Drummond and Lance, 1984), cluster headache (Lance and Anthony, 1971; Ekbom, 1975), chronic paroxysmal hemicrania (CPH) (Sjaastad et al., 1979), short-lasting unilateral neuralgiform headache attacks with conjunctival injection and tearing (SUNCT) syndrome (Pareja and Sjaastad, 1994), cervicogenic headache (Fredriksen et al., 1987), hemicrania continua (Sjaastad and Spierings, 1984), and supraorbital neuralgia (Sjaastad et al., 2004; Pareja and Caminero, 2006). Stabbing paroxysms may also herald the onset of CPH attacks (Sjaastad et al., 1979) or they can occur at the end of cluster headache attacks (Lance and Anthony, 1971). Contrary to what is the case in adults, PSH in the pediatric age is not usually associated with other headaches (Soriani et al., 1996; Fusco et al., 2003).

DIAGNOSIS

Diagnosis is based on the clinical features and the distinction from other similar headaches. There are neither biological markers nor neuroimaging findings, so diagnosis is entirely based upon assessment of the clinical features. The typical spatial and temporal development of the symptoms provides a safe basis for the diagnosis (Table 39.2). The straightforwardness of the PSH diagnosis is also illustrated by the blinded validation of: (1) 100 records in the Vågå study (with 37 PSH+ cases), 100% concurrence; and (2) 41 parishioners, with 18 PSH+ cases, kappa value of 0.841 (Sjaastad et al., 2001).

Since etiology and pathogenesis of PSH are uncertain, it is considered a primary headache. Indeed, in the majority of cases, attacks are not attributable to another disorder. However, similar symptoms as in PSH have been described in some patients with documented intracranial structural lesions or ocular conditions. Thus, PSH may be associated with intracranial structural lesions such as meningioma (Mascellino et al., 2001) and pituitary adenoma (Levy et al., 2003). It has also been associated with onset of cerebrovascular diseases (Pareja et al., 1996a; Piovesan et al., 2002), cranial and ocular trauma, and ophthalmic herpes zoster (Pareja et al., 1996a). A possible association with giant cell arteritis has also been proposed (Raskin and Schwartz, 1980), but this concept has not gained wide acceptance. In this context, it must be emphasized that PSH is ubiquitous and extremely frequent (Sjaastad et al., 2001). Therefore, concurrency of PSH with any other disorder may likely occur just by chance. Additional data, such as complete resolution of stabbing paroxysms after surgical/medical treatment of any structural lesion/disturbance, may be needed to strengthen the presumption of a symptomatic case.

Table 39.2

Diagnostic criteria for primary stabbing headache

A. Head pain occurring as a single stab or a series of stabs and fulfilling criteria B–D
B. Exclusively or predominantly felt in the distribution of the first division of the trigeminal nerve (orbit, temple, and parietal area)
C. Stabs last for up to a few seconds and recur with irregular frequency ranging from one to many per day
D. No accompanying symptoms
E. Not attributed to another disorder

(From Headache Classification Committee of the International Headache Society, 2004.)

Differential diagnosis

With attacks in the neighbourhood of 1 s duration and with a unilateral, mainly anterior localization, one may, in theory, be faced with three primary headache categories: PSH; first branch trigeminal (V1) neuralgia; or SUNCT syndrome (Table 39.3). In the very exceptional case, one may also have to deal with the most short-lasting CPH attacks. The main differential diagnosis will be V1 neuralgia. Stabbing pain occasionally concurs with CPH and SUNCT.

SUNCT and PSH show deviating features: SUNCT is generally confined to an orbital/periorbital location; PSH is characterized by a multidirectional, erratic attack pattern. PSH usually last from 1 s to a few seconds. SUNCT attacks, on the other hand, last 10 s in only 0.6% of cases (Pareja et al., 1996b). This is a decisive point. Moreover, contrary to what is the case in SUNCT, PSH is a female-predominant disorder, with spontaneous attacks, and these are not accompanied by autonomic signs.

V1 neuralgia paroxysms generally last less than 10 s (Sjaastad et al., 1997; Pareja et al., 2005). In V1 neuralgia, attacks always recur within the V1 territory; furthermore, the presence of trigger points and the carbamazepine effect are valuable distinguishing features.

Supraorbital neuralgia (SON), characterized by pain in the territory supplied by the supraorbital nerve, a terminal branch of the V1 nerve, does not usually pose any diagnostic problems. SON is mainly frontal, whereas PSH is mainly temporal. Also the temporal aspects of the symptoms generally differ: chronic-continuous in SON, and sporadic/paroxysmal and shortlasting in PSH. The fact that SON patients may experience superimposed jabs (Sjaastad et al., 2004; Pareja and Caminero, 2006) poses only minor diagnostic difficulties. SON patients show tenderness over the emergence of the nerve (supraorbital notch: Sjaastad et al., 2004) and occasionally over the supraorbital nerve branches. Generally, an absolute but transitory relief follows an anesthetic block of the supraorbital nerve.

Table 39.3

Primary, unilateral, short-lived headache syndromes

Category	Usual duration
Primary stabbing headache	≤1–3 s (or more)
First-division trigeminal neuralgia	1–10 s
SUNCT	10–120 s
Chronic paroxysmal hemicrania	2–30 min
Cluster headache	15–180 min

SUNCT: short-lasting unilateral neuralgiform headache attacks with conjunctival injection and tearing.

PATHOGENESIS

Frequently, unilateral headaches are caused by an ipsilateral disorder. PSH may come into another category: lack of topographic stereotype in PSH may reflect a shifting origin of paroxysms. The paroxysms may possibly be elicited in single fibers of pericranial nerves. In fact, the pain is felt superficially, and the profile of the single attack is spike-like, both features pointing to a peripheral origin of attacks.

Even in peripheral sensory disorders, the origin of the process may be anywhere alongside the sensory unit (from the ganglionic sensory neuron to the distal part of its dendrites/axon), but with a distal production of signs and symptoms. Loss of control from supraspinal sensitive centers may liberate the sensory units, thus producing "sensitive twitches" that could be perceived as stabbing or jabbing pain.

In SON in particular, the fact that superimposed jabs occur in the symptomatic area indeed points to a peripheral origin. The co-localization of PSH with cluster headache/migraine may suggest that all these headaches share a pathogenetic mechanism, possibly a disturbance alongside the trigeminal sensory branches, or it may indicate a more "central" origin.

TREATMENT

Treatment is rarely necessary. Owing to the mildness of the attacks and the benign course, reassurrance suffices in most cases. With frequent attacks, drug therapy may possibly be indicated. In Vågå, however, even those with ≥100 paroxysms per day were not interested in therapy. Indomethacin, 75–150 mg daily, seemed to be of some avail (Mathew, 1981; Pareja et al., 1996a) in that one-third seemed to get complete relief, whereas another third showed a partial response. Celecoxib (Piovesan et al., 2002), nifedipine (Jacome, 2001), melatonin (Rozen, 2003), and gabapentine (França et al., 2004) have been reported as effective in isolated cases/small series of patients.

Finally, we would like to stress the following two points: (1) the extremely erratic pattern of PSH makes the assessment of drug effect highly problematic in most cases; and (2) the potentially ominous aspects of indomethacin therapy make it ethically dubious to use it in a pain condition which is far from being life-threatening.

References

Dangond T, Spierings ELH (1993). Idiopathic stabbing headaches lasting a few seconds. Headache 33: 257–258.

Drummond PD, Lance JW (1984). Neurovascular disturbances in headache patients. Clin Exp Neurol 20: 93–99.

Ekbom K (1975). Some observations on pain in cluster headache. Headache 14: 219–225.

França MC Jr, Costa ALC, Maciel JA Jr (2004). Gabapentine-responsive idiopathic stabbing headache. Cephalalgia 24: 993–996.

Fredriksen TA, Hovdal H, Sjaastad O (1987). "Cervicogenic headache": clinical manifestations. Cephalalgia 7: 147–160.

Fusco C, Pisani F, Faienza C (2003). Idiopathic stabbing headache: clinical characteristics of children and adolescents. Brain Dev 25: 237–240.

Headache Classification Committee of the International Headache Society (1988). The international classification of headache disorders, 1st edition. Cephalalgia 8 (Suppl. 7): 1–96.

Headache Classification Subcommittee of the International Headache Society (2004). The international classification of headache disorders, 2nd edition. Cephalalgia 24 (Suppl. 1): 9–160.

Jacome DE (2001). Exploding head syndrome and idiopathic stabbing headache relieved by nifedipine. Cephalalgia 21: 617–618.

Klee A (1968). A clinical study of migraine with particular reference to the most severe cases. Thesis. Munksgaard, Copenhagen.

Lance JW, Anthony M (1971). Migrainous neuralgia or cluster headache? J Neurol Sci 13: 401–414.

Lansche RK (1964). Ophthalmodynia periodica. Headache 4: 247–249.

Levy MJ, Matharu MS, Goadsby PJ (2003). Prolactinomas, dopamine agonists and headache: two case reports. Eur J Neurol 10: 169–171.

Martins IP, Parreira E, Costa I (1995). Extratrigeminal icepick status. Headache 35: 107–110.

Mascellino AM, Lay CL, Newman LC (2001). Stabbing headache as the presenting manifestation of intracranial meningioma: a report of two patients. Headache 41: 599–601.

Mathew NT (1981). Indomethacin responsive headache syndromes. Headache 21: 147–150.

Monteiro JM (1995). Cefaleias. Estudio epidemiologico e clinico de uma população urbana. Thesis. Porto.

Pareja JA, Caminero AB (2006). Supraorbital neuralgia. Curr Pain Headache Rep 10: 302–305.

Pareja JA, Sjaastad O (1994). SUNCT syndrome in the female. Headache 34: 217–220.

Pareja JA, Ruiz J, de Isla C et al. (1996a). Idiopathic stabbing headache (jabs and jolts syndrome). Cephalalgia 16: 93–96.

Pareja JA, Shen JM, Kruszewski P et al. (1996b). SUNCT syndrome. Duration, frequency and temporal distribution of attacks. Headache 36: 161–165.

Pareja JA, Kruszewski P, Caminero AB (1999). SUNCT syndrome versus idiopathic stabbing headache (jabs and jolts syndrome). Cephalalgia 19 (Suppl. 25): 46–48.

Pareja JA, Cuadrado ML, Caminero AB et al. (2005). Duration of attacks of first division trigeminal neuralgia. Cephalalgia 25: 305–308.

Piovesan EJ, Kowacs P, Lange M et al. (2001). Prevalencia e caracteristicas de cefaleia idiopatica em punhaladas em uma população de migranoses. Arq Neuropsychiatr 59: 201–225.

Piovesan EJ, Zuckerman E, Kowacs PA et al. (2002). COX-2 inhibitor for the treatment of idiopathic stabbing headache secondary to cerebrovascular diseases. Cephalalgia 22: 197–200.

Raskin NH, Schwartz RK (1980). Icepick-like pain. Neurology 3: 203–205.

Rasmussen BK (1994). Epidemiology of headache. Thesis. Kobenhavns Universitet, Copenhagen.

Rozen TD (2003). Melatonin as treatment for idiopathic stabbing headache. Neurology 61: 865–866.

Sjaastad O, Bakketeig LS (2006). Migraine with aura: visual disturbances and interrelationship with the pain phase. J Headache Pain 7: 127–135.

Sjaastad O, Spierings E (1984). "Hemicrania continua": another headache absolutely responsive to indomethacin. Cephalalgia 4: 65–70.

Sjaastad O, Egge K, Horven I et al. (1979). Chronic paroxysmal hemicrania. Mechanical precipitation of attacks. Headache 19: 31–36.

Sjaastad O, Pareja JA, Zuckerman E et al. (1997). Trigeminal neuralgia. Clinical manifestations of 1. Branch involvement. Headache 37: 346–357.

Sjaastad O, Pettersen H, Bakketeig LS (2001). The Vågå study; epidemiology of headache I: The prevalence of ultrashort paroxysms. Cepahalalgia 21: 207–215.

Sjaastad O, Pettersen H, Bakketeig LS (2002). The Vågå study of headache epidemiology II. Jabs: clinical manifestations. Acta Neurol Scand 105: 25–31.

Sjaastad O, Pettersen H, Bakketeig LS (2003). Extracephalic jabs/idiopathic stabs. Vågå study of headache epidemiology. Cephalalgia 23: 50–54.

Sjaastad O, Petersen HC, Bakketeig LS (2004). Supraorbital neuralgia. Vågå study of headache epidemiology. Cephalalgia 25: 296–304.

Sjaastad O, Pettersen H, Bakketeig LS (2005). Long-lasting cephalic jabs (?). The Vågå study of headache epidemiology. Cephalalgia 25: 581–592.

Soriani S, Battistella PA, Arnaldi C et al. (1996). Juvenile idiopathic stabbing headache. Headache 36: 565–567.

Vieira JP, Salgueiro AB, Alfaro M (2006). Short-lasting headaches in children. Cephalalgia 26: 1220–1224.

Zacaria A, Graber M, Davis P (2000). Idiopathic stabbing headache associated with monocular vision loss. Arch Neurol 57: 745–746.

Handbook of Clinical Neurology, Vol. 97 (3rd series)
Headache
G. Nappi and M.A. Moskowitz, Editors

Chapter 40

Primary cough headache, primary exertional headache, and primary headache associated with sexual activity

JULIO PASCUAL,[1]* ANDRÉS GONZÁLEZ-MANDLY,[2] AGUSTÍN OTERINO,[3] AND RUBÉN MARTÍN[4]
[1]*Service of Neurology, University Hospital "Central de Asturias", Oviedo, Spain*
[2]*Neuroradiology Section, University Hospital Marqués de Valdecilla, Santander, Spain*
[3]*Service of Neurology, University Hospital Marqués de Valdecilla, Santander, Spain*
[4]*Neurosurgery Service, University Hospital Marqués de Valdecilla, Santander, Spain*

Activity-related headaches can be brought on by Valsalva maneuvers ("cough headache"), prolonged exercise ("exertional headache"), and sexual excitation ("orgasmic headache"). These entities are a challenging diagnostic problem as they can be primary or secondary and as their etiologies differ depending on the headache type. Until recently, cough headache was included in the broader context of exercise-induced headache, but clinical features of cough headache are clearly different from those of exertional and sexual headache, which do have many properties in common (Silbert et al., 1991).

In 1932, Tinel presented several patients with intermittent, paroxysmal headaches following exertion and maneuvers that increased intrathoracic pressure. Later, Symonds (1956) called the disorder "cough headache" and demonstrated that it may be a benign syndrome without demonstrable cause. Before this report, cough and exertional headaches were always considered ominous symptoms, and there was no clear recognition that benign types of these headache existed. The first large series published on exertional headache or head pain related to exertion came from the Mayo Clinic. This paper, however, still combined all exercise-induced headache, which contributed to the lack of differentiation among these provoked subtypes and included the following statement: "in every patient with this complaint, an intracranial lesion of potentially serious nature, such as a brain tumor, aneurysm, or vascular anomaly, has been suspected; and even when no such lesion could be identified, an uneasy uncertainty usually remained" (Rooke, 1968). It was not until modern neuroimaging techniques became available that these activity-related headaches were clinically differentiated.

PRIMARY COUGH HEADACHE

In the latest International Headache Society (IHS) classification, primary cough headache is included within "other primary headaches" and defined as that headache precipitated by coughing or straining in the absence of any intracranial disorder (Headache Classification Subcommittee of the International Headache Society, 2004). IHS diagnostic criteria appear in Table 40.1.

Epidemiology

Cough headache is considered a rare entity. In a wide (1838 participants) epidemiological survey in Norway, however, 12.3% referred to "exertional" headache (Sjaastad and Bakketeig, 2003). Rasmussen and Olesen (1992) have shown that the lifetime prevalence of cough headache is 1% (95% confidence interval 0–2%). Over 15 years, of the 3498 patients attending our neurology department due to headache, 20 (0.6%) consulted because of cough headache (Pascual et al., 1995, 2008).

Etiology

Cough headache can be either a primary benign condition or secondary to structural cranial disease. From older case series (prior to computed tomography (CT) and magnetic resonance imaging (MRI)) it was

*Correspondence to: Dr. Julio Pascual, Director, Area of Clinical Neuroscience, Service of Neurology, University Hospital "Central de Asturias", Oviedo, Spain, E-mail: juliopascual@telefonica.net

Table 40.1

Diagnostic criteria for primary cough headache

A.	Headache fulfilling criteria B and C
B.	Sudden onset, lasting from 1 s to 30 min
C.	Brought on by and occurring in association with coughing, straining, and/or Valsalva maneuver

concluded that about 20% of patients with cough headache had structural lesions, most of them a Chiari type I deformity (Symonds, 1956; Rooke, 1968; Nick, 1980; Sands et al., 1991). However, with modern neuroradiological techniques, it is clear that almost half of cough headache patients have symptomatic cough headache due to tonsillar descent or, more rarely, to other space-occupying lesions in the posterior fossa/foramen magnum area (Pascual et al., 1996). Around 30% of patients with Chiari type I malformation experience headache aggravated by Valsalva maneuvers, mainly cough (Pascual et al., 1992) (Figure 40.1). In summary, it can be concluded that about 50% of patients with cough headache will show no demonstrable etiology, while the other half will be secondary to structural lesions, mostly at the foramen magnum level (Pascual et al., 1996, 2008; Pascual, 2005).

Pathophysiology

The pathophysiology of secondary cough headache is reasonably well understood. This headache seems to be secondary to a temporary impact of the cerebellar tonsils below the foramen magnum (Tinel, 1932; Williams, 1976, 1980; Nightingale and Williams, 1987; Sansur et al., 2003). In 2 patients with cough headache and tonsillar herniation, Williams demonstrated a pressure difference between the ventricle and the lumbar subarachnoid space during coughing (Williams, 1976). The pressure difference, named craniospinal pressure dissociation, displaced the cerebellar tonsils into the foramen magnum. Williams also observed that the headache disappeared after decompressive craniectomy. Subsequently, Nightingale and Williams (1987) described 4 more patients who had headache due to episodic impact of the cerebellar tonsils in the foramen magnum after abrupt Valsalva maneuvers. In our series, not only was it demonstrated that tonsillar descent is the actual cause of cough headache, but it was also shown that the presence of cough headache in Chiari type I patients correlated only with the degree of tonsillar descent (Pascual et al., 1992, 1996).

Clear alterations in posterior fossa cerebrospinal dynamics in symptomatic patients with Chiari type I with abnormal pulsatile motion of the cerebellar tonsils

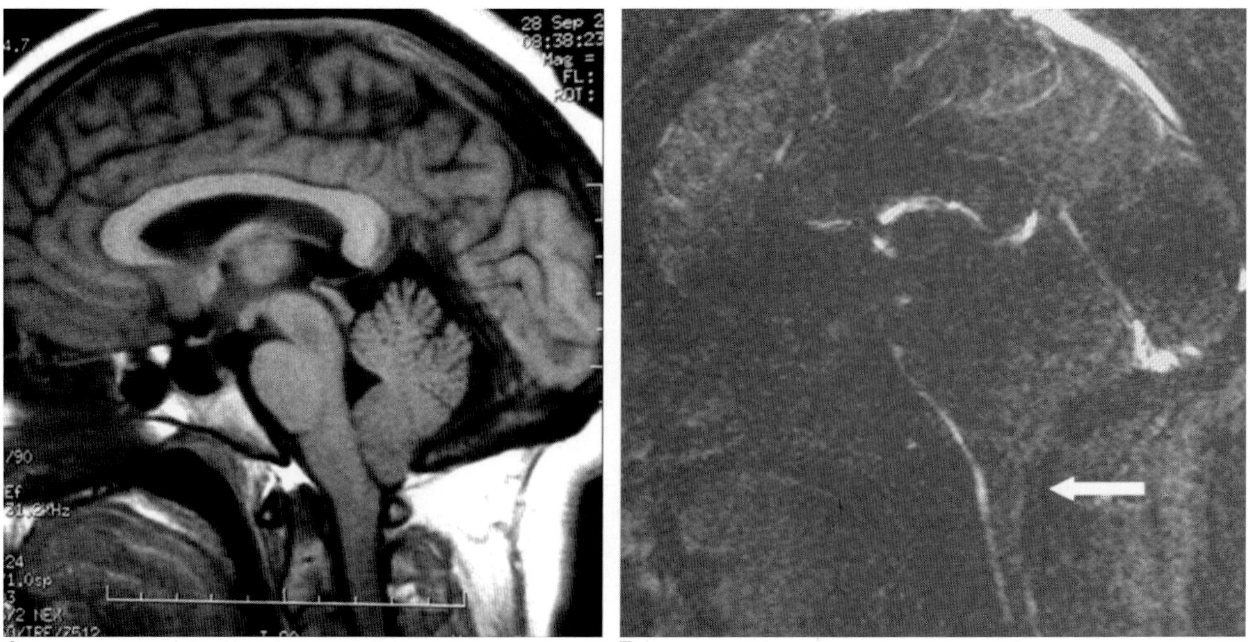

A B

Fig. 40.1. (A) Magnetic resonance imaging (MRI) of a 33-year-old female with Chiari type I presenting as cough headache. (B) Sagittal cine phase-contrast MRI showing difficulties in cerebrospinal fluid circulation posteriorly in the foramen magnum region (arrow).

have been described (Pujol et al., 1995; Quigley et al., 2004) (Figure 40.1). This movement produced a selective obstruction of the cerebrospinal fluid flow from the cranial cavity to the spine. The amplitude of the tonsillar pulsation and the severity of the arachnoid space reduction were associated with cough headache (Quigley et al., 2004). All these data confirm that symptomatic cough headache is secondary to Chiari type I deformity and that this pain is due to compression or traction of the caudally displaced cerebellar tonsils on pain-sensitive dura and other anchoring structures around the foramen magnum innervated by the first cervical roots.

The pathophysiology of primary cough headache is not known. The possibility of a sudden increase in venous pressure being sufficient in itself to cause headache due to an increase in brain volume has been proposed (Wang et al., 2000). There should be other contributing factors, however, such as a hypersensitivity of some receptors, sensitive to pressure, hypothetically localized on the venous vessels (Raskin, 1995). One of the potential etiologies for this transient receptor sensitization could be a hidden or previous infection. Finally, Chen and co-workers (2004b) have found that patients with primary cough headache are associated with a more crowded posterior cranial fossa, which may be a further contributing factor for the pathogenesis of this headache syndrome.

Clinical manifestations

Primary cough headache is defined as that head pain precipitated by coughing or other Valsalva maneuvers in the absence of any intracranial disorder. According the IHS diagnostic criteria, primary cough headache is a sudden-onset headache lasting from 1 s to 30 min, brought on by and occurring only in association with coughing, straining, and/or Valsalva maneuvers.

The clinical picture of primary cough headache is very characteristic, which allows its differentiation from secondary cases (Sands et al., 1991; Pascual et al., 1996, 2008; Boes et al., 2002; Pascual, 2005, 2009). Primary cough headache does not begin earlier than 40 years; its mean age of onset in the modern series is 67 years (range 44–81 years). Some 80% of patients suffering from primary cough headache have been shown to be males, even though, as also seems to be happening in other male-predominant headaches such as cluster headache, this male predominance is not dramatic in the patients seen by us in the last decade. Primary cough headache is an episodic disease, ranging from 2 months to a maximum of 2 years in our experience. The pain begins immediately or within seconds of the precipitants. Such precipitants include coughing, sneezing, nose blowing, laughing, crying, singing, lifting a weight, straining at stool, and stooping. Sustained physical exercise is not a precipitating factor for primary cough headache, which is moderate to severe in intensity, with a sharp, stabbing, splitting, or even explosive quality. Most patients have bilateral headaches all the time. The pain is usually maximal in the occipital region, but also in the frontal or temporal region or at the vertex. This headache typically lasts a few seconds or several minutes. In some patients, a dull, aching pain follows the paroxysm for several hours (Diamond, 1982). Primary cough headache is not associated with other clinical manifestations, not even nausea or vomiting, and responds to indomethacin (Pascual et al., 1996).

Differential diagnosis

Cough headache can be either a primary benign condition or secondary to structural cranial disease. By definition, primary cough headache can only be diagnosed if neuroimaging studies are normal. From the old series, before CT and MRI were available, it was concluded that only around 20% of patients with cough headache had structural lesions, most of them a Chiari type I deformity (Symonds, 1956; Rooke, 1968; Sands et al., 1991) (Figure 40.1). Half of cough headache patients initially studied with neuroradiological techniques such as CT scan and/or metrizamide myelography, however, were shown to have symptomatic cough headache due to tonsillar descent or, very rarely, to other space-occupying lesions in the posterior fossa/foramen magnum area (Pascual et al., 1992, 1996).

Our recent experience after the generalized availability of MRI in 50 new cases of cough headache indicates that only one-third are in fact primary cases. Within secondary cough headaches almost 90% are due to tonsillar descent, while the remaining cases are due to other structural, space-occupying posterior fossa lesions. Therefore, the presence of a Chiari type I malformation or any other lesion causing obstruction of cerebrospinal fluid pathways or displacing cerebral structures must be excluded before cough headache is assumed to be benign.

Around 30% of patients with Chiari type I malformation experience headache aggravated by Valsalva maneuvers, mainly cough. Cough headache may be the only clinical manifestation of Chiari type I malformation for several years in about one-fifth of symptomatic patients (Pascual et al., 1992). In our experience, however, most, if not all, patients with symptomatic cough headache finally develop posterior fossa symptoms or signs, mainly dizziness/vertigo,

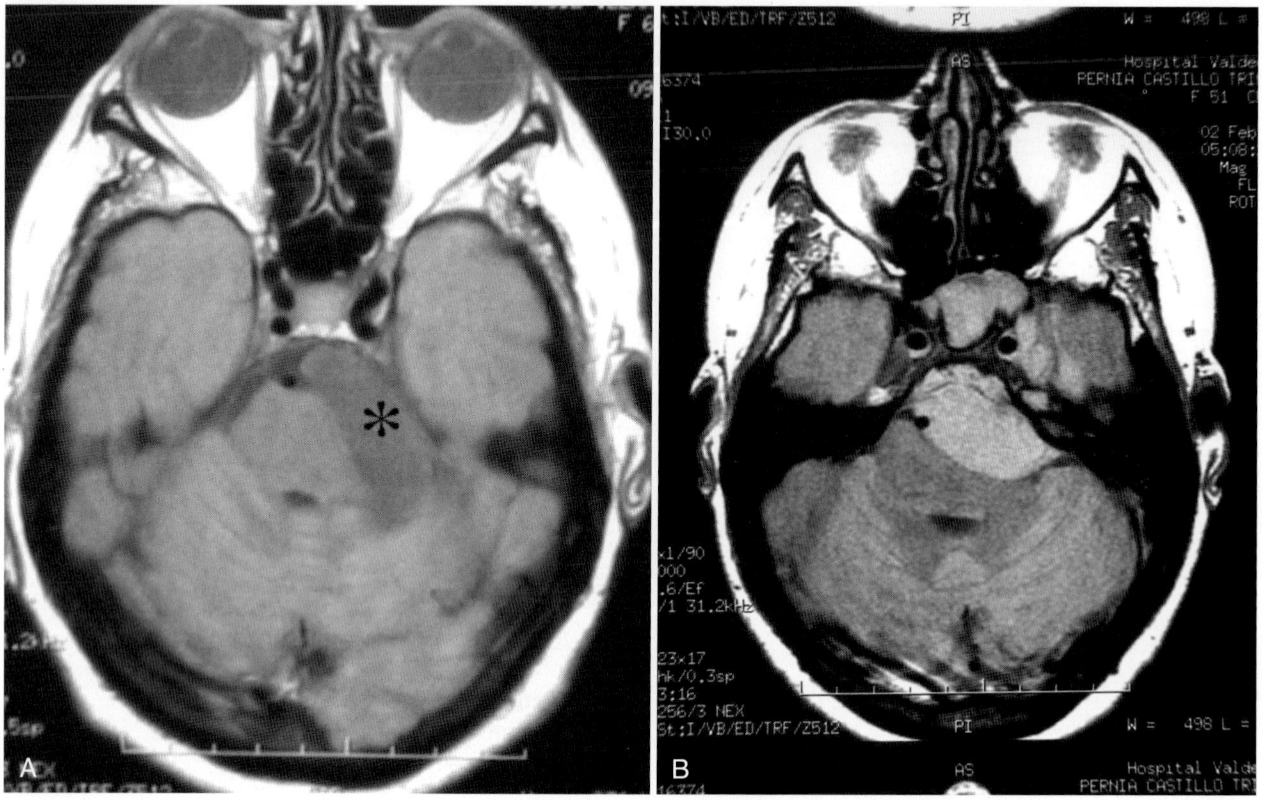

Fig. 40.2. Magnetic resonance imaging scans of 2 patients presenting with cough headache showing posterior fossa dermoid tumor (A) and meningioma (B).

unsteadiness, and syncopes. Symptomatic cough headache begins three decades earlier, on average, than primary cough headache, and does not show a clear male predominance or respond to indomethacin (Pascual et al., 1996) (Figure 40.2).

There are several clinical clues which can be of great help for the etiological diagnosis of cough headache. As compared with primary cough headache, secondary cough headache begins earlier (average 40 versus 60 years old), is located in the occipital region, lasts longer (5 years versus 11 months), is associated with posterior fossa symptoms/signs, and does not respond to indomethacin (Pascual et al., 2008).

Differential diagnosis with primary exertional headache is easy already on clinical grounds as this headache is not brought on by Valsalva maneuvers but by prolonged physical exercise. In addition, and in contrast to primary cough headache, primary exertional headache is typical of young people (range 10–48 years in our series) and contains a lot of migrainous characteristics. The same is true in general for primary sexual headache, which shares a lot of properties with exertional headache (Pascual et al., 1996). As sexual intercourse is a prolonged exercise also with Valsalva maneuvers, orgasm can also be seen as a precipitant factor for "cough" headache in a few patients (Evans and Pascual, 2000).

Migraine, cluster headache, postlumbar puncture headache, and idiopathic intracranial hypertension can be aggravated, but not elicited, by cough (Figure 40.3). Recently, we have seen a few cases of patients with low-pressure headache complaining of both orthostatic and cough headaches. In these patients, a transient pseudo-Chiari due to brain sagging could be clearly seen in the MRI study. Given the differential diagnosis outlined above, every patient with cough headache should have MRI of the brain to rule out a posterior fossa lesion. In spite of scattered reports, there is not enough scientific background to support unruptured aneurysms (Smith and Messing, 1993), carotid stenosis (Britton and Guiloff, 1988; Rivera et al., 1991), or vertebrobasilar disease (Satikov and Mattle, 1978) as specific causes of cough headache. Therefore, an MR angiography (MRA) study is not mandatory in these patients.

Treatment

Acute treatment is impractical because of the short duration and multiplicity of cough headaches. Potential precipitants, for instance lung infections or

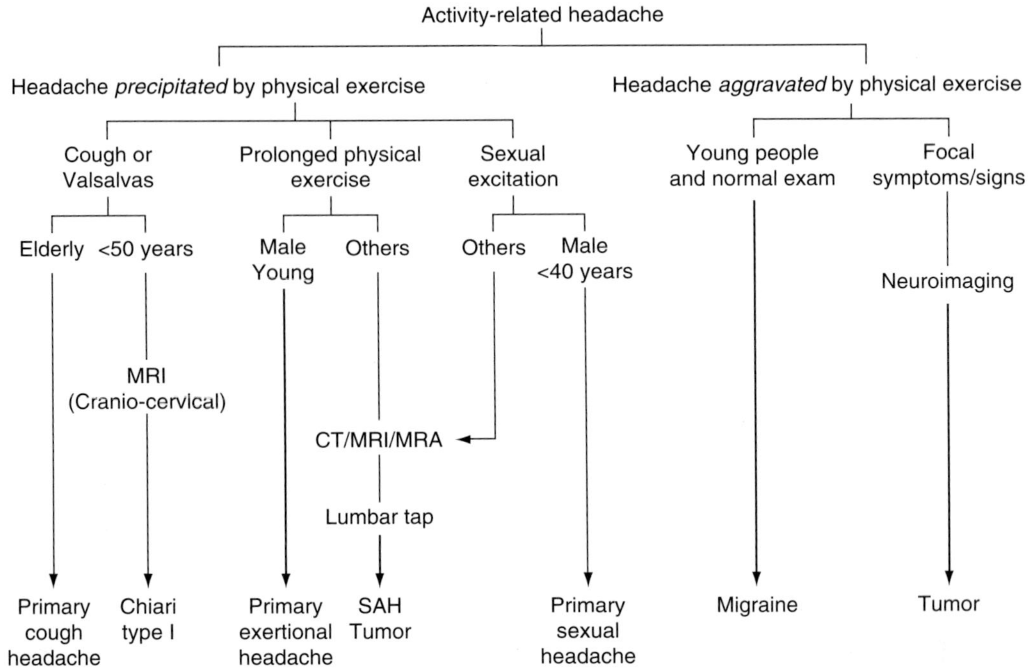

Fig. 40.3. Activity-related headache differential diagnosis. MRI: magnetic resonance imaging; CT, computed tomography; MRA, magnetic resonance angiography; SAH: subarachnoid hemorrhage. (Modified from Pascual, 2009.)

cough-inducing medications, must be treated or withdrawn. Primary cough headache responds to indomethacin, given prophylactically at doses usually ranging from 25 to 150 mg daily (Diamond and Medina, 1979; Mathew, 1981). The mechanism of action of this drug is unknown, but could include a decrease in intracranial pressure (Slavik and Rhoney, 1999). This would explain the benefits seen with lumbar puncture or acetazolamide in some patients with primary cough headache (Raskin, 1995; Chalaupka, 2000; Wang et al., 2000).

Patients with symptomatic cough headache do not consistently respond to any known pharmacological treatment, including indomethacin, and need specific surgical treatment. It has been shown that suboccipital craniectomy has relieved cough headache in Chiari type I malformation patients (Pascual et al., 1992, 1996, 2008).

PRIMARY EXERTIONAL HEADACHE

Exertional headache is precipitated by any form of prolonged exercise. Subforms such as "weightlifter's headache" are recognized. IHS diagnostic criteria for this entity appear in Table 40.2.

Epidemiology

Rasmussen and Olesen (1992) have assessed the lifetime prevalences of headache disorders in a cross-sectional epidemiologic survey of a representative 25–64-year-old general population. They found a lifetime prevalence of 1% for benign exertional headache. Judging from the number of cases of cough headache in the literature, the problem is probably an unusual one (Chakravarty, 2006). A survey, however, of 165 patients studied because of cough revealed that 19.3% had cough headache (Ozge et al., 2005). In a wide (1838 participants) epidemiological survey in Norway, 12.3% referred to exertional headache (Sjaastad and Bakketeig, 2002, 2003), while, in a further survey in Taiwan carried out in 1963 adolescents, the prevalence of exertional headache was as high as 30.4% (Chen et al., 2009). Benign exertional headache appears to be more frequent in men (Symonds, 1956; Rooke, 1968). Although benign cough headache characteristically begins after the fifth decade of life, benign exertional and sexual headaches are typical of young people (Pascual et al., 1996, 2008).

Pathophysiology

The pathophysiology of primary exertional headache remains speculative. The development of headache after sustained exertion, particularly after a hot day, is more likely caused by arterial dilation, but objective evidence is lacking. The etiology of benign exertional headache is presumed to be related to cerebral vasodilation, both extracranial and intracranial in nature. In these patients, cerebral blood flow velocity increases

Table 40.2

Diagnostic criteria for primary exertional headache

A. Pulsating headache fulfilling criteria B and C
B. Lasting from 5 min to 8 h
C. Brought on by and occurring only during or after physical exertion

and the pulsatility index decreases as compared with controls (Evers et al., 2003). Exertional headache in this respect may resemble headaches associated with high altitude and fever. Of interest, hexamethylpropylene amine oxime single-photon emission CT of a young man with exertional headache revealed transient hypoperfusion in the frontal lobes bilaterally (Basoglu et al., 1996). Since patients with primary exertional headache show an increased frequency of both migraine and orgasmic headache, they could also share some pathophysiological mechanisms (Silbert et al., 1991; Frese et al., 2003b). The acute onset of headache with straining and breath-holding, as in weight lifter's headache, is most likely explained by acute venous distension similar to what happens in cough headache (Lance, 1991).

Two recent reports have suggested that, in some patients, primary exertional headache could in fact be a venous disease. First, exertional headache disappeared in a young woman with bilateral transverse sinus stenosis after local venous stenting was carried out. Second, the prevalence of jugular valve incompetence (leading to transient increased intracranial pressure during exertion) has been shown to be much higher (70%) in patients with primary exertional headache when compared to controls (20%), which suggests that intracranial venous congestion caused by retrograde jugular venous flow may play a role in the pathophysiology of this condition, at least in some patients (Doepp et al., 2007; Donnet et al., 2008).

Clinical features

In contrast to primary cough headache, primary exertional headache is typical of young people (range 10–48 years in our series). As occurs with primary cough headache, primary exertional headache is more common in males. The majority of cases occur in patients who have a personal and/or family history of migraine (Pascual et al., 1996). Primary exertional headache occurs in both untrained people and trained athletes. Heat, humidity, barometric changes, high altitude, caffeine, hypoglycemia, and alcohol usage have been described as contributing factors (Dalessio, 1974). This headache may be triggered by any kind of prolonged physical exercise (Dalessio, 1974; Paulson, 1983; Indo and Takahashi, 1990), or at least exercise sufficient to double the resting pulse for over 10 s, but ordinarily for minutes or even hours. Headache usually occurs at the peak of the exercise and subsides when the activity ceases, even though on some occasions headache can last up to 2 days. Exertional headache is described as aching, pounding, or throbbing and has many migraine characteristics, with associated nausea, vomiting, and photophobia and some phonophobia. It may be bilateral (about 60% of cases) or unilateral (Pascual et al., 1996).

Differential diagnosis

Even in the presence of a typical clinical picture, the diagnosis of primary exertional headache can only be made after a thorough investigation. For typical patients (middle-aged men with normal exam), it is mandatory to exclude any kind of intracranial space-occupying lesion and sentinel hemorrhage due to vascular malformations (Pascual et al., 1996). Very rarely, exertional headache is a symptom of middle cerebral artery dissection or pheochromocytoma (Paulson, 1983). Nowadays, MRI followed by MRA should be the screening procedure. In doubtful cases, a lumbar tap could also be considered (Figure 40.3). A number of papers have documented exertional (Lefkowitz and Biller, 1982; Fleetcroft and Maddocks, 1985; Blacky et al., 1987; Bowen and Oppenheimer, 1993; Vernay et al., 1993; Lipton et al., 1997; Lance and Lambros, 1998; Chen et al., 2004a; Sathirapanya, 2004), and recently non-exertional (Gutiérrez-Morlote and Pascual, 2002), vascular headaches as the presenting symptoms of cardiac ischemia ("cardiac cephalalgia"). In these rare cases, cardiac enzymes and electrocardiography are indicated. The 34 patients with cardiac cephalalgia reported in the literature from 1966 to the present have been reviewed recently (Wei and Wang, 2008).

Management

For non-incapacitating cases or for those with a low exercise frequency, the first, and sometimes the only, recommendation should be transient exercise moderation or abstinence. Lambert and Burnet (1985) described how a prescribed warm-up period prevented swimmer's headache. Leaving exercise abstinence aside, there is no absolute evidence of the value of pharmacological treatments in the management of primary exertional headache. In general, however, migraine-preventive medications show some benefit. For most patients, beta-blockers at the usual antimigraine doses seem useful (Pascual et al., 1996; Evans and Pascual, 2000). There are well-documented cases of patients with exertional headache who did not improve or could not tolerate beta-blockers. Some of these patients seem to improve on indomethacin in doses varying from 25 to 150 mg a day (Diamond, 1982). There is no consensus on the treatment duration in these cases. Primary exertional headache is usually transient, lasting less than 3 months and rarely longer than 6 months. Therefore, we recommend stopping the preventive treatment after 3–6 months to check for headache recurrence.

Acute therapy, immediately before physical exercise, may be a reasonable alternative for some patients. Simple analgesics and non-steroidal anti-inflammatory drugs (NSAIDs) do not seem to prevent the development of exertional headaches. Ergotamine may be useful and triptans could theoretically be an alternative treatment to ergotamine, but, again, there is no scientific evidence to support the use of triptans in the acute or pre-emptive treatment of exertional headache (Evans and Pascual, 2000).

PRIMARY HEADACHES ASSOCIATED WITH SEXUAL ACTIVITY

Headaches may occur during sexual activities associated with intercourse or independent of intercourse (e.g., masturbation) or orgasm. Classically three types of sexual headache have been described. The so-called type 1, preorgasmic or dull type, resembles muscle contraction headache, whereas postural sexual headache is a low-cerebrospinal-fluid pressure-type headache resulting from a tear of the dura during sexual intercourse (Evans and Pascual, 2000; Mokri, 2002; Frese et al., 2003a). The most common is the type 2 explosive type, now called orgasmic headache. Its current IHS diagnostic criteria appear in Table 40.3. The third type, postural sexual headache, is very rare and must be regarded as a symptomatic headache and does not appear in the revised IHS classification. In 1986, Johns reviewed 110 published patients (24% dull type, 69% explosive type, and 7% postural type). Most subsequent publications have concerned the explosive type.

Table 40.3

Diagnostic criteria for headache attributed to sexual activity

Preorgasmic headache

A. Dull ache in the head and neck associated with awareness of neck and/or jaw muscle contraction fulfilling criterion B

B. Occurs during sexual activity and increases with sexual excitement

Orgasmic headache

A. Sudden severe ("explosive") headache fulfilling criterion B

B. Occurs at orgasm

Epidemiology

The prevalence of sexual headache is unknown. In the only population-based epidemiological study, the lifetime prevalence was 1% with a broad confidence interval and similar to that of primary cough and exertional headaches (Rasmussen and Olesen, 1992). The prevalence of this headache may be underestimated, since patients often feel embarrassed about reporting it. In terms of consultation in headache clinics, it accounts for 0.2–1.3% of all headache patients (Pascual et al., 1995; Frese et al., 2003a).

Pathophysiology

As a result of its semiology, the dull type has been related to muscle contraction or tension-type headache. The pathophysiology of primary orgasmic headache remains speculative. There is no evidence that this headache is primarily genetic, although a family with 4 affected sisters has been published (Johns, 1986). Vasospasm and impairment of cerebrovascular autoregulation have been proposed as pathophysiological explanations (Heckmann et al., 1997). Segmental spasms were observed in 3 patients in the days after the headaches, but these changes were still present months after in 2 cases, and were not confirmed in a series of 9 patients who had normal angiography (Silbert et al., 1989; Kapoor et al., 1990; Valenca et al., 2004). Regarding a possible impairment in autoregulation, Evers et al. (2003) showed that under conditions of sexual excitement the cerebral vessel walls respond to a pH decrease with impaired vasodilation compared to healthy subjects. Hypertension and migraine history had been related to orgasmic headache. Hypertension is not a major risk factor for this headache (Frese et al., 2003a), even though such patients usually show a higher increase of arterial blood pressure under physical stress (Evers et al., 2003). A comorbidity with migraine has been observed in several series (Johns, 1986; Pascual et al., 1996; Frese et al., 2003a). As with migraine, patients with orgasmic headache show a loss of cognitive habituation in symptomatic periods. There was no correlation, however, with the coexistence of migraine in these patients (Frese et al., 2003b).

Frese et al. (2003a) concluded that type 1 and type 2 sexual headaches are different manifestations of the same disorder rather than separate entities as both clinical comparison (see below) and experimental data have not shown any clear evidence that these are pathophysiologically distinct disorders.

Clinical manifestations

More than 90% of episodes of sexual headache occur during sexual intercourse with the usual partner. The rate of this headache does not seem to increase when the partner changes. About one-third also experience headache during masturbation (Vincent, 1982).

The age of onset of patients consulting due to this headache is 35–39 years (range 20–50 years). Similar to exertional headache, the male-to-female ratio is 3–4/1. The dull type occurs in less than one-quarter of patients. Two-thirds of patients have their headache in a bout: at least two attacks occurring in over 50% of sexual activities and then none for more than 2 weeks. The only clear difference between type 1 and type 2 sexual headaches is the onset time related to orgasm. Median onset time in type 1 is 150 s before orgasm and up to 5 s for type 2. The number of attacks per bout ranges from 2 to 50 and the mean duration of the symptomatic period is 3 months, though a minority of patients suffer from sexual headache for several years without apparent remission. Most of these patients experience infrequent (<20% of sexual activities) attacks (Paulson and Klawans, 1974; Lance, 1976; Silbert et al., 1991; Ostergaard and Kraft, 1992; Pascual et al., 1996; Frese et al., 2003a).

Pain characteristics are also similar to those described for primary exertional headache. The duration of pain is heterogeneous, ranging from 1 min to 24 h. Most patients have severe pain for between 1 and 3 h followed by mild pain for about 4 h. Pain is bilateral in two-thirds of patients, usually occipital or diffuse, and of a dull (47%), throbbing (47%), or stabbing (45%) quality (Evers and Lance, 2006).

Patients with sexual headache are usually healthy people, with no vascular disease. Two-thirds, however, suffer from other headache disorders such as episodic tension-type headache (35%), migraine (25%), and chronic tension-type headache (10%). Comorbid migraine and exertional headache are more frequent in orgasmic headache (Evers and Lance, 2006).

Differential diagnosis

Diagnostic work-up in patients with orgasmic headache is similar to that for exertional headache (see above) and includes subarachnoid hemorrhage, arterial dissection, and intracranial space-occupying lesions (Figure 40.3). Subarachnoid hemorrhage occurs during sexual activity in 4–12% of cases (Lundberg and Osterman, 1974; Evers and Lance, 2006). Rare cases of cerebral or brainstem infarction at the time of orgasm have been reported (Levy, 1981; Martínez et al., 1988; Lance, 1992). Orgasmic headaches disappeared in 1 patient with an intraventricular arachnoid cyst after its removal. Decreased levels of consciousness, vomiting, meningeal signs, focal symptoms, and severe pain lasting more than 24 h should be interpreted as "red flags" requiring immediate diagnostic work-up as described for exertional headaches. A minority of patients experiencing cough headache due to Chiari type I malformation or some other posterior fossa abnormality also notice head pain during orgasm. This is logical if we consider that sexual intercourse is a mixture of prolonged physical exercise and Valsalva maneuvers. In these cases, diagnostic investigations must follow the recommendations already given in this chapter for cough headache.

Treatment

There are no large clinical studies on the management of this condition. It seems reasonable to advise patients to remain sexually inactive as long as they are not completely free of symptoms (usually 3 months). About half of the patients can either terminate their headache by stopping sexual activity or ease the pain by taking a more passive role during coitus (Silbert et al., 1991; Frese et al., 2003a). Analgesics, NSAIDs, ergotamine, and benzodiazepines do not seem to be of great value if given before sexual activity. A recent report has shown the efficacy of triptans taken prior to headache intercourse in preventing the development of this headache (Frese et al., 2006). For those patients with longer-lasting bouts or with repeated attacks, preventive treatment can be indicated. For most patients treatment with a beta-blocker, at antimigraine dosages, seems very useful, even though the capricious nature of these headaches precludes the drawing of definite conclusions. Flunarizine, 5–10 mg at night, or indomethacin, 75–150 mg daily, are the options to try in those patients who do not respond to beta-blockers (Pascual et al., 1996, 2008; Evans and Pascual, 2000; Evers and Lance, 2006; Pascual, 2009).

References

Basoglu T, Ozbenli T, Bernay I et al. (1996). Demonstration of frontal hypoperfusion in benign exertional headache by technetium-99m-HMPAO SPECT. J Nucl Med 37: 1172–1174.

Blacky RA, Rittlemeyer JT, Wallace MR (1987). Headache angina. Am J Cardiol 60: 730.

Boes CJ, Matharu MS, Goadsby PJ (2002). Benign cough headache. Cephalalgia 22: 772–779.

Bowen J, Oppenheimer G (1993). Headache as presentation of angina: reproduction of symptoms during angioplasty. Headache 33: 238–239.

Britton TC, Guiloff RJ (1988). Carotid artery disease presenting as cough headache. Lancet 1: 1406–1407.

Chakravarty A (2006). Primary headaches associated with sexual activity – some observations in Indian patients. Cephalalgia 26: 202–207.

Chalaupka FD (2000). Therapeutic effectiveness of acetazolamide in hindbrain hernia headache. Neurol Sci 21: 117–119.

Chen SP, Fuh JL, Lu SR et al. (2009). Exertional headache – a survey of 1963 adolescents. Cephalalgia 29: 401–407.

Chen YY, Lirng JF, Yu WC et al. (2004a). Cardiac cephalgia. Case report and review of the literature with new ICHD-II criteria revisited. Eur Neurol 51: 221–226.

Chen YY, Lirng JF, Fuh JL et al. (2004b). Primary cough headache is associated with posterior fossa crowdedness: a morphometric MRI study. Cephalalgia 24: 694–699.

Dalessio DJ (1974). Effort migraine. Headache 14: 53.

Diamond S (1982). Prolonged benign exertional headache: its clinical characteristics and response to indomethacin. Headache 22: 96–98.

Diamond S, Medina JL (1979). Benign exertional headache: successful treatment with indomethacin. Headache 19: 249.

Doepp F, Valdueza JM, Schreiber SJ (2007). Incompetence of internal jugular valve in patients with primary exertional headache: a risk factor? Cephalalgia 28: 182–185.

Donnet A, Dufour H, Levrier O et al. (2008). Exertional headache: a new venous disease. Cephalalgia 28: 1201–1203.

Evans RW, Pascual J (2000). Orgasmic headaches: clinical features, diagnosis and management. Headache 40: 491–494.

Evers S, Lance JW (2006). Primary headache attributed to sexual activity. In: J Olesen, PJ Goadsby, P Tfelt-Hansen et al. (Eds.), The Headaches. 3rd edn. Lippincott Williams & Wilkins, Philadelphia, pp. 841–845.

Evers S, Schmidt O, Frese A et al. (2003). The cerebral hemodynamics of headache associated with sexual activity. Pain 102: 73–78.

Fleetcroft R, Maddocks JL (1985). Headache due to ischaemic heart disease. J R Soc Med 78: 676.

Frese A, Eikermann A, Frese K et al. (2003a). Headache associated with sexual activity: demographics, clinical features, and comorbidity. Neurology 23: 796–800.

Frese A, Frese K, Ringelstein EB et al. (2003b). Cognitive processing in headache associated with sexual activity. Cephalalgia 23: 543–551.

Frese A, Gantenbein A, Marziniak M et al. (2006). Triptans in orgasmic headache. Cephalalgia 26: 1458–1461.

Gutiérrez-Morlote J, Pascual J (2002). Cardiac cephalgia is not necessarily an exertional headache. Cephalalgia 22: 765–766.

Headache Classification Subcommittee of the International Headache Society (2004). The international classification of headache disorders, 2nd edn. Cephalalgia 24 (Suppl. 1): 1–160.

Heckmann JG, Hilz MJ, Muck-Weymann M et al. (1997). Benign exertional headache/benign sexual headache: a disorder of myogenic cerebral autoregulation? Headache 37: 597–598.

Indo T, Takahashi A (1990). Swimmer's migraine. Headache 30: 485–487.

Johns DR (1986). Benign sexual headache within one family. Arch Neurol 43: 1158–1160.

Kapoor R, Kendall BE, Harrison MJD (1990). Persistent segmental cerebral artery constriction in coital cephalgia. J Neurol Neurosurg Psychiatry 53: 266–270.

Lambert RW, Burnet DL (1985). Prevention of exercise-induced migraine by quantitative warm-up. Headache 25: 317–319.

Lance JW (1976). Headaches related to sexual activity. J Neurol Neurosurg Psychiatry 39: 1226–1230.

Lance JW (1991). Solved and unsolved headache problems. Headache 31: 439–445.

Lance JW (1992). Benign coital headache. Cephalalgia 12: 339.

Lance JW, Lambros J (1998). Unilateral exertional headache as a symptom of cardiac ischemia. Headache 38: 315–316.

Lefkowitz D, Biller J (1982). Bregmatic headache as a manifestation of myocardial ischemia. Arch Neurol 39: 120.

Levy RL (1981). Stroke and orgasmic headache. Headache 21: 12–13.

Lipton RB, Lowenkopf T, Bajwa ZH et al. (1997). Cardiac cephalgia: a treatable form of exertional headache. Neurology 49: 813–816.

Lundberg PO, Osterman PO (1974). The benign and malignant forms of orgasmic cephalgia. Headache 14: 164–165.

Martínez JM, Roig C, Arboix A (1988). Complicated coital cephalgia. Three cases with benign evolution. Cephalalgia 8: 265–268.

Mathew NT (1981). Indomethacin responsive headache syndromes. Headache 21: 147–150.

Mokri B (2002). Spontaneous CSF leaks mimicking benign exertional headaches. Cephalalgia 22: 780–783.

Nick J (1980). La céphalée d'effort. A propos d'une série de 43 cas. Semin Hop Paris 56: 525–531.

Nightingale S, Williams B (1987). Hindbrain hernia headache. Lancet 1: 731–734.

Ostergaard JR, Kraft M (1992). Benign coital headache. Cephalalgia 12: 353–355.

Ozge C, Atis S, Ozge A et al. (2005). Cough headache: frequency, characteristics and the relationship with the characteristics of cough. Eur J Pain 9: 383–388.

Pascual J (2005). Primary cough headache. Curr Pain Headache Rep 9: 272–276.

Pascual J (2009). Activity-related headache. In: S Gilman (Ed.), MedLink Neurology. MedLink, San Diego.

Pascual J, Oterino A, Berciano J (1992). Headache in type I Chiari malformation. Neurology 42: 1519–1521.

Pascual J, Combarros O, Leno C et al. (1995). Distribución por diagnósticos del dolor de cabeza como motivo de consulta neurológica. Med Clin (Barc) 104: 161–164.

Pascual J, Iglesias F, Oterino A et al. (1996). Cough, exertional, and sexual headaches. An analysis of 72 benign and symptomatic cases. Neurology 46: 1520–1524.

Pascual J, González-Mandly A, Martín R et al. (2008). Headaches precipitated by cough, prolonged exercise or sexual activity: a prospective etiological and clinical study. J Headache Pain 9: 259–266.

Paulson G, Klawans HL (1974). Benign orgasmic cephalgia. Headache 13: 57–60.

Paulson GW (1983). Weightlifter's headache. Headache 23: 193–194.

Pujol A, Roig C, Capdevila A et al. (1995). Motion of the cerebellar tonsils in Chiari type I malformation studied by cine-phase contrast MRI. Neurology 45: 1746–1753.

Quigley MF, Iskandar B, Quigley ME et al. (2004). Cerebrospinal fluid flow in foramen magnum: temporal and spatial patterns at MR imaging in volunteers and in patients with Chiari type I malformation. Radiology 232: 229–236.

Raskin NH (1995). The cough headache syndrome: treatment. Neurology 45: 1784.

Rasmussen BK, Olesen J (1992). Symptomatic and nonsymptomatic headaches in a general population. Neurology 42: 1225–1231.

Rivera M, del Real MA, Teruel JL et al. (1991). Carotid artery disease presenting as cough headache in a patient with haemodialysis. Postgrad Med J 67: 702.

Rooke ED (1968). Benign exertional headache. Med Clin North Am 52: 801–808.

Sands GH, Newman L, Lipton R (1991). Cough, exertional and other miscellaneous headaches. Med Clin North Am 75: 733–747.

Sansur CA, Heiss JD, DeVroom LH et al. (2003). Pathophysiology of headache associated with cough in patients with Chiari malformation. J Neurosurg 98: 453–458.

Sathirapanya P (2004). Anginal cephalgia: a serious form of exertional headache. Cephalalgia 24: 231–234.

Satikov IN, Mattle HP (1978). Vertebrobasilar dolicoectasia and exertional headache. J Neurol Neurosurg Psychiatry 41: 930–933.

Silbert PL, Hankey GP, Prentice DA et al. (1989). Angiographically demonstrated arterial spasm in a case of benign sexual headache and benign exertional headache. Aust N Z J Med 19: 466–468.

Silbert PL, Edis RH, Stewart-Wynne EG et al. (1991). Benign vascular sexual headache and exertional headache: interrelationships and long term prognosis. J Neurol Neurosurg Psychiatry 54: 417–421.

Sjaastad O, Bakketeig LS (2002). Exertional headache. I. Vaga study of headache epidemiology. Cephalalgia 22: 784–790.

Sjaastad O, Bakketeig LS (2003). Exertional headache. II. Clinical features of Vaga study of headache epidemiology. Cephalalgia 23: 803–807.

Slavik RS, Rhoney DH (1999). Indomethacin: a review of its cerebral blood flow effects and potential use for controlling intracranial pressure in traumatic brain injury patients. Neurol Res 21: 491–499.

Smith WS, Messing RO (1993). Cerebral aneurysm presenting as cough headache. Headache 33: 203–204.

Symonds C (1956). Cough headache. Brain 79: 557–568.

Tinel J (1932). La céphalée a l'effort. Syndrome de distension douloureuse des veines intracraniennes. Médecine (Paris) 13: 113–118.

Valenca MM, Valenca LP, Bordini CA et al. (2004). Cerebral vasopasm and headache during sexual intercourse and masturbatory orgasms. Headache 44: 244–248.

Vernay D, Deffond D, Fraysse P et al. (1993). Walk headache: an unusual manifestation of ischemic heart disease. Headache 29: 350–351.

Vincent FM (1982). Benign masturbatory cephalalgia. Arch Neurol 39: 673.

Wang SJ, Fuh JL, Lu SR (2000). Benign cough headache is responsive to acetazolamide. Neurology 55: 149–150.

Wei JH, Wang HF (2008). Cardiac cephalalgia: case reports and review. Cephalalgia 28: 892–896.

Williams B (1976). Cerebrospinal fluid changes in response to coughing. Brain 99: 331–346.

Williams B (1980). Cough headache due to craniocerebrospinal pressure dissociation. Arch Neurol 37: 226–230.

Handbook of Clinical Neurology, Vol. 97 (3rd series)
Headache
G. Nappi and M.A. Moskowitz, Editors

Chapter 41

Hypnic headache

RAFFAELE MANNI[1]* AND NATASCIA GHIOTTO[2]
[1]*Sleep Medicine and Epilepsy Unit, IRCCS "C. Mondino Institute of Neurology" Foundation, Pavia, Italy*
[2]*University Centre for Adaptive Disorders and Headache (UCADH), IRCCS "C. Mondino Institute of Neurology" Foundation, Pavia, Italy*

Hypnic headache (HH) is a new clinical entity included in ICHD-II (Headache Classification Subcommittee of the International Headache Society, 2004), in the section "other primary headaches." Originally described by Raskin in 1988 as a late-onset, "curious sleep-related headache syndrome," it has also been called "alarm-clock headache" (Dodick et al., 1998) as it regularly awakens subjects from sleep at a set time of night.

EPIDEMIOLOGY

At present about 100 HH cases have been reported in the literature. In a large tertiary-referred headache population, HH reportedly accounted for 0.07% of referrals (Dodick et al., 1998). However, this figure, although certainly precise, relates to an investigation of referrals to a specialist headache center, and therefore is likely not to reflect the true prevalence of this disorder in the general population.

With the exception of a few cases with onset before the age of 50 years, including a questionable case with onset at the age of 9 (Grosberg et al., 2005), HH generally has onset late in life, at a mean age of 63 ± 9 years (range 50–83 years). A review of the "other" primary headaches in children and adolescents did not mention HH (Lewis et al., 2005).

Hypnic headache is more frequent in females (70%) than in males, showing a male-to-female ratio of 1:3. Generally, HH has been reported to remain undiagnosed for several years (up to 6 years) and to show a chronic course, albeit sometimes with a relapsing–remitting pattern (Lisotto et al., 2004). However, studies with longer follow up are needed to establish whether HH really is a chronic disorder.

CLINICAL FEATURES

Table 41.1 summarizes the Second Edition of the International Classification of Headache Disorders (ICHD-II) diagnostic criteria for HH. The most important characteristics for HH, according to the seminal description by Raskin (1988), are: occurrence exclusively during sleep, chronic pattern of attacks ($\geq$ 15 per month), short duration, dull pain, absence of autonomic signs and symptoms.

The criteria adopted by the ICHD-II do not take into account the location, duration, and intensity of the pain. This is probably because the pain features and patterns are quite variable. Pain intensity, for instance, has been reported as severe in 31% of patients, moderate to severe in 12%, moderate in 45%, mild to moderate in 2%, and mild in 10%. Pain is unilateral in about one-third of subjects, with the attack always occurring on the same side in 67% of these cases. Generally the duration of the pain is shorter than 180 min; however, longer-lasting attacks (range: 15–600 min) have been reported. The clinical features of HH are shown in Table 41.2.

Autonomic signs are anecdotally reported in HH (unilateral ptosis in 1 case, bilateral lacrimation in 2 cases, unilateral lacrimation and rhinorrhea in 2 cases, nasal congestion in another) (Dodick et al., 1998, 2000; Centonze et al., 2001; Evers et al., 2003; Lisotto et al., 2004), as are autonomic symptoms: nausea in 19% of subjects, and photophobia ± phonophobia ± nausea in 5% of patients (Gould and Silberstein, 1997; Dodick et al., 1998, 2000; Dodick, 2000; Centonze et al., 2001; Martins and Gouveia, 2001; Ghiotto et al., 2002; Vieira Dias and Esperanca, 2002; Pinessi et al., 2003; Lisotto et al., 2004; Manni et al., 2004; Buzzi et al., 2005; Guido and Specchio, 2006; Kerr et al., 2006).

*Correspondence to: Dr. Raffaele Manni, Sleep Medicine and Epilepsy Unit, IRCCS "C. Mondino Institute of Neurology" Foundation, Via Mondino 2, 27100 Pavia, Italy, Tel: +390382380l, Fax: +390382380286, E-mail: raffaele.manni@mondino.it

Table 41.1

The International Classification of Headache Disorders, 2nd edn. (ICDH-II) diagnostic criteria for hypnic headache (Headache Classification Subcommittee of the International Headache Society, 2004)

A. Dull headache fulfilling criteria B–D
B. Develops only during sleep, and awakens patient
C. At least two of the following characteristics:
   1. Occurs >15 times per month
   2. Lasts ≥15 min after waking
   3. First occurs after age of 50 years
D. No autonomic symptoms and no more than one of nausea, photophobia, or phonophobia
E. Not attributed to another disorder

Table 41.2

Clinical findings in patients with hypnic headache (n = 96*)

Frequency of attacks	% of patients
≥15/month	83%
≤15/month	17%
Type of pain	
Dull/fixed/pressure	51%
Pulsating/throbbing	30%
Non-pulsating	7%
Dull and throbbing	6%
Stabbing	4%
Boring	2%
Side of pain	
Bilateral	65%
Unilateral	35%
Intensity of pain	
Mild	10%
Mild to moderate	2%
Moderate	45%
Moderate to severe	12%
Severe	31%
Duration of attack	
<60 min	52%
<120 min	26%
<180 min	6%
>180 min	16%
Autonomic symptoms	
Nausea	19%
Photophobia ± phonophobia ± nausea	5%
Autonomic signs	
Bilateral lacrimation/ptosis/ lacrimation and ipsilateral rhinorrhea/nasal congestion	5%

*Not all data are available for all subjects.

HH is considered a primary form of headache. However, as it is also a late-onset form, exclusion of an underlying disorder is mandatory. In particular, nocturnal headaches secondary to increased intracranial pressure, arterial hypertension, sleep apnea (Dodick, 2000), or pain-killing medication overuse must be ruled out (Rains and Poceta, 2005). Other symptomatic headaches should be also taken into account when diagnosing HH as, to date, 2 cases mimicking it have been described in the literature: the first was a case of nocturnal headache secondary to posterior fossa meningioma (Peatfield and Mendoza, 2003) and the second a case of nocturnal headache following an ischemic lesion in the pontine reticular formation. This latter case could indicate an involvement, in HH, of the neural networks involved in sleep–wake regulation (Moon et al., 2006).

Finally, HH must be differentiated from other primary headache forms that can also occur, although not exclusively, in sleep: migraine, tension-type headache, trigeminal-autonomic cephalalgias (cluster headache, paroxysmal hemicrania, short-lasting unilateral neuralgiform headache attacks with conjunctival injection and tearing (SUNCT)), primary thunderclap headache, and hemicrania continua (Cohen and Kaube, 2004; Nappi et al., 2005).

The concurrence of other types of primary headache in the same period or in different periods of life has been reported in 39% of HH patients. Migraine without aura was present in 16% of cases (Dodick et al., 1998, 2000; Martins and Gouveia, 2001; Ghiotto et al., 2002; Vieira Dias and Esperanca, 2002; Fukuhara et al., 2006; Ulrich et al., 2006), migraine with aura in 3% (Raskin, 1988; Dodick et al., 1998), tension-type headache (either chronic or episodic) in 12% (Dodick et al., 1998, 2000; Dodick, 2000; Relja et al., 2002; Pinessi et al., 2003; Fukuhara et al., 2006; Schurks et al., 2006), a coexistence of migraine and tension-type headache in 4% (Centonze et al., 2001; Ghiotto et al., 2002; Fukuhara et al., 2006), cervicogenic headache in 3% (Pinto et al., 2002; Evers et al., 2003), and a non-specific hemicrania in 1% (Gould and Silberstein, 1997).

PATHOPHYSIOLOGICAL HYPOTHESIS

The clinical observation of strict and sometimes cyclical occurrence of HH attacks during nocturnal sleep made most researchers think that HH was likely to be a phenomenon related to rapid eye movement (REM) sleep. Most polysomnographic studies show that about 69% of HH attacks occur during REM sleep (Dodick, 2000; Evers et al., 2003; Pinessi et al., 2003; Manni et al., 2004; Patsouros et al., 2004; Capuano et al., 2005).

Accordingly, HH attacks were hypothesized to be associated with REM-related inhibition of the activity of the locus coeruleus and of the dorsal raphe, and with brain serotonin reduction (Dodick et al., 2003). However, the fact that cases of HH attacks have been reported in non-REM (NREM) sleep, during both NREM stage 2 and stages 3–4, seems to rule out an exclusive relationship between HH and REM sleep.

Interestingly, a low level of arousability has been documented during both NREM and REM sleep in subjects with headache attacks occurring exclusively during nocturnal sleep (Capuano et al., 2005). It has been suggested that such a pattern of blunted arousal responses may indicate the existence of a hypothalamic or brainstem dysfunction in these patients (Della Marca et al., 2006).

The observation that most patients suffering from HH report attacks occurring regularly at the same time of night ("alarm-clock headache") has prompted the hypothesis that this peculiar type of headache may be regarded as a chronobiological disorder. This suggestion is further supported *ex adiuvantibus* by reports describing the efficacy of lithium salt (a drug with a proven role in the treatment of definite chronobiological disorders, such as cluster headache and bipolar disorder) in preventing the recurrence of HH attacks (Newman et al., 1990; Costa and Nappi, 2003; Sandrini et al., 2006).

Finally, the Pavia group has advanced the intriguing hypothesis that HH could represent a phenotypical variation of migraine occurring over time (Ghiotto et al., 2002). This hypothesis is based on several factors: the partial overlapping of clinical features between HH and migraine; the tendency of migraine to disappear in elderly people; the typical onset of HH after the age of 50; and the observation that about 20% of patients suffering from HH have a past history of migraine. According to this line of reasoning, one may hypothesize that changes in external factors, ranging from hormonal patterns to lifestyle (in relation to the menopause, retirement, etc.), may act upon a predisposed terrain and, over time, trigger the appearance of different clinical characteristics ("phenotypical heterochronia").

THERAPY

Several different treatments have been tried in HH (Evers and Goadsby, 2003). Lithium salts (300–900 mg/day) were first used by Raskin (1988) and remain the most suitable preventive treatment for HH (Gould and Silberstein, 1997; Morales-Asin et al., 1998; Perez-Martinez et al., 1999; Vieira-Dias and Esperanca, 2001; Ghiotto et al., 2002; Pinto et al., 2002; Pinessi et al., 2003; Kocasoy et al., 2004; Kerr et al., 2006).

Indomethacin (50–150 mg/day) is another interesting prophylactic choice, particularly effective in unilateral forms of HH (Ivanez et al., 1998; Dodick, 2000; Dodick et al., 2000; Centonze et al., 2001; Sibon et al., 2003; Buzzi et al., 2005; Peters et al., 2006). The role of this drug is of particular interest as indomethacin is effective in the trigeminal autonomic headaches (Goadsby and Lipton, 1997).

Flunarizine (5–10 mg/day) proved to be useful in some cases of HH (Morales-Asin et al., 1998; Klimek and Sklodowski, 1999; Pinto et al., 2002; Domitrz, 2005; Schurks et al., 2006).

Caffeine (40–60 mg or 1–2 cups of coffee) at bedtime, sometimes in association with melatonin (3–6 mg), was successfully used by some authors (Dodick et al., 1998, 2000; Ghiotto et al., 2002).

In anecdotal reports, antiepileptic drugs, such as topiramate (Guido and Specchio, 2006), gabapentin (Arjona et al., 2000; Ghiotto et al., 2002) and pregabalin (Ulrich et al., 2006), have apparently been useful in preventing HH attack recurrence in a few cases.

There are only few reports dealing with the symptomatic treatment of HH. Generally, subcutaneous sumatriptan (Dodick et al., 2000; Evers et al., 2003; Pinessi et al., 2003) and oxygen inhalation (Evers et al., 2003; Schurks et al., 2006) proved to be ineffective, and there are also two reports of successful use of the triptans (Dodick et al., 1998; Schurks et al., 2006). In some HH sufferers, pain relief has been reported following oral consumption of acetylsalicylic acid or drinking a cup of coffee. Finally, getting out of bed and walking around was found to improve the pain in others (Pinto et al., 2002).

REFERENCES

Arjona JA, Jimenez-Jimenez FJ, Vela-Bueno A et al. (2000). Hypnic headache associated with stage 3 slow wave sleep. Headache 40: 753–754.

Buzzi MG, Cologno D, Formisano R et al. (2005). Hypnic headache responsive to indomethacin: second Italian case. Funct Neurol 20: 85–87.

Capuano A, Vollono C, Rubino M et al. (2005). Hypnic headache: actigraphic and polysomnographic study of a case. Cephalalgia 25: 466–469.

Centonze V, D'Amico D, Usai S et al. (2001). First Italian case of hypnic headache, with literature review and discussion of nosology. Cephalalgia 21: 71–74.

Cohen AS, Kaube H (2004). Rare nocturnal headaches. Curr Opin Neurol 17: 295–299.

Costa A, Nappi G (2003). Cluster headache as a disorder of inner temporal organization. In: O Sjaastad, G Nappi (Eds.), Cluster Headache Syndrome in General Practice. Smith-Gordon, London, pp. 25–34.

Della Marca G, Vollono C, Rubino M et al. (2006). Dysfunction of arousal systems in sleep-related migraine without aura. Cephalalgia 26: 857–864.

Dodick DW (2000). Polysomnography in hypnic headache syndrome. Headache 40: 748–752.

Dodick DW, Mosek AC, Campbell JK (1998). The hypnic ("alarm clock") headache syndrome. Cephalalgia 18: 152–156.

Dodick DW, Jones JM, Capobianco DJ (2000). Hypnic headache: another indomethacin-responsive headache syndrome? Headache 40: 830–835.

Dodick DW, Eross EJ, Parish JM et al. (2003). Clinical, anatomical, and physiologic relationship between sleep and headache. Headache 43: 282–292.

Domitrz I (2005). [Hypnic headache as a primary short-lasting night headache: a report of two cases.] Neurol Neurochir Pol 39: 77–79.

Evers S, Goadsby PJ (2003). Hypnic headache: clinical features, pathophysiology, and treatment. Neurology 60: 905–909.

Evers S, Rahmann A, Schwaag S et al. (2003). Hypnic headache – the first German cases including polysomnography. Cephalalgia 23: 20–23.

Fukuhara Y, Takeshima T, Ishizaki K et al. (2006). [Three Japanese cases of hypnic headache.] Rinsho Shinkeigaku 46: 148–153.

Ghiotto N, Sances G, Di Lorenzo G et al. (2002). Report of eight new cases of hypnic headache and mini-review of the literature. Funct Neurol 17: 211–219.

Goadsby PJ, Lipton RB (1997). A review of paroxysmal hemicranias, SUNCT syndrome and other short-lasting headaches with autonomic feature, including new cases. Brain 120: 193–209.

Gould JD, Silberstein SD (1997). Unilateral hypnic headache: a case study. Neurology 49: 1749–1751.

Grosberg BM, Lipton RB, Solomon S et al. (2005). Hypnic headache in childhood? A case report. Cephalalgia. 25: 68–70.

Guido M, Specchio LM (2006). Successful treatment of hypnic headache with topiramate: a case report. Headache 46: 1205–1206.

Headache Classification Subcommittee of the International Headache Society (2004). The international classification of headache disorders, 2nd edn. Cephalalgia 24: 1–160.

Ivanez V, Soler R, Barreiro P (1998). Hypnic headache syndrome: a case with good response to indomethacin. Cephalalgia 18: 225–226.

Kerr E, Hewitt R, Gleadhill I (2006). Benign headache in the elderly – a case report of hypnic headache. Ulster Med J 75: 158–159.

Klimek A, Sklodowski P (1999). [Night headache: report of 2 cases.] Neurol Neurochir Pol 33 (Suppl. 5): 49–54.

Kocasoy OE, Kayrak EN, Orhan KS et al. (2004). Hypnic headache syndrome: excessive periodic limb movements in polysomnography. Agri 16: 28–30.

Lewis DW, Gozzo YF, Avner MT (2005). The "other" primary headaches in children and adolescents. Pediatr Neurol 33: 303–313.

Lisotto C, Mainardi F, Maggioni F et al. (2004). Episodic hypnic headache? Cephalalgia 24: 681–685.

Manni R, Sances G, Terzaghi M et al. (2004). Hypnic headache: PSG evidence of both REM- and NREM-related attacks. Neurology 62: 1411–1413.

Martins IP, Gouveia RG (2001). Hypnic headache and travel across time zones: a case report. Cephalalgia 21: 928–931.

Moon HS, Chung CS, Hong SB et al. (2006). A case of symptomatic hypnic headache syndrome. Cephalalgia 26: 81–83.

Morales-Asin F, Mauri JA, Iniguez C et al. (1998). The hypnic headache syndrome: report of three new cases. Cephalalgia 18: 157–158.

Nappi G, Sandrini G, Ghiotto N et al. (2005). Other primary headaches: old concepts and new views. In: J Olesen (Ed.), Classification and Diagnosis of Headache Disorders. Oxford University Press, Oxford, pp. 120–128.

Newman LC, Lipton RB, Solomon S (1990). The hypnic headache syndrome: a benign headache disorder of the elderly. Neurology 40: 1904–1905.

Patsouros N, Laloux P, Ossemann M (2004). Hypnic headache: a case report with polysomnography. Acta Neurol Belg 104: 37–40.

Peatfield RC, Mendoza ND (2003). Posterior fossa meningioma presenting as hypnic headache. Headache 43: 1007–1008.

Perez-Martinez DA, Berbel-Garcia A, Puente-Munoz AI et al. (1999). [Hypnic headache: a new case.] Rev Neurol 28: 883–884.

Peters N, Lorenzl S, Fischereder J et al. (2006). Hypnic headache: a case presentation including polysomnography. Cephalalgia 26: 84–86.

Pinessi L, Rainero I, Cicolin A et al. (2003). Hypnic headache syndrome: association of the attacks with REM sleep. Cephalalgia 23: 150–154.

Pinto CA, Fragoso YD, Souza Carvalho D et al. (2002). Hypnic headache syndrome: clinical aspects of eight patients in Brazil. Cephalalgia 22: 824–827.

Rains JC, Poceta JS (2005). Sleep-related headache syndromes. Semin Neurol 25: 69–80.

Raskin NH (1988). The hypnic headache syndrome. Headache 28: 534–536.

Relja G, Zorzon M, Locatelli L et al. (2002). Hypnic headache: rapid and long-lasting response to prednisone in two new cases. Cephalalgia 22: 157–159.

Sandrini G, Tassorelli C, Ghiotto N et al. (2006). Uncommon primary headaches. Curr Opin Neurol 19: 299–304.

Schurks M, Kastrup O, Diener HC (2006). Triptan responsive hypnic headache? Eur J Neurol 13: 666–667.

Sibon I, Ghorayeb I, Henry P (2003). Successful treatment of hypnic headache syndrome with acetazolamide. Neurology 61: 1157–1158.

Ulrich K, Gunreben B, Lang E et al. (2006). Pregabalin in the therapy of hypnic headache. Cephalalgia 26: 1031–1032.

Vieira-Dias M, Esperanca P (2001). Hypnic headache: report of two cases. Headache 41: 726–727.

Vieira Dias M, Esperanca P (2002). [Hypnic headache: a report of four cases.] Rev Neurol 34: 950–951.

Handbook of Clinical Neurology, Vol. 97 (3rd series)
Headache
G. Nappi and M.A. Moskowitz, Editors

Chapter 42

Primary thunderclap headache

F.H.H. LINN*

Department of Neurology, Central Military Hospital and Rudolf Magnus Institute of Neuroscience, University Medical Center, Utrecht, The Netherlands

INTRODUCTION AND DEFINITION

The term "thunderclap headache" was first used by Day and Raskin in 1986 as a symptom of unruptured cerebral aneurysm. In 2004, the International Headache Society published the diagnostic criteria for primary thunderclap headache (Table 42.1) (Headache Classification Subcommittee of the International Headache Society, 2004). In a patient with thunderclap headache, first and foremost intracranial hemorrhage or other serious brain disorder should be excluded. The percentage of patients with sudden headache with a serious underlying brain disorder depends on the design of the study and the referred population: in primary care practice this proportion was 1 in 3 (Linn et al., 1994), whereas in the emergency room this proportion was 1 in 6 (Fodden et al., 1989; Morgenstern et al., 1998; Landtblom et al., 2002). But in a hospital-based series of patients referred to the neurology department, two-thirds had subarachnoid hemorrhage (SAH) (van der Wee et al., 1995; van Gijn, 1999) (Table 42.2).

In this chapter, primary thunderclap headache together with secondary underlying causes of thunderclap headache will be discussed and radiological techniques will be reviewed. In addition, conditions associated with thunderclap headache, such as unruptured aneurysm and cerebral vasoconstriction, will be discussed.

CAUSES OF THUNDERCLAP HEADACHE

Primary headache disorders or secondary symptomatic headache disorders, most frequently vascular disorders or non-vascular intracranial disorders, are the most important causes of thunderclap headache (Dalessio, 1994; Evans, 1996; Mayer et al., 1996) (Table 42.3). In particular SAH, other intracranial hemorrhage and cerebral venous thrombosis or intracranial hypotension should be excluded (Dalessio, 1994; Ramirez-Lassepas et al., 1997). After exclusion of a serious underlying brain disorder, acute severe headache most likely represents a primary headache syndrome, migraine, or primary thunderclap headache (Green, 2003).

Primary headache disorders

PRIMARY THUNDERCLAP HEADACHE

Primary thunderclap headache is a severe headache with a sudden onset of less than 1 min, lasting 1 h to 10 days. The headache is not attributed to another disorder (normal cerebrospinal fluid (CSF) and normal brain imaging are needed) (Headache Classification Subcommittee of the International Headache Society, 2004) (Table 42.1). The search for an underlying cause should be expedient and exhaustive. Primary thunderclap headache is thus a diagnosis of exclusion. Other synonyms are idiopathic thunderclap headache, benign thunderclap headache (BTH), and crash migraine (Fisher, 1984). Primary thunderclap headache occurs without provocative circumstances. In patients with thunderclap headache it is important to ask in detail about the speed of onset of the headache, whether the headache occurred in a split second or in a few minutes (Adams et al., 1980; Dalessio, 1994; Mayer et al., 1996; van Gijn, 1997). The severity of the headache should be quantified if possible on a scale from 0 to 10 (Linn et al., 1998). Features in the patient's history that indicate a possible serious underlying brain disorder are: "first" headache, headache during exertion, symptoms and signs such as fever, stiff neck, vomiting, transient loss or clouding of consciousness, focal symptoms, and loss of vision.

*Correspondence to: F.H.H. Linn, MD, Department of Neurology, Central Military Hospital and Rudolf Magnus Institute of Neuroscience, University Medical Center, Heidelberglaan 100, 3584 CX Utrecht, The Netherlands, Tel: +31-88-7557975, Fax: +31-30-2542100, E-mail: f.h.h.linn@umcutrecht.nl

Table 42.1

The International Headache Society's diagnostic criteria for primary thunderclap headache

A. Severe head pain fulfilling criteria B or C
B. Both of the following characteristics:
  1. Sudden onset, reaching maximum intensity in <1 min
  2. Lasting from 1 h to 10 days
C. Does not recur regularly over subsequent weeks or months (although headache may recur within the first week after onset)
D. Not attributed to another disorder (normal cerebrospinal fluid and brain imaging are required)

Table 42.2

Causes of sudden headache in primary care (Linn et al., 1994) and in hospital (van der Wee et al., 1995)

	Primary care	Hospital series (neurology referrals)
Intracranial hemorrhage	25%*	67%
Other severe cerebral disorders	12%	
Primary headache syndromes	63%	33%

*12% if headache is the only symptom.

Table 42.3

Main and rare causes of thunderclap headache

Main causes	Rare causes
Vascular disorders	
Subarachnoid hemorrhage	Pituitary apoplexy
	Arteritis/angiitis
Intracerebral hemorrhage	Unruptured vascular malformation/aneurysm
Cerebral venous thrombosis	Arterial hypertension
Spontaneous intracranial hypotension	Cerebral segmental vasoconstriction
Cervical artery dissection	
Non-vascular disorders	
	Greater occipital neuralgia
	Intermittent hydrocephalus by colloid cyst
Infections	
Meningitis/encephalitis	Erve virus
	Sinusitis
Primary headache disorders	
Migraine	Cluster headache
Primary thunderclap headache	Tension headache/ new daily persistent headache
Primary exertional headache	
Primary cough headache	
Primary headache associated with sexual activity	

The characteristics of headache in thunderclap headache without underlying cause do not differ substantially from SAH (Wijdicks et al., 1988; Harling et al., 1989; Markus, 1991; Linn et al., 1998; Morgenstern et al., 1998; Landtblom et al., 2002); neither symptoms nor signs can be used to distinguish BTH from aneurysmal SAH (Linn et al., 1998). Vomiting occurred in 43% of patients with BTH and in 70% of SAH patients (Markus, 1991; Linn et al., 1998). Transient loss of consciousness and focal symptoms occurred with equal frequency in patients with BTH and in patients with SAH (Linn et al., 1998).

On physical examination, subtle focal neurological signs and papilledema may be detected. The absence of neck stiffness does not exclude a serious brain disorder, particularly if the patient is examined shortly after the thunderclap headache. It may take hours before neck stiffness is evident in cases of SAH (Vermeulen and van Gijn, 1990).

Currently, there is no clear concept on pathogenesis of thunderclap headache. The sympathetic nervous system may play an important role in the pathophysiology of thunderclap headache. Secondary thunderclap headache in patients with hypertensive crises, eclampsia, or pheochromocytoma, or in patients who use sympathomimetic drugs (Singhal et al., 2002) suggests excessive sympathetic activity or a heightened response to endogenous catecholamines, drug-influenced sympathetic receptors, or autonomic dysreflexia (Chen et al., 2006; Schwedt et al., 2006). The occurrence of reversible vasospasm in reversible vasoconstriction syndromes reflects localized contraction of the smooth muscle in the vessel wall, influenced by the sympathetic nerves containing neuropeptides. In migraine, recent functional imaging studies show that changes in the dorsolateral pons are pivotal in the phenotypic expression of migraine. Changes in the brain activation in the pons persist after the migraine attack, and suggest a disorder of brain function rather than of the blood vessels (Goadsby, 2006).

Studies on thunderclap headache showed that 40% of patients had a history of migraine or tension headache (Wijdicks et al., 1988; Markus, 1991; Linn et al., 1999) and many others develop these types of headache at later stages (Harling et al., 1989; Linn et al., 1999). Whether thunderclap headache in a patient with previous migraine or tension headache is an unusual rare manifestation of these headaches or a distinct clinical entity remains uncertain. One should also realize the epidemiological principle that rare variants of common conditions (such as migraine or tension headache) often outnumber regular presentations of uncommon conditions such as SAH. Interestingly, in 10% of patients with thunderclap headache, recurrent thunderclap headaches occur, without any evidence for serious brain disease at long-term follow-up (Wijdicks et al., 1988; Markus, 1991; Linn et al., 1994). These data indicate that patients with thunderclap headache are sensitive to headache attacks. The fact that thunderclap headache is experienced and classified as different from other headaches (with most patients seeking medical advice) supports the argument that thunderclap headache is a distinct clinical entity. Follow-up on absence of work or further medical consultations was not uniformly excellent (Linn et al., 1999). Prognosis is excellent regarding subsequent SAH (Wijdicks et al., 1988; Harling et al., 1989; Linn et al., 1999; Landtblom et al., 2002).

It is mandatory to exclude SAH or other serious brain disorders with computed tomography (CT) or lumbar puncture. In case of negative findings, further investigations with magnetic resonance imaging (MRI), magnetic resonance venography (MRV), or cerebral angiography are warranted if clinical suspicion for a serious brain disease is high.

Reversible vasoconstriction syndromes

Sometimes thunderclap headache is associated with transient focal neurological symptoms and signs, as well as seizures, altered mental status, and often cortical visual disturbances. On angiography some of these patients have diffuse segmental vasoconstriction in the proximal or distal arteries around the circle of Willis (Call et al., 1988; Silbert et al., 1989; Slivka and Philbrook, 1995). The clinical symptoms and signs as well as the angiographic findings are often reversible. MRI may be normal, but white-matter abnormalities consistent with the posterior reversible leukoencephalopathy syndrome (Chen et al., 2006) are described. These reversible vasoconstriction syndromes involve the Call–Fleming syndrome, and are associated with the puerperium (postpartum angiopathy), benign angiopathy of the central nervous system (CNS) (Hajj-Ali et al., 2002), drugs (triptans, bromocriptine) (Singhal et al., 2002), hypertension (Tang-Wai et al., 2001), or migraine, sexual or exertional headache (Silbert et al., 1989). They should be differentiated from primary angiitis of the CNS. In this disease, the start of the headache is often more insidious, the neurological signs are progressive, and the laboratory investigations (sedimentation rate, leukocyte count) are abnormal, as well as CSF analysis. Brain MRI shows multifocal abnormalities in the white matter and cortical infarctions.

Unruptured aneurysms

In some patients with thunderclap headache with normal CT and lumbar puncture, an (asymptomatic) aneurysm was found accidentally by angiography (Day and Raskin, 1986; Clarke et al., 1988). The frequency of an asymptomatic cerebral aneurysm in the general population is 3.6–6% (Wardlaw and White, 2000). Because of the benign outcome in these patients with thunderclap headache during long-term follow-up (Wijdicks et al., 1988; Markus, 1991; Linn et al., 1999) and the potentially serious complications of angiography (Cloft et al., 1999), routine angiography is not recommended for patients with thunderclap headache (Schwedt et al., 2006). Therapeutic dilemmas may occur in cases of thunderclap headache in combination with an aneurysm that has not (yet) ruptured, but there is a tendency to clip the aneurysm (Day and Raskin, 1986; The International Study of Unruptured Intracranial Aneurysms Investigators, 1998; Johnston et al., 1999; Witham and Kaufmann, 2000).

Other primary headache disorders

The hallmark of some primary headache disorders is the occurrence of repeated attacks of sudden headache, often precipitated by the same mechanism (exercise, coughing, sexual activity). Of course, the first attack of such a sudden headache is alarming, and a serious underlying brain disease should then be excluded (Lance, 1976; Finelli, 1993; Pascual et al., 1996). Most patients have migraine or non-specific headache (Fodden et al., 1989; Ward et al., 2001). Tension-type headache and new daily persistent headache may present as sudden headache. Primary exertional headache has a short duration in general but can last up to 48 h (Rooke, 1968; Lane and Gulevich, 2002). On first occurrence it is mandatory to exclude SAH or arterial dissection (Rooke, 1968; Sands et al., 1991; Pascual et al., 1996). Primary cough headache (Pascual et al., 1996) lasts less than 30 min and has a stabbing and sharp character. Cough headache is symptomatic in 40% of cases and in the large majority presents with Arnold–Chiari malformation type I (Pascual et al., 1996). Primary headache associated with sexual activity usually disappears within 3 h, mostly in the absence of an intracranial disorder (Lance, 1976; Frese et al., 2003), but may mimic SAH. Hemorrhage in the basal ganglia has been reported (Finelli, 1993). Cluster headache and clusterlike headache syndromes are all quite uncommon (Fodden et al., 1989). The hypnic headache syndrome is another rare primary headache disorder (Newman et al., 2001).

Secondary or symptomatic headache disorders

Vascular disorders

Subarachnoid hemorrhage: clinical features

Aneurysmal rupture is characterized by a sudden, excruciating headache (Dalessio, 1994; Ramirez-Lassepas et al., 1997; Morgenstern et al., 1998). Other accompanying symptoms in SAH are loss of consciousness (Vermeulen et al., 1984), seizures (6–9%) (Pinto et al., 1996), delirium, or focal stroke (caused by an intracerebral hematoma). In the large majority, SAH is caused by a ruptured aneurysm, and 5% of patients have a rare cause for SAH (Table 42.3) (Rinkel et al., 1993). Previous sudden headaches, "sentinel headaches" in patients with aneurysmal SAH, were attributed to a so-called warning leak in older hospital-based and retrospective studies (King and Saba, 1974). In a systematic review, sentinel headaches in aneurysmal SAH occurred in the range of 10–43% (Polmear, 2003), varying by region. The cause of a previous sudden severe headache could be due to stretching or dissection in the wall of the aneurysm or earlier bleeding (SAH) (Ball, 1975; Day and Raskin, 1986), a diagnosis other than SAH (Mayer et al., 1996; van Gijn, 1999; Edlow and Caplan, 2000), or recall bias (overinterpretation of an episode of headache in the context of a serious brain disease) (Linn et al., 1994).

Perimesencephalic hemorrhage is a more benign type of SAH, caused by a possible venous (instead of arterial aneurysmal) rupture in the cisterns around the midbrain (Rinkel et al., 1991; Schwartz and Solomon, 1996). The clinical features are less impressive than in aneurysmal SAH: the start of the headache occurs in minutes rather than seconds, loss of consciousness is exceptional, and neurological abnormalities are generally not found (Rinkel et al., 1991).

In a minority of patients, history and/or physical examination are helpful in pointing to other causes of SAH. Prominent neck pain is suggestive for a dissection of the vertebral artery, in general in its extracranial course. If the dissection extends to the intradural portions of the vessel or begins intradurally, it may rupture into the subarachnoid space and cause SAH (Caplan et al., 1988; Saeed et al., 2000). Rupture of a mycotic aneurysm might be the first manifestation of endocarditis (Hart et al., 1990; Ferro et al., 1995). The aneurysms are often associated with headache, aseptic meningitis, cranial nerve palsies, or transient focal signs. When thunderclap headache occurs with a sudden decrease in vision, pituitary apoplexy in a preexistent tumor, often an adenoma, must be excluded (Dodick and Wijdicks, 1998; Semple et al., 2005).

On physical examination, neck stiffness may be present as well as ocular palsies, caused by compression of the nerves in the adjacent cavernous sinus (McFadzean et al., 1991). MRI is the investigation of choice (Dodick and Wijdicks, 1998). Patients who use cocaine have a higher chance of developing an aneurysm and SAH (Levine et al., 1990; Neiman et al., 2000). Sudden headache combined with severe back pain, root pain, or symptoms and signs of spinal cord dysfunction all point to a spinal cause of SAH (Kai et al., 2005). In some patients with trauma in combination with SAH, it may be impossible to diagnose the cause, in particular with of predominant headache or neck stiffness (Sakas et al., 1995; Cummings et al., 2000). Isolated angiitis of the CNS can present with SAH, in general without neurological abnormalities on initial examination (Kumar et al., 1997).

Other brain hemorrhages

The majority of patients with thunderclap with a hemorrhage have SAH, but it is impossible to distinguish clinically between other brain hemorrhages. Up to half of patients with intracerebral hemorrhage have headache at onset (Gorelick et al., 1986; Jorgensen et al., 1994; Melo et al., 1996; van Gijn, 1997; Tentschert et al., 2005), especially those with cerebellar or lobar hematoma (Melo et al., 1996; Tentschert et al., 2005; Schwedt and Dodick, 2006). Clinical presentations of cerebellar hemorrhage and SAH are often rather similar because of the prominent headache and the relatively mild focal deficits. Vomiting or vertigo is frequently another early symptom of cerebellar hematoma (Gerritsen van der Hoop et al., 1988). Most patients have a slightly impaired level of consciousness, and half of them have cerebellar or brainstem signs (Mathew et al., 1995). Chronic subdural hematomas may resemble SAH starting with sudden headache (Kotwica and Brzezinski, 1985). A retroclival hematoma is a rare cause of thunderclap headache (Schievink et al., 2001a).

Cerebral venous sinus thrombosis

Severe headache increasing gradually in days occurs in 90% of patients with cerebral venous sinus thrombosis (CVST) (Cumurciuc et al., 2005; Stam, 2005). Thunderclap headache was present in a large study (de Bruijn et al., 1996) in 10 out of 71 patients, with neurological signs at that time in only 1 patient. CT scan on admission was interpreted as normal in half the patients. The authors suggested that, in cases of thunderclap headache with normal CT scan, CSF pressure should be determined in addition to the routine CSF examinations. CVST occurs predominantly in young women (Bousser and Ross Russell, 1997) and oral contraceptives, pregnancy, and the puerperium are common risk factors (van den Bergh et al., 2005). Headache may develop because of intracranial hypertension caused by thrombosis in the major sinus.

Cervical artery dissection

Dissection of the extracranial carotid artery should be considered if thunderclap headache is followed after an interval of hours to days by Horner's syndrome, focal cerebral ischemia, or cranial nerve palsies (Silbert et al., 1995; Mokri et al., 1996; Leys et al., 1997; Schievink, 2001). Pain is felt on one side of the face, around the eye, or in the neck. Trauma, neck movement, and connective tissue disorders like fibromuscular dysplasia, Marfan's syndrome, or cystic medial necrosis are possible causes, but often no cause is found (Leys et al., 1997). Dissections occur predominantly in young people (Schievink et al., 1994). The dissection of the internal carotid artery is characteristically a few centimeters distal to the bifurcation, in contrast to atherosclerotic lesions (Leys et al., 1997).

Non-vascular disorders

Patients with spontaneous intracranial hypotension from a spinal fluid leak may also experience thunderclap headache. In one study (Schievink et al., 2001b), 4 of 28 patients with spontaneous intracranial hypotension had thunderclap headaches, and on physical examination 3 had a stiff neck. CT scan was normal and lumbar puncture in 3 patients showed an opening pressure of, at most, 10 cmH_2O. On MRI diffuse pachymeningeal enhancement, brain sagging, or subdural collections were visualized (Mokri et al., 1997). The spinal leak can be detected by CT myelography, radionuclide cisternography, or MRI. All patients have orthostatic headaches, and in the vast majority recumbency relieves the headache (Schievink et al., 1996; Mokri et al., 1997). Pitfalls in differential diagnosis are the occurrence of cranial nerve palsies or CSF xanthochromia due to increased subdural vascular permeability. SAH must be excluded in these cases (Schievink et al., 2001b).

Severe sudden short headache attacks can follow after intermittent obstruction of CSF by a colloid cyst moving in and out of the foramen of Monro on its pedicle (Antunes et al., 1980; Young and Silberstein, 1997). Nausea, vomiting, or even deterioration in level of consciousness is caused by increased intracranial pressure. MRI is the investigation of choice, because on CT 30% of these cysts can be isodense (Young and Silberstein, 1997). The onset of headache in bacterial or viral meningitis is typically gradual, but is occasionally reported as sudden (Linn et al., 1994). Erve virus is described as a rare cause of thunderclap headache (Treib et al., 1998). Sinusitis may also cause headache within seconds (McGeeney et al., 2006).

RADIOLOGICAL INVESTIGATIONS

CT scan of the brain is the first investigation to rule out SAH or another hemorrhage in a patient with thunderclap headache. CT scanning is preferred over MRI in the acute setting because of the wide availability of CT, low costs, and the fast scanning time (Evans, 2001; Ward et al., 2001; Boesiger and Shiber, 2005). In cases of SAH, the blood in the basal cisterns is easily visible as hyperdense. However, the detection of subarachnoid blood depends on the interval from the onset of symptoms, decreasing to 82–98% within 12 h to 50% after 1 week and to nil after 3 weeks (van Gijn and van Dongen, 1982; van der Wee et al., 1995; Sidman et al., 1996; Evans, 2001).

MRI of the brain could be performed in patients with thunderclap headache when CT shows no abnormalities. MRI detects SAH in the posterior fossa easier because there are no beam-hardening artefacts (Ward et al., 2001). MRI is superior to CT in detecting SAH after an interval of 3 days up to 45 days after the ictus (Ogawa et al., 1995; Noguchi et al., 1997) and is useful in late referrals with a negative CT scan but xanthochromia in the CSF. MRI with gradient echo T_2 can reliably demonstrate SAH in the acute phase with a sensitivity of 94%, and 100% in the subacute phase, and fluid-attenuated inversion recovery (FLAIR) techniques with values of 81% and 87% respectively (Noguchi et al., 1995; Mitchell et al., 2001). Other indications for MRI are vascular anomalies such as pituitary apoplexy, arterial dissection, arteriovenous malformation (AVM), and cerebral venous thrombosis (Ward et al., 2001), and MRI is useful to detect diffuse meningeal enhancement in spontaneous intracranial hypotension.

One of the main indications for CT angiography (CTA) is the detection of an intracranial aneurysm. Compared to magnetic resonance angiography (MRA), CTA is more rapid. Available data suggest that CTA has an equal sensitivity (85–98%) to MRA for detecting aneurysms compared to the gold standard, intra-arterial digital subtraction angiography (Wardlaw and White, 2000). With standard time-of-flight MRA techniques, flow-related artifacts may interfere with anatomical details. Other indications to perform MRA are vascular anomalies such as arterial dissection, AVM, or venous thrombosis (Evans, 2001). MRV is useful in the evaluation of patients with suspected cerebral venous thrombosis (Ward et al., 2001), with higher sensitivity compared to MRI (Raizer and DeAngelis, 2000). Cerebral angiography/digital subtraction angiography have been considered the gold standard to detect cerebral aneurysms. Other indications are diagnostic work-up of an AVM, vasculitis, or arterial dissection (Evans, 2001). Disadvantages of this investigation are that it is invasive, expensive, and harbors a (small) risk of complications (Cloft et al., 1999).

Lumbar puncture

All patients with a negative CT scan but a history of acute severe headache should have lumbar puncture to exclude SAH, even if the CT is obtained within the first hours after the onset of hemorrhage. The risk for SAH is 2–3% (van der Wee et al., 1995; Morgenstern et al., 1998) (95% confidence interval 0.4–12%) (van der Wee et al., 1995) in patients who have had an early (negative) CT scan within 12 h of onset of headache (van der Wee et al., 1995). Lumbar puncture should not be done within the first 6 (preferably 12) h after the onset of headache. If there are red cells in the CSF, sufficient lysis will have taken place in this period to detect bilirubin and oxyhemoglobin (Vermeulen and van Gijn, 1990). These pigments give the CSF a yellow color after centrifugation (xanthochromia), and are detectable up to 3 weeks later. Even after 4 weeks the probability of detecting xanthochromia was more than 40% (Vermeulen et al., 1989). Spinning down the CSF should be done immediately, otherwise oxyhemoglobin will form *in vitro*. Absence of blood pigments should be confirmed by spectrophotometry (Vermeulen and van Gijn, 1990; Beetham et al., 1998). The "three-tube test" (a decrease in red cells in three consecutive tubes) is unreliable and may give false-positive results (Heasley et al., 2005). Other important reasons to perform lumbar puncture in patients with thunderclap headache are exclusion of an infectious disorder or cerebral venous thrombosis.

SUMMARY

Thunderclap headache is an uncommon type of headache, but recognition and diagnosis are important because of the possibility of a serious underlying brain disorder. Most importantly, SAH, other intracranial hemorrhages, or cerebral venous thrombosis should be excluded by CT, or, if the CT scan is negative, by examining the CSF. When an underlying intracranial disorder is still suspected, MRI is the investigation of choice. The remaining patients with thunderclap headache have a primary headache disorder, most frequently migraine or primary thunderclap headache. Primary thunderclap headache is a distinct clinical entity and has a relationship with other headaches.

References

Adams HP, Jergenson DD, Kassell NF et al. (1980). Pitfalls in the recognition of subarachnoid hemorrhage. JAMA 244: 794–796.

Antunes JL, Louis KM, Ganti SR (1980). Colloid cysts of the third ventricle. Neurosurgery 7: 450–455.

Ball MJ (1975). Pathogenesis of the "sentinel headache" preceding berry aneurysmal rupture. CMAJ 112: 78–79.

Beetham R, Fahie-Wilson MN, Park D (1998). What is the role of CSF spectrophotometry in the diagnosis of subarachnoid haemorrhage? Ann Clin Biochem 35: 1–4.

Boesiger BM, Shiber JR (2005). Subarachnoid hemorrhage diagnosis by computed tomography and lumbar puncture: are fifth generation CT scanners better at identifying subarachnoid hemorrhage? J Emerg Med 29: 23–27.

Bousser MG, Ross Russell RW (1997). Cerebral Venous Thrombosis. WB Saunders, London.

Call GK, Fleming MC, Sealfon S et al. (1988). Reversible cerebral segmental vasoconstriction. Stroke 19: 1159–1170.

Caplan LR, Baquis GD, Pessin MS et al. (1988). Dissection of the intracranial vertebral artery. Neurology 38: 868–877.

Chen SP, Fuh JL, Lirng JF et al. (2006). Is vasospasm requisite for posterior leukoencephalopathy in patients with primary thunderclap headaches? Cephalalgia 26: 530–536.

Clarke CE, Shepherd DI, Chishti K et al. (1988). Thunderclap headache. Lancet ii: 625.

Cloft HJ, Joseph GJ, Dion JE (1999). Risk of cerebral angiography in patients with subarachnoid hemorrhage, cerebral aneurysm, and arteriovenous malformation. A meta-analysis. Stroke 30: 317–320.

Cummings TJ, Johnson RR, Diaz FG et al. (2000). The relationship of blunt head trauma, subarachnoid hemorrhage, and rupture of pre-existing intracranial saccular aneurysms. Neurol Res 22: 165–170.

Cumurciuc R, Crassard I, Sarov M et al. (2005). Headache as the only neurological sign of cerebral venous thrombosis: a series of 17 cases. J Neurol Neurosurg Psychiatry 76: 1084–1087.

Dalessio DJ (1994). Diagnosing the severe headache. Neurology 44 (Suppl. 3): S6–S12.

Day JW, Raskin NH (1986). Thunderclap headache: symptom of unruptured cerebral aneurysm. Lancet ii: 1247–1248.

de Bruijn SFTM, Stam J, Kappelle LJ et al. (1996). Thunderclap headache as first symptom of cerebral venous sinus thrombosis. Lancet 348: 1623–1625.

Dodick DW, Wijdicks EFM (1998). Pituitary apoplexy presenting as a thunderclap headache. Neurology 50: 1510–1511.

Edlow JA, Caplan LR (2000). Avoiding pitfalls in the diagnosis of subarachnoid hemorrhage. N Engl J Med 342: 29–36.

Evans RW (1996). Diagnostic testing for the evaluation of headaches. Neurol Clin 14: 1–26.

Evans RW (2001). Diagnostic testing for headache. Med Clin North Am 85: 865–885.

Ferro JM, Melo TP, Oliveira V et al. (1995). A multivariate study of headache associated with ischemic stroke. Headache 35: 315–319.

Finelli PF (1993). Coital cerebral hemorrhage. Neurology 43: 2683–2685.

Fisher CM (1984). Painful states: a neurological commentatory. Clin Neurosurg 31: 32–53.

Fodden DI, Peatfield RC, Milsom PL (1989). Beware the patient with a headache in the accident and emergency department. Arch Emerg Med 6: 7–12.

Frese A, Eikermann A, Frese K et al. (2003). Headache associated with sexual activity: demography, clinical features, and comorbidity. Neurology 61: 796–800.

Gerritsen van der Hoop R, Vermeulen M, van Gijn J (1988). Cerebellar hemorrhage: diagnosis and treatment. Surg Neurol 29: 6–10.

Goadsby PJ (2006). Recent advances in the diagnosis and management of migraine. BMJ 332: 25–29.

Gorelick PB, Hier DB, Caplan LR et al. (1986). Headache in acute cerebrovascular disease. Neurology 36: 1445–1450.

Green MW (2003). The emergency management of headaches. Neurologist 9: 93–98.

Hajj-Ali RA, Furlan A, Bou-Chebel A et al. (2002). Benign angiopathy of the central nervous system: cohort of 16 patients with clinical course and long-term followup. Arthritis Rheum 47: 662–669.

Harling DW, Peatfield RC, van Hille PT et al. (1989). Thunderclap headache: is it migraine? Cephalalgia 9: 87–90.

Hart RG, Foster JW, Luther MF et al. (1990). Stroke in infective endocarditis. Stroke 21: 695–700.

Headache Classification Subcommittee of the International Headache Society (2004). The international classification of headache disorders, 2nd edn. Cephalalgia 24 (Suppl. 1): 1–151.

Heasley DC, Mohamed MA, Yousem DM (2005). Clearing of red blood cells in lumbar puncture does not rule out ruptured aneurysm in patients with suspected subarachnoid hemorrhage but negative head CT findings. AJNR Am J Neuroradiol 26: 820–824.

Johnston CS, Dudley RA, Gress DR et al. (1999). Surgical and endovascular treatment of unruptured cerebral aneurysms at university hospitals. Neurology 52: 1799–1805.

Jorgensen HS, Jespersen HF, Nakayama H et al. (1994). Headache in stroke: The Copenhagen Stroke Study. Neurology 44: 1793–1797.

Kai Y, Hamada J, Morioka M et al. (2005). Arteriovenous fistulas at the cervicomedullary junction presenting with subarachnoid hemorrhage: six case reports with special reference to the angiographic pattern of venous drainage. AJNR Am J Neuroradiol 26: 1949–1954.

King RB, Saba MI (1974). Forewarnings of major subarachnoid hemorrhage. N Y State J Med 74: 638–639.

Kotwica Z, Brzezinski J (1985). Chronic subdural hamatoma presenting as spontaneous subarachnoid hemorrhage. Report of six cases. J Neurosurg 63: 691–692.

Kumar R, Wijdicks EFM, Brown RD Jr et al. (1997). Isolated angiitis of the CNS presenting as subarachnoid haemorrhage. J Neurol Neurosurg Psychiatry 62: 649–651.

Lance JW (1976). Headaches related to sexual activity. J Neurol Neurosurg Psychiatry 39: 1226–1230.

Landtblom AM, Fridriksson S, Boivie J et al. (2002). Sudden onset headache: a prospective study of features, incidence and causes. Cephalalgia 22: 354–360.

Lane JC, Gulevich S (2002). Exertional, cough, and sexual headaches. Curr Treat Options Neurol 4: 375–381.

Levine SR, Brust JC, Futrell N et al. (1990). Cerebrovascular complications of the use of the 'crack' from of alkaloidal cocaine. N Engl J Med 323: 699–704.

Leys D, Lucas C, Gobert M et al. (1997). Cervical artery dissections. Eur Neurol 37: 3–12.

Linn FHH, Wijdicks EFM, van der Graaf Y et al. (1994). Prospective study of sentinel headache in aneurysmal subarachnoid haemorrhage. Lancet 344: 590–593.

Linn FHH, Rinkel GJE, Algra A et al. (1998). Headache characteristics in subarachnoid haemorrhage and benign thunderclap headache. J Neurol Neurosurg Psychiatry 65: 791–793.

Linn FHH, Rinkel GJ, Algra A et al. (1999). Follow-up of idiopathic thunderclap headache in general practice. J Neurol 246: 946–948.

Markus H (1991). A prospective follow up of thunderclap headache mimicking subarachnoid haemorrhage. J Neurol Neurosurg Psychiatry 54: 1117–1118.

Mathew P, Teasdale G, Bannan A et al. (1995). Neurosurgical management of cerebellar haematoma and infarct. J Neurol Neurosurg Psychiatry 59: 287–292.

Mayer PL, Awad IA, Todor R et al. (1996). Misdiagnosis of symptomatic cerebral aneurysm. Prevalence and correlation with outcome at four institutions. Stroke 27: 1558–1563.

McFadzean RM, Doyle D, Rampling R et al. (1991). Pituitary apoplexy and its effect on vision. Neurosurgery 29: 669–675.

McGeeney BE, Barest G, Grillone G (2006). Thunderclap headache from complicated sinusitis. Headache 46: 517–520.

Melo TP, Pinto AN, Ferro JM (1996). Headache in intracerebral hematomas. Neurology 47: 494–500.

Mitchell P, Wilkinson ID, Hoggard N et al. (2001). Detection of subarachnoid haemorrhage with magnetic resonance imaging. J Neurol Neurosurg Psychiatry 70: 205–211.

Mokri B, Silbert PL, Schievink WI et al. (1996). Cranial nerve palsy in spontaneous dissection of the extracranial internal carotid artery. Neurology 46: 356–359.

Mokri B, Piepgras DG, Miller GM (1997). Syndrome of orthostatic headaches and diffuse pachymeningeal gadolinium enhancement. Mayo Clin Proc 72: 400–413.

Morgenstern LB, Luna-Gonzales H, Huber JC et al. (1998). Worst headache and subarachnoid hemorrhage: prospective, modern computed tomography and spinal fluid analysis. Ann Emerg Med 32: 297–304.

Neiman J, Haapaniemi HM, Hillbom M (2000). Neurological complications of drug abuse: pathophysiological mechanisms. Eur J Neurol 7: 595–606.

Newman LC, Goadsby P, Lipton RB (2001). Cluster and related headaches. Med Clin North Am 85: 997–1016.

Noguchi K, Ogawa T, Inugami A et al. (1995). Acute subarachnoid hemorrhage: MR imaging with fluid-attenuated inversion recovery pulse sequences. Radiology 196: 773–777.

Noguchi K, Ogawa T, Seto H et al. (1997). Subacute and chronic subarachnoid hemorrhage: diagnosis with fluid-attenuated inversion-recovery MR imaging. Radiology 203: 257–262.

Ogawa T, Inugami A, Fujita H et al. (1995). MR diagnosis of subacute and chronic subarachnoid hemorrhage: comparison with CT. Am J Radiol 165: 1257–1262.

Pascual J, Iglesias F, Oterino A et al. (1996). Cough, exertional, and sexual headaches: an analysis of 72 benign and symptomatic cases. Neurology 46: 1520–1524.

Pinto AN, Canhao P, Ferro JM (1996). Seizures at the onset of subarachnoid hemorrhage. J Neurol 243: 161–164.

Polmear A (2003). Sentinel headaches in aneurysmal subarachnoid haemorrhage: what is the true incidence? A systematic review. Cephalalgia 23: 935–941.

Raizer JJ, DeAngelis LM (2000). Cerebral venous thrombosis diagnosed by MRI and MR venography in cancer patients. Neurology 54: 1222–1226.

Ramirez-Lassepas M, Espinosa CE, Cicero JJ et al. (1997). Predictors of intracranial pathologic findings in patients who seek emergency care because of headache. Arch Neurol 54: 1506–1509.

Rinkel GJE, Wijdicks EFM, Vermeulen M et al. (1991). The clinical course of perimesencephalic nonaneurysmal subarachnoid hemorrhage. Ann Neurol 29: 463–468.

Rinkel GJE, van Gijn J, Wijdicks EFM (1993). Subarachnoid hemorrhage without detectable aneurysm. A review of the causes. Stroke 24: 1403–1409.

Rooke ED (1968). Benign exertional headache. Med Clin North Am 52: 801–808.

Saeed AB, Shuaib A, Al-Sulaiti G et al. (2000). Vertebral artery dissection: warning symptoms, clinical features and prognosis in 26 patients. Can J Neurol Sci 27: 292–296.

Sakas DE, Dias LS, Beale D (1995). Subarachnoid haemorrhage presenting as head injury. BMJ 310: 1186–1187.

Sands GH, Newman L, Lipton R (1991). Cough, exertional, and other miscellaneous headaches. Med Clin North Am 75: 733–747.

Schievink WI (2001). Spontaneous dissection of the carotid and vertebral arteries. N Engl J Med 344: 898–906.

Schievink WI, Mokri B, Piepgras DG (1994). Spontaneous dissections of cervicocephalic arteries in childhood and adolescence. Neurology 44: 1607–1612.

Schievink WI, Meyer FB, Atkinson JLD et al. (1996). Spontaneous spinal cerebrospinal fluid leaks and intracranial hypotension. J Neurosurg 84: 598–605.

Schievink WI, Thompson RC, Loh CT et al. (2001a). Spontaneous retroclival hematoma presenting as a thunderclap headache. J Neurosurg 95: 522–524.

Schievink WI, Wijdicks EFM, Meyer FB et al. (2001b). Spontaneous intracranial hypotension mimicking aneurysmal subarachnoid hemorrhage. J Neurosurg 48: 513–517.

Schwartz TH, Solomon RA (1996). Perimesencephalic nonaneurysmal subarachnoid hemorrhage: review of the literature. Neurosurgery 39: 433–440.

Schwedt TJ, Dodick DW (2006). Thunderclap stroke: embolic cerebellar infarcts presenting as thunderclap headache. Headache 46: 520–522.

Schwedt TJ, Matharu MS, Dodick DW (2006). Thunderclap headache. Lancet Neurol 5: 621–631.

Semple PL, Webb MK, de Villiers JC et al. (2005). Pituitary apoplexy. Neurosurgery 56: 65–72.

Sidman R, Connolly E, Lemke T (1996). Subarachnoid hemorrhage diagnosis: lumbar puncture is still needed when the computed tomography scan is normal. Acad Emerg Med 3: 827 831.

Silbert PL, Hankey G, Prentice DA et al. (1989). Angiographically demonstrated arterial spasm in a case of benign sexual headache and benign exertional headache. Aust N Z J Med 19: 466–468.

Silbert PL, Mokri B, Schievink WI (1995). Headache and neck pain in spontaneous internal carotid and vertebral artery dissections. Neurology 45: 1517–1522.

Singhal AB, Caviness VS, Begleiter AF et al. (2002). Cerebral vasoconstriction and stroke after use of serotonergic drugs. Neurology 58: 130–133.

Slivka A, Philbrook B (1995). Clinical and angiographic features of thunderclap headache. Headache 35: 1–6.

Stam J (2005). Thrombosis of the cerebral veins and sinuses. N Engl J Med 352: 1791–1798.

Tang-Wai DF, Phan TG, Wijdicks EFM (2001). Hypertensive encephalopathy presenting with thunderclap headache. Headache 41: 198–200.

Tentschert S, Wimmer R, Greisenegger S et al. (2005). Headache at stroke onset in 2196 patients with ischemic stroke or transient ischemic attack. Stroke 36: e1–e3.

The International Study of Unruptured Intracranial Aneurysms Investigators (1998). Unruptured intracranial aneurysms – risk of rupture and risks of surgical intervention. N Engl J Med 339: 1725–1733.

Treib J, Dobler G, Haass A et al. (1998). Thunderclap headache caused by Erve virus? Neurology 50: 509–511.

van den Bergh WM, van der Schaaf I, van Gijn J (2005). The spectrum of presentations of venous infarction caused by deep cerebral vein thrombosis. Neurology 65: 192–196.

van der Wee N, Rinkel GJE, Hasan D et al. (1995). Detection of subarachnoid haemorrhage on early CT: is lumbar puncture still needed after a negative scan? J Neurol Neurosurg Psychiatry 58: 357–359.

van Gijn J (1997). Slip-ups in diagnosis of subarachnoid haemorrhage. Lancet 63: 1492.

van Gijn J (1999). Pitfalls in the diagnosis of sudden headache. Proc R Coll Physicians Edinb 29: 21–31.

van Gijn J, van Dongen KJ (1982). The time course of aneurysmal haemorrhage on computed tomograms. Neuroradiology 23: 153–156.

Vermeulen M, van Gijn J (1990). The diagnosis of subarachnoid haemorrhage. J Neurol Neurosurg Psychiatry 53: 365–372.

Vermeulen M, Lindsay KW, Cheah F et al. (1984). Antifibrinolytic treatment in subarachnoid hemorrhage. N Engl J Med 311: 432–437.

Vermeulen M, Hasan D, Blijenberg BG et al. (1989). Xanthochromia after subarachnoid hemorrhage needs no revisitation. J Neurol Neurosurg Psychiatry 52: 826–828.

Ward TN, Levin M, Phillips JM (2001). Evaluation and management of headache in the emergency department. Med Clin North Am 85: 971–985.

Wardlaw JM, White PM (2000). The detection and management of unruptured intracranial aneurysms. Brain 123: 205–221.

Wijdicks EF, Kerkhoff H, van Gijn J (1988). Long-term follow-up of 71 patients with thunderclap headache mimicking subarachnoid haemorrhage. Lancet ii: 68–70.

Witham TF, Kaufmann AM (2000). Unruptured cerebral aneurysm producing a thunderclap headache. Am J Emerg Med 18: 88–90.

Young WB, Silberstein SD (1997). Paroxysmal headache caused by colloid cyst of the third ventricle: case report and review of the literature. Headache 37: 15–20.

Handbook of Clinical Neurology, Vol. 97 (3rd series)
Headache
G. Nappi and M.A. Moskowitz, Editors

Chapter 43

Hemicrania continua

FABIO ANTONACI [1] AND OTTAR SJAASTAD [2]*

[1]*University Centre for Adaptive Disorders and Headache (UCADH) Pavia, Headache Medicine Centre, Department of Neurology Policlinic of Monza, Monza, Italy*

[2]*Department of Neurology, St. Olavs Hospital, Trondheim University Hospitals, Trondheim, Norway*

Hemicrania continua (HC), like chronic paroxysmal hemicrania (CPH), is an indomethacin-responsive headache. While other unilateral headaches accompanied by local autonomic phenomena are intermittent, short-lasting headaches, HC is characterized by a continuous course. HC varies in intensity, but, in the form observed in practice, it does not usually disappear entirely. HC was first described by Sjaastad and Spierings (1984). Since that initial description, more than 130 cases have been described.

EPIDEMIOLOGY

Neither the incidence nor the prevalence of HC is known exactly. Generally, HC has been regarded as a rare syndrome; however, some headache clinics that have systematically searched for HC have reported a considerable number of patients; this suggests that the condition may be underdiagnosed (Peres et al., 2001; Wheeler et al., 2001). The fact that HC was not detected among 1838 parishioners in Vågå (Norway) shows that there are certain limitations. There is a female preponderance: the sex ratio is approximately 5. Age of onset varied between 19 and 58 years, with a mean of 35.2 years (Bordini et al., 1991). The range may probably be wider.

CLINICAL FEATURES

HC is basically a continuous headache; HC is also in principle a unilateral headache (Sjaastad and Spierings, 1984). In unilateral headaches, there is a minor tendency to bilaterality, e.g., in CPH about 3–4%. One case of bilaterality (Pasquier et al., 1987) and a couple of cases of side-shift that have been described (Newman et al., 1992) are possibly acceptable. These occasional exceptions should be regarded as oddities. The forehead and temporo-orbital area are the principal sites of pain, although any part of the head can be affected (Bordini et al., 1991). Typically, the pain is mild to moderate in intensity. Pain quality is dull, aching, or pressing. Exacerbations are super imposed upon the continuous pain. Exacerbations can last 20 min to several days. Nocturnal exacerbations can be mistaken for cluster headache or hypnic headache. Exacerbations may be associated with cranial autonomic and migrainous features.

Local autonomic symptoms, mostly ipsilateral lacrimation and conjunctival injection and nasal stuffiness (Bordini et al., 1991), are present in approximately one-third of HC patients but are not as prominent as in cluster headache or CPH. Migrainous features (photophobia, phonophobia, nausea, and throbbing) are common during exacerbations. Migrainous visual aura may occur in association with exacerbations of HC (Peres et al., 2002). There is a paucity of precipitating factors: menses and alcohol have been mentioned (Bordini et al., 1991). Neck movements do not trigger exacerbations, although occipital tenderness has been claimed to be present in about 70% of patients (Newman et al., 1994; Peres et al., 2001). These are apparently uncontrolled data.

The extent to which cervicogenic headache (CEH) is intermingled with HC is unknown (Sjaastad et al., 1993). Primary stabbing headaches may occur (41%), predominantly during the exacerbations (Peres et al., 2001). This figure should be compared with the figure of 35% in the general population (Sjaastad et al., 2001). The diagnostic criteria of HC according to the International Classification of Headache Disorders (ICDH-II: Headache Classification Subcommittee of the International Headache Society, 2004) are presented in Table 43.1. It is worrying that our first case (Sjaastad and Spierings, 1984) would not have been

*Correspondence to: Ottar Sjaastad, Department of Neurology, St. Olavs Hospital, Trondheim University Hospitals, 7006 Trondheim, Norway, Fax: +47 73 525276, E-mail: tora.rui@ntnu.no

Table 43.1

Diagnostic criteria for hemicrania continua according to the International Classification of Headache Disorders, 2nd edition (Headache Classification Subcommittee of the International Headache Society, 2004)

A. Headache for >3 months fulfilling criteria B–D
B. All of the following characteristics:
  1. Unilateral pain without side-shift
  2. Daily and continuous pain without pain-free periods
  3. Moderate intensity, but with exacerbations of severe pain
C. At least one of the following autonomic features occurs during exacerbations and ipsilateral to the side of pain:
  1. Conjunctival injection and/or lacrimation
  2. Nasal congestion and/or rhinorrhea
  3. Ptosis and/or miosis
D. Complete response to therapeutic doses of indomethacin
E. Not attributed to another disorder

recognized if "the autonomic features section" of the criteria had existed at the time. In other words, the criteria have regrettable shortcomings.

PATHOGENESIS

Matharu et al. (2004) demonstrated activation of the contralateral posterior hypothalamus and ipsilateral dorsal rostral pons in indomethacin-sensitive HC ($n = 7$). There are several issues that remain unresolved in the understanding of HC and similar headache pathophysiology. To the best of our knowledge, it has not been demonstrated where indomethacin or active metabolites have their effect in the central nervous system. Cerebrospinal fluid in the dog contained much lower concentrations of radioactivity after labeled indomethacin administration than plasma. The same was true in 1 human subject (Hucker et al., 1966).

Orbital phlebography ($n = 10$), blockade of the greater/minor occipital and supraorbital nerves ($n = 7$), and forehead sweating were all without gross pathology. Pupillometry did not show any gross abnormalities of sympathetic function (Antonaci, 1998). Quantification of lacrimation, nasal secretion, and salivation ($n = 2$) showed no asymmetries (Sjaastad et al., 1984). End-tidal carbon dioxide monitoring and vagal nerve function tests ($n = 2$) were normal. Corneal indentation pulse amplitudes showed a slight asymmetry (<15%; most marked on the symptomatic side) in 1 patient, whereas intraocular pressure was normal in both (Sjaastad et al., 1984).

TEMPORAL PATTERN

Like cluster headache and CPH, HC can also be classified in an episodic and chronic form. HC is frequently primary chronic. Prior to the chronic stage, there may be a recurrent stage, observed already in our third case (Sjaastad and Tjörstad, 1987). Although 10 of 18 HC patients had started out with a recurrent pattern, only 2 remained in this stage at examination (Bordini et al., 1991; Sjaastad and Antonaci, 1993). A transition from chronic to remitting stage has also been observed (Pareja, 1995). In some patients, the remitting stage may be long lasting.

SECONDARY HEMICRANIA CONTINUA AND ASSOCIATED DISORDERS

C7 root irritation caused by a cervical disc herniation seemed to have aggravated the condition in one case (Sjaastad et al., 1995). A patient with human immunodeficiency virus (HIV) developed HC, by chance or not (Brilla et al., 1998). A patient in whom the indomethacin response faded after 2 months proved to have a mesenchymal tumor in the sphenoid bone (Antonaci and Sjaastad, 1992). Patients with escalating indomethacin requirement or loss of efficacy should be re-evaluated (Sjaastad et al., 1995). Two patients developed secondary HC after internal carotid artery dissection (Rogalewski and Evers, 2004).

In 8 cases of "posttraumatic HC," the temporal relationship between trauma and HC onset was variable (Lay and Newman, 1999). Cases of HC with aura and side-shift of pain (Peres et al., 2006); migraine with aura, transformed into HC with aura (Palmieri et al., 2004); HC originating within the postpartum period (Spitz and Peres, 2004); HC with contralateral episodic cluster headache (Lisotto et al., 2003); HC evolved from episodic paroxysmal hemicrania (Castellanos-Pinedo et al., 2006); and a clinical picture resembling HC, but attributed to an unruptured saccular aneurysm (Vikelis et al., 2005) have been reported. Relating these constellations does not imply that we in any way commit ourselves as to the messages conveyed.

DIFFERENTIAL DIAGNOSES

Differential diagnoses of long-lasting unilateral headache include: (1) HC (primary and symptomatic forms); (2) so-called unilateral chronic migraine; (3) CEH; and (4) CPH and other similar headaches that can be associated with interictal, dull ache.

HC can be readily differentiated from unilateral chronic migraine by the responsiveness to indomethacin. CEH is characterized by: (1) unilateral pain, initially in the neck/occipital region, the pain eventually radiating anteriorly; (2) precipitation/aggravation of headache by neck movements/sustained uncomfortable neck posture or external pressure; (3) limitation of neck movements; and (4) discomfort in the ipsilateral neck and shoulder, none of which applies in HC. Moreover, the response to indomethacin is absolute in HC, but not in CEH (Sjaastad et al., 1993). Various clinical features help to distinguish HC from CPH. First, in CPH exacerbations are short-lasting (mean: 13 min; range: 2–45 min), whereas those in HC are longer-lasting. Secondly, the intensity in CPH is excruciating, whereas in HC it is moderate (or severe). A biological marker will be required to gain insight into how best to differentiate between these syndromes (Antonaci, 1998).

INVESTIGATIONS

Diagnosis is based on clinical history, neurological examination, and a therapeutic trial of indomethacin. Cases of unilateral, chronic headache should have an indomethacin trial. Brain computed tomography and magnetic resonance imaging (MRI) of brain/cervical spine have demonstrated cervical degeneration changes, but no systematic, grave pathology. Four-vessel angiography has revealed no pathology ($n = 3$) (Bordini et al., 1991). An MRI brain scan is a reasonable screening investigation to exclude a symptomatic form of HC. If there is no response to indomethacin, further work-up should be carried out.

TREATMENT

Indomethacin is the drug of choice in HC as well as CPH. Sumatriptan is without effect in HC (Antonaci, 1998). Prophylatic therapy gives a prompt, complete, and enduring response. The effective dose of indomethacin ranges from 25 to 150 mg/day (Bordini et al., 1991). Dosage titration is necessary to cope with clinical fluctuations. Skipping or delaying doses may result in recurrence. “Indotest,” i.e., indomethacin 50–100 mg intramuscularly, has been proposed as a diagnostic test for HC (Antonaci et al., 1998). The Indotest has the advantage that the diagnosis can be rapidly established, with complete pain relief occurring within 2 h. Indotest is likely to become the test of choice in chronic unilateral headache.

Concurrent treatment with gastric mucosa-protective agents is probably obligatory with courses of indomethacin of some length. Indomethacin does not exert any curative effect upon the basic disorder; it keeps the situation at bay, without any tachyphylaxis. Besides the indomethacin test, indomethacin discontinuation verification plays a crucial role for the diagnosis. The fact that the pain returns upon indomethacin discontinuation is a strong testimony, as regards HC, perhaps even stronger than that of the Indotest itself. It is only when this test is positive that the diagnosis can be considered as finally being established. If pain does not recur upon indomethacin discontinuation, this indicates that either: the pain has disappeared spontaneously, or: the diagnosis is wrong. In the first case, the HC may be in a recurring stage. Another indomethacin discontinuation test must then be carried out, during another bout, to verify the diagnosis. Cases to be reported in the future should follow this standard; they have not invariably done that in the past.

The site of action of indomethacin may be in the periphery or centrally. Kuritzky (1992) has described 4 cases of HC, non-responsive to indomethacin. Indomethacin response is an indisputable requirement in HC. The Kuritzky cases are accordingly unacceptable as HC; there is no proof for HC in Kuritzky’s cases. One or more of them may have CEH. Since indomethacin response is a fundamental quality of HC, the Goadsby–Lipton proposal (1997) to accommodate indomethacin-negative cases is, therefore, beside the point. Indomethacin-resistant patients are not likely to be true cases of HC. Until the underlying pathophysiology of HC and the mode of action of indomethacin are better understood, it is prudent in clinical practice to diagnose HC only in patients with an unquestionable response to indomethacin.

There seems to have been a recent wave of revisionism, to the effect that HC was described in 1982 as “atypical cluster headache,” a syndrome responsive to indomethacin (Diamond et al., 1982). Indomethacin response is a hallmark of the HC. HC is, according to Matharu et al. (2004), “exquisitely responsive to indomethacin.” It is, therefore, highly surprising to know that only 50% of Diamond’s cases showed a complete indomethacin response, and that in 17% there was no response at all. And with the most pure form of “background vascular headache” (solely together with “multiple jabs”), only 1 of 8 patients responded “excellently” to indomethacin. Unilaterality of headache is another characteristic of HC. In only 67% of the “atypical cluster headache” cases was there unilaterality – and even side-shift in 30%.

Other drugs reported to have been partially or even completely effective, frequently in isolated cases, include ibuprofen, piroxicam, betadextrin, naproxen, aspirin, paracetamol with caffeine, and melatonin. Other non-steroidal anti-inflammatory drugs are generally less efficient than indomethacin. A positive response to verapamil was apparently observed in 2 patients, and in 2 patients there was a response to topiramate (Matharu et al., 2005). Occipital nerve stimulation was reported to improve pain in 1 case (Schwedt et al., 2006). This patient might not be a genuine case of HC.

NATURAL HISTORY AND PROGNOSIS

HC is a recently described disorder; its natural history is still being outlined. At this stage, it may seem to be a lifelong disorder in most cases. Patients should discontinue indomethacin at least every 6 months to ensure that they still have headache. The titrated dose should be the minimum effective one. Some patients prefer to use a rather low dosage and have a little pain, as a "sentinel" against overuse. The first case of HC described was treated with indomethacin for 19 years (Sjaastad, 2006). There was no tachyphylaxis, and intensity and other headache characteristics were unchanged.

As with CPH, patients with HC can thus expect an enduring response to indomethacin without developing tachyphylaxis. Almost a quarter develop gastrointestinal adverse effects (Pareja et al., 2001). Indomethacin does not seem to alter the long-term course; some patients experience a decrease in indomethacin requirement over time.

References

Antonaci F (1998). Chronic paroxysmal hemicrania and hemicrania continua: two different entities? Thesis. Tapir, NTNU publisher, Trondheim.

Antonaci F, Sjaastad O (1992). Hemicrania continua: a possible symptomatic case due to mesenchymal tumor. Funct Neurol 7: 471–474.

Antonaci F, Pareja JA, Caminero AB et al. (1998). Chronic paroxysmal hemicrania and hemicrania continua: parenteral indomethacin: the "Indotest". Headache 38: 122–128.

Bordini C, Antonaci F, Stovner LJ et al. (1991). "Hemicrania continua": a clinical review. Headache 31: 20–26.

Brilla R, Evers S, Soros P et al. (1998). Hemicrania continua in an HIV-infected outpatient. Cephalalgia 18: 287–288.

Castellanos-Pinedo F, Zurdo M, Martinez-Acebes E (2006). Hemicrania continua evolving from episodic paroxysmal hemicrania. Cephalalgia 26: 1143–1145.

Diamond S, Magabgab E, Diamond M (1982). Cluster headache variant: spectrum of a new headache syndrome responsive to indomethacin. In: FC Rose (Ed.), Advances in Migraine Research and Therapy. Raven Press, New York, pp. 57–65.

Goadsby PJ, Lipton RB (1997). A review of paroxysmal hemicranias. SUNCT syndrome and other short-lasting headaches with autonomic features including new cases. Brain 120: 193–209.

Headache Classification Subcommittee of the International Headache Society (2004). The international classification of headache disorders, 2nd edn. Cephalalgia 24: 1–195.

Hucker HB, Zacchei AG, Cox SV et al. (1966). Studies of the absorption, distribution, and excretion of indomethacin in various species. J Pharmacol Exp Ther 153: 237–249.

Kuritzky A (1992). Indomethacin-resistant hemicrania continua. Cephalalgia 12: 57–59.

Lay C, Newman LC (1999). Posttraumatic hemicrania continua. Headache 39: 275–279.

Lisotto C, Mainardi F, Maggioni F et al. (2003). Hemicrania continua with contralateral episodic cluster headache: a case report. Cephalalgia 23: 929–930.

Matharu MS, Cohen AS, McGonigle DJ et al. (2004). Posterior hypothalamic and brainstem activation in hemicrania continua. Headache 44: 747–761.

Matharu MS, Bradbury P, Swash M (2005). Hemicrania continua: side alternation and response to topiramate. Cephalalgia 26: 341–344.

Newman LC, Lipton RB, Russell M et al. (1992). Hemicrania continua: attacks may alternate sides. Headache 32: 237–238.

Newman LC, Lipton RB, Solomon S (1994). Hemicrania continua: ten new cases and a review of the literature. Neurology 44: 2111–2114.

Palmieri A, Mainardi F, Maggioni F et al. (2004). Hemicrania continua evolving from migraine with aura: clinical evidence of a possible correlation between two forms of primary headache. Cephalalgia 24: 1007–1008.

Pareja JA (1995). Hemicrania continua: remitting stage evolved from the chronic form. Headache 35: 161–162.

Pareja JA, Caminero AB, Franco E et al. (2001). Dose, efficacy and tolerability of long-term indomethacin treatment of chronic paroxysmal hemicrania and hemicrania continua. Cephalalgia 21: 906–910.

Pasquier F, Leys D, Petit H (1987). Hemicrania continua: the first bilateral case. Cephalalgia 7: 169–170.

Peres MFP, Silberstein SD, Nahmias S et al. (2001). Hemicrania continua is not that rare. Neurology 57: 948–951.

Peres MFP, Siow HC, Rozen TD (2002). Hemicrania continua with aura. Cephalalgia 22: 246–248.

Peres MFP, Masruha MR, Young WB (2006). Side-shifting hemicrania continua with aura (migraine with aura with autonomic symptoms responsive to indomethacin?). Cephalalgia 26: 917–919.

Rogalewski A, Evers S (2004). Symptomatic hemicrania continua after internal carotid artery dissection. Headache 45: 167–169.

Schwedt TJ, Dodick DW, Trentman TL et al. (2006). Occipital nerve stimulation for chronic cluster headache and hemicrania continua: pain relief and persistence of autonomic features. Cephalalgia 26: 1025–1027.

Sjaastad O (2006). Chronic paroxysmal hemicrania, hemicrania continua and SUNCT: the fate of the three first described cases. J Headache Pain 7: 151–156.

Sjaastad O, Antonaci F (1993). Chronic paroxysmal hemicrania (CPH) and hemicrania continua: transition from one stage to another. Headache 33: 551–554.

Sjaastad O, Spierings EL (1984). Hemicrania continua: another headache absolutely responsive to indomethacin. Cephalalgia 4: 65–70.

Sjaastad O, Tjörstad K (1987). Hemicrania continua: a third Norwegian case. Cephalalgia 7: 175–177.

Sjaastad O, Spierings EL, Saunte C et al. (1984). "Hemicrania continua". An indomethacin responsive headache. II. Autonomic function studies. Cephalalgia 4: 265–273.

Sjaastad O, Joubert J, Elsås T et al. (1993). Hemicrania continua and cervicogenic headache: separate headaches or two faces of the same headache? Funct Neurol 8: 79–83.

Sjaastad O, Stovner LJ, Stolt-Nielsen A et al. (1995). CPH and hemicrania continua: requirements of high dose indomethacin dosages: an ominous sign? Headache 35: 363–367.

Sjaastad O, Pettersen H, Bakketeig LS (2001). The Vågå study; epidemiology of headache I: the prevalence of ultrashort paroxysms. Cephalalgia 3: 207–215.

Spitz M, Peres MFP (2004). Hemicrania continua postpartum. Cephalalgia 24: 603–604.

Vikelis M, Xifars M, Magoufis G et al. (2005). Headache attributed to unruptured saccular aneurysm, mimicking hemicrania continua. J Headache Pain 6: 156–158.

Wheeler SD, Allen KF, Pusey T (2001). Is hemicrania continua a migraine variant? Cephalalgia 21: 508.

Handbook of Clinical Neurology, Vol. 97 (3rd series)
Headache
G. Nappi and M.A. Moskowitz, Editors

Chapter 44

New daily persistent headache

TODD D. ROZEN*
Department of Neurology, Geisinger Headache Center, Geisinger Medical Center, Wilkes-Barre, PA, USA

INTRODUCTION

New daily persistent headache (NDPH) was first described by Vanast in 1986 as a benign form of chronic daily headache (CDH) that improved without therapy. In the headache specialist's office NDPH is anything but benign and is felt to be one of the most treatment-refractory of all headache conditions. Very little is known about this syndrome. It is unique in that the headache begins daily from onset, typically in a patient with no prior headache history, and can continue for years, without any sign of alleviation, despite aggressive treatment. It seems that only in the last several years has NDPH been recognized as a distinct headache syndrome by the headache community. NDPH is one of the primary headache disorders in that no underlying secondary cause can be identified. However, there are secondary conditions that can present as a daily headache from onset, which must be ruled out before a diagnosis of primary NDPH can be made.

DIAGNOSTIC CRITERIA

NDPH has been included in the second edition of the International Classification of Headache Disorders (ICHD-II) criteria (Table 44.1; Headache Classification Subcommittee of the International Headache Society, 2004). As there have been only a few studies looking at the clinical characteristics of NDPH, these consensus criteria may not reflect what is seen in everyday practice and they will most likely need to be modified over time, as more data on this syndrome are published. The ICHD-II criteria reflect almost a daily form of tension-type headache, although migrainous features have certainly been identified in this patient population (see below).

It appears that there are two subtypes of NDPH: a self-limited form which typically goes away within several months without any therapy and never presents to a physician's office (at least a neurologist or headache specialist's office), and a refractory form which is basically resistant to aggressive outpatient and inpatient treatment. In Vanast's original description of NDPH (Vanast, 1986), he described the self-limited subtype and referred to NDPH as a benign daily headache.

EPIDEMIOLOGY

Even though NDPH has probably been around for centuries, it has only recently been diagnosed as an entity separate from chronic tension-type headache, hemicrania continua, and chronic migraine. The prevalence of CDH from population-based studies in the USA, Asia, and Europe is about 4% (Silberstein and Lipton, 2001). In those epidemiological investigations, primary CDH subtypes are sometimes not mentioned in the analysis and NDPH is rarely stratified out from the data. Several studies have documented the prevalence of NDPH. Castillo et al. (1999) looked at 2252 subjects in Spain and found that 4.7% of the population had CDH, of whom 0.1% had NDPH. Bigal et al. (2002) noted that 10.8% of 638 patients with CDH in a headache specialty clinic had NDPH. Koenig et al. (2002) found that 13% of a pediatric CDH population, surveyed from selected pediatric headache specialty clinics, had NDPH. Meineri et al. (2004) from Italy diagnosed NDPH in 18 of 265 CDH patients (6.8%) while Wang et al. (2006) did not find a single adolescent with NDPH in a survey of 122 children from Taiwan with CDH, although this population was very age-restricted (12–14 years).

CLINICAL FEATURES

There are only four case series in the literature dedicated to describing the clinical characteristics of NDPH: Vanast's initial description in 1986, Li and Rozen's

*Correspondence to: Todd D. Rozen, MD, FAAN, Department of Neurology, Geisinger Headache Center, Geisinger Medical Center, Geisinger Wyoming Valley, 1000 E. Mountain Drive, MC 37-31, Wilkes-Barre, PA 18711, USA, Tel: 570-808-6026, Fax: 570-808-7943, E-mail: tdrozmigraine@yahoo.com

Table 44.1

International Headache Society criteria for new daily persistent headache

A. Headache for >3 months fulfilling criteria B–D
B. Headache is daily and unremitting from onset or <3 days from onset
C. At least two of the following pain characteristics:
   1. Bilateral location
   2. Pressing/tightening (non-pulsating) quality
   3. Mild or moderate intensity
   4. Not aggravated by routine physical activity such as walking or climbing stairs
D. Both of the following:
   1. No more than one of photophobia, phonophobia, or mild nausea
   2. Neither moderate or severe nausea nor vomiting
E. Not attributed to another disorder

(2002) manuscript, Meineri et al.'s investigation from 2004, and Takase et al's study from Japan (2004). Vanast (1986) noted in 45 patients, whom he identified with NDPH over a 2-year period, a female predominance to the syndrome (26 women and 19 men). There was an earlier age of onset of NDPH in women compared to men and the age of onset of NDPH in women ranged from 16 to 35 years, while in men it ranged from 26 to 45 years. Seventy-two percent of patients stated the pain of NDPH was constant. Pain location was temporal in 9 of 45 patients, temporal plus other areas in 14 patients, occipital and extra sites in 20 patients, and holocranial in 5 patients. "Migrainous" associated symptoms were noted in a large percentage of patients: nausea 55%, vomiting 12%, photophobia 34%, and phonophobia 37%. Other associated symptoms included drowsiness and lethargy in 15%, vertigo in 13%, and near-fainting spells in 1%.

The Li and Rozen (2002) article is the largest study to date describing the syndrome of NDPH. A retrospective chart review was carried out using a computerized database of patients from the Jefferson Headache Center (a large university-based headache specialty unit). All patients who were seen at Jefferson between August 1997 and May 2000 and diagnosed with NDPH were included. Secondary headache disorders were excluded (via laboratory and neuroimaging studies) before a diagnosis of primary NDPH was made. Patients with other forms of CDH, including hemicrania continua, chronic migraine, and chronic tension-type headache, were excluded from the study.

Forty women and 16 men were identified (female-to-male ratio was 2.5:1). Age of onset ranged from 12 to 78 years. Peak age of onset was the second and third decade in women and the fifth decade in men. Eighty-two percent of patients were able to pinpoint the exact day their headache started. Headache onset occurred in relation to an infection or flu-like illness in 30%, extracranial surgery (e.g., hysterectomy) in 12%, and a stressful life event in 12%. Over 40% of patients could not identify any precipitating event. A previous headache history was found in 38% of patients (episodic migraine 19%, episodic tension-type headache 2%, non-specific headache 17%). No patient had a prior history of CDH or an increasing frequency of episodic headache just prior to the onset of NDPH. The duration of the daily headache ranged from 1.5 to 24 h. In 79% of patients the pain was continuous throughout the day with no pain-free time noted. Baseline average pain intensity was moderate (4–6 out of 10 on a visual analogue pain scale) in 61% of patients while 21% experienced severe pain (≥7 out of 10) all of the time.

Headache location was bilateral in 64% of patients. Almost 60% of patients had some pain localized to the occipital-nuchal region, while 44% experienced retro-orbital pain and 18% had holocranial pain. Headache quality was described as a throbbing sensation in 55% and pressure-like in 54%; other descriptions included stabbing 45%, achy 43%, dull 37%, tightness 36%, burning 23%, and searing 4%. Headaches were aggravated by stress in 40%, physical exertion in 32%, and bright light in 29%. Headaches were relieved by lying down in 66%, being in a dark room 48%, with massage 23%, and with sleep 9%. In regard to associated symptoms nausea occurred in 68% of patients, photophobia in 66%, phonophobia in 61%, lightheadedness in 55%, sore/stiff neck in 50%, blurred vision in 43%, vomiting in 23%, osmophobia in 23%, and vertigo in 11%. Aura-type symptoms were also present in some patients, including visual photopsias in 9%, and seeing zigzag lines in 5%. A family history of headache was documented in 29% of patients.

Meineri et al. (2004) documented the clinical characteristics of 18 NDPH patients (11 female, 7 male) diagnosed in an Italian headache specialty clinic. Females had a younger age of onset of NDPH. A previous personal headache history was noted in 33%, while a family history of headache was noted in 33% of NDPH patients. All patients had bilateral pain, which was of moderate intensity in most, while some had mild daily pain. Severe pain was not noted in this population. Migrainous features were noted in 14 of 18 NDPH sufferers. With regard to triggering events, NDPH started with a flu-like illness in 11% while another 11% had their headaches begin after a surgical procedure.

Finally Takase et al. (2004) looked at the clinical characteristics of NDPH in 30 Japanese patients. In this study there was a male predominance (17 men and 13 women). Age of onset of NDPH ranged from 13 to 73 years. Headache onset was associated with a stressful life event in

Table 44.2

Clinical characteristics of new daily persistent headache

- Gender: female predominance noted in three out of four studies (gender ratio range 1.4–2.5:1)
- Age of onset: younger in women, many in their 20s and 30s
- Location: bilateral in most
- Intensity: moderate to severe in most patients
- Pain duration: constant without pain-free time
- Associated symptoms: migrainous features are common
- Recognized triggering event in <50%

20%, while the remainder could not identify a probable cause. The headache was of severe intensity in all patients. Headache was present throughout the entire day with little, if any, headache-free time. Headache quality was pressure or tightening in 73%, pulsating in 10%, and both pressing and pulsating in 5%. Associated symptoms were rare, with mild nausea occurring in 10 patients, while only 1 patient had photophobia.

Table 44.2 presents an overview of the clinical characteristics of NDPH patients.

ETIOLOGY OF NDPH

As a number of NDPH patients state that they had a cold or flu-like illness when their headache began, an infectious etiology for NDPH can be hypothesized. Some authors have linked Epstein–Barr virus (EBV) infection with NDPH. Diaz-Mitoma et al. (1987) identified oropharyngeal secretions of EBV in 20 of 32 patients with NDPH compared with 4 of 32 age and gender-matched controls. A history of mononucleosis was identified in 12 of the patients with NDPH. Almost 85% of the NDPH patients were found to have an active EBV infection, as opposed to 8 in the control group. The authors hypothesized that activation of a latent EBV infection may have been the trigger for the development of a CDH from onset. EBV titers were tested in 7 patients from the Li and Rozen (2002) investigation, of whom 5 had positive titers indicating past but not active infection. Meineri et al. (2004) did not find an EBV infection in any NDPH patient but did note that 6/18 patients had elevated IgM titers for HSV while 2/18 patients had elevated immunoglobulin M cytomegalovirus titers, all indicating recent infection.

Santoni and Santoni-Williams (1993) demonstrated evidence of systemic infection in 108 patients with NDPH, including *Salmonella*, adenovirus, toxoplasmosis, herpes zoster, EBV, and *Escherichia coli* urinary tract infections.

An infectious etiology is not the presumed cause of NDPH in every patient, as almost 40–60% of NDPH sufferers have no recognized trigger. A stressful life event has been shown to trigger NDPH in a subset of patients. Stewart et al. (2001) documented that stressful life events are a risk factor for CDH in the general population. In the year before or same year of onset of CDH, individuals who developed headache compared to controls more likely had a change in personal relationships, had moved, had a problem with their children, or had an extremely stressful ongoing situation. The study did not define CDH subtypes, so the number of patients who developed NDPH after a stressful life event could not be ascertained.

The only study to date looking at the possible cause of NDPH in children was completed at the Mayo Clinic in 2003. Mack (2003) identified 41 children with NDPH, of whom 15 patients had their onset of headache during a viral infection. A positive EBV titer was found in 60% of these patients. Of the remaining children, 8 had their headaches begin after mild head injury, 3 patients after a surgical procedure, and 1 patient during high-altitude camping. In 5 patients no inciting event was identified, while in 4 patients an initial diagnosis of intracranial hypertension was made but the headache persisted after treatment and normalization of pressures.

LABORATORY STUDIES IN NDPH

In most instances general laboratory and neuroimaging studies in NDPH patients are normal. Elevation of EBV titers has been identified but the significance of this is unknown. In the Li and Rozen (2002) investigation brain magnetic resonance imaging (MRI) or computed tomography was completed in 49 patients, of whom 66% had normal studies while the remainder had non-specific imaging findings felt not to be related to the headache condition (e.g., nasal polyps). Cerebrospinal fluid (CSF) data are sparse. Rozen et al. (2004) reported the first observation of CSF from adolescents with NDPH. A lumbar puncture was completed in 4 adolescent patients with NDPH who were admitted to an inpatient headache unit. CSF evaluation included opening pressures, cell count, total protein, glucose, Gram stain, and bacterial cultures. A low and almost nonexistent CSF protein level was documented in 4 out of 4 adolescent patients with NDPH. The cause of the low CSF protein level was unknown. Low CSF protein has been associated with hyperthyroidism, leukemia, and intracranial hypertension (recent reports have refuted this), and in children between the ages of 6 months and 2 years. One patient did have an elevated opening pressure but had no papilledema and no response to CSF-lowering agents. No other pertinent medical conditions were identified in any patient. Serum protein levels were normal in all patients (CSF protein does not decrease if serum protein levels are above 4 g/dl). The authors stated that further study looking into the cause of the low CSF protein is needed and elucidation of the cause may lead to a better understanding of the pathogenesis of NDPH.

SECONDARY MIMICS OF NDPH

A diagnosis of primary NDPH is made only after secondary causes have been ruled out. Two disorders in particular can mimic the presentation of NDPH: spontaneous CSF leak and cerebral venous sinus thrombosis. Spontaneous CSF leaks typically present as a daily headache with a positional component. However, the longer a patient suffers with a CSF leak-induced headache the less pronounced the positional component becomes. Thus if a patient is seen in a physician's office months to years after onset of a CSF leak, that patient may not even divulge a history of positional headaches as that trigger may not have been evident to the patient for a very long time. In this setting the CSF leak headache may mimic a primary NDPH picture.

In the patient who presents with new daily headache and is subsequently found to have cerebral venous thrombosis, in many instances none of the typical features recognized for cerebral venous thrombosis is present, including: no history of new-onset seizures, focal neurological deficits, change of consciousness, cranial nerve palsies, bilateral cortical signs, and no evidence of papilledema on fundoscopic examination. A recent patient of the author presented with a daily headache from onset of 4 months' duration with mostly occipital-nuchal discomfort. Her examination was normal and she had no prior coagulopathy history. She obtained complete headache relief with occipital nerve blockade and the headache never returned after only a single nerve block. On subsequent magnetic resonance venography she was found to have an extremely large transverse sinus thrombosis. The presentation of NDPH is unique so, even if patients readily improve with therapy, investigative studies still must be completed. Other recognized secondary causes of NDPH are noted in Table 44.3.

The evaluation of a NDPH patient should include neuroimaging, specifically brain MRI and with gadolinium, and magnetic resonance venography (MRV). Gadolinium must be given to look for the pachymeningeal enhancement associated with spontaneous CSF leaks, while MRV will help make the diagnosis of venous sinus thrombosis. If those studies are negative then a lumbar puncture should be considered, especially in a patient who is treatment-refractory. The lumbar puncture can rule out an indolent infection and can also determine CSF pressures. In some instances a patient may have a CSF leak without typical MRI changes and with a loss of a positional headache; thus an opening CSF pressure on lumbar puncture is the only way in which to diagnose a low CSF pressure syndrome.

Table 44.3

Secondary mimics of new daily persistent headache

- Low cerebrospinal fluid pressure
- Cerebral vein thrombosis
- High cerebrospinal fluid pressure
- Carotid or vertebral artery dissection
- Giant cell arteritis
- Meningitis
- Sphenoid sinusitis
- Cervical facet syndrome
- Intranasal contact (contact point headache): pain caused by contact of intranasal structures (e.g., nasal septum and nasal turbinate)
- Intracranial neoplasm or mass lesion

A syndrome of idiopathic intracranial hypertension may also mimic NDPH. Papilledema on fundoscopic examination would be a major reason to search for this diagnosis, although some individuals may have elevated spinal pressure without papilledema and may not resemble the typical pseudotumor cerebri patient of a young obese woman with CDH, tinnitus, and visual obscurations (Marcelis and Silberstein 1991). CSF analysis would be the only way to determine the presence of elevated spinal pressure.

TREATMENT

NDPH can continue for years to decades after onset and be extremely disabling to the patient. Even with aggressive treatment many NDPH patients do not improve. Primary NDPH is felt to be the most treatment-refractory of all headache disorders by many headache specialists. Patients with NDPH will fail every possible class of abortive and preventive medications without any sign of pain relief. Typically, NDPH patients will start to overuse medications as they have a daily chronic headache, but unlike with chronic migraine from analgesic overuse, getting NDPH patients out of analgesic rebound typically does nothing to help in relieving their pain. Rozen (2002) presented 5 patients in whom successful treatment of NDPH was obtained with gabapentin or topiramate, but these agents do not work in the majority of cases.

At present no specific treatment strategy can be suggested for primary NDPH based on clinical evidence. Most headache specialists will treat NDPH with the same acute and preventive medications that they use to treat chronic migraine, although, based on non-response to these medications, NDPH and chronic migraine are two disparate syndromes.

As a number of NDPH patients appear to have cervicogenic signs on examination (even without a history of head or neck trauma), sending them for anesthesiology/pain evaluation for nerve blocks and facet blocks is recommended when medication is not helping. Anecdotally, the author has had several NDPH patients achieve significant pain relief after cervical facet blocks or selective nerve blocks (greater occipital, auriculotemporal, supraorbital/trochlear). As this can be a refractory syndrome, any pain relief is welcomed by the patient.

PROGNOSIS

The self-limited form of NDPH has a good prognosis as patients appear to improve without any intervention. In Vanast's (1986) initial description of NDPH, 30% of the men affected were headache-free at 3 months, and 86% were headache-free at 2 years. In women, 30% were headache-free at 3 months, while 73% were pain-free at 2 years. In the patients who have the refractory form of NDPH their syndrome can go on unabated for years to decades even with aggressive treatment. Takase et al. (2004) evaluated the effect of treatment utilizing muscle relaxants, tricyclic antidepressants, selective serotonin reuptake inhibitors, and valproic acid on NDPH. In 8 of 30 patients treatment was deemed very effective (daily headache intensity 3/10 or less), 1 patient had a moderately effective response (daily headache intensity 4–5/10), in 6 patients it was mildly effective (daily headache intensity 6–7/10), while 15 patients showed no response to treatment. Only 2 patients developed headache-free time after therapy; the remainder continued with daily head pain although some had an improved quality of life. The authors concluded that NDPH is, overall, unresponsive to typical headache treatment.

Newer insight

As NDPH is really in its infancy compared to the other primary headache syndromes very little research has been completed looking at the pathogenesis of this syndrome. This section will look at two new studies which have helped to unravel some of the mysteries of this complicated headache condition.

Cervical spine joint hypermobility as a predisposing factor for the development of NDPH

Rozen and colleagues (2005) noticed a similar body habitus in NDPH patients at a headache specialty clinic of tall height, low weight, and a long neck, reminiscent of the physical characteristics seen in individuals with hereditary connective tissue disorders. In addition, on examination NDPH patients also appeared to have lax joints, suggesting underlying joint hypermobility. As joint hypermobility is recognized as a predisposing factor for the development of chronic pain in the rheumatology literature, Rozen et al. (2005) looked for the presence of joint hypermobility in NDPH patients, hypothesizing that joint hypermobility, especially of the cervical spine, may be a predisposing factor for the development of NDPH. Twelve individuals (10 female, 2 male) with primary NDPH were evaluated by one of two physical therapists. Each patient was tested for active cervical range of motion and for the presence of excessive intersegmental vertebral motion in the cervical spine. All patients were screened utilizing the Beighton score, which determines degree of systemic hypermobility. Eleven of the 12 NDPH patients were found to have cervical spine joint hypermobility. Ten of the 12 NDPH patients had evidence of widespread joint hypermobility with the Beighton score. The authors concluded that joint hypermobility specifically of the cervical spine may be a predisposing factor for the development of NDPH.

How joint hypermobility in the cervical spine can lead to persistent daily head pain can only be hypothesized. Evidence exists that there is a convergence of trigeminal and cervical afferents in the trigeminal nucleus caudalis (Piovesan et al., 2003). Thus, cervical spine pathology can present as head pain typically in a trigeminal nerve V1 distribution (Piovesan et al., 2001). Cervical spine joint hypermobility in some manner may influence cervical afferent input into the trigeminal nucleus caudalis with the subsequent development of head pain. Limitations to the study included a small sample size, lack of a double-blinded examination by both physical therapists, and no age- and gender-matched control group population.

Elevation of CSF tumor necrosis factor-alpha levels in NDPH patients

As a certain percentage of NDPH patients have their headaches start after an infection, the possibility of a persistent state of systemic or central nervous system (CNS) inflammation comes into question. Tumor necrosis factor-alpha (TNF-alpha) is a proinflammatory cytokine involved in brain immune and inflammatory activities, as well as in pain initiation. Rozen et al. (2006) looked at TNF-alpha levels in the CSF of primary NDPH patients from an inpatient headache unit. Twenty patients with NDPH were studied and TNF-alpha levels were elevated in 19 of the 20 CSF samples. Serum TNF-alpha levels, however, were normal in most of the study subjects. The authors, based on their results, suggested a role for proinflammatory cytokines (specifically TNF-alpha) in the pathogenesis of NDPH. As serum TNF-alpha levels were not elevated in most NDPH patients, NDPH does not appear to be a disorder derived from systemic inflammation, but rather inflammation solely involving the CNS. Glial cells are known manufacturers of cytokines in the CNS. Interestingly, in laboratory animals, recognized triggers of glial cell activation and thus cytokine production include infection, stress, and surgical procedures (Bigal et al., 2002; Koenig et al., 2002; Meineri et al., 2004). These are the recognized triggering events of NDPH in humans.

How elevated TNF-alpha levels can produce head pain can only be postulated. There is recent evidence that TNF-alpha will induce calcitonin gene-related peptide production, which is a known factor in the pathogenesis of other primary headaches, including migraine and cluster headache (Durham, 2006). Interestingly, as most of the positive tested patients showed minimal to no improvement during aggressive inpatient treatment, this suggested that persistent elevation of CSF TNF-alpha levels may be one of the causes of treatment refractoriness in patients with NDPH. It also suggests that specific TNF-alpha inhibitors may have an important future role in the treatment of NDPH and this needs to be investigated.

CONCLUSION

NDPH is a newly recognized form of CDH. It is unique in its presentation and course. Many NDPH patients can state the exact date their headache began. NDPH is marked by a continuous daily head pain of varying intensity which may be associated with migrainous symptoms. Further research must be invested into studying NDPH as it is becoming more prevalent in the physician's office and in many instances is refractory to many of the known CDH preventive and abortive treatment strategies.

References

Bigal ME, Sheftell FD, Rapoport AM et al. (2002). Chronic daily headache in a tertiary care population: correlation between the International Headache Society diagnostic criteria and proposed revisions of criteria for chronic daily headache. Cephalalgia 22: 432–438.

Castillo J, Munoz P, Guitera V et al. (1999). Epidemiology of chronic daily headache in the general population. Headache 38: 497–506.

Diaz-Mitoma F, Vanast WJ, Tyrell DL (1987). Increased frequency of Epstein–Barr virus excretion in patients with new daily persistent headaches. Lancet 1: 411–415.

Durham PL (2006). Calcitonin gene-related peptide (CGRP) and migraine. Headache 46 (Suppl. 1): 3–8.

Headache Classification Subcommittee of the International Headache Society (2004). The international classification of headache disorders, 2nd edn. Cephalalgia 24: 1–160.

Koenig MA, Gladstein J, McCarter RJ et al. (2002). Chronic daily headache in children and adolescents presenting to tertiary headache clinics. Headache 42: 491–500.

Li D, Rozen TD (2002). The clinical characteristics of new daily persistent headache. Cephalalgia 22: 66–69.

Mack K (2003). What causes new daily persistent headache in children? Cephalalgia 23: 609.

Marcelis J, Silberstein SD (1991). Idiopathic intracranial hypertension without papilledema. Arch Neurol 48: 392–399.

Meineri P, Torre E, Rota E et al. (2004). New daily persistent headache: clinical and serological characteristics in a retrospective study. Neurol Sci 25 (Suppl. 3): S281–S282.

Piovesan EJ, Kowacs PA, Tatsui CE et al. (2001). Referred pain after painful stimulation of the greater occipital nerve in humans: evidence of convergence of cervical afferences on trigeminal nuclei. Cephalalgia 21: 107–109.

Piovesan EJ, Kowacs PA, Oshinsky ML (2003). Convergence of cervical and trigeminal sensory afferents. Curr Headache Rep 2: 155–161.

Rozen TD (2002). Successful treatment of new daily persistent headache with gabapentin and topiramate. Headache 42: 433.

Rozen T, Haynes G, Range C et al. (2004). Low cerebrospinal fluid protein levels in adolescents with new daily persistent headache. Neurology 63: 1432–1438.

Rozen TD, Roth JM, Denenberg N (2005). Joint hypermobility as a predisposing factor for the development of new daily persistent headache. Headache 45: 828–829.

Rozen TD, Swidan Rozen TD, Swidan S (2006). Elevation of CSF tumor necrosis factor alpha levels in NDPH and treatment refractory chronic daily migraine. Headache 46: 897.

Santoni JR, Santoni-Williams CJ (1993). Headache and painful lymphadenopathy in extracranial or systemic infection: etiology of new daily persistent headaches. Intern Med 32: 530–533.

Silberstein SD, Lipton RB (2001). Chronic daily headache, including transformed migraine, chronic tension-type headache and medication overuse. In: SD Silberstein, RB Lipton, DJ Dalessio (Eds.), Wolff's Headache and Other Head Pain. Oxford University Press, Oxford, pp. 247–282.

Stewart WF, Scher AI, Lipton RB (2001). Stressful life events and risk of chronic daily headache: results from the frequent headache epidemiology study. Cephalalgia 21: 278–280.

Takase Y, Nakano M, Tatsumi C et al. (2004). Clinical features, effectiveness of drug based treatment and prognosis of new daily persistent headache: thirty cases in Japan. Cephalalgia 24: 955–959.

Vanast WJ (1986). New daily persistent headaches: definition of a benign syndrome. Headache 26: 317.

Wang SJ, Fuh JL, Lu SR et al. (2006). Chronic daily headache in adolescents: prevalence, impact, and medication overuse. Neurology 66: 193–197.

Section 5

Secondary headaches

Handbook of Clinical Neurology, Vol. 97 (3rd series)
Headache
G. Nappi and M.A. Moskowitz, Editors

Chapter 45

Secondary headaches: introduction

GIUSEPPE NAPPI,[1*] AND MICHAEL A. MOSKOWITZ,[2]

[1]*Chair of Neurology, "Sapienza" University of Rome and IRCSS "C. Mondino Institute of Neurology" Foundation, Pavia, Italy*

[2]*Stroke and Neurovascular Regulation Laboratory, Departments of Radiology and Neurology, Massachusetts General Hospital, Harvard Medical School, Charlestown, MA, USA*

GENERAL DESCRIPTION

Secondary headaches, which are characterized by high epidemiological impact (Rasmussen and Olesen, 1992; Bigal et al., 2000), are certainly of multidisciplinary interest. Headache is sometimes the only sign of a severe underlying disease that must be identified as quickly as possible through a diagnostic process that can potentially involve any of the specialized medical or surgical fields, from general medicine to intensive care. In primary care settings secondary headaches account for around 44% of all headaches, and in 5% of cases they derive from neurological disorders (Bigal et al., 2000). Headache, presenting as an isolated or as an accompanying symptom, can signal the onset of a number of systemic and neurological diseases. Inflammatory, metabolic, and vascular causes, in that order of frequency, can cause the appearance of headache through mechanisms involving, respectively, the nerve endings of meningeal nociceptors, the neurotransmitter balance, and control of cerebrospinal fluid pressure. It follows that early detection and correct systemic contextualization of the symptom will yield the first information useful for interpreting the whole clinical picture.

STRUCTURE OF THE BOOK

Basically, this book follows the nosological categories set out in the revised International Headache Classification (ICHD-II: Headache Classification Subcommittee of the International Headache Society, 2004). In some cases (diseases that generally imply a degree of urgency), in order to facilitate the diagnostic course after the initial assessment of the patient, the etiological classification criteria are integrated with "symptom-based" algorithms.

CLASSIFICATION

Despite the considerable social impact of secondary headaches, the first systematic attempt to classify headache disorders (ICHD-I) was not published until as recently as 1988 (Headache Classification Subcommittee of the International Headache Society, 1988). The ICHD-I was structured as a single body, divided into 13 chapters, of which six (chapters 5–10) dealt with secondary headaches. The ICHD-II was published in 2004 following an extensive revision of the original classification which led to substantial changes being made to the main body of the work, to the general criteria, and to the disease-specific criteria. This new version is divided into three main parts: the primary headaches (chapters 1–4), the secondary headaches (chapters 5–12), and "cranial neuralgias, central and primary facial pain, other headaches" (chapter 13). The classification criteria are different for each of these parts, being, respectively, "symptom-based", "etiological", and "distribution-based". The following definition of secondary headache is introduced: "a *de novo* headache occurring with another disorder recognized to be capable of causing it", regardless of the phenomenological presentation. Basically, the ICHD-I and ICHD-II differ in structure and content as well as in the inclusion, in the updated version, of new topics.

ICHD-I VERSUS ICHD-II

Headache is an extremely prevalent condition, which means that it can occur simultaneously with another disorder without a causal relationship. Therefore, a headache can only be diagnosed definitively as a secondary headache when an explicit cause-and-effect relationship has been established in scientific studies

*Correspondence to: Professor Giuseppe Nappi, Chair of Neurology, "Sapienza" University of Rome and IRCSS "C. Mondino Institute of Neurology" Foundation, Pavia, Italy, E-mail: giuseppe.nappi@mondino.it

between the underlying disorder and the headache. The best way of establishing a causal relationship is to document a close temporal association between the onset and disappearance of headache and of the causative disorder in large series of patients. Indeed, the authors of the ICHD-II, as one of their main objectives, set out to define as clearly as possible the strength of the link between headache and the underlying disease. The two versions of the classification differ from one another both structurally and in terms of content. In the ICHD-II the term "associated with", used in the old version, has been replaced with the stronger "attributed to", to underline the link between the original cause and the headache.

The classification criteria are standardized, following a fixed format based on four fundamental points. Point A lists the salient features of the symptoms for descriptive purposes without making any mention of the possible weight or hierarchy of these symptoms for that particular headache type; point B establishes the presence of a new condition whose potential to induce headache has already been demonstrated; point C establishes the presence of a temporal criterion linking the onset of the symptom (headache) with the underlying disease, while point D requires resolution of the headache within a variable period of time, depending on the partial or complete resolution of the underlying disease. If this final criterion D is not met, then the relationship between cause and effect is classified as "probable".

This format, which has made an important contribution to defining many forms of secondary headache, is also open to a number of criticisms. In some cases, the underlying disease can persist for a long time; this may be because of a poor response to treatment or because of the intrinsic nature of the disease, as in the case of some systemic infections. In these cases it can prove impossible, for a long time, to arrive at a nosological categorization of the headache; this is why the term "chronic post other disease headache" has been coined. Some experts believe that these situations call for the addition of a further criterion, E, which would rule out other diseases that can cause that same type of headache. This would strengthen the pathogenetic link between the headache and the underlying disease.

Compared with the previous classification, the groups into which the secondary headaches were divided in the ICHD-II have been refined through the incorporation of new elements to aid diagnosis. Some chapters have been reorganized and renamed ("Headache attributed to head and neck trauma", "Headache attributed to cranial or cervical vascular disorders", "Headache attributed to disorders of homeostasis"), some are new chapters ("Headache attributed to psychiatric disorders"), and others have been considerably modified, as in the case of "Headache attributed to infection". In the first classification, this latter group was divided into "intracranial" forms (listed in chapter 7: "Headache associated with non-vascular intracranial disorders") and "systemic" forms (described in chapter 9: "Headache associated with non-cephalic infection"). In the revised classification, on the other hand, it is covered in a single chapter (ICHD-II Chapter 9). Moreover, all the paragraphs dealing with secondary headaches have been considerably enriched with information regarding both the characteristics of the pain and the salient features of the causative disease. This process of enrichment has had some important therapeutic implications, particularly in some sections, e.g., "Headache attributed to cranial or cervical vascular disorders", in which many details have been added on the diagnosis of arteritis, and "Headache attributed to infection", which has been completely revised and updated.

One new feature of the ICHD-II is the addition of an appendix in which the authors have included some recently reported variants of primary and, above all, secondary headache forms for which there is still no definite evidence in the literature.

Another new feature is the possibility of classifying some conditions with more than one code. Patients presenting a pre-existing primary headache have to be assigned two codes, the first indicating the previous, primary headache diagnosis and the second the current, secondary headache diagnosis. The onset of a new type of headache, potentially attributable to a new disease, can manifest itself in two ways: either through a worsening of the pre-existing headache (in this case the quality of the headache remains the same), or through the onset of a new type of pain with its own distinct characteristics. According to the ICHD-II, both conditions can be classified as "secondary headaches", providing the criteria establishing a temporal link between the headache and the original cause, both during onset (criterion C) and resolution (criterion D), are fulfilled. This new approach, entirely different from that of the ICHD-I, reflects the authors' intention to found the classification of secondary headaches primarily on etiological criteria.

A good example of this situation is that of the onset of a daily headache theoretically due to an overuse of analgesics. In the first diagnostic phase this condition could be classified using three codes: primary headache (specific code), plus probable chronic headache (specific code), plus probable medication overuse headache (MOH, code: 8.2). Fulfilment of criterion D, which requires that the headache should resolve within 2 months of the discontinuation of the analgesics, would strongly support a diagnosis of MOH as opposed to chronic headache.

Table 46.1

International Headache Society criteria of acute posttraumatic headache

5.1.1 With moderate or severe head injury
- A. New headache appearing after head trauma and fulfilling criteria B–D
- B. Head trauma with at least one of the following:
  1. Loss of consciousness >30 min
  2. Glasgow Coma Scale <13
  3. Posttraumatic amnesia >48 h
  4. Imaging demonstration of a traumatic brain lesion (cerebral hematoma, brain contusion, or skull fracture)
- C. Headache occurs less than 7 days after head trauma or after regaining consciousness or memory
- D. Headache lasts <3 months after regaining consciousness or memory

5.1.2 With mild head injury
- A. New headache appearing after head trauma and fulfilling criteria B–D
- B. Head trauma with all the following:
  1. No loss of consciousness, or loss of consciousness of <30 min duration
  2. Glasgow Coma Scale >13
  3. Symptoms or signs diagnostic of concussion
- C. Headache occurs less than 7 days after head trauma or after regaining consciousness or memory
- D. Headache lasts <3 months after regaining consciousness or memory

(Reproduced from Headache Classification Subcommittee of the International Headache Society, 2004.)

Table 46.2

International Headache Society criteria of chronic posttraumatic headache

5.2.1 With moderate or severe head injury
- A. New headache appearing after head trauma and fulfilling criteria B–D
- B. Head trauma with at least one of the following:
  1. Loss of consciousness >30 min
  2. Glasgow Coma Scale <13
  3. Posttraumatic amnesia >48 h
  4. Imaging demonstration of a traumatic brain lesion (cerebral hematoma, brain contusion, or skull fracture)
- C. Headache occurs less than 7 days after head trauma or after regaining consciousness or memory
- D. Headache lasts >3 months after regaining consciousness or memory

5.2.2 With mild head injury
- A. New headache appearing after head trauma and fulfilling criteria B–D
- B. Head trauma with all the following:
  1. No loss of consciousness, or loss of consciousness of <30 min duration
  2. Glasgow Coma Scale >13
  3. Symptoms or signs diagnostic of concussion
- C. Headache occurs less than 7 days after head trauma or after regaining consciousness or memory
- D. Headache lasts >3 months after regaining consciousness or memory

(Reproduced from Headache Classification Subcommittee of the International Headache Society, 2004.)

Epidemiology of acute PTH

Almost all headache subtypes have been described after head trauma: headache with characteristics of tension-type headache, migraine, cervicogenic headache, elevated intracranial pressure headache, cluster headache, and the headache of intracranial hemorrhage (Keidel et al., 2006). Thus, acute PTH is not uniform in its clinical presentation and subsequent epidemiology.

The frequency of this type of headache varies between different series, but to summarize: tension-type headache is the most frequent, with an incidence of 85% (Evans, 1992, 2004; Haas, 1993, 1996); post-whiplash unilateral cervicogenic headache occurs in 8% at 6 weeks, 4% at 6 months, and 3% at 1 year (with a female-to-male ratio of 3:2) (Drottning et al., 2002; Drottning, 2003); and migraine-like headache occurs in 2.5%, and is more common in children and teenagers (Guthkelch, 1977; Snoek et al., 1984; Vohanka and Zouhar, 1990). The approximate prevalence of migraine associated with head trauma is 14% (Russell, 1932; Evans, 2004; Pascual-Lozano et al., 2005). The exact frequency of posttraumatic cluster-like headache is not determined because this type of headache remains rare (Reik, 1987; Turkewitz et al., 1992). Basilar migrainelike PTH (Jacome, 1986, Haas, 1996) and PTH associated with sexual activity (Denny-Brown, 1945) have also been reported.

The incidence of head trauma is approximately 180–220 per 100 000 people in North America and 350 per 100 000 in Europe, comparable with cerebrovascular ischemia (Frommelt, 1995).

The relative incidence of acute PTH in head trauma is up to 200 per 100 000 in the USA and nearly 315 per 100 000 in Europe (it is more common in Germany) (Cartlidge, 1981; Minderhoud et al., 1980; Levin et al., 1987; Denker, 1994).

An interesting fact is that the severity of the head injury is inversely proportional to the occurrence of both acute and chronic PTH: 72% in mild head injury and 33% in severe head injury (Couch and Bearss,

2001). There is also an inverse relationship between the duration of the LOC, the duration of PTA, and the incidence of both acute and chronic PTH (Brenner et al., 1944; Cartlidge and Shaw, 1981).

Pathophysiology of acute PTH

The exact pathophysiology of acute PTH is unknown. Probably there are different mechanisms implicated in its origin, because, as we know, it could mimic migraine, tension-type, cluster, and other subtypes of headache. Thus, the mechanisms of primary headaches may help us to understand each subtype of acute PTH.

Factors that play a role in the pathophysiology (provided by animal models and functional brain imaging studies) are:

- Referred pain from nociceptive input caused by direct lesions in musculoskeletal, discoligamentous, and other soft-tissue structures. Cervicogenic acute PTH is related to the multisegmental pain impulses generated by nociceptive afferents in stretched tendons, ligaments, and intervertebral discs, as well as sympathetic nerve fibers of arterial vessels entering the cervical spinal cord via dorsal C fibers (Pfaffenrath et al., 1987; Pöllmann et al., 1997). The explanation of the referred pain to the frontal area is from the convergence of the upper cervical roots and the spinal nucleus of the trigeminal nerve (Kerr, 1972, Bogduk, 1986). Other rare mechanisms proposed are direct compression of C2 fibers in the lateral atlantoaxial joint, sympathetic vertebral nerve irritation, and ischemia of vertebral artery (Bärtschi-Rochaix, 1949; Bogduk, 1993)
- Activation of meningeal nociceptive afferents due to traumatic meningeal bleeding: epidural, subdural, and subarachnoid
- Stretching of pain-sensitive intracranial structures from increased intracranial pressure
- Intracranial hypotension (Ramadan, 1996)
- Activation of the trigeminovascular system by posttraumatic sinus venous thrombosis.

Other factors related to the pathophysiology of the two most important primary headaches, tension-type and migraine, include:

- Transient impairment of serotoninergic fibers implicated in the inhibitory pain system (Keidel, 2000)
- Increase in general pain sensitivity (Nebel et al., 2005; Stude et al., 2004)
- Neurochemical changes described in head injury, similar to primary migraine and aura. These include elevated concentrations of extracellular K, intracellular Na, Ca and Cl, reduced intracellular and total brain amount of Mg, influx of extracellular Ca in axolemmas, accumulation of platelet-derived 5-hydroxytryptamine in the central nervous system, release of excitatory amino acids like glutamate, cortical spreading depression, decreased levels of endogenous opioids, and increased nitric oxide activity (Yamaguchi, 1992; Packard and Ham, 1997; Young and Packard, 1997).

Clinical presentation

Headache is a cardinal symptom of the posttraumatic syndrome (Young et al., 2001; Láinez and Piera, 2006) caused by head trauma and whiplash injury in a similar way. In the acute phase, there are autonomic symptoms like dizziness, nausea, and vomiting, orthostatic dysregulation and thermodysregulation, accompanied by some degree of cognitive disturbance or other neuropsychological indeterminate deficits, irritability, and excessive sensitivity to light and noise (Keidel, 2000).

Clinical characteristics of acute PTH are similar to those of primary headache disorders:

- Acute PTH tension-type headache (90% of patients): a dull pressing, dragging, or pulling pain, mainly holocephalic, band or helmet-like, usually occipital, seldom episodic, and often continuous (Stude et al., 2004)
- Cervicogenic acute PTH: headache that radiates from occipital to frontal, not holocephalic, strongly unilateral without side change, and commonly associated with a limited mobility of the cervical spine; thus, the pain can be triggered by turning the head and sometimes in a position which results in pressure on the occipital nerve points. This diagnosis can be reached because of traumatic antecedent spine injury and improvement after local anesthetic infiltration of the tender greater occipital nerve of C2 root (Pöllmann et al., 1997).
- Acute PTH migraine-like headache: a pulsating, hemicranial, and side-changing headache in almost all cases. It can be accompanied by vegetative symptoms such as nausea, vomiting, dizziness, photophobia, and phonophobia (Winston, 1987; Weiss et al., 1991; Haas, 1993, 1996). Posttraumatic aura (isolated or accompanied by headache) may also occur and, rarely, posttraumatic basilar migraine is diagnosed, with vertigo, nausea, vomiting, and cranial nerve disorders (Jacome, 1986; Haas, 1996).
- Cluster-like acute PTH headache: similar to cluster-type headache, this is a unilateral, periorbital, and frontotemporal pressing or throbbing pain, accompanied by local autonomic signs such as ptosis, miosis, enophthalmos, lacrimation, conjunctival injection, and rhinorrhea (Reik, 1987; Turkewitz et al., 1992).

Acute PTH due to traumatic intracranial bleeding in traumatic brain injury, such as epidural, subdural, subarachnoid, intracerebral, or intraventricular hematoma, can mimic acute PTH of tension type and occurs in 11–53% of cases (Headache Classification Subcommittee of the International Headache Society, 2004). This is a frequent complication of elderly patients, patients on anticoagulants or antiplatelet medication, or patients with alcohol abuse. The most important differentiating features from acute PTH tension-type headache are focal neurological signs, altered LOC, lethargy, and signs of meningeal irritation.

Diagnosis

The usual technique used in the emergency room in the diagnosis of head trauma is cranial computed tomography (CCT) with bone window to screen fractures too. CCT is useful to identify hematomas, focal contusion, and any potential complications. In cervical spine injuries, computed tomograhy (CT) is also used to identify fractures, luxations, and kinking of the spine, as well as X-rays.

Other procedures could be conducted depending on the symptom complex and the neurological signs that accompany acute PTH (Keidel, 1997, 2000). Sometimes repeated studies may be necessary if there is a change in the localization and character of the headache, new associated symptoms, or new or emergent focal neurological signs.

Management strategies of acute PTH

Treatment guidelines are all based on clinical experience rather than on controlled studies (Keidel, 1997, 2000; Radanov et al., 2001; Seferiadis et al., 2004). Treatment could differ depending on the type of acute PTH.

Tension-type acute PTH

Analgesics and non-steroidal antiinflammatory drugs (NSAIDs) are appropiate, for no longer than 4 weeks. Examples include ibuprofen (maximum 1500 mg/day), naproxen (500–1000 mg/day), and dexketoprofen (25–75 mg/day). Analgesics are less effective but could be useful in some patients, e.g., paracetamol (1–6 g/day). Myorelaxants could be associated with tension-type acute PTH, with the same time pattern; examples include tizanidine (2–8 mg/day).

Migraine-like acute PTH

Treatment is similar to that for migraine attacks, usually with NSAIDs, associated with antiemetic drugs like domperidone or metoclopramide (10–20 mg orally). Triptans are also useful. In cases of severe, long-lasting, or frequent attacks, prophylactic treatment with beta-blockers, such as propranolol, and neuromodulators, such as topiramate or amitriptyline, could be used.

Cluster-type acute PTH

Cluster-type acute PTH is treated like cluster headache: sumatriptan subcutaneously and high-flow oxygen therapy are elective therapy for attacks. In these cases, prophylactic treatment with a short course of steroids and other preventives such as verapamil should be started.

Acute PTH should not be usually treated with opioid analgesics because of the risk of dependency and substance overuse, as well as benzodiazepines and muscle relaxants. Therapies like plaster collars, manual traction, massage, and local unguent treatment are not usually effective.

Prognosis

Almost all patients with mild concussion (without LOC) have a full recovery within a few days (Barth et al., 1989). In head trauma with concussion, with minimum LOC and amnesia of less than 60 min duration, patients generally improve in approximately 6–12 weeks. If there is severe concussion with a prolonged LOC (more than 10 min and prolonged amnesia of 4–6 h), improvement could take a long time, from several months to years (Gronwall and Wrightson, 1974; Levin et al., 1987).

However, generally, more than 75% of patients are free of symptoms after 6 months (Denny-Brown, 1945; Rutherford et al., 1978; Minderhoud et al., 1980; Cartlidge and Shaw, 1981; Binder, 1986; Edna and Cappelen, 1987; Levin et al., 1987; Marshall and Ruff, 1989; Rutherford, 1989; Mazzuchi et al., 1992; Denker, 1994).

CHRONIC POSTTRAUMATIC HEADACHE

Headache after head injury was described many centuries ago. PTH is, usually, a cardinal symptom of the "postconcussion syndrome" and therefore may be accompanied by somatic, psychological, or cognitive disturbances (Evans, 1996). PTH may result from brain, head, and sometimes neck injury and simulates the clinical characteristics of several primary headaches. Severe, moderate, and mild head injuries have been related to the beginning of new headaches (Ramadan, 2000; Solomon, 2001). The mechanisms of headache are still poorly understood: biological, psychological, and social factors have been implicated (Martelli et al., 1999). Similarly, the pathophysiology of symptoms in individuals with postconcussive syndrome continues to be a subject of controversy, ranging from neural damage to malingering (Keidel and Diener, 1997).

It is easy to establish the relationship between a headache and head or neck trauma when the headache develops immediately or in the first days after trauma has occurred. However it is very difficult when a headache develops weeks or even months after trauma, especially when most of these headaches have the pattern of tension-type headache and the prevalence of this type of headache in the population is very high. In accordance with ICHD-II (Headache Classification Subcommittee of the International Headache Society, 2004), PTH develops within 7 days of head trauma or regaining consciousness following head trauma, and resolves within 3 months. If such headaches persist beyond the first 3 months postinjury, they are subsequently referred to as chronic PTH.

Several months after the beginning of a PTH, some patients develop a new daily headache that can have features of migraine, tension-type headache, or both. In the majority of patients with episodic headaches after head injury, this condition is self-limited, but a minority of individuals may develop persistent headaches (Ramadan and Láinez, 2006). Neurological factors have been implicated in the initial phase, as well as psychological and legal factors (litigation and expectations for compensation) in the maintenance of a chronic PTH. Complementary studies (neuroimaging, electroencephalography, evoked potentials, cerebrospinal fluid examination, vestibular function test) should also be considered for patients with ongoing PTHs, especially for research purposes. The relationship to severity of injury has not been conclusively established. Surprisingly, the risk of developing chronic symptoms seems also to be greater for mild to moderate head injury (Yamaguchi, 1992; Couch and Bearss, 2001).

For patients with symptoms after 6 months to several years, there is a strong probability that emotional, motivation, and premorbid personality factors could support this residual symptomatology (Yamaguchi, 1992; Lanz and Bryant, 1996).

Epidemiology

Mild head injury accounts for more than 75% of brain injuries (Kraus and Nourjah, 1988). The annual incidence of mild head injury varies from 131 to 511 per 100 000 subjects (Evans, 1996). PTH follows head trauma and whiplash injury in 30–90% of patients (Evans, 1992; Keidel and Diener, 1997). The reported incidence of chronic PTH also varies from one study to another, partly because of disagreement on the duration of symptoms from the time of injury. The new International Headache Society diagnosis criteria defined chronic PTH as involving symptoms that persist beyond 3 months after the original insult (Headache Classification Subcommittee of the International Headache Society, 2004). Up to 32% of patients with head injury report persistent headaches 3 months after trauma, and approximately 1 in 4 continues to report headache at 4 years (Brenner et al., 1944; Cartlidge and Shaw, 1981; Edna and Cappelen, 1987; Keidel and Diener, 1997). International Headache Society criteria require the onset of PTH to be within 1 week of head trauma (Headache Classification Subcommittee of the International Headache Society, 2004). Late-acquired headaches have been recognized in children (Lanser et al., 1988) and in adults (Nick and Sicard-Nick, 1965; Cartlidge and Shaw, 1981; De Benedittis and De Santis, 1983). Some studies indicate that late-acquired headaches (starting more than 2 weeks after the trauma) are as common (Cartlidge and Shaw, 1981; Lanser et al., 1988), or more common (De Benedittis and De Santis, 1983), as those of early onset, but there is no evidence for this in case–control studies.

Clinical presentation

A great variety of headache patterns has been described after head injury and may closely resemble primary headache disorders (Hachinski, 2000). Previous reviews about the clinical presentation of PTH revealed that tension-type headache was the most common variety (De Benedittis and De Santis, 1983). In one of the first prospective studies, Haas (1996) followed 48 patients with PTH and the same number of controls with similar "natural" or primary headache 3 months after a traumatic event. According to previous International Headache Society criteria (Headache Classification Committee of the International Headache Society, 1988), 75% of patients with PTH had a tension-type headache, 21% had migraine without aura, and 4% had an unclassified headache a control group, showed that the headache pattern after head injury may be variable, and tension-type, cervicogenic, and migrainous headaches are the most usual (Bettuci et al., 1998; De Souza et al., 1999). Posttraumatic migraine represents a variable percentage (3–28%) of PTH depending on the series. When posttraumatic migraine appears it is usually a migraine without aura, often in children, adolescents, and young adults with a family history of migraine but without history of previous headache (Evans, 1996; Haas, 1996; Margulies, 2000). Trauma acts as a triggering factor of migraine (Haas and Lourie, 1988; Evans, 1996), whereas family history is a predisposing factor. Migraine attacks with visual or sensorial aura, dizzines, or mental confusion have been described in only a few patients (Weiss et al., 1991; Hachinski, 2000). Cluster-like headache, supraorbital neuralgia, occipital neuralgia, exertional headache, and headache associated with sexual activity have been described occasionally (Evans, 1996; Haas, 1996; Packard and Ham, 1997; Bettuci et al., 1998).

The diagnosis of a secondary headache requires a close temporal relationship between the head injury and the beginning of the headache. Evans's review (1992) had demonstrated that headache presentation was highest within the first month (90%) after head or neck trauma, especially within the first week (71%). In other more recent studies, both observational and prospective, PTH after MHT habitually began in the first week (De Souza et al., 1999; Van der Naalt et al., 1999).

The relationship between severity of injury and severity of PTH has not been conclusively established. Moreover, there are some controversial data. Frequently MTH is related to severe and chronic PTH, more than moderate or severe cranial traumas. In prospective studies (Evans, 1992; Packard and Ham, 1993; Moore, 1997), patients with a history of MHT have shown a longer maintenance of postconcussion symptoms. Chronic PTH maintains the clinical characteristics of acute headaches (tension, cervicogenic, or migrainous headache) but is prolonged for more than 3 months. Although the pathophysiological mechanisms of chronic PTH are still not known, its prevalence seems to grow. This prevalence is between 32% and 44% at 6 months after head trauma (Russell, 1932; Brenner et al., 1944; Martelli et al., 1999) and 10–15% at 4 years (Edna and Cappelen, 1987; Van der Naalt et al., 1999).

Risk factors

Jensen and Nielsen (1990) conducted a study to examine the risk factors for chronic PTH. They found that patients with pre-existing headaches (i.e., before head trauma) had a similar incidence of chronic PTH to those who reported no history of headache before the accident. Of note is that the prevalence of headache increased in that cohort from 40% pretrauma to 64% after the injury. Most of the increase was in significant headaches, that is, those occurring 1–2 days per week or more. Also, Jensen and Nielsen found that more women (49%) than men (30%) were affected, confirming the results of an earlier study indicating an increased incidence of chronic PTH in women 2 years posttrauma but not at 6 months (Cartlidge and Shaw, 1981). Neither of these studies noted whether the headaches began in the early posttraumatic period or later.

Posttraumatic migraine was more frequent in men in one study of 35 patients (Weiss et al., 1991). Older age was not a risk factor for chronic PTH in one study (Jensen and Nielsen, 1990) and was associated with slower and incomplete recovery in two subsequent studies (McClelland et al., 1994; Ponsford et al., 2000). A commonly held view is that chronic PTH is more common in people who sustain mild injury compared with those who suffer a major insult; that is, there is an inverse relationship between the severity of the head injury and the occurrence of chronic PTH (Evans, 1992; Packard and Ham, 1993; Moore, 1997). Only in some old studies as the one published by Brenner and associates (1944) reported the opposite. They noted that headaches lasting longer than 2 months after accidents affected 10% of patients who were merely dazed by their trauma and 34% of patients rendered unconscious.

Poor outcome has also been related to long duration of unconsciousness or neurological deficits after the head or neck injury. Cartlidge and Shaw (1981) found that, among 372 patients, chronic headaches were more common in those whose PTA had a duration of less than 1 h than in those who had more prolonged amnesia. At 6 months, 34% of patients with short-duration amnesia and 19% of those with prolonged amnesia reported headache; at 1 year, 21% and 14%; and at 2 years, 24% and 19%, respectively. In agreement with these findings are those of Jensen and Nielsen (1990), who interviewed patients 9–12 months after their head injuries. They observed chronic PTH in 42% of 48 patients who had not lost consciousness, in 38% of 74 patients unconscious for less than 15 min, and in 23% of 30 patients unconscious for 15 min to 24 h.

Mechanical impact factors such as an abnormal head position (rotation or inclined) also increase the risk of PTH (Lanz and Bryant, 1996; Keidel and Diener, 1997; Van der Naalt et al., 1999). Other predictive factors for a bad prognosis are: low intellectual, educational, and socioeconomic level, previous history of headache or alcohol abuse, presence of skull fracture, reduced GCS score, elevated serum protein S-100B, and dizziness, headache, and nausea in the emergency room (De Kruijk et al., 2002; Savola and Hillbom, 2003).

Pathophysiology of PTH

The mechanisms of headache following mild head injury are varied. Axonal injury, soft-tissue damage, cerebral metabolic derangements, and altered cerebral hemodynamics have been implicated in the genesis of symptoms, including headache, following head trauma. In the pathogenesis, common headache pathways with the primary headaches have been proposed.

During typical migraine, cerebral cortical and brainstem changes occur. The activation of the brainstem monoaminergic nuclei has been demonstrated with functional imaging studies (Bahra et al., 2001; May, 2003). Disturbed neuronal calcium influx or hemostatic alterations have also been involved (Kors et al., 2002);

however, these events have not yet been admitted for posttraumatic migraine.

In recent years, several researchers have implicated in both typical migraine and experimental traumatic brain injury similar neurochemical changes: excessive release of excitatory amino acids; alterations of serotonin; abnormalities in catecholamines and endogenous opioids; decline in magnesium levels; abnormalities in nitric oxide formation; and alterations in neuropeptides (Packard and Ham, 1997; Solomon, 1998). It is still unknown whether these changes are determining, contributing, or precipitating factors for headache. Besides, in patients with posttraumatic migraine a sensitization phenomenon is possible. In some patients without previous migraine and a history of a recent mild head injury, the trigeminal neuron sensitization could have a non-central cause in relation to focal lesions (Láinez et al., 2003). Central and peripheral sensitization has been proposed (Malick and Burstein, 2000; Packard, 2002; Buzzi et al., 2003; Láinez, 2005).

Further research is still necessary to clarify the relationship between chronic symptoms after mild head trauma and neuroimaging abnormalities. These abnormalities could provide a pathological basis for long-term neurological disability in patients with chronic PTH. New magnetic resonance imaging techniques are useful for detecting small parenchymal brain lesions, diffuse axonal injury secondary to disruption of axonal membranes, or delayed cerebral atrophy (especially, diffusion tensor imaging and magnetization transfer ratio) (Arfanakis 2001; Volter et al., 2001; Hofman et al., 2002). In normal-appearing white matter, magnetic resonance spectroscopy studies detect metabolic brain changes (an early reduction in *N*-acetyl aspartate and an increase in choline compounds) that correlate with head injury severity (Garnett et al., 2000; Son et al., 2000). Positron emission tomography (PET), single-photon emission computed tomography (SPECT), and ^{133}Xe CT may show evidence of brain perfusion abnormalities after MHT and chronic posttraumatic symptoms (Ramadan, 1996; Aumile et al., 2002).

To date, the cause of chronic PTH remains unknown. Advances in electrophysiological, hemodynamic, and neuroimaging techniques are progressing towards establishing an organic etiology for chronic PTH and postconcussive syndrome. Cortical dysfunction with resultant alteration in neuronal threshold for pain, axonal injury with subsequent dysregulation of brainstem nociceptive pathways, and unstable cerebral hemodynamics (Ramadan et al., 1995) may provide the basis for the organicity of chronic PTH. The inverse relationship between the severity of the injury and the persistence of chronic symptoms and the psychosocial risk factors speak against the hypothesis of an organic basis for the chronic symptoms that follow a head injury. We believe that an intricate interplay between the physical injury of the brain, however minimal; psychological disturbances generated by the physical and emotional stresses of the accident and perpetuated by persistent individual concerns regarding the injury suffered and the ability to work; and the patient's premorbid disposition all contribute to chronic PTH (Packard and Ham, 1993; Ham et al., 1994; Evans, 1996; Martelli et al., 1999; Solomon, 2001). The desire for financial compensation may play a role in some cases, but not in all.

Many patients with posttraumatic migraine but also with tension-type PTH suffer frequent generalized headaches and analgesic overuse (Weeks, 1992; Warner and Fenichel, 1996). The role of analgesic overuse in perpetuating chronic PTH is a relevant factor that can contribute to the development of daily headache in many patients.

Management strategies

Trauma-induced headaches are usually heterogeneous in nature, including both tension-type and intermittent migraine attacks. Over time, PTH may take on a pattern of daily occurrence. If aggressive treatment is initiated early, PTH is less likely to become a permanent problem. Adequate treatment typically requires both central and peripheral measures. Delayed recovery from PTH may be a result of inadequately aggressive or ineffective treatment, overuse of analgesic medications resulting in analgesia rebound phenomena, or comorbid psychiatric disorders (posttraumatic stress disorder, insomnia, substance abuse, depression, or anxiety) (Lane and Arciniegas, 2002).

In general, treatment strategies are based upon studies of non-traumatic headache types. Acute PTH may be treated with analgesics, anti-inflammatory agents, and physiotherapy. Posttraumatic migraine may also be treated with ergotamine or triptans. Chronic PTH needs prophylactic medication using chronic posttraumatic migraine-specific antimigraine medications. Previously amitriptyline or propranolol, used alone or in combination, and verapamil have been demonstrated to improve all symptoms of postconcussive syndrome, especially migraine (Tyler et al., 1980; Moore, 1997; Solomon, 2001). Packard (2000) has published very good results with divalproex sodium as a preventive option in the treatment of posttraumatic migraine. Additional physical therapy, psychotherapy (biofeedback), appropriate educational support, and cutaneous stimulation can be performed, particularly in patients with risk factors for poor prognosis (Medina, 1992; Evans, 1996). An explanation of the headache's nature could also improve the patient's recovery (Packard and Ham, 1993). In some cases, when a posttraumatic lesion is identified as a peripheral triggering factor for headache, specific treatment of the triggering lesion can resolve the pain (Láinez et al., 2003). The role of botulinum toxin type A has not been established in chronic PTH, although some studies suggest efficacy in a variety of chronic headache disorders; thus it might be reasonable to assume that in PTH which presents characteristics that satisfy criteria for a particular headache disorder, the use of agents that are effective for those disorders might be useful (Sheftell et al., 2007). Poorly treated posttraumatic migraine will affect family life, recreation, and employment. Cognitive difficulties and psychological symptoms (depression, anxiety) may need specific treatment (rehabilitation, pharmacology).

HEADACHE POSTWHIPLASH

As mentioned above, the term "whiplash" commonly refers to symptoms and signs associated with a mechanical event such as a sudden acceleration and deceleration of the neck (in most cases, due to a road accident). Clinical manifestations after whiplash include symptoms related to the neck, as well as somatic extracervical, neurosensory, behavioral, cognitive, and affective disorders, whose appearance and mode of expression can vary widely over time. Postwhiplash headache (headache attributed to neck injury or whiplash) is usually accompanied by neck pain and often has a tensional or cervicogenic pattern (Table 46.3). Whiplash is commonly evaluated in medicolegal practice (Bono et al., 2000). Several social-demographic and crash-related factors, as well as a combination of specific musculoskeletal and neurological signs, have been identified as predictive factors for a longer recovery.

Table 46.3

Acute headache attributed to whiplash injury

A. Headache, no typical characteristics known, fulfilling criteria C and D
B. History of whiplash (sudden and significant acceleration/deceleration movement of the neck) associated at the time with neck pain
C. Headache develops within 7 days of whiplash injury
D. One or other of the following:
   1. Headache resolves within 3 months of whiplash injury
   2. Headache persists but 3 months have not yet passed since whiplash injury

Epidemiology

Headache occurs in 50–90% of patients within 1 month of a whiplash injury, and 8–30% continue to complain of headache 3–6 months later (Stovner, 1996). Schrader et al. (1996) reported that, outside the medicolegal context and compared with 202 control subjects, patients with whiplash injury had a similar incidence of headaches 1–3 years after the accident. Infrequent headaches (less than 1 day per month), those recurring more than 7 days per month, and chronic daily headaches were similar among patients and controls.

Similar to chronic PTH, there are no distinguishing features of headache after whiplash. Cervical pain is the most prominent symptom of the whiplash syndrome. Stovner (1996) emphasized, however, that up to 80% of patients are asymptomatic at that stage.

Clinical presentation

Several prospective studies have shown prevalence figures and the clinical presentation patterns of headache postwhiplash. After the article of Evans in 1992, many authors have followed different groups of patients with whiplash injury for several months to years. For Foletti and Regli (1995), 74% of 63 patients with headache and neck pain after whiplash complained of characteristics of tension-type headache and around 10% reported migraine with or without aura. Tension-type headache was the most frequent type of PTH in Evans's second study (1996) (85%), followed by cervicogenic (10%). Headache due to common whiplash was located occipitally (67%), was of dull pressing or dragging character (77%), and lasted on average 3 weeks. In 80% of patients postwhiplash headache showed remission within 6 months. Posttraumatic migraine and cluster-like headache was observed in rare cases (Keidel and Diener, 1997). In a new report, Pearce (2001) described the follow-up of 48 patients with headache 1 month after whiplash injury. Twenty-five of these 48 patients suffered a tension-type headache; only 3 (6%) fulfilled migrainous characteristics. Headache onset was maximal in the first 24 h after injury. Constant headaches disappeared within 3 weeks in 85% of subjects. In a prospective study Radanov et al. (2001) followed a cohort of 112 patients with a whiplash injury for 2.5 years. A total of 37% of patients had tension-type headache, 27% suffered from migraine, and 18% had cervicogenic headache. The rest were unclassified. In 104 (93%) neck pain was associated in time with headache.

In relation to these data we can conclude that the occurrence of headache attributed to whiplash injury is around 80–90%, with an early start after cervical trauma (usually within the first 6 h). Headache has mainly an occipital localization, a dull or pressing character, and is usually associated with neck pain. The pain is predominantly felt in the evening and usually resolves in 3–4 weeks (Keidel, 2000). Less than 20% of cases continue for more than 6 months.

The severity of neck injury is usually evaluated with the Quebec Classification. In 1995, a task force from Quebec, Canada, developed this classification to assist healthcare workers in making therapeutic decisions. The classification was applied to an inception cohort of patients presenting for emergency medical care following their involvement in a rear-end motor vehicle collision.

The Quebec Whiplash-Associated Disorders (WAD) Task Force evaluated whiplash injury severity (neck pain, neck muscle contraction, neck mobility, and other additional symptoms presenting in the emergency medical care) and proposed five grades that may be useful in prospective studies (WAD grades 0–IV). Grade 0 indicates no lesion, grades I and II refer to mild whiplash injury, and grades III and IV to moderate and severe whiplash injury, respectively (Spitzer et al., 1995). An adequate multiparametric procedure is required to study WAD, which takes into account the patient's main details; an exact reconstruction of the event; description and analysis of the signs and symptoms, with various complications and correlated dysfunctions; an objective neurological and neck and shoulder examination; and a battery of complementary instrumental tests (manual palpation, algometry, electromyography, kinematic analysis of the cervical spine, neuropsychological and psychological evaluations, and evaluation of disability). The Quebec classification may predict the duration of work disability and the long-term health damage caused by the injury (Hartling et al., 2001; Miettinen et al., 2002). Subsequently, other questionnaires have been developed to evaluate whiplash injury severity (Hoving et al., 2003).

Chronic postwhiplash headache has been described in several prospective studies (see new diagnosis criteria in Table 46.4). According to these studies, after mild whiplash injury chronic postwhiplash headache has shown variable presentation: 25–90% within a few days of whiplash, 12–44% within the first year, and 3–24% within 2–4 years (Radanov et al., 1994, 1995; Sturzenegger et al., 1995; Pearce, 2001; Suissa et al., 2001). Only the studies of H. Kasch, J.M. Pearce and D. Obelieniene had a control group. Particularly interesting is the work of Obelieniene et al. (1999), because the authors analyzed the presence and duration of neck pain and headache, day to day, during the first 29 days after whiplash. Most patients developed headache in the first 24 h after neck trauma.

Table 46.4

Chronic headache attributed to whiplash injury

A.	Headache, no typical characteristics known, fulfilling criteria C and D
B.	History of whiplash (sudden and significant acceleration/deceleration movement of the neck) associated at the time with neck pain
C.	Headache develops within 7 days of whiplash injury
D.	Headache persists for >3 months after whiplash injury

Risk factors

Stovner (1996) reviewed the literature on the whiplash syndrome and reported that pretrauma headaches, insurance claims, neurological findings, and degenerative changes on initial radiological studies correlated highly ($P < 0.001$) with chronic complaints posttrauma, including headache. In other recent prospective studies, women, older patients, previous cervical disturbance, lower educational or economical levels, and the absence of employment have been identified as factors of poor outcome (Radanov et al., 1995; Pujol et al., 2003; Scholten-Peeters et al., 2003; Sterner et al., 2003). Finally, some mechanical factors have also been related to the development of chronic symptoms (velocity of impact, grade of deformity of the neck at the moment of the collision) (Sturzenegger et al., 1995; Suissa et al., 2001; Nederhand et al., 2003).

Pathophysiology of postwhiplash headache

In animal studies, retropharyngeal hematomas and lesions in anterior longitudinal ligaments during acceleration injuries have been observed in monkeys (Macnab and Mc Culloch, 1994). Other authors have reported membrane leakage in cervical spinal ganglia in pigs sustaining experimental hyperextension and hyperflexion trauma of the neck (Örtengren et al., 1996).

With regard to human studies, the strain of anterior structures and compression of posterior elements like spinous processes and apophyseal joints may occur during forced extension of the neck. In addition, there is a potential strain of posterior structures (nuchal ligament, posterior neck muscles, and apophyseal joint capsules) and a compression of anterior structures (intervertebral discs and vertebral bodies) during forced flexion (Bogduk and Aprill, 1993; Barnsley et al., 1994; Garcia and Ravani 2003; Tong and Barest, 2003). Moreover, a lesion of cervical apophyseal joints has been proposed as a possible pain source (Bogduk and Aprill, 1993) and might be the cause of eye dysfunction. It is well known that painful stimulation of superficial nociceptors in the neck and head induces ipsiolateral pupil dilation by the ciliospinal reflex; thus deep nociceptors near apophyseal joints may have the same properties (Bogduk and Aprill, 1993). Indeed, in clinical practice, pain relief is obtained in whiplash patients after diagnostic blockade to apophyseal joints and following radiofrequency medial Branco neurotomy (Barnsley et al., 1993; Sapir and Gorup, 2001). On the other hand, good pain relief can be obtained in over 70% of patients with whiplash injury and deep occipital aching pain by occipital nerve release (Magnusson et al., 1996). This fact is explained by the anatomical convergence of deep and superficial nociceptive information to the dorsal horn (Mense, 1993; Hoheisel et al., 1994) or the trigeminal subnucleus caudalis located at C2–C3 level (Sessle et al., 1993). Moreover, some anatomic studies support the theory that injuries in the second cervical ganglion and nerve cause occipital headache in whiplash (Keith, 1986; Sterling et al., 2003). Other possible sources for dysfunction/damage after whiplash injury are strain of cervical (Macnab and Mc Culloch, 1994) and alar (Dvorak et al., 1987) ligaments, disc protrusions (Jonsson et al., 1991, 1994), and reduced cerebral blood flow in posterior regions (Otte et al., 1996, 1997; Bicik et al., 1998; Tercer et al., 2003).

In a prospective study, Hildingsson (1990) reported an oculomotor test: a smooth pursuit test with pathological result in 8 of 40 patients. All 8 patients and a further 5 patients at a 15-month follow-up had abnormal test results. All patients with abnormal oculomotor mobility had persisting symptoms. In addition, the smooth pursuit test and the modified smooth pursuit neck torsion test can be abnormal in chronic whiplash patients both with and without complaints of dizziness and visual disturbance (Gimse et al., 1996; Tjell and Rosenhall, 1998). Dysfunction of proprioceptors in the neck is a proposed cause of dizziness and eye mobility deficiency. However, some argue that the abnormal eye movements could be the result of hyperventilation when performing that test (Fischer et al., 1995a, b).

The main question is: why does pain develop after an acute whiplash injury? At the time of acceleration of the trunk and shoulders when a car is rear-ended, there are no direct forces on the head, which is in a greater inertial state than the neck, shoulder, or trunk. This results in neck hyperextension. After the head's inertia is overcome, the head accelerates, facilitated by decompression of a previously compressed neck structure and with the neck acting as a lever for the head. Deceleration, thus, is due to a difference in inertia, which is slower in the head than in the neck and trunk. This results in a neck hyperflexion. Autopsies indicate that structures at risk are cervical discs, facet joints, and soft-tissue structures in the neck (Bogduk, 1986; Jonsson, 1991; Taylor and Finch, 1993; Panjabi et al., 1998; Winkelstein et al., 2000). However, CT, PET, and SPECT scans have not revealed any visible structural changes after common whiplash lesions (Petterson et al., 1994; Ronnen et al., 1996; Karlsborg et al., 1997; Alexander 1998; Borchgrevink et al., 1998).

Management strategies

No universal guidelines have been published for the treatment of this condition. In acute whiplash injury, short-term active exercise and physiotherapy (Giebel et al., 1997; Borchgrevink et al., 1998; Rosenfeld et al., 2000) and short-term use of NSAIDs as well as myorelaxants are recommended (Spitzer et al., 1995; Ferrari et al., 1999). Application of a soft collar, immobilization, and more than 3 days of rest should be avoided (Spitzer et al., 1995; Borchgrevink et al., 1998; Ferrari et al., 1999).

In the management of chronic whiplash syndrome, no studies have described the long-term effectiveness of physiotherapy, interdisciplinary approach, ultrasound, or other passive treatments (Spitzer et al., 1995; Ferrari et al., 1999). The therapeutic strategy must be individualized. Myorelaxants, NSAIDs, physiotherapy, nerve blockades, and local anesthetic infiltrations could be useful; likewise, in some cases transcutaneous stimulation could improve the pain (Ferrari et al., 1999).

LITIGATION IN CHRONIC POSTTRAUMATIC HEADACHE

In our increasingly litigious society there persists an attitude that PTH and other injuries will either improve or disappear following resolution of a claim. The role of litigation in the persistence of PTH is still discussed. Nowadays, the relationship between legal settlements and the temporal profile of chronic PTH is still not clearly established. In relation to this question it is important to assess carefully patients who may be malingering or seeking enhanced compensation.

In general, there is no good evidence that litigation and economic expectations are associated with prolongation of headaches; however, the aim of all specialists in medicine is to solve medicolegal issues as soon as possible.

In fact some patients improved whilst still involved in litigation and, on the other hand, the resolution of litigation or compensation claims was not enough for headache resolution in another group of patients (Weiss et al., 1991; Evans, 1992). For Packard and Ham (1993), all 50 patients interviewed 1 year or more following a legal settlement continued to report persistent headache symptoms. Other authors have proposed that insurance and compensation systems have a significant impact on recovery from posttraumatic and postwhiplash headaches (Cote et al., 2001). In a prospective, controlled inception cohort study, 210 victims of a rear-end collision from Lithuania were consecutively identified and followed by Obelieniene et al. (1999). Neck pain and headache were evaluated shortly after the accident, after 2 months, and at 1 year. One year later, there were no significant differences between the accident victims and the control group concerning frequency and intensity of these symptoms. The authors concluded that in a country where there is no preconceived notion of chronic pain arising from rear-end collision, insurance companies, or litigation, symptoms after an acute whiplash injury are self-limiting, brief, and do not seem to correspond to the so-called late whiplash syndrome (Ferrari et al., 1999; Obelieniene et al., 1999). These data were corroborated by other groups (Schrader et al., 1996; Cassidy et al., 2000) and make us think about the contribution of an intensive and early treatment of these patients to the development of more frequent chronic posttraumatic symptoms (Borchgrevink et al., 1998).

CONCLUSIONS

PTH is the most common postconcussive symptom and most frequent type of posttraumatic pain associated with MHT. Tension-type headache is the usual presentation of PTH but other heterogeneous patterns can appear. Temporal diagnostic criteria have been reviewed with the purpose of gaining specificity. The pathogenesis of chronic symptoms is not known: neurological, psychological, and legal factors are involved.

PTH and headache attributed to whiplash may be treated early or associated complications will appear (daily occurrence of headache, overuse of analgesic medication, and comorbid psychiatric disorders). Preventive and symptomatic treatments may be prescribed in relation to clinical patterns of headache (tension-type, migraine, cluster, or cervicogenic headaches), as a primary headache. Physiotherapy, psychotherapy, and resolution of litigation can be contributing factors for recovery.

References

American Congress of Rehabilitation Medicine (1993). Definition of mild traumatic brain injury. J Head Trauma Rehabil 8(3): 86–87.

Arfanakis K, Haughton VM, Carew JD et al. (2002). Diffusion tensor MR imaging in diffuse axonal injury. AJNR Am J Neuroradiol 23: 794–802.

Alexander MP (1998). In the pursuit of proof of brain damage after whiplash injury. Neurology 51: 345–350.

Aumile EM, Sandel ME, Alavi A et al. (2002). Dynamic imaging in mild traumatic brain injury support for the theory of medial temporal vulnerability. Arch Phys Med Rehabil 83: 1506–1513.

Baandrup L, Jensen R (2005). Chronic post-traumatic headache – a clinical analysis in relation to the International Headache Classification, 2nd edition. Cephalalgia 25: 132–138.

Bahra A, Matharu MS, Buchel C et al. (2001). Brainstem activation specific to migraine headache. Lancet 357: 1016–1017.

Barnsley L, Lord S, Bogduk N (1993). Comparative local anaesthesic blocks in the diagnosis of cervical zygapophysial joint pain. Pain 55: 93–106.

Barnsley L, Lord S, Bogduk N (1994). Whiplash injury. Pain 58: 283–307.

Barth JT, Alves WM, Ryan TV et al. (1989). Mild head injury in sports: neuropsychological sequelae and recovery of function. In: HS Levin, HM Eisenberg, AL Benton (Eds.), Mild Head Injury. Oxford University Press, New York, pp. 257–273.

Bärtschi-Rochaix W (1949). Migraine cervicale, das encephale Syndrom nach Halswirbelsäulentrauma. Huber, Berne.

Bettuci D, Aguggia M, Bolamperti L et al. (1998). Chronic post-traumatic headache associated with minor cranial trauma: a description of cephalalgic patterns. Ital J Neurol Sci 19: 20–24.

Bicik I, Radanov BP, Schäfer N et al. (1998). PET with 18-fluorodeoxyglucose and hexamethylpropylene amine oxime SPECT in late whiplash syndrome. Neurology 51: 345–350.

Binder LM (1986). Persisting symptoms after mild head injury: a review of the postconcussive syndrome. J Clin Exp Neuropsychol 8: 323–346.

Bogduk N (1986). The anatomy and pathophysiology of whiplash. Clin Biomech 1: 92–101.

Bogduk N, Aprill C (1993). On the nature of neck pain, discography and cervical zygapophysial joint blocks. Pain 54: 213–217.

Bono G, Antonaci F, Ghirmai S et al. (2000). Whiplash injuries: clinical picture and diagnostic work-up. Clin Exp Rheumatol 18 (Suppl. 19): S23–S28.

Borchgrevink GE, Kaasa A, McDonagh D et al. (1998). Acute treatment of whiplash neck sprain injuries. A randomized trial of treatment during the first 14 days after a car accident. Spine 23: 25–31.

Brenner C, Friedman AP, Merritt HH et al. (1944). Posttraumatic headache. J Neurosurg 1: 379–391.

Buzzi MG, Tassorelli C, Nappi G (2003). Peripheral and central activation of trigeminal pain pathway in migraine: data from experimental animal models. Cephalalgia 23 (Suppl. 1): 1–4.

Cartlidge NEF, Shaw DA (1981). Posttraumatic headache. In: Head Injury. WB Saunders, London, pp. 95–154.

Cassidy JD, Carrol LJ, Cote P et al. (2000). Effect of eliminating compensation for pain and suffering on the outcome of insurance claims for whiplash injury. N Engl J Med 342: 1179–1186.

Cote P, Cassidy JD, Carroll L et al. (2001). A systematic review of the prognosis of acute whiplash and a new conceptual framework to synthesize the literature. Spine 26: E445–E458.

Couch JR, Bearss C (2001). Chronic daily headache in the posttrauma syndrome: relation to extent of head injury. Headache 41: 559–564.

De Benedittis G, De Santis A (1983). Chronic posttraumatic headache: clinical, psychopathological features and outcome determinants. J Neurosurg Sci 27: 177–186.

De Kruijk JR, Leffers P, Menheere PP et al. (2002). Prediction of posttraumatic complaints after mild traumatic brain injury: early symptoms and biochemical markers. J Neurol Neurosurg Psychiatry 73: 727–732.

De Souza JA, Moreira Filho PF, Jevoux Cda C (1999). [Chronic post-traumatic headache after mild head injuries]. Arq Neuropsiquiatr 57: 243–248.

Denker PG (1994). The postconcusion syndrome. Prognosis and evaluation of the organic factors. N Y State J Med 44: 379–384.

Denny-Brown D (1945). Disability arising from closed head injury. JAMA 127: 429–436.

Drottning M (2003). Cervicogenic headache after whiplash injury. Curr Pain Headache Rep 7: 384–386.

Drottning M, Staff PH, Sjaastad O (2002). Cervicogenic headache (CEH) after whiplash injury. Cephalalgia 22: 165–171.

Dvorak J, Panjabi M, Gerber M et al. (1987). CT functional diagnostics of the rotatory instability of upper cervical spine. An experimental study on cadavers. Spine 12: 197–205.

Edna TH, Cappelen J (1987). Late postconcussional symptoms in traumatic head injury. An analysis of frequency and risk factors. Acta Neurochir 86: 12–17.

Evans RW (1992). The postconcussion syndrome and the sequelae of mild head injury. Neurol Clin 10: 815–847.

Evans RW (1996). The postconcussion syndrome and the sequelae of mild head injury. In: RW Evans (Ed.), Neurology and Trauma. WB Saunders, Philadelphia, pp. 91–116.

Evans RW (2004). Posttraumatic headaches. Neurol Clin 22: 237–249.

Ferrari R, Kwan O, Russel AS et al. (1999). The best approach to the problem of whiplash? One ticket to Lithuania, please. Clin Exp Rheumatol 17: 321–326.

Fischer AJ, Huygen PL, Folgering HT et al. (1995a). Hyperactive VOR and hyperventilation after whiplash injury. Acta Otolaryngol Suppl 520: 49–52.

Fischer AJ, Huygen PL, Folgering HT et al. (1995b). Vestibular hyperreactivity and hyperventilation after whiplash injury. J Neurol Sci 132: 35–43.

Foletti G, Regli F (1995). Characteristics of chronic headaches after whiplash injury. Presse Med 24: 1121–1123.

Frommelt P (1995). Neurologische Erkrankungen. Sozialmedizinische Begutachtung in der gesetzlichen Rentenversicherung. Fischer, Stuttgart, pp. 409–451.

Garcia T, Ravani B (2003). A biomechanical evaluation of whiplash using a multi-body dynamic model. J Biomech Eng 125: 254–265.

Garnett MR, Blamire AM, Rajagopalau B et al. (2000). Evidence for cellular damage in normal-appearing white matter correlates with injury severity in patients following traumatic brain injury: a magnetic resonance spectroscopy study. Brain 123: 1043–1049.

Gfeller JD, Chibnall JT, Duckro PN (1994). Postconcussion symptoms and cognitive functioning in posttraumatic headache patients. Headache 34: 503–507.

Giebel GD, Edelmann M, Huser R (1997). Sprain of the cervical spine: early functional vs immobilization treatment. Zentralbl Chir 122: 517–521.

Gilkey SJ, Ramadan NM, Aurora TK et al. (1997). Cerebral blood flow in chronic posttraumatic headache. Headache 37: 583–587.

Gimse R, Tjell C, Bjørgen IA, Saunte C (1996). Disturbed eye movements after whiplash due to injuries to the posture control system. J Clin Exp Neuropsychol 18: 178–186.

Gronwall D, Wrightson P (1974). Delayed recovery after mild head injury. Lancet 2: 605–609.

Guthkelch AN (1977). Benign post-traumatic encephalopathy in young people and its relation to migraine. Neurosurgery 1: 101–105.

Haas DC (1993). Acute posttraumatic headache. In: J Olesen, P Tfelt-Hansen, KMA Welch (Eds.), The Headaches. Raven, New York, pp. 629–637.

Hass DC (1996). Chronic posttraumatic headaches classified and compared with natural headaches. Cephalalgia 16: 486–493.

Hass DC, Lourie H (1988). Trauma-triggered migraine: an explanation for common neurological attacks following mild head injury. J Neurosurg 68: 181–188.

Hachinski W (2000). Posttraumatic headache. Arch Neurol 57: 1780.

Ham LP, Andras KF, Packard RC et al. (1994). Psychopathology in individuals with posttraumatic headache and other pain types. Cephalalgia 14: 118–126.

Hartling L, Brison RJ, Ardem C et al. (2001). Prognosis value of the Quebec: classification of whiplash-associated disorders. Spine 26: 36–41.

Headache Classification Committee of the International Headache Society (1988). Classification and diagnostic criteria for headache disorders, cranial neuralgias and facial pain. Cephalalgia 8 (Suppl. 7): 1–96.

Headache Classification Subcommittee of the International Headache Society (2004). The international classification of headache disorders, 2nd edition. Cephalalgia 24 (Suppl. 1): 9–160.

Hildingsson C (1990). Soft-Tissue Injury of the Cervical Spine. New Series No. 296. Umea University Medical Dissertations, Umea.

Hofman PA, Verhey FR, Wilmink JT et al. (2002). Brain lesions in patients visiting a memory clinic with postconcussional sequelaes after mild to moderate brain injury. J Neuropsychiatry Clin Neurosci 14: 176–178.

Hoheisel U, Koch K, Mense S (1994). Functional reorganization in the rat dorsal horn during an experimental myositis. Pain 59: 111–118.

Hoving JL, O'Leary EF, Niere KR et al. (2003). Validity of the neck disability index, Northwick Park neck pain questionnaire, and problem elicitation technique for measuring disability associated with whiplash-associated disorders. Pain 102: 273–281.

Jacome DE (1986). Basilar artery migraine after uncomplicated whiplash injuries. Headache 26: 515–516.

Jensen OK, Nielsen FF (1990). The influence of sex and pre-traumatic headache on the incidence and severity of headache after head injury. Cephalalgia 10: 285–293.

Jonsson H, Bring G, Rauschning W et al. (1991). Hidden cervical spine injuries in traffic accidents with skull fractures. J Spinal Disord 4: 251–263.

Jonsson H, Cesarini K, Sahlstedt B et al. (1994). Findings and outcome in whiplash-type neck distortions. Spine 19: 2733–2741.

Karlsborg M, Smed A, Jespersen H et al. (1997). A prospective study of 39 patients with whiplash injury. Acta Neurol Scand 95: 65–72.

Kasch H, Qerama E, Kongsted A et al. (2008). Clinical assessment of prognostic factors for long-term pain and handicap after whiplash injury: a 1-year prospective study. Eur J Neurol 15(11): 1222–1230.

Keidel M (2000). Posttraumatic headache. In: HC Diener (Ed.), Drug Treatment of Migraine and Other Frequent Headaches. Monographs in Clinical Neuroscience, Vol. 17. Karger, Basel, pp. 329–336.

Keidel M, Ramadan NM (2006). Acute posttraumatic headaches. In: J Olesen, PJ Goadsby, NM Ramadan, P Tfelt-Hansen, KMA Welch (Eds.), The Headaches. 3rd edn. Lippincott, Williams and Wilkins, Philadelphia, pp. 863–872.

Keidel M, Diener HC (1997). Posttraumatic headache. Nervenarzt 68: 769–777.

Keith WS (1986). "Whiplash" – injury of the 2nd cervical ganglion and nerve. Curr J Neurol Sci 13: 133–137.

Kerr FW (1972). Central relationships of trigeminal and cervical primary afferents in the spinal cord and medulla. Brain Res 43: 561–572.

Kors E, van der Maagdenberg AM, Plomp JJ et al. (2002). Calcium channel mutations and migraine. Curr Opin Neurol 15: 311–316.

Kraus JF, Nourjah P (1988). The epidemiology of mild uncomplicated brain injury. J Trauma 28: 1637–1643.

Láinez JM (2005). Cefalea atribuída a traumatismo craneal y cervical. In: F Gómez, MD Jiménez (Eds.), Diagnóstico y tratamiento de la cefalea. Ergon, Madrid, pp. 233–248.

Láinez MJA, Pascual A (2005). A young man with new headache after mild head trauma. In: A Purdy, A Rapoport, F Sheftell, S Tepper (Eds.), Advanced Therapy of Headache, 2nd edn. BC Decker, Hamilton, Ontario, pp. 269–274.

Láinez JM, Piera A (2006). Cefalea postraumática. In: J Pascual, JM Láinez (Eds.), Manejo de las cefaleas refractarias. Ergon, Madrid, pp. 99–113.

Láinez JM, Pascual A, Salvador A (2003). Migraña postraumática crónica con desencadenante periférico: un caso de sensibilización no central. Neurologia 18: 71–72.

Lane J, Arciniegas DB (2002). Post-traumatic headache. Curr Treat Options Neurol 4: 89–104.

Lanser JBK, Jennekens-Schinkel A, Peters ACB (1988). Headache after closed head injury in children. Headache 28: 176–179.

Lanz S, Bryant RA (1996). Incidence of chronic pain following traumatic brain injury. Arch Phys Med Rehabil 77: 889–891.

Lenaerts ME, Couch JR (2004). Posttraumatic headache. Curr Treat Options Neurol 6: 507–517.

Levin HS, Mattis S, Ruff RM et al. (1987). Neurobehavioral outcome following minor head injury. A three-center study. J Neurosurg 66: 234–243.

Macnab I, McCulloch J (1994). Whiplash injury of the cervical spine. In: WM Passano (Ed.), Neck Ache and Shoulder Pain. Williams and Wilkins, Baltimore, pp. 140–159.

Magnusson T, Ragnarsson T, Bjornsson A (1996). Occipital nerve release in patients with whiplash trauma and occipital neuralgia. Headache 36: 32–36.

Malick A, Burstein R (2000). Peripheral and central sensitization during migraine. Funct Neurol 15 (Suppl. 3): 28–35.

Margulies S (2000). The postconcussion syndrome after mild head trauma, part II: is migraine underdiagnosed? J Clin Neurosci 7: 495–499.

Marshall LF, Ruff RM (1989). Neurosurgeon as victim. In: HS Levin, HM Eisenberg, AL Benton (Eds.), Mild Head Injury. Oxford University Press, New York, pp. 276–280.

Martelli MF, Grayson RL, Zasler ND (1999). Posttraumatic headache: neuropsychological and psychological effects and treatment implications. J Head Trauma Rehabil 14: 49–69.

May A (2003). Headache: lessons learned from functional imaging. Br Med Bull 65: 223–234.

Mazzuchi A, Cattelani R, Missale G et al. (1992). Head-injured subjects aged over 50 years: correlations between variables of trauma and neuropsychological follow-up. J Neurol 239: 256–260.

McClelland RJ, Fenton GW, Rutherford W (1994). The post-concussion syndrome revisited. J R Soc Med 87: 508–510.

Medina JL (1992). Efficacy of an individualized outpatient program in the treatment of chronic posttraumatic headache. Headache 32: 180–183.

Mense S (1993). Spinal mechanisms of muscle pain and hyperalgesia. In: L Vecchiet, D Albe-Fessard, U Lindblom (Eds.), New Trends in Referred Pain and Hyperalgesia. Elsevier, Amsterdam, pp. 25–35.

Miettinen T, Lindgren KA, Airaksinen O et al. (2002). Whiplash injuries in Finland: a prospective 1-year follow-up study. Clin Exp Rheumatol 20: 399–402.

Minderhoud JM, Boelens MEM, Huizenga J (1980). Treatment of minor head injuries. Clin Neurol Neurosurg 82: 127–140.

Moore KL (1997). Headache associated with head trauma. In: Neurobase. 3rd edn. Arbor Publishing, San Diego, p. 90.

Nebel K, Stude P, Lüdecke C et al. (2005). Prospective PC-interactive pressure algesimetry of post-traumatic neck pain after whiplash injury. Cephalalgia 25: 205–213.

Nederhand MJ, Hermens HJ, Ijzerman MJ et al. (2003). Chronic neck pain disability due to an acute whiplash injury. Pain 102: 63–71.

Nick J, Sicard-Nick C (1965). Late posttraumatic headache. Symptomatologic, physiopathological and therapeutic study. A propos of 240 cases. Presse Med 73: 2587–2592.

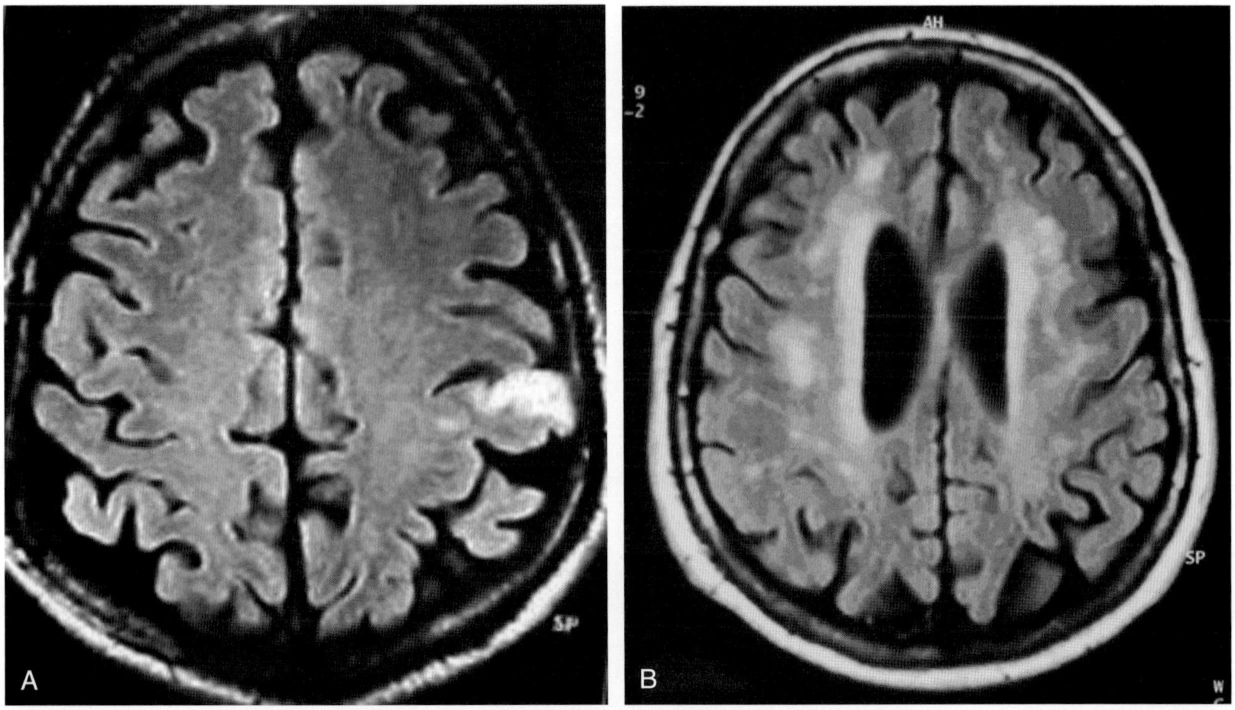

Fig. 47.1. (A) Brain magnetic resonance imaging (MRI) showing a cortical area of increased signal on fluid-attenuated inversion recovery (FLAIR) sequences indicating ischemic stroke. (Courtesy of Professor Stefano Bastianello.) (B) Brain MRI showing subcortical areas of increased signal on FLAIR sequences indicating confluent ischemic lacunar and periventricular white-matter lesions. (Courtesy of Professor Stefano Bastianello.)

with the stroke in 30%, and initiates after the stroke in 27% of patients (Vestergaard et al., 1993). When headache anticipates stroke onset, the time interval differs from a few hours to several weeks before stroke. The mean duration of the headache is 25 h (Arboix et al., 1994). The intensity of headache is reported as variable, from severe to moderate or mild. Headache severity is not related to size of infarction or to localization of stroke, but headache is more severe when the lesion is lateralized occipitally than frontally (Vestergaard et al., 1993).

The observation that headache is not related to the size of the ischemic lesion suggests that ischemia and parenchymatous damage are not the main factors for the presence of headache (Jørgensen et al., 1994). Patients with a positive history of migraine have a 1.7-fold increased risk of developing headache at stroke onset compared with patients with a negative history (Mitsias et al., 2005; Tentschert et al., 2005). Increased intracranial pressure is observed in 4.5% of patients with IS (Arboix et al., 1994).

Headache attributed to transient ischemic attack

Headache is present in 24–36% of patients with TIA and a sentinel headache in 6.5% (Table 47.1) (Grindal and Toole, 1974; Edmeads, 1979; Portenoy et al., 1984; Arboix et al., 1994; Ferro et al., 1995a). In approximately 25% of patients with TIA, headache is a prominent symptom and is the presenting complaint. Diagnostic criteria are reported in Table 47.3.

Headache is more common in TIA, occurring in the vertebrobasilar (58%) rather than in the carotid (5%) territory (Arboix et al., 1994). Among patients with TIA in the carotid distribution, the headache can be predominantly frontal or retro-orbital, being more commonly ipsilateral to the symptomatic internal carotid artery than contralateral or bifrontal. Among patients with amaurosis fugax, an ipsilateral frontal or orbital pain following the disturbance of vision may be reported. The headache occurring among patients with transient vertebrobasilar symptoms is primarily occipital or nuchal in location but it can also be diffuse or bifrontal. The mean duration of headache is 17 h (Arboix et al., 1994).

HEADACHE ATTRIBUTED TO NON-TRAUMATIC INTRACRANIAL HEMORRHAGE

Hemorrhage into the substance of the brain is a condition which most clinicians regard as prominently associated with the occurrence of a secondary headache.

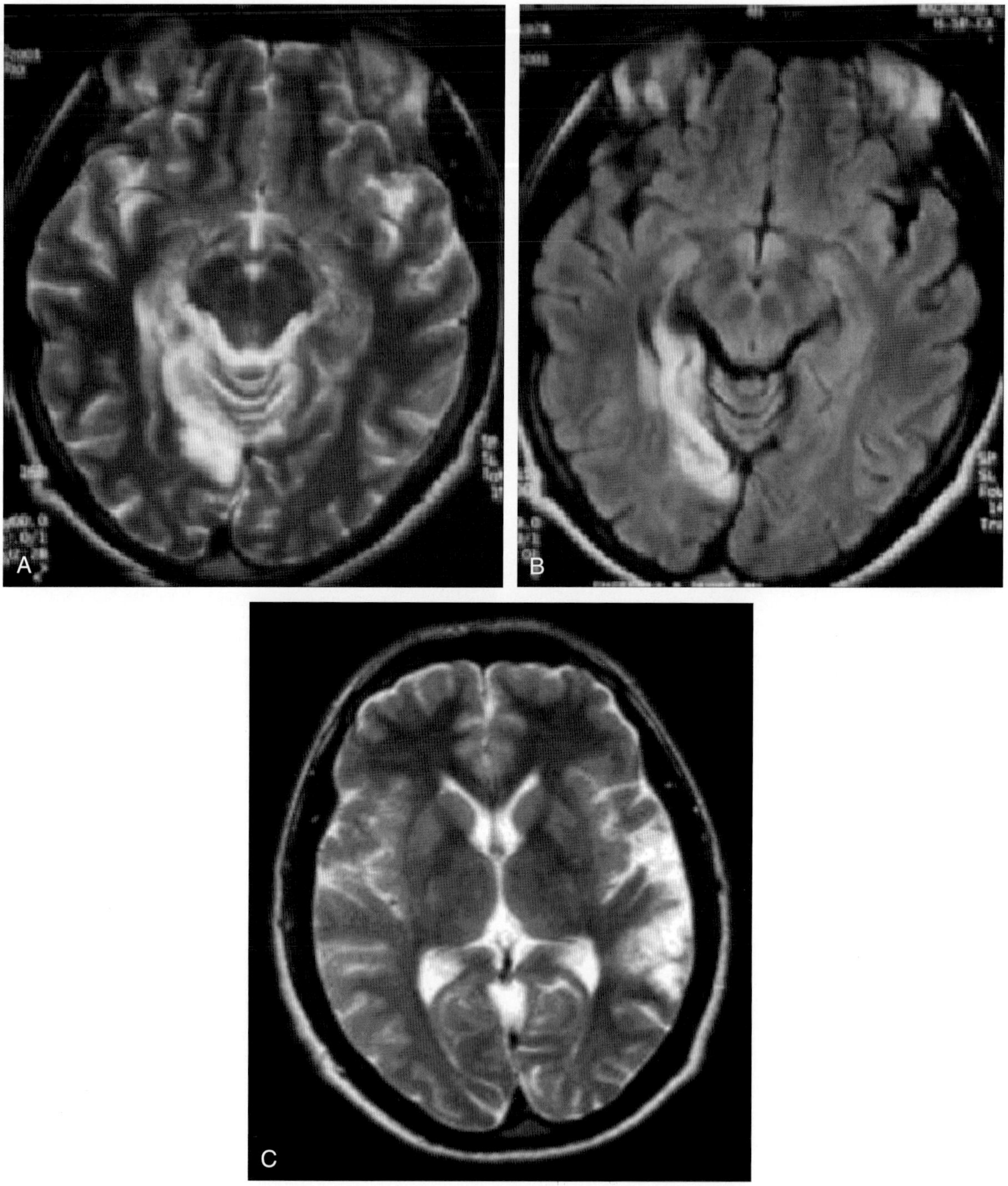

Fig. 47.2. (A and B) Brain magnetic resonance imaging (MRI) showing an area of increased signal on T_2-weighted and fluid-attenuated inversion recovery (FLAIR) sequences indicating ischemic stroke in the right posterior cerebral artery (PCA) territory involving the calcarine branches. (Courtesy of Professor Stefano Bastianello.) (C) Brain MRI showing a cortical area of increased signal on T_2-weighted sequences indicating chronic cerebral ischemia in the left middle cerebral artery territory, involving the insular and posterior temporal branches. (Courtesy of Professor Stefano Bastianello.)

Headache attributed to intracerebral hemorrhage

Primary ICH accounts for around 15% of all first-ever strokes (Carolei et al., 1997). The incidence is around 41 per 100 000 per year. Headache is reported in 33–88% of patients at the onset of the ICH (Mohr et al., 1978; Caplan et al., 1983) (Table 47.1). Diagnostic criteria are reported in Table 47.4. Headache frequency varies widely depending upon location and size of the hemorrhage

Table 47.3

Diagnostic criteria for headache attributed to transient ischemic attack

A. Any new acute headache fulfilling criteria C and D
B. Focal neurological deficit of ischemic origin lasting <24 h
C. Headache develops simultaneously with onset of focal deficits
D. Headache resolves within 24 h

Table 47.4

Diagnostic criteria for headache attributed to intracerebral hemorrhage

A. Any new acute headache fulfilling criterion C
B. Neurological signs and/or neuroimaging evidence of a recent non-traumatic intracerebral hemorrhage
C. Headache develops simultaneously with or in very close temporal relation to intracerebral hemorrhage

(Fisher, 1968). In ICH, headache is usually unilateral, focal, and of mild or moderate severity (Gorelick et al., 1986). When the hemorrhage is small, headache may be entirely absent (Weisberg and Wall, 1984).

Increased intracranial pressure headache is observed in 51.5% of patients with ICH (Arboix et al., 1994). The mean duration of the headache is 64 h (Arboix et al., 1994). In putaminal and thalamic hemorrhages, the headache, usually severe, is presumably caused by the intraventricular and subarachnoid extension of the hematoma. Often the headache is bilateral and dreadful, resembling that of a ruptured saccular aneurysm. Less commonly the headache is less severe, less abrupt in onset, and may be localized in the forehead ipsilateral to the hemorrhage. Uncommonly there is no headache at all; lack of headache tends to be associated with small hemorrhages that do not rupture in the ventricular system (Edmeads, 1986). In cerebellar hemorrhage, the headache is often acute and may be maximal at onset and severe, mimicking a SAH. Headache is reported in 13% of patients with putaminal hemorrhage (Fisher, 1968), 46–68% with lobar hemorrhage (Ropper and Davis, 1980; Kase et al., 1982), 30% with thalamic hemorrhage (Barraquer-Bordas et al., 1981), 35% with pontine hemorrhage (Silverstein, 1967), and 48–80% with cerebellar hemorrhage (Freeman et al., 1973; Little et al., 1978; Melamed and Satya-Murti, 1984).

Headache features have been identified for specific lobar hemorrhage sites: the occipital lobe is associated with severe pain, localized in and around the ipsilateral eye; the temporal lobe with mild to moderate pain, localized around the ear or just anterior to it; the frontal lobe with moderately severe pain, localized bifrontally but predominantly on the side of the hemorrhage; and the parietal lobe with severe pain, localized to the anterior temporal region (Ropper and Davis, 1980). In cerebellar hemorrhages, the characteristics of the headache depend on the size. Smaller hemorrhages may present with headache localized to the ipsilateral suboccipital region or retroauricular area. Larger hemorrhages may present with more diffuse and sometimes frontal headaches (Edmeads, 1986).

In patients with ICH the headache is related to its mass effect into the brain parenchyma with local distension, distortion, deformation, or stretching of pain-sensitive intracranial structures (Edmeads, 1986; Melo et al., 1996; Jensen and Gorelick, 2000) and is more likely to occur with larger hemorrhages than with smaller hemorrhages. Headache may be produced by the escape of blood into the subarachnoid space via the ventricular system. This may occur when the site of the primary ICH is paraventricular, as in thalamic and putaminal hemorrhage. Direct rupture of blood through the cortex in the subarachnoid space is rare. Headaches may also be caused by acute distension of the ventricular system through engorgement of the ventricles with blood under arterial pressure (as in putaminal or thalamic hemorrhages) or as acute hydrocephalus produced by obstruction of the aqueductus or of the fourth ventricle (as in some pontine or cerebellar hemorrhages). In all these instances, loss of consciousness may happen so rapidly that the history of headache may be lost. The headache may also be caused by tearing of the pain-sensitive vessel wall where the hemorrhage occurs.

The organization of the trigeminovascular system might explain the ipsilateral and sometimes the bilateral location of pain and the high frequency of headache in the presence of occipital and cerebellar hematomas (Melo et al., 1996). For this reason, the occurrence and severity of headache depend largely on the location, rate of evolution, and size of the hemorrhage (Edmeads, 1986).

Headache attributed to subarachnoid hemorrhage

SAH accounts for around 3% of all first-ever strokes (Carolei et al., 1997). In most populations the incidence is 6–7 per 100 000 per year, but it is around 20 per 100 000 in Finland and Japan (Linn et al., 1996). Ruptured aneurysms are the cause of SAH in 85% of patients, 10% are non-aneurysmal perimesencephalic hemorrhages, and the remaining 5% are caused by vasculitis, arterial dissection, arteriovenous malformations (AVMs), tumors, coagulopathies, venous thrombosis, sickle-cell disease, and Moyamoya disease (Suarez et al., 2006; van Gijn et al., 2007).

Diagnostic criteria are reported in Table 47.5. Of all types of stroke, SAH is the most prominently associated with a severe headache (Table 47.1). The typical presentation of SAH includes the sudden onset of severe headache with nausea, vomiting, neck pain, photophobia, and loss of consciousness (Suarez et al., 2006). Headache is the only symptom in about a third of patients in general practice. Conversely, in patients who present with sudden headache alone in general practice, SAH is the cause in 1 in 10 patients (Linn et al., 1994). Headache from SAH is generally diffuse and often described by patients as the most severe headache they have ever had. Patients use the terms tremendous, awful, excruciating, bursting, crushing, and unbearable. It is, however, not the severity but the suddenness of onset that is the characteristic feature, which patients often forget to mention because it is the severity of the pain for which they seek medical attention. The headache usually lasts 1–2 weeks, sometimes longer. It is atypical for the headache to resolve in less than 2 h.

The onset headache is non-lateralized in 70% of cases and lateralized in 30% (Fisher, 1968). When non-lateralized, headache is distributed diffusely over the cranium and is usually caused by rupture of anterior communicating artery aneurysms. Lateralized headaches are almost all frontal or frontoparietal, occur chiefly with carotid posterior communicating and middle cerebral artery aneurysms, and are located on the side of the aneurysmal rupture. Pain in, behind, or around the eye has often been reported in the region of carotid and posterior communicating artery aneurysms (Fisher, 1968). Pain often radiates posteriorly and down into the neck (as blood enters through the cervical subarachnoid space). In non-aneurysmal perimesencephalic hemorrhage, the onset of headache is more often gradual (in minutes rather than seconds) than in patients with aneurysmal rupture (Schwartz and Solomon, 1996; Linn et al., 1998).

Table 47.5

Diagnostic criteria for headache attributed to subarachnoid hemorrhage

A. Severe headache of sudden onset fulfilling criteria C and D
B. Neuroimaging (computed tomography or magnetic resonance imaging T_2 or fluid attenuated inversion recovery) or cerebrospinal fluid evidence of non-traumatic subarachnoid hemorrhage with or without other clinical signs
C. Headache develops simultaneously with hemorrhage
D. Headache resolves within 1 month

When sudden severe headache is the only symptom, 1 in 10 cases turns out to be a SAH, so the absence of other symptoms cannot be used to rule out the condition. Conversely, other symptoms of SAH may accompany other causes of sudden severe headache, so they cannot reliably help to distinguish SAH. No single or combined features of the headache exist that distinguish reliably, and at an early stage, between SAH and non-hemorrhagic thunderclap headache. Vomiting is not a distinctive feature because almost half of the patients with non-hemorrhagic thunderclap headache also report vomiting at onset (van Gijn et al., 2007). Seizures at onset occur in about 7% of patients with SAH (Pinto et al., 1996; Linn et al., 1998). Other symptoms suggesting the presence of a SAH are coma, various degrees of lethargy, confusion, agitation, obtundation, or acute confusional state. Neck stiffness is a common sign in SAH. Fundoscopy examination may reveal intraocular hemorrhage. Focal neurological deficits occur when an aneurysm compresses a cranial nerve or bleeds into the brain parenchyma, or from focal ischemia due to acute vasoconstriction immediately after aneurysmal rupture. Sometimes, the clinical manifestations of a ruptured aneurysm are indistinguishable from a stroke due to ICH or IS. Because no clinical feature is sufficiently reliable to make the diagnosis, SAH must be excluded in patients presenting with sudden severe headache that is maximal within minutes, lasts for more than an hour, and has no alternative explanation.

The presence of a severe, sudden headache, often referred to as a warning leak, minor leak, or sentinel headache, during the days or weeks before SAH has been reported in 15–95% of all patients eventually admitted with a SAH (Gorelick et al., 1986; Linn et al., 1994). Sentinel headache has been described as sudden, severe, or disabling and is unlike any headache the patient had experienced previously. It is located in the occipital region in 31% of cases, frontally in 26%, and retro-orbital in 14%, and usually subsides over several hours to days. With the exception of posterior communicating artery aneurysms, premonitory headache is a poor localizing symptom of the site of the aneurysm. In addition to sentinel headache, two-thirds of patients had other signs and symptoms, including vomiting (19%), meningism or neck pain (35%), syncope or brief coma (26%), visual symptoms (17%), and motor or sensory manifestations (20%) (Gorelick et al., 1986).

In the absence of the classic signs and symptoms, SAH may be misdiagnosed (Edlow and Caplan, 2000). The most common incorrect diagnoses are migraine or tension-type headaches (Suarez et al., 2006). Other primary headache syndromes that can resemble headache caused by SAH include thunderclap headache, cluster headache, and headache associated with sexual activity or exertion. Secondary headache syndromes that can resemble a headache caused by SAH include cerebral venous thrombosis, ICH, extradural or subdural hemorrhage, IS, arterial dissection, vasculitis, infections such as meningitis or encephalitis, acute hydrocephalus, intracranial tumours, pituitary apoplexy, spontaneous intracranial hypotension or post-lumbar puncture hypotension, metabolic diseases such as pheochromocytoma, or tyramine ingestion combined with monoamine oxidase inhibitors.

The exact pathogenesis of onset headache is unclear, but it has been plausibly suggested that the initial pain is produced by stretching and tearing of the distended vessel and its adjacent arachnoid and that pain is perpetuated through chemical irritation by blood of the pain-sensitive meninges directly surrounding the vessels. To this may contribute increased intracranial pressure headache as blood under arterial pressure extravasates into the intracranial compartment. The pathophysiology of sentinel headache has been a matter of debate. The proposed explanations for sentinel headache range from changes in the wall of the aneurysm without rupture or rupture of an intracranial aneurysm causing minor SAH to recall bias, which is unreleted to SAH (Ball, 1975; Linn et al., 1994).

HEADACHE ATTRIBUTED TO UNRUPTURED VASCULAR MALFORMATIONS

Headache attributed to saccular aneurysm

Intracranial aneurysms are common lesions. The best estimate of their frequency for an average adult without specific risk factors is 2.3%; this proportion increases with age. Saccular aneurysms arise at sites of arterial branching, usually at the base of the brain, either on the circle of Willis itself or at a nearby branching point. The majority of intracranial aneurysms (80–85%) are located in the anterior circulation, most commonly at the junction of the internal carotid artery and the posterior communicating artery, the anterior communicating artery complex, or the trifurcation of the middle cerebral artery. Aneurysms of the posterior circulation are most frequently located at the bifurcation of the basilar artery or at the junction of a vertebral artery and the ipsilateral posterior inferior cerebellar artery (Schievink, 1997).

Most intracranial aneurysms will never rupture, remaining clinically silent (van Gijn et al., 2007). Other aneurysms will start to produce mass-effect symptoms that, in most cases, indicate a near rupture. The frequency of these prerupture symptoms varies from 10% to 60%. The most common symptom of an aneurysmal mass effect is headache, and the most common sign is a palsy of the third nerve. Third cranial nerve palsy is a classic presentation of an unruptured or slowly or intermittently leaking aneurysm originating at the junction of the carotid artery and the posterior communicating artery, or an aneurysm of the upper end of the basilar artery. The typical presentation consists of a slowly or quickly evolving unilateral third-nerve palsy, with a dilated and unresponsive pupil, downward and outward deviation of the eye, ptosis, diplopia, and pain behind the eye or in the ipsilateral forehead and/or temple. Without treatment, after a period of days, weeks, or even months the patient suffers an overt SAH. Depending on the location of the aneurysm, other manifestations of a mass effect include brainstem dysfunction, visual field defects, trigeminal neuralgia, a cavernous sinus syndrome, seizures, and hypothalamic–pituitary dysfunction.

Much more difficult to assess are those patients with isolated severe headache, no other symptoms, and no abnormal signs. Also these headaches, named also as premonitory headache, sentinel headache, and warning leaks, may represent a prelude to SAH. Problems, when faced with a patient with headache, rely on trying to identify those with an unruptured intracranial aneurysm. Brain neuroimaging examination should be performed in the presence of a new-onset headache without the characteristics of a primary headache; a headache changing its characteristics in a patient suffering from a primary headache; headache in a patient suffering from one of the numerous heritable disorders that have been associated with intracranial aneurysms such as autosomal-dominant polycystic kidney disease, Ehlers–Danlos syndrome type IV, neurofibromatosis type 1, Marfan's syndrome; and a positive family history of intracranial aneurysms. Diagnostic criteria are reported in Table 47.6.

Headache and nerve palsies in the case of unruptured intracranial aneurysms may be caused by little hemorrhages involving the nerve, destruction of the aneurysmal sac, pressure on the adjacent free edge of

Table 47.6

Diagnostic criteria for headache attributed to saccular aneurysm

A. Any new acute headache, including thunderclap headache and/or painful third-nerve palsy fulfilling criteria C and D
B. Neuroimaging evidence of saccular aneurysm
C. Evidence exists of causation by the saccular aneurysm
D. Headache resolves within 72 h
E. Subarachnoid hemorrhage, intracerebral hemorrhages and other causes of headache ruled out by appropriate investigations

the tentorium, or direct pressure on nerves or pain structures (Edmeads, 1986). Giant aneurysms, particularly if their location permits them to distort the ventricular system, may produce the progressively worsening diffuse headaches reminiscent of increased intracranial pressure.

Headache attributed to arteriovenous malformation

AVMs are lesions that are defined by the presence of arteriovenous shunting through a nidus of coiled and tortuous vascular connections that link feeding arteries to draining veins (Fleetwood and Steinberg, 2002). An important anatomical feature of this vascular nidus is the lack of a capillary bed as arteries feeding the nidus are directly connected to the draining veins (shunting) (Choi and Mohr, 2005). Technical advances in neuroimaging have increased the rate of detection of AVMs to the extent that they now pose a frequent management problem.

Brain AVMs come to clinical attention mainly in young adults, typically before the age of 40 years (Marini et al., 2001). Intracranial hemorrhage is the most frequently (53%) recorded type of AVM presentation. Other symptoms include generalized (30%) or focal (10%) seizures, chronic headache (14%), and progressive (5%), persistent (7%), or reversible (8%) neurological deficits (Hofmeister et al., 2000). Diagnostic criteria are reported in Table 47.7. Headache is the presenting symptom in 7–48% of patients, with no distinctive features such as frequency, duration, or severity. In a study of 700 patients with AVM who were treated with radiosurgery, 109 (16%) had headache; headaches were isolated in 6% of cases (i.e., not related to hemorrhage, seizure, or neurological deficit), predominant in female patients, mostly non-pulsating, and on the same side as the lesion (Ghossoub et al., 2001).

Distinctive characteristics to identify AVM-related headache types have not been established. No side

Table 47.7

Diagnostic criteria for headache attributed to arteriovenous malformation

A. Any new acute headache fulfilling criteria C and D
B. Neuroimaging evidence of arteriovenous malformation
C. Evidence exists of causation by the arteriovenous malformation
D. Headache resolves within 72 h
E. Subarachnoid hemorrhage, intracerebral hemorrhage, and other causes of headache ruled out by appropriate investigations

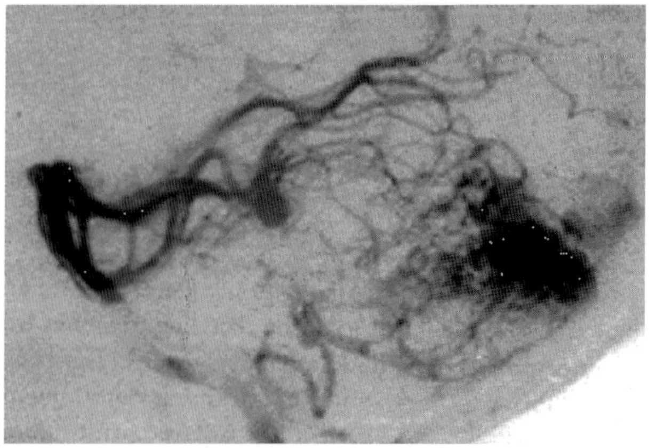

Fig. 47.3. Conventional angiography of the posterior circulation showing an arteriovenous vascular malformation. (Courtesy of Dr Giorgio Minonzio.)

preference is reported for symptoms. In the general population AVMs are an extremely infrequent cause of headache and are found in around 1% of patients with migraine (Bruyn, 1984). However, headache is a well-known symptom of occipital AVM (Figure 47.3). Migraine-like ophthalmic symptoms are present in 15% of patients (Nagata et al., 2006). Also the association of headache and epilepsy raises the possibility of AVM. A headache may also represent the symptom of bleeding from an AVM; in such circumstances it is rarely isolated and more commonly accompanied by focal neurological signs or symptoms.

The pathogenesis of headache is unclear, but large nidus volume, a tortuous feeding artery, and cortical drainage with reflux in the superior sagittal sinus are associated with a higher incidence of headache (Kurita et al., 2000).

Headache attributed to dural arteriovenous fistula

Dural arteriovenous fistulas (DAVFs) are abnormal arteriovenous connections that are located within the dura mater and involve a dural sinus and/or cortical veins. DAVFs are thought to be acquired through trauma, sinus occlusion, or chronic venous hypertension (Chaudhary et al., 1982). Although most DAVFs have a benign course, they can result in life-threatening hemorrhage and venous hypertension. It is interesting to note that most DAVFs involve the left-side transverse and sigmoid sinus. When located in the cavernous sinus (Figure 47.4), the DAVFs may produce a typical cavernous sinus syndrome with headache mostly retro-orbital and accompanied by a variable degree of ocular and visual symptoms (Theaudin et al., 2007). Diagnostic criteria are reported in Table 47.8.

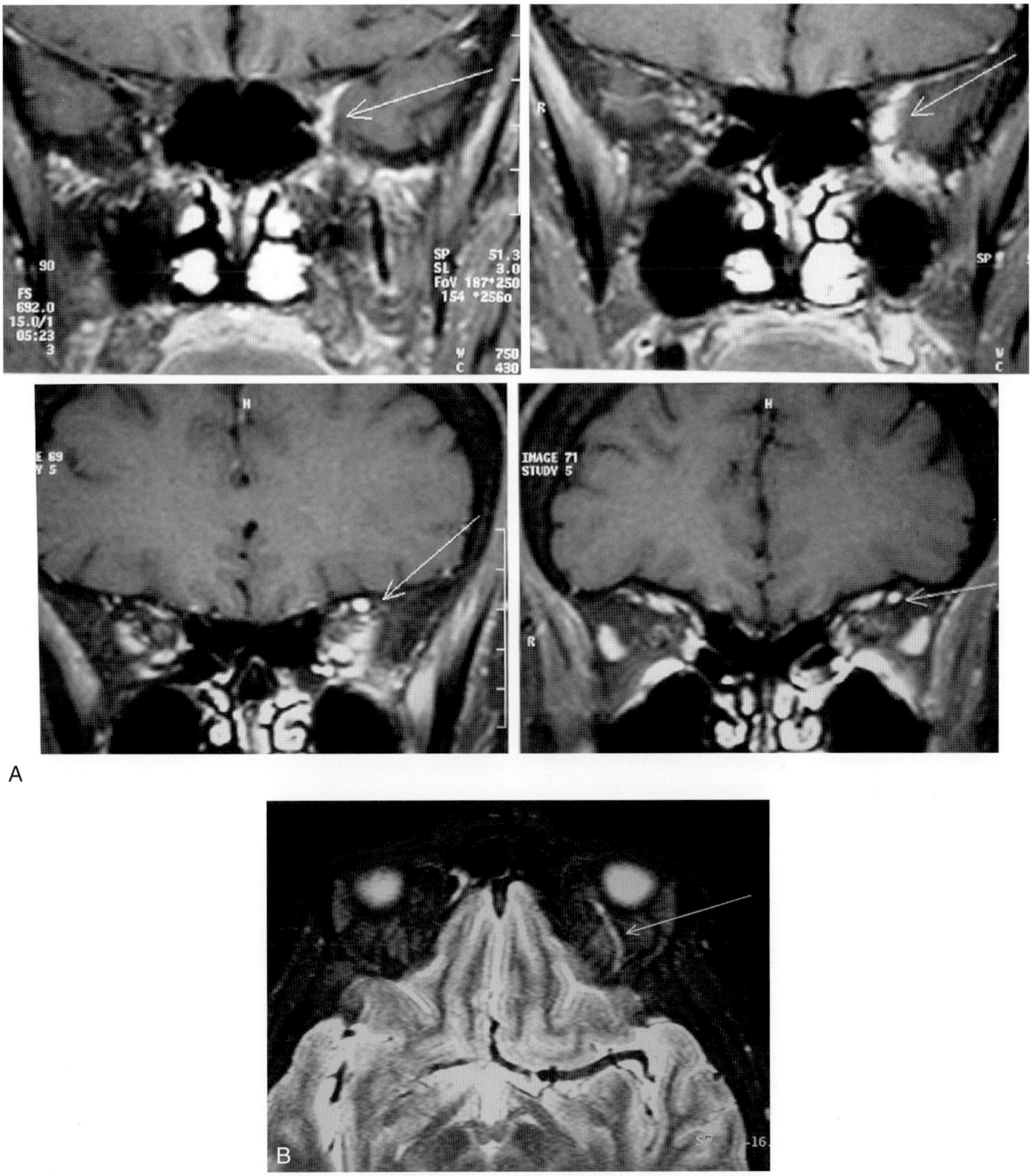

Fig. 47.4. Brain magnetic resonance imaging (MRI)-enhanced T_1-weighted sequences on coronal planes (A) and T_2-weighted sequences on axial plane (B) of a traumatic left carotid cavernous fistula; a dilation of the superior ophthalmic vein is typically present. (Courtesy of Professor Stefano Bastianello.)

Table 47.8

Diagnostic criteria for headache attributed to dural arteriovenous fistula

A. Any new acute headache fulfilling criterion C
B. Neuroimaging evidence of dural arteriovenous fistula
C. Evidence exists of causation by the fistula
D. Subarachnoid hemorrhage, intracerebral hemorrhage, and other causes of headache ruled out by appropriate investigations

Headache attributed to dural cavernous angioma

Headache in such conditions may be associated with rupture of the angioma. However, no studies are available reporting the frequency of the headache. Diagnostic criteria are reported in Table 47.9.

Headache attributed to encephalotrigeminal or leptomeningeal angiomatosis (Sturge–Weber syndrome)

Sturge–Weber syndrome (SWS) is a rare, sporadic neurocutaneous syndrome affecting the cephalic venous microvasculature. One per 50 000 live births has SWS, although more people might have the disorder without a proper diagnosis. The hallmark intracranial vascular anomaly is leptomeningeal angiomatosis, most often involving the occipital and posterior parietal lobes. A typical characteristic is an ipsilateral facial cutaneous vascular malformation usually affecting the upper face in the ophthalmic division of the trigeminal nerve. Other clinical findings include seizures, glaucoma, headache, transient stroke-like neurological deficits, and behavioral problems. Hemiparesis, hemiatrophy, and hemianopia may occur contralateral to the cortical abnormality (Thomas-Sohl et al., 2004).

Diagnostic criteria for headache attributed to SWS are reported in Table 47.10. The frequency and severity of headaches are higher in SWS than in the general population. Headache occurs in 30–45% of patients and may be debilitating (Klapper, 1994). The headache often presents with the characteristics of a migraine attack (symptomatic migraine) which may be accompanied by a prolonged aura (Bousser et al., 2001). Many children report a temporal relationship between their headaches and seizure activity.

The leptomeningeal angioma in patients with SWS may predispose to neuronal hyperexcitability, causing changes in cortical perfusion and oxygenation. An alternative hypothesis aimed at explaining the migraine-like attacks with aura suggests that chronic focal oligemia and ensuing tissue hypoxia might precipitate severe, prolonged deficits without cerebral infarctions, bearing striking similarities to those reported in some varieties of familial hemiplegic migraine (Bousser et al., 2001).

Table 47.9

Diagnostic criteria for headache attributed to dural cavernous angioma

A. Any new acute headache fulfilling criterion C
B. Neuroimaging evidence of cavernous angioma
C. Evidence exists of causation by the cavernous angioma
D. Subarachnoid hemorrhage, intracerebral hemorrhage, and other causes of headache ruled out by appropriate investigations

Table 47.10

Diagnostic criteria for headache attributed to encephalotrigeminal or leptomeningeal angiomatosis (Sturge–Weber syndrome)

A. Any new acute headache fulfilling criterion C
B. Facial angioma, seizures, and neuroimaging evidence of meningeal angioma ipsilateral to the facial angioma
C. Evidence exists of causation by the angioma
D. Other causes of headache ruled out by appropriate investigations

References

Allen MC (1983). Clinical diagnosis of the acute stroke syndrome. Am J Med 208: 515–523.

André C, Neves FF, Vincent MB (1996). Headache in transient ischaemic attack. Funct Neurol 11: 195–200.

Arboix A, Massons J, Oliveres M et al. (1994). Headache in acute cerebrovascular disease: a prospective clinical study in 240 patients. Cephalalgia 14: 37–40.

Ball MJ (1975). Pathogenesis of the "sentinel headache" preceding berry aneurysm rupture. Can Med Assoc J 112: 78–79.

Barraquer-Bordas L, Illa I, Escartin A et al. (1981). Thalamic hemorrhage: a study of 23 patients with diagnosis by computed tomography. Stroke 12: 524–527.

Bogousslavsky J, Van Melle G, Regli F (1988). The Lausanne Stroke Registry: analysis of 1,000 consecutive patients with first stroke. Stroke 19: 1083–1092.

Bousser MG, Good J, Kittner SJ et al. (2001). Headache associated with vascular disorders. In: SD Silberstein, RB Lipton, DJ Dalessio (Eds.), Wolff's Headache and Other Head Pain. 7th edn. Oxford University Press, New York, pp. 349–392.

Bruyn GW (1984). Intracranial arteriovenous malformation and migraine. Cephalalgia 4: 191–207.

Caplan LR, Hier DB, D'Cruz I (1983). Cerebral embolism in the Michael Reese Stroke Registry. Stroke 14: 530–536.

Carolei A, Marini C, Di Napoli M et al. (1997). High stroke incidence in the prospective community-based L'Aquila registry (1994–1998). First year's results. Stroke 28: 2500–2506.

Chaudhary MY, Sachdev VP, Cho SH et al. (1982). Dural arteriovenous malformation of the major venous sinuses: an acquired lesion. Am J Neuroradiol 3: 13–19.

Choi JH, Mohr JP (2005). Brain arteriovenous malformations in adults. Lancet Neurol 4: 299–308.

Edlow JA, Caplan LR (2000). Avoiding pitfalls in the diagnosis of subarachnoid hemorrhage. N Engl J Med 342: 29–36.

Edmeads J (1979). The headaches of ischemic cerebrovascular disease. Headache 19: 345–349.

Edmeads J (1986). Headache in cerebrovascular disease. In: PJ Vinken, GW Bruyn, HL Klawans (Eds.), Handbook of Clinical Neurology: Headache (revised series 4), Vol. 48. Elsevier, Amsterdam, pp. 273–290.

Ferro JM, Costa I, Melo TP et al. (1995a). Headache associated with transient ischemic attacks. Headache 35: 544–548.

Ferro JM, Melo TP, Oliveira V et al. (1995b). A multivariate study of headache associated with ischemic stroke. Headache 35: 315–319.

Fisher CM (1968). Headache in acute cerebrovascular disease. In: PJ Vinken, CW Bruyn (Eds.), Headaches and Cranial Neuralgias, Vol. 5. John Wiley, New York, pp. 124–156.

Fleetwood IG, Steinberg GK (2002). Arteriovenous malformations. Lancet 359: 863–873.

Freeman RE, Onofrio BM, Okazaki H et al. (1973). Spontaneous intracerebellar hemorrhage. Neurology 23: 84–90.

Gawel M, Burkitt M, Rose FC (1979). The platelet release reaction during migraine attacks. Headache 19: 323–327.

Ghossoub M, Nataf F, Merienne L et al. (2001). Characteristics of headache associated with cerebral arteriovenous malformations. Neurochirurgie 47: 177–183.

Gorelick PB, Hier DB, Caplan LR et al. (1986). Headache in acute cerebrovascular disease. Neurology 36: 1445–1450.

Grindal AB, Toole JF (1974). Headache and transient ischemic attacks. Stroke 5: 603–606.

Headache Classification Subcommittee of the International Headache Society (2004). The international classification of headache disorders, 2nd edition. Cephalalgia 24 (Suppl. 1): 1–160.

Hofmeister C, Stapf C, Hartmann A et al. (2000). Demographic, morphological, and clinical characteristics of 1289 patients with brain arteriovenous malformation. Stroke 31: 1307–1310.

Jensen TS, Gorelick PB (2000). Headache associated with ischemic stroke and intracranial hematoma. In: J Olesen, P Tfelt-Hansen, KMA Welch (Eds.), The Headaches. Lippincott Williams & Wilkins, Philadelphia, pp. 781–787.

Jørgensen HS, Jespersen HF, Nakayama H et al. (1994). Headache in stroke: The Copenhagen Stroke Study. Neurology 44: 1793–1797.

Kase CS, Williams JP, Wyatt DA et al. (1982). Lobar intracerebral hematomas: clinical and CT analysis of 22 cases. Neurology 32: 1146–1150.

Klapper J (1994). Headache in Sturge–Weber syndrome. Headache 34: 521–522.

Koudstaal PJ, van Gijn J, Kappelle LJ (1991). Headache in transient or permanent cerebral ischemia. Dutch TIA Study Group. Stroke 22: 754–759.

Kumral E, Bogousslavsky J, Van Melle G et al. (1995). Headache at stroke onset: the Lausanne Stroke Registry. J Neurol Neurosurg Psychiatry 58: 490–492.

Kurita H, Shin M, Kirino T (2000). Resolution of migraine with aura caused by an occipital arteriovenous malformation. Arch Neurol 57: 1219–1220.

Leira R, Castellanos M, Alvarez-Sabín J et al. (2005). Stroke Project, Cerebrovascular Diseases Group of the Spanish Neurological Society. Headache in cerebral hemorrhage is associated with inflammatory markers and higher residual cavity. Headache 45: 1236–1243.

Linn FHH, Wijdicks EFM, van der Graaf Y et al. (1994). Prospective study of sentinel headache in aneurysmal subarachnoid haemorrhage. Lancet 344: 590–593.

Linn FHH, Rinkel GJE, Algra A et al. (1996). Incidence of subarachnoid hemorrhage: role of region, year, and rate of computed tomography: a meta-analysis. Stroke 27: 625–629.

Linn FHH, Rinkel GJE, Algra A et al. (1998). Headache characteristics in subarachnoid haemorrhage and benign thunderclap headache. J Neurol Neurosurg Psychiatry 65: 791–793.

Little JR, Tubman DE, Ethier R (1978). Cerebellar hemorrhage in adults: diagnosis by computerized tomography. J Neurosurg 48: 575–579.

Marini C, Totaro R, De Santis F et al. (2001). Stroke in young adults in the community-based L'Aquila registry: incidence and prognosis. Stroke 32: 52–56.

Melamed N, Satya-Murti S (1984). Cerebellar hemorrhage: a review and reappraisal of benign cases. Arch Neurol 41: 425–428.

Melo TS, Pinto AN, Ferro JM (1996). Headache in intracerebral hematomas. Neurology 47: 494–500.

Mitsias PD, Ramadan NM, Levine SR et al. (2005). Factors determining headache at onset of acute ischemic stroke. Cephalalgia 26: 150–157.

Mohr JP, Caplan LR, Melski JW et al. (1978). The Harvard Cooperative Stroke Registry: a prospective registry. Neurology 28: 754–762.

Moskowitz MA, Buzzi G, Sakas DE et al. (1989). Pain mechanisms underlying vascular headaches. Rev Neurol 145: 181–193.

Nagata S, Morioka T, Natori Y et al. (2006). Surgical treatment of non-ruptured giant occipital arteriovenous malformations with frequent migraine-like headache. Neurol Med Chir 46: 441–445.

Pinto AN, Canhao P, Ferro JM (1996). Seizures at the onset of subarachnoid haemorrhage. J Neurol 243: 161–164.

Portenoy RK, Abissi CJ, Lipton RB (1984). Headache in cerebrovascular disease. Stroke 15: 1009–1012.

Ropper AH, Davis KR (1980). Lobar cerebral hemorrhages: acute clinical syndromes in 26 cases. Ann Neurol 8: 141–147.

Schievink WI (1997). Intracranial aneusyms. N Engl J Med 336: 28–40.

Schwartz TH, Solomon RA (1996). Perimesencephalic nonaneurysmal subarachnoid hemorrhage: review of the literature. Neurosurgery 39: 433–440.

Silverstein A (1967). Primary pontine hemorrhage: a review of 50 cases. Confin Neurol 29: 33–46.

Suarez JI, Tarr RW, Selman WR (2006). Aneurysmal subarachnoid hemorrhage. N Engl J Med 354: 387–396.

Tentschert S, Wimmer R, Greisenegger S et al. (2005). Headache at stroke onset in 2196 patients with ischemic stroke or transient ischemic attack. Stroke 36: e1–e3.

Theaudin M, Saint-Maurice JP, Chapot R et al. (2007). Diagnosis and treatment of dural carotid-cavernous fistulas: a consecutive series of 27 patients. J Neurol Neurosurg Psychiatry 78: 174–179.

Thomas-Sohl KA, Vaslow DF, Maria BL (2004). Sturge–Weber syndrome: a review. Pediatr Neurol 30: 303–310.

van Gijn J, Kerr RS, Rinkel GEJ (2007). Subarachnoid haemorrhage. Lancet 369: 306–318.

Vestergaard K, Andersen G, Nielsen MI et al. (1993). Headache in stroke. Stroke 24: 1621–1624.

Weisberg LA, Wall M (1984). Small capsular hemorrhages. Arch Neurol 41: 1255–1257.

Wells C (1961). Premonitory symptoms of cerebral embolism. Arch Neurol 5: 490–496.

Handbook of Clinical Neurology, Vol. 97 (3rd series)
Headache
G. Nappi and M.A. Moskowitz, Editors

Chapter 48

Headache attributed to arteritis, cerebral venous thrombosis, and other vascular intracranial disturbances

ANTONIO CAROLEI* AND SIMONA SACCO
Department of Neurology, University of L'Aquila, L'Aquila, Italy

HEADACHE ATTRIBUTED TO ARTERITIS, CEREBRAL VENOUS THROMBOSIS, AND OTHER VASCULAR INTRACRANIAL DISTURBANCES

Headache attributed to arteritis

Arteritis is an inflammation of the vessel wall. Vessels of any type and in any organ may be involved, resulting in a wide variety of signs and symptoms. Arteritides in which the central nervous system is the main target organ are classified as primary even if the central nervous system may also be involved by systemic primary or secondary arteritis (Jennette and Falk, 1997; Weyand and Goronzy, 2003). Headache with variable characteristics and associated signs and symptoms may occur in all kinds of arteritis.

Giant cell arteritis

Giant cell arteritis, one of the most common arteritides, is also known as cranial arteritis, temporal arteritis, or Horton's disease. It consists of a large and medium-sized granulomatous arteritis involving branches of the external and, more rarely, of the internal carotid arteries. The highest incidence rates are described in Scandinavia and North America (Calvo-Romero, 2003). Giant cell arteritis is more common among women than men. Some familial accumulation and the association with the human leukocyte antigen (HLA)-DR4 haplotype indicate a genetic predisposition (Salvarani et al., 1991), where epidemiological observations and studies using DNA detection techniques suggest an infectious origin (*Mycoplasma pneumoniae*, *Chlamydia pneumoniae*, and parvovirus B19) (Gabriel et al., 1999; Rimenti et al., 2000). The etiology remains unknown despite recent encouraging contributions.

Giant cell arteritis occurs exclusively in patients over the age of 50. Fever, new-onset headache, prominence and tenderness of the temporal artery, claudication of the muscles of mastication with chewing, amaurosis fugax, and visual loss are among the most common neurological manifestations. Other associated conditions and symptoms include polymyalgia rheumatica, weight loss, absent temporal artery pulse, peripheral joint pain, tongue claudication, pain on swallowing, limb claudication, and stroke (Carolei and Sacco, 2003; Ward and Levin, 2005).

Headache in giant cell arteritis is the initial symptom in 48% of patients and is eventually found in 90%. Headache may be of any type, constant or intermittent, may mimic tension-type headache, migraine, or even cluster headache, and may be of variable location and severity (Ward and Levin, 2005). The pain in giant cell arteritis is felt in the scalp, especially in the region of the inflamed blood vessels (Ross Russell, 1986). Mild pressure on the scalp, such as that caused by wearing a hat or resting the head on a pillow, may be unbearable. Ischemic changes in the skin with hair loss and occasionally gangrene may also occur. The usual location is temporal and the patient may notice localized swelling and tenderness along the course of the superficial temporal artery and its branches. Similar symptoms may occur in the occipital region.

The pain is of variable severity but is often bad enough to disturb sleep. It has a constant boring quality and analgesics give temporary relief. Muscular aching affecting shoulders and hips is a common complaint, and it may precede the headache by several months.

*Correspondence to: Professor Antonio Carolei, MD, FAHA, Department of Neurology, University of L'Aquila, L'Aquila, Italy, Tel. and Fax: +39.0862.64153, E-mail: a_carolei@yahoo.com

The muscles may be tender to palpation, often with a mild degree of weakness, but muscle atrophy is exceptional (Ross Russell, 1986).

Recent investigations support the hypothesis that polymyalgia rheumatica and giant cell arteritis are two different expressions of the same underlying vasculitic disorder (Cantini et al., 2004). Jaw claudication refers to pain in the muscles of mastication coming on when the patient chews and eased by rest. It is caused by restriction of the blood supply to the temporalis and masseter muscle when arteritis involves branches of the maxillary and facial arteries. Painful swelling of the tongue with induration and restriction of movements, sometimes with ulceration, may also occur (Ross Russell, 1986).

Amaurosis fugax and blindness reflect end-organ ischemia causing anterior ischemic optic neuropathy, posterior ischemic optic neuropathy, or central retinal artery occlusion. Pain in one or both orbits is an occasional symptom. It may be accompanied by visual loss and ophthalmoplegia. The most common cause of visual loss in patients with giant cell arteritis is ischemic damage to the optic nerve and retina on one or both sides. Loss of vision in the other eye may occur within a few days of the first. The prognosis for recovery of loss of vision of more than a few hours' duration is very poor.

In some patients partial or complete occlusion of the internal carotid or vertebral arteries may occur, causing hemispheric or brainstem infarction. A lateral medullary infarct is the most common type. There is another mechanism which accounts for cerebral ischemia: mural thrombosis has been shown to occur in inflamed arteries and portions of thrombus may embolize in the distal intracranial circulation. This is particularly likely to affect the vertebral distribution since vertebral arteries are favored sites for inflammation. The resulting embolic infarct may be hemorrhagic in type and affects the posterior cerebral artery territory on one or both hemispheres. Bilateral visual loss can thus be caused either by ocular or by bilateral occipital damage.

Laboratory tests reveal an erythrocyte sedimentation rate above 50 mm/h. Only in particular circumstances and early in the disease may this parameter be normal. C-reactive protein is also constantly elevated. Temporal artery biopsy remains the gold standard for diagnosis, allowing granulomatous inflammation with multinucleated giant cells to be revealed (Carolei and Sacco, 2003). Diagnostic criteria are otherwise reported in Table 48.1.

Table 48.1

Diagnostic criteria for headache attributed to giant cell arteritis

A. Any new persisting headache fulfilling criteria C and D
B. At least one of the following:
   1. Swollen tender scalp artery with elevated erythrocyte sedimentation rate and/or C-reactive protein
   2. Temporal artery biopsy demonstrating giant cell arteritis
C. Headache develops in close temporal relation to other symptoms and signs of giant cell arteritis
D. Headache resolves or greatly improves within 3 days of high-dose steroid treatment

Primary central nervous system angiitis

Primary central nervous system angiitis is a rare, male predominant, and highly fatal disease that has been reported in a wide range of age groups. It is a leptomeningeal and cortical vasculitic disease involving small and medium-sized leptomeningeal cortical arteries and, less frequently, veins and venules. The histological pattern consists of the classic granulomatous angiitis together with a polyarteritis nodosa-type necrotizing vasculitis, and with normal arteries and veins nearby (Carolei and Sacco, 2003). Both foreign-body and Langhans' giant cells may be present in granulomatous angiitis, or there may be only a necrotizing lymphocytic vasculitis. The etiology and pathogenesis are unknown. Particles resembling *Mycoplasma* or virus-like structures have been described (Rehman, 2000).

The majority of patients develop a variety of focal neurological deficits, mostly in the presence of diffuse neurological signs, such as decreased mentation or altered level of consciousness. Since the manifestations of primary angiitis of the central nervous system are highly variable, unusual presentations are expected to occur. Simple stroke as well as pure dementia are distinctively uncommon presentations, only occasionally reported. Headache is one of the most frequent symptoms, being present in 50–78% of cases (Calabrese and Mallek, 1987; Calabrese et al., 1997; Chu et al., 1998). The headache is usually acute, it may be severe at onset or may worsen over time, and it may also be referred as neck pain (Lanthier et al., 2001). Given its non-specific characteristics, headache is of little diagnostic relevance. The pathogenesis of headache is multifactorial and includes inflammation of pain-sensitive vessels, meningeal inflammation, stroke, and raised intracranial pressure. Clinical findings of transient ischemic attack, stroke, spinal cord involvement (paraparesis, quadriparesis), cranial neuropathies, seizures, and ataxia have occasionally been described. Diagnosis may be supported by the typical angiographic features of vasculitis with multiple segmental narrowing of cerebral arteries, but biopsy represents the gold standard. Diagnostic criteria are reported in Table 48.2.

Table 48.2

Diagnostic criteria for headache attributed to primary central nervous system (CNS) angiitis

A.	Any new persisting headache fulfilling criteria D and E
B.	Encephalic signs of any type (e.g., stroke, seizures, disorders of cognition or conciousness)
C.	CNS angiitis proven by cerebral or meningeal biopsy or suspected on angiographic signs in the absence of systemic arteritis
D.	Headache develops in close temporal relation to encephalic signs
E.	Headache improves within 1 month of steroid and/or immunosuppressive treatment

Secondary central nervous system angiitis

In secondary central nervous system angiitis the brain involvement is associated with signs and symptoms of a systemic arteritis.

Behçet disease

In Behçet disease, headache is the most common neurological symptom, in patients both with and without neurological involvement (Sakane et al., 1999). The prevalence of migraine and tension-type headache is close to that commonly found in the general population (14.9% and 23.6%, respectively) but a non-structural migrainous headache, which is commonly associated with exacerbations with some of the systemic symptoms of the syndrome (recurrent ulcers in the mouth and on the genitals, and eye inflammation, skin lesions, arthritis, bowel inflammation, meningitis, and cranial nerve palsies), is noteworthy in patients with Behçet syndrome. The headache may be vascular in origin or triggered by the immune-mediated disease activity. In 5.2% of patients, the headache is associated with neurological involvement and in 3.9% with uveal inflammation (Saip et al., 2005). A predominantly frontal, bilateral, paroxysmal, throbbing pain of moderate severity was reported in 18.4% of the patients with Behçet disease who do not fulfill the International Headache Society (IHS) criteria for any of the primary headaches (Headache Classification Subcommittee of the International Headache Society, 2004). Other series reported recurrent headache in 82.5% of patients with Behçet disease; the majority exhibited symptoms that fulfilled the IHS criteria for migraine, with a 52% higher than normal prevalence of visual or sensory aura (Kidd, 2006). However, since headache has no specific features it is of little diagnostic value until other signs of systemic disease appear.

Takayasu disease

Takayasu disease, an uncommon indolently progressive inflammation of the aortic arch and its branches, is associated with headaches in one-third to one-half of patients (Edmeads, 1986). The headaches are seldom severe, and may be difficult to distinguish from tension-type headache or migraine depending on their higher frequency in the young female population characteristically affected by Takayasu disease. Associated features, such as persistent malaise, sweating, fever, myalgia, arterial hypertension, and stroke, indicate that these headaches are part of a serious disease even if their mechanism remains quite obscure (Numano and Kobayashi, 1999; Johnston et al., 2002; Kobayashi and Numano, 2002).

Polyarteritis nodosa

Polyarteritis nodosa consists of a progressive inflammation of small and medium-sized arteries producing segmental necrosis of the media with either thrombosis or hemorrhages caused by aneurysmal rupture (Colmegna and Maldonado-Cocco, 2005). In the brain small meningeal arteries are commonly involved, small parenchymal arteries less frequently, and medium-sized arteries are more rarely involved. Central nervous system manifestations include encephalopathy, focal neurological deficits, and seizures (Rosenberg et al., 1990). About 35% of patients with polyarteritis nodosa complain of headache in the course of the disease (Edmeads, 1986). The headache may be isolated and without any consequences or may be sudden and associated with nausea, vomiting, and diplopia, suggesting a central nervous system involvement (Song et al., 2005). In some cases, clinical manifestations may be similar to a meningoencephalitis and in those cases headache is associated with prolonged fever, decreased level of consciousness, neck stiffness, and papilledema (Paula De Carvalho et al., 2004). The mechanism of headache is uncertain but may be related to inflammation of pain-sensitive vessels, meningeal irritation from perivascular inflammation, subarachnoid blood, or vascular hypertension.

Kawasaki disease

Kawasaki disease is an acute vasculitis of childhood whose etiology remains unknown, although an infectious agent is strongly suspected, based on clinical and epidemiological features (Freeman and Shulman, 2006; Kim, 2006). A genetic predisposition is also likely, based on varying incidences among ethnic groups, with higher rates in Asians (Falcini, 2006; Freeman and Shulman, 2006; Kim, 2006). Symptoms include fever, conjunctival injection, erythema of the lips and oral mucosa, rash, and cervical lymphadenopathy (Falcini, 2006). In Kawasaki disease, an aseptic meningitis with associated headache may be the presenting symptom in about 5% of cases (Edmeads, 1986).

Wegener's granulomatosis

Wegener's granulomatosis is an uncommon condition characterized by necrotizing granulomatosis of the upper and lower respiratory tract and glomerulonephritis. The central nervous system is rarely affected and generally consists of a meningeal involvement (Specks et al., 2000; Di Comite et al., 2006). Headache is almost always the first symptom of this involvement. Later in the course of the disease other abnormalities may develop, such as cranial nerve palsy, seizures, and encephalopathy (Specks et al., 2000). Fever may be associated with other neurological symptoms (Tojo et al., 1998). Headache has also been reported as the possible presenting symptom in Wegener's granulomatosis. In this case the headache has been described as migratory, throbbing, and accentuated with head movements (Lim et al., 2002). At autopsy, the dura mater and meninges present a fibrous thickening with scarring of segmental arteries. Some granulomatous lesions may be observed around the arterioles of the dura mater associated with extensive scarring fibrosis. Meningeal inflammation may be responsible for cerebral vein or sinus obstruction (Tojo et al., 1998).

Systemic lupus erythematosus

In systemic lupus erythematosus about 25–46% of patients complain of headache (Edmeads, 1986; Mitsikostas et al., 2004; Bernatsky et al., 2006). The headaches may have the characteristics of migraine, tension-type, or mixed headaches (Weder-Cisneros et al., 2004; Lessa et al., 2006). Of the patients with migraine, 56% have criteria for migraine without aura and 44% have criteria for migraine with aura (Glanz et al., 2001). Headache occurrence is often associated with the presence of Raynaud's phenomenon (Mitsikostas et al., 2004; Weder-Cisneros et al., 2004; Lessa et al., 2006). The presence of migraine has been associated with a higher disease activity (Appenzeller and Costallat, 2004). However, the proportion of pre-existing headache which could be attributed to the disease and whether the proportion is higher than in the general population is debated. For this reason it has been suggested that headaches occurring in patients with systemic lupus erythematosus should be considered and managed as primary headaches (Mitsikostas et al., 2004). However, this suggestion was not implemented by the IHS Committee and such headaches are still classified as secondary headaches (Headache Classification Subcommittee of the International Headache Society, 2004).

Patients with systemic lupus erythematosus may present with headache also in the context of a posterior reversible encephalopathy syndrome; in such cases, seizures, loss of vision, altered mental function, and a pattern on magnetic resonance imaging (MRI) studies of predominantly transient posterior cerebral hyperintensities on T_2-weighted images are associated (Kur and Esdaile, 2006). No pathogenic mechanism has so far been described that can fully explain the headache. The role of circulating cytokines, vascular injury, neuronal damage, or antiphospholipid antibodies in the development of the headache is still a matter of debate (Cuadrado and Sanna, 2003).

Secondary vasculitides

Many organisms, including viruses, bacteria, fungi, rickettsiae, and protozoa, are associated with systemic and central nervous system vasculitis. In many instances the organism may be angioinvasive, but in others the vascular inflammatory reaction may result from alterations in host defenses with secondary damage to tissues. Also a variety of drugs, particularly those with sympathomimetic properties, have been associated with central nervous system vasculitis. Pathologists have described findings ranging from perivascular cuffing of small cerebral vessels to frank vasculitis, with or without necrosis (Carolei and Sacco, 2003). Central nervous system vasculitis has also been reported in association with Hodgkin's and non-Hodgkin's lymphoma and angioimmunolymphoproliferative lesions (Carolei and Sacco, 2003).

Identification of a secondary vasculitis may be clinically important, and removal of the specific inducing agent or control of the associated systemic disease may result in amelioration of the vasculitis. Though biopsy of the leptomeninges and brain is the gold standard of diagnosis, a presumptive diagnosis of central nervous system vasculitis is frequently made on the basis of a compelling clinical picture and angiograms consistent with vasculitis (Carolei and Sacco, 2003). The decision to perform invasive diagnostic tests is inevitably based on the results of non-invasive tests, such as lumbar puncture, brain computed tomography (CT) and MRI. Cerebrospinal fluid analysis shows a modest pleocytosis with elevated protein levels. Increased immunoglobulin G synthesis with oligoclonal bands is occasionally detected. At brain MRI the most common findings are multiple, bilateral, supratentorial infarcts distributed in the cortex and/or deep white matter (Figure 48.1). With the use of contrast agents,

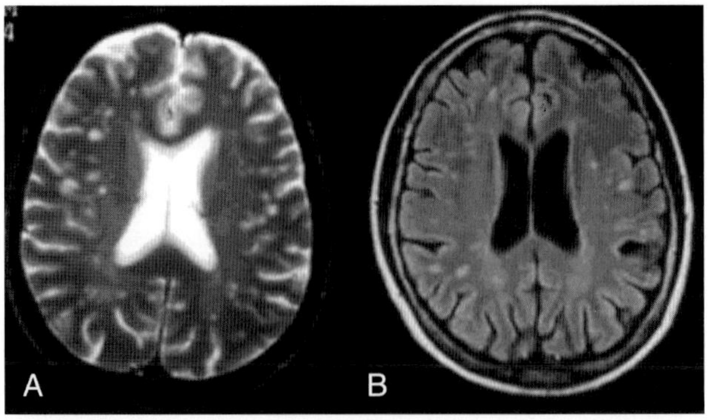

Fig. 48.1. Brain magnetic resonance imaging showing small, punctate, bright areas of increased signal on (A) T_2-weighted and (B) fluid-attenuated inversion recovery (FLAIR) sequences subcortically located, indicating vasculitis. (Courtesy of Professor Stefano Bastianello.)

enhancement of the lesions may be seen, but this finding is not specific. However, in patients with positive angiograms, brain CT and brain MRI may be normal. Angiographic findings of vasculitis include multiple alternating areas of stenosis and ectasia. Histological confirmation remains the standard for diagnosis of all forms of vasculitis whose diagnostic criteria are reported in Table 48.3.

Headache attributed to cerebral venous thrombosis

Thrombosis of the cerebral veins and sinuses is a distinct cerebrovascular disorder that, unlike arterial stroke, most often affects young adults and children. It accounts for 0.5% of all strokes (Bousser and Ferro, 2007). The incidence is around 3–4 per 1 000 000 per year and up to 7 per 1 000 000 per year among children. About 75% of the adult patients are women (Stam, 2005). Thrombosis may involve the cerebral veins, with local effects, or major sinuses, causing intracranial hypertension. In the majority of patients, these two processes occur simultaneously. The venous obstruction may be the cause of a venous infarction,

Table 48.3

Diagnostic criteria for headache attributed to secondary central nervous system angiitis

A.	Any new persisting headache fulfilling criteria D and E
B.	Encephalic signs of any type (e.g., stroke, seizures, disorders of cognition or consciousness)
C.	Evidence of systemic arteritis
D.	Headache develops in close temporal relation to encephalic signs
E.	Headache improves within 1 month of steroid and/or immunosuppressive treatment

which usually involves an atypical arterial district and is frequently associated with hemorrhagic transformation. Many causes or predisposing risk factors have been identified for intracranial venous thrombosis in general. They include oral contraceptive use, pregnancy, puerperium, infections of the nervous system, neighboring infections, systemic inflammatory disease, cancer, hematological disorders, and thrombophilia (van den Bergh et al., 2005; Bousser and Ferro, 2007). The clinical presentation may be variable, including headache, seizures, focal neurological deficits, altered consciousness, and papilledema. The most frequent but least specific symptom of sinus thrombosis is severe headache, which is present in more than 90% of adult patients (Cumurciuc et al., 2005; Stam, 2005). The headache is probably underestimated since some comatose or aphasic patients are unable to report the disturbance.

Headache has no specific features: it can be of any grade of severity and is slightly more frequently diffuse (58%) than localized (42%). The onset of headache can be progressive over a few days (65%), acute (17.5%), or sudden (17.5%) (Cumurciuc et al., 2005; Stam, 2005). Pain is mostly persistent (88%) but can occasionally be intermittent; it is typically worse on recumbence and present on awakening. The headaches are exacerbated by transient increases in intracranial pressure that occur during coughing, sneezing, or other equivalents of the Valsalva maneuver. Nausea, vomiting, and/or phono- and photophobia may be present in around half of patients. Headache may be the sole clinical manifestation of cerebral venous thrombosis in up to 23% of patients, but in most cases it is associated with other typical signs or symptoms. In almost all patients with severe headache who survive, the pain starts to improve within a few days; it disappears within 2 weeks in two-thirds and within 1 month in a third of patients (Cumurciuc et al., 2005).

The headache is sometimes a misleading symptom, mimicking migraine when unilateral and/or intermittent, and with associated visual phenomena mimicking aura. In patients with a history of migraine the headache is usually different from the usual migraine attack, although it can also be similar but more persistent. Moreover, cerebral venous thrombosis should be considered in the etiological diagnosis of thunderclap headache, as some authors reported cases of this headache due to cerebral venous thrombosis (de Bruijn et al., 1996; Cumurciuc et al., 2005; Schwedt et al., 2006). About 2–10% of patients with cerebral venous sinus thrombosis present with thunderclap headache as their predominant clinical sign. This may constitute a diagnostic challenge, as thunderclap headache can be associated with other severe conditions or may also be idiopathic (benign thunderclap headache) (Schwedt et al., 2006).

In patients with cerebral venous thrombosis, thunderclap headache may be an isolated clinical disturbance or it may be associated with warning signs or symptoms, thus raising the suspicion of a non-idiopathic thunderclap headache (de Bruijn et al., 1996). The headache may also present with cluster-like attacks of severe orbital pain lasting around 30 min (Cumurciuc et al., 2005). Headache may also mimic post lumbar puncture headache since lumbar puncture has been reported as a possible cause of cerebral venous thrombosis. Patients with isolated intracranial hypertension have headache but no other neurological symptoms, with the exception of diplopia due to involvement of the sixth cranial nerve when the intracranial pressure increases. Funduscopic examination reveals papilledema. Migrainous patients usually continue to present with migraine attacks even after the cerebral vein thrombosis, but a new tension-type headache may also be initiated. A new-onset migraine with aura in non-migraineur patients has also been observed in cerebral venous thrombosis.

In thrombosis of the superior sagittal sinus, not infrequently the only clinical manifestations may be those of increased intracranial pressure (headache, papilledema, and obtundation), though if the clot extends into the larger cerebral venous sinuses causing hemorrhagic infarction, focal signs such as hemiplegia, crural monoplegia or diplopia, or convulsions may occur. Cavernous sinus thrombosis is usually a complication of an infection in the upper half of the face. In cavernous sinus thrombosis, ocular signs dominate the clinical picture, with orbital pain, chemosis, proptosis, and oculomotor palsies. In unilateral lateral sinus thrombosis the headache is more commonly unilateral and ipsilateral to the thrombosis, and may often become bilateral due to propagation of the clot through the circular sinus around the hypophysis (Cumurciuc et al., 2005). In thrombosis of the transverse and lateral sinuses the symptoms and signs are typically those of increased intracranial pressure. Some patients with the occlusion of this venous channel may complain of pain behind the ipsilateral ear and/or in the ipsilateral side of the neck, possibly due to propagation of the clot in the jugular venous system. Such lateralized pain is uncommon (Edmeads, 1986) because patients with jugular vein thrombosis usually present with ipsilateral neck pain (Cumurciuc et al., 2005).

Headache in cerebral venous thrombosis may be produced by several mechanisms, such as increased intracranial pressure due to generalized intracranial venous engorgement or to swelling of a venous infarct of the brain, meningeal irritation due to purulent meningitis complicating septic thrombosis or to contamination of cerebrospinal fluid by blood from hemorrhagic infarction, systemic factors due to fever and inflammation, and local factors due to the involvement of the trigeminal nerve from inflammation in the veins and sinuses. Such mechanisms may together play an important role but may be isolated causes in different phases of the diseases and in different pathological variations, as headache has also been reported in patients without parenchymal lesions, intracranial hypertension, or meningeal infection.

Although the clinical presentation is highly variable, the diagnosis should be considered in young and middle-aged patients with recent unusual headache or with stroke-like symptoms in the absence of the common vascular risk factors, in patients with intracranial hypertension, and in patients with brain CT evidence of hemorrhagic infarct, especially if the infarcts are multiple and not confined to the arterial vascular territories. The average delay from the onset of symptoms to diagnosis is 7 days. The most sensitive diagnostic protocol requires a combination of brain MRI (Figure 48.2) and MR venography. The outcome of patients with cerebral venous thrombosis is usually favourable, with mortality well below 10% (Cumurciuc et al., 2005). Diagnostic criteria are reported in Table 48.4.

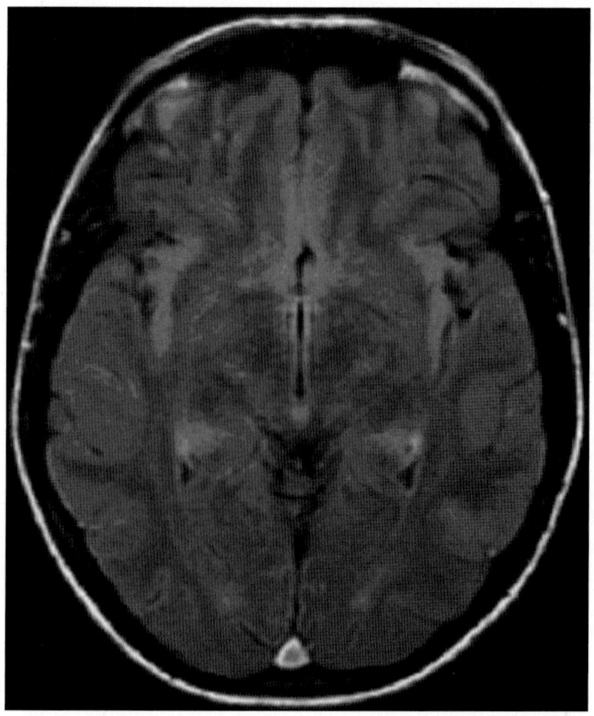

Fig. 48.2. Fluid-attenuated inversion recovery (FLAIR) magnetic resonance imaging sequences showing a longitudinal sinus thrombosis evident as a hyperintense delta sign signal. (Courtesy of Professor Stefano Bastianello.)

Table 48.4

Diagnostic criteria for headache attributed to cerebral venous thrombosis

A. Any new headache, with or without neurological signs, fulfilling criteria C and D
B. Neuroimaging evidence of cerebral venous thrombosis
C. Headache (and neurological signs if present) develops in close temporal relation to cerebral venous thrombosis
D. Headache resolves within 1 month of appropriate treatment

Cerebral autosomal-dominant arteriopathy with subcortical infarcts and leukoencephalopathy (CADASIL)

CADASIL is a rare autosomal-dominant genetic disorder clinically characterized by a variety of symptoms, including migraine, recurrent ischemic strokes, mood disorders, progressive cognitive impairment resulting in dementia, and premature death (Desmond et al., 1999). CADASIL is an inherited disease with mutations in the transmembrane receptor of the *Notch3* gene on chromosome 19q12 (Joutel et al., 1996). CADASIL usually manifests itself in early or middle adulthood with the onset of migraine or with an ischemic event. A migraine-like headache is the presenting symptom in 40% of patients, occurring at a mean age of 28 years. Migraine-like attacks take place, often with a typical aura, although patients can also present with migraine aura without headache, migraine without aura, basilar migraine, hemiplegic migraine, acute-onset aura without migraine headache, and migraine with acute-onset aura (Vahedi et al., 2004). The most common aura type is the visual one but it may also be sensory and visual, only sensory, and sensory, visual, and dysphasic. Different varieties of visual aura symptoms are reported: most commonly scintillating scotomas or photophobia followed by blurred vision and lateral homonymous hemianopia. Other visual aura symptoms include kaleidoscopic vision, diplopia, optic ataxia, and prosopagnosia. The various types of visual symptom may occur in combination. The location of the sensory aura involves predominantly the face and arm, whereas motor aura involves mainly the arm. Speech disturbances consist of an expressive aphasia with reduced fluency and paraphasia. Other symptoms present during migraine attacks are fatigue and gait ataxia or vertigo (Vahedi et al., 2004). The migraine attack may also be accompanied by brief confusional episodes lasting minutes to hours. Few patients with late-onset migraine have been described, suggesting that migraine is unlikely to occur if it is not the presenting symptom. The frequency of migraine attacks is variable, from 2 per week to 1 every 3–4 years or less. Triggering factors are occasionally reported and consist of stress, flashing lights, fatigue, physical exercise, vacation, head trauma, strong smells, angiography, postpartum, insomnia, missing meals, and cold temperature.

The underlying mechanisms of migraine in CADASIL remain unknown. Migraine with aura has been considered as directly due to an ischemic event but this seems unlikely because infarcts in CADASIL are subcortical with a typical presentation as lacunar syndromes, whereas the migraine disturbances are cortical, as suggested by the very high frequency of visual aura symptoms such as progressive scintillating scotoma and/or photopsia. Furthermore, the first attack of migraine precedes the onset of the ischemic strokes by 10–15 years. It is more likely that the genetic alteration on chromosome 19 might be responsible for both migraine and CADASIL (Sacco and Carolei, 2007).

Brain MRI plays a central role in the diagnosis and evaluation of CADASIL, showing diffuse hyperintensities on T_2-weighted images that are consistently found in the white matter and are particularly frequent in the periventricular areas, although they also occur in the basal ganglia and pons, and hypointensities on T_1-weighted images may also be found in the same areas (Markus et al., 2002) (Figure 48.3).

However, T_2 hyperintensities occur in the absence of T_1 hypointensities in up to one-third of affected individuals. Unfortunately, the MRI features are nonspecific, as they are also observed in other conditions. Patients with a suspicious clinical history and specific abnormal MRI findings in the absence of vascular risk factors should be considered for genetic testing to rule out CADASIL syndrome. The differential diagnosis of CADASIL includes diseases that have clinical characteristics and MRI findings resembling those of CADASIL, such as Binswanger's disease, multiple sclerosis, metachromatic leukodystrophy, and primary central nervous system angiitis. However, these diseases are not familiar and findings such as arterial hypertension in Binswanger's disease and involvement of the spinal cord or optic nerves, or oligoclonal bands in the spinal fluid in multiple sclerosis, will be lacking in patients with CADASIL. Diagnostic criteria are reported in Table 48.5.

Mitochondrial encephalopathy, lactic acidosis, and stroke-like episodes (MELAS)

MELAS is a mitochondrial encephalomyopathy characterized by recurrent stroke-like episodes, epilepsy, and migrainous headache (Pavlakis et al., 1984). The genetic abnormality in most cases consists of the 3243-point

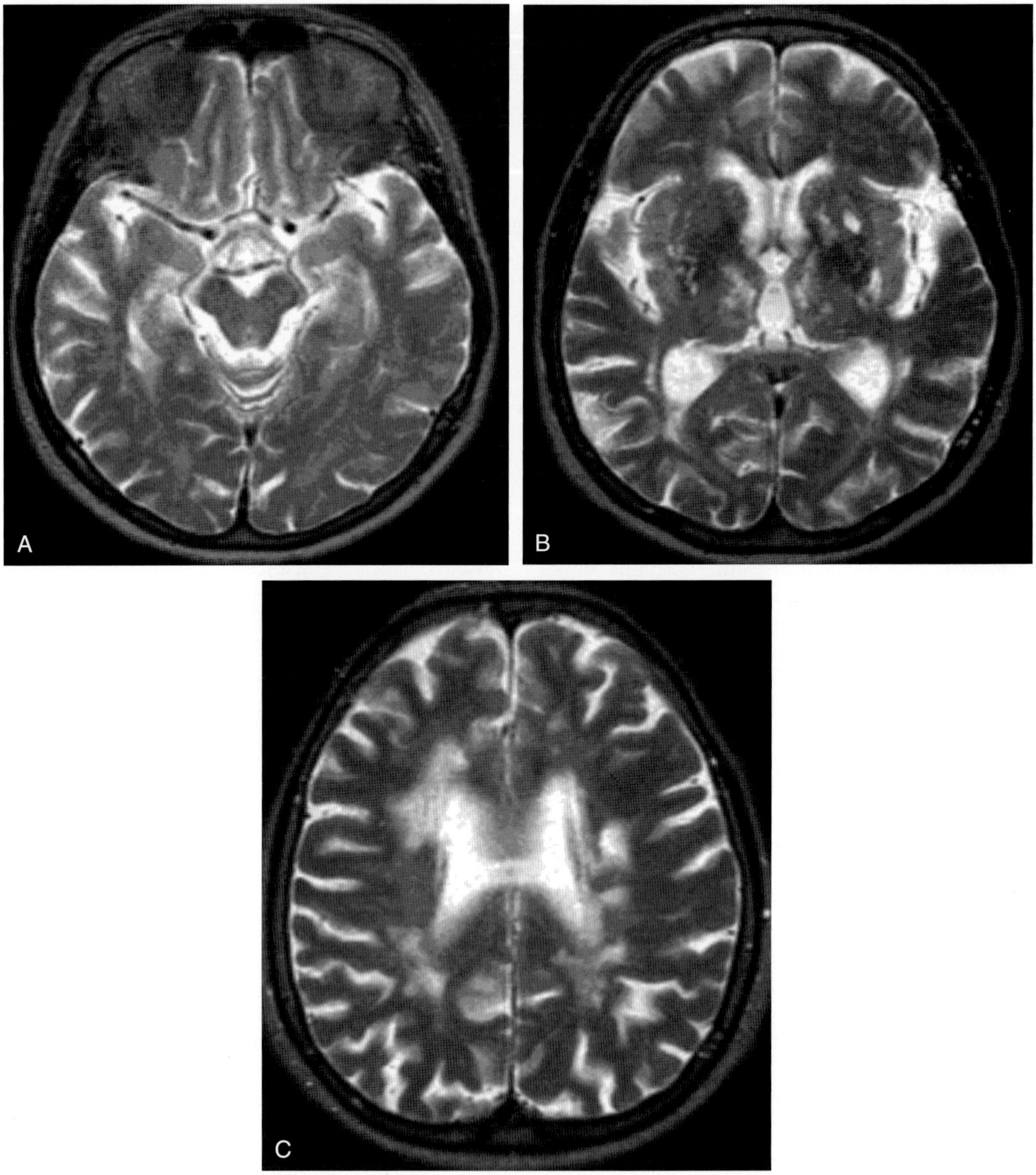

Fig. 48.3. (A–C) Brain magnetic resonance imaging showing multiple areas of increased signal on T_2-weighted sequences indicating multiple ischemic vascular involvement in cerebral autosomal-dominant arteriopathy with subcortical infarcts and leukoencephalopathy (CADASIL). (Courtesy of Professor Stefano Bastianello.)

mitochondrial DNA mutation in the tRNALeu gene, but other DNA MELAS point mutations may be responsible for the disease.

Age at the first stroke-like episode ranges from 23 to 68 years (Iizuka et al., 2002). The initial symptoms may include headache with nausea and vomiting (50%), convulsions (32.5%), visual disturbances (7.5%), numbness (5%), and hemiplegia and aphasia in a minority of patients (Goto et al., 1992; Iizuka et al., 2002). Headache in MELAS may develop without stroke-like lesions or may be the presenting symptom of a stroke-like lesion. Headache is frequently throbbing in nature,

Table 48.5

Diagnostic criteria for cerebral autosomal-dominant arteriopathy with subcortical infarcts and leukoencephalopathy (CADASIL)

A. Attacks of migraine with aura, with or without other neurological signs
B. Typical white-matter changes on magnetic resonance imaging T_2-weighted image
C. Diagnostic confirmation from skin biopsy evidence or genetic testing (*Notch3* mutations)

Table 48.6

Diagnostic criteria for mitochondrial encephalopathy, lactic acidosis, and stroke-like episodes (MELAS)

A. Attacks of migraine with or without aura
B. Stroke-like episodes and seizures
C. Genetic abnormality (3243-point mitochondrial DNA mutation in the tRNALeu gene or other DNA MELAS point mutation)

similar to a migraine attack. Unformed visual hallucinations may also be present in association with headache. Pain may be severe and localized in the retro-orbital and temporal areas and may be associated with visual field defects. Focal and generalized convulsions may occur during the episodes of headache with vomiting, and also independently. After these episodes, transient hemiplegia or hemianopia lasting from a few hours to several weeks has been recognized in 25% of patients (Goto et al., 1992). The worsening of the encephalopathy which can also lead to death is often preceded by severe and prolonged migraine-like headache with nausea and vomiting, which sometimes occurs in clusters lasting a few days (Montagna et al., 1988). Mental deterioration progresses and neurological deficits increase with repeated attacks of stroke-like episodes. This fact led to the hypothesis that the reduction of the episodic attacks might be important in preventing disease progression (Montagna et al., 1988). However, headache may more properly be considered an epiphenomenon of the pathogenic mechanism rather than as pathogenic itself (Sacco and Carolei, 2007).

The mechanisms of migraine-like headache remain to be elucidated. Three important features proposed as migraine pathophysiology include neuronal hyperexcitability, peripheral pain mechanisms activated by the trigeminovascular system, and central processing of the transduction of the pain signal (Moskowitz, 1984; Welch et al., 1990). In MELAS, some triggering metabolic changes in the cerebral cortex, which lower the threshold of the cortical excitability, may cause neuronal hyperexcitability activating the trigeminovascular fibers innervating cortical blood vessels, causing headache as proposed in the mechanisms of migraine (Moskowitz, 1984). Alternatively, headache as a presenting symptom of stroke-like lesions might be triggered by pericapillary plasma extravasation, leading to activation of the first division of the trigeminal nerve fibers innervating the small vessels around the stroke-like lesion. Diagnostic criteria for MELAS are reported in Table 48.6.

Headache attributed to benign (or reversible) angiopathy of the central nervous system

The disease is characterized by acute onset of headache and other acute neurological deficits which correspond to angiographic findings of reversible segmental vasoconstriction (Calabrese, 1999). A form of benign angiopathy of the central nervous system is the one which develops in the postpartum and is named postpartum cerebral angiopathy (Bousser et al., 2001). The nature of the angiopathy is not always benign, as patients with segmental arterial vasoconstriction present a risk of developing posterior reversible encephalopathy syndrome or ischemic stroke (Chen et al., 2006).

Headache is present in almost all cases. It is usually severe, diffuse, and pulsating. The headache can be abrupt in onset, mimicking subarachnoid hemorrhage, or progressive over hours or days. It is one of the identified causes of thunderclap headache (Call et al., 1988; Dodick et al., 1999; Schwedt et al., 2006) and is generally self-limited since attacks subside within 3 months, and the accompanying MR angiography segmental vasoconstrictions, if present, resolve after headache resolution. Headache may be the only symptom or may be associated with seizures or fluctuating focal neurological signs.

It has recently been postulated that primary thunderclap headache and benign (or reversible) angiopathy of the central nervous system might represent spectra of the same disorder (Chen et al., 2006). The exact underlying mechanisms of thunderclap headache and its relationship with vasoconstriction are unknown. The finding that nimodipine is effective in patients both with and without vasoconstriction suggests that vasoconstriction might not be the sole mechanism underlying the headaches. In contrast, the blood pressure surge and the triggers with elevated sympathetic tone indicated that heightened sympathetic activities were involved in the pathogenesis, which was coherent with the previously proposed neurogenic mechanism stressing the role of aberrant central sympathetic response (Dodick, 2002). Diagnostic criteria are reported in Table 48.7.

Table 48.7

Diagnostic criteria for headache attributed to benign (or reversible) angiopathy of the central nervous system

A. Diffuse, severe headache of abrupt or progressive onset, with or without focal neurological deficits and/or seizures and fulfilling criteria C and D
B. "Strings and beads" appearance on angiography and subarachnoid hemorrhage ruled out by appropriate investigations
C. One or both of the following:
   1. Headache develops simultaneously with neurological deficits and/or seizures
   2. Headache leads to angiography and discovery of "string and beads" appearance
D. Headache (and neurological deficit if present) resolves spontaneously within 2 months

Table 48.8

Diagnostic criteria for headache attributed to pituitary apoplexy

A. Severe acute retro-orbital, frontal, or diffuse headache accompanied by at least one of the following and fulfilling criteria C and D:
   1. Nausea and vomiting
   2. Fever
   3. Diminished level of consciousness
   4. Hypopituitarism
   5. Hypotension
   6. Ophthalmoplegia or impaired visual acuity
B. Neuroimaging evidence of acute hemorrhagic pituitary infarction
C. Headache develops simultaneously with acute hemorrhagic pituitary infarction
D. Headache and other symptoms and/or signs resolve within 1 month

Headache attributed to pituitary apoplexy

Pituitary apoplexy is represented by hemorrhage and/or infarction of the pituitary gland (Figure 48.4). Although pituitary apoplexy is rarely encountered in the clinical setting, autopsy evidence of infarction of more than 25% of the pituitary gland is found in 1–3% of the population (Reid et al., 1985). Apoplexy may occur in the setting of a pituitary adenoma but associations with pregnancy, puerperium, general anesthesia, bromocriptine therapy, and pituitary irradiation have been reported (Mohr and Hardy, 1982; Sibal et al., 2004). Furthermore, it may be caused by cerebral aneurysms and idiopathic thrombocytopenic purpura (Maiza et al., 2004; Chuang et al., 2006; Romano et al., 2006).

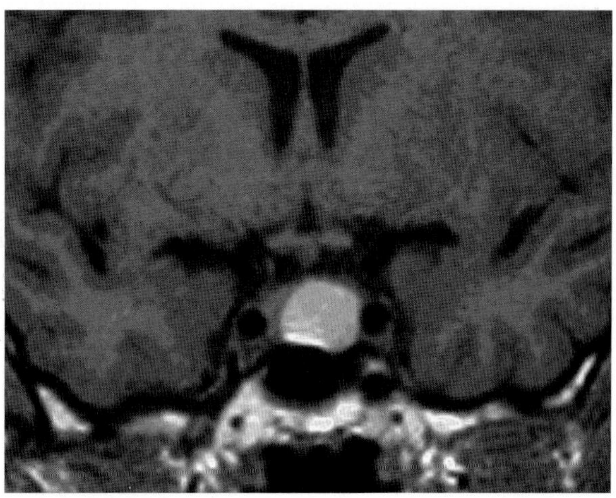

Fig. 48.4. Sellar region magnetic resonance imaging showing a rounded area of increased signal on T_1-weighted sequences in the left portion of the hypophysis related to intraparenchymal hemorrhage. (Courtesy of Professor Stefano Bastianello.)

There is a wide variation in the severity of clinical symptoms in patients with pituitary apoplexy, from relatively mild symptoms to adrenal crisis, coma, and sudden death. Patients with pituitary apoplexy most commonly present with a combination of acute headache, nausea, decreased visual acuity, ophthalmoplegia, and reduction in visual fields (Randeva et al., 1999; Crowder and Rothrock, 2006). Headache, usually of sudden and severe onset, is the most common presenting symptom and may be the predominant presenting feature. Severe sudden headache occurs simultaneously with visual failure and often a loss of consciousness. The headache may be bifrontal, retrosinusal, localized at the vertex, or diffuse. It is probably caused by upward stretching or tearing of the diaphragma sellae, pressure on the adjacent first trigeminal branch, or extension of blood into the basal cisterns (Edmeads, 1986). It is a possible cause of thunderclap headache (Schwedt et al., 2006). Diagnostic criteria are reported in Table 48.8.

References

Appenzeller S, Costallat LT (2004). Clinical implications of migraine in systemic lupus erythematosus: relation to cumulative organ damage. Cephalalgia 24: 1024–1030.

Bernatsky S, Pineau CA, Lee JL et al. (2006). Headache, Raynaud's syndrome and serotonin receptor agonists in systemic lupus erythematosus. Lupus 15: 671–674.

Bousser MG, Ferro JM (2007). Cerebral venous thrombosis: an update. Lancet Neurol 6: 162–170.

Bousser MG, Good J, Kittner SJ et al. (2001). Headache associated with vascular disorders. In: SD Silberstein,

RB Lipton, DJ Dalessio (Eds.), Wolff's Headache and Other Head Pain. 7th edn. Oxford University Press, New York, pp. 349–392.

Calabrese LH (1999). Angiographically defined primary angiitis of the CNS: is it really benign? Neurology 52: 1302.

Calabrese LH, Mallek JA (1987). The treatment of vasculitis of the central nervous system. JAMA 258: 778.

Calabrese LH, Duna GF, Lie JT (1997). Vasculitis in the central nervous system. Arthritis Rheum 40: 1189–1201.

Call GK, Fleming MC, Sealfon S et al. (1988). Reversible cerebral segmental vasoconstriction. Stroke 19: 1159–1170.

Calvo-Romero JM (2003). Giant cell arteritis. Postgrad Med J 79: 511–515.

Cantini F, Niccoli L, Storri L et al. (2004). Are polymyalgia rheumatica and giant cell arteritis the same disease? Semin Arthritis Rheum 33: 294–301.

Carolei A, Sacco S (2003). Central nervous system vasculitis. Neurol Sci 24 (Suppl. 1): S8–S10.

Chen SP, Fuh JL, Lirng JF et al. (2006). Is vasospasm requisite for posterior leukoencephalopathy in patients with primary thunderclap headaches? Cephalalgia 26: 530–536.

Chu CT, Gray L, Goldstein LB et al. (1998). Diagnosis of intracranial vasculitis: a multi-disciplinary approach. J Neuropathol Exp Neurol 57: 30–38.

Chuang CC, Chen YL, Pai PC (2006). A giant intracavernous carotid artery aneurysm embedded in pituitary macroadenoma presenting with pituitary apoplexy. Cerebrovasc Dis 21: 142–144.

Colmegna I, Maldonado-Cocco JA (2005). Polyarteritis nodosa revisited. Curr Rheumatol Rep 7: 288–296.

Crowder JW, Rothrock JF (2006). Pituitary tumor and apoplexy. Headache 46: 1587–1588.

Cuadrado MJ, Sanna G (2003). Headache and systemic lupus erythematosus. Lupus 12: 943–946.

Cumurciuc R, Crassard I, Sarov M et al. (2005). Headache as the only neurological sign of cerebral venous thrombosis: a series of 17 cases. J Neurol Neurosurg Psychiatry 76: 1084–1087.

De Bruijn SF, Stam J, Kappelle LJ (1996). Thunderclap headache as first symptom of cerebral venous sinus thrombosis. CVST Study Group. Lancet 348: 1623–1625.

Desmond D, Moroney J, Lynch T et al. (1999). The natural history of CADASIL: a pooled analysis of previously published cases. Stroke 30: 1230–1233.

Di Comite G, Bozzolo EP, Praderio L et al. (2006). Meningeal involvement in Wegener's granulomatosis is associated with localized disease. Clin Exp Rheumatol 24 (Suppl. 41):S60–S64.

Dodick DW (2002). Thunderclap headache. J Neurol Neurosurg Psychiatry 72: 6–11.

Dodick DW, Brown RD Jr, Britton JW et al. (1999). Nonaneurysmal thunderclap headache with diffuse, multifocal, segmental, and reversible vasospasm. Cephalalgia 19: 118–123.

Edmeads J (1986). Headache in cerebrovascular disease. In: PJ Vinken, GW Bruyn, HL Klawans (Eds.), Handbook of Clinical Neurology: Headache (Revised series 4). Vol. 48. Elsevier, Amsterdam, pp. 273–290.

Falcini F (2006). Kawasaki disease. Curr Opin Rheumatol 18: 33–38.

Freeman AF, Shulman ST (2006). Kawasaki disease: summary of the American Heart Association guidelines. Am Fam Physician 74: 1141–1148.

Gabriel SE, Espy M, Erdman DD et al. (1999). The role of parvovirus B19 in the pathogenesis of giant cell arteritis: a preliminary evaluation. Arthritis Rheum 42: 1255–1258.

Glanz BI, Venkatesan A, Schur PH et al. (2001). Prevalence of migraine in patients with systemic lupus erythematosus. Headache 41: 285–289.

Goto Y, Horai S, Matsuoka T et al. (1992). Mitochondrial myopathy, encephalopathy, lactic acidosis, and stroke-like episodes (MELAS): a correlative study of the clinical features and mitochondrial DNA mutation. Neurology 42: 545–550.

Headache Classification Subcommittee of the International Headache Society (2004). The International Classification of Headache Disorders, 2nd edition. Cephalalgia 24 (Suppl. 1): 1–160.

Iizuka T, Sakai F, Suzuki N et al. (2002). Neuronal hyperexcitability in stroke-like episodes of MELAS syndrome. Neurology 59: 816–824.

Jennette JC, Falk RJ (1997). Small-vessel vasculitis. N Engl J Med 337: 1512–1523.

Johnston SL, Lock RJ, Gompels MM (2002). Takayasu arteritis: a review. J Clin Pathol 55: 481–486.

Joutel A, Corpechot C, Ducros A et al. (1996). Notch3 mutations in CADASIL, a hereditary adult-onset condition causing stroke and dementia. Nature 383: 707–710.

Kidd D (2006). The prevalence of headache in Behcet's syndrome. Rheumatology (Oxford) 45: 621–623.

Kim DS (2006). Kawasaki disease. Yonsei Med J 47: 759–772.

Kobayashi Y, Numano F (2002). Takayasu arteritis. Intern Med 41: 44–46.

Kur JK, Esdaile JM (2006). Posterior reversible encephalopathy syndrome – an underrecognized manifestation of systemic lupus erythematosus. J Rheumatol 33: 2178–2183.

Lanthier S, Lortie A, Michaud J et al. (2001). Isolated angiitis of the CNS in children. Neurology 56: 837–842.

Lessa B, Santana A, Lima I et al. (2006). Prevalence and classification of headache in patients with systemic lupus erythematosus. Clin Rheumatol 25: 850–853.

Lim IG, Spira PJ, McNeil HP (2002). Headache as the initial presentation of Wegener's granulomatosis. Ann Rheum Dis 61: 571–572.

Maiza JC, Bennet A, Thorn-Kany M et al. (2004). Pituitary apoplexy and idiopathic thrombocytopenic purpura: a new case and review of the literature. Pituitary 7: 189–192.

Markus HS, Martin RJ, Simpson MA et al. (2002). Diagnostic strategies in CADASIL. Neurology 59: 1134–1138.

Mitsikostas DD, Sfikakis PP, Goadsby PJ (2004). A meta-analysis for headache in systemic lupus erythematosus: the evidence and the myth. Brain 127: 1200–1209.

Mohr G, Hardy J (1982). Hemorrhage, necrosis, and apoplexy in pituitary adenomas. Surg Neurol 18: 181–189.

Handbook of Clinical Neurology, Vol. 97 (3rd series)
Headache
G. Nappi and M.A. Moskowitz, Editors

Chapter 50

Headache attributed to non-vascular intracranial disorder

HANS-CHRISTOPH DIENER,[1]* U. JOHANSSON,[1] AND DAVID W. DODICK[2]
[1]*Department of Neurology, University of Duisburg-Essen, Essen, Germany*
[2]*Department of Neurology, Mayo Clinic Arizona, Phoenix, AZ, USA*

INTRODUCTION

In this chapter are the headaches attributed to changes in intracranial pressure. Both increased and decreased cerebrospinal fluid (CSF) pressure can lead to headache. Other causes of headache here are non-infectious inflammatory diseases, intracranial neoplasia, seizures, rare conditions such as intrathecal injections and Chiari malformation type I, and other non-vascular intracranial disorders.

Compared to those on primary headaches, there are few epidemiological studies on these headache types. Controlled trials of therapy are almost non-existent. Headache persisting for more than 1 month after successful treatment or spontaneous resolution of the intracranial disorder usually has other mechanisms. Chronic headache persisting for >3 months after treatment or remission of intracranial disorders exist but have been poorly studied

GENERAL COMMENT

Primary or secondary headache, or both?

When a new headache occurs for the first time in close temporal relation to a non-vascular intracranial disorder, it is regarded as a secondary headache attributed to the intracranial disorder (Headache Classification Subcommittee of the International Headache Society, 2004). This is also true if the headache has the characteristics of migraine, tension-type headache, or cluster headache. When a pre-existing primary headache is made worse in close temporal relation to an intracranial disorder, there are two possibilities, and judgment is required. The patient can either be given only the diagnosis of the pre-existing primary headache or be given both this diagnosis and the diagnosis of headache attributed to the intracranial disorder. Factors that support adding the latter diagnosis are: a very close temporal relation to the intracranial disorder, a marked worsening of the pre-existing headache, very good evidence that the intracranial disorder can aggravate the primary headache, and, finally, improvement or resolution of the headache after relief from the intracranial disorder.

Definite, probable, or chronic?

A diagnosis of *Headache attributed to non-vascular intracranial disorder* usually becomes definite only when the headache resolves or greatly improves after effective treatment or spontaneous remission of the causative disorder. If the intracranial disorder cannot be treated effectively or does not remit spontaneously, or when there has been insufficient time for this to happen, a diagnosis of *Headache probably attributed to a non-vascular intracranial disorder* is usually applied.

The alternative, when the causative disorder is effectively treated or remits spontaneously but headache does not resolve or markedly improve after 3 months, is a diagnosis of *Chronic post-intracranial disorder headache.*

HEADACHE ATTRIBUTED TO HIGH CEREBROSPINAL FLUID PRESSURE

Headache attributed to idiopathic intracranial hypertension (IIH)

Previously used terms

Benign intracranial hypertension (BIH), pseudotumor cerebri, meningeal hydrops, serous meningitis.

*Correspondence to: Hans-Christoph Diener, MD, Department of Neurology, University of Duisburg-Essen, Hufelandstrasse 55, 45122 Essen, Germany, Tel: +49 201 723 2460/61, Fax: +49 201 723 5901, E-mail: hans.diener@uni-duisburg-essen.de

History and older nomenclature

In 1897 Quincke first described a syndrome of papilledema and raised intracranial pressure, which he attributed to impaired cerebrospinal fluid circulation. In 1904 Nonne coined the term "pseudotumor cerebri". In 1937 Dandy suggested increased cerebral blood volume as a possible etiology. In 1955 Foley proposed the term "benign intracranial hypertension." Reports of severe visual loss and the not so benign nature of the condition in the 1980s led to the modification of "Idiopathic intracranial hypertension".

Definition

Idiopathic intracranial hypertension is a diagnosis of exclusion. The criteria as currently formulated in the International Headache Society's (IHS) classification of headache disorders (Headache Classification Subcommittee of the International Headache Society, 2004) are:

1. Alert patient with neurological examination that either is normal or demonstrates any of the following abnormalities:
   a. Papilledema
   b. Enlarged blind spot
   c. Visual field defect
   d. Sixth nerve palsy
2. Increased CSF pressure (>200 mmH_2O in the non-obese, >250 mmH_2O in the obese) measured by lumbar puncture in the recumbent position or by epidural or intraventricular pressure monitoring.
3. Normal CSF chemistry (low CSF protein is acceptable) and cellularity.
4. Intracranial disease (including venous sinus thrombosis) ruled out by appropriate investigation.
5. No metabolic, toxic, or hormonal cause of intracranial hypertension.

A presenting headache is attributed to idiopathic intracranial hypertension when the headache develops in close temporal relation to the increased intracranial pressure and improves after withdrawal of CSF. The headache should be progressive with at least one of the following:

- Daily occurrence
- Diffuse and/or constant non-pulsating pain
- Aggravated by coughing or straining.

Epidemiology

Idiopathic intracranial hypertension is a disease with an incidence of 0.9 per 100 000 in the general population, rising to 3.5 per 100 000 for females aged 15–44 years. In US studies, approximately 70% of females with IIH are obese (body mass index >26) (Durcan et al., 1988; Radhakrishnan et al., 1993). In the last decade the incidence of IIH has at least doubled; therefore the incidence of IIH seems to reflect the prevalence of obesity in the population. The female:male ratio is about 8:1 (Durcan et al., 1988; Kesler and Gadoth, 2001). Familial occurrence has been reported in few cases (Kharode et al., 1992) but has not been evaluated. The incidence of asymptomatic cases is not known. These patients are found on routine ophthalmological examination (Galvin et al., 2004). In a series of 62 patients with chronic migraine, six had increased opening pressure at lumbar puncture (Vieira et al., 2008).

Etiology

The etiology of IIH is unknown. All cases with a known etiology should be classified as secondary intracranial hypertension. Obesity and female gender are the only factors shown in case–control studies to be significantly more common in IIH patients than in controls (Ireland et al., 1990). Nevertheless, in case reports there are a number of other exogenous and endogenous factors such as medications, vitamin A, endocrine abnormalities, and other diseases reported (Digre and Corbett, 1988; Friedmann, 2004). Medications associated with IIH are tetracyclines, nitrofurantoin, nalidixic acid, sulfamethoxazole, corticosteroids, lithium, ciclosporin, vitamin A, growth hormone, and thyroid hormone (Digre and Corbett, 1988; Friedmann, 2004). Systemic retinoids (isotretinoin, all-*trans* retinoic acid), corticosteroid withdrawal, human growth hormone, cerebral venous sinus thrombosis, mastoiditis, Behçet's disease, renal failure, and obstructive sleep apnea have also been associated with elevated intracranial pressure. Prospective studies are needed to establish these associations clearly.

Pathogenesis

The pathogenesis remains unclear. There may be several contributing factors. Theories have included: (1) parenchymal edema, (2) increased cerebral blood volume, (3) excessive CSF production, (4) compromised CSF resorption, and (5) venous outflow obstruction. Factors 1–3 have not been confirmed in newer MRI studies. Factor 4 applies mostly in few symptomatic cases. Venous outflow obstruction is the currently favoured concept by most authors (Karahalios et al., 1996). In a retrospective study of 188 patients with IIH investigated over the period 1968–1999, 37 patients (20%) had evidence of cranial venous outflow abnormality (Johnston et al., 2002).

Tumors that occlude the cerebral venous sinuses may cause increased intracranial pressure. Septic or aseptic thrombosis of the cavernous sinus, lateral, sigmoid, or superior sagittal sinus, ligation of one or both jugular veins (e.g., during radical neck dissection for regional tumors), thrombosis of a central intravenous catheter in the chest or neck, subclavian vein catheterization and arteriovenous fistula, hemodynamically significant left-to-right cardiac shunt from a cardiac septal defect, the superior vena cava syndrome, or a glomus jugulare tumor impairing venous drainage have also been associated with increased intracranial pressure (Kiers and King, 1991; Ageli et al., 1994; Ansari et al., 2002; Jicha and Suarez, 2003).

Venous sinus thrombosis can present with an isolated syndrome of increased intracranial pressure that is clinically indistinguishable from IIH. In one study of 59 patients, 37% presented with what appeared to be IIH (Biousse et al., 1999). Cerebral venous sinus thrombosis accounted for 9.4% of patients with presumed IIH in three tertiary care neuro-ophthalmology services (Lin et al., 2006).

The prevalence and nature of sinovenous structural abnormalities in 29 patients with IIH and 59 control subjects was determined in a study using auto-triggered elliptic-centric-ordered three-dimensional gadolinium-enhanced MR venography (ATECO MRV) (Farb et al., 2003), a technique that offers considerable benefits over time-of-flight and phase-contrast techniques commonly employed in clinical practice currently. Significant bilateral sinovenous stenoses were seen in 27 of 29 patients with IIH and in only 4 of 59 control patients. The authors speculated that the venous sinus stenosis may be related to congenital narrowing of the transverse sinus, or intracranial hypertension may create create a flow-limiting stenosis and resultant pressure gradient in a collapsible venous sinus. There have been subsequent examples in the literature of both reversible and persistent transverse venous sinus stenosis after normalization of CSF pressure and small case series of clinical improvement after stenting of the stenotic transverse venous sinus (Corbett and Digre, 2002; King et al., 2002; Bono et al., 2005). While most clinicians would agree with the need for imaging of the cerebral venous sinuses to exclude thrombosis, further study is required to clarify the relationship between venous sinus stenosis and IIH, and certainly whether and in whom interventional treatment is indicated.

Symptoms

Headache

Headache is present in 90% of patients (Friedmann, 2004) and is usually characterized as a daily pain of moderate intensity. There is a variety of locations reported such as holocranial as well as hemicranial, retrobulbar, temporal, or occipital. The pain quality is also variable being pulsatile, pressing, or alternating. There even has been a case report of cluster-like headache due to IIH (Volcy and Tepper, 2006). In a retrospective study of 82 patients with treated IIH, 68% additionally had definable headache disorders, including episodic tension-type headache (30%) and migraine without aura (20%), chronic tension-type headache (20%), and analgesic overuse headache (8%) (Friedmann and Rausch, 2002). Nausea occurs in 20–40% of patients with IIH while vomiting is less common (Skau et al., 2006).

Cranial nerve dysfunction

Three-fourths of patients describe transient visual disturbances such as blurring or total loss of light perception lasting from seconds to minutes, so-called transient visual obscurations (TVOs) (Wall and George, 1991). TVOs are thought to represent brief episodes of optic nerve head ischemia caused by papilledema, though they do not correlate with the severity of papilledema and do not predict visual loss. They are often precipitated by arising from a stooped position or rolling the eyes. In severe cases visual loss may be acute and dramatic, leading to profound visual loss or blindness (Rowe and Sarkies, 1998).

The increased intracranial pressure can also lead to diplopia, pulsatile tinnitus, neck stiffness or shoulder pain (Round and Keane, 1988). Diplopia is generally binocular and horizontal, resulting from unilateral or bilateral sixth nerve palsy, a non-localizing sign of increased intracranial pressure. Pulsatile tinnitus occurs in 60% of patients and is often described as a *whooshing* sound in one or both ears.

Diagnosis

The ophthalmological examination should be performed by a trained neuro-ophthalmologist, since it can sometimes be challenging to differentiate between papilledema and pseudopapilledema of optic disc drusen or tilted optic discs. In most patients, papilledema precedes or coincides with symptom onset, but some patients may become symptomatic shortly before appreciable disc swelling is seen on ophthalmoscopy, while in others, papilledema may evolve over hours or days to weeks. There are cases of IIH without papilledema reported in the literature, which in the acute phase may occur because papilledema has not yet developed. The diagnosis of IIH without papilledema is very likely erroneous in patients with chronic daily headache and elevated cerebrospinal pressure, most of whom have medication overuse.

Visual field defects, such as an enlargement of the blind spot, inferonasal defects, arcuate scotomas, and concentric constrictions, occur in about 96% of patients during the course of IIH (Rowe and Sarkies, 1998). Central acuity is usually preserved in early papilledema, so a decline in acuity early in the course of the disease is an ominous sign. Automated or Goldmann perimetry is necessary to detect and quantify these defects as well as to follow the course of the disease and response to therapy. Follow-up examinations are important to detect and prevent visual loss.

Lumbar puncture in the lateral decubitus position is required to show an increased CSF pressure of 200 mmH_2O in non-obese and 250 mmH_2O in obese patients. Many authors consider the pressure interval between 200 and 250 mmH_2O a non-diagnostic gray zone. Since intracranial pressure in IIH has fluctuations, there also can be normal or even low pressure. Therefore occasionally it may be necessary to repeat lumbar punctures or even measure CSF pressure by a lumbar drain or intracranial transducer monitoring (Johnston and Paterson, 1974; Gjerris and Borgesen, 2000). CSF chemistry is normal without pleocytosis, but the protein level can be below the normal range (Johnston et al., 1991).

Neuroimaging is crucial. Standard MRI and magnetic resonace venography (MRV) should be carried out in any patient to evaluate an IIH. Unenhanced CT scan discloses space-occupying mass lesions, but to exclude venous sinus thrombosis, spiral-CT venography is an excellent tool. Elliptic-centric-ordered three-dimensional gadolinium-enhanced MRI increases the sensitivity of MRV for detecting intracranial sinovenous stenosis. Signs of raised intracranial pressure can infrequently be seen on MRI, such as an empty sella (70%), flattening of the posterior sclera (80%), dilation (45%) or tortuosity (40%) of the optic nerve sheet, or gadolinium enhancement of the optic disc (50%) (Broadsky and Vaphiades, 1998; Said and Rosman, 2004).

Differential diagnosis

The most common differential diagnosis is secondary intracranial hypertension due to cerebral venous sinus thrombosis, which has to be considered especially in all cases of ophthalmoparesis. There may also be evidence of transverse sinus stenosis, which is most likely a result of increased intracranial pressure rather than the cause (King et al., 2002). Other causes include infection, malignancy, and toxicity (Skau et al., 2006). There may be pre- or co-existing tension-type headache, migraine headache, analgesic rebound headache, and depression.

Treatment

Since the cause of idiopathic intracranial hypertension remains unknown, therapy has to be symptomatic to lower intracranial pressure and prevent complications. There are no evidence-based treatment guidelines. Recommendations are empiric. Usually a supervised weight loss program is mandatory (Kupersmith et al., 1998). Carbonic anhydrase inhibitors (acetazolamide 1000–1250 mg daily) and diuretics (furosemide 40–120 mg daily) are helpful. However, while acetazolamide may reduce CSF production by up to 50%, the reduction does not occur until over 99.5% of choroid plexus carbonic anhydrase is inhibited. This physiological effect requires a dose beyond which most patients can tolerate (4 g per day). The side-effects of acetazolamide, such as paresthesias, taste perversion, somnolence, and depression, often limit its use. Topiramate has been helpful in alleviating headaches in small patient numbers and seems to be as effective as acetazolamide (Celebisoy et al., 2007; Wall, 2008). Weight loss is a favourable side-effect (Pagan et al., 2002) of topiramate in this patient population. Steroids may be helpful in the acute phase, but worsening intracranial pressure may occur with steroid withdrawal, and weight gain associated with steroid treatment may worsen the clinical course. They should no longer be recommended. Traditionally repeated lumbar punctures are performed especially in patients with infrequent severe flare-ups. Currently they are not recommended as a isolated treatment option because the effect is short-lasting.

In case of vision deterioration and refractory headache, immediate surgical intervention is necessary. Traditionally, optic nerve sheet decompression has been performed with success, with improvement or stabilization of vision (Agarwal and Yoo, 2007). Most patients experience a relief of headache, although probably the intracranial hypertension persists in most patients (Spoor and McHenry, 1993). Therefore most authors prefer CSF shunting. Traditionally lumboperitoneal shunting (LPS) has been preferred, because cannulation of slim ventricles was considered difficult. Today most patients undergo ventriculoperitoneal shunting (VPS), since the rate of shunt obstructions and revisions as well as iatrogenic Chiari I malformation is lower than with LPS (Burgett et al., 1997; Bynke et al., 2004; McGirt et al., 2004).

Prognosis and complications

While no long-term natural history data are available, about 70–80% of IIH patients recover spontaneously (Sorensen et al., 1988). While most patients with IIH will have a monophasic course, some will have recurrences that may happen years after the initial presentation (Kesler et al., 2004). Papilledema does not always completely resolve. The most common complication is permanent visual field defects (Rowe and Sarkies, 1998). Unfortunately permanent visual loss due to intracranial hypertension occurs in approximately 25–30% of patients. The risk of total blindness of one or both eyes in patients is about 5% and related to duration of papilledema; therefore any progress in visual defects has to involve a more aggressive treatment (Corbett et al., 1982). Other complications are disabling severe headache and cognitive dysfunction.

Headache attributed to intracranial hypertension secondary to metabolic, toxic, or hormonal causes

Headache attributed to increased intracranial pressure due to head trauma, vascular disorder, or intracranial infection is coded to whichever one of those disorders is present. Headache attributed to raised intracranial pressure occurring as a side-effect of medication is coded as headache as an adverse event attributed to chronic medication (Headache Classification Subcommittee of the International Headache Society, 2004).

Headache attributed to intracranial hypertension secondary to metabolic, toxic, or hormonal causes is the most important differential diagnosis to benign intracranial hypertension. Raised intracranial pressure is found in patients with renal failure and hypoparathyroidism, as well as systemic lupus erythematodes. Increased intake of vitamin A, steroids, amiodarone, lithium, tetracyclines or and minocycline may also lead to raised intracranial pressure (Table 50.1).

Diagnostic criteria

A. Headache with at least one of the following characteristics and fulfilling criteria C and D:
   1. daily occurrence
   2. diffuse and/or constant (non-pulsating) pain
   3. aggravated by coughing or straining

Table 50.1

Causes of pseudotumor cerebri

Raised intracranial pressure due to disease	Renal failure Hypoparathyroidism Systemic lupus erythematosus
Drug-induced intracranial hypertension	Hypervitaminosis A Anabolic steroids Amiodarone Tetracycline Minocycline Rapidly lowered corticosteroids Lithium

B. Intracranial hypertension fulfilling the following criteria:
   1. alert patient with neurological examination that either is normal or demonstrates any of the following abnormalities:
      a) papilledema
      b) enlarged blind spot
      c) visual field defect (progressive if untreated)
      d) sixth nerve palsy
   2. increased CSF pressure (>200 mmH_2O in the non-obese, >250 mmH_2O in the obese) measured by lumbar puncture in the recumbent position or by epidural or intraventricular pressure monitoring
   3. normal CSF chemistry (low CSF protein is acceptable) and cellularity
   4. intracranial diseases (including venous sinus thrombosis) ruled out by appropriate investigations
C. Headache develops after weeks or months of endocrine disorder, hypervitaminosis A, or intake of substances (other than medications) that can elevate CSF pressure
D. Headache resolves within 3 months after removal of the cause.

Headache attributed to intracranial hypertension secondary to hydrocephalus

Diagnostic criteria

A. Headache with at least two of the following characteristics and fulfilling criteria C and D:
   1. diffuse pain
   2. worse in the morning
   3. worse with Valsalva-like maneuvers
   4. accompanied by vomiting
   5. associated with papilledema, sixth nerve palsy, altered level of consciousness, gait instability, and/or increased head circumference (in children <5 years old)
B. High-pressure hydrocephalus fulfilling the following criteria:
   1. ventricular enlargement on neuroimaging
   2. intracranial pressure >200 mmH_2O in the non-obese or >250 mmH_2O in the obese
   3. no other intracranial disorder causing increased CSF pressure
C. Headache develops in close temporal relation to increased CSF pressure
D. Headache resolves within 72 h of normalization of CSF pressure.

Historical and present nomenclature

Hydrocephalus cases were regularly described by Hippocrates, Galen, and early medieval Arabian physicians, who believed that this disease was caused by an extracerebral accumulation of water. Vesalius (1514–64) first recognized hydrocephalus as an accumulation of fluid within the cerebral ventricles. For the first time, the types internal and external hydrocephalus, meaning an abnormal accumulation of cerebrospinal fluid (CSF) within the internal and external ventricles, were differentiated by Whytt 1768. Hydrocephalus is characterized by increased cerebrospinal fluid (CSF) and dilation of the cerebral ventricles.

Definition

Headache attributed to intracranial hypertension secondary to hydrocephalus is defined in the International Headache Society's (IHS) classification of headache disorders (2004) with the following diagnostic criteria. The headache has to develop in close temporal relation to increased CSF pressure and to be resolved within 72 h of normalization of CSF pressure. Furthermore the headache should accomplish at least two of the following criteria:

- diffuse pain
- worse in the morning
- worse with Valsalva-like maneuvers
- accompanied by vomiting
- associated with papilledema, sixth nerve palsy, altered level of consciousness, gait instability, and/or increased head circumference (in children <5 years old).

"High-pressure hydrocephalus" is identified by the following criteria:

- ventricular enlargement on neuroimaging
- intracranial pressure >200 mmH_2O in the non-obese or >250 mmH_2O in the obese
- no other intracranial disorder causing increased CSF pressure.

Epidemiology

Recent studies of the prevalence of infantile hydrocephalus indicate a rate between 0.64 and 0.81 per 1000 live births (Fernell et al., 1990; Stoll et al., 1992). About one-half of these cases are the result of premature birth, with almost 90% of these cases caused by intraventricular hemorrhage.

In a study group of 20 children with hydrocephalus, secondary headache due to intracranial hypertension occurred in 5% of cases, whereas secondary headache due to other reasons was much more frequent, occurring in 20% of cases (Matta and Carod-Artal, 2004). Chronic headaches in adults with spina bifida and associated hydrocephalus were found in 55% of the patients (Edwards et al., 2003). In a study of 130 children with shunted hydrocephalus the incidence of migrainous headache was documented in 9% and non-migrainous headache in 15% of cases (Stellman-Ward et al., 1997).

Classification

Hydrocephalus is occult when there are no clinical symptoms of intracranial hypertension. It is active when the disease is progressive and there is increased intracranial pressure. Hydrocephalus is arrested when ventricular enlargement has ceased. The terms communicating and non-communicating hydrocephalus were introduced by Dandy and Blackfan to describe the flow of CSF. Non-communicating hydrocephalus denotes a blockade of CSF pathways at, or proximal to, the outlet foramina of the fourth ventricle. Communicating hydrocephalus denotes a blockade distal to this point, in the basal subarachnoid cisterns and in the subarachnoid spaces over the brain surface (McCullough, 1989). The term obstructive hydrocephalus is used to describe conditions after obstruction of either intraventricular or extraventricular pathways. In communicating hydrocephalus no obstruction can be demonstrated by standard tests. Hydrocephalus with normal pressure at lumbar puncture and absence of papilledema led to the term normal pressure hydrocephalus. These forms of hydrocephalus are distinguished from hydrocephalus ex vacuo, in which CFS volume increases without change in CFS pressure because brain tissue has been lost.

Pathogenesis

The pathogenesis of hydrocephalus is related to any pathophysiological process capable of altering CSF production, circulation, or absorption in such a way as to allow an increased accumulation of CSF in a brain unable to compensate for the resulting increase in CSF volume (Hamlat et al., 2006). Molecular genetic findings have implicated mutations of the *L1CAM* gene in some inherited forms of hydrocephalus (Graf et al., 2000) and a gene which is responsible for causing hydrocephalus in the mouse (Davy and Robinson, 2003). Experiments in animal models are advancing our understanding of cellular damage in this condition and its similarities to ischemic white matter injury (Del Bigio, 2004). Potential causes of non-communicating hydrocephalus are aqueductal stenosis, Chiari malformation, Dandy–Walker malformation, atresia of the foramen of Monroe, skull base anomalies, mass effect from neoplasias, and inflammatory ventriculitis from infection, hemorrhage, chemical irritation, and ruptured cysts. Communicating hydrocephalus is often the result of congenital anomalies and leptomeningeal inflammation.

Clinical presentations

Headache

Chronic headache is reported frequently amongst children with shunted hydrocephalus (Stellman-Ward et al., 1997). Headache is a common symptom of intracranial hypertension. The etiology plays an important role in determining the presentation of hydrocephalus. Depending on the time course of the underlying disease process causing hydrocephalus, the clinical manifestations of hydrocephalus can present in an acute, subacute, or chronic manner. Severe headache can be the only symptom of a long-standing shunt dysfunction (Dahlerup et al., 1985). Heat-triggered episodes of headache were reported in a boy with postinfectious internal hydrocephalus (Wamsler et al., 2006). In 46 adults with hydrocephalus, primary symptoms were related to gait (70%), cognition (70%), urinary urgency (48%), and headaches (56%) (Cowan et al., 2005).

Other clinical presentations

The usual presentation of hydrocephalus in infants is head enlargement. Signs and symptoms of intracranial hypertension such as vomiting, irritability, lethargy, poor feeding, and changes in muscle tone accompany ventriculomegaly. In a newborn this is regularly accompanied by a bulging fontanel and separation of the sutures. Some newborns present with forced downward deviation of the eyes ("sunset sign"). Hydrocephalus of acute onset in older children usually presents with headaches worsening in the morning, vomiting, disturbances of eye movements (particularly sixth nerve palsy and gaze palsies), and altered levels of consciousness. In children with cerebral palsy, hydrocephalus may be asymptomatic (Albright et al., 2005). Memory deficits, discourse and pragmatic abnormalities (Vachha and Adams, 2003), executive dysfunction, and cognitive visual problems may also occur in association with hydrocephalus (Barnes and Dennis, 1998; Scott et al., 1998). In adults the common presentations include epilepsy, rhinorrhea, ataxia, tremor, dementia, incontinence, nystagmus, or other eye movement disorder (Shelden et al., 1930; McMillan and Williams, 1970; Bret et al., 1977; Phadke et al., 1981). Selective compression of posterior brain regions in hydrocephalic patients seems to impair visuospatial and visuomotor performance.

Diagnosis

Magnetic resonance imaging (MRI) and computed tomography (CT) are the gold standard tests to evaluate a patient for the presence of hydrocephalus (El Gammal et al., 1987). MRI is particularly important because of its ability to accurately image hindbrain structures as well as to identify areas of CSF flow. Sometimes lumbar puncture is indicated to measure an increased CSF pressure of 200 mmH_2O in non-obese and 250 mmH_2O in obese patients and to determine the presence of blood or signs of inflammatory or infectious disease. Continuous monitoring of intraventricular pressure may differentiate arrested from progressive disease when lumbar CSF pressure is normal and may not assess the intraventricular pressure.

In infants ultrasonography is an alternative diagnostic method in evaluating ependymal and intraventricular hemorrhage in high-risk and and premature infants (Callen et al., 1986). Occasionally cerebral angiography is indicated for diagnostic problems of hydrocephalus owing to intracranial mass lesions (Morrison et al., 1984).

Differential diagnosis

The differential diagnosis of non-hydrocepahlic macroencephaly includes thick calvarium, degenerative disorders such as Canavan disease (Srikanth et al., 2007), and benign familial megaencephaly (Day and Schutt, 1979). The presentation of hydrocephalus is similar to that of other situations that result in increased intracranial pressure such as brain tumors and benign intracranial hypertension. There is overlap with the differential diagnosis of various headache syndromes such as migraine headache, tension-type headache, medication overuse headache, and depression, because headache is a frequent symptom of hydrocephalus.

Treatment

Since the 1950s, valve-regulated shunt systems by Nulsen and Spitz have become the standard of care. Numerous CFS shunting procedures have been advocated to effect CFS removal from one portion of the craniospinal space to another (ventriculocisternal shunting) or from the craniospinal space to an extracranial reservoir (ventriculoperitoneal shunting). Increasingly, pediatric neurosurgeons are considering the use of neuroendoscopically guided third ventriculostomy as an alternative to shunting, and even the procedure of choice for hydrocephalus (de Ribaupierre et al., 2007). Although the procedure is considered safe by neurosurgeons, significant complications, such as basilar artery perforation, have been reported

(Abtin et al., 1998). Awareness and recognition, as well as prevention and treatment of repeated shunt failures, of slit ventricle syndrome (McLaurin, 1989) and shunt infections is emerging (Drake et al., 2000). Antibiotic-impregnated shunts are available, but data thus far have not demonstrated a reduction in shunt infection in hydrocephalus patients (Ritz et al., 2007). A few studies have reported effective medical treatments of certain forms of infantile hydrocephalus using isosorbide or furosemide and acetazolamide (Skinner et al., 1985).

Prognosis

The prognosis for individuals with most forms of hydrocephalus has radically changed with the valve-regulated shunt system. In a series of 182 untreated individuals, Laurence and Coates (1967) illustrated the natural history and prognosis of this disorder. Adulthood was reached by only 20% of infants. Many of the deaths occurred in the first 1.5 years of life. Of those who survived with untreated hydrocephalus, 60% had intellectual impairment and 25% were "completely ineducable." Some patients with compensated hydrocephalus had sudden death. The most important prognostic factors are the underlying etiology of hydrocephalus, the duration of the condition before shunting, and the associated structural brain lesions. Shunt infections are obviously a risk factor for below normal IQ scores (McLone et al., 1982).

HEADACHE ATTRIBUTED TO LOW CEREBROSPINAL FLUID PRESSURE

Post-dural (post-lumbar) puncture headache

Diagnostic criteria

A. Headache that worsens within 15 min after sitting or standing and improves within 15 min after lying, with at least one of the following and fulfilling criteria C and D:
   1. neck stiffness
   2. tinnitus
   3. hypacusia
   4. photophobia
   5. nausea

B. Dural puncture has been performed

C. Headache develops within 5 days after dural puncture

D. Headache resolves either:
   1. spontaneously within 1 week
   2. within 48 h after effective treatment of the spinal fluid leak (usually by epidural blood patch).

Epidemiology

Post-dural puncture headache is the most frequent complication of major conduction anesthesia and lumbar puncture for diagnostic or therapeutic reasons.

There is controversy over whether age and gender are independent risk factors for the development of post-dural puncture headache. The earlier studies mainly included parturient and thus mostly younger women (Gaiser, 2006; Wu et al., 2006). Despite this controversy it is in general more common in younger people than in children or the elderly. Females are more often affected than males. A lower body mass index (BMI) is also associated with a higher risk for post-dural puncture headache (Raskin, 1990; Kuntz et al., 1992; Vilming and Kloster, 1997; Vilming et al., 2001; Wadud et al., 2006). It is more common in patients who are suffering from other primary headaches such as migraine or chronic tension-type headache.

Clinical manifestations

Post-dural puncture headache is a postural headache. It worsens within 15 min after assuming an upright position and improves within 15 min after assuming a supine position. Most patients describe this as a bilateral, throbbing, mostly occipitally and/or frontally localized headache. This headache is accompanied by at least with one of the following symptoms: neck stiffness, tinnitus, hypacusia, photophobia, or nausea. Other less frequent symptoms include vertigo, gait imbalance, nuchal pain, diplopia (caused by affected CN III, IV, VI) or other (mostly caudal) cranial nerve deficits. In rare cases galactorrhea and increased serum prolactin levels are described (Yamamoto et al., 1993). The pain intensity is classified as moderate to severe. It can be aggravated by Valsalva-type maneuvers.

In 5% of patients paradoxical postural headache may be observed. In this case the headache relieves when in an upright position (Mokri et al., 2004). Some patients are even free of headache in the morning and an increasing headache develops over the course of the day (Mokri et al., 2004).

Vilming and Kloster (1997) examined the time interval in 293 patients when changing from recumbent to upright position and vice versa with regard to onset and relief of headache respectively. The median interval was 20 s for both positional changes.

This headache develops in less than 24 h in 65% of patients and in less than 48 h in 90% (Lybecker et al., 1995). Some 72% of post-dural puncture headaches resolve spontaneously within 7 days and 87% within 6 months (Dripps and Vandam, 1954). Usually after several months this headache changes its character.

It becomes a more lingering chronic daily headache with fluctuating intensity and attenuated orthostatic symptoms (Mokri et al., 1997).

Pathophysiology

Post-dural puncture headache results from a leakage of cerebral spinal fluid (CSF) through the dural hole caused by the needle. The consequence of the loss of CSF is a decrease in pressure, as shown on MRI (Vakharia et al., 1997). There are two diverging hypotheses. One postulates a caudal displacement of the brain and therefore traction of dural structures with blood vessels and attending pain-sensitive trigeminal nerve branches (Mokri et al., 1997; Bartsch and Goadsby, 2003; Miyazawa et al., 2003). However, at least one study does not support this theory, because displacement of intracranial structures was not visible on MRI (Grant et al., 1991). The alternate hypothesis is that headache may be due to dilation of cerebral veins and venous plexus which results from an increase in blood volume to compensate for a loss of CSF volume.

The development of post-dural puncture headache does not depend on the quantity of CSF withdrawn by diagnostic lumbar puncture (Dieterich, 2003). In experimental settings this headache is observed after loss of 20 ml of CSF (Kunkle et al., 1943).

Diagnostic workup

Most important for diagnosis is the history of a dural puncture. If in doubt, radioisotope cisternography, CT (myelography), and MRI may be diagnostic.

Therapy

Often a spontaneous remission is observed and intervention is not required. Bed rest is the most common recommended treatment, but rest after lumbar puncture is not useful in preventing post-dural puncture headache (Dieterich and Brandt, 1985; Mokri, 2003). While often recommended and widely considered to be effective, there is no evidence to support the effectiveness of hydration (Dieterich and Brandt, 1988), caffeine, or theophylline (Feuerstein and Zeides, 1986; Jarvis et al., 1986; Camann et al., 1990; Halker et al., 2007). The effectiveness of corticosteroids is anecdotal (Pascual et al., 2002; Gentile et al., 2004).

If spontaneous improvement does not occur, autologous epidural blood patch is the treatment of choice. This has been shown in randomized controlled trial (van Kooten et al., 2008). In more than 85% the first blood patch (10–20 ml) is effective. For some patients repeated patching is necessary. The patient's own blood will be injected epidurally under sterile conditions at the position of lumbar puncture. This results in a compression of the dura by the injected volume and presumably sealing of the dura. The response rate is up to 90% (Olsen, 1987; Seebacher et al., 1989; Heide and Diener, 1990; Duffy and Crosby, 1999; Sencavoka et al., 2001; Berroir et al., 2004).

Electrical epidural stimulation (Tsui test) could be used to confirm accurate placement of a thoracic epidural catheter for administration of a blood patch (Morley-Forster et al., 2006).

If epidural blood patch fails, epidural injections of fibrin glue – requiring exact knowledge of the site of leakage – may be effective (Gerritse et al., 1997; Crul et al., 1999). Fibrin glue could be applied by CT guidance (Rai et al., 2005; Savoiardo et al., 2006). This is effective in 30% of patients with failure of epidural blood patch (Schievink, 2006). Even epidural application of dextran or saline has been reported (Gibson et al., 1988; Barrios-Alarcon et al., 1989; Bel et al., 2006).

Open surgical repair of the leak may be necessary in patients who fail to respond to epidural blood patches or targeted percutaneous approaches with fibrin glue (Schievink et al., 1998). Meningeal diverticula can be ligated with a suture or aneurysm clip. In contrast dural rents or holes are repaired with a suture or placement of a muscle pledget along with gelfoam and fibrin sealant (Schievink, 2006).

Prevention

The most essential predictor for development of post-dural puncture headache is needle size. Needles with a lower diameter are associated with a lower incidence of headache (Diener et al., 1985; Lynch et al., 1991). Several studies reveal a lower incidence of post-dural puncture headache when using atraumatic ("Sprotte") needles (Halpern and Preston, 1994; Strupp et al., 2001). It is also recommended to insert the needle in a parallel rather than a perpendicular orientation with respect to the alignment of the dural fibers and to re-insert the stylet (Strupp et al., 1998; Wu et al., 2006).

CSF fistula headache

Diagnostic criteria

A. Headache that worsens within 15 min after sitting or standing, with at least one of the following and fulfilling criteria C and D:
   1. neck stiffness
   2. tinnitus
   3. hypacusia
   4. photophobia
   5. nausea

B. A known procedure or trauma has caused persistent CSF leakage with at least one of the following:
   1. evidence of low CSF pressure on MRI (e.g., pachymeningeal enhancement)
   2. evidence of CSF leakage on conventional myelography, CT myelography, or cisternography
   3. CSF opening pressure <60 mmH_2O in sitting position
C. Headache develops in close temporal relation to CSF leakage
D. Headache resolves within 7 days of sealing the CSF leak.

Epidemiology

Prevalence and incidence are not kown. Most fistulas are due to trauma, particularly of the skull base, or iatrogenic as a complication of neurosurgical procedures that require penetration of the dura. Some are spontaneous. The literature consists of case reports or studies with cohorts of less than 10 patients.

Clinical manifestations

CSF fistula could present as oculorrhea or rhinorrhea depending on localization of the fistula (Salame et al., 2000; Schmerber et al., 2001).

Diagnostic workup

MRI and CT are most widely used to identify fistulas (Shetty et al., 2000). Intrathecal gadolinium may help to identify the CSF leak (Albayram et al., 2008).

Therapy

Surgical treatment performed either endoscopically or conventionally is usually employed. Closure of the fistula reduces the risk for developing meningitis.

Prevention

The risk of CSF fistula following laminectomy was reduced in a porcine model when hemostat devices were used (Robertson et al., 2003). Alternatively dural substitutes with polyglycolic acid mesh and fibrin glue may be employed (Shimada et al., 2006).

Headache attributed to spontaneous (or idiopathic) low CSF pressure

Previously used terms

Spontaneous intracranial hypotension, primary intracranial hypotension, low CSF volume headache, hypoliquorrheic headache

Diagnostic criteria

A. Diffuse and/or dull headache that worsens within 15 min after sitting or standing, with at least one of the following and fulfilling criterion D:
   1. neck stiffness
   2. tinnitus
   3. hypacusia
   4. photophobia
   5. nausea
B. At least one of the following:
   1. evidence of low CSF pressure on MRI (e.g., pachymeningeal enhancement)
   2. evidence of CSF leakage on conventional myelography, CT myelography, or cisternography
   3. CSF opening pressure <60 mmH_2O in sitting position
C. No history of dural puncture or other cause of CSF fistula
D. Headache resolves within 72 h after epidural blood patching.

Comments

The underlying disorder may be low CSF volume. A history of a trivial increase in intracranial pressure (e.g., on vigorous coughing) is often elicited. In other cases a sudden drop in atmospheric pressure has occurred. Postural headache resembling that of low CSF pressure has been reported after coitus. Such headache should be coded here because it is due to CSF leakage.

Many patients with spontaneous low CSF pressure headache respond to conservative therapy or epidural blood patching. Some have spontaneous resolution of their headache, while others relapse after initial successful treatment. Cases of dural sleeve herniation, particularly in the thoracic area, have been reported and have been successfully treated surgically.

Dural puncture should be avoided in patients with positive MRI signs such as meningeal enhancement with contrast.

Epidemiology

The prevalence was estimated in a community-based study conducted in 1994 at 1 per 50 000 (Schievink et al., 1998). An annual incidence for spontaneous intracranial hypotension was reported as 5 per 100 000 (Schievink, 2006). It is also not clearly determined if age and gender are risk factors for development of this headache.

Etiology

Spontaneous CSF leaks are the most common cause of spontaneous CSF volume depletion causing orthostatic headaches. The vast majority of spontaneous leaks occur at the spinal level, particularly the thoracic spine or cervicothoracic junction. While the exact cause of spontaneous CSF leak remains unknown in the majority of patients, weakness of the meningeal sac in certain regions and trivial trauma are considered to be important contributing factors. Meningeal diverticulae are frequently seen in these patients and areas of attenuated dura have been noted in patients who have undergone surgery to repair the leak. Spontaneous CSF leaks have also been observed in patients with inherited disorders of the connective tissue, such as Marfan syndrome, and abnormalities of elastin or fibrillin, or both, are suspected in these patients (Davenport et al., 1995; Mokri et al., 1997, 2002; Milledge et al., 2005; Schievink, 2006). Occasional dural tears resulting from spondylotic spurs or disc herniation may lead to CSF leak (Eross et al., 2002). Many patients report a history of trivial trauma, exertion, or Valsalva maneuvers (Schievink, 2000; Mokri, 2003). Some authors observed this headache following chiropractic spinal manipulation (Albayram, 2006; Prasad et al., 2006).

Diagnostic workup

Computed tomography of the head is often not useful, but may demonstrate the presence of a subdural fluid collection (Schievink, 2006), increased tentorial enhancement, or small ventricular size. Magnetic resonance imaging of the brain with gadolinium is the most useful diagnostic study in patients with spontaneous CSF leak (Fishman and Dillon, 1993; Mokri et al., 1997; Schievink, 2006). Diffuse pachymeningeal enhancement is the most common abnormality without any evidence of leptomeningeal involvement. The enhancement is smooth, linear, and involves both the supertentorial and infratentorial dura mater. Pachymeningeal enhancement may be absent in up to one-third of cases, when imaging is performed well after the onset of symptoms (Mokri et al., 1999; Schievink and Tourje, 2000).

Sagging or descent of brain structures is also a common finding and may take the form of cerebellar tonsillar descent (mimicking a Chiari type I malformation), a reduction in the size of the prepontine cistern, inferior displacement of the optic chiasm, effacement of perichiasmatic cisterns, and crowding of the posterior fossa.

Also uni- or bilateral subdural fluid collections are reported in up to 50% of patients (Pavlin et al., 1979; Schievink et al., 2005). Engorgement or even thrombosis of the cerebral sinus is a possible complication and may be seen on MRI and conventional angiography (Koss et al., 2003; Roll et al., 2003; Savoiardo et al., 2006). Enlargement and diffuse enhancement of the pituitary gland may also be seen, mimicking a pituitary tumor (Alvarez-Linera et al., 2000; Mokri and Atkinson, 2000). Due to collapse of the ventricular system, a collapse of the ventricle is seen sometimes (Murros and Fogelholm, 1983).

MRI of the spine may reveal an extra-arachnoid fluid collection without revealing the site of CSF leakage (Rabin et al., 1998; Chiapparini et al., 2002). Single or multiple meningeal diverticula of variable size are identified frequently on MRI without necessarily being the site of leakage (Mokri, 1999). Spinal pachymeningeal enhancement and engorgement of spinal venous plexus are less often observed than with intracranial imaging (Chen et al., 2002; Chiapparini et al., 2002).

In most patients the CSF opening pressure is low, even not measurable. However, the opening pressure may be within the normal range in up to 40% of patients (Atkinson et al., 1998; Mokri et al., 1998). Analysis of CSF is usually normal, but may reveal xanthochromia, protein concentrations of up to 200 mg/dl or greater, CSF erythrocyte counts up to several hundred, and CSF leukocyte counts (typically lymphocytes) as high as 200/mm^3 reported.

Most important for therapy of spontaneous intracranial hypotension is to localize the leakage of CSF if conservative measures and autologous blood patching fails. The most accurate test to localize leakage of CSF is thin-cut CT myelography with water-soluble contrast (Schievink et al., 2005). The leak may vary from a small amount of contrast along a single nerve root to extensive paraspinal enhancement. Meningeal diverticula may also be detected. Mostly the leakage is found at the cervicothoracic junction or along the thoracic spine. Delayed imaging is required to visualize slow or intermittent leaks, whereas early ultra-fast scanning is needed to capture rapid high-volume leaks (Schievink, 2006).

Alternatively MRI myelography could be employed, which also requires a lumbar puncture and consecutive intrathecal injection of gadolinium (Tali et al., 2002; Liong et al., 2006).

Radionuclide cisternography with intrathecally applied indium-111 is useful for detection of CSF leakage in up to 50% of patients, particularly when diagnosis is in doubt or myelography results are normal (Chung et al., 2000). Scanning is performed at various time intervals for up to 24 or 48 h. Normally radioactivity should be detected over the cerebral convexities before 24 or at least 48 h after intrathecal administration. In patients with CSF leaks, radioactivity extends only to basal cisterns, or sometimes only paraspinal activity is seen. Early activity (in first 4 h) in the urinary bladder, compared to the normal appearance between 6 to 24 h, is also suggestive of CSF leakage. If diagnosis is in doubt, cisternograpy could be supplemented with analysis of the radioisotope clearance (Moriyama et al., 2004). If meningeal diverticula are large enough they could appear as foci of radioactivity and thus indicate the site of CSF leakage (Molins et al., 1990; Bai et al., 2002).

Therapy

While many patients may improve spontaneously, a substantial number will require autologous epidural blood patching (EPB) (Chung et al., 2005; Kong et al., 2005). EPB may have an immediate effect related to volume replacement and a delayed effect related to sealing of the dural defect (Sencavoka et al., 2001). In spontaneous CSF leaks, the success of EPB is less successful than with post-dural puncture headache (Sencavoka et al., 2001; Udommongkol et al., 2005). Many patients require more than one blood patch and some may require up to six blood patches. This difference may be related to the fact that, with spontaneous CSF leaks, the level of the epidural blood patch may be distant from the level of the leak, and in many spontaneous CSF leaks the nature and anatomy of the leak are much different from those of a simple hole or rent produced by the spinal tap needle. In spontaneous CSF leaks, many of the dural defects are in the anterior aspect of the dura or in the root sleeves.

While the rate of recurrence is not known, recurrent CSF leaks may occur within weeks to years after the initial leak. Patients with multiple meningeal diverticula and underlying disorders of connective tissue matrix may be more susceptible to recurrence of CSF leakage either from one site or from multiple sites, although this has not been formally studied.

HEADACHE ATTRIBUTED TO NON-INFECTIOUS INFLAMMATORY DISEASE

Headache attributed to neurosarcoidosis

Definition and epidemiology

Sarcoidosis is a multi-systemic granulomatous disease of unknown origin. The term "sarcoid", or sarcoma-like, was proposed by a Norwegian dermatologist, Caesar Peter Moeller Boeck, after detailed histological studies of skin plaques (Boeck, 1899). Recognition of the multi-system nature of the disease is generally credited to Jorgen Schaumann, a Swedish dermatologist who in 1936 described involvement of the liver, spleen, lungs, and the bones. Most commonly the disease affects young adults, with predominance in women and North Americans of African descent (Newman et al., 1997). Sarcoidosis is usually diagnosed between the ages of 20 and 40 years (Newman et al., 1997). The prevalence is estimated at 20–50 per 100 000 in the Caucasian population, and the incidence at 20 per 100 000 among Caucasians (Stern et al., 1985).

Neurological symptoms due to involvement of the central nervous system (CNS) develop in about 5% of patients with systemic sarcoidosis (Delaney, 1977). Ricker and Clark (1949) found a 14% prevalence of CNS involvement in a series of 300 autopsy cases with a premortem diagnosis of systemic sarcoidosis. Thus silent CNS involvement is present in approximately 10% of patients with systemic disease. In 10–30% of patients with systemic sarcoidosis there are initial signs and symptoms of neurosarcoidosis at presentation (Stern et al., 1985). Very rarely sarcoid granulomatosis is strictly confined to the CNS (Cariski, 1981). The incidence of isolated neurosarcoidosis is estimated at less than 0.2 per 100 000 among Caucasians (Nowak and Widenka, 2001).

Because of its non-specific clinical presentation and neuroradiological imaging characteristics, intracranial neurosarcoidosis remains a very difficult diagnosis, particularly in the absence of systemic signs of the disease. Intracranial neurosarcoidosis has a predilection for the basal leptomeninges, commonly affecting the cranial nerves, but any part of the brain may be involved, resulting in a wide spectrum of clinical syndromes.

Imaging evidence of neurosarcoidosis may include cranial nerve lesions, intracranial space-occupying lesions on magnetic resonance imaging (MRI), aseptic meningitis, and/or periventicular inflammatory focal lesions and homogeneously enhancing mass lesions that are confirmed on biopsy as non-caseating granulomas.

Sarcoid lesions are non-caseating epitheloid granulomas. Intracranial lesions, detectable by MRI, appear as nodular or diffuse leptomeningeal thickening, mimicking various forms of meningitides, including neoplastic or carcinomatous meningitis. MRI findings have been included in the diagnostic criteria (Zajicek et al., 1999).

Pathogenesis

There is still no precise understanding of the pathogenesis of sarcoidosis. The origin of the disease remains unknown, although it seems that a genetic predisposition for an exaggerated immune response to specific antigens causes inflammatory ganuloma formation and progressive fibrosis (Newman et al., 1997). Newman et al. emphasize the particular role of T-lymphocytes in the development of sarcoidosis. These authors suggest that, following exposure to an unknown antigen and acquisition of a cellular immunity directed against the antigen, T-lymphocytes amplify the local cellular immune response. Mycobacteria and propionibacteria are considered to contribute to the pathogenesis of sarcoidosis (Saboor et al., 1992; Ishige et al., 1999).

Histopathogenesis of CNS sarcoidosis is thought to be primarily leptomeningeal with inflammatory exudate extending from the subarachnoid space along the Virchow–Robin spaces into brain parenchyma (Mirfakhraee et al., 1986). The Virchow–Robin spaces are especially large at the base of the brain, which may explain the predilection of sarcoid lesions for the basal leptomeninges with frequent involvement of the hypothalamus, third ventricle, and optic and other cranial nerves. The pattern of granulomatous inflammation spreading from the Virchow–Robin spaces into the brain can be analyzed histologically and visualized on contrast-enhanced MRI (Williams et al., 1990).

Clinical manifestations

Cranial nerves

Facial nerve dysfunction is one of the most common neurological abnormalities and may occur either in isolation or in combination with other cranial neuropathies. Zajicek et al. (1999) reported cranial neuropathies in 72% of 68 patients who were thought to "very likely" have neurosarcoidosis. Facial nerve dysfunction is one of the most common neurological abnormalities. Colover (1948) examined 118 patients and found facial paresis or palsy in 49%. Of these, 65% showed unilateral involvement. Distinction from idiopathic Bell's palsy may be difficult. Although the pathophysiology of facial nerve dysfunction remains unclear, frequent association with hyperacusis, abnormal lacrimation, and taste disturbance seems to suggest a more proximal involvement.

The optic nerve may be involved in up to 38% of patients suspected of neurosarcoidosis (Zajicek et al., 1999). Symptoms and signs tend to evolve subacutely and include enlargement of the blind spot, field defect, blurred vision, and pupillary dysfunction. Examination may reveal anterior uveitis, papillitis, papilledema, and optic atrophy. Retrobulbar optic neuritis may mimic a common finding in multiple sclerosis and confuse the clinician. Variable mechanisms are responsible for optic nerve dysfunction. Papilledema, which results from increased intracranial pressure, can be caused by hydrocephalus and parenchymal mass lesions; both granulomatous infiltration and direct compression of the nerve can cause optic atrophy. Less frequently reported is involvement of oculomotor nerves, trigeminal nerve, vestibular, auditory, and other lower cranial nerves.

Central nervous system

Clinical signs of parenchymal involvement depend on the location and the size of the lesions. Granulomas mimicking neoplasms and demyelinating plaques have been found in virtually all regions of the neuraxis. Large or strategically located lesions can cause increased intracranial pressure with headache and papilledema. Seizures of various types are seen in up to 20% of those with intra-axial lesions, and the association with prognosis is unclear (Delaney, 1980).

Involvement of basal ganglia, brainstem, cerebellum, and spinal cord may result in a movement disorder, cranial nerve dysfunction, ataxia, or progressive myelopathy. Spinal lesions may be solitary or multiple and can cause back and leg pain, paraparesis, quadriparesis, and sphincter dysfunction. A well-recognized target is the hypothalamic–pituitary axis, characteristically resulting in diabetes insipidus. The clinical presentation can range from panhypopituitarism to selective disturbances of anterior or posterior pituitary function. Leptomeningeal disease with or without aseptic meningitis and communicating and non-communicating hydrocephalus are other potential manifestations of neurosarcoidosis.

Other neurological manifestations

Neuropsychiatric dysfunction in neurosarcoidosis includes psychoses, bipolar disorder, depression, amnestic syndrome, dementia, and encephalopathy. Gilmore et al. (1980) described a case of acute agitated depression in a man with known systemic sarcoidosis. Although rarely described, vascular involvement due to extension of the granulomas into the wall of the blood vessels may lead to subarachnoid or intraparenchymal hemorrhage, and ischemic stroke (Delaney, 1977; Oksanen, 1986).

Peripheral spinal nerves are frequently involved. Mononeuritis, which may progress to a multiplex picture, was reported with an incidence of 17% in one series (Chapelon et al., 1990). Clinically, patients are typically found to have a mixed sensorimotor deficit, although pure motor and sensory types have been described. The pure motor manifestation may be clinically and electrophysiologically identical to Guillain–Barré syndrome. The mechanism of nerve injury is unclear, with evidence for both axonal injury and demyelination (Oh, 1980; Galassi et al., 1984). The sequence of damage to myelin and axons, which may result from compression and ischemia, is not conclusively known.

Muscle may be affected alone or in combination with peripheral nerves. Reports of symptomatic myopathy range from less than 1% to 26% (Oksanen, 1986; Chapelon et al., 1990).

Clinical aspects with focus on headache

As described above, any part of the CNS may be involved in neurosarcoidosis. This fact results in a wide spectrum of clinical symptoms. With a prevalence of 50% in patients with neurosarcoidosis, cranial nerve palsies are the most common disorder. Headache follows wih a prevalence of 30% in affected subjects (Nowak and Widenka, 2001). Headache type will depend on the nature of the neuropathological involvement: focal lesions, meningitis, and cranial nerve palsies.

For the diagnosis of a "headache attributed to neurosarcoidosis" the International Headache Society (IHS) demands the development of a headache, with no typical characteristics known, in temporal relation to the development of evidence of neurosarcoidosis. Evidence of neurosarcoidosis includes cranial nerve lesions, intracranial space-occupying lesions on magnetic resonance imaging (MRI), aseptic meningitis, and/or periventicular inflammatory focal lesions and homogeneously enhancing mass lesions that are confirmed on biopsy as non-caseating granulomas. Finally, the headache should resolve within 3 months after successful treatment of neurosarcoidosis. Although no typical characteristics of headache are known, detailed information on these aspects is occasionally reported in published studies.

Intractable occipital headache with radiation to the frontal head region and associated with nausea and visual disturbances has been reported in patients with isolated supratentorial tumor-like lesions (Vannemreddy et al., 2002). Diffuse or bifrontal pain is a more typical symptom of leptomeningeal involvement, with or without papilledema (Zouaoui et al., 1992; Katz et al., 2003). Other forms of cranial pain may be related to trigeminal or optic nerve involvement. Migrainc has also been reported (Dizdarevic et al., 1998). In another case report (La Mantia and Erbetta, 2004) a 56-year-old woman presented with a painful paresis of the third cranial nerve, neuropapillitis, and transient trigeminal neuralgia on the right side. MRI showed a granulomatous lesion of the right cavernous sinus. Steroid treatment provided pain remission within 3 months, but without improvement of the neurological deficits. MRI showed a significant reduction of the lesion after therapy. The diagnostic workup (angiotensin-converting enzyme level, chest CT scan, bromcho-alveolar lavage, gallium scintigraphy) allowed the diagnosis of probable neurosarcoidosis (Zajicek et al., 1999).

Progress

Clinical symptoms may develop acutely or subacutely and may also progress in a chronic fashion. Spontaneous remissions are more frequent than progressive neurological deterioration (Luke et al., 1987). Patients in whom neurological signs resolve spontaneously may develop further neurological symptoms years later (Delaney, 1977). This indicates that sarcoid granulomas within the CNS can subsequently occur and disappear at various intracranial locations and thus mimic the clinical and radiological pictures of encephalomyelitis disseminata (Lexa and Grossman, 1994). Every part of the brain can be involved, and intracranial neurosarcoidosis substantially increases both morbidity and mortality compared to sarcoidosis without CNS involvement.

Therapy

The success concerning treatment of headache attributed to neurosarcoidosis is, next to symptomatic treatment, directly related to successful treatment of the causative neurosarcoidosis. The treatment of neurosarcoidosis for the most part consists of immunosuppression and is largely adopted from the pulmonary experience. Various modalities are routinely employed, but a controlled trial has yet to be performed.

Corticosteroid use in various schedules is the standard therapy. Oral prednisone ranging from 40 to 80 mg/day is generally sufficient to gain control of the disease and reverse symptoms. If successful in controlling the disease, it can later be reduced to a lower dose. The recommended time of treatment ranges from months to years and should be decided on a case-by-case basis. Some patients may require higher doses of oral or intravenous steroids to gain control of symptoms. Those with intractable disease or dependence on high doses of chronic steroids may benefit from other classes of drugs.

Chloroquine has demonstrated efficacy in a controlled trial of pulmonary sarcoid (Baltzan et al., 1999). Serial ophthalmological examination is recommended due to its association with retinopathy. Several authors have reported success with low doses (4 to 6 mg/kg per day) of cyclosporine; steroid-dependent patients with neurosarcoidosis were able to substantially reduce the dose (Chapelon et al., 1990; Stern et al., 1992). Because cyclosporine acts by inhibiting T-cell proliferation by interfering with the phosphatase activity of calcineurin, its effectiveness in treating refractory neurosarcoidosis argues in favour of a role for cell-mediated immunity in the pathogenesis.

Methotrexate, an antimetabolite, can also be effective in achieving stabilization of symptoms (Chapelon et al., 1990). Tikoo and colleagues (2004) reported response of a patient with suprasellar disease to cladribine (2-chlorodeoxyadenosine), a purine analog used in the treatment of hairy cell leukemia. Therapeutic use of other immunosuppressants, such as azathioprine, chlorambucil, cyclophosphamide, and mycophenolate mofetil, may prove worthwile in appropriate cases (Zajicek et al., 1999).

Targeted therapy to a specific component of the immune response is illustrated by the promising effects of infliximab, a chimeric IgG monoclonal antibody directed against tumor necrosis factor (TNF)-alpha, and thalidomide, an agent reputed to attenuate release of TNF-alpha (Yee and Pochapin, 2001; Baughman et al., 2002). Anecdotal reports of infliximab in neurosarcoidosis are encouraging (Pettersen et al., 2002; Katz et al., 2003). The National Heart, Lung, and Blood Institute is currently conducting a phase II trial of pentoxifylline, a xanthine derivative known to inhibit TNF-alpha release by peripheral blood mononuclear cells, as an adjunct to steroid therapy in systemic sarcoidosis.

Non-pharmacological strategies include irradiation for drug-resistant disease and surgical approaches. Neurosurgical intervention is directed at relieving hydrocephalus by insertion of a shunt and excision of large, accessible, parenchymal lesions. Remaining management issues relate to controlling seizures, correcting endocrine abnormalities when necessary, and neuropsychiatric therapy.

According to the IHS criteria, the headache should resolve within 3 months after successful treatment of neurosarcoidosis.

Headache attributed to aseptic (non-infectious) meningitis

Diagnostic criteria

A. Diffuse headache fulfilling criterion D
B. Examination of CSF shows lymphocytic pleocytosis, mildly elevated protein, and normal glucose in the absence of infectious organisms
C. Use of one of the following: ibuprofen, immunoglobulins, penicillin or trimethoprim, intrathecal injections, or insufflations
D. Headache resolves within 3 months after withdrawal of the offending substance.

History and background

The most common forms of aseptic meningitis are drug-induced meningitis and benign recurrent aseptic meningitis or Mollaret disease.

Drug-induced aseptic meningitis (DIAM) is a rare idiosyncratic event and may occur after local or systemic drug administration. The data on this adverse reaction are predominantly collated from anecdotal case reports and case series. The major categories of causative agents are non-steroidal anti-inflammatory drugs, antimicrobials, intravenous immunoglobulin, intrathecal agents, vaccines, and a number of other less frequently reported agents (Table 50.2). The first diagnositic criteria for drug-induced aseptic meningitis were described by Wallgren in 1925:

- Acute onset of signs and symptoms of meningeal involvement such as headache, fever, and stiff neck.
- Changes in CSF typical of meningitis (e.g., pleocytosis).
- Absence of infectious organisms in CSF
- Short and benign course of the illness; the patient recovers within a matter of days
- Absence of local parameningeal infection (e.g., otitis media)
- Absence from the community of epidemic disease of which meningitis is a feature.

Mollaret meningitis was first described by Pierre Mollaret in 1944 under the title "benign recurrent endothelial-leukocytic meningitis" but came quickly recognized as Mollaret meningitis. The initial description included clinical manifestations as well as CSF findings of a particular type of cell of endothelial origin thought to be pathognomonic for the disorder and later classified as monocytic. It is no longer regarded to be pathognomonic. Mollaret meningitis today is considered to be a recurrent form of aseptic meningitis, due to the close similarities between the descriptions of Walgren and Mollaret. The interval between the attacks in Mollaret meningitis is usually symptom-free (Frederiks and Bruyn, 1989). In one case of Mollaret meningitis, 2 attacks of the 5 attacks were drug-induced (Thilmann et al., 1991). It was originally thought to be idiopathic, but with increasing case reports several causes have been delineated (Table 50.3).

Epidemiology

The incidence of aseptic meningitis can only be estimated by the frequency of occurrence as reported by case reports for different drugs. No clear-cut evidence is available of this rare disorder. In a retrospective analysis of a prospective cohort study to determine the incidence of aseptic meningitis in patients treated with high-dose intravenous immunoglobulin, 6 (11%) of 54 patients developed aseptic meningitis within 24 h after completion of the infusions, lasting from 3 to 5 days (Scribner et al., 1994). The total number of cases now exceeds 100. Fifty-four cases of aseptic meningitis following mumps vaccine were reported in France during a 9-year period, which represents a mean incidence of 0.82 cases per 100 000 doses of vaccine (Jonville-Bera et al., 1996). No racial or ethnic preponderance has been reported with aseptic meningitis, generally

Table 50.2

Drugs and substances associated with aseptic meningitis

Drug	Example	Reference
Antimicrobial drugs		
Sulfonamides	Sulfanilamide	Fisher and Sydney, 1939
	Trimethoprim/sulfamethoxazole	Wambulwa et al., 2005
	Sulfasalazine	Barrett and Thier, 1963
Cephalosporin		Creel and Hurtt, 1995
Ciprofloxacin		Kepa et al., 2005
Isoniazid		
Ornidazole		Mondon et al., 2002
Penicillin	Amoxicillin	River et al., 1994; Czerwenka et al., 1999; Jacobsson and Elowson, 1999
Antivirals	Valacyclovir	Olin and Gugliotta, 2003
Antineoplastics		
Cytosine arabinoside		
Corticosteroids		
Methylprednisolone acetate		Karmochkine et al., 1993
Hydrocortisone sodium succinate		
Non-steroidal anti-inflammatory drugs		
Celecoxib		Papaioannides et al., 2004
Diclofenac		
Ibuprofen		Nguyen and Juurlink, 2004
Naproxen		Kepa et al., 2005
Sulindac		Greenberg, 1988
Tolmetin		
Ketoprofen		
Salicylates		
Piroxicam		
Rofecoxib		Bonnel et al., 2002; Ashwath and Katner 2003; Ashton et al., 2004
Intraventricular drugs		
Gentamicin		Haase et al., 2001
Antineoplastic drugs		
Spinal intrathecal drugs		
Antineoplastics	Cytosine arabinoside	
	Methotrexate	
Antimicrobials		
Baclofen		Naveira et al., 1996
Steroids		
Spinal anesthesia		Aldrete, 2003
Intrathecal diagnostic agents		
Radiological contrast media	Iophendylate	Navani et al., 2006
	Metrizamide	
Radiolabeled albumin		
Miscellaneous drugs		
Allopurinol		Dumouchel-Champagne et al., 2004
Azathioprine		
Carbamazepine		
Lamotrigine		Kilfoyle et al., 2005
Famotidine		
Infliximab		
Metaraminol		Barakat et al., 1988
Intravenous immune globulin		Jain, 2001, Wright et al., 2008
Muromonab CD-3		Thomas et al., 1999; Jain, 2001
Phenazopyridine		
Pyrazinamide		

Table 50.2

Continued

Drug	Example	Reference
Ranitidine		
Vaccines	Polio	
	Measles, mumps, rubella	Ueda et al., 1995, Jonville-Bera et al., 1996, Kimura et al., 1996
	Hepatitis B	
Wood preservatives		Rottach et al., 1996

Table 50.3

Etiologies of recurrent aseptic meningitis

	Viral	References
Infectious	Epstein–Barr	Graman, 1987
	Herpes simplex	Skoldenberg et al., 1975; Steel et al., 1982; Yamamoto et al., 1991; Tang et al., 2000
	Human herpesvirus-6	
	Other viruses	
	Lyme disease	
Inflammatory	Mixed connective tissue disease	Greenberg, 1988; Chez et al., 1989; Moris and Garcia-Monco, 1999
	Recurrent hereditary polyserositis	Barakat et al., 1988
	Relapsing polychondritis	
	Systemic lupus erythematosus	Sands et al., 1988; Kilfoyle et al., 2005
	Multiple sclerosis	Bornke et al., 1999
Structural	Craniopharyngioma	
	Dermoid cyst	Schwartz and Balentine, 1978; Crossley and Dismukes, 1990
	Ependymoma	
	Glioma	
	Hemangioma (cavernous)	
	Neuroepithelial cyst	Kuroda et al., 1991
	Pineal cyst	
	Pituitary abscess	
	Teratoma	
	Vein of Galen aneurysm	Collins and Fisher, 1990
Medication and toxins (Table 50.1)		
Miscellaneous	Complement factor 1 and 7 deficiency	Bonnin et al., 1993; Corvini et al., 2004
	Lymphoma	Swithinbank and Rake, 1978

occurring in young and middle-aged adults. However, the reported age groups affected range from 14 months (Schwartz and Balentine, 1978) to 72 years (Sundaram and Siemens, 1986).

Pathophysiology

The exact pathomechanism underlying aseptic meningitis is still unknown. Most likely immunological mechanisms play a major role (Nettis et al., 2003). The proposed mechanisms of drug-induced aseptic meningitis fall into two categories: hypersensitivity reactions and direct irritation of the meninges.

Current understanding is in favour of the hypersensitivity hypothesis, most likely type III and IV, as symptoms develop rapidly following drug ingestion, with progressively shorter periods in recurrent cases, and development of classic hypersensitivity features such as facial edema, conjunctivitis, and pruritus, while direct irritation of the meninges usually involves direct instillation of an agent into the meninges (Jolles et al., 2000). Reports of elevated levels of immune complexes in the CSF of patients with drug-induced aseptic meningitis further support the hypersensitivity reaction theory (Hopkins and Jolles, 2005). Patients that initially tolerated a drug well may develop drug-induced aseptic meningitis on subsequent administration. This phenomenon could be explained by the hapten theory: a drug could act as a hapten that binds to intravascular proteins, prompting the immune system to subsequently recognize those proteins as foreign antigens. Drug-induced aseptic meningitis due to direct irritation may be delayed for up to several weeks following the administration of the drug and is related to the following criteria:

- Concentration of the drug or the chemical in the CSF
- Lipid solubility and particle size of the substance
- Ability to ionize the CSF
- Duration of contact with CSF.

Several predisposing factors in patients with drug-induced aseptic meningitis have been identified. Patients that suffer from autoimmune disorders (such as SLE) or immunodeficiency conditions (such as AIDS) may be at greater risk for the development of drug-induced aseptic meningitis (Kilfoyle et al., 2005). Regulator protein factor I deficiency usually leads to an increased risk of pyogenic bacterial infections as result of reduced complement-dependent ability to opsonize and kill bacteria but may also lead to recurrent aseptic meningitis (Bonnin et al., 1993). The mechanism underlying the administration of intravenous immunoglobulin (IVIG) is not well understood but it has been hypothesized that IVIG may breech the blood–brain barrier in patients with autoimmune disorders and thus allow entry of even bigger molecules into the CSF causing cytokine-mediated progressive damage to the endothelial cells. This may result in an inflammatory reaction as evidenced by CSF pleocytosis. IVIG-associated aseptic meningitis is presumed to be an acute hypersensitivity reaction limited to the leptomeninges without systemic anaphylaxis. Patients with migraine are more likely to develop aseptic meningitis when receiving IVIG. This may be due to increased cerebrovascular sensitivity or damaged blood–brain barrier in migraineurs.

The pathophysiology of Mollaret meningitis has frequently been associated with reactivation of herpes simplex virus type 1 but also type 2 and other herpes viruses. Elevated CSF concentration of T-lymphocytes was interpreted as evidence for HSV-1 reactivation and these identified cells showed high resemblance to the endothelial cell that Mollaret described himself and believed to be pathognomonic for this disease (Goldstein et al., 1986). In different investigations a strong intrathecal humoral immune response was observed but with fewer active T-cells in the CSF (Kinnman et al., 1979). Gene abnormalities associated with severe or recurrent microbial infection might play a role in Mollaret meningitis. Polymorphisms were noted in 40% of cases infected with HSV type 2 in the mannose-binding lectin gene but in interferon-g receptor sequences (Tang et al., 2000). A connection of Mollaret meningitis to the underlying pathophysiological mechanism of drug-induced meningitis has been proposed by reports of cysts responsible for the development of Mollaret meninigitis. This leakage from a neuroepidermal cyst suggested that the fluid elicits a predominant initial infiltration of T-helper cells possibly due to blood–brain barrier dysfunction similar to what might be seen in exacerbations of multiple sclerosis (Kuroda et al., 1991). The role of immune complexes and autoantibodies has also been postulated for Mollaret meningitis (Creel and Hurtt, 1995).

Clinical presentation and diagnostic workup

Cardinal features include signs and symptoms of meningeal irritation such as nuchal rigidity, headache, often Kernig and Brudzinski signs usually with fever accompanied by CSF pleocytosis without readily identifiable cause. Somatic complaints may include malaise, nausea, and muscular pains. Neurological findings include photophobia, clouding of consciousness, transient focal or non-localizing signs (Parinaud syndrome, slight aphasia, abnormal reflexes, coma, seizures, hallucinations, hemiparesis, ptosis, abducens, and facial nerve palsies). In cases of Mollaret meningitis, these symptoms may be recurrent with full remission between attacks. These episodes of meningitis resolve spontaneously in 2–4 days without remaining neurological deficit and are separated by asymptomatic periods lasting weeks to months, even years. Most cases seem to resolve spontaneously within a few years with the longest-lasting case reported to be 28 years (Tyler and Adler, 1983).

Laboratory investigations including white blood count and lumbar puncture are relevant tests but may be normal. White blood count may be normal or elevated. Serum procalcitonin might be able to discriminate between bacterial and chemical causes of meningitis in postmyelographic meningitis (Bender et al., 2004). CSF pleocytosis may range from a hundred to several thousand cells. Predominance of mononuclear cells in the CSF is characteristic of chronic recurrent meningitis. Rarely, lymphocytic and eosinophilic forms of aseptic meningitis have been reported. Eosinophils in the CSF are characteristic of drug-induced aseptic meningitis due to intravenous immunoglobulin. CSF proteins are usually elevated while glucose and lactic acid is normal. CSF culture results are always unremarkable. Lumbar puncture usually reveals high opening pressure. EEG is generally normal or diffusely slow (in 1 case triphasic waves were reported) (Sundaram and Siemens, 1986).

Magnetic resonance imaging could be a valuable diagnostic procedure in aseptic meningitis. Transient diffuse meningeal enhancement and diffuse supratentorial white matter abnormalities were reported in drug-induced aseptic meningitis that completely resolved after recovery (Eustace and Buff, 1994; Blumenfeld et al., 1996).

Management and prognosis

Management depends entirely on the particular cause. Most cases of unknown cause are self-limiting and benign, and require no specific treatment other than symptomatic relief for pain, nausea, or fever. In idiopathic cases, steroids may shorten the episode in recurrent cases, as may indomethacin. If drug-induced meningitis is suspected, the drug should be discontinued, if possible. Prednisone has been an effective preventive agent for recurrent aseptic meningitis in some cases (Coleman et al., 1975), but not in others (Kinnman et al., 1979). Colchicine has been reported to help in some cases associated with Epstein–Barr virus (Mora and Gimeno, 1980; Graman, 1987) but did not help in others (Stamm et al., 1984). In herpetic outbreaks, acyclovir was reported to be an effective preventive agent (Limburg et al., 1985).

By definition this syndrome has a benign course and resolves spontaneously without residual deficit. One case of recurrent meningitis related to an epidermoid cyst resulted in the death of a 2-year-old after 10 episodes (Schwartz and Balentine, 1978); another from squamous cell carcinoma converted from an epidermoid cyst (Crossley and Dismukes, 1990).

Headache attributed to other non-infectious inflammatory disease

Diagnostic criteria

A. Headache, no typical characteristics known, fulfilling criteria C and D
B. Evidence of one of the inflammatory diseases known to be associated with headache
C. Headache develops in close temporal relation to the inflammatory disorder
D. Headache resolves within 3 months after successful treatment of the inflammatory disorder.

Inflammatory diseases known to be associated with headache are:

- acute demyelinating encephalomyelitis (ADEM)
- systemic lupus erythematosus (SLE)
- Behçet's syndrome
- anti-phospholipid antibody syndrome
- Vogt–Koyanagi–Harada syndrome

These disorders can be associated with headache but it is not usually a presenting or dominant symptom of the underlying disorder. Investigations on incidence or prevalence of headache associated with non-infectious inflammatory disorders are not available. Headache therapy is symptomatic and will always have to concentrate on the underlying disease. Headache can be associated with, but is not usually a presenting or dominant symptom of, acute demyelinating encephalomyelitis (ADEM), systemic lupus erythematosus (SLE), Behçet's syndrome, anti-phospholipid antibody syndrome, or Vogt–Koyanagi–Harada syndrome.

Headache attributed to lymphocytic hypophysitis

Diagnostic criteria

A. Headache, no typical characteristics known, fulfilling criterion C
B. Hypopituitarism fulfilling the following criteria:
   1. MRI demonstrates symmetrical pituitary enlargement with homogeneous contrast enhancement
   2. Biopsy confirmation of lymphocytic hypophysitis
C. Headache develops in close temporal relation to hypopituitarism.

Lymphocytic hypophysitis is often accompanied by hyperprolactinemia (50% of cases) or autoantibodies against hypophyseal cytosol protein (20%). This disorder typically develops at the end of pregnancy or during the postpartum period, but it can occur in men.

History and background

Typical pathological findings of the pituitary gland associated with panhypopituitarism were described by Bellastella et al. (2003), and Asa et al. (1981) postulated an autoimmune pathogenetic mechanism. They reported on a young postpartum woman with Hashimoto's thyroiditis and amenorrhea who died from progressive hypopituitarism. Since then several cases have been reported. Lymphocytic hypophysitis is a rare neuroendocrine disorder characterized by autoimmune inflammation of the pituitary gland. It is believed to be associated with the expression of anti-pituitary cytosolic protein and anti-nuclear antibodies (Tanaka et al., 2002). It predominantly affects young women in the peripartum period. Its clinical presentation varies remarkably and there is no single characteristic feature that is diagnostic of the disease.

Epidemiology

Epidemiological data of lymphocytic hypophysitis are scarce. Existing data are based upon reported cases. About 80–90% of the reported cases of lymphocytic hypophysitis are in women; 90% of these women were premenopausal and, of these, 50–70% suffered disease during the peripartum period (Heinze and Bercu, 1997; Cheung et al., 2001; Bellastella et al., 2003). Familial predisposition or ethnic preference has not been reported.

Pathophysiology

Several facts support an autoimmune etiology of the lymphocytic hypophysitis.

- It is frequently associated with other autoimmune disorders.
- The histopathological findings in impaired tissues.
- The presence of pituitary autoantibodies in serum from impaired patients.

Some research groups isolated anti-GH and anti-prolactin antibodies in serum from patients with lymphocytic hypophysitis (Takahashi et al., 1999; O'Dwyer et al., 2002). Further research showed that autoantibodies found in the serum of lymphocytic hypophysitis patients show a cross-reaction with neuron-specific enolase (NSE), which is restricted to neural tissue. Since NSE is also expressed in placental tissue it may play a potential role in the pathogenesis of lymphocytic hypophysitis with pregnancy.

Clinical presentation

Headache and visual impairment are the most frequent complaints reported (50–70%) (Thodou et al., 1995; Bellastella et al., 2003). The headache is attributed to structural (e.g., mass effect) lesions. However, even small pituitary lesions can cause headache (Levy et al., 2004b, 2005). Thus the pathophysiology of the latter case is not understood completely. Mostly the headache is located frontal, retro-orbital, or temporal. Nausea and vomiting can be present in about 25% of the cases (Hashimoto et al., 1997). Visual impairment (temporal hemianopsia, superior quadrantopsias) and decrease in visual acuity or diplopia were reported earlier (Kristof et al., 1999). Besides neurological disorders partial or total hypopituitarism, hyperprolactinemia, and neurohypophysiological impairment are frequently associated with lymphocytic hypophysitis.

Treatment

The treatment of the lymphocytic hypophysitis is not evidence based but rather based upon reported cases. Glucocorticoids seem to be effective, as reviewed cases have shown (Hashimoto et al., 1997; Kristof et al., 1999). Treatment with glucocorticoids is still controversial as reported cases showed recurrence of symptoms after cessation of therapy (Cemeroglu et al., 1997; Tubridy et al., 2001). If poor response to glucocorticoid occurs, immunosuppressive treatment with azathioprine, methotrexate, or cyclosporin A may be an alternative strategy. Transsphenoidal surgery or stereotactic radiotherapy may be advised if symptoms do not improve with conservative management.

HEADACHE ATTRIBUTED TO INTRACRANIAL NEOPLASM

Headache attributed to increased intracranial pressure or hydrocephalus caused by neoplasm

Headache following organic brain diseases concerns less than 10% of recorded headaches (Pfund et al., 1999). Headache as a common symptom of brain tumors has previously been described due to clinical characteristics. Based on modern imaging techniques and earlier diagnosis, the spectrum of headache associated with increased intracranial pressure or hydrocephalus caused by neoplasm has changed. Brain tumor-associated headache, despite variation, presents mainly as diffuse, non-pulsating headache (Forsyth and Posner, 1993), as pressure headache in 77%, throbbing in 63%, or shooting headache in 38% (Pfund et al., 1999), with at least one of the following characteristics: in up to 60% of patients nausea and/or vomiting are reported and in 23% exacerbation and/or worsening of headache by Valsalva maneuvers or physical activity, coughing or sneezing, known to increase intracranial pressure. In 7–9% of patients headache occurs in attack-like episodes resembling migraine headache, usually with atypical features (Rushton and Rooke, 1962; Pfund et al., 1999). Headache is intermittent in up to 88% of patients and moderate to severe in intensity. Nocturnal or morning headaches are reported in 25–36% of the patients. A higher rate of nocturnal headache or headache upon awakening, associated with nausea and vomiting, is reported in children with brain tumors (Rossi and Vassella, 1989). Nausea and vomiting are more frequent in children than in adults, and have been reported in 72% of children with supratentorial and 86% with infratentorial tumors (Childhood Brain Tumor Consortium, 1991).

For diagnosis of headache attributed to increased intracranial pressure or hydrocephalus, the following characteristics should be fulfilled: by definition headache develops and/or deteriorates in close temporal relation to the hydrocephalus and improves within 7 days after surgical removal or volume reduction of the tumor. The etiology of brain tumor-associated headache is multifactorial. Several studies revealed evidence for raised intracranial pressure as a cause for headache due to high CSF pressure, traction on brain-sensitive structures, and mass effect.

A colloid cyst of the third ventricle, for example, may present with paroxysmal or positional headache, not associated with focal neurological symptoms but possibly with acute deterioration or loss of consciousness following obstruction of the foramen of Monroe (Filkins et al., 1996). Though the classical description of headache caused by a colloid cyst was one that improved with changes in head position (Harris, 1944), in a recent study 92% of patients reported generalized, intermittent headache and a postural component was uncommon (Desai et al., 2002).

Headache attributed directly to neoplasm

The prevalence of headache associated with brain tumors varies depending on location, tumor type, and age, and ranges from 48% to 71% (Rushton and Rooke, 1962; Childhood Brain Tumor Consortium, 1991; Forsyth and Posner, 1993; Suwanwela et al., 1994; Davies and Clarke, 2004). A prior history of headache may predict an increased risk of headache in patients with brain tumors. In patients with known systemic malignancies, about one-third with a new or different headache were found to have intracranial metastases (Christiaans et al., 2002). Commonly, headache is more frequent in patients with infratentorial than with supratentorial tumors. The elderly and young children are less likely to present with headache associated with brain tumor (Lowry et al., 1998). Isolated headache with no other symptoms is less likely to be associated to brain tumor. In both adults and children, only a few patients present with isolated headache and nearly all develop neurological symptoms within 2.5–4 months (Rossi and Vassella, 1989).

Headache attributed directly to neoplasm is characterized by a progressive, localized headache, often worse in the morning and aggravated by coughing and bending forward. Diagnostic criteria are defined by at least one of these features in patients with intracranial neoplasm shown by cranial imaging. Headache develops in temporal and spatial relationship to the tumor.

Headache lateralization predicted tumor location in only one-third of the patients, but 12% with unilateral headache showed a tumor contralaterally (Pfund et al., 1999). Others found a more reliable prediction of tumor location in patients with unilateral headaches with correct lateralization in 80% of supratentorial and 62% of infratentorial tumors (Suwanwela et al., 1994). Only 27% of patients with infratentorial tumors presented with nuchal or occipital pain, while 73% of them reported supratentorial headaches (Forsyth and Posner, 1993; Pfund et al., 1999). Frontal headaches were the most unreliable in predicting tumor location.

Further factors that predict headache in patients with brain tumors are intracranial pressure, midline shift, and brain edema. Although there is no clear evidence from clinical studies, headache intensity commonly increases with tumor size, but the relation between tumor size and the likelihood of headache remains unclear. No association between tumor size and headache was found by Levy et al. (2004b), while another study reported increasing headache associated with increasing tumor size (Forsyth and Posner, 1993).

Possible mechanisms of headache attributed directly to neoplasm are traction on the veins with resulting displacement of venous sinuses, traction on the middle meningeal artery and on arteries at the base of the brain, direct pressure to cranial nerves with afferent pain fibers, or distension of intracranial and extracranial arteries, and possibly inflammation around pain-sensitive structures of the head (Forsyth and Posner, 1993).

Treatment of headache associated with brain tumor depends on the tumor pathology, location and accompanying symptoms. Following treatment with corticosteroids there is symptomatic headache relief due to reduction of raised intracranial pressure and mass effect secondary to tumor-associated edema. After surgical removal or volume reduction, headache resolves by definition within 7 days. Following palliative radiotherapy of brain metastases, headache resolved in 82% of patients (Borgelt et al., 1980). Surgical resection or stereotactic radiotherapy may be equally effective in reducing headache. Palliative care should include pain control using corticosteroids, simple analgesics, or narcotics, and radiotherapy in patients with cerebral metastases. In recurrent gliomas, headache recurrence has been observed in about half of the patients (Osoba et al., 2000).

Headache in patients with brain tumors can also be an adverse event from radiation or chemotherapy or postcraniotomy pain. Persistent postcraniotomy headache is uncommon; 83% of patients are free from headache 4 months after surgery (Kaur et al., 2000). In 82% of patients without headache preoperatively, headache resolved within the following 1–3 years (Gee et al., 2003). The prevalence of postoperative headache is higher after suboccipital craniotomies and has been observed in 64% of patients with acoustic neuromas, with headache persistence in 84% of these patients (Schessel et al., 1992). Replacing the bone flap has been reported to reduce postoperative headache (Schessel et al., 1993; Soumkeh et al., 1996; Santarius et al., 2000). Pharmacotherapy in patients with brain tumors can also cause headache. In the treatment of malignant gliomas, temozolomide has been reported to cause headache in 25% of the patients (Middleton et al., 2000; Yung et al., 2000). Chemical meningitis has been found in 25% of patients following intrathecal chemotherapy (Glantz et al., 1999). Moreover headache may be caused by corticosteroid withdrawal. Radiotherapy has been reported to cause headache both during the stage of acute irradiation at the onset of therapy or following demylelinating radiation encephalopathy up to 6 months later.

Headache attributed to carcinomatous meningitis

Headache is a common feature in carcinomatous meningitis. Although systematic analyses of headache characteristics are lacking, several cases have been reported showing that the presentation of the headache may differ. Chan (2006) reported a case of carcinomatous meningitis with ipsilateral headache mimicking symptoms of a giant cell arteritis. In a patient with severe refractory headache that did not improve with administration of oral analgesics including morphine, further investigation revealed carcinomatous meningitis and underlying breast cancer. The headache responded finally to whole-brain radiotherapy (Jain et al., 2005). Following pulmonary adenocarcinoma, carcinomatous meningitis initially presented with headache as the only clinical symptom (Outteryck et al., 2004). Because of the non-specific nature of the headache, carcinomatous meningitis is often misdiagnosed in the early stages, especially when headache is the only clinical manifestation. Wang et al. (2003) reported on a woman who was initially treated for a migraine and then for viral meningitis as her headache worsened, until carcinomatous meningitis was detected after 3 weeks of persistent headache.

Carcinomatous meningitis is caused by invasion of neoplastic cells into the leptomeninges. The most common origins of the neoplastic cells from systemic tumors are lung cancer and breast cancer (Perez de Colosia et al., 1994). A solid tumor is revealed in about 10% of the cases. Carcinomatous meningitis may also occur with intracerebral tumors such as medulloblastoma, germinoma, ependymoma, and glioblastoma. The diagnosis is made by brain MRI with gadolinium demonstrating leptomeningeal enhancement, and cerebrospinal fluid (CSF) examination. In the CSF, elevated tumor markers in comparison to serum levels and pathological cells may be seen.

Headache attributed to hypothalamic or pituitary hyper- or hyposecretion

Headache is a common feature in pituitary tumors, occuring with a prevalence of 33–75% (Abe et al., 1998). A higher prevalence is described in women than in men (Levy et al., 2005). In addition, a positive family history of headache appears to be a risk factor for developing headache in those with pituitary tumors (Levy et al., 2005). Particular tumor subgroups are highly associated with headache. It is a common feature in acromegaly, where it is decribed in 55–85% of the patients (Nabarro, 1987; Ezzat et al., 1994; Hennessey and Jackson, 1995), and prolactinoma (Abe et al., 1998). These subtypes seem to be particularly pro-nociceptive tumors.

The underlying mechanisms causing pain are still unclear. Forsyth and Posner (1993) suggested that dural stretch and cavernous sinus invasion might be considered as a main predicting factor for developing headache, but pain is also seen in small, non-invasive, functional pituitary tumors (Abe et al., 1998; Millan-Guerrero and Isaia-Cardenas, 1999). Arafah et al. (2000) reported that intrasellar pressure might be the main factor for developing pituitary-related headache. Neuropeptides are involved in the development of primary headache (Edvinsson and Goadsby, 1995), so it is hypothesized that they are also involved in pituitary-related pain. The hypothalamic–pituitary axis is known to play a main role in different types of headache. Activation of the ipsilateral hypothalamus in all of the trigeminal autonomic cephalalgias has been demonstrated (Goadsby, 2002; Cohen and Goadsby, 2006). In addition, dysfunction in a hypothalamic circuit which projects to the medullary dorsal horn, specifically the orexinergic system, which inhibits nociceptive processing through the trigeminal nucleus caudalis, may be one mechanism by which hypothalmic dysfunction may lead to the generation of certain primary headache disorders (Holland and Goadsby, 2007).

Futhermore the additional symptoms preceding the headache in migraine, including polyuria, polidipsia, food cravings and mood disturbances (Giffin, 2002), might result from hypothalamic dysfunction (Levy et al., 2006). Calcitonin gene-related peptide (CGRP) and substance P (SP) were two neuropeptides that were considered to play an important role in the pathophysiology of pituitary-related pain. An elevation of CGRP during migraine (Gallai et al., 1995) and cluster headache (Goadsby and Edvinsson, 1994; Fanciullacci et al., 1995) was reported previously. SP and CGRP play a role in the paracrine regulation of the anterior pituitary and were isolated from pituitary tissue (Roth and Krause, 1990; Wimalawansa, 1994). Levy et al. (2004a) could not demonstrate an association between the presence of CGRP or SP in a pituitary specimen and the prevalence of headache. Neuropeptide Y (NPY) is a neuropeptide that plays a paracrine role within the anterior pituitary gland, influencing different hormone axes. In acromegaly (Watanobe and Tamura, 1997) and in prolactinoma (Watanobe and Tamura, 1996), NPY affects the growth hormone release. Levy et al. (2006) found, in 26 pituitary tumor specimens, that there was no significant association between the amount of NPY expression and the presence of headache. The same group could not find an association between vasoactive intestinal polypeptide and pituitary-related headache (Nathoo et al., 2005). Because the observation that small, funcionally active tumors are more often associated with headache (Williams et al., 1987; Ferrari et al., 1988; Millan-Guerrero and Isaia-Cardenas, 1999; Massiou et al., 2002; Levy et al., 2003), the hypothesis of secretion of an unknown nociceptive peptide remains. Further studies are required to analyze the possible role of other influencing physical, biochemical, or genetic features.

Headache associated with pituitary tumors is a heterogeneous entity. Abe et al. (1998) described generalized and predominantly bilateral frontal headache. Levy et al. (2005) described a predominance of strictly unilateral and side-locked pain in more than half of the cases. Another common site is orbital and retro-orbital pain. In more than two-thirds of patients, the trigeminal territory is exclusively involved (Levy et al., 2005). Levy and colleagues investigated 84 patients with pituitary tumor and analyzed the clinical characteristics of the headache. Forty-six percent of the patients were suffering from chronic and 30% from episodic migraine. Other common headache subtypes included primary stabbing headache (27%), short-lasting unilateral neuralgiform headache attacks with conjunctival injection and tearing (SUNCT; 5%), cluster headache (4%), and hemicrania continua (1%). Seven percent of the headaches could not be classified. Half of the patients were suffering from chronic daily headache (>15 headache days or more per month) (Levy et al., 2005). SUNCT was seen just in tumors with secretion of prolactin or growth hormone. SUNCT and cluster headache are rare features in the normal population, indicating a higher prevalence in headache associated with pituitary tumors. The headache is often associated with other symptoms including photophobia (71%) and nausea (58%). About two-thirds of patients preferred to lie still during a headache attack. Several trigger factors of the headache were observed including stress (64%), exertion (26%), hunger (40%), alcohol (26%), and bright lights (18%) (Levy et al., 2005).

There is little information regarding the severity of the headache seen in patients with pituitary tumors. Most of the studies simply describe the quality but not the magnitude or severity of the pain. In the study by Levy et al. (2005) most of the patients reported severe headache (65%). The median duration of the headache was 7 h. Headache attacks were observed with a frequency of 20 per month (Levy et al., 2005). Non-pharmacological factors that alleviated the headache were seen in few patients: fresh air (1%), warm bath (2%), caffeine ingestion (1%), sleep (1%), and acupuncture (1%) (Levy et al., 2005).

Other symptoms that reflect the histology and secretory activity of the tumor may also be seen in patients with headache due to pituitary tumors. Galactorrhea, oligo- and amenorrhea, and gynecomastia may be seen in patients with prolactinomas, With macroadenomas the extend out of the sella turcica, visual impairment and field deficits (bitemporal hemianopia) may be seen. Other disorders that may be seen with hypersecretory pituitary tumors include acromegaly, sweating, arterial hypertension and diabetes mellitus.

Cranial autonomic symptoms are a common feature. About one-third of the patients demonstrated lacrimation and conjunctival injection in association with ipsilateral headache. Ptosis, eyelid edema, nasal blockage, rhinorrhea, facial sweating, and facial flushing were also reported but with a smaller prevalence (Levy et al., 2005).

Pituitary tumors may be treated medically, surgically, or with radiotherapy. The medications used in this disease include somatostatin analogs, dopamine agonists, and serotonin $5HT_{IB/ID}$ receptor agonists. The somatostatin analogues octreotide and lanreotide may have a positive therapeutic impact on pituitary-related headache, especially in patients with acromegaly. About two-thirds of patients report a significant benefit with this medication (Levy et al., 2005). The mechanism of the analgesic effect is still unclear A significant side-effect of somatostatin analogs is rebound headaches (Levy et al., 2005). Medication overuse is a common feature of chronic headache in general and also in headaches associated with pituitary tumors

(Levy et al., 2005). Dopamine agonists are also used in therapy of pituitary-related headache, especially with prolactin-secreting pituitary tumors. Dopamine agonists have been reported to both relieve completely and lead to severe exacerbations in patients with SUNCT syndrome (Ferrari et al., 1988; Massiou et al., 2002; Levy et al., 2003). The improvement or worsening of pain attacks in SUNCT emphasizes additionally that the hypothalamic–pituitary axis might be important in the genesis of this particular type of pituitary-related headache. Furthermore, phenotype-driven treatment including triptans was reported to be a beneficial therapy in many patients (Shah and Freij, 1999; Pascual, 2000; Levy et al., 2005). Sinus cavernous invasion is more often seen in patients that did not respond to pharmacotherapy (Levy et al., 2005). Sarov et al. (2006) indicated that patients with chronic paroxysmal hemicrania due to a macroprolactinoma may benefit from indomethacin.

Half of the cases improved after surgery (transsphenoidal or transcranial approach) (Levy et al., 2005). There are some case reports emphasizing that surgery remains a possible option if medical intervention fails. Leroux et al. (2006) reported a patient with a 14-year history of SUNCT who suffered from medically and surgically resistant SUNCT syndrome. In this patient, dopamine agonists significantly worsened the frequency and severity of symptoms, requiring hospitalization twice. However, transsphenoidal resection of the microademona resulted in the patient being pain-free during a 4-year follow-up period. Pituitary hormone levels, including testosterone, normalized after surgery. However, after radiotherapy just 1 of 16 patients reported improvement of the headache (Levy et al., 2005).

Headache attributed to intrathecal injection

Diagnostic criteria

A. Diffuse headache remaining present in the recumbent position and fulfilling criteria C and D
B. Intrathecal injection has been given
C. Headache develops within 4 h after intrathecal injection
D. Headache resolves within 14 days.

Intrathecal injection refers to accessing the subarachnoid space, usually by means of a needle and/or catheter, to administer a therapeutic or diagnostic substance.

The first perforation of the dura mater dates back to the New York physician John Corning in 1885, who applied cocaine for spinal anesthesia (Gorelick and Zych, 1987). In 1891, Winter and Quincke used the new technique for diagnostic purposes to lower increased intracranial pressure in patients with tuberculous meningitis (Pearce, 1994). The first myelography was performed in 1921 by Athanase Sicard, who injected lipiodol into the subarachnoid space and observed the radio-opaque contrast agent moving on radiography (Sicard and Forestler, 1926). The first report of headache associated with intrathecal injection was published in 1898, when the German surgeon Karl August Bier performed spinal anesthesia in patients and himself (Wulf, 1998). He assumed that the headache developed as a result of CSF loss. Around that time headache was reported to occur in about 50% of patients (Lee, 1979). Other early reports of neurological complications included oculomotor palsy, cauda equina syndrome, and paraplegia (Blanluet and Caron, 1907; Lusk, 1911). The technique was subsequently improved and has become a standard tool in therapy and diagnosis. The first implantable pump for intrathecal and intraventricular morphine application was introduced in 1978 (Lazorthes et al., 1991).

Application of intrathecal injection

The three most common areas where intrathecal injections are used are anesthesia and pain management, myelography, and chemotherapy. Experimentally this route is also used for gene therapy within the central nervous system (Meuli-Simmen et al., 1999; Ishii et al., 2000). For anesthesia, short-term pain management, myelography, and chemotherapy drugs are usually administered via a thin catheter by lumbar puncture. On the other hand, pumps, often implanted, are used for chronic pain management (e.g., patient-controlled analgesia), which allows this highly effective intrathecal analgesia to be continued in the outpatient setting (Kaplan and Brose, 2004). One study has shown that an implantable intrathecal drug delivery system is superior to conventional pain management with regard to pain control, toxicity, and overall survival (Smith et al., 2002). The advantages of intrathecal drug administration over systemic administration are multiple. First, it allows a drug to bypass the blood–brain barrier. Since some drugs penetrate the blood–brain barrier poorly or not at all, intrathecal application allows for higher concentrations in the CSF and facilitates focused nervous system treatment. Secondly, it allows for a marked reduction in the dose of the drug required for a therapeutic effect, for example morphine is usually administered at 1/100 the dose of the intravenous dose. Thirdly, systemic toxicity, particularly in the case of anesthesia and chemotherapy, can be considerably reduced. However, despite these advantages, the potential dangers must not be overlooked. Headache is one of the most frequent symptoms in patients undergoing intrathecal injections. Apart from iatrogenic infections (section 9 of the ICHD II), which are to be avoided by sterile technical procedures, and bleeding (section 6 of the ICHD II), headache may be a sign of local irritation of the meninges or aseptic meningitis. Every drug or substance administered intrathecally has the potential to cause headaches (Hodgson et al., 1999). Table 50.4 lists commonly used drugs for intrathecal administration and Table 50.5 a number of other substances and experimental drugs that have been used for intrathecal injection recently.

Epidemiology

There are no systematic investigations regarding the incidence of headache following intrathecal injections in certain clinical settings. Several reasons account for this. First, not all studies record side-effects in general or headache in particular (Smith et al., 2002; Guglielmino et al., 2006). Secondly, if headaches occur, the nature often remains obscure. Headaches *following* an intrathecal injection may be due to the procedure (post-dural puncture headache), the drug administered, the underlying disorder, or a combination of these factors. Hence, the exact reason cannot always be discerned. Third, most studies do not follow patients up for their adverse events, nor do they apply the criteria of the International Headache Society (2004) to characterize the headache. The best data are available regarding post-dural puncture headache. In case of an accidental post-dural puncture, headaches are estimated to occur in about 50% of patients (Gaiser, 2006). However, this headache is differentiated from headache following intrathecal injection, as it decreases or disappears in the recumbent position.

Table 50.4

Examples of drugs commonly used for intrathecal administration and drug-specific adverse effects with a focus on the central nervous system

Drug	Indication	Drug-specific adverse effects	Reference
Baclofen	Spasticity	Dry mouth, drowsiness, dizziness, constipation, tiredness, headache 4–8%	Hodgson et al., 1999; www.drugs.com
Local anesthetics, e.g., bupivacaine	Peri- and postoperative pain	Allergy, paresthesia, paralysis, headache, seizures, restlessness, anxiety, tinnitus	Hodgson et al., 1999; www.drugs.com
Ketamine	Postoperative pain Neuropathic pain	Blood pressure and pulse changes, change in respiration, myoclonus, nausea and vomiting	Hodgson et al., 1999; www.drugs.com
Clonidine	Postoperative pain Neuropathic pain Cancer pain Bladder hyperreflexia	Dry mouth, drowsiness, dizziness, constipation, blood pressure and pulse changes, nausea and vomiting, headache ~1%	Hodgson et al., 1999; www.drugs.com
Opioids	Postoperative pain Cancer pain	Pruritus 30–100% Urinary retention ~35% Nausea and vomiting ~30% Respiratory depression <1% Headache ~40% (various dugs, mostly opioids)	Etches et al., 1989; Chaney, 1995; Wheeler et al., 2002; Rathmell et al., 2005; www.drugs.com
Ziconotide	Neuropathic pain	Depression, cognitive impairment, hallucinations, depressed levels of consciousness, headache ~15%, creatinine kinase elevation	Lynch et al., 2006; www.drugs.com
Chemotherapy with methotrexate and cytosinarabinoside	Lymphomatous meningitis	Aseptic chemical meningitis, myelopathy, leukencephalopathy, headache ~10–20%, nausea and vomiting, dizziness, fever	Glantz et al., 1999; www.drugs.com
Methylprednisolone	Multiple sclerosis	Chemical meningitis, transverse myelitis, cauda equina syndrome, lumbar radiculitis, headache	Nelson and Landau, 2001; www.drugs.com

Table 50.5

Examples of other substances and experimental drugs for intrathecal administration

Substance	Indication	Reference
Preservatives (e.g., benzyl alcohol, polyethylene glycol)	Should not be used	Hetherington and Dooley, 2000; Jolles et al., 2000
Adenovirus–thymidine kinase complexes	Experimental gene therapy for leptomeningeal metastases and pain management	Driesse et al., 2000; Beutler et al., 2005
Recombinant human superoxide dismutase	Experimental treatment of amyotrophic lateral sclerosis	Cudkowicz et al., 1997
Insulin-like growth factor-1	Experimental treatment of amyotrophic lateral sclerosis	Nagano et al., 2005
Encapsulated bovine adrenal cell subarachnoid implant secreting catecholamines and opioids	Cancer pain refractory to conventional therapy	Lazorthes et al., 1991
Methylprednisolone	Intractable postherpetic neuralgia	Kotani et al., 2000
Combined morphine and clonidine	Post spinal cord injury	Siddall et al., 2000
Nicardipine by portable infusion pump	Vasospasm due to subarachnoid hemorrhage	Fujiwara et al., 2001
Antitetanus immunoglobulin	Tetanus	Miranda-Filho Dde et al., 2004
Liposomal neostigmine	Postoperative pain	Grant et al., 2002

Pathophysiology

Two main reasons may account for headache following intrathecal injection. First, the change in volume and pressure in the subarachnoid space, and secondly, a toxic effect of the drug administered. In the case of increased or low CSF pressure. When the headache is related to the administration of the drug, the headache may occur as a drug-specific effect or the headache may be due to meningeal irritation with clinical signs of aseptic chemical meningitis (Jolles et al., 2000). Drugs like methotrexate, cytosine arabinoside, methylprednisolone, preservatives, and biologicals may cause both.

Clinical presentation

The headache is usually diffuse, develops within 4 h after the intrathecal administration of a drug and resolves spontaneously within 14 days. However, as with every new-onset headache, other symptomatic causes need to be excluded by careful history taking, clinical examination, as well as laboratory tests and imaging techniques if necessary. In the case of aseptic meningitis, the clinical picture may also include fever, meningismus, somnolence, photo- and phonophobia (Jolles et al., 2000). Hence lumbar puncture and microbial analyses are necessary to exclude an infectious cause of the meningitis. Local erythema, edema, or pain after intrathecal injections or after the surgical implantation of catheter should alert the physician to an infectious process such as an abscess or staphylococcal epidermidis meningitis. Clinically, headache following intrathecal injection is distinguished from post-dural lumbar headache because it persists after lying down. A persistent CSF leak needs to be considered if the headache does not resolve within 14 days (see section 7.2.2 *CSF fistula headache*). An extradural hematoma is usually accompanied by a progressive local tenderness and progressive sensory or motor deficit.

Clinical course and therapy

By definition the headache is self-limited and spontaneously remits in 14 days. If repetitive injections are planned or continuous application is performed, discontinuation of the drug is usually necessary to terminate symptoms. Often no specific therapy is necessary. If the patient does not tolerate the pain, an empirical symptomatic treatment is recommended. Acetylsalicylic acid, acetaminophen, and NSAIDs should be the drugs of first choice provided there are no contraindications. Symptomatic pain management should not exceed 2 weeks to avoid the development of medication overuse headache, which would obscure the course of the underlying headache. No systematic trial has investigated any of these therapeutic concepts. If more serious side-effects like aseptic meningitis develop, the patient needs to be supervised, other causes of meningitis must be excluded, and treatment needs to be started accordingly.

B. Evidence of an intracranial disorder other than those described above
C. Headache develops in close temporal relation to the intracranial disorder
D. Headache resolves within 3 months after cure or spontaneous remission of the intracranial disorder.

Acknowledgment

The authors want to thank the following individuals for their help with this chapter: G Gerwig, N Hansen, D Holle, O Kastrup, M Küper, D Müller, M Obermann, F Poitz, C Schorn, M Schuerks, M Slomke, all at the Department of Neurology, University of Duisburg-Essen, Germany. This study was supported by the German Ministry of Education and Research Grant 01 EM 0117.

References

Abe T, Matsumoto K, Kuwazawa J et al. (1998). Headache associated with pituitary adenomas. Headache 38: 782–786.

Abtin K, Thompson BG, Walker ML (1998). Basilar artery perforation as a complication of endoscopic third ventriculostomy. Pediatr Neurosurg 28: 35–41.

Agarwal MR, Yoo JH (2007). Optic nerve sheath fenestration for vision preservation in idiopathic intracranial hypertension. Neurosurg Focus 23: E7.

Ageli SI, Sato Y, Gantz BJ (1994). Glomus jugulare tumors masquerading as benign intracranial hypertension. Arch Otolaryngol 120: 1277–1280.

Albayram S (2006). Intracranial hypotension syndrome following chiropratic manipulation of the cervical spine. J Headache Pain 7: 369–370.

Albayram S, Kilic F, Ozer H et al. (2008). Gadolinium-enhanced MR cisternography to evaluate dural leaks in intracranial hypotension syndrome. AJNR Am J Neuroradiol 29: 116–121.

Albright AL, Ferson S, Carlos S (2005). Occult hydrocephalus in children with cerebral palsy. Neurosurgery 56: 93–96: discussion 96–7.

Aldrete JA (2003). Neurologic deficits and arachnoiditis following neuroaxial anethesia. Acta Anaesthesiol Scand 43: 3–12.

Alvarez-Linera J, Escribano J, Benito-Leon J et al. (2000). Pituitary enlargement in patients with intracranial hypotension syndrome. Neurology 55 (12): 1895–1897.

Alzate JC, Kothbauer KF, Jallo GI et al. (2001). Treatment of Chiari I malformation in patients with and without syringomyelia: a consecutive series of 66 cases. Neurosurg Focus 11: E3.

Andermann F (1987). Migraine–epilepsy relationships. Epilepsy Res 1: 213–226.

Ansari I, Crichlow B, Gunton KB et al. (2002). A child with venous sinus thrombosis with initial examination findings of pseudotumor syndrome. Arch Ophthalmol 120: 867–869.

Apostol G, Cady RK, Laforet GA et al. (2008). Divalproex extended-release in adolescent migraine prophylaxis: results of a randomized, double-blind, placebo-controlled study. Headache 48: 1012–1025.

Arafah BM, Prunty D, Ybarra J et al. (2000). The dominant role of increased intrasellar pressure in the pathogenesis of hypopituitarism, hyperprolactinemia, and headaches in patients with pituitary adenomas. J Clin Endocrinol Metab 85: 1789–1793.

Asa SL, Bilbao JM, Kovacs K et al. (1981). Lymphocytic hypophysitis of pregnancy resulting in hypopituitarism: a distinct clinicopathologic entity. Ann Intern Med 95: 166–171.

Ashton D, Kim P, Griffiths N et al. (2004). Cognitive decline with chronic meningitis secondary to a COX-2 inhibitor. Age Ageing 33: 408–409.

Ashwath ML, Katner HP (2003). Recurrent aseptic meningitis due to different non-steroidal anti-inflammatory drugs including rofecoxib. Postgrad Med J 79: 295–296.

Atkinson JL, Weinshenker BG, Miller GM et al. (1998). Acquired Chiari I malformation secondary to spontaneous spinal cerebrospinal fluid leakage and chronic intracranial hypotension syndrome in seven cases. J Neurosurg 88 (2): 237–242.

Bai J, Yokoyama K, Kinuya S et al. (2002). Radionuclide cisternography in intracranial hypotension syndrome. Ann Nucl Med 16: 75–78.

Baltzan M, Mehta S, Kirkham TH et al. (1999). Randomized trial of prolonged chloroquine therapy in advanced pulmonary sarcoidosis. Am J Respir Crit Care Med 160: 192–197.

Barakat MH, Mustafa HT, Shakir RA (1988). Mollaret's meningitis. A variant of recurrent hereditary polyserositis, both provoked by metaraminol. Arch Neurol 45: 926–927.

Bartleson JD, Swanson JW, Whisnant JP (1981). A migrainous syndrome with cerebrospinal fluid pleocytosis. Neurology 31: 1257–1262.

Barnes MA, Dennis M (1998). Discourse after early-onset hydrocephalus: core deficits in children of average intelligence. Brain Language 61: 309–334.

Barrett PV, Thier SO (1963). Meningitis and pancreatitis associated with sulfamethizole. N Engl J Med 268: 36–37.

Barrios-Alarcon J, Aldrete JA, Paragas-Tapia D (1989). Relief of post-lumbar puncture headache with epidural dextran 40: a preliminary report. Reg Anesth 14: 78–80.

Bartsch T, Goadsby P (2003). Increased responses in trigeminocervical nociceptive neurons to cervical input after stimulation of the dura mater. Brain 126: 1801–1813.

Baughman RP, Judson MA, Teirstein AS et al. (2002). Thalidomide for chronic sarcoidosis. Chest 122: 227–232.

Bel I, Moreno LA, Gomar C (2006). Epidural dextran-40 and paramethasone injection for treatment of spontaneous intracranial hypotension. Can J Anaesth 53: 591–594.

Bellastella A, Bizzarro A, Coronella C et al. (2003). Lymphocytic hypophysitis: a rare or underestimated disease? Eur J Endocrinol 149: 363–376.

Bender A, Elstner M, Paul R et al. (2004). Severe symptomatic aseptic chemical meningitis following myelography: the role of procalcitonin. Neurology 63: 1311–1313.

Berg MJ, Williams LS (1995). The transient syndrome of headache with neurologic deficits and CSF lymphocytosis. Neurology 45: 1648–1654.

Bernasconi A, Andermann F, Bernasconi N et al. (2000). Lateralizing value of peri-ictal headache: a study of 100 patients with partial epilepsy. Neurology 56: 130–132.

Berroir S, Loisel B, Ducros A et al. (2004). Early epidural blood patch in spontaneous intracranial hypotension. Neurology 63: 1950–1951.

Beutler AS, Banck MS, Walsh CE et al. (2005). Intrathecal gene transfer by adeno-associated virus for pain. Curr Opin Mol Ther 7: 431–439.

Biousse V, Ameri A, Bousser MG (1999). Isolated intracranial hypertension as the only sign of cerebral venous thrombosis. Neurology 53: 1537–1542.

Blanluet C, Caron P (1907). Paralysie de la vie paire apres rachistovainisation. Ann d'Oculistique 137: 62–65.

Blumenfeld H, Cha JH, Cudkowicz ME (1996). Trimethoprim and sulfonamide-associated meningoencephalitis with MRI correlates. Neurology 46: 556–558.

Boeck C (1899). Multiple benign sarkoid of the skin. J Cutan Gen Urin Dis 17: 543–550.

Bonnel RA, Villalba ML, Karwoski CB et al. (2002). Aseptic meningitis associated with rofecoxib. Arch Intern Med 162: 713–715.

Bonnin AJ, Zeitz HJ, Gewurz A (1993). Complement factor I deficiency with recurrent aseptic meningitis. Arch Intern Med 153: 1380–1383.

Bono F, Giliberto C, Mastrandrea C et al. (2005). Transverse sinus stenoses persist after normalization of the CSF pressure in IIH. Neurology 65: 1090–1093.

Borgelt B, Gelber R, Kramer S et al. (1980). The palliation of brain metastases: final results of the first two studies by the Radiation Therapy Oncology Group. Int J Radiat Oncol Biol Phys 6: 1–9.

Bornke C, Przuntek H, Postert T et al. (1999). Atypical multiple sclerosis presenting as chronic-progressive encephalomyelitis with polyneuritis and recurrent aseptic meningitis. J Neurol 246: 136–139.

Boyles AL, Enterline DS, Hammock PH et al. (2006). Phenotypic definition of Chiari type I malformation coupled with high-density SNP genome screen shows significant evidence for linkage to regions on chromosomes 9 and 15. Am J Med Genet A 140: 2776–2785.

Brandes J, Saper J, Diamond M et al. (2004). Topiramate for migraine prevention: a randomized controlled trial. JAMA 291: 965–973.

Bret P, Lapras C, Lecuire J et al. (1977). Les oblitérations tumorales de l'aqueduc de Sylvius à révélation tardive. Lyon Med 238: 357–364.

Broadsky MC, Vaphiades M (1998). Magnetic resonance imaging in pseudotumor cerebri. Ophthalmology 105: 1686–1693.

Burgett RA, Purvin VA, Kawasaki A (1997). Lumboperitoneal shunting for pseudotumor cerebri. Neurology 49: 734–739.

Bynke G, Zemack G, Bynke H et al. (2004). Ventriculoperitoneal shunting for idiopathic intracranial hypertension. Neurology 63: 1314–1316.

Callen PW, Hashimoto BE, Newton TH (1986). Sonographic evaluation of cerebral cortical mantle thickness in the fetus and neonate with hydrocephalus. J Ultrasound Med 5: 251–255.

Camann WR, Murray S, Mushlin PS et al. (1990). Effects of oral caffeine on postural puncture headache. A double-blind, placebo-controlled trial. Anesth Analg 70: 181–184.

Caminero AB, Pareja JA, Arpa J et al. (1997). Migrainous syndrome with CSF pleocytosis. SPECT findings. Headache 37: 511–515.

Cariski AT (1981). Isolated CNS sarcoidosis. JAMA 245: 62–63.

Castels-van Daele M, Standaert L, Boel M et al. (1981). Basilar migraine and viral meningitis. Lancet 6: 1366.

Celebisoy N, Gokcay F, Sirin H et al. (2007). Treatment of idiopathic intracranial hypertension: topiramate vs acetazolamide, an open-label study. Acta Neurol Scand 116: 322–327.

Cemeroglu AP, Blaivas M, Muraszko KM et al. (1997). Lymphocytic hypophysitis presenting with diabetes insipidus in a 14-year-old girl: case report and review of the literature. Eur J Pediatr 156: 684–688.

Chan JW (2006). Acute monocular visual loss in carcinomatous hypertrophic pachymeningitis mimicking giant cell arteritis. J Clin Rheumatol 12: 30–31.

Chaney MA (1995). Side effects of intrathecal and epidural opioids. Can J Anaesth 42: 891–903.

Chapelon C, Ziza JM, Piette JC et al. (1990). Neurosarcoidosis: signs, course and treatment in 35 confirmed cases. Medicine (Baltimore) 69: 261–276.

Chen CJ, Lee TH, Hsu HL et al. (2002). Spinal MR findings in spontaneous intracranial hypotension. Neuroradiology 44: 996–1003.

Cheung CC, Ezzat S, Smyth HS et al. (2001). The spectrum and significance of primary hypophysitis. J Clin Endocrinol Metab 86: 1048–1053.

Chez M, Sila CA, Ransohoff RM et al. (1989). Ibuprofen-induced meningitis: detection of intrathecal IgG synthesis and immune complexes. Neurology 39: 1578–1580.

Chiapparini L, Farina L, D'Incerti L et al. (2002). Spinal radiological findings in nine patients with spontaneous intracranial hypotension. Neuroradiology 44: 143–150; discussion 151–152.

Childhood Brain Tumor Consortium (1991). The epidemiology of headache among children with brain tumor. Headache in children with brain tumors. J Neurooncol 10: 31–46.

Christiaans MH, Kelder JC, Arnoldus EP et al. (2002). Prediction of intracranial metastases in cancer patients with headache. Cancer 94: 2063–2068.

Chung SJ, Kim JS, Lee M (2000). Syndrome of cerebral fluid hypovolemia. Clinical and imaging features and outcome. Neurology 55: 1321–1327.

Chung SJ, Lee JH, Im JH et al. (2005). Short- and long-term outcomes of spontaneous CSF hypovolemia. Eur Neurol 54: 63–67.

Cohen AS, Goadsby PJ (2006). Functional neuroimaging of primary headache disorders. Exp Rev Neurother 6: 1159–1171.

Coleman WS, Lischner HW, Grover WD (1975). Recurrent aseptic meningitis without sequelae. J Pediatr 87: 89–91.
Collins JJ, Fisher WS (1990). Vein of Galen aneurysm presenting with recurrent aseptic meningitis and subsequent spontaneous thrombosis. Surg Neurol 3: 325–328.
Colover J (1948). Sarcoidosis with involvement of the nervous system. Brain 71: 451–475.
Corbett JJ, Digre K (2002). Idiopathic intracranial hypertension. An answer to, "the chicken or the egg?" Neurology 58: 5–6.
Corbett JJ, Savino PJ, Thompson HS et al. (1982). Visual loss in pseudotumor cerebri. Follow-up of 57 patients from five to 41 years and a profile of 14 patients with permanent severe visual loss. Arch Neurol 39: 461–474.
Corning J (1885). Spinal anesthesia and local medication of the cord. N Y Med J 42: 483–485.
Corvini M, Randolph C, Aronin SI (2004). Complement C7 deficiency presentino as recurrent aseptic meningitis. Ann Allergy Athma Immunol 93: 200–205.
Cowan JA, McGirt MJ, Woodworth G et al. (2005). The syndrome of hydrocephalus in young and middle-aged adults. Neurol Res 27: 540–547.
Creel GB, Hurtt M (1995). Cephalosporin-induced recurrent aseptic meningitis. Ann Neurol 37: 815–817.
Crossley GH, Dismukes WE (1990). Central nervous system epidermoid cyst: a probable etiology of Mollaret's meningitis. Am J Med 89: 805–806.
Crul BJ, Gerritse BM, van Dongen RT et al. (1999). Epidural fibrin glue injection stops persistent postdural puncture headache. Anesthesiology 91: 576–577.
Cudkowicz ME, Warren L, Francis JW et al. (1997). Intrathecal administration of recombinant human superoxide dismutase 1 in amyotrophic lateral sclerosis: a preliminary safety and pharmacokinetic study. Neurology 49: 213–222.
Czerwenka W, Gruenwald C, Conen D (1999). Aseptic meningitis after treatment with amoxicillin. BMJ 318: 1521.
Dahlerup B, Gjerris F, Harmsen A et al. (1985). Severe headache as the only symptome of long-standing shunt dysfunction in hydrocephalic children with normal or slit ventricles revealed by computed tomography. Childs Nerv Syst 1: 49–52.
Davenport RJ, Chataway SJ, Warlow CP (1995). Spontaneous intracranial hypotension from a CSF leak in a patient with Marfan's syndrome. J Neurol Neurosurg Psychiatry 59: 516–519.
Davies E, Clarke C (2004). Early symptoms of brain tumours. J Neurol Neurosurg Psychiatry 75: 1205–1206.
Davy BE, Robinson ML (2003). Congenital hydrocephalus in hy3 mice is caused by a frameshift mutation in Hydin, a large novel gene. Hum Mol Genet 12: 1163–1170.
Day RE, Schutt WH (1979). Normal children with large heads – benign familial megalencephaly. Arch Dis Child 54: 512–517.
de Ribaupierre S, Rilliet B, Vernet O et al. (2007). Third ventriculostomy vs ventriculoperitoneal shunt in pediatric obstructive hydrocephalus: results from a Swiss series and literature review. Childs Nerv Syst 23: 527–533.
Del Bigio MR (2004). Cellular damage and prevention in childhood hydrocephalus. Brain Pathol 14: 317–324.
Delaney P (1977). Neurological manifestations in sarcoidosis: review of the literature, with report of 23 cases. Ann Intern Med 87: 336–345.
Delaney P (1980). Seizures in sarcoidosis: a poor prognosis. Ann Neurol 7: 494.
Desai KI, Nadkarni TD, Muzumdar DP et al. (2002). Surgical management of colloid cyst of the third ventricle – a study of 105 cases. Surg Neurol 57: 295–302.
Di Trapani G, Mei D, Marra C et al. (2000). Gabapentin in the prophylaxis of migraine: a double-blind, randomized, placebo-controlled study. Cephalalgia 20: 345.
Diener HC, Bendig M, Hempel V (1985). Der postpunktionelle Kopfschmerz [postpuncture headache]. Fortschr Neurol Psychiatr 53: 344–349.
Diener HC, Tfelt-Hansen P, Dahlöf C et al. (2004). Topiramate in migraine prophylaxis: results from a placebo-controlled trial with propranolol as an active control. J Neurol 251: 943–950.
Dieterich M (2003). Spontanes und postpunktionelles Liquorunterdrucksyndrom. In: T Brandt, J Dichgans, HC Diener (Eds.), Therapie und Verlauf neurologischer Erkrankungen. Kohlhammer, Stuttgart, pp. 88–94.
Dieterich M, Brandt T (1985). Is obligatory bed rest after lumbar puncture obsolete? Eur Arch Psychiatr Neurol Sci 235: 71–75.
Dieterich M, Brandt T (1988). Incidence of post-lumbar puncture headache is independent of daily fluid intake. Eur Arch Psychiatry Neurol Sci 237: 194–196.
Digre KB, Corbett JJ (1988). Pseudotumor cerebri in men. Arch Neurol 45: 866–872.
Dizdarevic K, Dizdarevic S, Dizdarevic Z (1998). Neurosarcoidosis presenting with transitory neurodeficit and generalized epileptic seizures associated with migraine. Med Arh 52: 159–162.
Drake JM, Kestle JR, Tuli S (2000). CSF shunts 50 years on – past, present and future. Childs Nerv Syst 16: 800–804.
Driesse MJ, Esandi MC, Kros JM et al. (2000). Intra-CSF administered recombinant adenovirus causes an immune response-mediated toxicity. Gene Ther 7: 1401–1409.
Dripps RD, Vandam LD (1954). Long-term follow-up of patients who received 10 098 spinal anesthetics: failure to discover major neurological sequelae. JAMA 156: 1486–1491.
Duffy PJ, Crosby ET (1999). The epidural blood patch. Resolving the controversies. Can J Anaesth 46: 878–886.
Dumouchel-Champagne H, Ferry T, Bouhour D et al. (2004). Allopurinol-induced aseptic meningitis. Presse Med 33: 1008–1009.
Durcan FJ, Corbett JJ, Wall M (1988). The incidence of pseudotumor cerebri: population studies in Iowa and Louisiana. Arch Neurol 45: 875–877.
Edvinsson L, Goadsby PJ (1995). Neuropeptides in the cerebral circulation: relevance to headache. Cephalalgia 15: 272–278.
Edwards RJ, Witchell C, Pople IK (2003). Chronic headaches in adults with spina bifida and associated hydrocephalus. Eur J Pediatr Surg 13: 13–17.

El Gammal T, Allen MD Jr, Brooks BS (1987). MRI evaluation of hydrocephalus. AJR 149: 807–813.

Eross EJ, Dodick DW, Nelson KD et al. (2002). Orthostatic headache syndrome with CSF leak secondary to bony pathology of the cervical spine. Cephalalgia 22: 439–443.

Etches RC, Sandler AN, Daley MD (1989). Respiratory depression and spinal opioids. Can J Anaesth 36: 165–185.

Eustace S, Buff B (1994). Magnetic resonance imaging in drug-induced meningitis. Can Assoc Radiol J 45: 463–465.

Ezzat S, Forster MJ, Berchtold P et al. (1994). Acromegaly. Clinical and biochemical features in 500 patients. Medicine (Baltimore) 73: 233–240.

Fanciullacci M, Alessandri M, Figini M et al. (1995). Increase in plasma calcitonin gene-related peptide from the extracerebral circulation during nitroglycerin-induced cluster headache attack. Pain 60: 119–123.

Farb RI, Vanek I, Scott JN et al. (2003). Idiopathic intracranial hypertension: the prevalence and morphology of sinovenous stenosis. Neurology 60: 1418–1424.

Fernell E, Hagberg G, Hagberg B (1990). Infantile hydrocephalus – the impact of enhanced preterm survival. Acta Paediatr Scand 79: 1080–1086.

Ferrari MD, Haan J, van Seters AP (1988). Bromocriptine-induced trigeminal neuralgia attacks in a patient with pituitary tumor. Neurology 38: 1482–1484.

Feuerstein TJ, Zeides A (1986). Theophylline relieves headache following lumbar puncture. Placebo-controlled, double-blind pilot study. Klin Wochenschr 64: 216–218.

Filkins JA, Cohle S, Levy BK et al. (1996). Unexpected deaths due to colloid cysts of the third ventricle. J Forensic Sci 41: 521–523.

Fisher JH, Sydney MB (1939). Encephalomyelitis following administration of sulfanilamide. Lancet 1: 301–305.

Fishman RA, Dillon WP (1993). Dural enhancement and cerebral displacement secondary to intracranial hypotension. Neurology 43: 609–611.

Forsyth PA, Posner JB (1993). Headaches in patients with brain tumors: a study of 111 patients. Neurology 43: 1678–1683.

Frederiks JA, Bruyn GW (1989). Mollaret's meningitis. In: RR McKendall (Ed.), Handbook of Clinical Neurology. Vol. 12: Viral Disease. Elsevier Science, Amsterdam, pp. 627–635.

Freitag F, Collins S, Carlson H et al. (2002). A randomized trial of divalproex sodium extended-release in migraine prophylaxis. Neurology 58: 1652–1659.

Friedmann DI (2004). Pseudotumor cerebri. Neurol Clin North Am 22: 99–131.

Friedmann DI, Rausch EA (2002). Headache diagnosis in patients with treated idiopathic intracranial hypertension. Neurology 58: 1551–1553.

Fuentes B, Diez Tejedor E, Pascual J et al. (1998). Cerebral blood flow changes in pseudomigraine with pleocytosis analyzed by single photon emission computed tomography. A spreading depression mechanism. Cephalalgia 18: 570–573.

Gaiser R (2006). Postdural puncture headache. Curr Opin Anaesthesiol 19: 249–253.

Galassi G, Gibertoni M, Mancini A et al. (1984). Sarcoidosis of the peripheral nerve: clinical, electrophysiological and histological study of two cases. Eur Neurol 23: 459–465.

Gallai V, Sarchielli P, Floridi A et al. (1995). Vasoactive peptide levels in the plasma of young migraine patients with and without aura assessed both interictally and ictally. Cephalalgia 15: 384–390.

Galvin JA, Van Stavern GP (2004). Clinical characterization of idiopathic intracranial hypertension at the Detroit Medical Center. J Neurol Sci 30; 223 (2): 157–160.

Gee JR, Ishaq Y, Vijayan N (2003). Postcraniotomy headache. Headache 43: 276–278.

Gentile S, Giudice RL, Martino PD et al. (2004). Headache attributed to spontaneous low CSF pressure: report of three cases responsive to corticosteroids. Eur J Neurol 11: 849–851.

Gerritse BM, van Dongen RT, Crul BJ (1997). Epidural fibrin glue injection stops persistent cerebrospinal fluid leak during long-term intrathecal catheterization. Anesth Analg 84 (5): 1140–1141.

Gibson BE, Wedel DJ, Faust RJ et al. (1988). Continuous epidural saline infusion for the treatment of low CSF pressure headache. Anesthesiology 68: 789–791.

Giffin N (2002). Surfing for headache. J Neurol Neurosurg Psychiatry 72 (Suppl. 2): ii9.

Gilmore K, Rudden M, Kalman TP (1980). Psychiatric manifestations of sarcoidosis. Can J Psychiatry 25: 329–331.

Gjerris F, Borgesen S (2000). Pathophysiology of the CSF circulation. In: A Crockard, R Hayward, J Hoff (Eds.), Neurosurgery – The Scientific Basis of Clinical Practice. 3rd edn. Blackwell Science, Boston, pp. 147–168.

Glantz MJ, Jaeckle KA, Chamberlain MC et al. (1999). A randomized controlled trial comparing intrathecal sustained-release cytarabine (Depocyt) to intrathecal methotrexate in patients with neoplastic meningitis from solid tumors. Clin Cancer Res 5: 3394–3402.

Goadsby PJ (2002). Pathophysiology of cluster headache: a trigeminal autonomic cephalgia. Lancet Neurol 1: 251–257.

Goadsby PJ, Edvinsson L (1994). Human in vivo evidence for trigeminovascular activation in cluster headache. Neuropeptide changes and effects of acute attacks therapies. Brain 117: 427–434.

Goldstein R, Guberman A, Izaguiree CA et al. (1986). Mollaret's meningitis: a case with increased circulating natural killer cells. Ann Neurol 20: 359–361.

Gomez-Aranda F, Canadillas F, Marti-Masso JF et al. (1997). Pseudomigraine with temporary neurological symptoms and lymphocytic pleocytosis: a report of fifty cases. Brain 120: 1105–1113.

Gorelick PB, Zych D (1987). James Leonard Corning and the early history of spinal puncture. Neurology 37: 672–674.

Graf WD, Born DE, Shaw DW et al. (2000). Diffusion-weighted magnetic resonance imaging in boys with neural cell adhesion molecule L1 mutations and congenital hydrocephalus. Ann Neurol 47: 113–117.

Graman PS (1987). Mollaret's meningitis associated with acute Epstein–Barr virus mononucleosis. Arch Neurol 44: 1204–1205.

Grant GJ, Piskoun B, Bansinath M (2002). Intrathecal administration of liposomal neostigmine prolongs analgesia in mice. Acta Anaesthesiol Scand 46: 90–94.

Grant R, Condon B, Hart I et al. (1991). Changes in intracranial CSF volume after lumbar puncture and their relationship to post-LP headache. J Neurol Neurosurg Psychiatry 54: 440–442.

Greenberg GN (1988). Recurrent sulindac-induced aseptic meningitis in a patient tolerant to other nonsteroidal anti-inflammatory drugs. South Med J 81: 1463–1464.

Guglielmino A, Sorbello M, Fazzio S et al. (2006). Continuous intrathecal baclofen administration by a fully implantable electronic pump for severe spasticity treatment: our experience. Minerva Anestesiol 72: 807–820.

Haase KK, Lapointe M, Haines SJ (2001). Aseptic meningitis after intraventricular administration of gentamicin. Pharmacotherapy 21: 103–107.

Halker RB, Demaerschalk BM, Wellik KE et al. (2007). Caffeine for the prevention and treatment of postdural puncture headache: debunking the myth. Neurologist 13: 323–328.

Halpern S, Preston R (1994). Postdural puncture headache and spinal needle design. Metaanalyses. Anesthesiology 81: 1376–1383.

Hamlat A, Adn M, Sid-ahmed S et al. (2006). Theoretical considerations on the pathophysiology of normal pressure hydrocephalus (NPH) and NPH-related dementia. Med Hypotheses 67: 115–123.

Harris W (1944). Paroxysmal and postural headaches from intraventricular cysts and tumors. Lancet 244: 654–655.

Hashimoto K, Takao T, Makino S (1997). Lymphocytic adenohypophysitis and lymphocytic infundibuloneurohypophysitis. Endocr J 44 (1): 1–10.

Headache Classification Subcommittee of the International Headache Society (2004). The international classification of headache disorders, second edition. Cephalalgia 24 (Suppl. 1): 1–160.

Heide W, Diener HC (1990). Epidural blood patch reduces the incidence of post lumbar puncture headache. Headache 30 (5): 280–281.

Heinze HJ, Bercu BB (1997). Acquired hypophysitis in adolescence. J Pediatr Endocrinol Metab 10: 315–321.

Hennessey JV, Jackson IM (1995). Clinical features and differential diagnosis of pituitary tumours with emphasis on acromegaly. Baillieres Clin Endocrinol Metab 9: 271–314.

Hetherington NJ, Dooley MJ (2000). Potential for patient harm from intrathecal administration of preserved solutions. Med J Aust 173: 141–143.

Hodgson PS, Neal JM, Pollock JE et al. (1999). The neurotoxicity of drugs given intrathecally (spinal). Anesth Analg 88: 797–809.

Holland P, Goadsby PJ (2007). The hypothalamic orexinergic system: pain and primary headaches. Headache 47: 951–962.

Hopkins S, Jolles S (2005). Drug-induced aseptic meningitis. Expert Opin Drug Saf 4: 285–297.

Ireland B, Corbett JJ, Wallace RB (1990). The search for causes of idiopathic intracranial hypertension. A preliminary case-control study. Arch Neurol 47 (3): 315–320.

Ishige I, Usui Y, Takemura T et al. (1999). Quantitative PCR of mycobacterial and propionibacterial DNA in lymph nodes of Japanese patients with sarcoidosis. Lancet 354: 120–123.

Ishii K, Isono M, Inoue R et al. (2000). Attempted gene therapy for intractable pain: dexamethasone-mediated exogenous control of beta-endorphin secretion in genetically modified cells and intrathecal transplantation. Exp Neurol 166: 90–98.

Jacobsson G, Elowson S (1999). Amoxicillin caused aseptic meningoencephalitis. Lakartidningen 96: 201–202.

Jain KK (2001). Drug-Induced Neurological Disorders. 2nd edn. Hogrefe & Huber, Seattle.

Jain PN, Kavishvar N, Jalali R (2005). Refractory headache in a patient with breast cancer and carcinomatous meningitis unresponsive to analgesics: case report. J Pain Palliat Care Pharmacother 19: 33–35.

Jarvis AP, Greenawalt JW, Fagraeus L (1986). Intravenous caffeine for postdural puncture headache. Anesth Analg 65: 316–317.

Jicha GA, Suarez GA (2003). Pseudotumor cerebri reversed by cardiac septal defect repair. Neurology 60: 2016–2017.

Johnston I, Paterson A (1974). Benign intracranial hypertension II. CSF pressure and circulation. Brain 97: 301–312.

Johnston I, Kollar C, Dunkley S et al. (2002). Cranial venous outflow obstruction in the pseudotumour syndrome: incidence, nature and relevance. J Clin Neurosci 9 (3):273–278.

Johnston PK, Corbett JJ, Maxner CE (1991). Cerebrospinal fluid protein and opening pressure in idiopathic intracranial hypertension (pseudotumor cerebri). Neurology 41: 1040–1042.

Jolles S, Sewell WA, Leighton C (2000). Drug-induced aseptic meningitis: diagnosis and management. Drug Saf 22: 215–226.

Jonville-Bera A, Autret E, Galy-Eyraud C et al. (1996). Aseptic meningitis following mumps vaccine: a retrospective survey by the French Regional Pharmacovigilance centres and by Pasteur-Mérieux Sérums & vaccins. Pharmacoepidemiol Drug Saf 5: 33–37.

Kaplan KM, Brose WG (2004). Intrathecal methods. Neurosurg Clin North Am 15: 289–296,vi.

Karahalios DG, Rekate HL, Khayata MH et al. (1996). Elevated intracranial venous pressure as a universal mechanism in pseudotumor cerebri of varying etiologies. Neurology 46: 198–202.

Karmochkine M, Chaibi P, Rogeux O et al. (1993). Meningite chimique simulant une minigite infectieuse apres infiltration intradurale de corticoides. Presse Med 22: 82.

Katz JM, Bruno MK, Winterkorn JMS et al. (2003). The pathogenesis and treatment of optic disk swelling in neurosarcoidosis: a unique therapeutic response to infliximab. Arch Neurol 60: 426–430.

Kaur A, Selwa L, Fromes G et al. (2000). Persistent headache after supratentorial craniotomy. Neurosurgery 47: 633–636.

Kepa L, Oczko-Grzesik B, Stolarz W et al. (2005). Drug-induced aseptic meningitis in suspected central nervous system infections. J Clin Neurosci 12: 562–564.

Kesler A, Gadoth N (2001). Epidemiology of idiopathic intracranial hypertension in Israel. J Neuroophthalmol 21 (1): 12–14.

Kesler A, Hadayer A, Goldhammer Y et al. (2004). Idiopathic intracranial hypertension: risk of recurrences. Neurology 63: 1737–1739.

Kharode C, McAbee G, Sherman J, Kaufman M (1992). Familial intracranial hypertension: report of a case and review of the literature. J Child Neurol 7 (2): 196–198.

Kiers L, King JO (1991). Increased intracranial pressure following bilateral neck dissection and radiotherapy. Aust N Z J Surg 61: 459–461.

Kilfoyle DH, Anderseon NE, Wallis WE et al. (2005). Recurrent severe aseptic meningitis after exposure to lamotrigine in a patient with systemic lupus erythematosus. Epilepsia 46: 327–328.

Kimura M, Kuno-Sakai H, Yamazaki S et al. (1996). Adverse events associated with MMR vaccines in Japan. Acta Paediatr Jpn 38: 205–211.

King JO, Mitchell PJ, Thompson KR et al. (2002). Monometry combined with cervical puncture in idiopathic intracranial hypertension. Neurology 58: 26–30.

Kinnman J, Kam-Hansen S, Link H et al. (1979). Studies of the humoral and cell-mediated immune response in a patient with Mollaret's meningitis. J Neurol Sci 43: 265–275.

Klapper J, on behalf of the Divalproex Sodium in Migraine Prophylaxis Study Group (1997). Divalproex sodium in migraine prophylaxis: a dose-controlled study. Cephalalgia 17: 103–108.

Kong DS, Park K, Nam DH et al. (2005). Clinical features and long-term results of spontaneous intracranial hypotension. Neurosurgery 57: 91–96.

Koss SA, Ulmer JL, Hacein-Bey L (2003). Angiographic features of spontaneous intracranial hypotension. AJNR Am J Neuroradiol 24 (4):704–706.

Kotani N, Kushikata T, Hashimoto H et al. (2000). Intrathecal methylprednisolone for intractable postherpetic neuralgia. N Engl J Med 343: 1514–1519.

Kovacs K, Bors L, Tothfalusi L et al. (1989). Cerebrospinal fluid (CSF) investigations in migraine. Cephalalgia 9: 53–57.

Kristof RA, Van Roost D, Klingmuller D et al. (1999). Lymphocytic hypophysitis: non-invasive diagnosis and treatment by high dose methylprednisolone pulse therapy? J Neurol Neurosurg Psychiatry 67: 398–402.

Kunkle EL, Ray BS, Wolff HG (1943). Experimental studies on headache: analysis of the headache associated with changes in intracranial pressure. Arch Neurol Psychiatry 49: 323–359.

Kuntz KM, Kokmen E, Stevens JC et al. (1992). Post-lumbar puncture headaches: experience in 501 consecutive procedures. Neurology 42: 1884–1887.

Kupersmith MJ, Gamell L, Turbin R et al. (1998). Effects of weight loss on the course of idiopathic intracranial hypertension in women. Neurology 50: 1094–1098.

Kuroda Y, Abe M, Nagumo F et al. (1991). Neuroepithelial cyst presenting as recurrent aseptic meningitis. Neurology 41: 1834–1835.

La Mantia L, Erbetta A (2004). Headache and inflammatory disorders of the central nervous system. Neurol Sci 25: 148–153.

Laurence KM, Coates S (1967). Spontaneously arrested hydrocephalus: results of re-examination of 82 survivors from a series of 182 unoperated cases. Dev Med Child Neurol 13: 4–13.

Lazorthes Y, Sallerin-Caute B, Verdie JC et al. (1991). Advances in drug delivery systems and applications in neurosurgery. Adv Tech Stand Neurosurg 18: 143–192.

Lee JA (1979). Arthur Edward James Barker 1850–1916. British pioneer of regional analgesia. Anaesthesia 34: 885–891.

Lennox WG, Lennox MA (1960). Epilepsy and Related Disorders. Little Brown, Boston.

Leroux E, Schwedt TJ, Black DE et al. (2006). Intractable SUNCT cured after resection of a pituitary microadenoma. Can J Neurol Sci 33: 411–413.

Levy MJ, Matharu MS, Goadsby PJ (2003). Prolactinomas, dopamine agonist and headache: two case reports. Eur J Neurol 10: 169–174.

Levy MJ, Classey JD, Maneesri S et al. (2004a). The association between calcitonin gene-related peptide (CGRP), substance P and headache in pituitary tumours. Pituitary 7: 67–71.

Levy MJ, Jager HR, Powell M et al. (2004b). Pituitary volume and headache: size is not everything. Arch Neurol 61: 721–725.

Levy MJ, Matharu MS, Meeran K et al. (2005). The clinical characteristics of headache in patients with pituitary tumours. Brain 128: 1921–1930.

Levy MJ, Classey JD, Maneesri S et al. (2006). The relationship between neuropeptide Y expression and headache in pituitary tumours. Eur J Neurol 13: 125–129.

Lexa FJ, Grossman RI (1994). MR of sarcoidosis in the head and spine: spectrum of manifestation and radiographic response to steroid therapy. AJNR AM J Neuroradiol 15: 973–982.

Limburg M, Feenstra L, Lecluse FL et al. (1985). Mollaret's meningitis responding to phenylbutazonum. A case report. Clin Neurol Neurosurg 87: 127–130.

Lin A, Foroozan R, Danesh-Meyer HV et al. (2006). Occurrence of cerebral venous sinus thrombosis in patients with presumed idiopathic intracranial hypertension. Ophthalmology 113: 2281–2284.

Liong WC, Constantinescu CS, Jaspan T (2006). Intrathecal gadolinium-enhanced magnetic resonance myelography in the detection of CSF leak. Neurology 67: 1522.

Lowry JK, Snyder JJ, Lowry PW (1998). Brain tumors in the elderly: recent trends in a Minnesota cohort study. Arch Neurol 55: 922–928.

Luke RA, Stern BJ, Krumholz A et al. (1987). Neurosarcoidosis: the long-term clinical course. Neurology 37: 461–463.

Lusk W (1911). The anatomy of spinal puncture with some considerations on technic and paralytic sequels. Ann Surg 54: 449–484.

Lybecker H, Djernes M, Schmidt JF (1995). Postdural puncture headache (PDPH): onset, duration, severity, and associated symptoms. An analysis of 75 consecutive patients with PDPH. Acta Anaesthesiol Scand 39: 605–612.

Lynch J, Krings-Ernst I, Strick K et al. (1991). Use of a 25-gauge Whitacre needle to reduce the incidence of postdural puncture headache. Br J Anaesth 67: 690–693.

Lynch SS, Cheng CM, Yee JL (2006). Intrathecal ziconotide for refractory chronic pain. Ann Pharmacother 40: 1293–1300.

Massiou H, Launay JM, Levy C et al. (2002). SUNCT syndrome in two patients with prolactinomas and bromocriptine-induced attacks. Neurology 58: 1698–1699.

Matta AP, Carod-Artal FJ (2004). [Primary headaches in children with hydrocephalus who have a ventriculoperitoneal bypass valve.] Rev Neurol 39: 1101–1104.

McCullough DC (1989). Hydrocephalus: etiology, pathologic effects, diagnosis, and natural history. In: RL McLaurin (Ed.), Pediatric Neurosurgery: Surgery of the Developing Nervous System. 2nd edn. Saunders, Philadelphia, pp. 180–199.

McGirt MJ, Woodworth G, Thomas G et al. (2004). Cerebrospinal fluid shunt placement for pseudotumor cerebri-associated intractable headache: predictors of treatment response and an analysis of longterm outcomes. J Neurosurg 101: 627–632.

McGirt MJ, Nimjee SM, Floyd J et al. (2005). Correlation of cerebrospinal fluid flow dynamics and headache in Chiari I malformation. Neurosurgery 56: 716–721.

McGirt MJ, Nimjee SM, Fuchs HE et al. (2006). Relationship of cine phase-contrast magnetic resonance imaging with outcome after decompression for Chiari I malformations. Neurosurgery 59: 140–146.

McLaurin RL (1989). Ventricular shunts: complications and results. In: RL McLaurin (Ed.), Pediatric Neurosurgery: Surgery of the Developing Nervous System. 2nd edn. Saunders, Philadelphia, pp. 219–229.

McLone DG, Czyzewski D, Raimondi AJ et al. (1982). Central nervous system infections as a limiting factor in the intelligence of children with myelomeningocele. Pediatrics 70: 338–342.

McMillan JJ, Williams B (1970). Aqueduct stenosis. Case review and discussion. J Neurol Neurosurg Psychiatry 40: 521–532.

Meadows J, Kraut M, Guarnieri M et al. (2000). Asymptomatic Chiari type I malformations identified on magnetic resonance imaging. J Neurosurg 92: 920–926.

Meuli-Simmen C, Liu Y, Yeo TT et al. (1999). Gene expression along the cerebral–spinal axis after regional gene delivery. Hum Gene Ther 10: 2689–2700.

Middleton MR, Grob JJ, Aaronson N et al. (2000). Randomized phase III study of temozolomide versus dacarbazine in the treatment of patients with advanced metastatic malignant melanoma. J Clin Oncol 18: 158–166.

Milhorat TH, Chou MW, Trinidad EM et al. (1999). Chiari I malformation redefined: clinical and radiographic findings for 364 symptomatic patients. Neurosurgery 44: 1005–1017.

Millan-Guerrero RO, Isaia-Cardenas MA (1999). Headache associated with pituitary adenomas. Headache 39: 522–523.

Milledge JT, Ades LC, Cooper MG et al. (2005). Severe spontaneous intracranial hypotension and Marfan syndrome in an adolescent. J Paediatr Child Health 41: 68–71.

Miranda-Filho Dde B, Ximenes RA, Barone AA et al. (2004). Randomised controlled trial of tetanus treatment with antitetanus immunoglobulin by the intrathecal or intramuscular route. BMJ 328: 615.

Mirfakhraee M, Crofford MJ, Guinto FC et al. (1986). Virchow–Robin space: a path of spread in neurosarcoidosis. Radiology 158: 715–720.

Miyazawa KSY, Hasegawa T, Endoh M et al. (2003). CSF hypovolemia vs intracranial hypotension in "spontaneous intracranial hypotension syndrome". Neurology 60: 941–947.

Mokri B (1999). Spontaneous cerebrospinal fluid leaks: from intracranial hypotension to cerebrospinal fluid hypovolemia – evolution of a concept. Mayo Clin Proc 74: 1113–1123.

Mokri B (2003). Headaches caused by decreased intracranial pressure: diagnosis and management. Curr Opin Neurol 16: 319–326.

Mokri B, Atkinson JL (2000). False pituitary tumor in CSF leaks. Neurology 55: 573–575.

Mokri B, Piepgras DG, Miller GM (1997). Syndrome of orthostatic headaches and diffuse pachymeningeal gadolinium enhancement. Mayo Clinic Proc 72: 400–413.

Mokri B, Hunter SF, Atkinson JL et al. (1998). Orthostatic headaches caused by CSF leak but with normal CSF pressures. Neurology 51: 786–790.

Mokri B, Atkinson JLD, Dodick DW et al. (1999). Absent pachymeningeal gadolinium enhancement on cranial MRI despite symptomatic CSF leak. Neurology 53: 402–404.

Mokri B, Maher CO, Sencavoka D (2002). Spontaneous CSF leaks: underlying disorder of connective tissue. Neurology 58: 814–816.

Mokri B, Aksamit A, Atkinson J (2004). Paradoxical postural headaches in spontaneous CSF leaks. Cephalalgia 24: 883–887.

Molins A, Alvarez J, Sumalla J et al. (1990). Cisternographic pattern of spontaneous liquoral hypotension. Cephalalgia 10: 59–65.

Mollaret MP (1944). La meningite endothelio-leucocytaire multirecurrente benigne syndrome nouveau ou maladie nouvelle. Rev Neurol 76: 57–76.

Mondon M, Ollivier L, Daumont A (2002). Aseptic meningitis ornidazole-induced in the course of infectious endocarditis. Rev Med Interne 23: 784–787.

Mora JS, Gimeno A (1980). Mollaret meningitis: report of a case with recovery after colchicines. Ann Neurol 8: 631–633.

Moris G, Garcia-Monco JC (1999). The challenge of drug-induced aseptic meningitis. Arch Intern Med 159: 1185–1194.

Moriyama E, Ogawa T, Nishida A et al. (2004). Quantitative analysis of radioisotope cisternography in the diagnosis of intracranial hypotension. J Neurosurg 101: 421–426.

Morley-Forster PK, Abotaiban A, Ganapathy S et al. (2006). Targeted thoracic epidural blood patch placed under electrical stimulation guidance (Tsui test). Can J Anaesth 53: 375–379.

Morrison DG, Phuah HK, Reddy AT et al. (2003). Ophthalmologic involvement in the syndrome of headache, neurologic deficits, and cerebrospinal fluid lymphocytosis. Ophthalmology 110: 115–118.

Morrison G, Sobel DF, Kelley WM et al. (1984). Intraventricular mass lesions. Radiology 53: 435–442.

Mulleners WM, Chronicle EP (2008). Anticonvulsants in migraine prophylaxis: a Cochrane review. Cephalalgia 28: 585–597.

Murros K, Fogelholm R (1983). Spontaneous intracranial hypotension with slit ventricles. J Neurol Neurosurg Psychiatry 46: 1149–1151.

Nabarro JD (1987). Acromegaly. Clin Endocrinol (Oxf) 26: 481–512.

Nagano I, Shiote M, Murakami T et al. (2005). Beneficial effects of intrathecal IGF-1 administration in patients with amyotrophic lateral sclerosis. Neurol Res 27: 768–772.

Nathoo S, Classey JD, Levy MJ et al. (2005). No relationship between vasoactive intestinal polypeptide expression and headache in pituitary tumours. Acta Neurol Scand 111: 317–322.

Navani A, Dominguez CL, Hald JK et al. (2006). An injection from the past: fluoroscopic evidence of remote injections of radiopaque substances. Reg Anesth Pain Med 31: 82–85.

Naveira FA, Speight KL, Rauck RL et al. (1996). Meningitis after injection of intrathecal baclofen. Anesth Analg 82: 1297–1299.

Nelson DA, Landau WM (2001). Intrathecal methylprednisolone for postherpetic neuralgia. N Engl J Med 344: 1019.

Nettis E, Calogiuri G, Colanardi MC et al. (2003). Drug-induced aseptic meningitis. Curr Drug Targets Immune Endocr Metabol Disord 3: 143–149.

Newman LS, Rose CS, Meier LA (1997). Review article. Sarcoidosis. N Engl J Med 336: 1224–1234.

Nguyen HT, Juurlink DN (2004). Recurrent ibuprofen-induced aseptic meningitis. Ann Pharmacother 38: 408–410.

Nohria V, Oakes WJ (1990). Chiari I malformation: a review of 43 patients. Pediatr Neurosurg 16: 222–227.

Nohria V, Oakes WJ (1993). Chiari headaches. Neurology 43: 1272.

Nowak DA, Widenka DC (2001). Neurosarcoidosis: a review of its intracranial manifestation. J Neurol 248: 363–372.

O'Dwyer DT, Smith AI, Matthew ML et al. (2002). Identification of the 49kDa autoantigen associated with lymphocytic hypophysitis as alpha-enolase. J Clin Endocrinol Metab 87: 752–757.

Oh SJ (1980). Sarcoid polyneuropathy: a historically proved case. Ann Neurol 7: 178–181.

Oksanen V (1986). Neurosarcoidosis: clinical presentations and course in 50 patients. Acta Med Scand 73: 283–290.

Olin JL, Gugliotta JL (2003). Possible valacyclovir-related neurotoxicity and aseptic meningitis. Ann Pharmacother 37: 1814–1817.

Olsen KS (1987). Epidural blood patch in the treatment of post-lumbar puncture headache. Pain 30: 293–301.

Osoba D, Brada M, Prados MD et al. (2000). Effect of disease burden on health-related quality of life in patients with malignant gliomas. Neuro-oncology 2: 221–228.

Outteryck O, Berteloot D, Senechal O et al. (2004). Carcinomatous meningitis presenting with isolated headache. Rev Neurol (Paris) 160: 949–951.

Pagan FL, Restrepo L, Balish M et al. (2002). A new drug for an old condition? Headache 42: 695–696.

Papaionnides DH, Korantzopoulos PG, Giotis CH (2004). Aseptic meningitis possibly associated with celecoxib. Ann Pharmacother 38: 172.

Pascual J (2000). Headache relief after sumatriptan in a patient with pituitary macroadenoma. Headache 40: 399–400.

Pascual J, Valle N (2003). Pseudomigraine with lymphocytic pleocytosis. Curr Pain Headache Rep 7: 224–228.

Pascual J, Oterino A, Berciano J (1992). Headache in type I Chiari malformation. Neurology 42: 1519–1521.

Pascual J, Iglesias F, Oterino A et al. (1996). Cough, exertional, and sexual headaches: an analysis of 72 benign and symptomatic cases. Neurology 46: 1520–1524.

Pascual J, Gonzalez-Mandly A, Martin R et al. (2008). Headaches precipitated by cough, prolonged exercise or sexual activity: a prospective etiological and clinical study. J Headache Pain 9: 259–266.

Pascual LF, Santos S, Escalza I et al. (2002). Spontaneous intracranial hypotension: quick clinical and magnetic resonance imaging response to corticosteroids. A case report. Headache 42: 359–361.

Pavlin DJ, McDonald JS, Child B et al. (1979). Acute subdural hematoma – an unusual sequela to lumbar puncture. Anesthesiology 51: 338–340.

Pearce JM (1994). Walter Essex Wynter, Quincke, and lumbar puncture. J Neurol Neurosurg Psychiatry 57: 179.

Perez de Colosia V, Tunon A, Pelaez I et al. (1994). Meningeal carcinomatosis. Review of 30 cases. Rev Clin Esp 194: 530–534.

Pettersen JA, Zochodne DW, Bell RB et al. (2002). Refractory neurosarcoidosis responding to infliximab. Neurology 59: 1660–1661.

Pfund Z, Szapary L, Jaszberenyi O et al. (1999). Headache in intracranial tumors. Cephalalgia 19: 787–790.

Phadke JG, Hern JE, Blaiklock CT (1981). Downbeat nystagmus – a false localising sign due to communicating hydrocephalus. J Neurosurg Psychiatry 44: 459.

Prasad S, El-Haddad G, Zhuang H et al. (2006). Intracranial hypotension following chiropractic spinal manipulation. Headache 46: 1456–1458.

Rabin B, Roychowdhury S, Meyer JR et al. (1998). Spontaneous intracranial hypotension: spinal MRI findings. AJNR Am J Neuroradiol 19: 1034–1039.

Radhakrishnan K, Ahlskog JE, Cross SA et al. (1993). Idiopathic intracranial hypertension (pseudotumor cerebri). Descriptive epidemiology in Rochester, Minn, 1976 to 1990. Arch Neurol 50 (1): 78–80.

Rai A, Rosen C, Carpenter J et al. (2005). Epidural blood patch at C2: diagnosis and treatment of spontaneous intracranial hypotension. AJNR Am J Neuroradiol 26: 2663–2666.

Raskin NH (1990). Lumbar puncture headache: a review. Headache 30: 197–200.

Rathmell JP, Lair TR, Nauman B (2005). The role of intrathecal drugs in the treatment of acute pain. Anesth Analg 101: S30–S43.

Ricker W, Clark M (1949). Sarcoidosis: a clinical pathologic review of 300 cases. Am J Clin Pathol 19: 725–749.

Ritz R, Roser F, Morgalia M et al. (2007). Do antibiotic-impregnated shunts in hydrocephalus therapy reduce the risk of infection? An observational study in 258 patients. BMC Infect Dis 7: 38.

River Y, Averbuch-Heller L, Weinberger M et al. (1994). Antibiotic-induced meningitis. J Neurol Neurosurg Psychiatry 57: 705–708.

Robertson JT, Soble-Smith J, Powers N et al. (2003). Prevention of cerebrospinal fistulae and reduction of epidural scar with new surgical hemostat device in a porcine laminectomy model. Spine 28: 2298–2303.

Roll JD, Larson TC3rd, Soriano MM (2003). Cerebral angiographic findings of spontaneous intracranial hypotension. AJNR Am J Neuroradiol 24: 707–708.

Rossi LN, Vassella F (1989). Headache in children with brain tumors. Childs Nerv Syst 5: 307–309.

Roth KA, Krause JE (1990). Substance-P is present in a subset of thyrotrophs in the human pituitary. J Clin Endocrinol Metab 71: 1089–1095.

Rottach K, Scheglmann K, Pfadenhauer K (1996). Mollaret's meningitis: a new aetiologic feature. Eur Neurol 36: 172–173.

Round R, Keane JR (1988). The minor symptoms of increased intracranial pressure: 101 patients with benign intracranial hypertension. Neurology 38: 1461–1464.

Rowe FJ, Sarkies NJ (1998). Assessment of visual function in idiopathic intracranial hypertension: a prospective study. Eye 12: 111–118.

Rushton JG, Rooke ED (1962). Brain tumor headache. Headache 2: 147–152.

Saboor SA, Johnson NM, McFadden J (1992). Detection of mycobacterial DNA in sarcoidosis and tuberculosis with polymerase chain reaction. Lancet 339: 1012–1015.

Said RR, Rosman NP (2004). A negative cranial computed tomographic scan is not adequate to support a diagnosis of pseudotumor cerebri. J Child Neurol 19: 609–613.

Salame K, Segev Y, Fliss DM et al. (2000). Diagnosis and management of posttraumatic oculorrhea. Neurosurg Focus 9: e3.

Sands ML, Ryczak M, Brown RB (1988). Recurrent aseptic meningitis followed by transverse myelitis as presentation of systemic lupus erythematosus. J Rheumatol 15: 862–864.

Santarius T, D'Sousa AR, Zeitoun HM et al. (2000). Audit of headache following resection of acoustic neuroma using three different techniques of suboccipital approach. Rev Laryngol Otol Rhinol (Bord) 121: 75–78.

Sarov M, Valade D, Jublanc C et al. (2006). Chronic paroxysmal hemicrania in a patient with a macroprolactinoma. Cephalalgia 26: 738–741.

Savoiardo M, De Simone T, Franzini A et al. (2006). Spontaneous CSF leak treated with percutaneous CT-guided fibrin glue. Neurology 66: 782.

Schaumann J (1936). Lymphogranuloma benigna in the light of prolonged clinical observations and autopsy findings. Br J Dermatol 48: 399.

Schessel DA, Nedzelski JM, Rowed D et al. (1992). Pain after surgery for acoustic neuroma. Otolaryngol Head Neck Surg 107: 424–429.

Schessel DA, Rowed DW, Nedzelski JM et al. (1993). Postoperative pain following excision of acoustic neuroma by the suboccipital approach: observations on possible cause and potential amelioration. Am J Otol 14: 491–494.

Schievink WI (2000). Spontaneous spinal cerebrospinal fluid leaks: a review. Neurosurg Focus 9: e8.

Schievink WI (2006). Spontaneous spinal cerebrospinal fluid leaks and intracranial hypotension. JAMA 295: 2286–2296.

Schievink WI, Tourje J (2000). Intracranial hypotension without meningeal enhancement on magnetic resonance imaging. Case report. J Neurosurg 92: 475–477.

Schievink WI, Morreale VM, Atkinson JLD et al. (1998). Surgical treatment of spontaneous spinal cerebrospinal fluid leaks. J Neurosurg 88: 243–246.

Schievink WI, Maya MM, Moser FG et al. (2005). Spectrum of subdural fluid collections in spontaneous intracranial hypotension. J Neurosurg 103: 608–613.

Schmerber S, Righini C, Lavielle JP et al. (2001). Endonasal endoscopic closure of cerebrospinal fluid rhinorrhea. Skull Base 11: 47–58.

Schon F, Blau JN (1987). Post-epileptic headache and migraine. J Neurol Neurosurg Psychiatry 50: 1148–1152.

Schwartz JF, Balentine JD (1978). Recurrent meningitis due to an intracranial epidermoid. Neurology 28: 124–129.

Scribner CL, Kapit RM, Phillips ET et al. (1994). Aseptic meningitis and intravenous immunoglobulin therapy. Ann Intern Med 121: 305–306.

Scott MA, Fletcher JM, Brookshire BL (1998). Memory functions in children with early hydrocephalus. Neuropsychology 12: 578–589.

Seebacher J, Ribeiro V, LeGuillou JL et al. (1989). Epidural blood patch in the treatment of post dural puncture headache: a double blind study. Headache 29: 630–632.

Sencavoka D, Mokri B, McClelland RL (2001). The efficacy of epidural blood patch in spontaneous CSF leaks. Neurology 57: 1921–1923.

Shah AK, Freij W (1999). Dramatic headache relief after sumatriptan in a patient with a pituitary macroadenoma. Headache 39: 443–445.

Shelden WD, Parker HL, Kemohan JW (1930). Occlusion of the aqueduct of Sylvius. Arch Neurol Psychiatry 23: 1183–1202.

Shetty PG, Shroff MM, Fatterpekar GM et al. (2000). A retrospective analysis of spontaneous sphenoid sinus fistula: MR and CT findings. AJNR Am J Neuroradiol 21: 337–342.

Shimada Y, Hongo M, Miyakoshi N et al. (2006). Dural substitute with polyglycolic acid mesh and fibrin glue for dural repair: technical note and preliminary results. J Orthop Sci 11: 454–458.

Sicard J, Forestler J (1926). Methode radiographique d'exploration de la cavite epidurale par la lipiodol. Rev Neurol (Paris) 28: 1264.

Siddall PJ, Molloy AR, Walker S et al. (2000). The efficacy of intrathecal morphine and clonidine in the treatment of pain after spinal cord injury. Anesth Analg 91: 1493–1498.

Silberstein SD, Neto W, Schmitt J et al. (2004). Topiramate in migraine prevention: results of a large controlled trial. Arch Neurol 61: 490–495.

Silberstein S, Saper J, Berenson F et al. (2008). Oxcarbazepine in migraine headache: a double-blind, randomized, placebo-controlled study. Neurology 70: 548–555.

Skau M, Brennum J, Gjerris F et al. (2006). What is new about idiopathic intracranial hypertension? An updated review of mechanism and treatment. Cephalalgia 26: 384–399.

Skinner S, Gammon K, Bergman E (1985). Management of hydrocephalus in infancy: use of acetazolamide and furosemide to avoid cerebrospinal fluid shunts. J Pediatr 107: 31–37.

Skoldenberg B, Jeansson S, Wolontis S (1975). Herpes simplex virus type 2 and acute aseptic meningitis. Clinical features of cases with isolation of herpes simplex virus from cerebrospinal fluids. Scand J Infect Dis 7: 227–232.

Smith TJ, Staats PS, Deer T et al. (2002). Randomized clinical trial of an implantable drug delivery system compared with comprehensive medical management for refractory cancer pain: impact on pain, drug-related toxicity, and survival. J Clin Oncol 20: 4040–4049.

Sorensen PS, Krogsaa B, Gjerris F (1988). Clinical course and prognosis of pseudotumor cerebri. A prospective study of 24 patients. Acta Neurol Scand 77: 164–172.

Soumekh B, Levine SC, Haines SJ et al. (1996). Retrospective study of postcraniotomy headaches in suboccipital approach: diagnosis and management. Am J Otol 17 (4): 617–619.

Spoor TC, McHenry JG (1993). Long-term effectiveness of optic nerve sheath decompression for pseudotumor cerebri. Arch Ophthalmol 111: 632–635.

Srikanth SG, Chandrashekar HS, Nagarajan K et al. (2007). Restricted diffusion in Canavan disease. Childs Nerv Syst 23: 465–468.

Stamm AM, Livingston WK, Cobbs CG et al. (1984). Failure of colchicine in the treatment of Mollaret's meningitis. Arch Intern Med 144: 2265–2266.

Steel JG, Dix RD, Baringer JR (1982). Isolation of herpes simplex virus type 1 in recurrent (Mollaret) meningitis. Ann Neurol 11: 17–21.

Stellman-Ward GR, Bannister CM, Lewis MA et al. (1997). The incidence of chronic headache in children with shunted hydrocephalus. Eur J Pediatr Surg 7: 12–14.

Stern BJ, Krumholz A, Johns C et al. (1985). Sarcoidosis and its neurological manifestations. Arch Neurol 42: 909–917.

Stern BJ, Schonfeld SA, Sewell C et al. (1992). The treatment of neurosarcoidosis with cyclosporine. Arch Neurol 49: 1065–1072.

Stoll C, Alembik Y, Dott B et al. (1992). An epidemiologic study of environmental and genetic factors in congenital hydrocephalus. Eur J Epidemiol 8 (6): 797–803.

Stovner LJ (1993). Headache associated with the Chiari malformation. Headache 33: 175–181.

Strupp M, Brandt T, Müller A (1998). Incidence of post-lumbar puncture syndrome reduced by reinserting the stylet: a randomized prospective study of 600 patients. J Neurol 245: 589–592.

Strupp M, Schueler O, Straube A et al. (2001). "Atraumatic" Sprotte needle reduces the incidence of post-lumbar puncture headaches. Neurology 57: 2310–2312.

Sundaram MB, Siemens P (1986). Triphasic waves of Mollaret's meningitis. J Neurol Neurosurg Psychiatry 49: 331–334.

Suwanwela N, Phanthumchinda K, Kaoropthum S (1994). Headache in brain tumor: a cross-sectional study. Headache 34: 435–438.

Swithinbank IM, Rake MO (1978). A case of Mollaret's meningitis associated with a lymphoma. Postgrad Med J 54: 682–685.

Takahashi M, Otsuka F, Miyoshi T et al. (1999). An elderly patient with transient diabetes insipidus associated with lymphocytic infundibuloneuro-hypophysitis. Endocr J 46: 741–746.

Tali ET, Ercan N, Krumina G et al. (2002). Intrathecal gadolinium (gadopentetate dimeglumine) enhanced magnetic resonance myelography and cisternography: results of a multicenter study. Invest Radiol 37: 152–159.

Tanaka S, Tatsumi KI, Kimura M et al. (2002). Detection of autoantibodies against the pituitary-specific proteins in patients with lymphocytic hypophysitis. Eur J Endocrinol 147: 767–775.

Tang Y-W, Cleavinger PJ, Li H et al. (2000). Analysis of candidate–host immunogenetic determinants in herpes simplex virus-associated Mollaret's meningitis. Clin Infect Dis 30: 176–178.

Thilmann AF, Möbius E, Thilmann RR et al. (1991). [Recurrent aseptic meningitis (Mollaret meningitis) – spontaneous and drug-induced origin.] Fortschr Neurol Psychiatr 59: 493–497.

Thodou E, Asa SL, Kontogeorgos G et al. (1995). Lymphocytic hypophysitis: clinicopathological findings. J Clin Endocrinol Metab 80: 2302–2311.

Thomas MC, Walker R, Wright A (1999). Handl syndrome after "benign" OKT3-induced meningitis. Transplantation 67: 1384–1385.

Tikoo RK, Kupersmith MJ, Finlay JL (2004). Treatment of refractory neurosarcoidosis with cladribine. N Engl J Med 350: 1798–1799.

Tubridy N, Saunders D, Thom M et al. (2001). Infundibulo-hypophysitis in a man presenting with diabetes insipidus and cavernous sinus involvement. J Neurol Neurosurg Psychiatry 71: 798–801.

Tyler KL, Adler D (1983). Twenty-eight years of benign recurring Mollaret meningitis. Arch Neurol 40: 42–43.

Udommongkol C, Rajchadara S, Choedamphai E (2005). Successful epidural blood patch treatment for spontaneous low cerebrospinal pressure headache with multiple leakages in lumbar spinal matter. J Med Assoc Thai 88 (Suppl. 3): S271–S274.

Ueda K, Miyazaki C, Hidaka Y et al. (1995). Aseptic meningitis caused by measles-mumps-rubella vaccine in Japan. Lancet 346: 701–702.

Vachha B, Adams R (2003). Language differences in young children with myelomeningocele and shunted hydrocephalus. Pediatr Neurosurg 39: 184–189.

Vakharia SB, Thomas PS, Rosenbaum AE et al. (1997). Magnetic resonance imaging of cerebrospinal fluid leak and tamponade effect of blood patch in postdural puncture headache. Anesth Analg 84: 585–590.

van Kooten F, Oedit R, Bakker SL et al. (2008). Epidural blood patch in post dural puncture headache: a randomised, observer-blind, controlled clinical trial. J Neurol Neurosurg Psychiatry 79: 553–558.

Vannemreddy PSSV, Nanda A, Reddy PK et al. (2002). Primary cerebral sarcoid granuloma: the importance of definite diagnosis in the high-risk patient population. Clin Neurol Neurosurg 104: 289–292.

Vieira DS, Masruha MR, Goncalves AL et al. (2008). Idiopathic intracranial hypertension with and without papilloedema in a consecutive series of patients with chronic migraine. Cephalalgia 28: 609–613.

Vilming ST, Kloster R (1997). Post-lumbar puncture headache: clinical features and suggestions for diagnostic criteria. Cephalalgia 17: 778–784.

Vilming ST, Kloster R, Sandvik L (2001). The importance of sex, age, needle size, height and body mass index in post-lumbar puncture headache. Cephalalgia 21: 738–743.

Volcy M, Tepper SJ (2006). Cluster-like headache secondary to idiopathic intracranial hypertension. A case report. Cephalalgia 26: 883–886.

Wadud R, Laiq N, Qureshi FA et al. (2006). The frequency of postdural puncture headache in different age groups. J Coll Physicians Surg Pak 16: 389–392.

Wall M (2008). Idiopathic intracranial hypertension (pseudotumor cerebri). Insight 33: 18–25.

Wall M, George D (1991). Idiopathic intracranial hypertension. Brain 114: 155–180.

Wambulwa C, Bwayo S, Laiyemo AO et al. (2005). Trimethoprin-sulfamethoxazole-induced aseptic meningitis. J Natl Med Assoc 97: 1725–1728.

Wamsler C, Schurmann S, Dubbel G et al. (2006). [Unique children – unique headaches. Case reports of pediatric headache patients from an outpatient children's pain department.] Schmerz 20: 17–23.

Wang VS, Tuch P, Wang CC (2003). An unusual case of headache. J Clin Neurosci 10: 612–616.

Watanobe H, Tamura T (1996). Stimulation by neuropeptide Y of growth hormone secretion in prolactinoma in vivo. Neuropeptides 30: 429–432.

Watanobe H, Tamura T (1997). Stimulatory and inhibitory effects of neuropeptide Y on growth hormone secretion in acromegaly in vivo. Neuropeptides 31: 29–34.

Wheeler M, Oderda GM, Ashburn MA et al. (2002). Adverse events associated with postoperative opioid analgesia: a systematic review. J Pain 3: 159–180.

Williams DW, Elster AD, Kramer SI (1990). Neurosarcoidosis: gadolinium enhanced MR imaging. J Comput Assist Tomogr 14: 704–707.

Williams G, Ball JA, Lawson RA et al. (1987). Analgesic effect of somatostatin analogue (octreotide) in headache associated with pituitary tumours. Br Med J (Clin Res Ed) 295: 247–248.

Wimalawansa S (1994). Expression of CGRP in pituitary and pituitary adenoma. 76th Annual Meeting of the Endocrine Society. Anaheim, CA.

Wright SE, Shaikh ZH, Castillo-Lugo JA et al. (2008). Aseptic meningitis and abducens nerve palsy as a serious side effect of high dose intravenous immunoglobulin used in a patient with renal transplantation. Transpl Infect Dis 10: 294–297.

Wu CL, Rowlingson AJ, Cohen SR et al. (2006). Gender and post-dural puncture headache. Anesthesiology 105: 613–618.

Wulf HF (1998). The centennial of spinal anesthesia. Anesthesiology 89: 500–506.

Yamamoto LJ, Tedder DG, Ashley R et al. (1991). Herpes simplex virus type 1 DNA in cerebrospinal fluid of a patient with Mollaret's meningitis. N Engl J Med 325: 1082–1085.

Yamamoto M, Suehiro T, Nakata H et al. (1993). Primary low cerebrospinal fluid pressure syndrome associated with galactorrhea. Intern Med 32: 228–231.

Yee AM, Pochapin MB (2001). Treatment of complicated sarcoidosis with infliximab anti-tumor necrosis factor-alpha therapy. Ann Intern Med 135: 27–31.

Yung WK, Albright RE, Olson J et al. (2000). A phase II study of temozolomide vs. procarbazine in patients with glioblastoma multiforme at first relapse. Br J Cancer 83: 588–593.

Zajicek JP, Scolding NJ, Foster O et al. (1999). Central nervous system sarcoidosis – diagnosis and management. Q J Med 92: 103–117.

Zouaoui A, Maillard JC, Dormont D et al. (1992). MRI in neurosarcoidosis. J Neuroradiol 19: 271–284.

Handbook of Clinical Neurology, Vol. 97 (3rd series)
Headache
G. Nappi and M.A. Moskowitz, Editors

Chapter 51

Headache attributed to a substance or its withdrawal

HANS-CHRISTOPH DIENER,[1*] ZAZA KATSARAVA,[1] AND VOLKER LIMMROTH[1,2]
[1]*Department of Neurology, University of Duisburg-Essen, Essen, Germany*
[2]*Department of Neurology, Kliniken Köln Merheim, Cologne, Germany*

DEFINITION

The International Headache Society (IHS) originally defined drug-induced headache as chronic headache which occurs on 15 or more days per month following overuse of any kind of acute headache medication and improves after withdrawal (Headache Classification Committee of the International Headache Society, 1988). This, however, was based on experience with overuse of analgesics and ergots only and did not cover triptan-induced medication overuse headache (MOH). After triptans were introduced, it became clear that they too can lead to MOH (Kaube et al., 1994; Limmroth et al., 1999, 2002). The second edition of the IHS classification criteria introduced the term "medication overuse headache," which replaced previous terms such as "drug-induced headache," "analgesic-induced headache," and "rebound headache" (Headache Classification Subcommittee of the International Headache Society, 2004). The classification further differentiated between MOHs induced by analgesics, ergots, triptans, and opioids (Olesen and Lipton, 2004). Although most experts agreed on thresholds for intake frequencies of acute headache drugs, the issue of MOH clinical characteristics is still under debate (Silberstein et al., 2005). Finally, a broader concept of MOH has been introduced. The diagnosis of MOH is based on headache frequency ($\geq$15 days/month) and medication overuse but does not require the headache to improve after withdrawal (Olesen et al., 2006) (Table 51.1).

MEDICATION OVERUSE HEADACHE (PREVIOUSLY USED TERMS: REBOUND HEADACHE, DRUG-INDUCED HEADACHE, MEDICATION MISUSE HEADACHE)

Clinical manifestations

Diener and Dahlof (1999) performed a meta-analysis summarizing 29 studies comprising a total of 2612 patients with chronic MOH. Sixty-five percent of patients reported migraine as their primary headache, 27% of patients reported tension-type headache as their primary headache, and 8% of patients reported mixed or other headaches as their primary headache. Women were more prone to MOH than men (3.5:1; 1533 women, 442 men). This ratio is slightly higher than would be expected from the gender differences in frequency of migraine. The mean duration of primary headache was 20.4 years. The mean admitted time of frequent drug intake was 10.3 years, and the mean duration of daily headache was 5.9 years.

Limmroth et al. (2002) performed a prospective study on 96 patients with MOH and analyzed clinical features of headache with regard to different overused substances. In this study, triptan overuse far outnumbered ergot overuse, reflecting the fact that, despite high costs, triptans have become widely used (but also overused). The study suggested that, unlike patients who suffer from MOH following ergot or analgesic overuse, migraine patients (but not patients with

*Correspondence to: Hans-Christoph Diener, MD, Department of Neurology, University of Duisburg-Essen, Hufelandstrasse 55, 45122 Essen, Germany, Tel: +49 201 723 2460/61, Fax: +49 201 723 5901, E-mail: h.diener@uni-essen.de

Table 51.1

Headache attributed to a substance or its withdrawal

Diagnostic criteria

A. Headache present on >15 days/month fulfilling criteria C and D*
B. Regular overuse for >3 months of one or more drugs that can be taken for acute and/or symptomatic treatment of headache
C. Headache has developed or markedly worsened during medication overuse
D. Headache resolves or reverts to its previous pattern within 2 months after discontinuation of overused medication*

*Removed in latest revision (Olesen et al., 2006).

tension-type headache) who overused triptans did not describe the typical tension-type daily headache but rather a migraine-like daily headache (unilateral, pulsating headache with autonomic disturbances) or a significant increase in migraine frequency. Furthermore, the delay between the start of frequent medication intake and the development of daily headache was shortest for triptans (1.7 years), longer for ergots (2.7 years), and longest for analgesics (4.8 years). The intake frequency (single dosages per month) was lowest for triptans (18 single dosages per month), higher for ergots (37 single dosages per month), and highest for analgesics (114 single dosages per month). In conclusion, the study suggested that overuse of triptans might lead to the development of chronic headache faster and with lower dosages than other substance groups.

Zeeberg and colleagues (2006) described a prospective cohort of 216 patients with MOH from the Danish Headache Center. Twenty-one percent of them had migraine, 43% had migraine and tension-type headache, and 14% had another headache type. Median headache duration was 17 years. The most frequently overused drugs were combination analgesics (42%), followed by simple analgesics (29%), triptans (20%), opioids (6%), and ergots (4%).

Meskunas and colleagues (2006) performed a retrospective analysis in order to evaluate the overuse of acute headache drugs in a US center over the previous 15 years. The proportion of subjects with a diagnosis of MOH remained stable over the years, varying from 64% of all cases seen in the center in 1990 to 59.3% in 2005. The authors found a significant decrease in the relative frequency of probable ergotamine overuse headache (from 18.6% to 0%) and in probable combination analgesic overuse headache (from 42.2% to 13.6%). The relative frequency increased significantly for the triptans (from 0% to 21.6%), for simple analgesics (from 8.8% to 31.8%), and for combinations of acute medications (from 9.8% to 22.7%). These data indicated that MOH remained an important problem in tertiary headache care but that the profile of medication overuse had dramatically changed (Meskunas et al., 2006).

Epidemiology

Epidemiological studies on the consumption of analgesics in the general population clearly indicate that antiheadache drugs are widely overused all over the world, in developed as well as developing countries. According to these surveys, between 1% and 3% of the general population take analgesics on a daily basis, and up to 7% take them at least once a week (Schwarz et al., 1985; Gutzwiller and Zemp, 1986).

Population-based studies were performed mostly in the USA and Europe, reporting the prevalence of chronic headache as about 3–4% and the prevalence of probable MOH as about 1–2% (Castillo et al., 1999; Lu et al., 2001; Prencipe et al., 2001; Lanteri-Minet et al., 2003; Colas et al., 2004). However, a recent study in Brazil found a significantly higher prevalence of 6% (Queiroz et al., 2008). A further study in a population of elderly (65 years or older) Chinese subjects revealed a prevalence of 1.3% for chronic daily headache in combination with analgesic overuse (Wang et al., 2000). Studies on incidence and prevalence of MOH among headache patients, however, were mostly conducted in or from specialized headache centers and these studies observed that up to 10% of their headache patients fulfilled the criteria of MOH (Granella et al., 1987; Micieli et al., 1988; Robinson, 1993). A survey among 174 general practitioners in the USA suggested that MOH had become the third most common cause of headache (Rapoport et al., 1996).

The vast majority of epidemiological studies investigated MOH following the overuse of analgesics or ergots according to the IHS criteria from 1988 (Headache Classification Committee of the International Headache Society, 1988). In recent years, however, triptans have become widely used and overused because of their high efficacy and low side-effects, but few studies have addressed the problem of triptan overuse. A study based on the prescription register in Denmark revealed the prevalence of sumatriptan use in the Danish population for 1995 to be 0.78%. Of these, up to 5% overused sumatriptan on a daily basis (Gaist et al., 1996). Evers and colleagues (1997) found that 4.7% of 320 sumatriptan users overused the drug by taking it at least every other day. A population-based study in France revealed a surprisingly low frequency (7.5%) of triptan use in migraine patients (Lucas et al., 2004). Data on the overuse of other newly approved triptans (zolmitriptan, naratriptan, rizatriptan, eletriptan, almotriptan) are not yet available.

Several studies addressed the prevalence of chronic headache in adolescents. One Taiwanese study revealed a prevalence of chronic daily headache in a population of adolescents (12–14 years of age) of 1.5%. Only 20% of them overused headache medication, confirming previous findings that medication overuse is less important in children and adolescents (Wang et al., 2006). A study from Canada reported a clinical analysis of 1669 children with headache seen in a neurology outpatient clinic. The prevalence of chronic headache was 3%. The prevalence of medication overuse, however, was significantly higher, about 52% (Moore and Shevell, 2004).

Etiology

Most headache experts agree that patients with migraine and tension-type headaches have a higher potential for MOH than patients who use drugs for other diseases. For example, patients who were consuming fairly large amounts of analgesics regularly for arthritis did not show an increased incidence of headache (Lance et al., 1988; Bahra et al., 2003).

A large, prospective, population-based study in Norway investigated the risk for chronic headache development in patients with headache and patients with back pain. The authors evaluated analgesic use by 32 067 adults in 1984 and again 11 years later. Those who used analgesics daily or weekly at baseline had a higher risk of developing chronic migraine (relative risk (RR) 13.3), of chronic non-migraine headache (RR 6.2), and of chronic neck pain (RR 2.4) at follow-up. This study's drawback is that, although information on medication use was collected at both baseline and follow-up, information on headache status was only collected at follow-up. Therefore, because the authors did not collect information on the headache status at baseline, they could not exclude the possibility that frequent analgesic use was simply a marker for frequent headache. Nor could they determine if baseline headache type predicted the development of chronic headache (Zwart et al., 2003).

Two more studies prospectively investigated the incidence and predictors for chronic headache development. In a prospective, population-based study, Scher and colleagues (2003) showed that 3% of individuals with episodic headache (headache frequency of 2–104 days per year) progressed to chronic headache over the course of 1 year. In this study higher headache frequency at baseline and medication overuse were risk factors for developing chronic headache. In the second study, Katsarava and colleagues (2004) prospectively followed a population of patients with episodic migraine (headache frequency fewer than 15 days per month) for 1 year to assess the incidence and to evaluate possible risk factors for headache becoming chronic. The 1-year incidence risk for headache becoming chronic was 14%. Patients who used acute headache medication frequently (more than 10 days per month) had a 20-fold increased risk for headache becoming chronic than patients who used acute headache medication fewer than 5 days per month. The risk increased twofold in patients who used two or more different headache drugs simultaneously. The first was a population-based investigation; the second studied the patient population of a tertiary headache center, which is the explanation for the higher incidence of headache chronicity in the last study.

Low socioeconomic status has been identified as a further risk factor for MOH (Hagen et al., 2002). Wiendels and colleagues (2006) found a threefold higher prevalence of chronic headache in immigrants than in a Dutch general population. Kavuk and colleagues (2006) observed a sevenfold higher prevalence of chronic headache (21%) in first-generation Turkish immigrants in Germany than in German natives (3.1%). Interestingly, prevalence of MOH in Turkish immigrants of the second generation (i.e., born in Germany) was 3.6%. This study clearly demonstrated that poor utilization of adequate medical care in first-generation Turkish immigrants in Germany was a major factor leading to a high prevalence of MOH (Kavuk et al., 2006).

A large ($n = 8219$) population-based prospective American Migraine Prevalence and Prevention study revealed that use of analgesics containing barbiturates or opioids, but not triptans, doubled the risk for developing chronic migraine (Bigal et al., 2008). Another population-based, case–control study revealed caffeine consumption to be a modest risk factor for chronic daily headache development (Scher et al., 2004). A French study compared patients with MOH with patients with migraine and found that mood disorders (odds ratio 4.5, 95% confidence interval 1.2–10.7) or use of psychoactive substances (odds ratio 7.6, 95% confidence interval 22.0–26.0) were associated with MOH (Radat et al., 2005). Another study from Turkey found mood disorders to be associated with MOH only in patients with pre-existing episodic tension-type headache (Atasoy et al., 2005).

Until recently it was assumed that patients with cluster headache are resistant to medication overuse. This, however, is only true for patients who do not also have migraine or a positive family history of migraine (Paemeleire et al., 2006).

Mechanisms by which headache becomes chronic

The pathophysiology of MOH is unknown. Until now, clarification of the underlying pathophysiology was hampered by the lack of experimental research or suitable animal models. During recent years, however, the number of animal studies has increased significantly, providing new insight into potential mechanisms that initiate and maintain chronic headache. Reuter and colleagues (2004) studied serotonin (5-HT) receptor expression and function in rats following chronic application of sumatriptan and zolmitriptan. The study demonstrated that chronic exposure of triptans causes a downregulation of receptors in trigeminal ganglion and, subsequently, a reduction of receptor function. Chronic administration of sumatriptan and zolmitriptan also caused a decrease in 5-HT synthesis in the dorsal raphe nuclei of the brainstem (Tohyama et al., 2002; Dobson et al., 2004).

An upregulation of pronociceptive 5-HT_{2A} receptors was observed in platelets of patients with drug-induced headache (Srikiatkhachorn and Anthony, 1996). Chronic application of non-narcotic analgesics in rats resulted in a significant decrease in the maximum number of 5-HT_{2A} binding sites and an increase in the maximum number of 5-HT transporter binding sites in the central nervous system (CNS) (Srikiatkhachorn et al., 2000). Ayzenberg et al. (2008) observed an increase in serotonin turnover in patients with MOH, disregarding the class of overused substance, which normalized after withdrawal. An association of a serotonin transporter protein gene polymorphism (short allele) with medication overuse in chronic tension-type headache has been described (Park et al., 2005). Rossi et al. (2008a) observed a decreased level of two main endocannabinoids, anandamide and 2-acylglycerol, in platelets of MOH patients, indicating an impairment of the endocannabinoid system in chronic migraine.

Growing evidence shows that central sensitization may play an important role in the pathophysiology of headache becoming chronic. A series of investigations using psychophysical and electrophysiological techniques clearly demonstrated a facilitation of trigeminal pain processing in patients with chronic headache. Decreased pain thresholds have been found in patients with chronic tension-type headache (Bendtsen et al., 1996). These findings have been confirmed by demonstrating increased amplitudes of laser-evoked cortical potentials in patients with chronic tension-type headache (de Tommaso et al., 2003). Ayzenberg and colleagues (2006) used a novel technique of simultaneous recording of blink reflex and nociceptive cortical potentials following nociceptive trigeminal stimulation. The authors were able to demonstrate at a supraspinal level a temporary facilitation of the trigeminal nociceptive system that normalized again after withdrawal.

Imaging studies provide further insights into the pathophysiology of MOH. A magnetic resonance imaging voxel-based morphometry study revealed structural brainstem changes in patients with chronic tension-type headache but not in patients with MOH (Schmidt-Wilcke et al., 2005). Another study investigated glucose metabolism in 16 patients with MOH before and after withdrawal and in 68 healthy controls. The authors found reversible hypometabolic changes in brain regions belonging to the general pain network. The orbitofrontal cortex, however, showed persistent hypometabolism before and after drug withdrawal, more so when patients were overusing combination analgesics (Fumal et al., 2006).

Psychological factors include the reinforcing properties of pain relief by drug consumption, a powerful component of positive conditioning. Many patients report that they take migraine drugs prophylactically because they are worried about missing work or an important social event, or they fear an imminent headache. They are often instructed by physicians or by the instructions supplied with the medication to take the migraine drug as early as possible at the start of either the aura or the headache phase of a migraine attack.

Withdrawal headache is an additional factor. When the patient tries to stop or reduce the medication, the preexisting headache worsens. Barbiturates that are contained in drugs used to treat tension-type headache have a high potency for addiction. The stimulating action of analgesics or migraine drugs and their psychotropic side-effects, such as sedation or mild euphoria, may lead to drug dependency. Barbiturates, codeine, other opioids, and caffeine are most likely to have this effect. Caffeine increases vigilance, relieves fatigue, and improves performance and mood (Griffiths and Woodson, 1988a, b). The typical symptoms of caffeine withdrawal, such as irritability, nervousness, restlessness, and "caffeine withdrawal headache" (van Dusseldorp and Katan, 1990; Silverman et al., 1992), which may last for several days, encourage patients to continue the overuse. Despite the fact that caffeine may enhance the analgesic action of acetylsalicylic acid and acetaminophen, caffeine-containing combinations should only be used in patients who do not respond to single analgesics. Caffeine and meprobamate, the main metabolite of carisoprodol, should be removed from ergotamine-containing formulations.

Headache patients can develop physical dependence on codeine and other opioids (Ziegler, 1994; Fisher and Glass, 1997). Although some headache patients have been on codeine for as long as 10 years, no studies have investigated the effects of codeine intake over this time period. It should be remembered that up to 10% of codeine is metabolized to morphine.

Ergotamine and dihydroergotamine may lead to physical dependency (Saper and Jones, 1986). Many migraineurs take ergotamine as prophylactic treatment. The reason for the physical dependency on ergotamine remains obscure. One study found that the tyramine-induced mydriasis after ergotamine administration was increased during abuse but not after withdrawal of ergotamine, which would indicate a central inhibition of pupillary sympathetic activity during abuse (Fanciullacci et al., 1992). Thus, a possible CNS effect of ergotamine can be observed after chronic use but not after a single dose of the drug. Other studies investigating the effect of chronic use of ergotamine on CNS regulation of the autonomic nervous system are needed.

The drugs that lead to chronic MOH vary considerably in different series depending probably on both selection of patients (e.g., "pure" ergotamine abusers being reported) and cultural factors. Each component contained in antimigraine drugs and analgesics can potentially induce headache. This is also true for acetylsalicylic acid and acetaminophen (Rapoport et al., 1985). It is difficult to identify a single substance, however, as 90% of patients take more than one compound at a time. Four studies investigating the frequency of the chemical compounds of various drugs have been performed (Diener et al., 1988; Micieli et al., 1988; Baumgartner et al., 1989; Mathew et al., 1990). Combination analgesics containing butalbital (short-acting barbiturate), caffeine, and aspirin with or without codeine were the leading candidates for MOH in one study (Mathew et al., 1990). Sumatriptan can also lead to MOH. This was first observed in patients who abused ergotamine (Catarci et al., 1994; Kaube et al., 1994). *De novo* cases were later reported (Pini and Trenti, 1994; Gaist et al., 1996, 1998). Patients who developed drug-induced headache from naratriptan and zolmitriptan have also been reported (Limmroth et al., 1999). Headache patients who have a previous history of analgesic or ergotamine misuse seem to be at higher risk. Results from headache diaries show that patients take an average of 4.9 tablets or suppositories per day (range 0.25–25) and on average 2.5–5.8 different pharmacological components simultaneously (range 1–14) (Diener and Dahlof, 1999). Patients who overuse triptans take fewer doses (Limmroth et al., 2002).

Differential diagnosis and diagnostic work-up

All conditions that lead to more than 10–12 headache days per month must be considered in the differential diagnosis of MOH. Careful inquiry regarding the course of the headache and acute medication use may suggest chronic migraine when the transformation is gradual over a period of many months or years. An abrupt increase in medication consumption may be caused by a spontaneous increase in the frequency of migraine or tension-type headache. Concomitant medical problems, stress, sleep disturbance, hormonal factors, depression, and certain non-headache medications can cause an increase in headache frequency. If no obvious non-organic cause exists for the change in headache pattern, clinical re-evaluation is advisable. If clinical re-evaluation suggests the possibility of serious medical or neurological illness, appropriate diagnostic testing, including imaging, is indicated.

Chronic tension-type headache is a diffuse, dull, non-localized headache with or without minimal autonomic features. Headache intensity is lower than that of migraine. Patients find it difficult to describe the character of the pain. Sometimes it is described as a feeling of a metal band around the head or a feeling of increased pressure. Many patients with chronic tension-type headache complain of mild autonomic disturbances such as nausea, photophobia, or phonophobia. The IHS definition of chronic tension-type headache requires head pain on at least 10 days per month for at least 3 months. Chronic tension-type headache has a prevalence of 2–3% (Schwartz et al., 1998; Castillo et al., 1999). Chronic tension-type headache with medication overuse can be differentiated from chronic tension-type headache without medication overuse only after drug withdrawal or a drug holiday. If the headache persists, chronic headache cannot be attributed to the analgesic intake.

Patients with chronic migraine have a history of episodic migraine attacks that increase in frequency over time. Chronic migraine is diagnosed if patients have daily or almost-daily headaches with migrainous features (e.g., unilateral throbbing pain, nausea or vomiting, photo- and phonophobia, and headache intensity that is increased by physical activity). The majority of patients are women, 90% of whom have a history of migraine without aura. About 80% of patients overuse medication. A few patients who do not overuse medication nevertheless develop chronic migraine. Chronic migraine has to be distinguished from combination headache, in which patients suffer from chronic tension-type headache along with the daily, pressing, tightening, and bilateral headache from intermittent migraine attacks. It is sometimes impossible to separate migraine from tension-type headache. In these cases, treating at least 3 headache days with a triptan is recommended. If the headache responds to the triptan, headache prophylaxis is performed as if a migraine exists (Diener and Wilkinson, 1988; Tfelt-Hansen, 1995;

Goadsby, 1997). The other patients are treated for chronic tension-type headache.

Hemicrania continua patients suffer from daily headache of moderate intensity. Superimposed exacerbation of severe headache with ipsilateral autonomic features such as ptosis, miosis, tearing, and sweating (Newman et al., 1992, 1993) may occur. Some patients have photo- and phonophobia or nausea. In some cases, the head pain alternates sides. Hemicrania continua is differentiated from cluster headache and chronic paroxysmal hemicrania by its continuous pain character; furthermore, the autonomic symptoms during acute pain exacerbations are less pronounced compared with cluster headache or chronic paroxysmal hemicrania. Hemicrania continua is frequently associated with jabs and jolts.

Patients with new daily persistent headache abruptly develop chronic headache without remission. Many patients remember the exact day the headache started. These patients did not have a previous history of migraine or episodic tension-type headache. In some patients a viral infection was suspected as causing this form of headache (Diaz-Mitoma et al., 1987). The headache does not usually respond to ergots, triptans, or simple analgesics.

Management

Abrupt drug withdrawal is the treatment of choice for MOH. However, no prospective and randomized trials comparing continuation of drug intake and drug withdrawal exist. A survey of 22 studies dealing with therapy of drug-induced headache shows that most centers use drug withdrawal as the primary therapy (Diener and Dahlof, 1999). Clinical experience indicates that medical and behavioral headache treatment will fail as long as the patient continues to take symptomatic drugs daily. The typical withdrawal symptoms last for 2–10 days (average 3.5 days) and include withdrawal headache, nausea, vomiting, arterial hypotension, tachycardia, sleep disturbances, restlessness, anxiety, and nervousness. The withdrawal phase is much shorter when patients are abusing only triptans (Katsarava et al., 2001). Seizures or hallucinations were only rarely observed, even in patients who were abusing barbiturate-containing migraine drugs.

Drug withdrawal is performed differently. Most prefer inpatient programs. Hering and Steiner (1991) abruptly withdrew the offending drugs on an outpatient basis utilizing adequate explanation of the disorder, regular follow-up, and amitriptyline (10 mg at night) and naproxen (500 mg) for relief of headache symptoms. A consensus paper by the German Migraine Society recommends outpatient withdrawal for patients who do not take barbiturates or tranquilizers with their analgesics and are highly motivated (Haag et al., 1999). Patients who take tranquilizers, codeine, or barbiturates and who failed to withdraw the drugs as outpatients or who have a high depression score should have inpatient treatment. A randomized study showed that detoxification can be performed successfully as an outpatient (Rossi et al., 2006).

Treatment recommendations for the acute phase of drug withdrawal vary considerably between studies. They include fluid replacement, analgesics, tranquilizers, neuroleptics, amitriptyline, valproate, intravenous dihydroergotamine, oxygen, and electrical stimulation. Valproate has been shown to have beneficial effects in the prophylactic treatment of chronic daily headache complicated by excessive analgesic intake (Mathew and Ali, 1991). A large open trial showed that cortisone effectively reduces withdrawal symptoms, including rebound headache (Krymchantowski and Barbosa, 2000). A recent double-blind placebo-controlled trial failed to support this concept (Bøe et al., 2007). A double-blind study showed a single subcutaneous dose of sumatriptan to be better than placebo in the treatment of ergotamine withdrawal headache, but the headache reappeared within 12 h (Diener et al., 1990). An open randomized study indicated that naproxen was better than symptomatic treatment with antiemetics and analgesics (Mathew, 1987). Further double-blind controlled trials are needed. Two randomized trials challenged the concept that preventive therapy in migraine is ineffective as long as daily intake of acute medication persists (Silvestrini et al., 2003; Diener et al., 2007). The study by Diener et al. showed that 50% of patients with migraine and MOH will improve with topiramate to a degree that they no longer fulfill the criteria for MOH. Therefore a trial of migraine-preventive medication using topiramate is recommended before the patient is referred for detoxification. In general, it seems to be important not to wait 1–2 months after withdrawal but rather to start the preventive therapy immediately, as demonstrated by a recent Norwegian study (Hagen et al., 2009).

When evaluating chronic headache patients, it is necessary to take a careful history. These patients frequently take several different substances daily despite the fact that their effect is negligible. This behavior is merely an attempt to avoid a disabling withdrawal headache. Patients should record their present and prior use of prescription drugs and non-prescription compounds and caffeine intake. Many patients also abuse other substances, such as tranquilizers, opioids, decongestants, and laxatives. It is often helpful for patients to keep a diagnostic headache diary for 1 month in order to record headache patterns and drug use. History and examination should also search for possible complications of regular drug intake, such as recurrent gastric ulcers, anemia, and ergotism. A good indicator is the number of physicians the patient has consulted and the number of previous unsuccessful therapies. One study showed that headache patients had consulted an average of 5.5 physicians who had prescribed 8.6 different therapies (Diener et al., 1989).

A short hospital stay or day care treatment is recommended if MOH has lasted more than 5 years when additional tranquilizer, barbiturate, or opioid intake exists. It is further indicated for patients who have failed outpatient withdrawal or have concomitant depression or anxiety disorder. In the hospital, all pain or headache medication is stopped abruptly. Fluids should be replaced by infusion if frequent vomiting occurs. Vomiting can be treated with antiemetics (e.g., metoclopramide or domperidone). The withdrawal headache can be treated with non-steroidal anti-inflammatory drugs (e.g., naproxen 500 mg twice daily). In some countries, aspirin is available in injectable form and 1000 mg is given every 8–12 h. If the headache has migrainous features and the patient has not abused ergotamine, intravenous dihydroergotamine 1–2 mg every 8 h is given (Raskin, 1986; Silberstein et al., 1990; Silberstein and Silberstein, 1992). Prednisone 100 mg on the first day, tapering by 20 mg for the next days, is highly effective (despite negative results from randomized trials). Symptoms of opioid withdrawal can be treated with clonidine. The initial dose is 0.1–0.2 mg 3 times daily, and this is titrated up or down based on withdrawal symptoms (tachycardia, tremor, sleeping disturbances). Some patients may require anxiolytic medication; this should be given for no longer than a week. Patients need the support of treating physicians and nurses as well as encouragement from family and friends. Behavioral techniques such as relaxation therapy and stress management should be initiated as soon as the withdrawal symptoms fade.

Outpatient treatment is advised for patients who take monosubstances or analgesic mixtures not containing barbiturates or codeine. Patients whose original headache is migraine can start prophylactic medication 4 weeks before withdrawal. Topiramate is recommended as treatment of first choice (Diener et al., 2007). Beta-blockers will improve withdrawal symptoms such as restlessness, tachycardia, or tremor. Patients who have chronic tension-type headache may be started on a tricyclic antidepressant 4 weeks before detoxification (e.g., amitriptyline 10 mg increasing to 25–75 mg at night-time). Ergots, triptans, and non-opioid drugs should be stopped abruptly. Opioids and barbiturates should be withdrawn more slowly depending on the dose and duration of intake. Withdrawal headache after ergots and triptans can be treated with oral or parenteral non-steroidal anti-inflammatory drugs (e.g., 500 mg naproxen 3 times daily for 5–7 days).

If a patient experiences more than 3 migraine attacks a month after withdrawal, medical and behavioral prophylaxis should be initiated. Clinical experience shows that many patients respond to prophylactic treatment with beta-blockers, flunarizine, valproic acid, or topiramate after drug withdrawal despite the fact that these drugs had been unsuccessful before (Coskun et al., 2007). Ergotamine, triptans, and possibly analgesics counteract the action of prophylactic therapy and will not improve drug-induced headache. The same phenomenon can be observed for the action of amitriptyline and behavioral therapy in patients with tension-type headache.

The most important preventive measure is proper instruction and appropriate surveillance of patients. Migraine patients at risk often have a mixture of migraine and tension-type headaches and should be carefully instructed to use specific antimigraine drugs for migraine attacks only. This point was already stressed in 1951 by Peters and Horton concerning ergotamine abuse. For example, complications can be avoided if enough time is taken to instruct the patient properly, so that he or she can distinguish between vasodilating and non-dilating headache (Peters and Horton, 1951).

Restricting the dose of ergotamine per attack (4 mg), per week (no more than twice per week), and per month (no more than 20 mg per month) also helps to avoid dependency. In a similar way, the number of doses of triptans should be limited per attack and to 10 intake days per month. Migraine drugs that contain barbiturates, caffeine, codeine, or tranquilizers, as well as mixed analgesics, should be avoided in all patients who suffer from MOH. Patients who take non-prescription medication should be advised to avoid caffeine combinations. Early migraine prophylaxis, by either medical or behavioral treatment, can be a preventive measure to avoid drug-induced headache.

Prognosis

Several studies have dealt with the long-term outcome of patients with MOH after successful withdrawal therapy. Success is defined as no headache at all or an improvement of more than 50% in terms of headache days. The success rate of withdrawal therapy within a time window of 1–6 months is 72.4% (17 studies, $n = 1101$ patients). Three further studies covered observation periods of 9 and 35 months (Baumgartner et al., 1989; Diener et al., 1989; Schnider et al., 1996; Grazzi et al., 2002; Williams and Stark, 2003). The success rates in these studies were 60%, 70%, and 73%, respectively. Long-term (4–6 years) follow-up studies

Table 51.2

Current studies on relapse in patients with medication overuse headache after withdrawal

Reference	Prospective/retrospective	Relapse	Follow-up in years
Ala-Hurula et al., 1982	Prospective	0.17	0.4
Andersson, 1988	Retrospective	0.09	0.5
Baumgartner et al., 1989	Prospective	0.24	1.4
Bigal et al., 2004	Retrospective	0.16	1
Dichgans et al., 1984	Prospective	0.11	1.3
Diener et al., 1989	Prospective	0.34	2.9
Drucker and Tepper, 1998	Prospective	0.15	0.5
Fritsche et al., 2001	Retrospective	0.48	4
Granella et al., 1987	Prospective	0.24	0.5
Grazzi et al., 2002*	Prospective	0.19	1
Grazzi et al., 2002*	Prospective	0.42	3
Hering and Steiner, 1991	Prospective	0.04	0.5
Katsarava et al., 2003	Prospective	0.38	1
Linton-Dahlof et al., 2000	Retrospective	0.44	0.4
Pini and Trenti, 1994*	Prospective	0.28	0.3
Pini et al., 2001*	Prospective	0.60	4
Rossi et al., 2008b	Prospective	0.0.2	1
Schnider et al., 1996	Prospective	0.39	5
Suhr et al., 1999	Prospective	0.21	5.9
Tribl et al., 2001	Prospective	0.33	5
Williams and Stark, 2003*	Retrospective	0.29	0.5
Williams and Stark, 2003*	Retrospective	0.42	1.33
Zidverc-Trajkovic J et al., 2007	Prospective	0.4	1

*Studies with two observation points are reported separately.

found relapse rates between 40% and 60% (Schnider et al., 1996; Evers et al., 1999; Pini et al., 2001; Tribl et al., 2001). Long-term (4–6 years) follow-up study performed by our group revealed a relapse rate of 48% (Fritsche et al., 2001). Predictors for relapses after successful withdrawal therapy remain difficult to analyze. Two aspects appear to be important: the type of primary headache (patients with tension-type headache or co-occurrence of migraine and tension-type headache have a higher relapse risk) (Diener et al., 1989; Schnider et al., 1996; Evers et al., 1999; Katsarava et al., 2003) and a longer duration of regular drug intake (Tfelt-Hansen and Krabbe, 1981; Pini et al., 2001). However, our group was unable to confirm the latter aspect in a 2003 study (Katsarava et al., 2003). In this study patients overusing triptans had a significantly lower relapse rate when compared with patients who were overusing other drugs. Because the predictors for high relapse rates are not fully revealed, further prospective long-term follow-up studies are needed, with a focus on newly developed triptans (Table 51.2).

References

Ala-Hurula V, Milia V, Hokkanen E (1982). Ergotamine abuse: results of ergotamine discontinuation, with special reference to the plasma concentrations. Cephalalgia 2: 189–195.

Andersson PG (1988). Ergotism – the clinical picture. In: HC Diener, M Wilkinson (Eds.), Drug-Induced Headache. Springer, Heidelberg, pp. 16–19.

Atasoy HT, Atasoy N, Unal AE et al. (2005). Psychiatric comorbidity in medication overuse headache patients with pre-existing headache type of episodic tension-type headache. Eur J Pain 9: 285–291.

Ayzenberg I, Obermann M, Nyhuis P et al. (2006). Central sensitization of the trigeminal and somatic nociceptive systems in medication overuse headache mainly involves cerebral supraspinal structures. Cephalalgia 26: 1106–1114.

Ayzenberg I, Obermann M, Leineweber K et al. (2008). Increased activity of serotonin uptake in platelets in medication overuse headache following regular intake of analgesics and triptans. J Headache Pain 9: 109–112.

Bahra A, Walsh M, Menon S et al. (2003). Does chronic daily headache arise de novo in association with regular analgesic use? Headache 43: 179–190.

Baumgartner C, Wessely P, Bingol C et al. (1989). Long-term prognosis of analgesic withdrawal in patients with drug-induced headaches. Headache 29: 510–514.

Bendtsen L, Jensen R, Olesen J (1996). Decreased pain detection and tolerance thresholds in chronic tension-type headache. Arch Neurol 53: 373–376.

Bigal ME, Rapoport AM, Sheftell FD et al. (2004). Transformed migraine and medication overuse in a tertiary headache center – clinical characteristics and treatment outcomes. Cephalalgia 24: 483–490.

Bigal ME, Serrano D, Buse D et al. (2008). Acute migraine medications and evolution from episodic to chronic migraine: a longitudinal population-based study. Headache 48: 1157–1168.

Bøe MG, Mygland A, Salvesen R (2007). Prednisolone does not reduce withdrawal headache: a randomized, double-blind study. Neurology 69: 26–31.

Castillo J, Munoz P, Guitera V et al. (1999). Epidemiology of chronic daily headache in the general population. Headache 39: 190–196.

Catarci T, Fiacco F, Argentino C et al. (1994). Ergotamine-induced headache can be sustained by sumatriptan daily intake. Cephalalgia 14: 374–375.

Colas R, Munoz P, Temprano R et al. (2004). Chronic daily headache with analgesic overuse: epidemiology and impact on quality of life. Neurology 27: 1338–1342.

Coskun O, Ucler S, Cavdar L et al. (2007). Effect of valproic acid on withdrawal therapy in patients with overuse of chronic daily headache medications. J Clin Neurosci 14: 334–339.

de Tommaso M, Libro G, Guido M et al. (2003). Heat pain thresholds and cerebral event-related potentials following painful CO_2 laser stimulation in chronic tension-type headache. Pain 104: 1111–1119.

Diaz-Mitoma F, Vanast WJ, Tyrrell DL (1987). Increased frequency of Epstein–Barr virus excretion in patients with new daily persistent headaches. Lancet 1: 411–415.

Dichgans J, Diener HC, Gerber WD et al. (1984). Chronic analgesic-induced headache. Dtsch Med Wochenschr 109: 369–373.

Diener HC, Dahlof CG (1999). Headache associated with chronic use of substances. In: J Olesen, P Tfelt-Hansen, KM Welch (Eds.), The Headaches. 2nd edn. Lippincott, Williams & Wilkins, Philadelphia, pp. 871–878.

Diener HC, Wilkinson M (1988). In: Drug-Induced Headache. Springer, New York, pp. 115–123.

Diener HC, Buhler K, Dichgans J et al. (1988). Analgetikainduzierter Dauerkopfschmerz. Existiert eine kritische Dosis? Arzneimitteltherapie 6: 156–164.

Diener HC, Dichgans J, Scholz E et al. (1989). Analgesic-induced chronic headache: long-term results of withdrawal therapy. J Neurol 236: 9–14.

Diener HC, Haab J, Peters C et al. (1990). Subcutaneous sumatriptan in the treatment of headache during withdrawal from drug-induced headache. Headache 31: 205–209.

Diener HC, Bussone G, Van Oene JC et al. (2007). Topiramate reduces headache days in chronic migraine: a randomized, double-blind, placebo-controlled study. Cephalalgia 27: 814–823.

Dobson CF, Tohyama Y, Diksic M et al. (2004). Effects of acute or chronic administration of anti-migraine drugs sumatriptan and zolmitriptan on serotonin synthesis in the rat brain. Cephalalgia 24: 2–11.

Drucker P, Tepper S (1998). Daily sumatriptan for detoxification from rebound. Headache 38: 687–690.

Evers S, Bauer B, Suhr B et al. (1997). The epidemiology of sumatriptan abuse. In: J Olesen, P Tfelt-Hansen (Eds.), Headache Treatment: Trial Methodology and New Drugs. Frontiers in Headache Research, Vol. 6. Lippincott Williams & Wilkins, Philadelphia, pp. 149–152.

Evers S, Suhr B, Bauer B et al. (1999). A retrospective long-term analysis of the epidemiology and features of drug-induced headache. J Neurol 246: 802–809.

Fanciullacci M, Alessandri M, Pietrini U et al. (1992). Long-term ergotamine abuse: effect on adrenergically induced mydriasis. Clin Pharm Ther 51: 302–327.

Fisher MA, Glass S (1997). Butorphanol (Stadol): a study in problems of current drug information and control. Neurology 48: 1156–1160.

Fritsche G, Eberl A, Katsarava Z et al. (2001). Drug-induced headache: long-term follow-up of withdrawal therapy and persistence of drug misuse. Eur Neurol 45: 229–235.

Fumal A, Laureys S, Di Clemente L et al. (2006). Orbitofrontal cortex involvement in chronic analgesic-overuse headache evolving from episodic migraine. Brain 129: 543–550.

Gaist D, Hallas J, Sindrup SH et al. (1996). Is overuse of sumatriptan a problem? A population-based study. Eur J Clin Pharmacol 3: 161–165.

Gaist D, Tsiropoulus I, Sindrup SH et al. (1998). Inappropriate use of sumatriptan: population based register and interview study. BMJ 316: 1352–1353.

Goadsby PJ (1997). How do the currently used prophylactic agents work in migraine? Cephalalgia 17: 85–92.

Granella F, Farina S, Malferrari G et al. (1987). Drug abuse in chronic headache: a clinico-epidemiologic study. Cephalalgia 7: 15–19.

Grazzi L, Andrasik F, D'Amico D et al. (2002). Behavioral and pharmacologic treatment of transformed migraine with analgesic overuse: outcome at 3 years. Headache 42: 483–490.

Griffiths RR, Woodson PP (1988a). Caffeine physical dependence: a review of human and laboratory animal studies. Psychopharmacology 94: 437–451.

Griffiths RR, Woodson PP (1998b). Reinforcing properties of caffeine: studies in humans and laboratory animals. Pharmacol Biochem Behav 29: 419–427.

Gutzwiller F, Zemp E (1986). Der Analgetikakonsum in der Bevölkerung und sozioökonomische Aspekte des Analgetikaabusus. In: MJ Mihatsch (Ed.), Das Analgetikasyndrom. Thieme, Stuttgart, p. 197.

Haag G, Baar H, Grotemeyer KH et al. (1999). Prophylaxe und Therapie des medikamenteninduzierten Dauerkopfschmerzes. Schmerz 13: 52–57.

Hagen K, Vatten L, Stovner LJ et al. (2002). Low socioeconomic status is associated with increased risk of frequent headache: a prospective study of 22718 adults in Norway. Cephalalgia 22: 672–679.

Hagen K, Albretsen C, Vilming S et al. (2009). Management of medication overuse headache: 1-year randomized multicentre open-label trial. Cephalalgia 29: 221–232.

Headache Classification Committee of the International Headache Society (1988). Classification and diagnostic criteria for headache disorders, cranial neuralgias and facial pain. Cephalalgia 8: 1–93.

Headache Classification Subcommittee of the International Headache Society (2004). The international classification of headache disorders, 2nd edn. Cephalalgia 24: 1–160.

Hering R, Steiner TJ (1991). Abrupt outpatient withdrawal of medication in analgesic-abusing migraineurs. Lancet 337: 1442–1443.

Katsarava Z, Fritsche G, Muessig M et al. (2001). Clinical features of withdrawal headache following overuse of triptans and other headache drugs. Neurology 57: 1694–1698.

Katsarava Z, Limmroth V, Finke M et al. (2003). Rates and predictors for relapse in medication overuse headache: a 1-year prospective study. Neurology 60: 1682–1683.

Katsarava Z, Schneeweiss S, Kurth T et al. (2004). Incidence and predictors for chronicity of headache in patients with episodic migraine. Neurology 62: 788–790.

Kaube H, May A, Diener HC et al. (1994). Sumatriptan misuse in daily chronic headache. BMJ 308: 1573.

Kavuk I, Weimar C, Kim BT et al. (2006). One-year prevalence and socio-cultural aspects of chronic headache in Turkish immigrants and German natives. Cephalalgia 26: 1177–1181.

Krymchantowski AV, Barbosa JS (2000). Prednisone as initial treatment of analgesic-induced daily headache. Cephalalgia 20: 107–113.

Lance F, Parkes C, Wilkinson M (1988). Does analgesic abuse cause headache de novo? Headache 38: 61–62.

Lanteri-Minet M, Auray JP, El Hasnaoui A et al. (2003). Prevalence and description of chronic daily headache in the general population in France. Pain 102: 143–149.

Limmroth V, Kazarawa S, Fritsche G et al. (1999). Headache after frequent use of new 5-HT agonists zolmitriptan and naratriptan. Lancet 353: 378.

Limmroth V, Katsarava Z, Fritsche G et al. (2002). Features of medication overuse headache following overuse of different acute headache drugs. Neurology 59: 1011–1014.

Linton-Dahlof P, Linde M, Dahlof C (2000). Withdrawal therapy improves chronic daily headache associated with long-term misuse of headache medication: a retrospective study. Cephalalgia 20: 658–662.

Lu SR, Fuh JL, Chen WT et al. (2001). Chronic daily headache in Taipei, Taiwan: prevalence, follow-up and outcome predictors. Cephalalgia 21: 980–986.

Lucas C, Auray JP, Gaudin AF et al. (2004). Use and misuse of triptans in France: data from the GRIM2000 population survey. Cephalalgia 24: 197–205.

Mathew NT (1987). Amelioration of ergotamine withdrawal with naproxen. Headache 27: 130–133.

Mathew NT, Ali S (1991). Valproate in the treatment of persistent chronic daily headache. An open labeled study. Headache 31: 71–74.

Mathew NT, Kurman R, Perez F (1990). Drug induced refractory headache – clinical features and management. Headache 30: 634–638.

Meskunas CA, Tepper SJ, Rapoport AM et al. (2006). Medications associated with probable medication overuse headache reported in a tertiary care headache center over a 15-year period. Headache 46: 766–772.

Micieli G, Manzoni GC, Granella F et al. (1988). Clinical and epidemiological observations on drug abuse in headache patients. In: HC Diener, M Wilkinson (Eds.), Drug-Induced Headache. Springer, New York, pp. 20–28.

Moore AJ, Shevell M (2004). Chronic daily headaches in pediatric neurology practice. J Child Neurol 19: 925–929.

Newman LC, Lipton RB, Russell M et al. (1992). Hemicrania continua: attacks may alternate sides. Headache 32: 237–238.

Newman LC, Lipton RB, Solomon S (1993). Hemicrania continua: 7 new cases and a literature review. Headache 32: 267.

Olesen J, Lipton RB (2004). Headache classification update. Curr Opin Neurol 17: 275–282.

Olesen J, Bousser MG, Diener HC et al. (2006). New appendix criteria open for a broader concept of chronic migraine. Cephalalgia 26: 742–746.

Paemeleire K, Bahra A, Evers S et al. (2006). Medication-overuse headache in patients with cluster headache. Neurology 67: 109–113.

Park JW, Kim JS, Kim YI et al. (2005). Serotonergic activity contributes to analgesic overuse in chronic tension-type headache. Headache 45: 1229–1235.

Peters GA, Horton BT (1951). Headache: with special reference to the excessive use of ergotamine preparations and withdrawal effects. Proc Staff Meet Mayo Clin 26: 153–161.

Pini LA, Trenti T (1994). Case report: does chronic use of sumatriptan induce dependence? Headache 34: 600–601.

Pini LA, Cicero AF, Sandrini M (2001). Long-term follow-up of patients treated for chronic headache with analgesic overuse. Cephalalgia 21: 878–883.

Prencipe M, Casini AR, Ferretti C et al. (2001). Prevalence of headache in an elderly population: attack frequency, disability, and use of medication. J Neurol Neurosurg Psychiatry 70: 377–381.

Queiroz LP, Peres MF, Kowacs F et al. (2008). Chronic daily headache in Brazil: a nationwide population-based study. Cephalalgia 28: 1264–1269.

Radat F, Creac'h C, Swendsen JD et al. (2005). Psychiatric comorbidity in the evolution from migraine to medication overuse headache. Cephalalgia 25: 519–522.

Rapoport A, Weeks R, Sheftell F (1985). Analgesic rebound headache: theoretical and practical implications. In: J Olesen, P Tfelt-Hansen, K Jensen (Eds.), Proceedings Second International Headache Congress. Scandinavian University Press, Oslo, pp. 448–449.

Rapoport A, Stang P, Gutterman DL et al. (1996). Analgesic rebound headache in clinical practice: data from a physician survey. Headache 36: 14–19.

Raskin NH (1986). Repetitive intravenous dihydroergotamine as therapy for intractable migraine. Neurology 36: 995–997.

Reuter U, Salomone S, Ickstein GW et al. (2004). Effects of chronic sumatriptan and zolmitriptan treatment on 5-HT receptor expression and function in rats. Cephalalgia 24: 398–407.

Robinson RG (1993). Pain relief for headaches. Is self-medication a problem? Can Fam Physician 39: 867–868.

Rossi P, Di Lorenzo C, Faroni J et al. (2006). Advice alone vs. structured detoxification programmes for medication overuse headache: a prospective, randomized, open-label trial in transformed migraine patients with low medical needs. Cephalalgia 26: 1097–1105.

Rossi P, Faroni JV, Nappi G (2008b). Medication overuse headache: predictors and rates of relapse in migraine patients with low medical needs. A 1-year prospective study. Cephalalgia 28: 1196–1200.

Rossi C, Pini LA, Cupini ML et al. (2008a). Endocannabinoids in platelets of chronic migraine patients and medication-overuse headache patients: relation with serotonin levels. Eur J Clin Pharmacol 64: 1–8.

Saper JR, Jones JM (1986). Ergotamine tartrate dependency: features and possible mechanisms. Clin Neuropharmacol 9: 244–256.

Scher AI, Stewart WF, Ricci JA et al. (2003). Factors associated with the onset and remission of chronic daily headache in a population-based study. Pain 106: 81–89.

Scher AI, Stewart WF, Lipton RB (2004). Caffeine as a risk factor for chronic daily headache: a population-based study. Neurology 63: 2022–2027.

Schmidt-Wilcke T, Leinisch E, Straube A et al. (2005). Gray matter decrease in patients with chronic tension type headache. Neurology 65: 1483–1486.

Schnider P, Aull S, Baumgartner C et al. (1996). Long-term outcome of patients with headache and drug abuse after inpatient withdrawal: five year follow-up. Cephalalgia 16: 481–485.

Schwartz BS, Stewart WF, Simon D et al. (1998). Epidemiology of tension-type headache. JAMA 279: 381–383.

Schwarz A, Farber U, Glaeske G (1985). Daten zu Analgetikakonsum und Analgetikanephropathie in der Bundesrepublik. Öffentliches Gesundheitswesen 47: 298.

Silberstein SD, Silberstein JR (1992). Chronic daily headache: long-term prognosis following inpatient treatment with repetitive intravenous DHE. Headache 32: 439–445.

Silberstein SD, Schulman EA, McFaden Hopkins M (1990). Repetitive intravenous DHE in the treatment of refractory headache. Headache 30: 334–339.

Silberstein SD, Olesen J, Bousser MG et al. (2005). The International Classification of Headache Disorders, 2nd Edition (ICHD-II) – revision of criteria for 8.2 Medication-overuse headache. Cephalalgia 25: 460–465.

Silverman K, Evans SM, Strain EC et al. (1992). Withdrawal syndrome after the double-blind cessation of caffeine consumption. N Engl J Med 327: 1109–1114.

Silvestrini M, Bartolini M, Coccia M et al. (2003). Topiramate in the treatment of chronic migraine. Cephalalgia 23: 820–824.

Srikiatkhachorn A, Anthony M (1996). Platelet serotonin in patients with analgesic-induced headache. Cephalalgia 16: 423–426.

Srikiatkhachorn A, Tarasub N, Govitrapong P (2000). Effect of chronic analgesic exposure on the central serotonin system: a possible mechanism of analgesic abuse headache. Headache 40: 343–350.

Suhr B, Evers S, Bauer B et al. (1999). Drug-induced headache: long-term results of stationary versus ambulatory withdrawal therapy. Cephalalgia 19: 44–49.

Tfelt-Hansen P (1995). Prophylactic treatment of migraine: evaluation of clinical trials and choice among drugs. Cephalalgia 15: 29–32.

Tfelt-Hansen P, Krabbe AA (1981). Ergotamine abuse: do patients benefit from withdrawal? Cephalalgia 1: 29–31.

Tohyama Y, Yamane F, Fikre Merid M et al. (2002). Effects of serotonin receptor agonists, TFMPP and CGS12066B, on regional serotonin synthesis in the rat brain: an autoradiographic study. J Neurochem 80: 788–798.

Tribl GG, Schnider P, Wober C et al. (2001). Are there predictive factors for long-term outcome after withdrawal in drug-induced chronic daily headache? Cephalalgia 21: 691–696.

van Dusseldorp M, Katan MB (1990). Headache caused by caffeine withdrawal among moderate coffee drinkers switched from ordinary to decaffeinated coffee: a 12 week double blind trial. BMJ 300: 1558–1559.

Wang SJ, Fuh JL, Lu SR et al. (2000). Chronic daily headache in Chinese elderly: prevalence, risk factors, and biannual follow-up. Neurology 54: 314–319.

Wang SJ, Fuh JL, Lu SR et al. (2006). Chronic daily headache in adolescents. Prevalence, impact, and medication overuse. Neurology 66: 193–197.

Wiendels NJ, Knuistingh Neven A, Rosendaal FR et al. (2006). Chronic frequent headache in the general population: prevalence and associated factors. Cephalalgia 26: 1434–1442.

Williams DR, Stark RJ (2003). Intravenous lignocaine (lidocaine) infusion for the treatment of chronic daily headache with substantial medication overuse. Cephalalgia 23: 963–971.

Zeeberg P, Olesen J, Jensen R (2006). Probable medication-overuse headache: the effect of a 2-month drug-free period. Neurology 66: 1894–1898.

Zidverc-Trajkovic J, Pekmezovic T, Jovanovic Z et al. (2007). Medication overuse headache: clinical features predicting treatment outcome at 1-year follow-up. Cephalalgia 27: 1219–1225.

Ziegler DK (1994). Opiate and opioid use in patients with refractory headache. Cephalalgia 14: 5–10.

Zwart JA, Dyb G, Hagen K et al. (2003). Analgesic use: a predictor of chronic pain and medication overuse headache: the Head-HUNT Study. Neurology 61: 160–164.

Handbook of Clinical Neurology, Vol. 97 (3rd series)
Headache
G. Nappi and M.A. Moskowitz, Editors

Chapter 52

Headache attributed to infections: nosography and differential diagnosis

E. MARCHIONI [1]* AND L. MINOLI [2]
[1]*Fondazione Istituto Neurologico Nazionale C. Mondino, IRCCS, Pavia, Italy*
[2]*Clinica di Malattie Infettive, Fondazione "Policlinico San Matteo", IRCCS, Pavia, Italy*

INTRODUCTION

Headache is a very frequent symptom of infection. It has many possible underlying mechanisms, of which two or more can coexist in a single patient. It can be caused by direct stimulation of intracranial pain-producing structures, as in the case of brain abscesses, by irritation of the pachy- and leptomeninges, as in cases of bacterial or viral meningitis, or by a state of intracranial hypertension, as seen in obstructive hydrocephalus. There are some difficulties inherent in the nosographic classification of all symptomatic headache forms and these are particularly apparent in the case of headaches attributed to infections, due to the extreme variety of conditions with which these headaches can be associated, the difficulty in defining specific clinical patterns for the different etiologies, and the intrinsic multidisciplinarity. There is no doubt that headache is often the first or the predominant symptom of serious, sometimes life-threatening, infectious diseases, or that it is, in any case, a condition frequently encountered in all epidemiological studies. Indeed, it is estimated that over 60% of people have, at some point in their lives, experienced headache during an infection (Rasmussen and Olesen, 1992). This evidence led to the need for a systematic approach to headache secondary to infection. Despite the encouraging attempts of the authors of the first and second versions of the International Classification of Headache Disorders (ICHD) (Headache Classification Committee of the International Headache Society 1988 and Headache Classification Subcommittee of the International Headache Society 2004) to develop criteria that are both exhaustive and readily usable for scientific and clinical purposes, there are still many problems, prominently related to the scarcity of good-quality material available in the literature. This is why Olesen (2006), in a recent editorial, highlighted the need to submit some chapters of the classification to critical review, in order to bring out their shortcomings, and to plan primary studies targeting some specific secondary headache forms. Of these, headaches attributed to infections are amongst the most complex and confused, given that they lack a structured historical framework of reference. Many topics should be submitted to regular review, given the rapid changes in the natural clinical course due to improvements in therapeutic regimens which, in some cases, such as human immunodeficiency virus (HIV) infection, have quickly and radically altered the disease's prognosis, and related neurological complications.

Structure and main aims

This chapter is divided into two parts. Section 1 aims to provide some elements on pain mechanisms in systemic and intracranial infections, and on the possible role of antimicrobial agents in the genesis of headache, and to provide a detailed "etiology-based" description of ICHD-II, and to compare it with ICHD-I. Section 2 aims to present a "symptom-based" algorithm applicable in the first diagnostic assessment, according to the headache features and to the most frequently associated clinical manifestations during infections of the central nervous system (CNS). It also describes the clinical pictures associated with the main infection-related headaches and their differential diagnosis.

SECTION 1: PAIN MECHANISMS

The mechanisms underlying the genesis of headache during systemic infections are still speculative and the role of fever is debated. Knowledge regarding the

*Correspondence to: Dr Enrico Marchioni, Fondazione Istituto Neurologico Nazionale C. Mondino, IRCCS, Pavia, Italy, E-mail: enrico.marchioni@mondino.it

origin of headache in CNS infections is poor and fragmentary. Headache has been linked, among other things, with intracranial hypertension syndrome, chemical meningeal irritation, and direct activation of pain-producing structures through stimulation of the trigeminovascular system (Strassman and Raymond, 1997; Headache Classification Subcommittee of the International Headache Society, 2004).

The increased intracranial pressure that is associated with brain edema, brain abscesses, and other space-occupying brain lesions can lead to mechanical stimulation of the meninges. Infectious diseases involving the CNS can result in different degrees of intracranial hypertension causing traction of the meninges and stimulation of mechanosensitive receptors. Meningeal irritation, instead, is mediated by activation of dural neurons through mechanical, thermal, and chemical stimuli. Intracranial bacterial infection is an example of both chemical and mechanical meningeal stimulation: on the basis of a series of findings derived from experimental studies, direct and indirect stimulation of the meningeal nerve fibers is due to the production of bacterial toxins and mediators of pain and inflammation, such as prostaglandins and nitric oxide (NO) (Olesen, 1993), and the secretion of neuropeptides (Hoffmann et al., 2002; Angstwurm et al., 2004); the latter can cause an increases in blood flow, probably mediated via local perivascular release of neuropeptides from afferent axons innervating the meninges (Williamson and Hargreaves, 2001; Hoffmann et al., 2002; Weber and Sakai, 2006). The role of the trigeminovascular system has been broadly studied in the genesis of migraine, but other mechanisms could also be invoked for headaches supported by an intracranial inflammatory/infectious stimulus.

Headache and antimicrobial agents

Some drugs used to treat infectious diseases can cause headache, usually as an immediate effect, more rarely as a consequence of prolonged treatment. Nearly all types of antimicrobial agent, whose mechanisms are diverse and not always known, can potentially be responsible for this effect: antiviral agents, antibiotics, antituberculous agents, antifungal agents, and antipyretic/anti-inflammatory agents. Overall, in this scenario, headaches show a frequency of occurrence of between 9% and 20%, and usually arise in association with other neurological and systemic manifestations. There exist different syndromes that include headache and these can be divided into three main groups: (1) classic flu-like syndrome; (2) a functional brainstem syndrome characterized by dizziness, tinnitus, postural disequilibrium, and sleep disturbances (in various combinations); and, more rarely, (3) aseptic meningitis.

The first syndrome is mainly linked to the use of certain antiviral agents, like standard and pegylated interferon-alpha, a leukocyte-derived cytokine used to treat hepatitis C virus infection (Perry and Wagstaff, 1998), some antiretroviral agents used in the treatment of HIV infection as part of the highly active antiretroviral therapy (HAART) complex, and amantadine (Muzi et al., 2005). Some antifungal agents, like griseofulvine and terbinafine (Elewski et al., 2008), and the antituberculous agent rifampicin can also cause this syndrome. Classic flu-like syndrome is characterized by fever, headache, chills, sweating, malaise, and myalgia. These effects are transient, dose-related, and reversible within 72 h of cessation of treatment. The headache, which has a rapid onset, is holocranial and sometimes disabling; it can be prevented or treated with acetaminophen. The pathogenetic mechanism underlying the syndrome, in the case of interferon and of some antiretroviral agents such as lopinavir, nelfinavir, zidovudine, and stavudine (Lagathu et al., 2007), could depend on increased production of some proinflammatory cytokines and, in particular, of tumor necrosis factor, which seems to be involved in the pathogenesis of some types of headache by itself (Covelli et al., 1991). In the treatment schedule for chronic hepatitis C virus infection interferon-alpha is often coadministered with ribavirin, another antiviral agent which could also be involved in the mechanism of headache induction. The second syndrome, which is the most heterogeneous and non-specific on account of the marked variability of symptoms and of the drug categories involved, is related above all to certain antiretroviral agents used, as part of the HAART complex, in the treatment of HIV infection. Some of the most important of these are: protease inhibitors, like lopinavir (Cvetkovic and Goa, 2003) and atazanavir (Busti et al., 2004), some nucleoside reverse transcriptase inhibitors, like the lamivudine/abacavir combination (Castillo et al., 2006), and several non-nucleosidic reverse transcriptase inhibitors. The cause of this type of headache remains unclear, even though it has been demonstrated that some antiretroviral agents are responsible for mitochondrial dysfunction, which seems to be involved in the genesis of some kinds of headache (Hulgan et al., 2008). The headache, usually a holocranial tension-type form, occurs with quite a high frequency and can require withdrawal of treatment. The same effects can be caused by some antibiotics and sulfamides (temafloxacin) (Iravani, 1991), by antimalarial drugs (mefloquine, chloroquine) (Albright et al., 2002), and by the antituberculous agent, isoniazid (Dutt et al., 1983).

The third syndrome is due to some non-steroidal anti-inflammatory drugs (NSAIDs), particularly ibuprofen (Cano Vargas-Machuca et al., 2006), which can cause aseptic meningitis and, more rarely, a form of meningoencephalitis, characterized mainly by neutrophil pleocytosis with blood–brain barrier (BBB) damage, which resembles a bacterial form. The same syndrome, although in a milder form, can (more rarely) be caused by antibiotic sulfamide therapy, for example, the trimethoprim–sulfamethoxazole combination (Capra et al., 2000).

The ICHD: an etiological approach

The first systematic classification of headache disorders (ICHD-I) was published by the International Headache Society in 1988 (Headache Classification Committee of the International Headache Society, 1988), and it included headaches associated with infections. The ICHD-I was structured as a single body, divided into 13 chapters, of which six (chapters 5–10) dealt with secondary headaches. Headaches secondary to infections were covered in chapters 7 and 9, devoted, respectively, to intracranial infections and systemic infections. The new classification, ICHD-II (Headache Classification Subcommittee of the International Headache Society, 2004), was published in 2004 following an extensive revision which led to substantial changes being made to the main body of the work, to the general criteria, and to the disease-specific criteria. This new version is divided into three main parts: the primary headaches (chapters 1–4), the secondary headaches (chapters 5–12), and "cranial neuralgias, central and primary facial pain, other headaches" (chapter 13). The classification of headaches attributed to infection, like that of all the secondary headaches, has undergone significant modifications to its structure and content. The whole area of headache attributed to infection is covered in chapter 9 which, in turn, is divided into four paragraphs dealing, respectively, with headache attributed to intracranial infection, headache attributed to systemic infection, headache attributed to HIV/acquired immune deficiency syndrome (AIDS), and chronic postinfection headache.

We now provide a brief descriptive analysis of each of these paragraphs, taking into account the suggestions derived from a recently published critical review (Marchioni et al., 2006).

Headache attributed to intracranial infections (ICHD-II 9.1)

ICHD-I dealt with all headaches related to intracranial infections (meningitis, encephalitis, subdural empyema, and cerebral abscess) in a single section (7.3). This was clearly an inadequate approach, given the clinical, physiopathogenetic, and, hence, therapeutic complexity of this whole area. In theory, ICHD-II was meant to reclassify all headaches attributed to intracranial infection according to their etiology. The new classification distinguishes encephalitis from meningitis and classifies these forms separately, even though clinical practice shows that these two diseases, particularly in their full-blown stages, are usually associated with one another, giving rise to complex clinical pictures. Headache, which is generally part of these pictures, is due to the interaction of various mechanisms linked to meningeal irritation, stimulation of the trigeminovascular system, intracranial hypertension, and hyperthermia.

Headache attributed to bacterial meningitis (ICHD-II 9.1.1)

In over 27% of cases of bacterial meningoencephalitis, headache is part of the syndromic picture (Carpenter and Petersdorf, 1962), and it can be the onset symptom. Section 2 describes in detail the various clinical pictures in relation to the various etiological agents involved. In general, the headache is holocranial, acute, and shows a worsening trend; it is invariably accompanied by severe nuchal rigidity and photo/phonophobia. It is regularly associated with consciousness disorders which progress rapidly from confusion to coma. Systemic disorders are associated with the neurological complaints in over half of all cases. Sometimes, however, the onset and evolution can be more insidious and take several days to develop. The agents most often responsible for bacterial meningitis are *Streptococcus pneumoniae* (50%), *Neisseria meningitidis* (25%), and *Haemophilus influenzae* (7%) (Solbrig et al., 2000). This latter form of bacterial meningitis was the most common form of meningitis in children until the advent of the *H. influenzae* b vaccine.

Headache attributed to lymphocytic meningitis (ICHD-II 9.1.2)

The term "lymphocytic meningitis" is a general definition that embraces all situations characterized by the presence, in the cerebrospinal fluid (CSF), of prevalently lymphocytic pleocytosis, irrespective of other etiopathogenetic or prognostic factors. The classification considers this CSF feature to be the most important finding and, as a result, includes in the same paragraph a series of conditions that are otherwise highly heterogeneous. These range from benign lymphocytic meningitis (Hirsch et al., 1974; Vanzee et al., 1975) to the very severe herpes simplex virus (HSV) meningitis (Whitley et al., 1977, 1981; Solbrig, 2000). It follows that the various associated clinical pictures (see Section 2) cannot easily be summarized in a single description. In general, headache is a constant accompanying symptom, but it presents with different features in different forms: acute, intense, and holocranial in HSV meningoencephalitis, and occipitonuchal in tuberculous meningitis and in aseptic meningitis. It is severe and progressively worsening in the former and mild and self-limiting in the latter. Vigilance disorders and focal symptoms (aphasia, hemiparesis, seizures) can: reach maximum intensity in the space of just a few days, as in HSV meningoencephalitis; develop gradually, as in tuberculous and fungal meningitis; or be entirely absent, as in aseptic meningitis.

Headache attributed to encephalitis (ICHD-II 9.1.3)

This paragraph sets out very clearly the characteristics of encephalitis. ICHD-II draws a rather scholastic distinction between headache attributed to meningitis and headache attributed to encephalitis, even though it is possible to observe mixed pictures of pain caused by irritation of the meninges, by cerebral edema, and by toxic substances produced by microorganisms.

Headache attributed to brain abscess (ICHD-II 9.1.4); headache attributed to subdural empyema (ICHD-II 9.1.5)

Both of these conditions are linked to the development of a space-occupying lesion generally secondary to an infection spreading from the paranasal sinuses, eyes, or ears. The diagnostic criteria for these headache forms share the following characteristics: increased intracranial pressure and irritation of the meninges and of the surrounding vessels.

Headache attributed to systemic infection (ICHD-II 9.2)

ICHD-II and ICHD-I use the same criteria to classify headache attributed to systemic infection. Headaches related to bacterial infection are considered distinct from those linked to viral (9.2.1) or to other (9.2.2) infections. Despite its frequency, the characteristics of this type of headache are not clearly delineated. The pain is generally diffuse, of variable intensity, and associated with other manifestations, such as malaise and myalgias, which accompany the onset of fever. It is not clear whether fever, *per se*, plays a role in the genesis of headache (De Marinis and Welch, 1992).

Headache attributed to HIV/AIDS (ICHD-II 9.3)

Headache (both primary and secondary forms) is one of the most frequent symptoms of HIV infection, showing a prevalence that ranges, in different studies, from 12.5% to 55% (Goldstein, 1990; Holloway and Kieburtz, 1995). Headache features may vary during different disease stages.

In clinical practice, it is useful to distinguish between three main types of headache which differ from one another in etiology, pain features, and associated instrumental findings:

1. HIV-related headache: the inclusion of headache attributed to HIV in chapter 9 of ICHD-II (Table 52.1) may be considered one of the most important aspects of the new classification, even though there is still debate over whether it actually exists as a distinct form (Table 52.2).
2. Headache attributed to aseptic meningitis, which can occur in all the stages of HIV infection. For more on the characteristics of this form, see Section 2.
3. Headache associated with opportunistic infections.

The first category is the one correlated with the infection itself, once other possible causes have been ruled out. To date, there do not exist adequate biological and instrumental data to allow a correlation to be established between HIV disease progression and the presence of headache; therefore the diagnosis is based

Table 52.1

Headache attributed to human immunodeficiency virus (HIV)/acquired immune deficiency syndrome (AIDS)

Diagnostic criteria

A. Headache with variable mode of onset, site, and intensity* fulfilling criteria C and D
B. Confirmation of HIV infection and/or of the diagnosis of AIDS, and of the presence of HIV/AIDS-related pathophysiology likely to cause headache†, by neuroimaging, cerebrospinal fluid examination, electroencephalography, and/or laboratory investigations
C. Headache develops in close temporal relation to the HIV/AIDS-related pathophysiology
D. Headache resolves within 3 months after the infection subsides

*Headache as a symptom of HIV infection is dull and bilateral; otherwise the onset, site, and intensity of headache vary according to the HIV/AIDS-related conditions (such as meningitis, encephalitis, or systemic infection) that are present.

†See comments.

Comments: dull, bilateral headache may be a part of the symptomatology of HIV infection. Headache may also be attributed to aseptic meningitis during HIV infection (but not exclusively in the AIDS stages) and to secondary meningitis or encephalitis associated with opportunistic infections or neoplasms (which mostly occur in the AIDS stages). The most common intracranial infections in HIV/AIDS are toxoplasmosis and cryptococcal meningitis. Headache occurring in patients with HIV/AIDS but attributed to a specific supervening infection is coded to that infection.

(Reproduced from Headache Classification Subcommittee of the International Headache Society, 2004.)

Table 52.2

Summary of principal *ad hoc* studies on human immunodeficiency virus (HIV)-related headache

	Lipton et al. (1991)	Brew and Miller (1993)	Berger et al. (1996)	Singer et al. (1996)	Mirsattari et al. (1999)	Evers et al. (2000)
Study design	Prospective	Retrospective controlled	Retrospective controlled	Prospective controlled	Retrospective	Retrospective and prospective
Basal population	HIV with headache	HIV outpatients and HIV inpatients undergoing lumbar puncture	HIV/AIDS with or without neurological complications	HIV/AIDS outpatients without severe immunosuppression	HIV outpatients and inpatients	HIV outpatients without evidence of central nervous system complications
Control group	No	Non-HIV inpatients with severe headache	Subjects with risk factors for HIV	Subjects with risk factors for HIV	No	No
Aim	Features of all headache patients	Comparative frequency of headache	Frequency and features of headache	Relationship between PH and occurrence of OND	Frequency, features, responsiveness to HAART and conventional headache therapy	Prevalence of PH and changes of pre-existing PH during follow-up
Number of HIV patients	49	312	193	229 (all men)	115	131
Percentage of "primary" headache	8/49 (16.3%)	HIV: 18/312 (5.3%) Controls: 2/971 (0.2%)	HIV: 91/193 (47.2%) Controls: 43/84 (51.2%)	HIV: 40/229 (17.5%) at baseline; 34/143 (23.8%) during 1-year follow-up. Controls: not reported	29/115 (25.2%): 19 new cases, 10 worsened	26/131 (19.8%)
Prevalent headache type:	Migraine	"Aseptic meningitis-like"	Undefined	Undefined	Migraine (13 became CDH)	Tension-type, migraine
Evidence of HIV-related headache	Not declared in the aims	Yes, but the study is retrospective	No evidence	Doubtful (unclear percentage in controls)	Yes, but the study is retrospective	Doubtful, no control group
Usefulness	Percentage and features of PH and SH in the whole group of HIV headache patients	Features of PH	No evidence of PH modifications during follow-up	Headache correlates with disease progression	No relationship with degree of immunosuppression, HAART and conventional headache therapy ineffective	Amelioration of migraine and deterioration of tension-type headache

PH: primary headache; SH: secondary headache; CDH: chronic daily headache; OND: other neurological disease; HAART: highly active antiretroviral treatment.

prevalently on clinical criteria that take into account the presence of any headache prior to the infection and the possible role of the antiretroviral therapy, which is also potentially implicated in the headache mechanism (see above, Headache and antimicrobial agents). Furthermore, the literature data do not allow a specific clinical profile to be established, even though in most cases the pain is holocranial, tensive, and only rarely hemicranial. The physiopathogenetic mechanism is not known.

Chronic postinfection headache (ICHD-II 9.4; chronic postbacterial meningitis headache ICHD-II 9.4.1)

Chronic postinfection headache, too, is an entity that appears for the first time in ICHD-II (Table 52.3). The term refers to chronic postbacterial meningitis headache, since this is the only form for which there currently exists evidence in the literature (Bohr et al., 1983; Neufeld et al., 1999). The pain is described as diffuse and continuous, but the literature also contains descriptions of migraine-like headaches. One of the criteria in the classification considers qualitative features of headache ("diffuse continuous pain") as an alternative to dizziness and difficulty in concentrating/memory loss and not as an essential characteristic. In our opinion, the list of symptoms should cite different patterns of quality of pain, otherwise the absence of diffuse continuous pain impedes the classification of this specific form of headache.

SECTION 2

Headache is a frequent symptom in the course of systemic and intracranial infections, and is often their presenting symptom. Rapid identification of the type of headache is the first step towards a correct interpretation of the whole syndrome picture and facilitates early diagnosis. It must be evaluated using specific semiological criteria for cranial pain, while also considering the complexity of the overall picture. During an infection, all headache types can, potentially, be present depending on the anatomical structures involved (i.e., meninges, trigeminovascular system, and other pain-producing structures), and sometimes the patient may complain of different modes of onset and development of the pain. The involvement of the CNS has a series of other consequences, too, that range from the simple appearance of mild focal signs to severe impairment of consciousness. The most important considerations, guiding the first choices in the diagnostic work-up, must be based on the following factors: characteristics of the headache (type, timing, and location of the pain), presence or absence of encephalopathy and focal signs, and presence or absence of clinical signs of increased intracranial pressure. A useful diagnostic approach could start from an evaluation of: (1) the clinical features of the headache at the time the patient is first seen; and (2) the general syndromic and neurological picture. For this reason, we propose a "symptom-based" algorithm designed to help the physician arrive at an initial diagnostic orientation considering the characteristics of the headache at onset. We define four main disease groups, which are in turn divided into subgroups (Figures 52.1–52.3 and Table 52.4):

1. Group 1: Acute headache with or without fever
   - Subgroup 1 (a) associated with encephalopathy and/or focal signs in the absence of signs of severe intracranial hypertension: severe bacterial or viral meningoencephalitis, septic cerebral vein thrombosis, brain abscess
   - Subgroup 1 (b) associated with encephalopathy and/or focal signs in the presence of signs of severe intracranial hypertension: ruptured brain abscess, septic obstructive hydrocephalus
   - Subgroup 1 (c) associated with neck stiffness, generally not associated with signs of encephalopathy and/or relevant focal signs: aseptic meningitis or benign lymphocytic meningitis, early borreliosis, meningitis attributed to HIV infection in the seroconversion period
   - Subgroup 1 (d) not associated with neck stiffness, encephalopathy or focal signs: flu-like syndrome, other systemic infections without significant CNS involvement
2. Group 2: Progressively worsening headache generally associated with signs of encephalopathy and/or focal signs. Fever may be present.

Table 52.3

Headache attributed to chronic postinfectious headache

Diagnostic criteria

A. Headache with at least one of the following characteristics and fulfilling criteria C and D:
   1. Diffuse continuous pain
   2. Associated with dizziness
   3. Associated with difficulty in concentrating and/or loss of memory
B. Evidence of previous intracranial bacterial infection from cerebrospinal fluid examination or neuroimaging
C. Headache is a direct continuation of 9.1.1 Headache attributed to bacterial meningitis
D. Headache persists for >3 months after resolution of infection

(Reproduced from Headache Classification Subcommittee of the International Headache Society, 2004.)

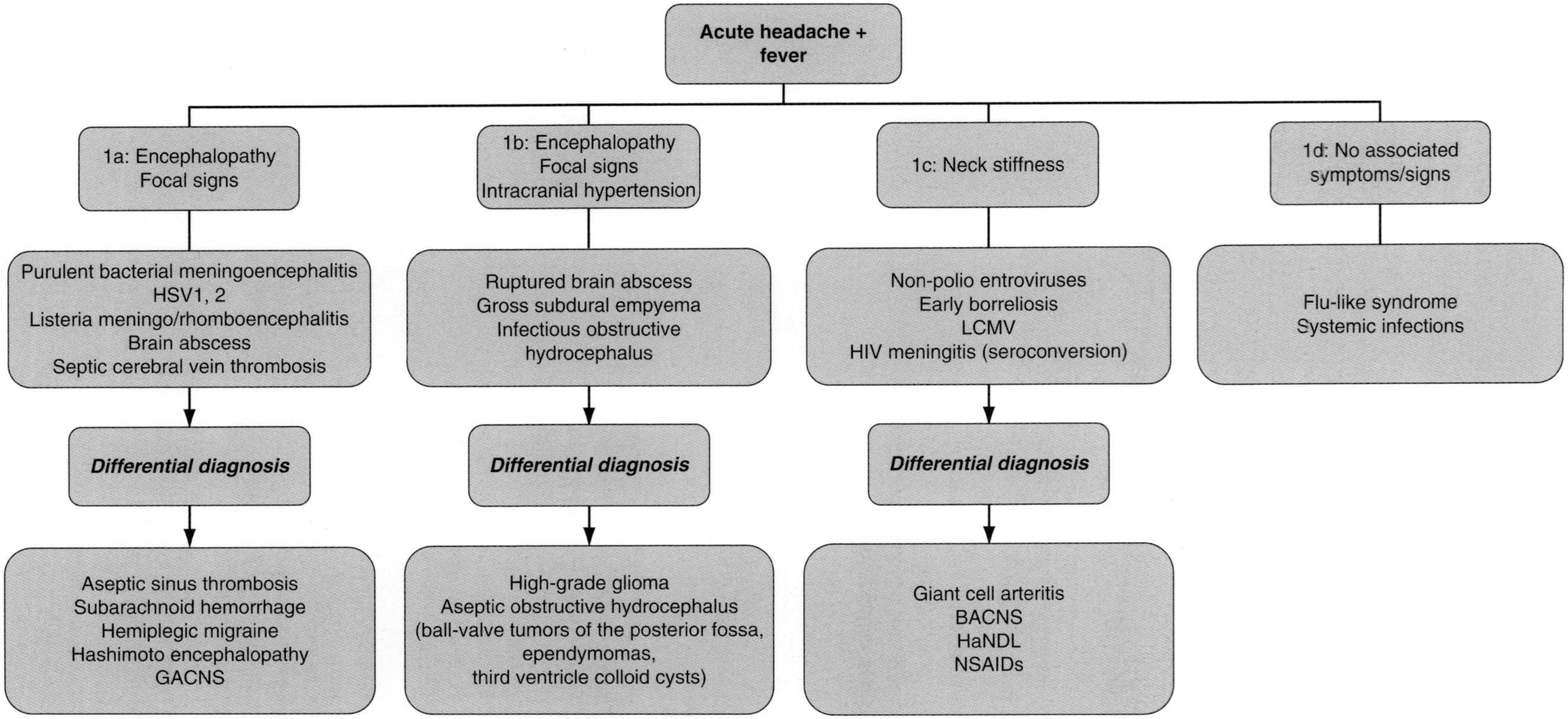

Fig. 52.1. Diagnostic algorithm for acute headache. HSV: herpes simplex virus; GACNS: granulomatous angiitis of the central nervous system; LCMV: lymphocytic choriomeningitis virus; BACNS: benign angiitis of the central nervous system; HaNDL: headache and neurological deficits with cerebrospinal fluid lymphocytosis; NSAIDs: non-steroidal anti-inflammatory drugs.

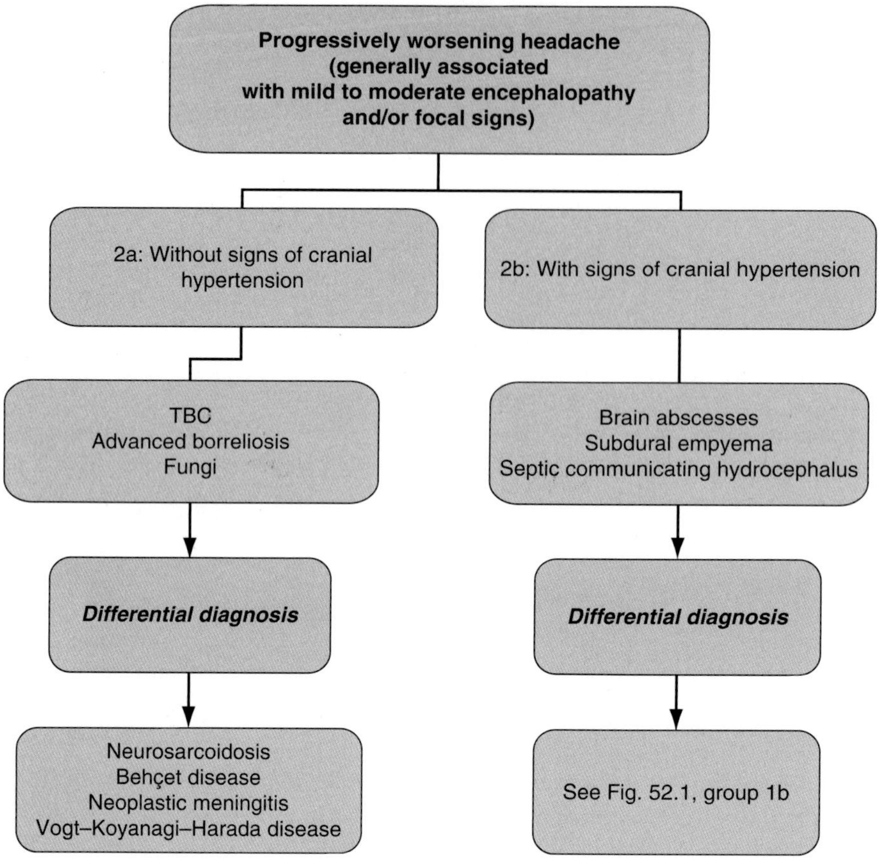

Fig. 52.2. Diagnostic algorithm for progressively worsening headache. TBC: tuberculosis.

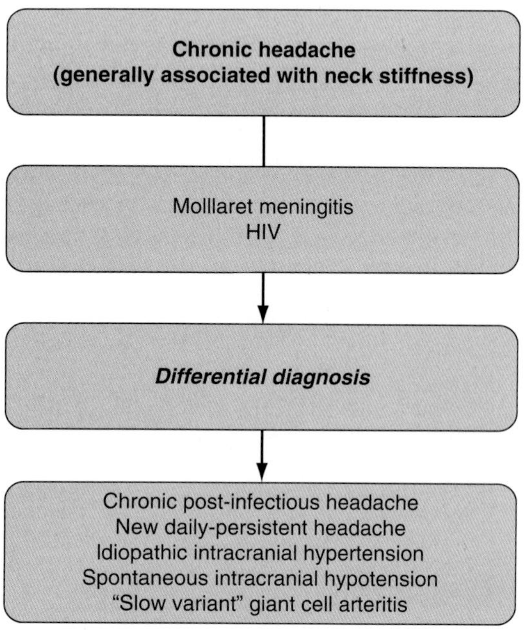

Fig. 52.3. Diagnostic algorithm for chronic headache. HIV: human immunodeficiency virus.

- Subgroup 2 (a) without signs of intracranial hypertension: tuberculosis, fungal infection, advanced borreliosis
- Subgroup 2 (b) with signs of intracranial hypertension: brain abscess, subdural empyema, septic communicating hydrocephalus

3. Group 3: Chronic or chronic-relapsing headache generally associated with neck stiffness (without or with only mild signs of encephalopathy and focal signs): headache attributed to HIV/AIDS infection not associated with opportunistic infections, Mollaret meningitis
4. Group 4: Headache localized in a specific part of the face frequently with asymmetrical distribution, not associated with encephalopathy or signs of CNS impairment (ear, nose, eye, tooth, mouth, and sinus infections). These conditions are illustrated in detail in chapter 54: "Headache or facial pain attributed to disorders of cranium, neck, eyes, ears, nose, sinuses, teeth, mouth, or other facial or cranial structures" (Headache Classification Subcommittee of the International Headache Society, 2004).

Table 52.4

Symptom-based classification of groups and subgroups: clinical features, diagnostic procedures, timing, and differential diagnosis

	Group 1				Group 2		Group 3
	a	b	c	d	a	b	/
CNS involvement	Enc ± FS + neck stiff	Enc ± FS + IH	Neck stiff		Enc ± FS + neck stiff	Enc ± FS + IH	Neck stiff + absent/ mild enc ± FS
Headache features	Holocranial/nuchal throbbing	Holocranial throbbing/ tension type	Nuchal	Holocranial	Progressively increasing, nuchal	Progressively increasing with acute worsening	Chronic tension type, nuchal
Urgent exams	Brain CT CSF	Brain CT				Brain CT	
Exams within 24 h	Brain MRI	Brain MRI + spectroscopy and DWI	Brain MRI CSF		Brain MRI CSF	Brain MRI	Brain MRI CSF
Principal CNS infections	Severe viral and bact ME, TBME, BA, septic cerebral vein thrombosis	Erupted BA, septic obstructive hydrocephalus, empyema	LCMV, non-polio EV meningitis, early Lyme, HIV seroconv meningitis	Flu-like syndrome, other systemic infections	TBC, fungi, advanced Lyme	BA, septic communicating hydrocephalus, empyema	HIV headache, Mollaret M
Principal differential diagnosis	Veins, sinuses, thrombosis, SH, FHM/SHM, SREAT, GACNS, ADEM	HGG, aseptic obstructive hydrocephalus	BACNS, GCA, HaNDL		CNS sarcoidosis, Behçet, VGH, NM	Aseptic obstructive hydrocephalus	NDPH, IIH, SIH, slow variant GCA

CNS: central nervous system; Enc: encephalopathy; FS: focal signs; neck stiff: neck stiffness; IH: intracranial hypertension; CT: computed tomography; CSF: cerebrospinal fluid; MRI: magnetic resonance imaging; DWI: diffusion-weighted imaging; bact: bacterial; ME: meningoencephalitis; TBME: tick-borne meningoencephalitis; BA: brain abscess; LCMV: lymphocytic choriomeningitis virus; EV: enterovirus; HIV: human immunodeficiency virus: seroconv: seroconversion; TBC: tuberculosis; SH: subarachnoid hemorrhage; FHM/SHM: familial/sporadic hemiplegic migraine; SREAT: steroid-responsive encephalopathy with autoimmunity of thyroid; GACNS: granulomatous arteritis of the central nervous system; ADEM: acute disseminated encephalomyelitis; HGG: high-grade glioma; BACNS: benign arteritis of the central nervous system; GCA: giant cell arteritis; HaNDL: syndrome of transient headache and neurological deficits with CSF pleocytosis; VGH: Vogt–Koyanagi–Harada disease; NM: neoplastic meningitis; NDPH: new daily-persistent headache; IIH: idiopathic intracranial hypertension; SIH: spontaneous intracranial hypertension;

Group 1

Subgroup 1a

This group includes conditions that share the following characteristics: moderate to severe hyperthermia, acute holocranial or occipital–nuchal pain that is accompanied within minutes/hours by severe neck stiffness, encephalopathy with focal signs, and/or epileptic seizures without signs of severe intracranial hypertension. It includes bacterial encephalitis with purulent CSF (caused by *Pneumococcus, Meningococcus*, *Haemophilus influenzae*), *Listeria* meningoencephalitis and rhombencephalitis, and viral encephalitis (caused by HSV-1, -2, varicella-zoster virus (VZV), arborviruses, West Nile encephalitis virus, or tick-borne encephalitis (TBE) virus).

Specific conditions

Bacterial meningitis (ICHD-II 9.1.1) Current data suggest that four major pathogens are involved in this often life-threatening illness: (1) *Streptococcus pneumoniae*; (2) *Neisseria meningitidis*; (3) *Haemophilus influenzae*; and (4) *Escherichia coli*. Almost 50% of cases are due to *S. pneumoniae*, which causes ear, sinus, or lung infections followed by bacteremia; *N. meningitidis* accounts for 25% of cases and begins with nasopharyngeal colonization (Durand et al., 1993). Epidemics usually occur in the winter and are spread from person to person through respiratory secretions. *H. influenzae* (7%) was the most common form of meningitis in children before the advent of the *H. influenzae* b vaccine. Other forms of bacterial meningitis in neonates reflect the organisms with which they come into contact in the birth canal, primarily *E. coli*, followed by group B streptococci (Roos et al., 2004). Nosocomially acquired meningitis is usually associated with neurosurgery and/or the placement of a ventricular shunt. Of the gram-negative bacilli, *E. coli* and *Klebsiella* spp. are the most common, while *Staphylococcus aureus*, enterococci, *S. epidermidis*, *Bacillus subtilis*, and corynebacteria are also frequent pathogens. The pathogenetic mechanism begins with the invasion of the subarachnoid space and the CSF, usually as a result of bacteremia or nasopharyngeal spreading via a CSF leak caused by a cribriform plate defect or basilar skull fracture. In the CSF, pathogens grow rapidly because the entry of immunoglobulins and complement is impeded by the BBB. Inflammation damages the BBB, increasing permeability, allowing entry of serum protein, and impairing glucose transport. Symptoms of an upper respiratory tract or ear infection often precede the abrupt onset of meningeal involvement. Petechial or purpuric skin lesions, usually considered bad prognostic signs, are most commonly observed with *N. meningitidis*.

In adults, bacterial meningitis typically presents with severe and acute systemic and CNS impairment characterized by severe headache, neck stiffness, nausea, vomiting, and consciousness disorders. In a classic description based on a large cohort of patients with bacterial meningitis, severe headache was the presenting symptom in 25% of cases and was rapidly associated with nuchal rigidity and altered mental status (Carpenter and Petersdorf, 1962). Headache can be due to meningeal irritation and diffuse cerebral edema and intracranial hypertension. The clinical presentation of *Streptococcus pneumoniae*, which is the most common bacterial meningitis in adults, is quite different from other types of bacterial meningitis. *S. pneumoniae* causes early consciousness impairment followed within a few hours by focal signs, recurrent seizures, and coma. It has the highest mortality rate of the major meningeal pathogens (Stanek and Mufson, 1999). The CSF is typically turbid with elevated opening pressure (up to 500 mmH_2O), marked polymorphonuclear pleocytosis (up to 10 000 cells/μl), low glucose level with low CSF to serum glucose ratio ($<40\%$), and moderate to marked BBB breakdown (Roos et al., 2004). Neuroimaging studies generally reveal diffuse cerebral edema, obstructive or communicating hydrocephalus, and venous sinus thrombosis. In some instances brain computed tomography (CT) and magnetic resonance imaging (MRI) may be within normal limits. Empirical antibiotics should be given within 30 min if bacterial meningitis is suspected. The recommended treatment is a combination of dexamethasone, ceftriaxone, or cefotaxime plus levoxacin. Ampicillin should be added in elderly or immunocompromised patients.

Listeria monocytogenes*-induced CNS complications (ICHD-II 9.1.2, 9.1.3)* *Listeria* is a common meningeal pathogen which generally causes CNS infections in immunocompromised patients and in newborns (Mylonakis et al., 1998). Separate variants of severe meningitis and encephalitis, each with a typical pattern of brainstem involvement, have also been described in immunocompetent hosts (Solbrig, 2000; Chan et al., 2001). The meningitis variant is characterized by acute neck pain and stiffness associated with varying degrees of impaired consciousness. It develops in 36% of cases of invasive listeriosis (Solbrig, 2000). The CSF profile differs from that normally observed in bacterial meningitis as *Listeria* causes marked lymphocytic pleocytosis with moderate to severe BBB damage. *Listeria*-induced encephalitis is characterized by significant neurological impairment with acute, severe, and diffuse headache, consciousness disorders of varying severity, seizures, and cranial nerve palsies. Its CSF features are unremarkable and, when present, not specific. Its *quoad valetudinem* prognosis is poor.

HSV meningoencephalitis (ICHD-II 9.1.2, 9.1.3) HSV infection of the CNS is a severe viral infection of the human brain (Solbrig, 2000; Whitley, 2004). Its estimated incidence is 1–2/500 000 persons/year. A distinction is drawn between HSV infection of the CNS in newborns, older children, and adults. Newborns may acquire a primary and disseminated infection with diffuse encephalitis during vaginal delivery from a mother shedding HSV-2 in the genital tract (Fleming et al., 1997), while HSV-1 is generally responsible for encephalitis in older children and adults. Only a minority of cases are due to a primary infection. Instead, the most frequently observed condition is HSV reactivation in the trigeminal ganglia, followed by spreading to the temporal lobe of the brain. Systemic prodromal signs, including fever, lassitude, myalgia, and gastrointestinal impairment, precede the neurological symptoms. HSV infection of the CNS has the classic characteristics of severe meningoencephalitis: acute onset, violent holocranial headache, neck stiffness, nausea, vomiting, and consciousness disorders leading to coma. Focal seizures with secondary generalization are common and difficult to treat. The CSF profile is not specific, showing moderate to severe lymphocytic pleocytosis (>100 cells/μl) and elevated protein (100–200 mg/dl) and slightly reduced glucose levels. Oligoclonal bands (OBs) are usually detectable, revealing anti-HSV IgG synthesis. Brain CT and MRI show the classic temporal involvement frequently associated with hemorrhagic foci. Edema and neuroradiological signs of mild intracranial hypertension are frequently observed. Unlike other conditions considered in differential diagnosis with HSV encephalitis, such as acute disseminated encephalomyelitis (ADEM) and primary angiitis of the CNS, brain CT scans could be useful for early diagnosis, although MRI is more sensitive. Polymerase chain reaction (PCR) detection of HSV DNA in the CSF is the most sensitive diagnostic method, showing sensitivity and specificity of 94% and 98% respectively (Lakeman and Whitley, 1995); however, the sensitivity of the method decreases progressively until it reaches zero (Revello et al., 1997). Without early and prolonged antiviral treatment (intravenous acyclovir for 14–28 days), mortality exceeds 70% and only 2.5% of all patients return to normal function after recovery.

Varicella-zoster virus-induced CNS complications (ICHD-II 9.1.2, 9.1.3) VZV is known to be responsible for a broad spectrum of neurological diseases, ranging from postherpetic neuralgia to forms of neuritis, encephalitis, myelitis, ventriculitis, and meningitis (Gilden et al., 2000; Kleinschmidt-DeMasters and Gilden, 2001). The target, spreading pathways, and clinical presentation of VZV-related CNS complications depend very much on the immune status of the patient. The CNS can be involved in two different ways: (1) immunocompetent patients usually present with a rash and local pain possibly followed by satellite focal large-vessel vasculitis and brain ischemia; or (2) immunocompromised subjects may show diffuse multifocal small-vessel vasculitis due to hematogenous spread, and do not usually exhibit cutaneous signs (Gray et al., 1994). In the latter, the meninges are always involved, giving rise to acute-onset severe headache, neck stiffness, consciousness disorders leading to coma, and seizures. The clinical spectrum resembles that of severe meningoencephalitis possibly associated with myelitis. Brain MRI shows diffuse pachy- and leptomeningeal enhancement with bilateral multifocal lesions. CSF analysis shows marked lymphocytic pleocytosis, severe BBB breakdown, with normal glucose levels and OBs. VZV-induced small-vessel vasculitis of the CNS has a severe prognosis with a high mortality rate.

Tick-borne encephalitis (ICHD-II 9.1.2, 9.1.3) TBE is an infectious zoonotic disease that originated in central Europe, subsequently spreading to other countries (Kaiser, 2002; Cruciatti et al., 2006). The disease typically shows a biphasic course, being characterized by neurological disorders of varying severity during its second phase. In a retrospective study of 850 patients, Kaiser (2002) found that TBE presented as meningitis in 400 patients (47%), as meningoencephalitis in 356 (42%), and as meningoencephalomyelitis in 93 (11%). Nine of the patients (1%) died. Impaired consciousness was the most frequent neurological symptom (31%). Laboratory investigations revealed leukocytosis in the peripheral blood in 74% of patients, elevation of the erythrocyte sedimentation rate (ESR) in 91%, increased C-reactive protein in 82%, pleocytosis in the CSF of all the patients tested, damage to the BBB in 79%, electroencephalogram (EEG) abnormalities in 77%, and MRI abnormalities in 18%.

Septic cerebral vein thrombosis See below.

Brain abscess See below.

Differential diagnosis with non-infectious diseases

The differential diagnosis includes sagittal sinus thrombosis or other cerebral vein thrombosis, subarachnoid hemorrhage, intracerebral hemorrhage, spinal epidural hemorrhage, hemiplegic migraine, steroid-responsive encephalopathy (Hashimoto's encephalopathy), lupus encephalopathy, isolated angiitis of the CNS, ADEM, Bickerstaff's brainstem encephalitis

(BBE), and mitochondrial encephalopathy, lactic acidosis, and stroke-like episodes (MELAS).

Sagittal sinus thrombosis or other cerebral vein thrombosis (ICHD-II 6.6) This is a severe condition which can be septic or, more frequently, aseptic. Indeed, the septic variant is rare and generally characterized by involvement of the cavernous sinus as a consequence of orbital or facial infections. Clinically it is characterized by sudden painful ophthalmoplegia, proptosis, and chemosis. Septic lateral sinus thrombosis is caused by otitis media or mastoiditis leading to lateralized headache, fever, earache, and abducens nerve palsy. Aseptic intracerebral venous thromboses can involve three anatomical districts: the dural venous sinus, the deep intracerebral veins, and the superficial cortical veins. Superior sagittal sinus thrombosis is the most frequent of these conditions and can be caused by a number of factors. Violent throbbing headache with acute or subacute onset is a cardinal symptom. Cerebral satellite infarction is a potentially serious consequence leading to hemiparesis, seizures, and severe consciousness disorders. Patients in whom sinus thrombosis is suspected should promptly be submitted to thrombophilia screening and MR venography.

Steroid-responsive encephalopathy with autoimmune thyroiditis (SREAT), Hashimoto's encephalopathy (ICHD-II 7.3.3) This is a rare encephalopathy associated with autoimmune thyroid disease (Tamagno et al., 2006; Mocellin et al., 2007). It consists of a subacute, relapsing–remitting, steroid-responsive encephalitis characterized by protean neurological and neuropsychiatric symptoms. Its clinical manifestations include headache, impaired consciousness, focal neurological signs, and altered cognitive function. Cerebral edema has also been described. MRI is aspecific, showing diffuse or focal white-matter involvement with possible meningeal enhancement. Vasculitis and autoimmunity directed against common brain thyroid antigens are possible etiological pathways, but features of a severe vasculitis are often absent (Mocellin et al., 2007). CSF examination often discloses an inflammatory process, with a mild increase in protein content and occasionally in lymphocyte count. The EEG shows diffuse abnormalities. Most patients presenting with this neurological complication are affected by Hashimoto's thyroiditis or, less frequently, by other autoimmune thyroid diseases, chiefly Graves' disease. The pathogenesis of this encephalopathy is still unknown and largely debated because of its extremely varied clinical presentation, possibly ascribable to different etiological and pathophysiological mechanisms. Treatment with corticosteroids is almost always successful.

Hemiplegic migraine (HM) (ICHD-II 1.2.4, 1.2.5) This is a rare variant of migraine with aura characterized by motor weakness preceding and accompanying a headache attack. Both familial (FHM) and sporadic (SHM) variants have been identified. The former is the only migraine subtype in which a monogenic mode of inheritance has been clearly established (Ducros and Thomsen, 2006). Genetic data allow the identification of two specific subtypes of FHM: FHM1 associated with mutations in the *CACNA1A* gene on chromosome 19 (Ophoff et al., 1996), and FHM2 associated with mutations in the *ATP1A2* gene on chromosome 1 (De Fusco et al., 2003). Various combinations of neurological deficits other than hemiparesis, such as aphasia, symptoms of brainstem impairment, prolonged consciousness disorders leading to coma (Fitzsimons and Wolfenden, 1985; Marchioni et al., 1995), and paroxysmal psychosis, have been described (Spranger et al., 1999) during HM attacks. Severe fever (up to 41°C), meningism, and coma can also be associated with the migraine attack (Ducros and Thomsen, 2006). These cases, which can require hospitalization in an intensive care unit, should be investigated for other causes such as meningoencephalitis. In FHM, the CSF profile is generally normal, but cases with lymphocytic pleocytosis (of varying degree) and mild BBB damage have been described (Schraeder and Burns, 1980; Motta et al., 1995). During the attacks the EEG is often characterized by slow-wave abnormalities over the contralateral hemisphere (Marchioni et al., 1995; Varkey and Varkey, 2004). Brain MRI is generally normal, even in severe variants of FHM (Marchioni et al., 1995), but one report describes hemispheric transient cerebral edema and decreased water diffusion not respecting vascular territories (Butteriss et al., 2003).

Systemic lupus erythematosus (SLE) (ICHD-II 6.4.3) This is a systemic inflammatory disease showing a clear female preponderance (a ratio of 9:1). Over 60% of patients with full-blown SLE show neurological complications and these complications are the first clinical manifestations of the disease in 5% of cases. SLE is the systemic autoimmune disease most frequently associated with neurological complications, whose nature is proteiform or, in some cases, unknown. Lupus encephalopathy, on account of its acute onset, type of symptoms, and initial course, can mimic other group 1 diseases. The clinical picture is characterized by acute/subacute onset of diffuse headache, possible neck stiffness, mild to moderate hyperthermia, psychotic disorders, cognitive impairment, and confusion that may be difficult to distinguish from steroid-induced behavioral abnormalities. These symptoms correspond to the typical pattern of lupus cerebritis that, although its pathogenesis is unknown, is probably related to the presence of antineural autoantibodies. The physiopathogenesis of the headache corresponds to that of a mild to moderate meningeal impairment. Focal neurological deficits and seizures may also be observed but, when present, they are due to cardioembolic stroke, antiphospholipid antibodies, or brain vasculitis. The antinuclear antibody titer and ESR are elevated but these findings do not appear to have a specific significance. Anti-double-stranded DNA and anti-Sm antibodies are more specific indicators of SLE. Classic lupus encephalopathy is characterized by non-specific brain MRI abnormalities with focal or multifocal lesions of gray and white matter, diffuse atrophy, and often slight meningeal contrast enhancement. In other instances the MRI pattern resembles that of typical cardiac embolism or multi-infarct encephalopathy. The CSF profile can be normal, but it generally shows moderate lymphocytic pleocytosis (no more than 50–100 cells/μl) and mild BBB damage.

Isolated angiitis of the CNS (ICHD-II 6.4.2) This is a rare and severe inflammatory disorder of unknown origin. It affects the CNS in the absence of an associated systemic disorder (Molloy and Hajj-Ali, 2007). Two variants have been described: granulomatous angiitis of the CNS (GACNS) and benign angiitis of the CNS (BACNS) (see subgroup 1c). GACNS is an acute, small-cell, vasculitic meningoencephalitis whose clinical pattern resembles that of severe viral encephalitis. Non-focal symptoms such as headache and confusion are the most common presenting features, but there are several exceptions, including patients who present with intracerebral hemorrhage or ischemic stroke. The headache is usually acute, violent, and holocranial, associated with confusion, neck stiffness, photo/phonophobia, and vomiting. There is no diagnostic laboratory test. The vascular inflammation is generally of a chronic granulomatous nature, with lymphocytes and plasma cells infiltrating arteries and veins of the leptomeninges. T_2-weighted brain MRI shows multiple bi-hemispheric lesions involving the cortical and subcortical areas. Tumor-like lesions are detectable in some instances. The CSF profile is non-specific with mild to moderate lymphocytic pleocytosis and varying degrees of BBB breakdown. The diagnosis should be confirmed by cerebral and meningeal biopsy (Nadeau, 1997). Pulsed high-dose steroids and chronic cyclophosphamide are the treatments of choice.

Acute disseminated encephalomyelitis (ICHD-II 7.3.3) ADEM is a usually monophasic postinfectious or postvaccinal disease of the CNS. The classic variant, found in 75% of patients, has the characteristics of acute encephalitis associated, in a third of these cases, with monomultifocal myelitis (Marchioni et al., 2005). In adults it can often follow a banal respiratory or gastrointestinal infection, whereas in children it can frequently follow an exanthematous disease (Anlar et al., 2003). MRI shows, in the classic form, multifocal bilateral involvement of white matter and basal ganglia. There also exist forms with pseudotumoral or hemorrhagic lesions (Tenembaum et al., 2007). Headache is not a predominant symptom in this disease, probably because the meninges are almost never involved; in any case the features of the headache, both qualitative and quantitative, change according to the particular form. When headache is present, the pain is characterized by an acute onset and is holocranial, moderately severe, and not associated with neck stiffness. It is more frequent in the postexanthematous forms more typically found in children. Disorders of consciousness and focal signs are almost always present, whereas epileptic seizures are infrequent. In general, the encephalitic disorders are transitory and resolve completely, whereas the inflammatory myelopathy carries a worse prognosis. Both brain and spine MRI should be performed in order to define the diagnosis, which is generally not supported by biological markers. Multiple T_2-weighted hyperintense lesions of the white matter and/or of the basal ganglia constitute the classic MRI pattern. Analysis of the CSF reveals mild lymphocytic pleocytosis, moderate BBB breakdown, and infrequent and transient OBs. High-dose steroids are usually employed as first-choice treatment (Tenembaum et al., 2007). Intravenous immunoglobulin has been shown to be effective in steroid-resistant cases (Marchioni et al., 2002; Ravaglia et al., 2007).

Bickerstaff's brainstem encephalitis (ICHD-II 7.3.3) BBE is a very uncommon CNS disease. Its etiology is unknown but it is postulated to have an autoimmunological origin. Almost all patients (92%) show a monophasic postinfectious course characterized by ophthalmoplegia, ataxia, and impaired consciousness (Odaka et al., 2003). The prognosis is generally good. Headache is frequently observed during the prodromal phase. Serum anti-GQ1b IgG antibody is positive in 66% of cases, and MRI shows brain abnormalities in 30%. There is frequent brainstem involvement.

Mitochondrial encephalomyopathy with lactic acidosis and stroke-like episodes (ICHD-II 6.7.2) MELAS is a non-inflammatory encephalopathy associated with muscular involvement, deafness, and cognitive impairment (Matsumoto et al., 2005). It is due to an A→G substitution at position 3243 of the mitochondrial DNA. The disease can have onset in adulthood, presenting with violent migrainous headache, seizures, and stroke, but the usual pattern of onset is that of recurrent episodes in childhood. Occipital infarcts are particularly frequent. Muscle biopsy reveals ragged-red fibers and most patients have lactic acidosis. The disease is characterized by frequent, often severe, relapses that, each time, leave permanent damage. The final outcome, usually reached in adulthood, consists of severe cognitive decline, epilepsy (poorly controlled with drugs), blindness, and other focal signs. The differential diagnosis of MELAS versus the other diseases in group 1 is easy if the entire spectrum of the disease is taken into consideration, but it can be difficult during the first episode, during a relapse, or if there are no available anamnestic data. The migrainous headache is a very common accompanying symptom, associated both with the seizures and with the episodes of metabolic acidosis that are frequently encountered in these patients and are often the cause of their death in adulthood.

MRI typically shows focal lesions in the parieto-occipital gray matter in both hemispheres. The EEG is characterized by multifocal epileptiform abnormalities and diffuse slowing of the basal rhythm. The CSF profile is generally unremarkable.

Subgroup 1b

This group includes conditions that have the same clinical manifestations listed under subgroup la, plus clinical signs of intracranial hypertension. It thus includes: ruptured brain abscess, rapidly evolving subdural empyema, and obstructive hydrocephalus induced by infection.

Specific conditions

Brain abscess (ICHD-II 9.1.4) Brain abscesses are localized suppurative processes affecting the brain parenchyma. They can be classified into four categories, on the basis of the pathogenesis:

1. Continuity with another infected cranial site (nose, ear, sinus, or teeth)
2. Secondary to open cranial trauma or neurosurgery
3. Hematogenous diffusion from a cardiac or pulmonary source. In these cases, due to the metastatization of infected microemboli, there are usually numerous cerebral localizations, and the clinical and neuroradiological pattern is variable (furthermore, there are no signs of intracranial hypertension)
4. Idiopathic cases. These cases account for around 20% of the total (Anderson, 1993).

The signs and symptoms associated with brain abscess are progressively worsening headache, nausea and vomiting, hemiparesis or other focal deficits, and focal seizures. Fever is present in less than 50% of cases. Rupture of the abscess is a dramatic complication associated with acute worsening of the headache, nuchal pain, neck stiffness, and consciousness disorders.

Subdural empyema (ICHD-II 9.1.5) Subdural empyema is a collection of pus between the dura and the arachnoid. It is caused by an ear, nose, or sinus infection, or, in other instances, can derive from cranial osteomyelitis, neurosurgery, or diffusion from peripheral infections. The symptoms differ from those observed in cerebral abscesses: acute and marked headache, fever, neck stiffness, nausea, hemiparesis, and disorders of vigilance.

Septic obstructive hydrocephalus due to progressive meningoencephalitis (ICHD-II 7.1.3) Ventricular obstruction after closure of the sutures leads to raised intracranial pressure. Headache is often worse on awakening, occipital in distribution, and associated with neck stiffness, vomiting, and blurred vision. Chronic progressive meningoencephalitis caused by tuberculosis or fungal infection frequently leads to hydrocephalus due to disorders of CSF absorption.

Differential diagnosis with non-infectious diseases

High-grade gliomas (ICHD-II 7.4) According to the World Health Organization classification (Louis et al., 2007), grade III (anaplastic astrocytoma) and grade IV (glioblastoma multiforme) gliomas belong to this category. The symptoms and signs are relatively uniform but non-specific. Glioblastomas can cause abrupt raised intracranial pressure phenomena leading to the classic clinical pattern of: violent and holocranial headache, nausea and vomiting, blurred or double vision, seizures, drowsiness, and consciousness disorders leading to coma (Parney and Prados, 2005). Typically these symptoms are most prominent in the morning and improve over the course of the day. Fever is usually absent. The occurrence of intratumoral hemorrhage could precipitate intracranial hypertension, leading to subtentorial herniation. As with many other urgent presentations in neuro-oncology, brain CT is frequently sufficient to confirm glioblastoma multiforme diagnosis (space-occupying low-density lesions with central hypodense area corresponding to necrosis). Commonly, the enhancement is associated with aggressiveness, but in some cases glioblastoma multiforme can be associated with minimal or no enhancement on CT imaging. Except in situations of urgency, conventional and non-conventional MRI techniques have largely replaced CT as the imaging method of choice for diagnostic work-ups in the field of neuro-oncology. CSF analysis is absolutely contraindicated.

Obstructive hydrocephalus (ICHD-II 7.1.3) Ball-valve tumors of the posterior fossa, ependymomas, and colloid cysts of the third ventricle lead rapidly to obstruction of CSF circulation. The clinical pattern is characterized by acute and violent headache, vomiting, and impaired consciousness leading to coma. This is a dramatic life-threatening condition and must be regarded as a neurosurgical emergency.

SUBGROUPS 1A AND 1B: TIMING AND PRIORITIES

General considerations

These are severe, sometimes life-threatening, diseases. They constitute genuine medical emergencies that demand an immediate diagnosis and the institution of appropriate treatment within hours. In the situations listed under the heading lb, the intracranial hypertension causes a headache of intolerable intensity, proportional to the severity of the general clinical picture. When these symptoms are present, it is mandatory to perform an urgent brain CT scan followed immediately by lumbar puncture for detection of herpes viruses (HSV, VZV, cytomegalovirus, Epstein–Barr virus), enterovirus and measles viral nucleic acid, using real-time PCR. Blood cultures, too, should be urgently performed. In the presence of clinical signs of intracranial hypertension, the CT must always be carried out before the lumbar puncture to avoid the very serious consequences of CSF depletion. This is nevertheless a rare occurrence in the field of neuroinfectious diseases. In all the forms of meningoencephalitis, both viral and bacterial, included in group la, the CSF pressure is raised (up to 500 mmH_2O) and the protein content (100–1000 mg/dl) reveals moderate to marked BBB breakdown. A decreased CSF to serum glucose ratio (<40%) and predominance of leukocytic pleocytosis (60% of cells or more) make it possible to distinguish bacterial from viral infections, while brain CT can allow identification of the possible cause of the intracranial hypertension syndrome, as well as its extent in the event of a ruptured abscess, empyema, or uncompensated obstructive hydrocephalus. This latter event certainly constitutes a medical–surgical emergency, but its appearance is generally preceded, months earlier, by forms of chronic or chronic-relapsing meningoencephalitis belonging to group 2.

Brain MRI is not generally an urgent requirement and can be postponed or even avoided if the CT, the blood cultures, and the PCR detection are able, in the space of a few hours, to determine the cause of the problem. MRI becomes fundamental when the results of the other investigations are doubtful or highly inconsistent. In such cases, it must be performed in less than 24 h due to the possibility of a venous sinus thrombosis, which is another medical emergency. In other situations, less urgent but nevertheless serious, it can reveal post- or parainfectious forms of encephalitis, belonging to the ADEM group, that prevalently affect the white matter. The clinical spectrum of ADEM, including headache, may be very similar to that observed during forms of encephalitis due to direct microbial damage and it is often confused with these forms. As indicated above, the acute forms of meningoencephalitis must also be distinguished from a series of non-infectious inflammatory disorders of the CNS (mainly vasculitis), both primary and subsequent to systemic diseases. In these cases, the headache can be the predominant symptom. MRI is very sensitive but generally lacks specificity. In most cases, it shows meningeal contrast enhancement and parenchymal lesions, mainly in the gray matter, with variable contrast enhancement. Analysis of the CSF is part of the diagnostic work-up and shows mild to moderate lymphocytic pleocytosis, mild BBB damage, and normal glucose and lactate levels. Screening for serum autoantibodies is mandatory.

Subgroup 1a: comments and "red flags"

Headache and signs of meningeal irritation play a fundamental diagnostic role provided they are interpreted within the correct clinical (systemic) context. As a rule, their intensity is proportional to the severity of the disease and is suggestive of an infectious form.

The non-infectious diseases we have described here must be taken into consideration when, albeit in the presence of typical symptoms and signs, the forms of meningoencephalitis listed in subgroup la are not confirmed by the presence of specific biological and instrumental markers. This is quite a rare situation and we can affirm, reasonably confidently, that severe bacterial and viral forms of meningoencephalitis constitute a group of pathologies that can be readily diagnosed using the currently available methods of investigation. A major reservation has to be expressed with regard to the diagnostic value of PCR analysis of the CSF: the longer it is since the onset of the disease, the more the sensitivity of this test is reduced.

GACNS, ADEM, and the other above-mentioned inflammatory diseases, while often appearing particularly aggressive and despite sometimes having a poor prognosis, show less dramatic clinical characteristics than the other infectious diseases included in this group. Hemiplegic migraine raises serious problems of differential diagnosis versus viral meningoencephalitis in cases – quite rare – characterized by impaired consciousness, fever, and CSF abnormalities. In these cases, the patient's own history and family history can obviously prove useful, since they may reveal similar episodes, even very remote in time.

Subgroup 1b: comments and "red flags"

The conventional and non-conventional neuroimaging techniques currently available make it possible to distinguish, relatively easily, brain abscess from high-grade glioma. It can be more difficult, however, if the clinical background of fever or the finding of a contiguous infection is lacking, or if the MRI picture of the abscess does not correspond to the usual criteria. While the features of the headache will not really help to eliminate any doubts, they are useful for drawing the physician's attention to situations that constitute medical–surgical emergencies.

Subgroup 1c

This subgroup includes diseases that present with mild to moderate fever, holocranial or occipital–nuchal subacute headache of generally mild to moderate intensity, mild neck stiffness, and mild or no clinical signs of encephalopathy, focal signs and epilepsy. It thus includes benign lymphocytic meningitis of viral origin, early Lyme disease, and, in general, so-called aseptic meningitis. The list of pathogenic agents that can cause this form of meningitis, albeit with widely varying frequency, is very long. In over 70% of cases a viral etiology can be demonstrated and the most common causal agents are non-polio enteroviruses (Coxsackie, Echovirus), early borreliosis, lymphocytic choriomeningitis virus (LCMV), and HIV during the seroconversion stage. This subgroup embraces conditions in which there is no clinical or instrumental evidence of parenchymal involvement. The meaning of the term "aseptic meningitis" is controversial. ICHD-II classifies "aseptic meningitis" in paragraph 7.3.2 ("Headache attributed to non-infectious inflammatory disease"), specifying in point C that the headache associated with aseptic meningitis is drug-induced. Both in the current literature (Sawyer and Rotbart, 2004) and in clinical practice this term describes conditions characterized by acute meningitis with a benign course, lymphocytic pleocytosis, probable but not proven viral etiology and exclusion of bacterial agents in the CSF. Our description of subgroup 1c refers to this latter meaning. CSF analysis reveals mild lymphocytic pleocytosis (generally no more than 100 cells/μl), slightly elevated opening pressure, and normal glucose and mildly raised protein levels. At onset, it is possible to detect a moderate polymorphonuclear pleocytosis which converts to lymphocytic pleocytosis in a matter of hours. The diagnosis is generally supported by PCR investigation of the CSF. Brain MRI is generally normal but can occasionally show slight meningeal enhancement. The persistence of headache, meningeal irritation, and CSF abnormalities beyond 20 days is suggestive of another diagnosis, such as brain vasculitis, meningeal carcinomatosis, or chronic granulomatous infection. Aseptic meningitis is a typical example of meningeal involvement without parenchymal involvement. For this reason, it is important to distinguish it from some of the forms of meningoencephalitis included in group 2 (in particular, those caused by advanced borreliosis, tuberculosis, and *Cryptococcus*) which, while sometimes showing a particularly benign picture, tending to chronicization, are invariably progressive. Consideration of the complete clinical, CSF, and MRI picture generally leads to the correct diagnosis.

Specific conditions

Lymphocytic choriomeningitis virus (ICHD-II 9.1.2) LCMV is an enveloped single-stranded RNA virus that belongs to the Arenaviridae family. The neurological pattern of LCMV infection corresponds to that of aseptic meningitis and it is observed in about 15% of patients with proven LCMV infection (Deibel et al., 1975; Vanzee et al., 1975). Diffuse or occipital headache is always present at disease onset. The recovery period can be prolonged, but permanent residual neurological deficits are infrequent. The CSF characteristics (lymphocytic pleocytosis, mild BBB breakdown, and normal glucose and lactate levels) resemble those of all forms of aseptic meningitis. Occasionally, LCMV provokes severe meningitis with encephalitis (Hirsch et al., 1974).

Non-polio enteroviruses (ICHD-II 9.1.2) Enterovirus meningitis is a generally benign form that lasts only a few days and often does not require admission to hospital. For this reason, its frequency is probably underestimated.

HIV meningitis during seroconversion (ICHD-II 9.1.2) This is a condition of little clinical significance that sometimes accompanies or follows the classic flu-like HIV seroconversion syndrome. HIV meningitis is characterized by mild hyperthermia, occipital headache, nausea, and meningism. Vigilance and consciousness are generally preserved. As a rule, no cranial nerve deficits or focal signs are observed. Patients suspected of having this syndrome and who have an initially negative HIV test require repeat testing, because HIV antibodies may be undetectable in this stage of the disease. Brain MRI scan is within normal limits and CSF analysis shows non-specific findings (mild lymphocytic pleocytosis and BBB damage). The finding of OBs, revealing anti-HIV IgG synthesis, when detectable, should alert the clinician to HIV seroconversion syndrome.

Early borreliosis (ICHD-II 9.1.2) In the USA many systemic clinical features of early borreliosis differ from those found in the European variant. Instead the neurological complications show a similar clinical profile. The aseptic meningitis typical of early borreliosis is characterized by mild headache with neck stiffness, frequently associated with diffuse radicular pain (Reik et al., 1986). The disease usually resolves spontaneously. Brain MRI scan is normal while CSF analysis shows moderate pleocytosis, BBB breakdown, and OBs with evidence of intrathecal production of specific antiborrelia antibodies.

Differential diagnosis with non-infectious diseases

The differential diagnosis includes giant cell arteritis (GCA: Horton's disease), BACNS, syndrome of transient headache and neurological deficits with CSF lymphocytosis (HaNDL), NSAIDs, and aseptic meningitis.

Giant cell arteritis (Horton's disease, temporal arteritis) (ICHD-II 6.4.1) GCA affects large and medium-sized arteries, especially those branching from the proximal aorta, that supply the neck, the extracranial structures of the head, and the arms.

It is one of the most frequently observed causes of headache in the elderly. About half of all patients affected by GCA experience polymyalgia rheumatica. The ESR is elevated (>70 mm/h) in more than 95% of cases. The clinical manifestations of GCA are various but headache is the most frequent symptom, present in at least 70% of cases (Caselli and Hunder, 1997). It may be focal or generalized, mild or severe, and there may be scalp tenderness over the arteries of the head or at other sites. Amaurosis fugax (10%) frequently precedes permanent visual loss due to ischemic unilateral or bilateral optic neuropathy. Another common symptom is jaw claudication, which can be observed in 40% of cases. Less commonly recognized neurological complications include transient ischemic attacks, cerebral infarctions, acute confusional states, multi-infarct dementia, ischemic cervical myelopathy, and ischemic mononeuropathies. The CSF profile is within normal limits and the brain MRI scan is unremarkable. Patients with GCA generally respond well to low doses of steroid therapy.

Benign angiitis of the CNS (ICHD-II 6.4.2) BACNS is the benign variant of isolated angiitis of the CNS (see above). It presents with subcontinuous headache of moderate intensity, tending towards chronicization. As the disease progresses, focal signs can appear, but consciousness, vigilance, and orientation are always preserved. There are no systemic abnormalities, given that this is an isolated small-cell vasculitis. The disease can also manifest as an extemporaneous, episodic form. The CSF is generally within normal limits and can present mild lymphocytic pleocytosis. MRI shows monofocal or multifocal abnormalities in both hemispheres that are often non-specific and can present contrast enhancement during relapses.

Syndrome of transient headache and neurological deficits with cerebrospinal fluid lymphocytosis (ICHD-II 7.8) ICHD-II classifies this entity under the heading "Headache attributed to non-vascular intracranial disorder" (code 7.8). It is characterized by prolonged and recurrent episodes of headache preceded by or associated with mild focal neurological symptoms (Lansberg et al., 1999; Fumal et al., 2005; Giorgetti et al., 2005). The CSF shows mild lymphocytic pleocytosis. The MRI scan is generally within normal limits.

Timing and priorities

The infections belonging to this group generally do not constitute medical emergencies. The onset is acute or subacute, while all the clinical signs and symptoms (fever, headache, neck stiffness) are mild to moderate. There follows a stabilization phase lasting a few days, after which the picture generally resolves gradually. In certain conditions, the headache may worsen somewhat, but it is never associated with clear encephalopathy and focal signs are extremely rare. In these situations, the results of the CT scan are often irrelevant; MRI can be carried out within the 24 h following the onset of the headache and is often found to be negative, too. On other occasions it might show slight lepto- and pachymeningeal enhancement. The CSF shows lymphocytic pleocytosis with normal or slightly raised protein levels (generally not in excess of 100 mg/dl). In any case, it is necessary to detect the viral genome in the patient's CSF, by means of the PCR technique.

Comments and "red flags"

The diseases in subgroup 1c are often difficult to tell apart and also to distinguish from other non-infectious diseases that present with some of the same characteristics. The etiological diagnosis is often hindered by failure to conduct prompt CSF analysis. In many cases, only a prolonged period of follow-up will make it possible to reach a definitive diagnosis, since the non-infectious inflammatory diseases listed above, unlike aseptic meningitis, tend to relapse. In these conditions, and on the basis of the current classification, the headache can be definitively coded only retrospectively. In the presence of headache and meningism presenting with the same characteristics as the diseases in group 1c, the clinician should look out for two situations in particular: (1) the presence of OBs in the CSF, which could point to HIV seroconversion syndrome or to paucisymptomatic HSV meningitis; and (2) the presence of very high inflammatory markers from the sixth decade of life onwards, since this would strongly suggest GCA which needs immediate steroid treatment.

Subgroup 1d: ICHD-II 9.2

This group includes conditions characterized by the presence of headache and fever, often associated with malaise and myalgias but without encephalopathy and/or focal signs. The flu-like syndrome and many other systemic infectious diseases are typically characterized by these symptoms (De Marinis and Welch, 1992; Montalto, 2003). Patients are generally unwell, to varying degrees, and nausea and vomiting can be observed, but little is known about the relationship between headache and these symptoms. The patient should be monitored and screened for systemic infections by means of laboratory examinations. Brain CT and CSF analysis are not indicated, at least not unless there appears to be encephalopathy or focal neurological signs.

Comments and "red flags"

Headache associated with systemic infectious diseases and particularly the flu-like syndrome is included in group 1d. It is one of the conditions most frequently encountered in primary care units (Bigal et al., 2000) and it does not constitute a medical emergency. The absence of neck stiffness, focal neurological signs, and encephalopathy can be regarded as a necessary and sufficient clinical criterion to exclude situations of significant CNS involvement. However, clinical and laboratory monitoring is warranted.

Group 2

Subgroup 2a

The diseases in this group have a subtle onset. Patients present with mild to moderate fever and a progression, from mild to severe, of the following conditions: occipital–nuchal headache, neck stiffness, encephalopathy with cranial nerve deficit, epileptic seizures, and frequent myeloradiculopathy. Generally patients do not come to medical attention until days after the onset of the symptoms. This group includes tuberculous meningitis, fungal meningitis, and advanced borreliosis.

Specific conditions

Tuberculous meningitis (ICHD-II 9.1.2) Tuberculosis is still the most common cause of chronic meningitis. Patients with tuberculous meningitis generally have a focus of infection elsewhere, but approximately 25% of cases may have no clinical evidence, or history, of systemic infection. The disease is usually the result of the breakdown of a long-standing granuloma or develops during miliary tuberculosis (>50%). Pulmonary disease is apparently absent in 50% of affected adults. Tuberculous meningitis generally has a subtle onset and a progressive pattern of development with possible accelerations of the symptoms that cause a rapid worsening of the clinical picture (Zuger, 2004). The onset is characterized by low-grade fever, headache, and mild neck stiffness. Over days or weeks the patient shows a progressive sluggishness and develops a severe meningoencephalitis syndrome associated with multiple cranial nerve palsies (III, VI, VII, and VIII), focal neurological deficits, and seizures (Verdon et al., 1996). The headache in tuberculous infection is normally associated with meningitis, less frequently being due to parenchymal dissemination of the disease (miliary disease), to the formation of space-occupying lesions (tumor-like tuberculomas), or to the formation of obstructive hydrocephalus. In these latter three cases, it assumes the characteristics of intracranial hypertension syndrome. On MRI, T_2-weighted images show typical pachy-leptomeningeal enhancement, and hyperintense multifocal lesions, which are ring-enhancing on T_1-weighted images after gadolinium injection. Analysis of the CSF shows normal or increased opening pressure, severe BBB breakdown, low CSF/serum glucose ratio (<40%), and marked pleocytosis ($\geq$300 cells/μl) with lymphocytic predominance. The treatment is based on the four first-line drugs: isoniazid, rifampicin, pyrazinamide, and ethambutol. The infection can be fatal within 5–8 weeks if not treated appropriately.

CNS complications of fungal infections (ICHD-II 9.1.2) Fungal infections can cause serious complications at the level of the CNS (McGinnis, 1983). For purely didactic purposes, these can be divided into three different conditions that, however, tend to overlap, in different ways, in individual patients: meningosis, vasculitis, and parenchymal syndromes. Generally, the full syndrome develops within the space of 3–4 weeks, but there also exist both slower and more aggressive variants. The clinical pattern is characterized by fever, progressive occipital or diffuse headache, neck stiffness, cranial nerve palsy, focal signs, and mentation and consciousness deficits. In the last stage it is possible to observe seizures and worsening of vigilance leading to coma. In rare cases, certain agents (*Cryptococcus, Aspergillus, Mucor, Candida*) can cause large brain abscesses that lead to clear states of intracranial hypertension (see paragraph 2b). Fungal infections rarely affect healthy subjects, as a rule appearing in the immunocompromised, diabetics, the elderly, and patients with lymphoproliferative syndromes under long-term treatment with antibiotics. Neuroimaging investigations show variable pictures reflecting the different ways in which the disease can affect the meninges and brain parenchyma. As a rule, mixed pictures emerge showing involvement of the lepto- and pachymeninges, signs of vasculitis with satellite ischemias, multiple small brain abscesses, or large parenchymal abscesses with a shift of the median line. CSF analysis reveals severe and mixed but prevalently lymphocytic pleocytosis, severe BBB damage, and a CSF/serum glucose ratio lower than 40%. Meningoencephalitis due to *Cryptococcus neoformans* has become much more common since the advent of the HIV era, and it can be the inaugural manifestation of AIDS. *Cryptococcus* has a marked tropism for the CNS and is the major cause of fungal meningitis. It is transmitted by pigeon excreta through inhalation and consequent infection of the lungs. The yeast-like fungus, which has several important virulence factors (polysaccharide capsule, melanin, mannitol), enters the bloodstream and disseminates to the meninges and brain. Treatment consists of amphotericin B and flucytosine followed by fluconazole.

So-called rhinocerebral syndrome warrants particular attention on account of the insidious nature of its initial manifestations and the severity it shows in the space of just a few days. It is a progressive and invasive fungal infection that affects the sinuses, orbits, and brain (de Shazo et al., 1997). The infection can spread to orbital and intracranial structures either by direct invasion or through the blood vessels (Auluck, 2007). The fungus invades the arteries, leading to thrombosis that subsequently causes necrosis of hard and soft tissues. The spread of the infection is associated with progressive facial pain and severe headache. Rhinocerebral syndrome is caused by saprophytic fungi of the order Mucorales and it is typically observed in diabetic ketoacidosis (Ameen et al., 2007).

Advanced borreliosis (ICHD-II 9.1.2) The most frequently observed late neurological complication of borreliosis is chronic progressive encephalomyelitis. It appears 6 weeks, or more, after disease onset and generally does not improve spontaneously (Logigian et al., 1990). Headache is uncommon but, when present, accompanies the progression of the brain encephalopathy, which is characterized by protean focal signs, seizures, ataxia, and hemiparesis. Meningitis is rare, while myelitis and polyradiculoneuritis are common. The CSF shows pleocytosis (100–200 cells/μl), moderate BBB damage, normal or low CSF/serum glucose ratio, and OBs with specific antiborrelia antibodies. Third-generation cephalosporin is the treatment of choice.

Differential diagnosis with non-infectious diseases

The differential diagnosis includes neurosarcoidosis, Behçet's disease, Vogt–Koyanagi–Harada disease, and neoplastic meningitis (primary or metastatic).

Neurosarcoidosis Sarcoidosis is a disorder characterized by multiorgan involvement (uveitis, pulmonary, cutaneous) and variable clinical presentation (Gullapalli and Phillips, 2004). Its cause is unknown. It is more frequently observed in black race and female gender. The disease affects the nervous system in up to 5% of cases, even though the estimations vary considerably in the different samples studied. In rare cases, neurosarcoidosis is the first manifestation of the systemic disease. Its main anatomical–pathological characteristic is the inflammatory granuloma that often affects the base of the skull causing chronic or chronic-relapsing meningitis. The features of the headache are essentially linked to this anatomical involvement which also leads to cranial multineuritis, often bilateral and involving the facial, optic, auditory, and trigeminal nerves. From a phenomenological point of view, the headache, at onset, has the characteristics of chronic meningosis, presenting with subcontinuous holocranial or occipital–nuchal pain, of varying intensity, which progressively worsens. In the full-blown phase, in relation to the presence of space-occupying granulomas, there may also be signs of intracranial hypotension with papilledema and persistent and violent headache that is aggravated by exertion. The chronic inflammation of the meninges can cause obstructive hydrocephalus. Neurosarcoidosis is difficult to diagnose; indeed, it may be impossible to diagnose in the absence of systemic signs. The tuberculin skin test and the blood and CSF concentration of angiotensin-converting enzyme are of little real use. It is often necessary to have recourse to a biopsy of seemingly unaffected tissue (lymph node, muscle, conjunctiva). Brain and spine MRI shows pachy- and leptomeningeal involvement with cranial nerves and multiradicular enhancing lesions at cervical, dorsal, and lumbar level. Obstructive hydrocephalus can be observed in the final stage of the disease. The CSF is generally characterized by mild to moderate lymphocytic pleocytosis, raised protein levels, and marked BBB damage.

Behçet's disease (ICHD-II 6.4.3) Behçet's disease is a systemic disease that in 5–20% of cases affects the CNS. It is more prevalent in Middle Eastern countries. It may be more frequent in young men and it is associated with human leukocyte antigen (HLA) B-51. Generally, its most frequent manifestations are uveitis and recurrent oral and vaginal ulcers. Headache is a frequent symptom; its features differ according to the type of CNS damage caused by the disease (Akman-Demir et al., 1999; Borhani-Haghighi et al., 2006). The most frequent neurological complication is meningitis or chronic meningoencephalitis which is associated with chronic-progressive occipital–nuchal headache of variable intensity as well as focal signs and possible focal epileptic seizures. The MRI pattern, in meningoencephalitis, is characterized by leptomeningeal enhancement with parenchymal lesions at brainstem, internal capsule, and basal ganglia level (Mnif et al., 2006). More rarely, the disease can cause venous sinus thrombosis with headache resembling that associated with intracranial hypertension. The appearance of the neurological complications is always associated with a reactivation of the signs and symptoms typical of the systemic disease. The CSF almost always shows an inflammatory profile with varying degrees of lymphocytic pleocytosis and hyperproteinorachia. There is no diagnostic biohumoral marker. Infliximab has proven to be effective in the treatment of both uveitis and extraocular manifestations of Behçet's disease, making possible a significant reduction in the daily dose of corticosteroids administered (Accorinti et al., 2007).

Vogt–Koyanagi–Harada disease (ICHD-II 6.4) Vogt–Koyanagi–Harada disease is a bilateral panuveitis associated with exudative retinal detachment. It typically affects young adults, and occurs most frequently among Asians. The disease is often associated with headache and meningism (Cho et al., 2008). Other usual conditions are dysacusia and vitiligo. CSF analysis, which should always be performed, is characterized by lymphocytic pleocytosis without BBB breakdown and a normal glucose level (Rao et al., 2007; Tsai et al., 2007). Steroid treatment may be effective.

Neoplastic meningitis (ICHD-II 7.4.3) Neoplastic meningitis or carcinomatous meningosis is due to the widespread multifocal involvement of brain, spine, and roots by a metastatic or primary brain tumor (Bleyer and Byrne, 1988). The clinical symptoms include severe headache, neck pain, somnolence, alteration of mental status, and cranial nerve palsies. Hydrocephalus and raised intracranial pressure can develop, leading to nausea, vomiting, and severe impairment of consciousness, ultimately resulting in coma. In 90% of cases the diagnosis of the primary tumor precedes that of the meningeal metastases. The prognosis is very severe: untreated patients usually die within 1–2 months. Intrathecal administration of chemotherapy (methotrexate or cytosine arabinoside, alone or in combination) increases the median survival time to between 4.5 and 7.2 months (Glantz and Walters, 1998). Liposomal cytarabine has recently been proven to prolong the time to neurological progression (Rueda Dominguez et al., 2005).

Neoplastic meningitis occurs in four main categories of malignant diseases: (1) solid tumors (breast, lung, melanoma); (2) leukemia; (3) non-Hodgkin lymphoma; and (4) primary brain tumors (mainly anaplastic oligodendrogliomas and anaplastic ependymomas). Differential diagnosis between neoplastic meningitis and infectious meningitis in subgroup 2a is often challenging. In both cases, the CSF shows severe BBB damage and a decreased CSF/serum glucose ratio, while the pleocytosis is generally mild in neoplastic meningitis and marked in infectious meningitis. The main problem concerns the difficulties detecting tumor cells in the CSF. A minimum of 8 ml of CSF on three separate occasions is required in order to reach a diagnostic sensitivity of over 80% (Glantz et al., 1998). CSF cytological examination, performed according to a rigorous protocol, may be the optimal diagnostic and outcome measure in neoplastic meningitis (MacKenzie, 1996). Contrast-enhanced brain and spine MRI show leptomeningeal involvement in 70% of patients. In neoplastic meningitis the leptomeningeal enhancement is usually patchy, while in infectious meningitis it is diffuse and uniform.

Timing and priorities

This is the group embracing the severe progressive forms of meningoencephalitis. Many cases of chronic-progressive meningoencephalitis are caused by opportunistic infections favored by immunosuppression. The headache and other clinical features of the disease have a subtle onset but generally become significant within days or weeks. A feature often associated with headache, even in the absence of focal signs, is mental sluggishness, or sometimes an out-and-out confusional state. In these forms there is no investigation that needs to be carried out urgently; instead the diagnostic process is long and complex and has to be conducted in stages. It is a good idea to start with brain and spine MRI, followed by lumbar puncture and blood and urine cultures. If these investigations fail to confirm the hypothesis of an infectious disease, the next condition to consider are non-infectious granulomatous (sarcoid) forms, several rare variants of vasculitis (e.g., Behçet's disease), or neoplastic meningosis. This last condition can arise in a phase of apparent long-lasting quiescence of the underlying disease, particularly in the presence of solid tumors (lung cancer, melanoma).

Comments and "red flags"

This is a difficult and controversial group. Many patients who present with the clinical characteristics of this group of diseases receive a late diagnosis and, in the most unfortunate cases, their condition worsens progressively as they fail to respond to empirical therapies. The characteristics of the headache, however, even at onset, make it possible to exclude diseases belonging to the group of acute forms of meningoencephalitis and can direct the physician's attention towards the progressive inflammatory encephalopathies. In our opinion, all patients with progressive headache and systemic signs of mild to moderate infectious disease could potentially be immunocompromised and should be screened for HIV infection. In particular, *Cryptococcus* and tuberculous meningitis are the two major causes of chronic progressive meningitis in AIDS. In some situations, such as tuberculous meningitis, neurosarcoidosis, and Behçet's disease, the diagnostic difficulties are, more than anything, due to the lack of reliable diagnostic markers. In these cases, too, it can be difficult to code the headache. Chronic, progressively worsening forms of meningoencephalitis have some characteristics in common with neoplastic meningitis, and headache is one of them. Many patients with solid neoplasias or leukemia/non-Hodgkin lymphoma, because of the immunosuppression induced by the neoplasia or by the chemo- or radiotherapy undertaken, can develop fungal meningitis. In these cases, differential diagnosis between meningoencephalitis and neoplastic meningitis is crucial, because of the very different therapeutic courses needed. Among the primary brain tumors, anaplastic oligodendroglioma is the CNS glioma that most frequently involves the leptomeninges (Kros et al., 2005).

Subgroup 2b

As above, but accompanied by signs of intracranial hypertension of varying severity. The group includes brain abscess and communicating hydrocephalus. See the section on group 1b for a detailed description, timing, and priorities.

Group 3

This group includes chronic, non-progressive, subcontinuous "benign" headache of moderate intensity, generally associated with neck stiffness but not with encephalopathy and/or focal signs. In some cases, the pattern can be relapsing or chronic-relapsing. Group 3 includes: headache attributed to HIV/AIDS uncomplicated by meningitis or opportunistic infections of the CNS; chronic postinfectious headache; and Mollaret meningitis (the latter presents features overlapping with group 1c).

Specific conditions

Headache attributed to HIV/AIDS See Section 1.

Chronic postinfectious headache See Section 1.

Mollaret meningitis In 1952 Mollaret described the first case of recurrent pleocytic meningitis (Mollaret, 1952). This is a benign illness characterized by severe headache, neck stiffness, and possible seizures. Considering its variable clinical course, this condition could be classified in both group 1b and group 3. The characteristics of this disease may be considered unique, since it is a subacute, relapsing condition. The disease resolves within 48 h with full recovery and it frequently recurs over a number of months or years. Analysis of the CSF analysis shows mixed pleocytosis, mild BBB damage, and peculiar large mononuclear "endothelial" cells. PCR has revealed that most cases of Mollaret meningitis are associated with HSV-2 infection (Gignoux et al., 1998; Tyler, 2004).

Differential diagnosis with non-infectious diseases

The differential diagnosis includes new daily-persistent headache (NDPH), idiopathic intracranial hypertension, spontaneous low CSF pressure headache, and "slow variant" GCA.

New daily-persistent headache (ICHD-II code 4.8) NDPH is a subtype of chronic daily headache. Diaz-Mitoma et al. (1987) found evidence of Epstein–Barr virus infection in NDPH patients. Li and Rozen (2002) retrospectively described a large cohort and found that age at onset ranged from 12 to 78 years. Eighty-two percent of patients were able to pinpoint the exact day their headache had started, and onset had occurred in relation to an infection or flu-like illness in 30%. A prior headache history was found in 38% of patients. Laboratory testing and neuroimaging in all patients were normal except for Epstein–Barr virus antibody titers, which were positive in 71% of 7 patients tested, indicating past infection with the virus.

Idiopathic intracranial hypertension (pseudotumor cerebri) (ICHD-II 7.1.1) This condition is characterized by increased intracranial pressure without MRI evidence of space-occupying lesions or hydrocephalus. In some instances, enlargement of the subarachnoid space around the optic nerve has been observed.

Clinical manifestations are holocranial headache of moderate intensity (throbbing or tension-type), neck stiffness, nausea, reversible loss of vision, and tinnitus. The headache generally increases in clinostatism. Bilateral papilledema is almost mandatory for diagnosis. CSF opening pressure is elevated (>250 mmH_2O).

Spontaneous low CSF pressure headache (ICHD-II 7.2.3) This condition is characterized by orthostatic tension-type headache associated with clear instrumental evidence of low pressure and CSF volume depletion (Miyazawa et al., 2003). A number of predisposing factors have been described, such as congenital weakness of the dural sac, connective tissue disorders, and meningeal diverticula. Previous trauma is frequent but not essential for the diagnosis, but other possibilities have been described. The most frequently observed symptoms are bilateral, non-throbbing headache, usually occurring within a few minutes of assuming the upright position. The headache can present in several other patterns and may be variably associated with nausea, vomiting, interscapular, neck, or low-back pain, sixth cranial nerve palsy, upper-limb pain, photophobia, and dizziness. Brain and cervical spine MRI are usually characterized by diffuse lepto-pachymeningeal enhancement, descent of cerebellar tonsils, obliteration of the prepontine and perichiasmatic cisterns, bilateral subdural fluid collection (hematoma/hygroma), and dilation of the cervical epidural venous plexus. The site of the CSF leakage (usually at the level of thoracic spines) can be detected by means of various techniques: CT, MR myelography, and indium-111 cisternography. CSF opening pressure is generally low (<60 mmH_2O) but can sometimes be normal. Mild BBB breakdown and lymphocytic pleocytosis can be detected.

"Slow variant" giant cell arteritis (ICHD-II 6.4.1) This condition is discussed in detail in the section on group 1c. In some cases the course of temporal arteritis may be particularly mild and slow, and in 10% of cases the ESR may be within normal limits.

Timing and priorities

Since this type of headache does not present aggressive characteristics, it does not usually generate alarm or create the need for urgent medical intervention. A few reports published in the past decade have raised the possibility of a relationship between a chronic form of this headache and HIV infection without evidence of concomitant opportunistic infections. In fact, to date, there are no epidemiological or biological data establishing a correlation between this symptom and the infection. This topic is discussed at length in the first part of this chapter.

Comments and "red flags"

The combination of chronic headache and low-grade fever should not initially prompt a hypothesis of an infectious disease, given that it is more frequently associated with systemic inflammatory diseases. Having said that, HIV testing and analysis of the CSF using the PCR technique to look for the possible viral genome should always be performed in the presence of any chronic neurological disease of unknown origin. The existence of NDPH and chronic postinfectious headache has been reported in the literature, but both of these are rare forms that should be considered only after the exclusion of other diseases. The diagnosis of the chronic headache form does not demand the application of urgent procedures, but it is complex and requires a series of separate investigations since the conditions that must be taken into consideration in the differential diagnosis, if untreated, will cause irreversible damage. The optic nerve is a potential target of both GCA and benign intracranial hypertension syndrome. The following examinations should always be performed: ESR, brain and spine MRI, MR angiography, CSF (routine examination and opening pressure), and complete ophthalmological evaluation.

Group 4

In this group there is pain/headache localized in a specific part of the face, frequently with asymmetrical distribution, not associated with encephalopathy or signs of CNS impairment (ear, nose, eye, tooth, mouth, and sinus infections). See chapter 54: "Headache or facial pain attributed to disorders of cranium, neck, eyes, ears, nose, sinuses, teeth, mouth, or other facial or cranial structures" (Headache Classification Subcommittee of the International Headache Society, 2004).

GENERAL CONCLUSIONS

In this chapter, we set out to illustrate the nosography of headaches attributed to infection and to discuss the main issues relating to their differential diagnosis. ICHD-II, which has furnished systematic diagnostic criteria based on etiological principles, may be regarded as an important evolution of ICHD-I. This new approach has undoubtedly helped headache researchers to carry their work forward; indeed, since 2004, the year in which it was first published, the new version has been cited repeatedly in the international literature. Obviously, ICHD-II has its flaws, already identified by leading experts in the field. Some of these flaws can probably be eliminated through the planning of further primary studies while others are intrinsic to the method. Some parts of the classification clearly feel the need for relevant, good-quality literature, currently lacking, and there thus exist forms that cannot be classified efficiently. Moreover, this classification model, based on an etiological approach, does not always accommodate real situations. For example, the section on lymphocytic meningitis lumps together a series of diseases of differing etiology which share only some physical–chemical characteristics of the CSF.

In the first part of this chapter, then, we concentrated on providing a description of ICHD-II together with a few critical observations based on the available literature. In the second section we suggested a different classification model based on a simple, "symptom-based" algorithm, the aim being to complement the first, shifting the focus from applied research to clinical practice. This model concentrates mainly on the first stage in the diagnostic process, where there automatically arises the difficult question of differential diagnosis. The infectious and non-infectious diseases considered in the differential diagnosis are nearly all characterized by potential clinical variability, which determines different courses and different prognoses. In the course of the same disease, the headache can improve, become chronic, or worsen. The criteria we have adopted reflect the most common features of the headache at onset in the various diagnostic groups and subgroups and the most frequent of the CNS manifestations that dominate the clinical picture.

Our aim was to provide the reader with a complete instrument that is easy to interpret and that meets the needs of both researcher and clinician.

References

Accorinti M, Pirraglia MP, Paroli MP et al. (2007). Infliximab treatment for ocular and extraocular manifestations of Behçet's disease. Jpn J Ophthalmol 51: 191–196.

Akman-Demir G, Serdaroglu P, Tasçi B (1999). Clinical patterns of neurological involvement in Behçet's disease: evaluation of 200 patients. The Neuro-Behçet Study Group. Brain 122: 2171–2182.

Albright TA, Binns HJ, Katz BZ (2002). Side effects of and compliance with malaria prophylaxis in children. J Travel Med 9: 289–292.

Ameen M, Arenas R, Martinez-Luna E et al. (2007). The emergence of mucormycosis as an important opportunistic fungal infection: five cases presenting to a tertiary referral center for mycology. Int J Dermatol 46: 380–384.

Anderson M (1993). Management of cerebral infection. J Neurol Neurosurg Psychiatry 56: 1243–1258.

Angstwurm K, Hanisch UK, Gassemi T et al. (2004). Tyrosine kinase inhibition reduces inflammation in the acute stage of experimental pneumococcal meningitis. Infect Immun 72 (6): 3294–3298.

Anlar B, Basaran C, Kose G et al. (2003). Acute disseminated encephalomyelitis in children: outcome and prognosis. Neuropediatrics 34: 194–199.

Auluck A (2007). Maxillary necrosis by mucormycosis. A case report and literature review. Med Oral Patol Oral Cir Bucal 12 (5): 360–364.

Berger JR, Stein N, Pall L (1996). Headache and human immunodeficiency virus infection: a case control study. Eur Neurol 36 (4): 229–233.

Bigal ME, Bordini CA, Speciali JG (2000). Etiology and distribution of headaches in two Brazilian primary care units. Headache 40 (3): 241–247.

Bleyer WA, Byrne TN (1988). Leptomeningeal cancer in leukemia and solid tumors. Curr Probl Cancer 12: 181–188.

Bohr V, Hansen B, Kjersem H et al. (1983). Sequelae from bacterial meningitis and their relation to the clinical condition during acute illness, based on 667 questionnaire returns. Part II of a three part series. J Infect 7 (2): 102–110.

Borhani-Haghighi A, Samangooie S, Ashjazadeh N et al. (2006). Neurological manifestations of Behçet's disease. Saudi Med J 27 (10): 1542–1546.

Brew BJ, Miller J (1993). Human immunodeficiency virus-related headache. Neurology 43 (6): 1098–1100.

Busti AJ, Hall RG, Margolis DM (2004). Atazanavir for the treatment of human immunodeficiency virus infection. Pharmacotherapy 24 (12): 1732–1747.

Butteriss DJ, Ramesh V, Birchall D (2003). Serial MRI in a case of familial hemiplegic migraine. Neuroradiology 45 (5): 300–303.

Cano Vargas-Machuca E, Mondéjar-Marín B, Navarro-Muñoz S et al. (2006). Recurrent aseptic meningitis secondary to taking ibuprofen and ketorolac. Rev Neurol 42 (4): 217–219.

Capra C, Monza GM, Meazza G et al. (2000). Trimethoprim-sulfamethoxazole-induced aseptic meningitis: case report and literature review. Intensive Care Med 26 (2): 212–214.

Carpenter RR, Petersdorf RG (1962). The clinical spectrum of bacterial meningitis. Am J Med 33: 262–275.

Caselli RJ, Hunder GG (1997). Giant cell (temporal) arteritis. Neurol Clin 15 (4): 893–902.

Castillo SA, Hernandez JE, Brothers CH (2006). Long-term safety and tolerability of the lamivudine/abacavir combination as components of highly active antiretroviral therapy. Drug Saf 29 (9): 811–826.

Chan YC, Ho KH, Tambyah PA et al. (2001). Listeria meningoencephalitis: two cases and a review of the literature. Ann Acad Med Singapore 30 (6): 659–663.

Cho JH, Ahn JY, Byeon SH et al. (2008). Thunderclap headache as initial manifestation of Vogt–Koyanagi–Harada disease. Headache 48: 153–155.

Covelli V, Massari F, Fallacara C et al. (1991). Increased spontaneous release of tumor necrosis factor-alpha/cachectin in headache patients. A possible correlation with plasma endotoxin and hypothalamic–pituitary–adrenal axis. Int J Neurosci 61 (1–2): 53–60.

Cruciatti B, Beltrame A, Ruscio M et al. (2006). Neurological manifestation of tick-borne encephalitis in North-Eastern Italy. Neurol Sci 27 (2): 122–124.

Cvetkovic RS, Goa KL (2003). Lopinavir/ritonavir: a review of its use in the management of HIV infection. Drugs 63 (8): 769–802.

De Fusco M, Marconi R, Silvestri L et al. (2003). Haploinsufficiency of ATP1A2 encoding the Na^+/K^+ pump alpha2 subunit associated with familial hemiplegic migraine type 2. Nat Genet 33 (2): 192–196.

De Marinis M, Welch KM (1992). Headache associated with non-cephalic infections: classification and mechanisms. Cephalalgia 12 (4): 197–201.

de Shazo RD, Chapin K, Swain RE (1997). Fungal sinusitis. N Engl J Med 337 (4): 254–259.

Deibel R, Woodall JP, Decher WJ et al. (1975). Lymphocytic choriomeningitis virus in man. Serologic evidence of association with pet hamsters. JAMA 232 (5): 501–504.

Diaz-Mitoma F, Vanast WJ, Tyrrell DL (1987). Increased frequency of Epstein–Barr virus excretion in patients with new daily persistent headaches. Lancet 1: 411–415.

Ducros A, Thomsen LL (2006). Sporadic and familial hemiplegic migraine. In: J Olesen, PJ Goatsby, NM Ramadan et al. (Eds.), The Headaches. Lippincott Williams & Wilkins, Philadelphia, pp. 577–593.

Durand ML, Calderwood SB, Weber DJ et al. (1993). Acute bacterial meningitis in adults. A review of 493 episodes. N Engl J Med 328 (1): 21–28.

Dutt AK, Moers D, Stead WW (1983). Undesirable side effects of isoniazid and rifampin in largely twice-weekly short-course chemotherapy for tuberculosis. Am Rev Respir Dis 128 (3): 419–424.

Elewski BE, Cáceres HW, Deleon L et al. (2008). Terbinafine hydrochloride oral granules versus oral griseofulvin suspension in children with tinea capitis: results of two randomized, investigator-blinded, multicenter, international, controlled trials. J Am Acad Dermatol 59: 41–54.

Evers S, Wibbeke B, Reichelt D et al. (2000). The impact of HIV infection on primary headache. Unexpected findings from retrospective, cross-sectional, and prospective analyses. Pain 85 (1–2): 191–200.

Fitzsimons RB, Wolfenden WH (1985). Migraine coma. Meningitic migraine with cerebral oedema associated with a new form of autosomal dominant cerebellar ataxia. Brain 108 (3): 555–577.

Fleming DT, McQuillan GM, Johnson RE et al. (1997). Herpes simplex virus type 2 in the United States, 1976 to 1994. N Engl J Med 337 (16): 1105–1111.

Fumal A, Vandenheede M, Coppola G et al. (2005). The syndrome of transient headache with neurological deficits and CSF lymphocytosis (HaNDL): electrophysiological findings suggesting a migrainous pathophysiology. Cephalalgia 25 (9): 754–758.

Gignoux L, Ryvlin P, Najioullah F et al. (1998). Recurrent Mollaret's meningitis of herpetic origin. Presse Med 27 (29): 1470–1472.

Gilden DH, Kleinschmidt-DeMasters BK, LaGuardia JJ et al. (2000). Neurologic complications of the reactivation of varicella-zoster virus. N Engl J Med 342 (9): 635–645.

Giorgetti A, Mariani G, Patruno GM et al. (2005). The transient syndrome of headache with neurological deficits, cerebrospinal fluid pleocytosis and acute confusional state: a case report. J Headache Pain 6 (6): 476.

Glantz MJ, Walters BC (1998). Diagnosis and outcome measures in trials for neoplastic meningitis: a review of the literature and clinical experience. Neurosurg Focus 4 (6): e4.

Glantz MJ, Cole BF, Glantz LK et al. (1998). Cerebrospinal fluid cytology in patients with cancer: minimizing false-negative results. Cancer 82 (4): 733–739.

Goldstein J (1990). Headache and acquired immunodeficiency syndrome. Neurol Clin 8 (4): 947–960.

Gray F, Bélec L, Lescs MC et al. (1994). Varicella-zoster virus infection of the central nervous system in the acquired immune deficiency syndrome. Brain 117 (Pt 5): 987–999.

Gullapalli D, Phillips LH 2nd (2004). Neurosarcoidosis. Curr Neurol Neurosci Rep 4 (6): 441–447.

Headache Classification Committee of the International Headache Society (1988). Classification and diagnostic criteria for headache disorders, cranial neuralgias and facial pain. Cephalalgia (Suppl. 7): 1–96.

Headache Classification Committee of the International Headache Society (2004). The International Classification of Headache Disorders: 2nd edition. Cephalalgia 24 (Suppl. 1): 9–160.

Hirsch MS, Moellering RC Jr, Pope HG et al. (1974). Lymphocytic-choriomeningitis-virus infection traced to a pet hamster. N Engl J Med 291 (12): 610–612.

Hoffmann O, Keilwerth N, Bille MB et al. (2002). Triptans reduce the inflammatory response in bacterial meningitis. J Cereb Blood Flow Metab 22 (8): 988–996.

Holloway RG, Kieburtz KD (1995). Headache and the human immunodeficiency virus type 1 infection. Headache 35 (5): 245–255.

Hulgan T, Tebas P, Canter JA et al. (2008). Hemochromatosis gene polymorphisms, mitochondrial haplogroups, and peripheral lipoatrophy during antiretroviral therapy. J Infect Dis 197 (6): 858–866.

Iravani A (1991). Comparative, double-blind, prospective, multicenter trial of temafloxacin versus trimethoprim-sulfamethoxazole in uncomplicated urinary tract infections in women. Antimicrob Agents Chemother 35 (9): 1777–1781.

Kaiser R (2002). Tick-borne encephalitis (TBE) in Germany and clinical course of the disease. Int J Med Microbiol 291 (Suppl. 33): 58–61.

Kleinschmidt-DeMasters BK, Gilden DH (2001). Varicella-zoster virus infections of the nervous system: clinical and pathologic correlates. Arch Pathol Lab Med 125 (6): 770–780.

Kros JM, Zeng P, Wolbers JG et al. (2005). Oligodendroglial tumors. In: MS Berger, MD Prados (Eds.), Textbook of Neuro-oncology. Elsevier-Saunders, Philadelphia, pp. 167–176.

Lagathu C, Eustace B, Prot M et al. (2007). Some HIV antiretrovirals increase oxidative stress and alter chemokine, cytokine or adiponectin production in human adipocytes and macrophages. Antivir Ther 12 (4): 489–500.

Lakeman FD, Whitley RJ (1995). Diagnosis of herpes simplex encephalitis: application of polymerase chain reaction to cerebrospinal fluid from brain-biopsied patients and correlation with disease. National Institute of Allergy and Infectious Diseases Collaborative Antiviral Study Group. J Infect Dis 171 (4): 857–863.

Lansberg MG, Woolfenden AR, Norbash AM et al. (1999). Headache with neurological deficits and CSF lymphocytosis: a transient ischemic attack mimic. J Stroke Cerebrovasc Dis 8 (1): 42–44.

Li D, Rozen TD (2002). The clinical characteristics of new daily persistent headache. Cephalalgia 22 (1): 66–69.

Lipton RB, Feraru ER, Weiss G et al. (1991). Headache in HIV-1-related disorders. Headache 31 (8): 518–522.

Logigian EF, Kaplan RF, Steere AC (1990). Chronic neurologic manifestations of Lyme disease. N Engl J Med 323: 1438–1444.

Louis, Ohgaki, Wiestler et al. (Eds.) (2007). WHO Classification of Tumours of the Central Nervous System. IARC, Lyon.

MacKenzie JM (1996). Malignant meningitis: a rational approach to cerebrospinal fluid cytology. J Clin Pathol 49 (6): 497–499.

Marchioni E, Galimberti CA, Soragna D et al. (1995). Familial hemiplegic migraine versus migraine with prolonged aura: an uncertain diagnosis in a family report. Neurology 45 (1): 33–37.

Marchioni E, Marinou-Aktipi K, Uggetti C et al. (2002). Effectiveness of intravenous immunoglobulin treatment in adult patients with steroid-resistant monophasic or recurrent acute disseminated encephalomyelitis. J Neurol 249 (1): 100–104.

Marchioni E, Ravaglia S, Piccolo G et al. (2005). Postinfectious inflammatory disorders: subgroups based on prospective follow-up. Neurology 65 (7): 1057–1065.

Marchioni E, Tavazzi E, Bono G et al. (2006). Headache attributed to infection: observations on the IHS classification (ICHD-II). Cephalalgia 26 (12): 1427–1433.

Matsumoto J, Saver JL, Brennan KC et al. (2005). Mitochondrial encephalomyopathy with lactic acidosis and stroke (MELAS). Rev Neurol Dis 2 (1): 30–34.

McGinnis MR (1983). Detection of fungi in cerebrospinal fluid. Am J Med 75 (1B): 129–138.

Mirsattari SM, Power C, Nath A (1999). Primary headaches in HIV-infected patients. Headache 39 (1): 3–10.

Miyazawa K, Shiga Y, Hasegawa T et al. (2003). CSF hypovolemia vs intracranial hypotension in "spontaneous intracranial hypotension syndrome". Neurology 60 (6): 941–947.

Mnif N, Rajhi H, Mlika N et al. (2006). MRI findings in neuro-Behçet's disease. J Neuroradiol 33 (4): 250–254.

Mocellin R, Walterfang M, Velakoulis D (2007). Hashimoto's encephalopathy: epidemiology, pathogenesis and management. CNS Drugs 21 (10): 799–811.

Mollaret P (1952). Benign recurrent pleocytic meningitis and its presumed causative virus. J Nerv Ment Dis 16 (6): 1072–1080.

Molloy ES, Hajj-Ali RA (2007). Primary angiitis of the central nervous system. Curr Treat Options Neurol 9 (3): 169–175.

Montalto NJ (2003). An office-based approach to influenza: clinical diagnosis and laboratory testing. Am Fam Physician 67 (1): 111–118.

Motta E, Rosciszewska D, Miller K (1995). Hemiplegic migraine with CSF abnormalities. Headache 35 (6): 368–370.

Muzi F, Orlando G, Ielpo B et al. (2005). Amantadine monotherapy is ineffective in the treatment of hepatitis C virus recurrence in the post-liver transplantation setting. Transplant Proc 37 (4): 1705–1707.

Mylonakis E, Hohmann EL, Calderwood SB (1998). Central nervous system infection with *Listeria monocytogenes*. 33 years' experience at a general hospital and review of 776 episodes from the literature. Medicine (Baltimore) 77 (5): 313–336.

Nadeau SE (1997). Diagnostic approach to central and peripheral nervous system vasculitis. Neurol Clin 15 (4): 759–777.

Neufeld MY, Treves TA, Chistik V et al. (1999). Postmeningitis headache. Headache 39 (2): 132–134.

Odaka M, Yuki N, Yamada M et al. (2003). Bickerstaff's brainstem encephalitis: clinical features of 62 cases and a subgroup associated with Guillain-Barré syndrome. Brain 126 (10): 2279–2290.

Olesen J (1993). IHS classification: present and future. Cephalalgia 13 (Suppl. 12): 94.

Olesen J (2006). International classification of headache disorders, second edition (ICHD-2): current status and future revisions. Cephalalgia 26 (12): 1409–1410.

Ophoff RA, Terwindt GM, Vergouwe MN et al. (1996). Familial hemiplegic migraine and episodic ataxia type-2 are caused by mutations in the Ca^{2+} channel gene CACNL1A4. Cell 87 (3): 543–552.

Parney IF, Prados MD (2005). Glioblastoma multiforme. In: MS Berger, MD Prados (Eds.), Textbook of Neuro-oncology. Elsevier-Saunders, Philadelphia, pp. 143–148.

Perry CM, Wagstaff AJ (1998). Interferon-alpha-n1: a review of its pharmacological properties and therapeutic efficacy in the management of chronic viral hepatitis. BioDrugs 9 (2): 125–154.

Rao NA, Sukavatcharin S, Tsai JH (2007). Vogt–Koyanagi–Harada disease diagnostic criteria. Int Ophthalmol 27 (2–3): 195–199.

Rasmussen BK, Olesen J (1992). Symptomatic and nonsymptomatic headaches in a general population. Neurology 42 (6): 1225–1231.

Ravaglia S, Piccolo G, Ceroni M et al. (2007). Severe steroid resistant post-infectious encephalomyelitis: general features and effects of IVIg. J Neurol 254: 1518–1523.

Reik L Jr, Burgdorfer W, Donaldson JO (1986). Neurologic abnormalities in Lyme disease without erytema chronicum migrans. Ann J Med 81: 73–78.

Revello MG, Baldanti F, Sarasini A et al. (1997). Quantitation of herpes simplex virus DNA in cerebrospinal fluid of patients with herpes simplex encephalitis by the polymerase chain reaction. Clin Diagn Virol 7 (3): 183–191.

Roos KL, Tunkel AR, Scheld M (2004). Acute bacterial meningitis. In: WM Scheld, RJ Whitley, CM Marra (Eds.), Infections of the Central Nervous System. Lippincott Williams & Wilkins, Philadelphia, pp. 347–422.

Rueda Domínguez A, Olmos Hidalgo D, Viciana Garrido R et al. (2005). Liposomal cytarabine (Depocyte) for the treatment of neoplastic meningitis. Clin Transl Oncol 7 (6): 232–238.

Sawyer MH, Rotbart HA (2004). Viral meningitis and aseptic meningitis sindrome. In: WM Scheld, RJ Whitley, CM Marra (Eds.), Infections of the Central Nervous System. Lippincott Williams & Wilkins, Philadelphia, pp. 75–93.

Schraeder PL, Burns RA (1980). Hemiplegic migraine associated with an aseptic meningeal reaction. Arch Neurol 37 (6): 377–379.

Singer EJ, Kim J, Fahy-Chandon B et al. (1996). Headache in ambulatory HIV-1-infected men enrolled in a longitudinal study. Neurology 47 (2): 487–494.

Solbrig MV (2000). Viral infections. In: WG Bradley, RB Daroff, GM Fenichel et al. (Eds.), Neurology in Clinical Practice, Vol. 2. Butterworth-Heinemann, Woburn, pp. 1353–1373.

Solbrig MV, Healy JF, Jay CA (2000). Bacterial infections. In: WG Bradley, RB Daroff, GM Fenichel et al. (Eds.), Neurology in Clinical Practice, Vol. 2. Butterworth-Heinemann, Woburn, pp. 1317–1351.

Spranger M, Spranger S, Schwab S et al. (1999). Familial hemiplegic migraine with cerebellar ataxia and paroxysmal psychosis. Eur Neurol 41 (3): 150–152.

Stanek RJ, Mufson MA (1999). A 20-year epidemiological study of pneumococcal meningitis. Clin Infect Dis 28 (6): 1265–1272.

Strassman AM, Raymond SA (1997). On the origin of headaches. Endeavour 21 (3): 97–100.

Tamagno G, Federspil G, Murialdo G (2006). Clinical and diagnostic aspects of encephalopathy associated with autoimmune thyroid disease (or Hashimoto's encephalopathy). Intern Emerg Med 1 (1): 15–23.

Tenembaum S, Chitnis T, Ness J et al. (2007). Acute disseminated encephalomyelitis. Neurology 68 (16 Suppl. 2): S23–S36.

Tsai JH, Sukavatcharin S, Rao NA (2007). Utility of lumbar puncture in diagnosis of Vogt–Koyanagi–Harada disease. Int Ophthalmol 27 (2–3): 189–194.

Tyler KL (2004). Herpes simplex virus infections of the central nervous system: encephalitis and meningitis, including Mollaret's. Herpes 11 (Suppl. 2): 57A–64A.

Vanzee BE, Douglas RG, Betts RF et al. (1975). Lymphocytic choriomeningitis in university hospital personnel. Clinical features. Am J Med 58 (6): 803–809.

Varkey B, Varkey L (2004). EEG in hemiplegic migraine. Neurol India 52 (1): 134.

Verdon R, Chevret S, Laissy JP et al. (1996). Tuberculous meningitis in adults: review of 48 cases. Clin Infect Dis 22 (6): 982–988.

Weber JR, Sakai F (2006). Headache attributed to infection. In: J Olesen, PJ Goatsby, NM Ramadan et al. (Eds.), The Headaches. Lippincott Williams & Wilkins, Philadelphia, pp. 981–987.

Whitley RJ (2004). Herpes simplex virus. In: WM Scheld, RJ Whitley, CM Marra (Eds.), Infections of the Central Nervous System. Lippincott Williams & Wilkins, Philadelphia, pp. 123–144.

Whitley RJ, Soong SJ, Dolin R et al. (1977). Adenine arabinoside therapy of biopsy-proved herpes simplex encephalitis. National Institute of Allergy and Infectious Diseases collaborative antiviral study. N Engl J Med 297 (6): 289–294.

Whitley RJ, Soong SJ, Hirsch MS et al. (1981). Herpes simplex encephalitis: vidarabine therapy and diagnostic problems. N Engl J Med 304 (6): 313–318.

Williamson DJ, Hargreaves RJ (2001). Neurogenic inflammation in the context of migraine. Microsc Res Tech 53 (3): 167–178.

Zuger A (2004). Tuberculosis. In: WM Scheld, RJ Whitley, CM Marra (Eds.), Infections of the Central Nervous System. Lippincott Williams & Wilkins, Philadelphia, pp. 441–459.

Handbook of Clinical Neurology, Vol. 97 (3rd series)
Headache
G. Nappi and M.A. Moskowitz, Editors

Chapter 53

Headache attributed to disorders of homeostasis

DAVID W. DODICK [1]* AND CARLOS A. BORDINI [2]
[1]*Department of Neurology, Mayo Clinic Arizona, Phoenix, AZ, USA*
[2]*Department of Neurology, Ribeirão Preto Medical School, São Paulo, Brazil*

INTRODUCTION

Headache associated with disorders of homeostasis has been defined using operational diagnostic criteria established by the revised International Classification of Headache Disorders (ICHD-II: Headache Classification Subcommittee of the International Headache Society, 2004), having previously been referred to as headache associated with metabolic or systemic disease. The use of the term "homeostasis" was felt to capture the range of disorders of homeostatic mechanisms affecting a variety of organ systems, including altered arterial blood gases, systemic arterial pressure, volume disturbances that occur as a result of dialysis, and disorders of endocrine function. Headache attributed to fasting and cardiac ischemia is also included in this category. This chapter will outline each disorder, as outlined by ICHD-II, define the operational diagnostic criteria associated with each, and provide updated information that has appeared subsequent to the evidence that served as the basis for these criteria.

HEADACHE ATTRIBUTED TO HYPOXIA AND/OR HYPERCAPNIA

Headache as a result of disturbances in arterial blood gas concentrations is well established, although it is often difficult to distinguish between the effects of hypoxia and hypercapnia.

High-Altitude Headache (HAH) (ICHD-II 10.1.1)

SHORT DESCRIPTION

The headache occurs within 24 h of acute onset of hypoxia with $Pa\text{O}_2$ <70 mmHg or in chronically hypoxic patients with $Pa\text{O}_2$ persistently at or below this level.

CLINICAL FEATURES

Diagnostic criteria

A. Headache with at least two of the following characteristics and fulfilling criteria C and D:
   1. Bilateral
   2. Frontal or frontotemporal
   3. Dull or pressing quality
   4. Mild or moderate intensity
   5. Aggravated by exertion, movement, straining, coughing, or bending
B. Ascent to altitude above 2500 m
C. Headache develops within 24 h of ascent
D. Headache resolves within 8 h of descent.

Headache is the most common symptom and complication that occurs during ascent to altitudes greater than 2500 m (Sharma et al., 1975; Hackett and Roach, 2001). In a prospective study involving members of an expeditionary unit to Kanchenjunga base camp in Nepal (5100 m), the incidence, risk factors, and clinical characteristics of HAH were evaluated (Silber et al., 2003). Participants were interviewed before the trip and while trekking: headaches experienced at altitudes above 3000 m were recorded using a structured questionnaire that incorporated the original diagnostic criteria for HAH and acute mountain sickness (AMS) from ICHD-I (Headache Classification Committee of the International Headache Society, 1988). In addition, clinical features of headaches in 19 trekkers from other groups above 3000 m were recorded using the same questionnaire.

This study demonstrated that 83% (50/60) reported at least 1 HAH (median 2, range 0–10) at a mean altitude of 4723 m. Those who developed HAH were significantly younger, suggesting that age-related

*Correspondence to: David W. Dodick, MD, Department of Neurology, Mayo Clinic Arizona, 5777 E Mayo Blvd, Phoenix, Arizona 85054, USA, Tel: 480-342-3078, Fax: 480-342-3083, E-mail: Dodick.David@mayo.edu

cerebral atrophy might allow a greater capacity to accommodate mild cerebral edema. Women and individuals with a history of recurrent headache were also more likely to report severe headaches at altitude. In this study, 95% of the women reported headaches compared to 82% of the men, and headaches were reported more frequently and were described as more severe in women compared with men. HAHs often awakened participants from sleep or occurred upon awakening, suggesting the possibility that sleep-related breathing disorders and subsequent hypoxia may be a contributing factor, compounding an already hypoxic state related to the high altitude. In addition, headaches were frequently exacerbated by bending, coughing, or sneezing, suggesting the possibility that intracranial pressure is elevated at high altitudes and any Valsalva maneuver that is associated with a brief and transient elevation in intracranial pressure magnifies the headache. In this study, headaches were bilateral, generalized, and described as a dull pressure. The duration was usually less than 1 day.

In another prospective cross-sectional study conducted in the Ecuadorian Andes, 98 mountain climbers underwent separate evaluations at 4700–5000 m and 5700–5800 m in an attempt to elicit the clinical features of HAH (Serrano-Dueñas, 2005). The headaches in this study were mainly holocranial (66%) and of pulsatile burst-type quality (75%), in contrast to the dull pressure quality seen in other studies. The headaches were also exacerbated by exercise in 50% of patients and relieved with rest in 42% of patients.

Persons rapidly ascending to high altitudes are also at risk of developing the syndrome of AMS, the principal symptom of which is moderate or severe headache. Individuals with AMS also experience some combination of nausea, anorexia, fatigue, dizziness, and sleep disturbances (Hackett and Roach, 2001). In extreme cases, AMS may progress to high-altitude cerebral edema (HACE), acute encephalopathy, ataxia, and a depressed level of consciousness (Hackett et al., 1998). This suggests that a proportion of headaches at altitude, and certainly AMS, may be part of a similar pathogenic process, with HACE at the extreme of the continuum.

Pathogenesis

The pathogenesis of HAH is not clear. The exacerbation during sleep and Valsalva maneuvers suggests that hypoxia and/or elevated intracranial or central venous pressure contribute to the symptoms. A recent study combined molecular and neuroimaging techniques to examine if free radical-mediated damage to blood–brain barrier function during hypoxia would result in extracellular edema and raised intracranial pressure and account for the neurological symptoms of HAH and AMS (Bailey et al., 2006). Twenty-two subjects underwent collection of venous blood at several time points (0, 8, 15, 18 h) and cerebrospinal fluid (CSF: 18 h) while being randomly exposed for 18 h to 12% (hypoxia) and 21% oxygen (O_2: normoxia). Electron paramagnetic resonance spectroscopy identified a significant increase in the blood and CSF concentration of O_2 and carbon-centered free radicals during hypoxia compared to the hypoxic state. In addition, brain magnetic resonance imaging (MRI) demonstrated a significant increase in brain volume in the hypoxic state that resolved within 6 h of normoxic recovery. However, there was no detectable evidence of disruption of the blood–brain barrier, elevated lumbar epidural opening pressures, T_2 prolongation on MRI or evidence of neuronal or astroglial damage. Clinical AMS was diagnosed in 50% of subjects during the hypoxic trial and corresponding headache scores were significantly and markedly elevated in this group. The authors concluded that mild brain swelling occurs during HAH, but that free radical-mediated vasogenic edema is not an important pathophysiological event.

Management

General and conservative strategies that can prevent or ameliorate the development of HAH include allowing 2 days of acclimatization before engaging in strenuous exercise at high altitudes, avoiding alcohol, and liberal fluid intake.

Previous controlled clinical trials have found that common non-steroidal anti-inflammatory drugs, including aspirin, naproxen, and ibuprofen, provide effective analgesia in patients with HAH (Broome et al., 1994; Burtscher et al., 1998). Acetazolamide and dexamethasone have also been found to be effective in prophylaxis or ameliorating AMS symptoms (Larson et al., 1982; Rock et al., 1987; Hackett et al., 1988; Levine et al., 1989). While sumatriptan has been shown in an isolated case report to provide relief of HAH (Bartsch et al., 1994), ibuprofen has been demonstrated to provide far superior relief to sumatriptan (Burtscher et al., 1995). In fact, in this study, not a single patient out of 6 had any relief of headache 2 h after a 100-mg dose whereas all 7 patients who received 600 mg ibuprofen had complete relief of headache within 2 h.

In a recent prospective, randomized, double-blind, clinical trial of ibuprofen versus acetaminophen in the Solu Khumbu, Nepal, Mount Everest base camp, Pheriche, Dingboche (4240–5315 m), 74 consecutive patients (aged 13–61 years) were randomized, assessed with the Lake Louise AMS criteria, and received a physical examination (Harris et al., 2003). Patients then received either 400 mg ibuprofen or 1000 mg acetaminophen. Baseline Lake Louise AMS scores were identical in the two groups and no difference in mean Visual Analog Scale (VAS) scores between the ibuprofen and acetaminophen groups were noted at time 0 (presentation), 30, 60, or 120 min. In this study population, acetaminophen was as effective as ibuprofen in relieving the pain of HAH.

Diving headache (ICHD-II 10.1.2)

Clinical features

Diagnostic criteria

A. Headache, no typical characteristics known, fulfilling criteria C and D
B. Diving to depth below 10 m
C. Headache develops during diving and is accompanied by at least one of the following symptoms of carbon dioxide (CO_2) intoxication in the absence of decompression illness:
   1. Light-headedness
   2. Mental confusion
   3. Dyspnea
   4. Flushed feeling in the face
   5. Motor incoordination
D. Headache resolves within 1 h after treatment with 100% O_2.

In a prospective study of Norwegian saturation divers, 4% reported having a headache during the first day of decompression, 23% on the last day of decompression, and 34% on the first day after reaching the surface (Englund and Risberg, 2003). The pain was located over the frontal or vertex regions, recorded as mild in severity with a median of 2.5 on a 10-point VAS (range 0.1–7.8), and lasted a median duration of 6 h (range 1–84 h).

Pathogenesis

Hypercapnia is felt to be a common cause of headache in divers, as well as a provocative trigger for migraine and cluster headache in susceptible divers (Hannerz and Jogestrand, 1995; Heckmann et al., 1998; Cheshire and Ott, 2001). CO_2 may accumulate in a diver who intentionally holds his or her breath intermittently (skip breathing) in a mistaken attempt to conserve air, or takes shallow breaths to minimize buoyancy variations in the narrow passages of a wreck or cave (Cheshire, 2004). Divers may also hypoventilate unintentionally when a tight wetsuit or buoyancy compensator jacket restricts chest wall expansion, or when ventilation is inadequate due to physical exertion. Strenuous exercise increases the rate of CO_2 production more than 10-fold, resulting in a transient elevation of $P\text{CO}_2$ to more than 60 mmHg (Cheshire, 2004). Diving headache usually intensifies during the decompression phase of the dive or upon resurfacing. A mechanism analogous to AMS has also been hypothesized to explain headaches affecting professional divers. Hypercapnia (arterial $P\text{CO}_2$ >50 mmHg) is known to cause relaxation of cerebrovascular smooth muscle and lead to vasodilation and increased intracranial pressure (Sliwka et al., 1998).

Other symptoms of CO_2 intoxication include lightheadedness, mental confusion, dyspnea, facial flushing, and motor incoordination. If CO_2 tension continues to rise after symptoms develop, central respiratory and cardiac depression may occur followed by loss of consciousness and seizures. Some individuals will have a markedly reduced ventilatory response to elevated $P\text{aCO}_2$ and are at greater risk of developing toxicity. Retention of CO_2 also potentiates O_2 toxicity or inert gas narcosis and may render the diver more susceptible to decompression illness (Cheshire, 2004).

Headache is also an early symptom of poisoning from carbon monoxide (CO), an odorless gas that rarely has contaminated a diver's compressed air supply when, during tank preparation, the air intake system was inadvertently positioned toward street traffic and exposed to the combustion engine exhaust of an idling vehicle (Clark and Thom, 1997). CO binds to hemoglobin with a 250-fold greater affinity than O_2, thereby resulting in tissue hypoxia and release of nitric oxide, which may dilate cerebral vessels and sensitize trigeminal sensory afferents. Frontal headache, dizziness, exertional dyspnea, and nausea result once blood carboxyhemoglobin levels exceed 10–15% (Clark and Thom, 1997). Treatment of CO poisoning consists of inhaling 100% O_2 or hyperbaric O_2 to hasten carboxyhemoglobin dissociation and should be administered without delay (Clark and Thom, 1997).

Management

The best treatment of headache in divers is education and taking the necessary precautions to avoid situations that increase the risk of hypercapnia or CO toxicity. The diver should take slow, deep breaths and avoid skip breathing or prolonged physical exertion under water. The regulator should be maintained to a satisfactory performance level in order to minimize breathing resistance. Treatment of hypercapnia consists of ensuring a patent airway, physical rest, and comfortable deep breathing. Non-steroidal anti-inflammatory and ergotamine preparations have been reported to be ineffective for the treatment of the headache experienced in divers (Cheshire and Ott, 2001).

Sedating medications, such as opioids, butalbital, or phenothiazines, should be avoided when diving because they can depress respiratory drive, increase CO_2 retention, and impair alertness and judgment, especially at depths beyond 20–30 m where inert gas narcosis may compound the diver's cognitive impairment. Beta-blockers for migraine prophylaxis in the diver should be prescribed cautiously because of their potential to unmask latent asthma and because they can reduce exercise capacity.

SLEEP APNEA HEADACHE (ICHD-II 10.1.3)

Short description

Although morning headache (nocturnal headache or headache upon awakening) may be seen in patients with obstructive or central sleep apnea, it is also a feature of a variety of primary headache disorders such as migraine, cluster headache, and other trigeminal autonomic cephalalgias, and hypnic headache. Morning headache may also be seen as part of a secondary headache syndrome such as medication overuse headache, in sleep-related breathing disorders other than sleep apnea (e.g., pickwickian syndrome, chronic obstructive pulmonary disorder), and in other primary sleep disorders such as periodic leg movements of sleep. A definitive diagnosis of sleep apnea headache (10.1.3) requires overnight polysomnography.

Epidemiology and clinical features

Diagnostic criteria

A. Recurrent headache with at least one of the following characteristics and fulfilling criteria C and D:
   1. Occurs on >15 days per month
   2. Bilateral, pressing quality and not accompanied by nausea, photophobia, or phonophobia
   3. Each headache resolves within 30 min
B. Sleep apnea (respiratory disturbance index ≥5) demonstrated by overnight polysomnography
C. Headache is present upon awakening
D. Headache ceases within 72 h, and does not recur, after effective treatment of sleep apnea.

Sleep apnea and headache are both very prevalent conditions in the population. In the general adult population, the prevalence of obstructive sleep apnea (OSA) syndrome is estimated to be 2% in women and 4% in men, applying the minimum diagnostic criteria of nocturnal apnea/hypopnea index >5/h and daytime sleepiness (Young et al., 1993). Sleep-associated disturbances of breathing without daytime sleepiness are even more frequent, demonstrating the importance of applying standardized diagnostic criteria (Young et al., 1993). Previous studies have suggested that headache in general, and morning headache in particular, is more common in patients with sleep apnea than in control subjects (Ulfberg et al., 1996; Paiva et al., 1997). On the other hand, others have reported that, although morning headache is common in OSA, it occurred just as frequently in other sleep-related disorders, and the headache characteristics are quite non-specific (Aldrich and Chauncey, 1990; Poceta and Dalessio, 1995; Neau et al., 2002). Furthermore, in a study involving tertiary care headache patients who reported heavy snoring and episodes of interrupted nocturnal breathing, only 1.5% who were examined with polysomnography had an apnea/hypopnea index of 5 or higher (Jensen et al., 2004).

However, Paiva et al. (1997) found not only that about half of the patients with nocturnal or early-morning headache suffered from a sleep disorder, including OSA, but also that headache relief was correlated with successful treatment of OSA. Headaches claimed to be associated with OSA are brief and headache severity has been correlated with the severity of OSA in one study (Loh et al., 1999). A series of 56 consecutive patients with OSA and 50 patients with insomnia underwent a detailed headache evaluation (Alberti et al., 2005). Headache was reported by 49% of OSA patients and 48% of insomnia patients. However, headache upon awakening occurred significantly more often in OSA patients (75%) compared to insomnia patients (40%) and the occurrence of morning headache was significantly correlated with nocturnal O_2 desaturation and OSA severity. These findings confirmed those from a previous study which also demonstrated an association between morning headache and the severity of OSA and nocturnal O_2 desaturation (Loh et al., 1999). Taken together, these results appear to demonstrate that headache is a common finding in both OSA and insomnia patients, but that morning headache appears to be more specific for OSA and the occurrence and severity of headache are associated with the severity of OSA.

Pathogenesis

The pathogenesis of headache in patients with OSA is not clear, but elevated intracranial pressure during apneic episodes and altered cerebrovascular reactivity have been implicated in patients with OSA. In one study, CSF pressure was measured continuously at the lumbar level during nocturnal sleep in 3 patients with OSA (Sugita et al., 1985). When the patients were awake and relaxed in the supine position, their CSF pressure was stable and within the normal range. Episodic marked elevations of CSF pressure occurred frequently during sleep, and each elevation was preceded and accompanied by an episode of sleep apnea or hypopnea. Significant correlations were found between both the duration of apneic episodes and decrease in O_2 saturation, and the corresponding increase in CSF pressure. The duration of sleep apnea was longer, the increase in CSF pressure greater, and O_2 desaturation more marked during rapid eye movement (REM) sleep than during non-REM sleep. The authors suggested that frequent marked episodic elevations of CSF pressure were caused by an increase in the intracranial vascular volume occurring mainly in response to transient hypercapnia and hypoxia, which were induced by pulmonary hypoventilation during the episodes of sleep apnea.

In another study, elevations of arterial pressure and intracranial pressure were related to the apneic episodes and there were highly significant correlations between duration of apnea and variation in arterial and intracranial pressure (Jennum and Borgesen, 1989). The highest values of intracranial pressure occurred during REM sleep. Vascular response was not changed during REM sleep, and the higher intracranial pressure during REM could only be explained by the longer apneas seen during REM sleep.

In addition to elevations in intracranial pressure during apnea episodes, significantly lower cerebrovascular reactivity has been demonstrated in the morning and afternoon in patients with OSA compared to control subjects (Diomedi et al., 1998). In addition, cerebrovascular reactivity was significantly higher in the afternoon than it was in the morning in both patients and controls. These data indicate that cerebrovascular reactivity is lowest in the morning in general, but significantly lower in patients with OSA compared to controls.

Management

OSA–hypopnea syndrome (OSA/HS) is a chronic disease that requires consultation and ongoing follow-up with a sleep medicine specialist, patient education, and alleviation of upper-airway obstruction. Because many patients with OSA/HS are overweight or have comorbid cardiovascular risk factors or diseases, they must be informed of the interaction of OSA and overall health. Prospective data on the cardiovascular and perioperative benefits of OSA/HS treatment are emerging, but the current, most widely accepted, patient and physician treatment target is hypersomnolence (Engleman, 2002; Olson et al., 2003).

In many patients, lifestyle modifications including weight loss, avoiding alcohol and other sedatives, smoking cessation, avoidance of sleep deprivation, and, if appropriate, sleep position restriction will decrease both the symptoms of OSA and the comorbid conditions.

Continuous positive airway pressure (CPAP) is the standard treatment for OSA. CPAP involves the use of a device that pneumatically splints the upper airway during inspiration and expiration. A placebo-controlled, randomized trial showed that CPAP decreases sleepiness and increases quality of life (Engleman, 2002). During polysomnography, CPAP is titrated to a level that eliminates snoring and apneas–hypopneas and is then most often prescribed at a "fixed" pressure level that will maintain airway patency during conditions of greatest vulnerability (REM sleep while supine). For most patients, the prescribed pressure is in the 7–11-cmH_2O range.

Compliance with CPAP continues to be a major issue limiting its use. Usage patterns and problems with CPAP vary among patients and patient characteristics that consistently predict CPAP compliance have not been identified. Only a few comprehensive, long-term compliance studies have been published, and they indicate that continuing CPAP use generally correlates with apnea–hypopnea index (AHI) severity, average nightly use of less than 2 h at 3 months predicts failure, and ongoing use at 5 years is 65–90% (Krieger, 1992; McArdle et al., 1999).

Alternative treatment options, including oral appliances, have been developed for mechanically enlarging or stabilizing the upper airway by advancing the mandible or tongue. Subjective improvements in snoring are reported in most case series with oral appliances. Approximately 50% of patients achieve an AHI lower than 10 with the use of oral appliances, and long-term compliance rates are 50–100% (Schmidt-Nowara et al., 1995). Randomized crossover comparisons reveal that CPAP devices are more effective at lowering the AHI than oral appliances, which are most appropriate for patients with mild to moderate OSA (White et al., 2002).

Uvulopalatopharyngoplasty, an operation that modifies the retropalatal airway by excision of the uvula, a portion of the soft palate, and tonsils (if present), produces mixed results. Although snoring is usually subjectively improved, objective improvements have not been well documented. Furthermore, less than 50% of patients achieve an apnea index lower than 10 and at least a 50% reduction in apneas (Sher et al., 1996). Laser-assisted uvulopalatoplasty is not currently recommended for the treatment of OSA/HS (Littner et al., 2001). Radiofrequency ablation techniques can be applied focally to reduce the size of the palate and base of tongue, but efficacy data are limited. Other surgical options include tracheostomy (used rarely) and oral maxillofacial procedures.

DIALYSIS HEADACHE (ICHD-II 10.2)

Short description

Headache commonly occurs in association with hypotension and dialysis disequilibrium syndrome. The disequilibrium syndrome may begin as headache and then progress to obtundation and finally coma, with or without seizures. This syndrome is relatively rare and may be prevented by changing dialysis parameters.

As caffeine is rapidly removed by dialysis, caffeine withdrawal headache should be considered in patients who consume large quantities of caffeine.

Clinical features

Diagnostic criteria

A. At least three attacks of acute headache fulfilling criteria C and D
B. Patient is on hemodialysis
C. Headache develops during at least half of hemodialysis sessions
D. Headache resolves within 72 h of each hemodialysis session and/or ceases altogether after successful transplantation.

Approximately 70% of patients receiving dialysis complain of headaches (Bana et al., 1972; Antoniazzi et al., 2003). Until recently, headaches in this population of patients have not been systematically evaluated. A prospective study of 123 patients with chronic renal failure from three Brazilian hemodialysis services reported headache in 87/123 (70.7%) (Antoniazzi et al., 2003). Before beginning dialysis, 48% had migraine, 19% had episodic tension-type headache, and 8% had both. Headache related to arterial hypertension was the second most frequent headache diagnosis in these patients (25.4%). Fifty patients (57.5%) experienced headache during the session of hemodialysis. Thirty-four were classified as dialysis headache, 7 were classified as migraine, 7 as episodic tension-type headache, and 2 were unclassified. Twenty-four patients (27.6%) reported dramatic improvement of their headaches after the beginning of the dialysis program.

Similar to other studies, there was a male preponderance in this study, and when headache occurred during hemodialysis, a higher incidence was observed between the third and fourth hour. Similarly, another recent study showed that the prevalence of headaches during hemodialysis was directly proportional to the number of hours in session (Brunet et al., 1996). The headaches that occurred during hemodialysis sessions resembled migraine without aura in 19 patients, tension-type headache in 13, probable migraine in 1, and tension-type headache disorder not fulfilling all criteria in 1 patient. They also observed a relative increase in the prevalence of tension-type headaches after the beginning of the dialysis program.

Pathogenesis

While it is clear that hemodialysis can be a trigger for antecendent headache disorders (migraine, tension-type headache), it is equally clear that headaches can occur *de novo* during hemodialysis. However, the clinical features and their pathogenesis have yet to be elucidated. A number of mechanisms may be involved, including hypoxemia that occurs at the beginning of the sessions, hyponatremia, changes in serotonin levels, alterations in levels of urea, aldosterone, and dialysis disequilibrium syndrome. Because these metabolic derangements do not resolve immediately, the resolution of dialysis headaches has been lengthened in ICHD-II from 24 h to 72 h after a hemodialysis session.

A recent study has suggested that elevated levels of calcitonin gene-related peptide (CGRP) in patients with dialysis headache may play a role in the generation of headaches associated with dialysis (Alessandri et al., 2006). Alessandri and colleagues obtained blood samples for radioimmunoassay of CGRP and substance P (SP) from the arteriovenous fistula before and after dialysis treatment in 12 patients with and 12 patients without dialysis headache. Basal plasma concentrations of CGRP, but not SP, were found to be higher in headache patients. However, dialysis significantly decreased CGRP concentrations in both groups, although plasma SP concentrations were reduced in headache-free patients but increased in headache patients. The significance of dialysis-induced elevations in SP is unclear, but raises the possibility that this too may play a role in dialysis headache, although this neuropeptide is not believed to play a role in the pathogenesis of primary headache disorders in humans.

HEADACHE ATTRIBUTED TO ARTERIAL HYPERTENSION (ICHD-II 10.3)

Short description

Mild (140–159/90–99 mmHg) or moderate (160–179/100–109 mmHg) chronic arterial hypertension does not appear to cause headache. Ambulatory blood pressure monitoring in patients with mild and moderate hypertension has shown no convincing relationship between blood pressure fluctuations over a 24-h period and the presence or absence of headache. However, headache related to various disorders that lead to abrupt and severe elevations in arterial blood pressure are associated with headache.

HEADACHE ATTRIBUTED TO PHEOCHROMOCYTOMA (ICHD-II 10.3.1)

Clinical features

Diagnostic criteria

A. Intermittent discrete attacks of headache accompanied by at least one of the following and fulfilling criteria C and D:
   1. Sweating
   2. Palpitations
   3. Anxiety
   4. Pallor
B. Pheochromocytoma demonstrated by biochemical investigations, imaging, and/or surgery
C. Headache develops concomitantly with an abrupt rise in blood pressure
D. Headache resolves or markedly improves within 1 h of normalization of blood pressure.

Pheochromocytomas are catecholamine-producing tumors that arise from chromaffin cells. Although rare, pheochromocytomas must be considered in patients with hypertension, autonomic disturbances, panic attacks, adrenal incidentalomas, or familial diseases (multiple endocrine neoplasia type II, von Hippel–Lindau disease, neurofibromatosis type 1, familial carotid body tumors) featuring a predisposition to develop pheochromocytoma. These tumors are mostly situated within the adrenal medulla, although in about 9–23% of cases tumors develop from extra-adrenal chromaffin tissue (adjacent to sympathetic ganglia of the neck, mediastinum, abdomen, and pelvis) and are often referred to as paragangliomas (Kudva et al., 2003). Sudden-onset headache is the most common symptom of pheochromocytoma, occurring in up to 80% of patients (Thompson, 2002). The headache is often severe, frontal, or occipital and generally described as either pulsating or steady in quality. An important feature of the headache is its short duration: <15 min in 50% and <1 h in 70% of patients. Hypertension is present in 80% and is paroxysmal in 50% of patients (Lance and Hinterberger, 1976). However, 13% have normal blood pressure, and 8% are completely asymptomatic. For these reasons, the definitive diagnosis of pheochromocytoma rests primarily on the demonstration of excessive and inappropriate catecholamine production. When paroxysms do occur, they may last 15–60 min and can occur several times per day or once or twice per year. They can occur spontaneously or may be provoked by physical exertion, emotional stress, pressor medications, changes in posture, or increases in intra-abdominal pressure. Symptoms and signs of adrenergic stimulation, such as sweating, palpitations, facial pallor or flushing, and tachycardia are each present in about 70% of patients, while other features, such as anxiety, sense of impending doom, tremor, visual disturbances, abdominal or chest pain, nausea, vomiting, and occasionally paresthesia may occur as well.

Diagnosis

The diagnosis is established by the demonstration of increased 24-h urinary excretion of metanephrine and normetanephrine (98%), vanillylmandelic acid (60%), and total catecholamines (60–80%) (Ilias and Pacak, 2004). Computed tomography (CT) and MRI of the neck, chest, abdomen, and pelvis have a sensitivity of 86–95% and 93–100% respectively, for detecting adrenal pheochromocytoma. CT is the imaging modality of first choice at most institutions, but if the CT is negative, in a patient with biochemically proven pheochromocytoma, MRI should be performed. MRI should be substituted for CT in children, pregnant women, and situations where radiation exposure must be minimized (Ilias and Pacak, 2004).

Adrenal masses are present in about 5–9% of the general population. Although most adrenal masses are benign, non-functional incidentalomas, about 6.5% of incidentally discovered adrenal masses are indeed pheochromocytoma (Ilias and Pacak, 2004). Thus, most adrenal abnormalities are not pheochromocytoma, highlighting the need for specific diagnostic imaging after anatomical studies are performed in patients with suspicion of pheochromocytoma. Additionally, there is no consensus on the existence of absolute clinical, imaging, or laboratory criteria to predict malignancy and multiplicity of pheochromocytoma (Pommier et al., 1993; van der Harst et al., 2000). Thus, in patients diagnosed with pheochromocytoma, the need to exclude metastatic disease or multiple tumors is important. This need might be fulfilled with functional imaging modalities using various radiopharmaceuticals that provide physicians with whole-body, pheochromocytoma-specific, scans. Pheochromocytoma cells usually abundantly express specific catecholamine plasma membrane and vesicular transporter systems, enabling imaging with [^{131}I] and [^{123}I]MIBG, as well as with several positron emission tomography (PET) ligands. [^{123}I]MIBG scintigraphy has a sensitivity ranging from 83% to 100% and a high specificity (95–100%) for pheochromocytoma (Nielsen et al., 1996; van der Harst E et al., 2001). [^{18}F]DOPA PET imaging may have a higher sensitivity and specificity than [^{123}I]MIBG scintigraphy, but further studies are needed to compare the two modalities (Ilias and Pacak, 2004).

Treatment

The management of pheochromocytoma has been dominated by efforts to prevent hypertensive episodes and associated complications and to diminish the magnitude of postoperative hypotension. For control of blood pressure, selective postsynaptic alpha-1 adrenergic receptor antagonists (prazosin, terazosin, doxazosin) have been used to circumvent some of the disadvantages of phenoxybenzamine (a non-specific alpha-blocking agent). Phenoxybenzamine produces significant orthostatic hypotension and reflex tachycardia and may prolong and contribute to the hypotension that follows removal of the tumor.

Labetalol, an alpha-adrenergic and beta-adrenergic blocker, was reported to be effective in the control of blood pressure and clinical manifestations associated with pheochromocytoma. Its safety has been questioned, however, because it has precipitated hypertensive crises in some patients (Ilias and Pacak, 2004).

Calcium channel blockers have also been successful in controlling blood pressure in pheochromocytoma. These agents do not produce hypotension or orthostatic hypotension and therefore may be used safely in patients who are normotensive but have occasional episodes of paroxysmal hypertension. Calcium channel blockers are useful agents in managing cardiovascular complications because they may also prevent catecholamine-induced coronary vasospasm and myocarditis. It is likely that they reduce arterial pressure by inhibiting the norepinephrine-mediated increase in intracellular calcium in vascular smooth muscle, not by decreasing catecholamine synthesis in tumors.

HEADACHE ATTRIBUTED TO HYPERTENSIVE CRISIS WITHOUT HYPERTENSIVE ENCEPHALOPATHY (ICHD-II 10.3.2)

Clinical features

Diagnostic criteria

A. Headache with at least one of the following characteristics and fulfilling criteria C and D:
    1. Bilateral
    2. Pulsating quality
    3. Precipitated by physical activity
B. Hypertensive crisis defined as a paroxysmal rise in systolic (to >160 mmHg) and/or diastolic (to >120 mmHg) blood pressure but no clinical features of hypertensive encephalopathy
C. Headache develops during hypertensive crisis
D. Headache resolves within 1 h of normalization of blood pressure
E. Appropriate investigations have ruled out vasopressor toxins or medications as causative factors.

Paroxysmal hypertension may occur in association with failure of baroreceptor reflexes. The arterial baroreceptors play a critical role in the control of arterial pressure in humans by buffering moment-to-moment changes so that acute and excessive fluctuations do not occur. Baroreceptors in each carotid sinus relay information regarding vessel distension via the glossopharyngeal nerves to the nucleus of the tractus solitarius which in turn activates cardiac parasympathetic outflow and inhibits sympathetic vasomotor outflow. Other mechanoreceptors in the aortic arch and great vessels of the thorax transmit similar information via the vagus nerves to the nucleus tractus solitarius and generate similar depressor responses. Because of this functional redundancy, bilateral lesions involving the carotid sinus are frequently required to produce baroreflex failure, although a central lesion in the region of the nucleus of the solitary tract can produce the same effect.

Baroreceptor reflex failure has been described in patients with bilateral lesions of the nucleus of the solitary tract or familial paraganglioma syndrome and after surgical resection of the glossopharyngeal nerves (Dodick, 2000). Idiopathic cases, referred to as Page syndrome, have been described (Robertson et al., 1993). The syndrome has also been well described as a delayed consequence in patients who have undergone radiation therapy to the neck for head and neck malignancies, as well as after carotid endarterectomy (Aksamit et al., 1987; Benzel and Hoppens, 1991). This may reflect the relative importance of carotid baroreceptor input over the cardiopulmonary afferents.

In patients with chronic baroreflex failure, the pressor episodes are associated with transient increases in plasma norepinephrine concentration (Benarroch, 1997). This correlation suggests that these episodes are caused by unrestrained activation of the sympathetic nervous system. A spectrum of symptoms may accompany these pressor episodes, including headache, palpitation, a hot sensation, diaphoresis, cutaneous flushing, and emotional lability (Robertson et al., 1993). The clinical presentation of baroreflex failure bears a striking resemblance to pheochromocytoma. However, although patients with baroreceptor failure may have elevated circulating levels of norepinephrine, urinary catecholamine and metanephrine levels and negative imaging studies for pheochromocytoma are usually sufficient to distinguish between the two entities. Furthermore, patients with baroreceptor failure have been reported to have a dramatic response to clonidine, a centrally acting sympathetic inhibitor (Dodick, 2000). Clonidine acts at the level of the rostral ventrolateral medulla to produce sympathoinhibition and, perhaps, at the level of the nucleus of the solitary tract, to sensitize baroreflex responses (Benarroch, 1997). Clonidine produces a significant decrease of arterial pressure in patients with baroreflex failure and autonomic dysreflexia, another centrally mediated hypertensive syndrome, but not in patients with pheochromocytoma.

HEADACHE ATTRIBUTED TO HYPERTENSIVE ENCEPHALOPATHY (ICHD-II 10.3.3)

Diagnostic criteria

A. Headache with at least one of the following characteristics and fulfilling criteria C and D:
   1. Diffuse pain
   2. Pulsating quality
   3. Aggravated by physical activity
B. Persistent blood pressure elevation to >160/100 mmHg with at least two of the following:
   1. Confusion
   2. Reduced level of consciousness
   3. Visual disturbances (other than those of typical migraine aura), including blindness
   4. Seizures
C. Headache develops in close temporal relation to blood pressure elevation
D. Headache resolves within 3 months of effective treatment and control of hypertension
E. Other causes of the neurological symptoms have been excluded.

Hypertensive encephalopathy is an acute cerebral syndrome caused by sudden severe hypertension. The rate and extent of the rise in blood pressure are the most important factors in the development of this syndrome. Encephalopathy may develop in previously normotensive persons at a level of 160/100 mmHg with no evidence of retinopathy at the time of clinical presentation. However, in patients with chronic hypertension, hypertensive encephalopathy is usually not observed until significant elevations in systolic (>250 mmHg) and diastolic (>120 mmHg) blood pressures occur. These patients often have grade 3 or 4 hypertensive retinopathy (Keith–Wagner classification) at the time of presentation.

Hypertensive encephalopathy has become part of an emerging clinical–neuroradiological entity referred to as posterior reversible leukoencephalopathy syndrome (PRES). PRES is a rapidly evolving neurological condition characterized by headache, nausea and vomiting, visual disturbances, altered mental status, decreased alertness, seizures, focal neurological signs, and a diagnostic MRI picture (Healton et al., 1982; Hinchey et al., 1996). PLES is associated with an abrupt and severe increase in blood pressure in most cases, including patients with pre-eclampsia, eclampsia, or renal disease with hypertension. Although hypertensive encephalopathy is the most common cause of PLES, there have been a number of cases described which occurred in the absence of severe hypertension. The syndrome is also seen in patients treated with immunosuppressive drugs such as intravenous immunoglobulin, cyclosporin A, tacrolimus, and interferon-alpha (Healton et al., 1982). The main finding in neuroimaging and autopsy studies is posterior white-matter edema, particularly involving the parietal and occipital lobes, which may spread to the basal ganglia, brainstem, and cerebellum (Chester et al., 1978; Hinchey et al., 1996; Schwartz et al., 1998). Complete clinical and radiological recovery often occurs with prompt antihypertensive treatment or withdrawal of the immunosuppressive drug. Occasionally, the clinical features and CT or standard MRI findings may be indistinguishable from a bilateral posterior cerebral artery stroke syndrome. Thus, early recognition of PLES is essential.

The pathogenesis is unclear, but a failure of cerebral autoregulation that may be facilitated in posterior brain regions due to a sparse sympathetic innervation of the vertebrobasilar vascular system has been proposed (Hinchey et al., 1996). In these cases, compensatory cerebrovascular vasoconstriction can no longer prevent cerebral hyperperfusion as blood pressure rises. As normal cerebral autoregulation of blood flow is overwhelmed, endothelial permeability increases and cerebral edema occurs.

HEADACHE ATTRIBUTED TO PRE-ECLAMPSIA (ICHD-II 10.3.4)

Clinical features and epidemiology

Diagnostic criteria

A. Headache with at least one of the following characteristics and fulfilling criteria C and D:
   1. Bilateral
   2. Pulsating quality
   3. Aggravated by physical activity
B. Pregnancy or puerperium (up to 4 weeks postpartum), and pre-eclampsia defined by both of the following:
   1. Hypertension (>140/90 mmHg) documented on two blood pressure readings at least 4 h apart
   2. Urinary protein excretion >0.3 g/24 h
C. Headache develops during periods of high blood pressure
D. Headache resolves within 7 days of effective treatment of hypertension
E. Appropriate investigations have ruled out vasopressor toxins, medications, or pheochromocytoma as causative factors.

HEADACHE ATTRIBUTED TO ECLAMPSIA (ICHD-II 10.3.5)

Diagnostic criteria

A. Headache with at least one of the following characteristics and fulfilling criteria C and D:
   1. Bilateral
   2. Pulsating quality
   3. Aggravated by physical activity
B. Pregnancy or puerperium (up to 4 weeks postpartum), and eclampsia defined by all of the following:
   1. Hypertension (>140/90 mmHg) documented on two blood pressure readings at least 4 h apart
   2. Urinary protein excretion >0.3 g/24 h
   3. A seizure has occurred
C. Headache develops during periods of high blood pressure
D. Headache resolves within 7 days of effective treatment of hypertension
E. Appropriate investigations have ruled out vasopressor toxins, medications, or pheochromocytoma as causative factors
F. Stroke has been excluded.

Pre-eclampsia is a multisystem disorder that usually occurs after 20 weeks' gestation. It was classically defined as a triad of hypertension, edema, and proteinuria, but a more modern definition of pre-eclampsia concentrates on a gestational elevation of blood pressure in combination with >0.3 g proteinuria per 24 h. Edema is no longer included because of the lack of specificity (Brown et al., 2000; Rachael and Nelson-Piercy, 2004). Eclampsia is defined as the occurrence of a generalized seizure in association with pre-eclampsia, although it may be the first presentation of the condition. Approximately 6.5% of patients have other neurological problems, including aphasia, paralysis, blindness, strokes, psychosis, or coma (Rachael and Nelson-Piercy, 2004). The headache associated with pre-eclampsia and eclampsia is often bilateral, pulsating, and aggravated by activity. Thunderclap headache has been described and reversible cerebral vasospasm in association with posterior leukoencephalopathy syndrome may also be seen (Van den Veyver et al., 1994; Apollon et al., 2000).

Pre-eclampsia and eclampsia complicate 5–6% and 1–2% of pregnancies, respectively. The incidence is significantly influenced by the presence of existing hypertension, although other risk factors are recognized, including nulliparity, multiple pregnancies, previous history or family history of pre-eclampsia, and chronic hypertension (Broughton Pipkin, 2001). An estimated 50 000 women die annually from pre-eclampsia worldwide and morbidity includes placental abruption, intra-abdominal hemorrhage, cardiac failure, intracerebral hemorrhage, and multi-organ failure (Broughton Pipkin, 2001; Royal College of Obstetricians and Gynaecologists, 2001). The risks to the fetus from pre-eclampsia include growth restriction secondary to placental insufficiency, and premature delivery.

Pathogenesis

Pre-eclampsia involves uteroplacental maladaption with failure of the normal cardiovascular changes of pregnancy, resulting in hypertension, reduction in plasma volume, and impaired perfusion to virtually every organ of the body. There is vasospasm and activation of platelets and the coagulation system, resulting in microthrombi formation. The link between the placenta and the systemic disorder appears to involve endothelial dysfunction and oxidative stress. The management of pre-eclampsia involves recognition of the syndrome and delivery of the placenta, which is curative. Since pre-eclampsia may arise with few symptoms, all women are screened during pregnancy through regular antenatal care. Those women who are recognized to be at increased risk have additional screening and more intensive monitoring.

Because of the circulating plasma volume contraction, women may be very sensitive to relatively small doses of antihypertensive agents (and diuretics), risking abrupt reductions in blood pressure. Good control of hypertension in severe pre-eclampsia can reduce the incidence of complications such as cerebral hemorrhage until delivery of the placenta. Management of severe hypertension involves adequate blood pressure control using parenteral hydralazine or labetalol. Hydralazine should be given after a colloid challenge to reduce the reflex tachycardia and abrupt hypotension, precipitated by vasodilation of a volume-contracted circulation. Both angiotensin-converting enzyme inhibitors and angiotensin receptor blockers are fetotoxic and the greatest risk to the fetus appears to be associated with exposure in the third trimester (Rachael and Nelson-Piercy, 2004). These drugs should therefore be avoided in the third trimester. These women are at high risk and should be managed in a high-dependency unit setting, because of the risk of non-cardiac pulmonary edema, through capillary leak, respiratory failure, or the development of a severe systemic inflammatory response syndrome. Seizure prophylaxis, with intravenous magnesium sulfate, may be required in these cases (Rachael and Nelson-Piercy, 2004).

HEADACHE ATTRIBUTED TO ACUTE PRESSOR RESPONSE TO EXOGENOUS AGENT (ICHD-II 10.3.6; CODED ELSEWHERE 8.1.6 COCAINE-INDUCED HEADACHE)

Diagnostic criteria

A. Headache, no typical characteristics known, fulfilling criteria C and D
B. An appropriate agent or toxin has been administered or ingested and an acute rise in blood pressure has occurred
C. Headache develops in close temporal relation to the acute rise in blood pressure
D. Headache resolves within 24 h of normalization of blood pressure
E. No other mechanism for the headache is apparent.

Apart from cocaine, agents that can produce acute elevations of blood pressure include sympathomimetics and amfetamines, and monoamine oxidase inhibitors when interactions with tyramine-containing foods or other drugs such as opioids occur. There is insufficient evidence to set criteria for how large an elevation in blood pressure is required to produce headache, and this may vary from person to person. Criterion D is arbitrary, but included to increase the specificity of the diagnostic criteria.

HEADACHE ATTRIBUTED TO HYPOTHYROIDISM (ICHD-II 10.4)

Clinical features

Diagnostic criteria

A. Headache with at least one of the following characteristics and fulfilling criteria C and D:
   1. Bilateral
   2. Non-pulsatile
   3. Continuous
B. Hypothyroidism is demonstrated by appropriate investigations
C. Headache develops within 2 months after other symptoms of hypothyroidism become evident
D. Headache resolves within 2 months after effective treatment of hypothyroidism.

Although headache has been associated with hypothyroidism since the 1940s (Fenichel, 1948), the only prospective trial evaluating patients with *de novo* hypothyroidism employing ICHD-I criteria was conducted in 1988 (Moreau, 1988). In this study, 31/102 (30.4%) newly identified patients with hypothyroidism were noted to have a recent history of headache. The major characteristics of the headache were: female predominance, bilateral localization (80%), non-pulsating quality (90%), continuous pain with no paroxysmal attacks (95%), mild intensity (95%), nausea, vomiting, or phonophobia, good response to salicylate therapy, and a duration greater than 72 h (82%). The headache decreased in intensity and duration near the 15th day after hormonal therapy in 18 patients, while in the remaining 13 patients the headache disappeared during a 12-month follow-up. A personal and family history of migraine was present in 39.8% and 12.6% of patients. The rate of migraine in hypothyroid patients who did not present with headache was 15.4%, whereas both headache and non-headache patients had equal rates of migraine in the family. The female predominance and the high rate of migraine in the hypothyroid patients with headache suggest that migraneurs are more susceptible to developing headache in the setting of hypothyroidism.

In a randomized, case–control study designed to identify somatic and lifestyle factors associated with the development of chronic migraine (CM) and new daily-persistent headache (NDPH), a strong correlation was found between hypothyroidism and NDPH (odds ratio 16.0 when compared with migraine controls, and 10.3 when compared with chronic posttraumatic headache) and CM (odds ratios of 8.4 and 5.4, respectively) (Bigal et al., 2002). The mechanism of headaches in hypothyroidism is not known.

HEADACHE ATTRIBUTED TO FASTING (ICHD-II 10.5; CODED ELSEWHERE HYPOGLYCEMIA-INDUCED MIGRAINE ACCORDING TO SUBTYPE UNDER 1. MIGRAINE, WITH HYPOGLYCEMIA CONSIDERED AS A PRECIPITATING FACTOR)

Clinical features

Diagnostic criteria

A. Headache with at least one of the following characteristics and fulfilling criteria C and D:
   1. Frontal location
   2. Diffuse pain
   3. Non-pulsating quality
   4. Mild or moderate intensity
B. The patient has fasted for >16 h
C. Headache develops during fasting
D. Headache resolves within 72 h after resumption of food intake.

Fasting is frequently reported by patients and noted in textbooks as a trigger for headache. A systematic study of the relationship between fasting and headache was conducted by Mosek and Korczyn (1995).

Headache history was documented in 370 hospital employees (60% female) before and immediately after a 25-h fast for the 1993 day of atonement (Yom Kippur). A history of recurrent headache was reported by 101 (29%) of those screened; 52 (15%) were migraineurs, 45 (13%) suffered from tension-type headache, and 4 (1%) had other types of headache. Of the 211 participants, 39% of those who fasted developed headache, compared with only 7% of non-fasters, a result that was highly significant. Headache was usually of a non-pulsating quality, mild to moderate in intensity, and bilateral and frontal in location. Subjects with a history of headache were more likely to develop fasting-induced headache than were those without such history (66% versus 29%; $P < 0.000002$). Moreover, photophobia, phonophobia, nausea, and vomiting accompanied the headache significantly more often among previous headache sufferers than among those not reporting a history of previous headache (39% versus 18%; $P < 0.05$). The number of headache sufferers increased in direct relation to the duration of the fast. Headaches first appeared after about 16 h of fasting (in the morning hours of the holiday), and additional headaches developed in other fasters at later time points after the fast began. However, 15 subjects developed their headache 30–60 min after the meal that concluded the fast. Caffeine and nicotine withdrawal, or oversleeping, did not appear to have an influence on the development of headache. The authors concluded that fasting is a strong trigger for headache, especially but not exclusively in those with a prior headache history.

In another study designed to estimate the frequency and characteristics of headaches occurring on the first day of Ramadan (Muslims' fasting month), headaches were reported by 37 (41%) of the 91 persons who had fasted compared to only 2 (8%) of those 25 who did not fast (Awada and Al Jumah, 1999). This difference was highly significant. The headache had a tension-type phenotype in 78% of cases. Headache frequency increased with the duration of fasting and affected mainly those prone to have tension-type headaches; the most important associated factor was caffeine withdrawal. Other factors such as lack of sleep, hypoglycemia, and dehydration may have been involved in a small number of cases.

The headache associated with fasting does not appear to be associated with hypoglycemia, although this relationship has not been systematically examined (Dalton, 1975; Dexter et al., 1978; Malouf and Brust, 1985). Fasting headache can occur in the absence of hypoglycemia, insulin-induced hypoglycemia does not precipitate headache in migraine sufferers, and headache is not a complaint of patients presenting to the emergency department with symptomatic hypoglycemia (Pearce, 1971; Dalton, 1975; Dexter et al., 1978; Malouf and Brust, 1985). The role of caffeine withdrawal as the main factor involved in the pathogenesis of headaches associated with fasting still needs to be systematically studied.

Treatment

The only treatment for fasting headache that has been subjected to a controlled trial is a recent study with rofecoxib. Drescher and Elstein (2006) performed a double-blind randomized prospective trial of rofecoxib 50 mg versus placebo, taken just prior to the onset of fasting, Yom Kippur 2004. Of those subjects receiving rofecoxib ($n = 53$), 10 or 18.9% versus 34 or 65.4% of the placebo group ($n = 52$) had headache at some point during the fast ($P < 0.0001$). Severity of headache was significantly less for the treatment group (3.45 versus 6.29 on a VAS of 10; $P = 0.009$). This study demonstrated that rofecoxib 50 mg taken before a 25-h ritual fast prevents and attenuates fasting headache. Although this medication is no longer available, other cyclooxygenase-2 inhibitors are available and are likely safe taken as a single dose prior to an annual 25-h fast.

CARDIAC CEPHALALGIA (ICHD-II 10.6)

Clinical features

Diagnostic criteria

A. Headache, which may be severe, aggravated by exertion and accompanied by nausea and fulfilling criteria C and D
B. Acute myocardial ischemia has occurred
C. Headache develops concomitantly with acute myocardial ischemia
D. Headache resolves and does not recur after effective medical therapy for myocardial ischemia or coronary revascularization.

Short description

Diagnosis must include careful documentation of headache and simultaneous cardiac ischemia during treadmill or nuclear cardiac stress testing. Failure to recognize and correctly diagnose cardiac cephalalgia (10.6) can have grave consequences. Therefore, distinguishing this disorder from migraine without aura (1.1) is of crucial importance, particularly since vasoconstrictor medications (e.g., triptans, ergots) are indicated in the treatment of migraine but contraindicated in patients with ischemic heart disease. Both disorders can produce severe head pain accompanied by nausea, and both disorders can be triggered by exertion. Migraine-like headache may be triggered by angina treatment such as nitroglycerine.

Headache occurring during acute myocardial ischemia (cardiac cephalalgia) has now been carefully documented in several cases (Lefkowitz and Biller, 1982; Fleetcroft and Maddocks, 1985; Blacky et al., 1987; Vernay et al., 1989; Bowen and Oppenheimer, 1993; Grace et al., 1997; Lipton et al., 1997). Cardiac cephalalgia can often be distinguished from other forms of exertional headache by the temporal profile of the pain. The headache typically begins in close proximity to the onset of vigorous exercise, and subsides with rest or with antianginal treatment. However, just as symptomatic myocardial ischemia can occur at rest, cardiac cephalalgia occurring at rest has been described (Guitierrez-Morlote and Pascual, 2002). The headache is often unilateral but may be located at the vertex, and is usually moderate or severe. Nausea is a frequent accompanying symptom, but other migrainous symptoms, such as vomiting, photophobia, and phonophobia, are absent. Valsalva maneuvers, such as coughing, sneezing, and bending, do not precipitate cardiac cephalalgia. The diagnosis should be suspected in patients with headache onset after age 50 and in patients with risk factors for cardiac disease. In such patients, a prompt cardiac evaluation is essential before a diagnosis of primary exertional headache, primary sexual headache, or migraine is diagnosed. This is especially important since treatment with specific antimigraine drugs has the potential to cause coronary vasoconstriction and could potentially lead to serious adverse outcomes in patients with unstable occlusive coronary disease. Headache onset must be demonstrated to occur with evidence of acute myocardial ischemia, and the headache should resolve after effective medical or endovascular therapy or surgical revascularization.

Pathogenesis

The mechanism of cardiac cephalalgia is speculative, but likely involves convergence of sympathetic or vagal input at the level of the trigeminal nucleus caudalis (Grace et al., 1997). However, there are other possibilities, such as raised intracranial pressure as a result of impaired cardiac venous return due to raised right heart pressures, or the result of an as yet unidentified mediator released secondary to cardiac ischemia that might act on intracranial pain-sensitive structures. Serotonin, bradykinin, histamine, and SP have been proposed as mediators of ischemic pain and may also have distant intracranial effects (Lipton et al., 1997).

Treatment

The management of cardiac cephalalgia involves coronary revascularization or treatment of the underlying cardiac condition. The alleviation of myocardial ischemia will alleviate the headache.

HEADACHE ATTRIBUTED TO OTHER DISORDERS OF HOMEOSTASIS (ICHD-II 10.7)

Diagnostic criteria

A. Headache fulfilling criteria C and D
B. Evidence of a disorder of homeostasis other than those described above
C. Headache develops within 2 months after onset of the disorder, and other evidence exists that the disorder can cause headache
D. Headache resolves within 3 months after relief from the disorder of homeostasis.

Although the relationship between headache and a variety of other systemic and metabolic diseases has been proposed, systematic evaluation of these relationships has not been performed and there is insufficient evidence to allow for operational diagnostic criteria. This is clearly an area with tremendous potential for future clinical and nosological research. The disorders for which there is insufficient evidence have been outlined in the appendix of the ICHD-II (A10.7.1). Headaches attributed to the following disorders are not sufficiently validated: anemia, hypercapnia, adrenocortical insufficiency, mineralocorticoid deficiency, hyperaldosteronism, polycythemia, hyperviscosity syndrome, thrombotic thrombocytopenic purpura, plasmapheresis-induced headache, anticardiolipin antibody syndrome, Cushing's disease, hyponatremia, hyperthyroidism, hyperglycemia, hypercalcemia, systemic lupus erythematosus, chronic fatigue syndrome, and fibromyalgia. Well-controlled prospective studies are needed to define more clearly the incidence and characteristics of headaches that occur in association with these disorders. In each case, only those patients who meet well-established diagnostic criteria for the disorders should be evaluated. In addition, there is insufficient evidence to validate the persistence of headache as a result of a disorder of homeostasis. Consequently, ICHD-II also includes a category in the appendix (A10.8 chronic post-homeostasis disorder headache). Operational criteria have been proposed to facilitate future nosological research in this area.

CHRONIC POSTHOMEOSTASIS DISORDER HEADACHE (ICHD-II 10.8)

Diagnostic criteria

A. Headache, no typical characteristics known, fulfilling criteria C and D
B. A disorder of homeostasis has been present but has been effectively treated or has remitted spontaneously

C. Headache has been attributed to the disorder of homeostasis
D. Headache persists for >3 months after treatment or remission of the disorder of homeostasis.

Short description

Some patients may suffer from persistent headache after resolution of a disorder of homeostasis. Such headache has never been the subject of systematic study.

References

Aksamit TR, Floras JS, Victor RG et al. (1987). Paroxysmal hypertension due to sinoaortic baroreceptor denervation in humans. Hypertension 9: 309–314.

Alberti A, Mazzotta G, Gallinella E et al. (2005). Headache characteristics in obstructive sleep apnea syndrome and insomnia. Acta Neurol Scand 111: 309–316.

Aldrich MS, Chauncey JB (1990). Are morning headaches part of obstructive sleep apnea syndrome? Arch Intern Med 150: 1265–1267.

Alessandri M, Massanti L, Geppetti P et al. (2006). Plasma changes of calcitonin gene-related peptide and substance P in patients with dialysis headache. Cephalalgia 26: 1287–1293.

Antoniazzi AL, Bigal ME, Bordini CA et al. (2003). Headache associated with dialysis. The IHS criteria revisited. Cephalalgia 23: 146–149.

Apollon KM, Robinson JN, Schwartz RB et al. (2000). Cortical blindness in severe preeclampsia: computed tomography, magnetic resonance imaging, and single-photon-emission computed tomography findings. Obstet Gynecol 95: 1017–1019.

Awada A, al Jumah M (1999). The first-of-Ramadan headache. Headache 39: 490–493.

Bailey DM, Roukens R, Knauth M et al. (2006). Free-radical mediated damage of barrier function is not associated with altered brain morphology in high-altitude headache. J Cereb Blood Flow Metab 26: 22–111.

Bana DS, Yap AU, Graham JR (1972). Headache during hemodialysis. Headache 12: 1–14.

Bartsch P, Maggi S, Kleger GR et al. (1994). Sumatriptan for high-altitude headache. Lancet 344: 1445.

Benarroch EE (1997). Central Autonomic Network: Functional Organization and Clinical Correlations. Futura, Armonk, NY.

Benzel EC, Hoppens KD (1991). Factors associated with postoperative hypertension complicating carotid endarterectomy. Acta Neurochir (Wien) 112: 8–12.

Bigal ME, Sheftell FD, Rapoport AM et al. (2002). Chronic daily headache: identification of factors associated with induction and transformation. Headache 42: 575–581.

Blacky RA, Rittlemeyer JT, Wallace MR (1987). Headache angina. Am J Cardiol 60: 730.

Bowen J, Oppenheimer G (1993). Headache as a presentation of angina: reproduction of symptoms during angioplasty. Headache 33: 238–239.

Broome JR, Stoneham JM, Beeley JS et al. (1994). High altitude headache: treatment with ibuprofen. Aviat Space Environ Med 65: 19–20.

Broughton Pipkin F (2001). Risk factors for pre-eclampsia. N Engl J Med 344: 925–926.

Brown MA, Hague WM, Higgins J (2000). The detection, investigation and management of hypertension in pregnancy: full consensus statement. Aust N Z J Obstet Gynaecol 40: 139–155.

Brunet P, Saingra Y, Leonetti F (1996). Tolerance of hemodialysis: a randomized cross-over trial of 5-h versus 4-h treatment time. Nephrol Dial Transplant 11: 46–51.

Burtscher M, Likar R, Nachbauer W et al. (1995). Ibuprofen versus sumatriptan for high-altitude headache. Lancet 346: 254–255.

Burtscher M, Likar R, Nachbauer W et al. (1998). Aspirin for prophylaxis against headache at high altitudes: randomized, double blind, placebo controlled trial. BMJ 316: 1057–1058.

Cheshire WP (2004). Headache and facial pain in scuba divers. Curr Pain Headache Rep 8: 315–320.

Cheshire WP, Ott MC (2001). Headache in divers. Headache 41: 235–247.

Chester EM, Agamanolis DP, Banker BQ et al. (1978). Hypertensive encephalopathy: a clinicopathologic study of 20 cases. Neurology 28: 928–939.

Clark JM, Thom SR (1997). Toxicity of oxygen carbon dioxide and carbon monoxide. In: AA Bove (Ed.), Diving Medicine. 3rd edn. WB Saunders, Philadelphia, pp. 131–145.

Dalton K (1975). Food intake prior to migraine attacks. Study of 2,313 spontaneous attacks. Headache 15: 188–193.

Dexter JD, Roberts J, Byer JA (1978). The five hour glucose tolerance test and effect of low sucrose diet in migraine. Headache 18: 91–94.

Diomedi M, Placidi F, Cupni LM et al. (1998). Cerebral hemodynamic changes in sleep apnea syndrome and effect of continuous positive airway pressure treatment. Neurology 51: 1051–1056.

Dodick DW (2000). Recurrent short-lasting headache associated with paroxysmal hypertension: a clonidine-responsive syndrome. Cephalalgia 20: 509–514.

Drescher MJ, Elstein Y (2006). Prophylactic COX 2 inhibitor: an end to the Yom Kippur headache. Headache 46: 1487–1491.

Engleman HM (2002). When does "mild" obstructive sleep apnea/hypopnea syndrome merit continuous positive airway pressure treatment? Am J Respir Crit Care Med 165: 743–745.

Englund M, Risberg J (2003). Self-reported headache during saturation diving. Aviat Space Environ Med 74: 236–241.

Fenichel NM (1948). Chronic headache due to masked hypothyroidism. Ann Intern Med 29: 456–460.

Fleetcroft R, Maddocks JL (1985). Headache due to ischaemic heart disease. J R Soc Med 78: 676.

Grace A, Horgan J, Breathnach K et al. (1997). Anginal headache and its basis. Cephalalgia 17: 195–196.

Guitierrez-Morlote J, Pascual J (2002). Cardiac cephalgia is not necessarily an exertional headache: case report. Cephalalgia 22: 765–766.

Hackett PH, Roach RC (2001). High-altitude illness. N Engl J Med 345: 107–114.

Hackett PH, Roach RC, Wood RA (1988). Dexamethasone for the prevention and treatment of acute mountain sickness. Aviat Space Environ Med 59: 950–954.

Hackett PH, Yarnell PR, Hill R et al. (1998). High-altitude cerebral edema evaluated with magnetic resonance imaging: clinical correlation and pathophysiology. JAMA 280: 1920–1925.

Hannerz J, Jogestrand T (1995). Provocation of unilateral pain in cluster headache patients by breathing CO_2. Headache 335: 38–43.

Harris NS, Wenzel RP, Thomas SH (2003). High altitude headache: efficacy of acetaminophen vs. ibuprofen in a randomized, controlled trial. J Emerg Med 24 (4): 383–387.

Headache Classification Subcommittee of the International Headache Society (1988). Classification and diagnostic criteria for headache disorders, cranial neuralgias and facial pain. Cephalalgia 8 (Suppl. 7): 1–96.

Headache Classification Committee of the International Headache Society (2004). The international classification of headache disorders, 2nd edition. Cephalalgia 24 (Suppl. 1): 1–195.

Healton E, Burst J, Feinfield D et al. (1982). Hypertensive encephalopathy and the neurologic manifestations of malignant hypertension. Neurology 32: 127–132.

Heckmann JG, Hilz MJ, Katalinic A (1998). Myogenic cerebrovascular autoregulation in migraine measured by stress transcranial Doppler sonography. Cephalalgia 18: 133–137.

Hinchey J, Chaves C, Appignani B et al. (1996). A reversible posterior leukoencephalopathy syndrome. N Engl J Med 334: 494–500.

Ilias I, Pacak K (2004). Current approaches and recommended algorithm for the diagnostic localization of pheochromocytoma. J Clin Endocrinol Metab 89: 479–491.

Jennum P, Borgesen SE (1989). Intracranial pressure and obstructive sleep apnea. Chest 95: 279–283.

Jensen R, Olsborg C, Salvesen R et al. (2004). Is obstructive sleep apnea syndrome associated with headache? Acta Neurol Scand 109: 180–184.

Krieger J (1992). Long-term compliance with nasal continuous positive airway pressure (CPAP) in obstructive sleep apnea patients and nonapneic snorers. Sleep 15: S42–S46.

Kudva YC, Sawka AM, Young WF Jr (2003). Clinical review 164: the laboratory diagnosis of adrenal pheochromocytoma: the Mayo Clinic experience. J Clin Endocrinol Metab 88: 4533–4539.

Lance JW, Hinterberger H (1976). Symptom of pheochromocytoma with particular reference to headache, correlated with catecholamine production. Arch Neurol 33: 281–288.

Larson EB, Roach RC, Schoene RB et al. (1982). Acute mountain sickness and acetazolamide: clinical efficacy and effect on ventilation. JAMA 288: 328–332.

Lefkowitz D, Biller J (1982). Bregmatic headache as a manifestation of myocardial ischemia. Arch Neurol 39: 130.

Levine BD, Yoshimura K, Kobayashi I et al. (1989). Dexamethasone in the treatment of acute mountain sickness. N Engl J Med 321: 1707–1713.

Lipton RB, Lowenkopf T, Bajwa ZH et al. (1997). Cardiac cephalalgia: a treatable form of exertional headache. Neurology 49: 813–816.

Littner M, Kushida CA, Hartse K (2001). Practice parameters for the use of laser-assisted uvulopalatoplasty: an update for 2000. Sleep 24: 603–619.

Loh NK, Dinner DS, Foldvary N et al. (1999). Do patients with obstructive sleep apnea wake up with headaches? Arch Intern Med 159: 1765–1768.

Malouf R, Brust JCM (1985). Hypoglycemia: causes, neurological manifestations, and outcome. Ann Neurol 17: 421–430.

McArdle N, Devereux G, Heidarnejad H et al. (1999). Long-term use of CPAP therapy for sleep apnea/hypopnea syndrome. Am J Respir Crit Care Med 159: 1108–1114.

Moreau T (1988). Headache in hypothyroidism. Prevalence and outcome under thyroid hormone therapy. Cephalalgia 18: 687–689.

Mosek AC, Korczyn AD (1995). Yom Kippur headache. Neurology 45: 1953–1955.

Neau JP, Paquereau J, Bailbe M et al. (2002). Relationship between sleep apnea syndrome, snoring and headaches. Cephalalgia 22: 333–339.

Nielsen JT, Nielsen BV, Rehling M (1996). Location of adrenal medullary pheochromocytoma by I-123 metaiodobenzylguanidine SPECT. Clin Nucl Med 21: 695–699.

Olson EJ, Moore WR, Morgenthaler TI et al. (2003). Obstructive sleep apnea-hypopnea syndrome. Mayo Clin Proc 78: 1545–1552.

Paiva T, Farinha A, Martins A et al. (1997). Chronic headache and sleep disorders. Arch Intern Med 157: 1701–1705.

Pearce J (1971). Insulin induced hypoglycaemia in migraine. J Neurol Neurosurg Psychiatry 34: 154–156.

Poceta JS, Dalessio DJ (1995). Identification and treatment of sleep apnea in patients with chronic headache. Headache 35: 586–589.

Pommier RF, Vetto JT, Billingsly K et al. (1993). Comparison of adrenal and extraadrenal pheochromocytomas. Surgery 114: 1160–1165.

Rachael JP, Nelson-Piercy C (2004). Management of hypertension before, during, and after pregnancy. Br Heart J 90: 1499–1504.

Robertson D, Hollister AS, Biaggioni I et al. (1993). The diagnosis and treatment of baroreflex failure. N Engl J Med 329: 1449–1455.

Rock PB, Johnson TS, Cymerman A et al. (1987). Effect of dexamethasone on symptoms of acute mountain sickness at Pikes Peak, Colorado (4300 m). Aviat Space Environ Med 58: 668–672.

Royal College of Obstetricians and Gynaecologists (2001). Confidential Enquiry into Maternal Deaths in the United Kingdom. Why Mothers Die. Royal College of Obstetricians and Gynaecologists, London.

Schmidt-Nowara W, Lowe A, Wiegand L et al. (1995). Oral appliances for the treatment of snoring and obstructive sleep apnea: a review. Sleep 18: 501–510.

Schwartz RB, Mulkern RV, Gudbjartsson H et al. (1998). Diffusion-weighted MR imaging in hypertensive encephalopathy: clues to pathogenesis. AJNR Am J Neuroradiol 19: 859–862.

Serrano-Dueñas M (2005). High altitude headache. A prospective study of its clinical characteristics. Cephalalgia 25: 1110–1116.

Sharma VM, Malhotra MS, Baskaran AS (1975). Variations in psychomotor efficiency during prolonged stay at high altitude. Ergonomics 18: 511–516.

Sher AE, Schechtman KB, Piccirillo JF (1996). The efficacy of surgical modifications of the upper airway in adults with obstructive sleep apnea syndrome. Sleep 19: 156–177.

Silber E, Sonnenberg P, Collier DJ et al. (2003). Clinical features of headache at altitude: a prospective study. Neurology 60: 1167–1171.

Sliwka U, Krasney JA, Simon SG (1998). Effects of sustained low-level elevations of carbon dioxide on cerebral blood flow and autoregulation of the intracerebral arteries in humans. Aviat Space Environ Med 69: 299–306.

Sugita Y, Iuima S, Teshima Y (1985). Marked episodic elevation of cerebrospinal fluid pressure during nocturnal sleep in patients with sleep apnea hypersomnia syndrome. Electromyogr Clin Neurophysiol 60: 214–219.

Thompson LD (2002). Pheochromocytoma of the Adrenal gland Scaled Score (PASS) to separate benign from malignant neoplasms: a clinicopathologic and immunophenotypic study of 100 cases. Am J Surg Pathol 26: 551–566.

Ulfberg J, Carter N, Talback M et al. (1996). Headache, snoring and sleep apnea. J Neurol 243: 621–625.

Van den Veyver IB, Belfort MA, Rowe TF et al. (1994). Cerebral vasospasm in eclampsia: transcranial Doppler ultrasound findings. J Matern Fetal Med 3: 9–13.

van der Harst E, Bruining HA, Jaap Bonjer H et al. (2000). Proliferative index in phaeochromocytomas: does it predict the occurrence of metastases? J Pathol 191: 175–180.

van der Harst E, de Herder WW, Bruining HA et al. (2001). [^{123}I]Metaiodobenzylguanidine and [^{111}In]octreotide uptake in benign and malignant pheochromocytomas. J Clin Endocrinol Metab 86: 685–693.

Vernay D, Deffond D, Fraysse P et al. (1989). Walk headache: an unusual manifestation of ischemic heart disease. Headache 29: 350–351.

White J, Cates C, Wright J (2002). Continuous positive airways pressure for obstructive sleep apnea. Cochrane Database Syst Rev (2)CD001106.

Young T, Palta M, Dempsey J et al. (1993). The occurrence of sleep-disordered breathing among middle-aged adults. N Engl J Med 328: 1230–1235.

Handbook of Clinical Neurology, Vol. 97 (3rd series)
Headache
G. Nappi and M.A. Moskowitz, Editors

Chapter 54

Headache or facial pain attributed to disorders of cranium, neck, eyes, ears, nose, sinuses, teeth, mouth, or other facial or cranial structures

STEVEN B. GRAFF-RADFORD *
The Pain Center, Cedars-Sinai Medical Center, Los Angeles, CA, USA

Chronic headache attributed to disorder of cranium, neck, eyes, ears, nose, sinuses, teeth, mouth, or other facial or cranial structures has been recently reclassified by the International Headache Society (IHS; Headache Classification Subcommittee of the International Headache Society, 2004). This classification system will be the structure of this chapter. The section is represented in the publication as section 11 and follows the following categories:

11.1. Cranial bone
11.2. Neck
- 11.2.1. Cervicogenic headache
- 11.2.2. Retropharyngeal tendinitis
- 11.2.3. Craniocervical dystonia

11.3. Eyes
- 11.3.1. Acute glaucoma
- 11.3.2. Refractive errors
- 11.3.3. Heterophoria or heterotropia (latent or manifest squint)
- 11.3.4. Ocular inflammatory disorders

11.4. Ears
- 11.4.1. Primary otalgia
- 11.4.2. Referred otalgia

11.5. Rhinosinusitis headache
11.6. Teeth, jaws, and related structures
11.7. Temporomandibular joint (TMJ) disease
11.8. Headache attributed to other disorder of cranium, neck, eyes, ears, nose, sinuses, teeth, mouth, or other cranial facial or cranial structures.

11.1. HEADACHE ATTRIBUTABLE TO DISORDERS OF CRANIAL BONE

Most disorders of the skull, e.g., congenital abnormalities, fractures, tumors, and metastases, are not usually accompanied by headache. Exceptions of importance are osteomyelitis, multiple myeloma, and Paget's disease. Other inflammatory processes, including mastoiditis and petrostitis, may cause pain. When pain occurs the periostium is usually involved. Multiple myloma presents with bone pain in the skull wherever there is a bony lesion. Pain in the oral cavity may present as toothache and lucent lesion may look like dental pathology. Imaging helps to define the extent and diagnosis of the lesion.

The IHS diagnostic criteria for cranial bone are as follows:

A. Pain in one or more regions of the head or face fulfilling criteria C and D
B. Clinical, laboratory, and/or imaging evidence of a lesion within the cranial bone, known to be, or generally accepted as, a valid cause of headache
C. Pain develops in close temporal relation to and is maximal over the bone lesion
D. Pain resolves within 3 months after successful treatment of bone lesion.

Management

Management of the cranial disorders is primarily surgical and may require a variety of different specialties

*Correspondence to: Steven B. Graff-Radford, DDS, The Pain Center, Cedars-Sinai Medical Center, 444 S. San Vicente Blvd., Suite 1101, Los Angeles, CA 90048, USA, Tel: 310 423 9600, Fax: 310 423 9610, E-mail: graffs@cshs.org

depending on the location. Often surgery is accompanied by pharmacological therapy. Opioid and non-opioid analgesics, especially anti-inflammatory agents, may serve for acute pain, and if chronicity develops the novel antiepileptic agents pregabalin and gabapentin, or tricyclic antidepressants, or selective serotonin/norepinephrine reuptake inhibitors may be added.

11.2. HEADACHE ATTRIBUTED TO NECK DISORDER

The IHS diagnostic categories for headache attributed to neck disorder are:

11.2.1. Cervicogenic headache
11.2.2. Headache attributed to retropharyngeal tendinitis
11.2.3. Headache attributed to craniocervical dystonia

11.2.1. Cervicogenic headache

Previously used terms include cervical headache and headache attributed to disorder of the cervical spine.

The IHS diagnostic criteria for cervicogenic headache are as follows:

A. Pain referred from a source in the neck and perceived in one or more regions of the head and/or face, fulfilling criteria C and D
B. Clinical, laboratory, and/or imaging evidence of a disorder or lesion within the cervical spine or in the soft tissues of the neck, known to be, or generally accepted as, a valid cause of headache
C. Evidence that the pain can be attributed to the neck disorder or lesion, based on at least one of the following criteria:
   1. Demonstration of clinical signs that implicate a source of pain in the neck
   2. Abolition of headache following diagnostic blockade of a cervical structure or its nerve supply using placebo or other adequate controls
D. Pain resolves within 3 months after successful treatment of the causative disorder or lesion.

Epidemiology

Estimates for the prevalence of cervicogenic headache range from 0.4% to 2.5% of the general population and increase to 15–20% in a chronic headache population. Cervicogenic headaches affect females more often than males in a 4:1 ratio and the mean age of sufferers is 42.9 years (Haldeman and Dagenais, 2001).

Anatomy and pathophysiology

Significant advances are being made in understanding the relationship between cervical inputs and trigeminal referral, or vice versa. The pain in primary headache is perceived in areas outside the forehead, including the face and cervical region. It is postulated that the referral to the face and neck is facilitated by an alteration in the trigeminal nociceptive system, requiring connectivity between the trigeminal sensory fields and cervical roots. It is also postulated that nociceptive input sensitizes central neurons to reduce the activation thresholds, increasing the responsiveness to afferent stimulation enlarging the receptive fields.

Bartsch and Goadsby (2003) investigated whether noxious dural stimulation evoked sensitization of second-order neurons that led to an increased responsiveness to stimulation of cervical afferents. Understanding this process is pivotal in explaining how therapies aimed at the cervical system alter headache, and similarly how treating pain originating from meningeal inflammation can reduce neck pain.

Diseases or dysfunctions of the cervical region may cause pain when the pathology involves pain-sensitive structures that refer in a physiologically based pattern. The structures known to cause pain include the facet joints, periosteum, ligaments, muscles, cervical nerve roots and nerves, and the vertebral arteries. The referral has been mapped by Bogduk and Marsland (1988).

The cervical causes of headache may include developmental anomalies of the craniovertebral junction and upper cervical spine, tumors, Paget's disease, osteomyelitis, rheumatoid arthritis, ankylosing spondylitis, traumatic subluxation, retropharyngeal tendinitis, and cervical dystonias. Cervical spina bifida does not cause headache unless associated with soft-tissue anomalies such as Arnold–Chiari malformation. Because cervical disc disease is so common, it is not usually accepted as a cause of headache. Typically, if it is to be implicated, the upper cervical segments (1–3) should be involved. An even more controversial cause of headache is cervical whiplash injury. Pain is usually self-limiting, should clear up in weeks, and is likely due to injury of ligaments and muscles. There is some evidence suggesting chronic pain may be secondary to shearing of long axons in the brainstem and upper cord, causing centrally mediated pain and headache (Hawkins, 1962; Weiss et al., 1991; Zwart, 1997). Sjaastad (1999) and Sjaastad and Bovim (1991) have suggested that patients with cervicogenic headache report a fairly uniform headache profile, with the implication that the pain emanates from cervical structures. Sjaastad emphasizes that this is not a disease but rather a reaction pattern. The profile he describes included: (1) unilaterality beginning in the neck and radiating to the oculofrontal area; (2) moderate non-throbbing pain, intermittent or continuous, and provoked by neck movement, or sustained awkward postures; (3) non-radicular pattern; (4) reduced range of motion in the cervical spine; (5) predominantly female; (6) history of trauma; and (7) transient relief with cervical block or C2 root block. Other migraine-associated symptoms or autonomic features are not necessary. Leone et al. (1998) performed a critical review of the current diagnostic criteria of cervicogenic headache. In their study of over 500 patients, only 2 patients had unilateral headache triggered by head/neck movements or posture, and no cases of neck pressure-induced headache. They conclude that neck structures may play a role in some headaches, but clinical patterns indicating a neck–headache relationship have not been sufficiently supported.

Management

There is no one specified therapy for cervicogenic headache. Cervical blockade, whether peripheral nerve block with steroid, facet block, or selective nerve root block, usually produces transient relief. Physical medicine techniques, including cervical mobilization and chiropractic manipulation, are not well studied. Although the complication rate is low, the risk of carotid disection from manipulation should deter cervical manipulation (Khan et al., 2005). Pharmacological intervention may be beneficial, using anti-inflammatory agents, muscle relaxants, tricyclic antidepressants, and selective serotonin/norepinepherine reuptake inhibitors, and novel antiepileptic agents. Bogduk and Marsland (1986, 1988), Bogduk (2003), and Schwedt et al. (2007) have postulated that zygoapophyseal joint disease at C2–C3 could produce headache. They stimulated the area creating pain and blocked the joints reducing pain. This does not imply the mechanism is joint-related, but could be a means of interrupting inhibiting trigeminal nociception.

11.2.2. Headache attributed to retropharyngeal tendinitis

This is an uncommon condition characterized by an acute onset of upper cervical and occipital pain, aggravated by movement and accompanied by pain on swallowing, tenderness in the sides of the neck, fever, and elevated erythrocyte sedimentation rate. Radiographic findings show thickened or calcified C1–C4 prevertebral soft tissue.

The IHS diagnostic criteria for retropharyngeal tendinitis are as follows.

A. Unilateral or bilateral non-pulsating pain in the back of the neck radiating to the back of the head or to the whole head and fulfilling criteria C and D
B. Swollen prevertebral soft tissues, in adults measuring >7 mm at the level between C1 and C4 (special X-ray technique may be required)
C. Pain is aggravated severely by bending the head backwards
D. Pain is alleviated within 2 weeks of treatment with non-steroidal anti-inflammatory drugs (NSAIDs) in their recommended doses.

The IHS comment

Body temperature and erythrocyte sedimentation rate are usually elevated. Although retroflexion most consistently aggravates pain, this also usually happens with rotation and swallowing. The transverse processes of the upper three vertebrae are usually tender to palpation. In several cases amorphous calcific material has been aspirated from the swollen prevertebral tissues. Thin calcification in prevertebral tissues is best seen on computed tomography. Upper carotid dissection should be ruled out.

Management

The symptoms and the swelling respond well and quickly to NSAIDs (Fahlgren, 1986).

11.2.3. Headache attributed to craniocervical dystonia

Dystonia can be primary (idiopathic) or secondary (symptomatic). Focal dystonias in the head and neck can be cranial, such as blepharospasm, spasmodic dysphonia, mandibular or lingual dystonia, and Meigs syndrome, or may be cervical, such as torticollis and retrocollis.

The IHS diagnostic criteria for craniocervical dystonia are as follows:

A. Sensation of cramp, tension, or pain in the neck, radiating to the back of the head or to the whole head and fulfilling criteria C and D
B. Abnormal movements or defective position of neck or head due to muscular hyperactivity
C. Evidence that pain is attributed to muscular hyperactivity, based on at least one of the following criteria:
   1. Demonstration of clinical signs that implicate a source of pain in the hyperactive muscle, e.g., pain is precipitated or exacerbated by muscle contraction, movements, sustained posture, or external pressure
   2. Simultaneous onset of pain and muscular hyperactivity
D. Pain resolves within 3 months after successful treatment of the causative disorder.

The clinical presentation depends on the muscle group involved. In mandibular dystonia the jaw opening and closing muscles create a malpositioned mandible, making chewing and talking uncomfortable. Often tooth grinding is persistent and tooth damage is significant. Resultant TMJ inflammation is not uncommon. In pharangeal dystonia, which usually occurs within the bigger picture of Meigs syndrome, there is spasmodic dysphagia and an annoying cramping sensation. Torticollis presents with abnormal movement or position of the head. The direction of head position defines the variant laterocollis, retrocollis, or anterocollis. Pain and head position are the primary complaints, caused by muscle contraction. Lingual dystonia presents with tongue movements, occasionally with pain.

Headache is a frequent presentation in focal dystonias, as are cervical pains. The pain may be secondary to the muscle straining, consciously or as a reflex to contraction; however, there is little correlation as to the degree of dystonia and the resultant pain.

Management

The primary therapy for cervical dystonia has been botulinum toxin since the early 1980s. Response rates have been reported as between 80% and 100% in both controlled and uncontrolled trials (Lorentz et al., 1991; Lew, 2002). The treatment results in pain reduction in addition to the changes in motor function and may be independent from the spasm. Surgical therapy such as peripheral nerve section may not reduce pain as effectively as microvascular decompression.

11.3. HEADACHE ATTRIBUTABLE TO OCULAR DISORDERS

11.3.1. Acute glaucoma
11.3.2. Refractive errors
11.3.3. Heterophoria or heterotropia (latent or manifest squint)
11.3.4. Ocular inflammatory disorders

Pain in and around the eye is usually caused by local disease but may also be referred from the teeth, jaw, or sinuses. In addition migraine and other neurovascular pains are often perceived in the eye. An inflammatory pseudotumor in the orbit associated with Tolosa–Hunt syndrome may produce eye pain. Psuedotumor cerebri, also called benign intracranial hypertension or idiopathic intracranial hypertension, classically presents with headache, associated with papilledema and sometimes sixth nerve palsy.

The eye and headache are often associated as they have common innervation. With few exceptions primary ocular causes of pain are associated with a red eye (Daroff, 2003). The primary ocular disorders causing headache as classified by the IHS will be listed below.

11.3.1. Acute glaucoma

The IHS diagnostic criteria for acute glaucoma are as follows:

A. Pain in the eye and behind or above it, fulfilling criteria C and D
B. Raised intraocular pressure, with at least one of the following:
   1. Conjunctival injection
   2. Clouding of the cornea
   3. Visual disturbances
C. Pain develops simultaneously with glaucoma
D. Pain resolves within 72 h of effective treatment of glaucoma.

Angle closure glaucoma is rare, occurring in 0.09% of US and European populations (Tasman and Jaeger, 2002). The pressure change is caused by a problem with drainage of fluid out of the eye through the trabecular meshwork, which lies in the angle formed by the intersection of the cornea and iris. A definitive diagnosis is made by measuring the intraocular pressure and observing the narrow or blocked filtration angle with gonioscopy. Acute angle closure glaucoma is an ophthalmic emergency. The pain may be severe, boring, and located in and around the eye; nausea and vomiting may accompany the pain. Vision deteriorates initially from corneal edema and may be permanent. Treatment must be immediate to decrease the risk of permanant visual loss.

11.3.2. Refractive errors

The IHS diagnostic criteria for refractive errors are as follows:

A. Recurrent mild headaches, frontal and in the eyes themselves, fulfilling criteria C and D
B. Uncorrected or miscorrected refractive errors (e.g., hyperopia, astigmatism, presbyopia, wearing of incorrect glasses)
C. Headache and eye pain first develop in close temporal relation to the refractive error, are absent on awakening, and are aggravated by the prolonged visual tasks at the distance or angle where vision is impaired
D. Headache and eye pain resolve within 7 days, and do not recur, after full correction of the refractive error.

Usually refractive errors cause a mild localized ocular pain and occasionally they can cause headache. When the patient has a primary headache, the refractive error may result in increased headache. The pain should quickly subside once the error is treated. The common problems described as causing pain are hyperopia (farsightedness), presbyopia, and astigmatism.

11.3.3. Heterophoria or heterotropia (latent or manifest squint)

The tendency for images to slip out of register is termed heterophoria. The normally single monocular vision does not overlap perfectly. Heterotropia presents as a diplopia and the image is seen in double. If this develops in childhood, suppression or amblyopia may cancel out the diplopia. The phorias or tropias can be constant or intermittent, and may be caused by disorders of the eye muscles and nerves, and problems with cranial pathways coordinating eye movement. Stress, fatigue, and medications may also be involved.

The IHS diagnostic criteria for heterophoria or heterotropia are as follows:

A. Recurrent, non-pusatile, mild to moderate frontal headache fulfilling criteria C and D
B. Heterophoria or heterotropia has been demonstrated with at least one of the following:
   1. Intermittent blurred vision or diplopia
   2. Difficulty in adjusting focus from near to distant objects or vice versa
C. At least one of the following:
   1. Headache develops or worsens during a visual task, especially one that is tiring
   2. Difficulty in adjusting focus from near to distant objects or vice versa
D. Headache resolves within 7 days, and does not recur, after appropriate correction of vision.

Headache associated with heterophorias may be intermittent or continuous. When diplopia is present headache is defined as a painful opthalmoplegia, whose differential diagnosis may include inflammatory, infectious, ischemic, neoplastic, and compressive causes. Treatment is aimed at correcting the underlying cause of the ocular manifestation.

11.3.4. Ocular inflammatory disorders

Ocular inflammation may be caused by immune disorders, infection, trauma, or neoplasm. Uveitis is a general term for inflammation, but when it involves the cornia the term "keratitis" is used, and when the sclera is involved, the term "scleritis" is used.

The IHS diagnostic criteria for ocular inflammatory disorders are as follows:

A. Pain in the eye and behind or around it
B. Ocular inflammation diagnosed by appropriate investigations
C. Headache occurs during inflammation
D. Headache resolves within 7 days, and does not recur, after elimination of the inflammatory disorder.

Ocular inflammation takes many forms, and may be categorized variously by anatomical site (i.e., iritis, cyclitis, pars planitis, choroiditis), by course (acute, subacute, chronic), by presumed cause (infectious agents that are endogenous or exogenous, lens-related, traumatic), or by type of inflammation (granulomatous, non-granulomatous). Ocular neuritis presents with eye pain aggravated by movement. It responds to steroid therapy. Other orbital conditions that cause pain include idiopathic orbital inflammation, cellulitis, hemorrhage, abscess, arteriovenous malformations, and neoplasms. When evaluating orbital pain it is suggested to evaluate the six Ps: periorbital changes, proptosis, progression, pain, palpation, and pulsation with postural change.

DISORDERS OF EAR, NOSE, AND SINUSES

11.4. Ears
   11.4.1. Primary otalgia
   11.4.2. Referred otalgia

Pain in the ear is often referred from musculoskeletal structures such as the TMJ or mastication muscles. Additionally the teeth or TMJ may refer pain to the ear. In these cases the pain is described as a dull achey, or stopped-up sensation. Because the ear is complexly innervated by cranial nerves V, VII, IX, and X, and cervical roots C2–C3, referred pain to the ear needs to be carefully considered. Ear pain may arise from the external ear canal as an acute inflammatory process, or due to an accumulation of wax, producing pressure. Middle-ear or mastoid problems are often due to infection of the mucous membranes, causing otitis media. If inflammation spreads to the petrous bones, a petrositis may develop or there may be meningitis. Acoustic neuroma, a benign tumor involving the neural sheath of cranial nerve VIII, is associated with hearing loss, a tingling sensation deep in the ear, and, if there is trigeminal nerve involvement, pain in the ear or face.

Local structural lesions in the region of the pinna, external ear canal, tympanic membrane, and middle ear may give rise to primary otalgia associated with headache. However, only about 50% of all earache is due to structural lesions of the external or middle ear. Disorders outside this region may lead to referred otalgia as a result of radiation of pain into the ear region. There is no evidence that problems of the ear can cause headache without otalgia.

11.4.1. Primary otalgia

The IHS diagnostic criteria for primary otalgia are as follows:

A. Headache accompanied by otalgia and fulfilling criteria C and D
B. Structural lesion of the ear diagnosed by appropriate investigations
C. Headache and otalgia develop in close temporal relation to the structural lesion
D. Headache and otalgia resolve simultaneously with remission or successful treatment of the structural lesion.

11.4.2. Referred otalgia

The IHS diagnostic criteria for referred otalgia are as follows:

A. Radiation of pain into the ear region
B. Structural lesions outside the external or middle ear diagnosed by appropriate investigations
C. Otalgia occurs in close temporal relation to the structural lesion
D. Headache and otalgia resolve simultaneously with remission or successful treatment of the structural lesion.

11.5. RHINOSINUSITIS HEADACHE

The IHS diagnostic criteria for rhinosinusitis headache are as follows:

A. Pain in one or more regions of the head, face, ears, or teeth
B. Clinical, laboratory, and/or imaging evidence of an acute rhinosinusitis, e.g., purulence in nasal cavitity, nasal obstruction, fever, hyposmia/anosmia, computed tomography imaging, magnetic resonance imaging (MRI), or fiberoptic nasal endoscopy findings
C. Simultaneous onset of headache and rhinosinusitis
D. Headache lasts <7 days after remission or successful treatment of the acute rhinosinusitis.

The IHS comment

Other conditions that are often considered to induce headaches are not sufficiently validated as a cause of headache. These include deviated nasal septum, hypertrophic turbinates, and atrophic sinus membranes. Chronic sinusitis is not validated as a cause of headache or facial pain unless relapsing into an acute stage. Migraine and tension-type headache are often confused with true rhinosinusitis headache because of similarity in location. A group of patients can be identified who, in addition to all the features of migraine without aura, may have clinical features such as location of head pain in the facial areas, associated congestion of the nose, and weather changes triggering headache. None of these patients has purulent nasal discharge or other abnormalities seen in acute rhinosinusitis. Therefore it is necessary to differentiate rhinosinusitis causing headaches versus so-called sinus headaches, which are headache attacks fulfilling the criteria of migraine without aura with prominent autonomic symptoms in the nose or of migraine without aura triggered by nasal changes.

11.6. TEETH, JAWS, AND RELATED STRUCTURES

Dental pain

The most common cause of intraoral pain is dental disease. Inflammatory dental disease may be pulpal, periodontal, or a combination of both. With limited capacity for repair, inflamed or damaged pulpal tissue frequently becomes necrotic. The management of irreversible pulpitis is root canal therapy (amputation of the symptomatic pulp) or extraction. Symptoms generally resolve but postoperative neurological change may lead to persistent pain or dysesthesia. Periodontal disorders involve the supporting structures of the teeth: the bone, periodontal ligament, and cementum.

Acute dental pain may lead to spread of pain unilaterally but, unlike headache, rarely crosses the midline. Convincing research on the epidemiology and qualitative characteristics of dental pain is lacking. However acute dental pain is generally intense, throbbing, poorly localized, but generally provoked by stimulation of the offending tooth (Sharav et al., 1984). Diagnostic problems are sometimes associated with a condition called "cracked-tooth syndrome." A crack which extends through enamel and dentine into pulpal tissue may arise during mastication or external trauma. Pain is usually poorly localized and radiographs are unhelpful (Homewood, 1998). In contrast, periodontal disease is normally associated with chronic discomfort or pain. It is clearly localized to the affected teeth (unlike pulpal pain), a characteristic attributed to the proprioceptive and mechanoreceptive sensibility of the periodontium.

Persistent tooth site or jaw pain in the absence of dental disease has been well described. The term "atypical facial pain" (AFP) has been defined (Headache Classification Committee of the International Headache Society, 1988) as persistent facial pain that does not have the characteristics of the cranial neuralgias and is not associated with physical signs or a demonstrable organic cause. While this diagnosis is a wastebasket for any pain in the face that the clinician cannot diagnose, the 1988 diagnostic criteria suggested by IHS are summarized below.

Diagnostic criteria for atypical facial pain

- Pain present daily and for most of the day
- Confined at onset to one side of face but may spread, deep and poorly localized
- Not associated with sensory loss or other physical signs
- Laboratory investigations, including radiographs, show no relevant abnormality.

Evidence regarding the etiology and epidemiology of AFP is scarce and unconvincing. Suggestions that this type of pain is psychogenic in origin have not been substantiated and probably represent biased clinical observation (Graff-Radford and Solberg, 1993). The relationship between headache and AFP has been reviewed and a neurovascular mechanism for the basis of AFP proposed. This belief is strengthened by the success of tricyclic antidepressants in managing AFP, but the relationship is obviously complex. Further evidence implicating a central headache mechanism was provided by Harrison et al. (1997), who produced pain relief in patients with AFP with a selective serotonin agonist (sumatriptan). Recently, Benoliel et al. (2008) called for expansion of the IHS classification system to include more orofacial pain problems, including neurovascular pain such as facial migraine.

Atypical odontalgia is considered to be a subcategory of AFP. Defined by Graff-Radford and Solberg (1992) as pain in a tooth or tooth site, it is characterized by a defined location. It is also linked to central mechanisms. Sicuteri and colleagues (1991) have suggested a neurovascular etiology for atypical odontalgia, but the evidence is not conclusive. Several authors have proposed a deafferentation mechanism as the cause (Graff-Radford and Solberg, 1991, 1992; Marbach, 1993a, b). Graff-Radford and Solberg (1991) implicate involvement of the sympathetic nervous system due to the high frequency of associated trauma, the equivocal effect of somatic block, and the positive effects of sympathetic block (Graff-Radford and Zarembinski, 2008). Unfortunately there are no epidemiological data on atypical odontalgia. Likely this is a form of deafferentation, and proposed criteria are listed below.

Criteria for trigeminal dysesthesia or deafferentation (Graff-Radford and Solberg, 1992)

- History of trauma
- Continuous pain
- Associated hyperalgesia
- Associated allodynia
- Temperature change
- Block effect (sympathetic versus somatic).

Management

Trigeminal dysesthesia or deafferentation is managed pharmacologically with tricyclic antidepressants, selective serotonin/norepinephrine reuptake inhibitors, antiepileptic agents, antidepressants, and alpha-blockers. Surgical options include sympathetic blockade, radiosurgical ablation, and neural stimulation. Topical therapy with local anesthetic and other agents may be useful.

Burning-mouth syndrome

Burning-mouth syndrome is characterized by a burning sensation in one or several oral structures (Tourne and Fricton, 1992). Although no obvious cause has been established, numerous possibilities exist. The pathogenesis may be summarized into local, systemic, and psychological etiologies. Local factors include contact allergy, denture irritation, oral habits, infection, and possible reflux esophagitis. The systemic factors include menopause, vitamin and mineral deficiency, diabetes, oral infection, and chemotherapy. Psychogenic factors have often been cited but are mostly anecdotal. An essential component to rule out is *Candida* infection. Patients with fungal infection respond quickly to antifungal preparations such as clotrimazole or fluconazole. Topical clonazepam (0.5 –1.0 mg three times per day) has been effective at reducing a burning oral pain (Woda et al., 1998). Patients are instructed to suck a tablet for 3 min (and then spit it out) three times per day for at least 10 days. Serum concentrations are minimal (3.3 ng/ml) 1 and 3 h after application. Woda hypothesized that clonazepam produced a peripheral, not central, action, disrupting the neuropathological mechanism. Additional treatments for burning-mouth syndrome include medications ranging from tricyclic antidepressants, antiepileptic drugs, benzodiazepines, to folic acid and oral rinses. Treatment outcome is varied.

11.7. TEMPOROMANDIBULAR DISORDERS (TMD)

TMDs are a collective term embracing a number of clinical problems that involve the masticatory musculature, the TMJ and associated structures, or both (Okeson, 1996).

Other terms

Other terms have included Costen's syndrome (Costen, 1934), craniomandibular disorders, oromandibular dysfunction and TMJ syndrome, and facial arthromyalgia (Harris, 1987).

11.7. HEADACHE OR FACIAL PAIN ATTRIBUTED TO TEMPOROMANDIBULAR JOINT DISORDER

The IHS diagnostic criteria for headache or facial pain attributed to TMJ disorder are as follows:

A. Recurrent pain in one or more regions of the head and/or face fulfilling criteria C and D
B. X-ray, MRI, and/or bone scintigraphy demonstrate TMJ disorder
C. Evidence that pain can be attributed to the TMJ disorder, based on at least one of the following:
   1. Pain is precipitated by jaw movements and/or chewing of hard or tough food
   2. Reduced range of or irregular jaw opening
   3. Noise from one or both TMJs during jaw movements
   4. Tenderness of the joint capsule(s) of one or both TMJs
D. Headache resolves within 3 months, and does not recur, after successful treatment of the TMJ disorder.

Epidemiology

Epidemiological studies suffer from lack of conformity in diagnostic criteria, data collection, and data interpretation. Agerberg and Carlsson (1972) showed in a TMD population study that 12% reported pain on wide opening of the mouth, 7% reported limitation of mouth opening, 39% had noise on opening the mandible, and 2% complained of joint pain and stiffness. Facial pain and headache were reported by 24% of respondents. Numerous studies have shown women to have more headache, TMJ clicking, TMJ tenderness, and muscle tenderness than men (Agerberg and Bergenholz, 1989; Salonen and Hellden, 1990; Lipton et al., 1993).

Anatomy and pathophysiology

The TMJ is unique in its bilateral location, with an upper and lower joint compartment separated by a fibrocartilaginous disc. This diarthroidial structure allows for both rotatory and translational movement of the mandible. Both joints move as a functional unit and are lined by a fibrous connective tissue which is more resistant to degenerative change than hyaline-lined joints, providing a greater capacity for repair. TMDs are generally divided into those that are joint-related (arthrogenous) and those that are muscular (myogenous). Clinically the two frequently occur together but this arbitrary separation facilitates research and discussion.

Sensory innervation of the TMJ is mediated through the mandibular division of the trigeminal nerve. Pain-sensitive elements within the TMJ include the joint capsule, the posterior attachment tissues, and the discal ligaments. The posterior attachment is highly innervated, richly vascularized, and frequently implicated in the pathophysiology of joint pain. In contrast the intra-articular disc is largely devoid of neural or vascular tissue, but plays a vital role in maintaining condylar stability during mandibular movement. Trauma to the TMJ may result in acute capsulitis but this inflammatory process tends to resolve quickly without complication. Chronic joint disorders are more frequently associated with painful derangement of the TMJ. Articular disc displacement frequently underlies the mechanism of joint derangement but the etiology is unclear. The remarkable adaptive capacity of the TMJ is well documented (Scapino, 1991; Kawamura et al., 1992). Failure of the TMJ adaptive mechanism may lead to tissue breakdown and disc displacement. This process is thought to be affected by age, stress, gender, systemic illness, and previous trauma. However, acute and chronic disc displacement is not always painful. MRI studies of the TMJ have shown a prevalence of 32% for anterior disc displacement in asymptomatic patients (Kircos et al., 1987).

Although the etiology of muscle pain in TMDs is unclear, putative mechanisms underlying the transition from acute to chronic muscle pain have been reviewed in detail. (Simons and Mense, 1998; Mense et al., 2001).

Factors implicated in this transition from acute to chronic muscle pain are summarized below:

- Chronic sensitization of nociceptors
- Changes in innervation density
- Reflex within the central nervous system
- Neuroplasticity
- Disturbance of the antinociceptive system
- Psychosomatic interactions
- Aggravating and perpetuating factors.

The most common form of TMD is myofascial pain. Myofascial pain is usually characterized as deep dull and aching pain referred from active trigger points. The trigger points may refer to muscular or non-muscular structures.

Muscle and other soft-tissue disorders are the most common source of pain in the general population. Much controversy still exists with nomenclature, making it difficult to differentiate accurately between splinting or spasm, myositis or localized myalgia, or myofascial pain due to trigger points. This area of controversy and confusion has been thoroughly reviewed and greatly clarified (Simons and Russell, 1999). The following clinical diagnostic criteria for myofascial pain due to trigger points are reiterated and their use is encouraged. These diagnostic criteria have been successfully used in previous studies (Jaeger and Reeves, 1986), and are a reasonable step towards separating simple local muscle tenderness (allodynia) from myofascial pain due to trigger points for research purposes.

Diagnostic criteria for myofascial trigger points

The diagnosis of myofascial pain due to trigger points depends on, at the very least, the presence of all of the following:

1. Regional or local pain situated in any structure of the body, typically with a deep, aching quality
2. Presence of a focally tender spot in a taut band of skeletal muscle (the trigger point), usually, but not invariably, distant from or outside the clinical pain site
3. The application of 2–4 kg/cm^2 of pressure on the trigger point will reproduce the clinical pain complaint within 10 s
4. Diminished range of motion of the involved muscle due to pain.

Common etiological factors for headache associated with TMD include bruxism, trauma, occlusal interferences, and emotional stressors and sleep disorders (Moldofsky, 1990).

Historically the dental profession has considered occlusal disharmony and variation as a potentially primary etiological factor in TMD. However, literature reviews and data from recent studies do not support occlusion as a significant etiological component to TMD (Pullinger and Seligman, 1991; Pullinger et al., 1993; Magnusson et al., 1994; Verdonck et al., 1994). Even loss of molar support, which seems to correlate with the occurrence of osteoarthritic changes in the TMJ, has no identifiable effect when age is controlled for, since loss of teeth and incidence of osteoarthritis both increase with age (Whittaker et al., 1990; Widmalm et al., 1994). At this time there is no evidence to support the role of occlusal therapy in the management of headache. It is not necessary to modify the occlusion permanently; rather stabilization splint therapy may be useful. Several authors doing systematic reviews of the TMD literature concluded that there is evidence to support the use of stabilization splints in patients with more severe TMD and weak evidence to support their use with mild TMD. Care should be taken to avoid repositioning therapy or partial coverage therapy as they may result in significant changes to the occlusion (Forssell et al., 1999; Kreiner et al., 2001; Al-Ani et al., 2004).

Clinical features of TMD

According to the IHS diagnostic criteria for TMJ disease (Headache Classification Committee of the International Headache Society, 1988), at least two of the following features are required to make the diagnosis:

1. Pain in the jaw precipitated by movement or clenching
2. Decreased range of movement
3. Noise during joint movement
4. Tenderness of the joint capsule
5. Positive radiographic or isotope scintigraphy findings
6. Mild to moderate pain located in the TMJ or radiating from it.

The most frequent presenting TMD symptom is pain, usually localized in the masticatory muscles, the preauricular area, or the TMJ. The pain is characteristically aggravated by jaw function. Additional characteristics are limited or asymmetrical jaw movements as well as joint noise on movement or locking on opening. Headache is a common associated complaint of TMD, and some studies report it to be the most common symptom of dysfunction (Gelb and Tarte, 1975). The association of TMD and headache is described by some to be directly related to the pathology of the TMJ (Scapino, 1991; Whitney and Von Korff, 1992). An alternate hypothesis is that headache in the presence of TMD is an associated symptom, possibly triggered but not related to etiology.

Prognosis

Most epidemiological studies confirm a decreasing prevalence in an elderly population. This evidence supports a widely held belief that TMD is self-limiting. A study by Whitney and Von Korff (1992) suggests that patients improve irrespective of treatment received. Symptom reduction can generally be achieved through conservative methods. Evidence for the use of invasive or irreversible treatment modalities is lacking.

Management

In general, treatment outcome studies of headache related to TMD use various methods of assessing pain reduction, seldom with the same outcome variables. One of the greatest problems is the generalization that if headache is decreased by treatment of TMD then the etiology of the pain is the TMD (Agerberg and Carlsson, 1974; Magnusson and Carlsson, 1980;

Forssell et al., 1986). Little comment is ever made of the role of the central nervous system or behavioral factors. The therapies described here may reduce headache that is aggravated by the coexistence of the TMD, but care should be exercised in assuming cause and effect.

The general principles of management include pain control, increased mandibular mobility where necessary, reduced joint loading, and resumption of normal functional activity of the mandible. These goals may be achieved through a structured, time-limited program that addresses the physical disorder and the perpetuating factors. The five basic areas that should be considered are summarized below and include: (1) patient education and self-care; (2) cognitive and behavioral intervention; (3) pharmacological management; (4) physical medicine techniques; and (5) surgery.

Patient education and self-care

Explanation and reassurance for the patient are prerequisites for satisfactory management. This approach is supported by the National Institutes of Health Technology Assessment Conference Statement (http://consensus.nih.gov/1996/1996TemporomandibularDisorders018html.htm). In susceptible patients persistent jaw joint noise may be interpreted as a sign of disease. Understanding that joint noise may occur in otherwise healthy joints may be difficult for a patient to accept. Likewise complaints of limited mouth opening and other signs of joint dysfunction must be interpreted and assessed in the context of patient age, gender, and general health. Expectations regarding treatment outcome must be realistic and provide reasonable goals for the patient. Simple modification of lifestyle and oral habits may be sufficient to alter symptom intensity. Ultimately treatment outcome will be contingent on patient compliance with the program offered.

Cognitive and behavioral intervention

Behavior modification programs are often accompanied by relaxation training, hypnosis, or biofeedback. Muscle relaxation training techniques are varied, and the choice of technique will depend on the skill of the therapist and suitability of the patient. This approach has been shown to be generally effective in reducing or controlling muscle pain. By teaching patients to relax their jaw muscles, pain levels may decrease and range of mouth opening may increase (Dohrman and Laskin, 1978).

Pharmacological management

A variety of medications are used in the management of TMD to control symptoms. These include anti-inflammatories (both steroidal and non-steroidal), muscle relaxants, and antidepressants. Sedative medications like muscle relaxants have popular clinical usage but have not been extensively researched. Jagger (1973) reported that diazepam was superior to placebo. In contrast tricyclic antidepressants have been used extensively for chronic musculoskeletal pain and numerous studies report on their efficacy (Feinmann, 1984; Sharav et al., 1987).

Physical therapy

Physical therapy modalities provide a popular and safe approach to the management of TMDs. However this area has not been well researched. Given that TMDs are generally self-limiting, physical therapy provides an acceptable, non-invasive, non-pharmacological, and reversible treatment for jaw joint and facial muscle pain (Clark et al., 1990).

Occlusal appliances have been the mainstay of dental therapies for TMD since Costen first published his report on jaw joint pain in 1934. Typically, occlusal appliances are made from rigid heat-cured acrylic which covers the occlusal surfaces of either the upper or lower dentition. The potential benefits of appliance use have been attributed to unloading of the joint surface, relaxation of masticatory muscles, and reduction or elimination of tooth clenching and grinding. These putative mechanisms of action are largely unsubstantiated in the literature; however, some studies have shown a reduction in TMD pain and an increase in function (Dahlstrom et al., 1982; Sheikholeslam et al., 1986). Clinically the most common type of occlusal device used is called a stabilization appliance. This design allows the mandible to open and close on a normal path of movement, leaving an even 4–5-mm layer of acrylic between the upper and lower teeth. As a result the condyle is suspended in a position that is inferior and anterior to its normal location. The joint can articulate freely in this position without restriction. Most patients with TMDs seem to benefit almost immediately from this appliance. Unfortunately excessive use of the appliance can result in occlusal changes, requiring further dental treatment. Thus patients are generally advised to use the appliances only when sleeping.

A second appliance design, called a repositioning device, is less commonly used. Its function is to reposition the mandible in a protrusion direction, theoretically to facilitate recovery of the inflamed retrodiscal tissues. The awkward nature of the appliance design coupled with the requirement to use the device both during the day and at night make it an unpopular mode of treatment with patients. The permanent articular and occlusal changes which may accompany use of this device increase the need for extensive dental reconstruction upon resolution of the joint symptoms.

Occulusal therapy

The association between occlusion and TMD is one of the most controversial topics in dentistry. Malocclusion or misalignment of the teeth is often purported to be a cause of headache in susceptible individuals. However, occlusal theories are weakly supported in the literature. The malocclusions which are seen in adults are probably of little consequence, as skeletal adaptation has already occurred. However, certain dental abnormalities, such as missing posterior teeth, cross-bite in the occlusion, or excessive vertical or horizontal discrepancy between the upper and lower anterior teeth may contribute in a small way to the development of TMD (Pullinger et al., 1993; Forssell et al., 1999).

Surgery

Given the self-limiting nature of most TMD, surgical intervention is rarely warranted. Joint injection with corticosteroid is frequently part of treatment programs but lacks literature support for its efficacy. Concerns have been expressed regarding the potential for condylar erosion due to repeated injection of corticosteroid. As a result clinicians have been urged to limit application of this modality for individual patients.

Re-establishment of mandibular mobility and reduction of joint pain have been reported with irrigation of the joint with lactated Ringer's solution or normal saline (Nitzan et al., 1991). Simple local anesthetic injection into the joint space may also provide short-term pain relief (Danzig et al., 1992). Arthroscopy is a more invasive approach than arthrocentesis but allows for direct visualization of the intra-articular surfaces. Its usefulness in the restoration of mouth opening is documented (Sanders, 1986; Murakami et al., 1996). The use of open-joint surgery is relatively rare but may be justified in cases where circumstances are extreme, and disability associated with joint disease has a great impact on quality of life.

References

Agerberg D, Carlsson GE (1974). Late results of treatment of functional disorders of the masticatory system: a follow-up by questionnaire. J Oral Rehabil 1: 309–316.

Agerberg G, Bergenholz A (1989). Craniomandibular disorders in adult populations of West Bothnia, Sweden. Acta Odontol Scand 47: 129–140.

Agerberg G, Carlsson GE (1972). Functional disorders of the masticatory system. Acta Odontol Scand 32: 597–613.

Al-Ani MZ, Davies SJ, Gray RJ et al. (2004). Stabilization splint therapy for temporomandibular pain dysfunction syndrome. Cochrane Database Syst Rev (1)CD002778.

Bartsch T, Goadsby PJ (2003). Increased responses in trigeminocervial nociceptive neurons to cervical input after stimulation of the dura mater. Brain 126: 1801–1813.

Benoliel R, Birman N, Eliav E et al. (2008). The international classification of headache disorders: accurate diagnosis of orofacial pain? Cephalalgia 28: 752–762.

Bogduk N (2003). The anatomy and pathophysiology of neck pain. Phys Med Rehabil Clin North Am 14: 455–472.

Bogduk N, Marsland A (1986). On the concept of third occipital headache. J Neurol Neurosurg Psychiatry 49: 775–780.

Bogduk N, Marsland A (1988). The cervical zygoapophyseal joints as a source of neck pain. Spine 13: 610–617.

Clark GT, Adachi NY, Dornan AR (1990). Physical medicine procedures affect temporomandibular disorders: a review. J Am Dent Assoc 121: 151–161.

Costen JB (1934). A syndrome of ear and sinus symptoms dependent upon disturbed function of the temporomandibular joint. Ann Rhinol Laryngol 43: 1–15.

Dahlstrom L, Carlsson GE, Carlsson SG (1982). Comparison of effects of electromyographic biofeedback and occlusal splint therapy on mandibular function. J Scand Dent Res 90: 151–156.

Danzig W, May S, McNeill C et al. (1992). Effect of an anesthetic into the joint space in patients with TMD. J Craniomandib Disord 6: 288–295.

Daroff RB (2003). Headaches and the eye: ocular and non ocular causes of eye and/or head pain and the ophthalmic manifestations of headache. Headache Pain 14: 87–92.

Dohrman RJ, Laskin DM (1978). An evaluation of electromyographic biofeedback in the treatment of myofascial pain-dysfunction syndrome. J Am Dent Assoc 96: 656–662.

Fahlgren H (1986). Retropharyngeal tendonitis. Cephalalgia 6: 169–174.

Feinmann C (1984). The diagnosis and management of psychogenic facial pain disorders. Clin Otolaryngol 9: 199–201.

Forssell H, Kiveskari P, Kangasniemi P (1986). Distinguishing between headaches responsive and irresponsive to treatment of mandibular dysfunction. Proc Finn Dent Soc 82: 219–222.

Forssell H, Kalso E, Koskela P et al. (1999). Occlusal treatments in temporomandibular disorders: a qualitative systematic review of randomized controlled trials. Pain 83: 549–560.

Gelb H, Tarte J (1975). A two year clinical dental evaluation of 200 cases of chronic headache: the cranio-cervical mandibular syndrome. J Am Dent Assoc 91: 1230–1236.

Graff-Radford SB, Solberg WK (1991). Differential neural blockade in atypical odontalgia. Cephalalgia (Suppl. 11): 289–291.

Graff-Radford SB, Solberg WK (1992). Atypical odontalgia. J Craniomandib Disord 6: 260–266.

Graff-Radford SB, Solberg WK (1993). Is atypical odontalgia a psychological problem? Oral Surg Oral Med Oral Pathol 75: 579–582.

Graff-Radford SB, Zarembinski C (2008). Sphenopalatine ganglion block compared with stellate ganglion block in patients with traumatic trigeminal neuralgia. 16th Annual Scientific Meeting, International Spinal Interventions Society, Las Vegas, July 2008, pp. 207–208.

Haldeman S, Dagenais S (2001). Cervicogenic headache: a critical review. Spine J 1: 31–46.

Harris M (1987). Medical versus surgical management of temporomandibular joint pain and dysfunction. Br J Oral Maxillofac Surg 25: 113–120.

Harrison SD, Balawi SA, Feinmann C et al. (1997). Atypical facial pain: a double blind placebo-controlled crossover pilot study of subcutaneous sumatriptan. Eur Neuropsychoparmacol 7: 83–88.

Hawkins GW (1962). Flexion and extension injuries of the cervicocapital joints. Clin Orthop 24: 22–33.

Headache Classification Committee of the International Headache Society (1988). Classification and diagnostic criteria for headache disorders, cranial neuralgias, and facial pain. Cephalalgia 8 (Suppl. 7): 1–96.

Headache Classification Subcommittee of the International Headache Society. (2004). The international classification of headache disorders, 2nd edition. Cephalalgia 24 (Suppl. 1): 1–160.

Homewood CI (1998). Cracked tooth syndrome – incidence, clinical findings and treatment. Aust Dent J 43: 217–222.

Jaeger B, Reeves JL (1986). Quantification of changes in myofascial trigger point sensitivity with the pressure algometer. Pain 27: 203–210.

Jagger RG (1973). Diazepam in the treatment of temporomandibular joint dysfunction syndrome: a double blind study. J Dent 2: 37–40.

Kawamura H, Qujada JG, Throckmorton GS et al. (1992). Temporomandibular joint adaptation following inferior repositioning of the maxilla in adult monkeys. Cranio 10: 51–58.

Khan AM, Ahmad N, Li X et al. (2005). Chiropractic sympathectomy: carotid artery dissection with oculosympathetic palsy after chiropractic manipulation of the neck. Mt Sinai J Med 72 (3): 207–210.

Kircos LT, Ortendahl DA, Mark AS et al. (1987). Magnetic resonance imaging of the TMJ disc in asymptomatic volunteers. J Oral Maxillofac Surg 45: 852–854.

Kreiner M, Betancor E, Clark GT (2001). Occlusal stabilization appliances. Evidence of their efficacy. J Am Dent Assoc 132 (6): 770–777.

Leone M, D'Amico D, Grazzi L et al. (1998). Cervicogenic headache: a critical review of the current diagnostic criteria. Pain 78 (1): 1–5.

Lew MF (2002). Review of the FDA-approved uses of botulinum toxins, including data suggesting efficacy in pain reduction. Clin J Pain 18: 142–146.

Lipton JA, Ship JA, Larach-Robinson D (1993). Estimated prevalence and distribution of reported orofacial in the United States. J Am Dent Assoc 125: 125–135.

Lorentz IT, Subramaniam SS, Yiannikas C (1991). Treatment of idiopathic spasmodic torticollis with botulinum toxin A: a double blind study on twenty three patients. Mov Disord 6: 145–150.

Magnusson T, Carlsson GE (1980). Changes in recurrent headache and mandibular dysfunction after various types of dental treatment. Acta Odontol Scand 38: 311–320.

Magnusson T, Carlsson GE, Egermark I (1994). Changes in clinical signs of craniomandibular disorders from the age of 15 to 25 years. J Orofacial Pain 8: 207–215.

Marbach JJ (1993a). Is phantom tooth pain a deafferentation (neuropathic) syndrome? Part I. Evidence derived from the pathophysiology and treatment. Oral Surg Oral Med Oral Pathol 75: 95–105.

Marbach JJ (1993b). Is phantom tooth pain a deafferentation (neuropathic) syndrome? Part II. Psychosocial considerations. Oral Surg Oral Med Oral Pathol 75: 225–232.

Mense S, Simons D, Russell JI (2001). Muscle Pain – Understanding its Nature, Diagnosis and Treatment. Lippincott Williams and Wilkins, Philadelphia, pp. 7–15.

Moldofsky H (1990). The contribution of sleep wake physiology to fibromyalgia. In: JR Fricton, EA Awad (Eds.), Advances in Pain Research and Therapy, Vol. 17: Myofascial Pain and Fibromyalgia. Raven Press, New York, pp. 227–240.

Murakami K Moriya Y, Foto K et al. (1996). Four year follow up study of temporomandibular joint arthroscopic surgery for advanced stage internal derangements. J Oral Maxillofac Surg 54: 285–290.

Nitzan DW, Dolwick MF, Martinez GA (1991). Temporomandibular joint arthrocentesis: a simplified treatment for severe, limited mouth opening. J Oral Maxillofac Surg 49: 163–167.

Okeson J (1996). Orofacial Pain: Guidelines for Assessment, Diagnosis and Management. 3rd edn. Quintessence, Chicago.

Pullinger AG, Seligman DA (1991). Trauma history in diagnostic groups of temporomandibular disorders. Oral Surg Oral Med Oral Pathol 71: 529–534.

Pullinger AG, Seligman DA, Gornbein JA (1993). A multiple logistic regression analysis of the risk and relative odds of temporomandibular disorders as a function of common occlusal features. J Dent Res 72: 968–979.

Salonen L, Hellden L (1990). Prevalence of signs and symptoms of dysfunction in the masticatory system: an epidemiologic study in an adult Swedish population. J Craniomandib Disord 4: 241–250.

Sanders B (1986). Arthroscopic surgery of the temporomandibular joint: treatment of internal derangement with persistent closed lock. Oral Surg Oral Med Oral Pathol 62: 361–372.

Scapino RP (1991). The posterior attachment: its structure, junction, and appearance in TMJ imaging studies, Part 1. J Craniomandib Disord 5: 83–95.

Schwedt TJ, Dodick DW, Trentman TL et al. (2007). Response to occipital nerve block is not useful in predicting efficacy of occipital nerve stimulation. Cephalalgia 27 (3): 271–274.

Sharav Y, Sleviner E, Tzukert A et al. (1984). The spatial distribution, intensity and unpleasantness of acute dental pain. Pain 20: 363.

Sharav Y, Singer E, Schmidt E et al. (1987). The analgesic effect of amitriptyline on chronic facial pain. Pain 31: 199–209.

Sheikholeslam M, Holmgren K, Riise C (1986). A clinical and electromyographic study of the long term effects of an occlusal splint of the temporal and masseter muscles in patients with functional disorders and nocturnal bruxism. J Oral Rehabil 13: 137–145.

Sicuteri F, Nicolodi M, Fusco BM et al. (1991). Idiopathic headache as a possible risk factor for phantom tooth pain. Headache 31: 577–581.

Simons DG, Mense S (1998). Understanding and measurement of muscle tone as related to clinical muscle pain. Pain 75: 1–17.

Simons S, Russell J (1999). Muscle Pain. Williams and Wilkins, Baltimore.

Sjaastad O (1999). Reliability of cervicogenic headache diagnosis. Cephalalgia 19: 767–768.

Sjaastad O, Bovim G (1991). Cervicogenic headache: the differentiation from common migraine. An overview. Funct Neurol 6: 93–100.

Tasman W, Jaeger EA (Eds.), (2002). Duanes's Clinical Ophthalmology (CD Rom). Williams and Wilkins, Baltimore.

Tourne LPM, Fricton JR (1992). Burning mouth syndrome: critical review and proposed clinical management. Oral Surg Oral Med Oral Pathol 74: 158–167.

Verdonck A, Takada K, Kitai N et al. (1994). The prevalence of cardinal TMJ dysfunction symptoms and its relationship to occlusal factors in Japanese female adolescents. J Oral Rehabil 21: 687–697.

Weiss RD, Stern BJ, Goldberg J (1991). Post traumatic migraine: chronic migraine precipitated by minor head or neck trauma. Headache 31: 451–456.

Whitney CW, Von Korff M (1992). Regression to the mean in treated versus untreated chronic pain. Pain 50: 281–286.

Whittaker DK, Jones JW, Edwards PW et al. (1990). Studies on the temporomandibular joints of an eighteenth century London population (Spitalfields). J Oral Rehabil 17: 89–97.

Widmalm SE, Westesson PL, Kim IK et al. (1994). Temporomandibular joint pathology related to sex, age and dentition in autopsy material. Oral Surg Oral Med Oral Pathol 78: 416–425.

Woda A, Navez ML, Picard P et al. (1998). A possible therapeutic solution for stomatodynia (burning mouth syndrome). J Orofac Pain 12: 272–278.

Zwart JA (1997). Neck mobility in different headache disorders. Headache 37: 6–11.

Handbook of Clinical Neurology, Vol. 97 (3rd series)
Headache
G. Nappi and M.A. Moskowitz, Editors

Chapter 55

Headache attributed to psychiatric disorders

VINCENZO GUIDETTI [1]* FEDERICA GALLI, [1] AND FRED SHEFTELL [2]

[1] *Department of Child and Adolescent Neurology, Psychiatry and Rehabilitation, "Sapienza", University of Rome, Rome, Italy*
[2] *New England Center for Headache, Stamford, CT, USA*

INTRODUCTION

The association between psychiatric illness and headache is widely recognized. "Headache attributed to psychiatric disorder" is a new category of secondary headache introduced in the second edition of the International Classification of Headache Disorders (ICHD-II) (Headache Classification Subcommittee of the International Headache Society, 2004). It represents a new, but not conclusive, step toward a better systematization of the topic "headache and psychological factors."

The interest in headache disorders from a psychiatric viewpoint is also growing, as described in recent papers on this topic (Cahill and Murphy, 2004; Allet and Allet, 2006). Neurology and psychiatry are progressively facing each other on this area, looking for likely shared mechanisms, diagnostic and therapeutic lines (Sheftell and Atlas, 2002; Low et al., 2003; Cologno et al., 2005; Hung et al., 2006).

From the early 1990s the involvement of psychological factors in headache disorders has been clearly identified as "psychiatric comorbidity." The term "comorbidity" is a general medical word that dates back to Feinsten (1970). Initially, it related to the occurrence of two distinct diseases in the same patient: "additional ailment in a patient with a particular index disease." The current conceptualization of the term implies an association which is more than casual, but likely not causal, between an index disease or disorder and one or more coexisting physical or psychological pathology. The adoption of Feinsten's definition does not imply *per se* the assumption of a hierarchy between the "index disorder" and the "additional" ones, whether in relation to our main focus, or considering a disease or disorder as the starting point of our analysis, or in terms of a time sequence. In part, the applicability of the definition to the medical field has been facilitated by the knowledge of biological mechanisms explaining the occurrence of some diseases (e.g., diabetes).

The transposition of the conceptualization to the psychiatric field is more recent, but not straightforward. Contents and implications of the concept of "comorbidity" have suggested reconsiderations and reframings over time.

Comorbidity refers to "disorders" (behavioral and psychological problems that are deviant from "normality") and/or "diseases" (well defined as clinical entities), not to the existence of related co-occurring symptoms (syndrome). However, recognizing comorbidities may be an initial step in identifying new syndromes.

Additionally, clarifying the direction, meaning, and weight of comorbidities has pathophysiological, nosological, course, and treatment implications. However, the study of comorbidity may present a series of difficulties related to the current understanding of etiology and pathophysiology of diseases at the center of our attention. Sometimes, as happens in the subject of headache, we proceed against a background where many issues need to be clarified. The question is amplified in psychiatry, and even more troublesome when the co-occurrence of psychiatric and no psychiatric variables is analyzed.

In the psychiatric field, we mainly deal with disorders, not diseases (Angold et al., 1999).

To date, knowledge of the etiology and pathophysiology of most psychiatric disorders is at best inferential. Research and clinical approaches to comorbidity need to take several issues into consideration.

*Correspondence to: Professor Vincenzo Guidetti, Department of Child and Adolescent Neurology, Psychiatry and Rehabilitation, "Sapienza", University of Rome, Via dei Sabelli 108, 00185 Rome, Italy, Tel: 0039-06-44712-255, Fax: 0039-06-4957857, E-mail: vincenzo.guidetti@uniroma1.it

Mental disorders such as comorbid diseases increase the risk for an impaired functional status or quality of life, as shown by different studies analyzing diverse disorders (Gijsen et al., 2001). These aspects, and related diagnostic and prognostic implications, suggest consideration of psychiatric disorders in the clinical setting.

FROM "MIGRAINE PERSONALITY" TO PSYCHIATRIC COMORBIDITY IN MIGRAINE

A characteristic set of psychological features has been observed among migraine sufferers since the last century. Moersch (1924) reported mild mental and physical depression, anxiety, apathy, lack of energy, and fatigue. Liveing (1978) considered depression and drowsiness as characteristics of migraineurs. Emotional disturbance is one of three causes of migraine, together with gastric and menstrual disturbances. Peters (1987) stated that migraine occurs "most frequently in delicate males and females of a highly nervous temperament ... apt to be reproduced by any unusual excitement, by joy, hope, fear, excessive pleasure, anxiety, fasting, fatigue". Anstie (1987) suggested that migraine follows a period of bodily changes, and then "the patient begins to suffer headache after any unusual fatigue or excitement".

Wolff (1937) proposed the definition of "migraine personality," mainly characterized by perfectionism and rigidity. Although his investigations concerned migrainous adults, he suggested that, as children, they were shy, withdrawn, and obedient, but occasionally could become inflexible, obstinate, and rebellious. Wolff's conclusions were based on his observations after a review of his patients' charts and his notes.

From the beginning of the 1990s, the subject began to undergo a systematic conceptualization in terms of "psychiatric comorbidity" by prospective population-based studies on young adults (Merikangas et al., 1990; Breslau et al., 1991; Breslau and Davis, 1993; Merikangas, 1994). Merikangas et al. (1993, 1994) suggested that many of the psychological features frequently related to migraine are more akin to psychopathological symptoms than to personality characteristics, so much so that a syndromic relationship with a peculiar time sequence (anxiety, migraine, and depression) has been suggested (Merikangas et al., 1990; Merikangas, 1994). Her conclusion is that Woff's description of the "migraine personality" may have reflected "subsyndromal" descriptions of anxiety and depressive symptomatology. This remark had been supported by Breslau and Davis's population-based study (1993), even though a bidirectional influence between migraine and depression has been suggested (Breslau and Davis, 1993; Breslau et al., 1994), with one increasing the first onset of the other.

The hypothesis of a shared biological predisposition between migraine and depression has been suggested on the basis of similarities in biological aspects (role of serotonergic system) (Glover et al., 1993; Haythornthwaite, 1993; Silberstein, 1994).

Initially, most studies on psychiatric comorbidity were in migraine. Further studies demonstrated that the presence of psychiatric disorders is related to severe and frequent headache (Breslau et al., 2000) rather than to migraine.

CHRONIC DAILY HEADACHE AND PSYCHIATRIC COMORBIDITY

More recently, attention has turned to the comorbid association between chronic daily headache (CDH) and psychiatric disorders. All studies agree that CDH patients demonstrate a higher number of psychiatric disorders than other headache subtypes.

Studies on CDH have been almost entirely based on a clinical population, with few exceptions (Guitera et al., 2002; Juang et al., 2004; Wang et al., 2006). The relatively low prevalence of CDH in the general population may explain the difficulty of carrying out a study on non-clinical samples, but doubts remain on likely biases of findings (the so-called Berkson's bias, namely the tendency of self-selected patients to consult specialists).

The prevalence of psychiatric disorders is higher in CDH patients than in other headache patients. Estimates of prevalence of psychiatric comorbidity in CDH patients range from 64–66.1% (Juang et al., 2000; Puca et al., 2000) to 90% (Verri et al., 1998), mostly anxiety and/or mood disorders, with higher scores in women than men with CDH (Mitsikostas and Thomas, 1999).

It is noteworthy that chronic pain in general is related to the co-occurrence of depression and anxiety, opening up diagnostic (Arnstein et al., 2004), treatment (Verma and Gallagher, 2001), and etiological (Gallagher and Verma, 1999; Blackburn-Munro and Blackburn-Munro, 2001) issues.

Studies on CDH patients are not always easy to compare since different classification systems have been used. Some studies deal with CDH only on the basis of a high "frequency" of crises or analyzing "severe headache without migrainous features" (not ICHD criteria). However, these studies contribute to emphasize the higher occurrence of psychiatric disorders in CDH than in migraine. The lifetime prevalence of major depression is three times higher in persons with migraine and in persons with "severe headaches" compared with controls (Breslau et al., 2000). Frequency of headache, but not headache severity, seems to be related to depression, anxiety, and high disability rate (Marcus, 2000). Similar findings refer to the occurrence of panic disorder, which is related not only to migraine headache, but also to "severe headache" without migrainous features (Breslau et al., 2001).

Attempts have been made to find specific relationships between CDH subtypes and different psychiatric disorders.

Transformed migraine seems to have the higher rates of psychiatric comorbidity (78%: 57% major depression, 11% dysthymia, 30% panic disorder, 8% generalized anxiety disorder) than chronic tension-type headache (64%: 51% major depression, 8% dysthymia, 22% panic disorder, 1% generalized anxiety disorder) (Juang et al., 2000). Another study (Puca et al., 2000) found the highest prevalence of psychiatric disorders in patients with coexisting migraine and chronic tension-type headache (72.2%) compared to chronic migraine (70.3%) and chronic tension-type headache (50%). However, studies are lacking of comparable diagnostic systems for the classification of both CDH and psychiatric disorders, and the results are currently unclear.

A new issue in the topic of CDH is represented by the role of psychiatric disorders in medication overuse headache (MOH). According to the ICHD-II (Headache Classification Subcommittee of the International Headache Society, 2004), MOH refers to headache attributed to abuse of abortive medications that may remit only when analgesics are withdrawn. Although there exists very little literature on this topic, we know that psychiatric comorbidity is an important factor for the transformation of sporadic headache into chronic headache. Atasoy et al. (2005) reported the involvement of psychiatric disorders in 68% of MOH patients evolving from episodic tension-type headache and 54% evolving from migraine (but in only 35% of chronic tension-type without analgesic overuse).

Radat et al. (2005) noted in their study that the onset of psychiatric comorbidity was likely to precede the onset of medication overuse, perhaps suggesting that patients may choose their medication of overuse to treat their psychiatric comorbidity (e.g., opiates/benzodiazepines, butalbital).

In regard to personality disorders, some studies are beginning to demonstrate the role of personality disorders in MOH (e.g., obsessive-compulsive personality disorder) (Atasoy et al., 2005), opening up the possibility of the likely role of substance dependence patterns (Lake, 2006).

Psychiatric comorbidity may represent an obstacle for drug treatment effectiveness (Curioso et al., 1999), but also another point on which to act when treating headaches. In fact, the occurrence of psychiatric disorders may influence the treatment, for instance by combining drug and non-drug therapy according to the whole case history. This aspect stresses the importance of multidisciplinary work with CDH patients, from diagnosis to therapy. Psychiatric comorbidity should be carefully analyzed in the diagnostic process, in order to choose the best treatment options. A psychological evaluation is the *conditio qua non* for a complete framing of the CDH patient and for tailoring the treatment according to the peculiarities of the case (Lebovits, 2000; London et al., 2001).

Pharmacological and non-pharmacological therapies should be combined in the treatment of CDH (Holroyd et al., 2001; Lake, 2001).

However, evidence-based data on non-pharmacological therapies are wanting, even if well-done studies have been realized in both adults and children or adolescents (Rockicki et al., 1997; Andrasik et al., 2002; Larsson and Andrasik, 2002). Studies should be performed to evaluate the effectiveness of such therapies and the different applications according to different CDH types and comorbid disorders.

On the pharmacological side, antidepressant medications have been the most widely studied in the prophylactic therapy of CDH (Redillas and Solomon, 2000) but their mechanism of action is unknown and likely not related to the antidepressive action.

The understanding of factors involved in the chronification and prognosis of headache is another point that should be analyzed. The role of analgesic overuse cannot explain all cases of CDH, as has been shown by the cases of CDH with onset in children or adolescents, in as much as only a minor percentage seems to be related to it. On the other hand, psychiatric disorders may be related to the chronification of headache (Guidetti et al., 1998; Galli et al., 2004), leading to the imperative need for assessing and treating it, from its onset at an early age.

An aspect to note, but still poorly understood, is that different kinds of chronic pain are related to the presence of psychiatric disorders (mainly anxiety and mood disorders) (Williams et al., 2006).

FROM PSYCHIATRIC COMORBIDITY TO HEADACHE ATTRIBUTED TO PSYCHIATRIC DISORDERS

ICHD-II (Headache Classification Subcommittee of the International Headache Society, 2004) advances an innovative categorization for headache related to psychological factors. The new classification is a first step toward a better systematization of the topic "headache and psychiatric disorders," even though, to date, there is limited evidence to support psychiatric causes of headache, as outlined in the general comment introducing the section of ICHD-II.

For the first time, there is a recognition of a "direction" (headache attributed to psychiatric disorders) in this relationship in the main body of the ICHD-II, even though it is only related to somatization and psychotic disorders. The previous classification (Headache Classification Committee of the International Headache Society, 1988) recognized psychosocial stress, anxiety, and depression as potential "causes" of headache, but only in regard to tension-type headache. The ICHD-II does not give criteria to diagnose headache characteristics ("no typical characteristics known"), stressing the fact that migraine, tension-type, and cluster headache may be attributed to psychiatric disorders.

A general rule allowing the attribution of headache to psychiatric disorder is the temporal connection, with head pain first appearing in close relationship to a psychiatric disorder, and resolving or improving when psychiatric disorder remits. When a pre-existing primary headache is made worse in close relation to psychiatric disorder, both diagnoses may be made. However, both the primary headache and headache attributed to psychiatric disorder may be diagnosed if clinical judgment deems it convenient.

The diagnostic categories provided by ICHD-II do not complete the list of the likely psychiatric disorders that may be causally related to headache, and do not overcome the concept of psychiatric comorbidity.

The appendix of the ICHD-II makes a list of various psychiatric disorders (major depressive disorder, panic disorder, generalized anxiety disorder, undifferentiated somatoform disorder, social phobia, separation anxiety disorder, and post-traumatic stress disorder) that are candidates to be inserted in the main body of the classification when a sufficient degree of scientific evidence is presented. However, the vast majority of headaches occurring in association with psychiatric disorders are not to be attributed to psychopathology (a close temporal relationship is not fitting), and we may only refer to comorbidity.

The mechanisms through which psychiatric disorders give rise to headache are not clear.

Several studies have clarified, though, that the most common relationship between psychiatric illness and headache is bidirectional and associational rather than causative (Breslau et al., 1991).

This relationship is especially clear in the case of mood disorders and migraine. The underlying neurochemistry of many primary headache disorders, especially migraine, has much in common with the neurochemistry (indole and biogenic amines) of various psychiatric illnesses (Breslau et al., 1991). The greater risk a patient with migraine or depression has of developing the other disorder seems related in most cases to shared underlying serotonergic abnormalities of the central nervous system (Glover et al., 1993). Even if association is the most common relationship between psychiatric illnesses and headache disorders, though, this does not preclude the possibility of a causal relationship in some conditions. Only such conditions are classified by criteria provided by the ICHD-II. However, further studies are warranted because headache disorders attributable to psychiatric conditions are probably more rarely diagnosed (Loder and Biondi, 2005) than they occur. The suspicion is that the ongoing understanding of the pathophysiological mechanisms of headache (mainly for migraine) is making it more difficult to give a diagnosis in terms of headache causally related to psychological/psychiatric factors.

The mechanisms through which psychiatric disorders give rise to headache are not clear. However, we can hypothesize a predisposition (genetic? environmental?) to develop headache of any kind, at the outset triggered by the occurrence of a psychiatric disorder. On the one hand, this interpretation may facilitate the overcoming of the mind–body dichotomy that seems to continue to permeate issues in regard to certain clinical approaches to headache disorders. On the other hand, the therapeutic implications must be taken into account to improve outcome. We know that the presence of psychiatric disorders predicts a worse prognosis for every headache subtype (Guidetti et al., 1998; Galli et al., 2004). It is clear that a complete diagnosis and treatment planning should not leave aside a psychiatric assessment as well. Patients with CDH with the absence of personality and mood/anxiety disorders are relatively easier to treat than patients with mood/anxiety and personality disorders (Sheftell and Atlas, 2002).

References

Allet JL, Allet RE (2006). Somatoform disorders in clinical practice. Curr Opin Psychiatry 19: 413–420.

Andrasik F, Larsson B, Grazzi L (2002). Biofeedback treatment of recurrent headaches in children and adolescents. In: V Guidetti, G Russell, M Sillanpää et al. (Eds.), Headache and Migraine in Childhood and Adolescence. Martin Dunitz, London, pp. 307–316.

Angold A, Costello JE, Erkanli A (1999). Comorbidity. J Child Psychol Psychiatry 40: 57–87.

Anstie FE (1987). Neuralgia and disease that resembles it. In: JN Blau (Ed.), Migraine. Chapman and Hall, London, pp. 17–33.

Arnstein P, Caudill M, Mandle CL et al. (2004). Self efficacy as a mediator of the relationship between pain intensity, disability and depression in chronic pain patients. Pain 80: 483–491.

Atasoy HT, Atasoy N, Unal AE et al. (2005). Psychiatric comorbidity in medication overuse headache patients with preexisting headache type of episodic tension-type headache. Eur J Pain 9: 285–291.

Blackburn-Munro G, Blackburn-Munro RE (2001). Chronic pain, chronic stress and depression: coincidence or consequence. J Neuroendocrinol 13: 1009–1023.

Breslau N, Davis G (1993). Migraine, physical health and psychiatric disorder: a prospective epidemiologic study in young adults. J Psychiatr Res 2: 211–221.

Breslau N, Davis GC, Andreski P (1991). Migraine, psychiatric disorders and suicide attempts: an epidemiological study of young adults. Psychiatry Res 37: 11–23.

Breslau N, Davis GC, Schultz LR (1994). Migraine and major depression: a longitudinal study. Headache 34: 387–393.

Breslau N, Schultz LR, Stewart LR et al. (2000). Headache and major depression: Is the association specific to migraine? Neurology 54: 308–312.

Breslau N, Schultz LR, Stewart WF et al. (2001). Headache types and panic disorder: directionality and specificity. Neurology 56: 350–354.

Cahill CM, Murphy KC (2004). Migraine: another headache for psychiatrists? Br J Psychiatry 185: 191–193.

Cologno D, Buzzi G, Carlesimo GA et al. (2005). Psychiatric disorders and pain location in unilateral migraineurs. J Head Pain 6: 227–230.

Curioso EP, Young WB, Shechter AL (1999). Psychiatric comorbidity predicts outcome in chronic daily headache patients. Neurology 52: A471.

Feinsten AR (1970). The pre-therapeutic classification of comorbidity in chronic disease. J Chronic Dis 23: 455–468.

Gallagher RM, Verma S (1999). Managing pain and comorbid depression: a public health challenge. Semin Clin Neuropsychiatry 4: 203–220.

Galli F, Patron L, Russo PM et al. (2004). Chronic daily headache in childhood and adolescence: clinical aspects and a 4-year follow-up. Cephalalgia 24: 850–858.

Gijsen R, Hoeymans N, Schellevis FG et al. (2001). Causes and consequences of comorbidity: a review. J Clin Epidemiol 54: 661–674.

Glover V, Jarman J, Sandler M (1993). Migraine and depression: biological aspects. J Psychiatr Res 2: 223–231.

Guidetti V, Galli F, Fabrizi P et al. (1998). Headache and psychiatric comorbidity: clinical aspects and outcome in an 8-year follow-up study. Cephalalgia 7: 455–462.

Guitera V, Munoz P, Castillo J et al. (2002). Quality of life in chronic daily headache: a study in a general population. Neurology 58: 1062–1065.

Haythornthwaite JA (1993). Migraine headaches and psychopathology: future directions. J Psychiatr Res 27: 183–186.

Headache Classification Committee of the International Headache Society (1988). Classification and diagnostic criteria for headache disorders, cranial neuralgias, and facial pain. Cephalalgia (Suppl. 7): 1–96.

Headache Classification Subcommittee of the International Headache Society (2004). The international classification of headache disorders, 2nd edition. Cephalalgia 24 (Suppl. 1): 1–151.

Holroyd KA, O'Donnell FJ, Stensland M et al. (2001). Management of chronic tension-type headache with tricyclic antidepressant medication, stress management therapy, and their combination: a randomized controlled trial. JAMA 285: 2208–2215.

Hung CI, Liu CY, Juang YY et al. (2006). The impact of migraine on patients with major depressive disorder. Headache 46: 469–477.

Juang KD, Wang SJ, Fuh JL et al. (2000). Comorbidity of depressive and anxiety disorders in chronic daily headache and its subtypes. Headache 40: 818–823.

Juang KD, Wang SJ, Fuh JL et al. (2004). Association between adolescent chronic daily headache and childhood adversity: a community-based study. Cephalalgia 24: 54–59.

Lake AE (2001). Behavioral and nonpharmacologic treatments of headache. Med Clin North Am 85: 1055–1075.

Lake AE (2006). Medication overuse headache: biobehavioral issues and solutions. Headache 46 (Suppl. 3): 88–97.

Larsson B, Andrasik F (2002). Relaxation treatment of recurrent headaches in children and adolescents. In: V Guidetti, G Russell, M Sillanpää et al. (Eds.), Headache and Migraine in Childhood and Adolescence. Martin Dunitz, London, pp. 307–316.

Lebovits AH (2000). The psychological assessment of patients with chronic pain. Curr Rev Pain 4: 122–126.

Liveing E (1978). On Migrim, Sick-Headache, and Some Allied Disorders: A Contribution to the Pathology of Nerve Storms. J & A Churchill, London.

Loder E, Biondi D (2005). Headache attributed to psychiatric disorder: a case series. Psychosomatics 46: 326–333.

London LH, Shulman B, Diamond S (2001). The role of psychometric testing and psychological treatment in tension-type headache. Curr Pain Headache Rep 5: 467–471.

Low NCP, Galbaud du Fort G, Cervantes P (2003). Prevalence, clinical correlates, and treatment of migraine in bipolar disorder. Headache 43: 940–949.

Marcus DA (2000). Identification of patients with headache at risk for psychological distress. Headache 40: 373–376.

Merikangas KR (1994). Psychopathology and headache syndromes in the community. Headache 34: S17–S26.

Merikangas KR, Angst J, Isler H (1990). Migraine and psychopathology. Results of the Zurich cohort study of young adults. Arch Gen Psychiatry 47: 849–853.

Merikangas KR, Merikangas JR, Angst J (1993). Headache syndromes and psychiatric disorders: association and familial transmission. J Psychiatr Res 2: 197–210.

Mitsikostas DD, Thomas AM (1999). Comorbidity of headache and depression. Cephalalgia 19: 211–217.

Moersch FP (1924). Psychic manifestations in migraine. Am J Psychiatry 3: 698–716.

Peters JC (1987). A treatise on headache. In: JN Blau (Ed.), Migraine. Chapman and Hall, London, pp. 367–386.

Puca F, Guazzelli M, Sciruicchio V (2000). Psychiatric disorders in chronic daily headache: detection by means of the SCID interview. J Headache Pain 1: S33–S37.

Radat F, Creach C, Swendsen JD et al. (2005). Psychiatric comorbidity in the evolution from migraine to medication overuse headache. Cephalalgia 24: 519–522.

Redillas C, Solomon S (2000). Prophylactic pharmacological treatment of chronic daily headache. Headache 40: 83–102.

Rockicki LA, Holroyd KA, France CR et al. (1997). Change mechanisms associated with combined relaxation/EMG biofeedback training for chronic tension headache. Appl Psychophysiol Biofeedback 22: 21–41.

Sheftell FD, Atlas SJ (2002). Migraine and psychiatric comorbidity: from theory and hypotheses to clinical application. Headache 42: 934–944.

Silberstein SD (1994). Serotonin (5-HT) and migraine. Headache 34: 408–417.

Verma S, Gallagher RM (2001). The psychopharmocologic treatment of depression and anxiety in the context of chronic pain. Curr Pain Headache Rep 6: 30–39.

Verri AP, Cecchini P, Galli C et al. (1998). Psychiatric comorbidity in chronic daily headache. Cephalalgia 18 (Suppl. 21): 45–49.

Wang SJ, Fuh JL, Lu SR et al. (2006). Daily headache in adolescents: prevalence, impact, and medication overuse. Neurology 66: 193–197.

Williams LJ, Jacka FN, Pasco JA et al. (2006). Depression and pain: an overview. Acta Neuropsychiatrica 18: 79–97.

Wolff HG (1937). Personality features and reactions of subjects with migraine. Arch Neurol Psychiatry 37: 895.

Handbook of Clinical Neurology, Vol. 97 (3rd series)
Headache
G. Nappi and M.A. Moskowitz, Editors

Chapter 56

Cranial neuralgias

G. CRUCCU,[1]* L.H. BONAMICO,[2] AND J.M. ZAKRZEWSKA[3]
[1]*Department of Neurological Sciences, La Sapienza University, Rome, Italy*
[2]*Neurological and Pain Department, FLENI Neurological Institute, Buenos Aires, Argentina*
[3]*Department of Oral Medicine, University College London Hospitals, NHS Foundation Trust, London, UK*

Perhaps because of the many peculiarities of the trigeminal system or because the facial region is extraordinarily rich in sensory receptors and sensory afferents, with a high density of small myelinated and unmyelinated fibers in the mouth area, facial pain is common. The trigeminal nerve mediates all cranial–facial pains, whether neuropathic (e.g., trigeminal neuralgia) or nociceptive (e.g., headache or dental pain). This chapter describes the most common cranial neuralgias and some other chronic pain conditions mediated by the trigeminal system, adhering to the recommendations of recent Euro-American guidelines (Cruccu et al., 2008; Gronseth et al., 2008).

ANATOMICAL–FUNCTIONAL ORGANIZATION OF THE TRIGEMINAL SYSTEM

Peripheral pathways

The trigeminal nerve is the fifth cranial nerve. It is the largest cranial nerve and its three major sensory branches are the ophthalmic (V1), maxillary (V2), and mandibular nerves (V3), which convey information about touch, temperature, pain, and proprioception from the mouth, face, and scalp to the brainstem. The trigeminal nerve originates in the posterior cranial fossa, emerging from the pons, with a small motor (portio minor, 7500 myelinated fibers) and a large sensory (portio major, 170 000 myelinated fibers) root (Pennisi et al., 1991).

The fibers of the sensory root arise from the pseudounipolar cells of the semilunar ganglion (gasserian ganglion) which is located in a dura mater cavity (Meckel's cave) in the middle cranial fossa. The three divisions depart from the convex border of the gasserian ganglion, heading toward their exits from the skull.

The ophthalmic nerve (25 000 fibers), the smallest of the three trigeminal divisions, is a purely sensory nerve. It runs along the lateral wall of the cavernous sinus, below the oculomotor and trochlear nerves. Just before entering the orbit through the superior orbital fissure, it divides into three branches – the lacrimal, frontal, and nasociliary nerves. These branches supply the cornea, nasal cavity, skin of the upper eyelid, dorsum of the nose, forehead, and scalp as far back as the border between the anterior two-thirds and the posterior third of the scalp (which is innervated by the great occipital nerve).

The maxillary nerve (50 000 fibers), again purely sensory, has an intermediate position and pathway between the ophthalmic and mandibular nerves. It originates at the middle of the semilunar ganglion and, running horizontally forward, exits the skull through the foramen rotundum, enters the orbit through the inferior orbital fissure and then the infraorbital canal on the floor of the orbit, and finally reaches the facial skin through the infraorbital foramen. The main terminal branches of the maxillary nerve convey sensory information from the lower eyelid, zygoma, nose, medial cheek, and upper lip. While running in the maxillary bone, the nerve also gives off a series of tiny branches to innervate the nasal and oral cavity, including upper teeth.

The mandibular nerve (78 000 fibers) is the largest of the trigeminal divisions and is a mixed nerve, made up of a large sensory root and a small motor root, which passes beneath the ganglion and unites with the sensory root immediately after their skull exit through the foramen ovale. In the infratemporal fossa,

*Correspondence to: Professor G. Cruccu, Department of Neurological Sciences, La Sapienza University, Rome, Italy, Tel: +39 06 49694209, Fax: +39 06 49914758, E-mail: cruccu@uniroma1.it

below the skull base, the nerve divides into several motor and sensory branches. Motor nerves innervate the jaw closers (masseter, temporalis, medial, and lateral pterygoid muscles) and jaw openers (mylohyoid and anterior belly of the digastric muscles), as well as the tensor veli palatini and the tensor tympani muscles. The main sensory nerves (buccal, lingual, inferior alveolar, mylohyoid, mental, and auriculotemporal nerves) innervate the mandibular portion of the oral cavity, including the anterior two-thirds of the tongue, teeth, and periodontium, the skin anterior to the ear, tympanic membrane, temporomandibular joint, the skin overlying the mandible, and lower lip.

Among the peculiarities of the trigeminal system, it is worth recalling that the corneal mucosa and the dental pulp have a special innervation, probably because their only sensory function is protective; they are exclusively provided with Aδ and C free nerve endings. The mechanical sensations projected to the teeth are mediated by periodontal mechanoreceptors. Corneal sensations are mostly unpleasant, if not frankly painful. Indeed, the corneal nerve endings are dense with substance P and calcitonin gene-related peptide, i.e., nociceptive neurotransmitters.

The proximal axons of the gasserian ganglion cells form the sensory root, which enters the mid-ventrolateral pons together with the motor root (which keeps a ventromedial position). The transition from Schwann cell myelination to oligodendroglial myelination begins a few millimeters from the root entry zone (Redlich–Obersteiner zone). The pathway of the sensory root, from the middle posterior fossa to the cerebellopontine angle, explains why trigeminal pain is often the presenting symptom of tumors of the skull base.

The intra-axial fibers of the primary neurons head toward the various nuclei that constitute the trigeminal brainstem complex, which extends from the midbrain to the C2 segment of the spinal cord.

Motor nucleus

The trigeminal motor nucleus is located in the dorsolateral pontine tegmentum, ventromedial to the trigeminal main sensory nucleus. Trigeminal motoneurons have been studied less extensively than spinal motoneurons and differ from them in several ways. They receive a strong inhibitory input from mechanoreceptors and free nerve endings (Nakamura, 1980). The powerful inhibition exerted by cutaneous and intraoral Aβ mechanoreceptors and Aδ nociceptors probably compensates for the unusual organization of the jaw-closing motoneurons because, unlike spinal motoneurons, they undergo neither reciprocal inhibition nor Renshaw inhibition: the jaw openers are devoid of muscle spindles and all trigeminal motoneurons lack recurrent axons (Darian Smith, 1966; Nakamura, 1980). This organization, particularly the inhibition arising from peri- and intraoral receptors, contributes to speech control, exerts a defensive action during mastication, and has been thought to play a role in masticatory myofascial pains.

Mesencephalic sensory nucleus

The mesencephalic nucleus of the trigeminal sensory complex is a thin column that extends in the dorsomedial tegmentum from the level of the trigeminal motor nucleus in the pons to the rostral midbrain. Unique in the nervous system, this sensory nucleus, rather than the ganglion, contains the cell bodies of primary sensory neurons; these convey information from proprioceptors of the oculomotor and masticatory systems. The Ia axons of mesencephalic neurons that innervate the muscle spindles of jaw-closing muscles, at a short distance from their cell bodies give off short collaterals that connect monosynaptically with jaw-closing motoneurons in the pons, and mediate the jaw jerk (or mandibular stretch reflex).

Principal sensory nucleus

Compared to the other trigeminal sensory nuclei, this is a small gray mass that lies in the dorsolateral pontine tegmentum, close to the motor nucleus. Although small-sized, it receives a most important input from the Aβ myelinated afferents that convey tactile information from capsulated mechanoreceptors in all trigeminal territories (Darian Smith, 1966).

Spinal trigeminal complex

This consists of the trigeminal descending tract (intra-axial primary afferents) and spinal nucleus (second-order neurons). The primary afferents descend caudally, always keeping lateral to the nucleus, down to the C2 spinal segment. The tract contains Aβ large myelinated, Aδ small myelinated, and unmyelinated (C) afferents conveying tactile, thermal, and nociceptive inputs from all trigeminal territories, as well as primary afferents of other cranial nerves (VII, IX, X) conveying sensory input from the ear, pharynx, and larynx. All these afferents connect with the second-order neurons in the spinal nucleus, which extends from mid-pons to C2 and is rostrocaudally divided into three subnuclei: oralis, interpolaris, and caudalis (Johnson et al., 1991). Nucleus oralis, the most rostral, merges in the pons with the main sensory nucleus. Nucleus interpolaris, located between the other two nuclei, extends from the rostral pole of the hypoglossal nucleus to the obex.

Nucleus caudalis merges with the spinal dorsal horn and, having a similar laminar organization, is also known as medullary dorsal horn. Gobel et al. (1977), incorporating the adjacent medullary reticular formation with the nucleus caudalis, divided this medullary dorsal horn in several layers: lamina I corresponds to the marginal layer and includes the interstitial nucleus of Cajal; lamina II corresponds to the substantia gelatinosa and contains a larger number of small-diameter axons than laminae III and IV, which correspond to the magnocellular layer and mostly contain large myelinated axons; lamina V corresponds to the subnucleus reticularis dorsalis and lamina VI to the subnucleus reticularis ventralis of the lateral reticular formation.

The trigeminal spinal nucleus has a multiple anatomical-functional organization, two dealing with somatotopy and one with sensory modality. It is traditionally accepted that the nucleus caudalis has an "onion peel" organization, with oral and perioral areas rostrally (rostrum), and then all the other lateral territories disposed progressively more caudally, with forehead and scalp reaching the first spinal segments. It is also known, however, that in the trigeminal spinal nucleus the somatotopic representation of the ophthalmic, maxillary, and mandibular regions follows a ventrolateral to dorsomedial disposition, with the ophthalmic region ventrolateral, the mandibular region dorsomedial, and the maxillary region in between (Johnson et al., 1991). Finally, it is generally agreed that the rostral subnuclei of the trigeminal spinal nucleus contribute with the main sensory nucleus to relay and modulation of the orofacial touch sense; they mostly contain low-threshold mechanoreceptive neurons that provide the higher brain levels with detailed information on tactile sensations (Darian Smith, 1966). In contrast, nucleus caudalis is universally considered as the main brainstem nucleus serving orofacial nociception.

In the nucleus caudalis, nociceptive terminals project to laminae I, II, V, and VI. Most neurons of the outer layers (I–II) are nociceptive-specific (NS); those in lamina V are wide dynamic range (WDR). The former respond selectively to noxious stimuli conveyed by small (Aδ and C) afferents. The latter, excited by both noxious and non-noxious stimuli, receive both large- (Aβ) and small-fiber terminals. WDR neurons can encode and project different types of sensory information, nociceptive and non-nociceptive, varying their firing rate (higher for noxious and lower for non-noxious stimuli). NS neurons have a fairly localized receptive field and probably play an important role in spatial detection of nociceptive stimuli. In contrast, since WDR neurons have a large receptive field and a stimulus–response function (the higher the stimulus intensity, the higher the firing rate of their output), their main function consists of detection and discrimination of intensity of the noxious stimuli (Dubner, 1985; Sessle, 1991).

Although nucleus caudalis is the most important trigeminal relay for pain transmission, it also contains low-threshold mechanoreceptive neurons, in laminae III and IV, mostly receiving tactile afferents from the ophthalmic division. Conversely, nucleus oralis and interpolaris receive small-diameter afferents and contain NS and WDR neurons. Hence, the whole trigeminal spinal complex probably contributes to orofacial nociception and may play a role in the pathophysiology of orofacial pains.

Central projections

Most axons of the trigeminal second-order neurons cross the midline and convey their signals through the trigeminothalamic pathways. The fibers arising from the main sensory nucleus and the rostral part of the spinal nucleus form the trigeminal lemniscus, which ascends with the medial lemniscus and projects to the ventral posteromedial nucleus (VPM) of the thalamus (Sessle, 1991). Those arising from the nucleus caudalis merge with the spinothalamic tract, which conveys thermal pain information, and project both to the lateral thalamus (VPM) and to the medial and intralaminar thalamic nuclei.

Similar to the spinal system, the trigeminal system finally projects to the somatosensory primary and secondary cortices (SI and SII) in the parietal lobe, and thermal nociceptive inputs also reach the insula and the anterior cingulated gyrus. In contrast with the classical description of the sensory homunculus, whereas the tactile input from the lower (V3) and upper (V1) facial territories are largely overlapped in SI, the lower territories are represented mostly contralaterally and the upper territories bilaterally in both SI and SII (Iannetti et al., 2003). Regarding the cortical processing of thermal pain sensations, the trigeminal system does not appear to differ from the spinal system: sensory discriminative aspects are probably processed in the opercular insular cortices, and affective motivational aspects in several areas, including the cingulate gyrus, for both the Aδ and C inputs (Cruccu et al., 2003).

TRIGEMINAL NEURALGIA (TN)

Definitions

TN or *tic douloureux* is most easily recognized in medical practice. The International Association for the Study of Pain defines TN as "a sudden, usually unilateral, brief stabbing recurrent pain in the distribution of one or more branches of the fifth cranial nerve" (Merskey and Bogduk, 1994). The disorder is more common in women than in men (female-to-male ratio 3:2).

TN may have no apparent cause (idiopathic, essential, or classical TN) or be secondary to multiple sclerosis, benign compressions in the posterior fossa, or arteriovenous malformations (symptomatic TN). Because the debate about the possible causes of the so-called idiopathic TN is still open, we believe that the terminology and definitions proposed by the International Headache Society, also adopted by recent Euro-American guidelines, are the most appropriate: classical TN (with no apparent cause other than vascular compressions) and symptomatic TN (pain indistinguishable from that of classical TN but caused by a demonstrable structural lesion other than vascular compressions) (Headache Classification Subcommittee of the International Headache Society, 2004; Cruccu et al., 2008; Gronseth et al., 2008).

The categorization of TN into typical and atypical forms is based on symptom constellation, and not etiology; thus typical TN must not be confused with classical TN. Although TN is classified as neuropathic pain because it is a direct consequence of a somatosensory system lesion, it has unique features that make it different from the other neuropathic pains.

Epidemiology

Until the last couple of years, the epidemiology of TN dated mainly from the 1980s (Zakrzewska and Hamlyn, 1999). Its incidence was estimated at 4.5 per 100 000, with a prevalence of 0.01%, and its peak incidence was in the 50–60-year age group. However, recent interest in neuropathic pain has resulted in several epidemiological studies which have among others looked at the prevalence and incidence of TN. In a community-based study involving 6.8 million patients in UK primary care centers, 8268 patients were reported to have TN, which gave an incidence of 26.8 per 100 000 persons per year. This study showed a higher incidence of females in all age groups and that the peak incidence of the disease appears to be falling, to between 45 and 59 years (Hall et al., 2006). A further study done in Europe, involving France, Germany, Italy, the Netherlands, Spain, and the UK, was part of a larger observational cross-sectional study of broad neuropathic pain syndromes. Eighty-two patients were identified with TN and in this sample the mean age was 62 years, with 46% of the patients being aged over 65. There was a predominance of females, at 67%. Over 50% of these patients reported having pain for over 3 years. Over two-thirds of the patients reported moderate to severe pain and this pain interfered significantly with their quality of life. Over 94% of the patients were on prescription medication and yet their pain appeared to be poorly controlled. The authors suggested that the burden of TN is significant and that many patients are treated suboptimally (Tolle et al., 2006). Occasionally, TN may occur in more than one member of the same family (Smyth et al., 2003).

Symptoms

TN symptoms are unmistakable and the condition is usually recognizable from the patient history alone.

Pain distribution is unilateral (bilateral TN may sometimes occur in multiple sclerosis) and follows the sensory distribution of the trigeminal divisions, typically radiating to the maxillary (V2) or mandibular (V3) territories. Ophthalmic (V1) on its own is less common and was considered indicative of symptomatic TN (see below). Strongly indicative of a symptomatic form, often a focal neuropathy, is pain in the tongue, which is very rarely affected in classical TN. The pain can be experienced extraorally, intraorally, or both. It is not felt in the teeth (Bowsher, 2000). The right side of the face is involved more frequently than the left. Pain, usually referred to as stabbing or electric shock-like, is brief and paroxysmal, lasting a few seconds, with no pain between paroxysms, although there is often an after-pain, described as burning or dull, which slowly fades away. Paroxysms may occur several times a day. Especially in the early years of the condition there can be long periods of no pain but these remission periods gradually become shorter and shorter. There is currently no method of determining when a patient will go into remission. The pain severity varies, but with time becomes worse and leads to reduced quality of life and depression, which can lead to suicide.

Pain can be evoked or spontaneous. Pain may be provoked by stimulating cutaneous or mucous trigeminal territories (trigger zones), regardless of the distribution of the perceived pain. Gently touching the face, washing or shaving, talking, brushing the teeth, chewing, swallowing, or even a slight breeze, but not thermal or painful stimuli, can trigger the paroxysms. Up to a third of patients will report the pain affecting their sleep. Adjunctive signs may occur during paroxysms. Pain provokes brief muscle spasms of the facial muscles, thus producing the tic. Lacrimation, rhinorrhea, or redness of the face is very rare.

Classical TN more often occurs in the sixth or seventh decade of life and is stereotyped in each individual.

Differential diagnosis between classical and symptomatic forms

About 15% of cases are secondary to major neurological disease such as tumors or multiple sclerosis (symptomatic TN) (Cruccu et al., 2008, 2009). How does one identify these patients? Many of these patients may have symptoms of typical TN (although both tumors and multiple sclerosis may induce other types of facial pain without the characteristics of typical TN). Traditionally, the clinical features that were considered indicators of probable symptomatic TN were:

- Bilateral pain
- Finding of sensory deficits
- Involvement of the ophthalmic division
- Unresponsiveness to medical treatment
- Onset age below 50 years.

In a recent, systematic review of the evidence-based literature, a joint Euro-American taskforce came to different conclusions (Cruccu et al., 2008; Gronseth et al., 2008). Bilateral pain has indeed 100% specificity, but its occurrence is rare, even in symptomatic TN (sensitivity 0–7%). Whereas quantitative sensory testing may disclose subclinical abnormalities (Nurmikko and Eldridge, 2001; Sinay et al., 2003), the finding of clinically manifest sensory deficits is highly specific (98%), but the sensitivity is only 37%. In other words, the finding of sensory deficits or bilateral pain is an excellent indicator of symptomatic TN but their absence does not indicate classical TN.

The involvement of the ophthalmic division is equally rare (21% and 23%) in the two forms. Similarly, there was no significant difference in response to treatment. The mean onset age was significantly lower in symptomatic (48 years) than in classical (57 years) TN, but the histogram of onset age distribution showed that there was considerable overlap in the age ranges of the two populations. Thus, although younger age increases the risk of finding symptomatic TN, the diagnostic accuracy of age as a predictor of symptomatic TN is too low to be clinically useful. Hence, this taskforce concluded that it is impossible to exclude a symptomatic form on clinical grounds alone (Cruccu et al., 2008; Gronseth et al., 2008). We recommend performing neuroimaging or neurophysiological investigations, at least once, in all patients (see below).

Etiology

Symptomatic TN can be related to slowly growing tumors, such as cholesteatomas, meningiomas, or neurinomas of the eighth nerve, which compress the trigeminal nerve root near the dorsal root entry zone. Tumors affecting the gasserian ganglion are rare, and neurinomas of the fifth nerve are never associated with typical TN. Rather, they cause sensory deficits and, if present, pain is constant (Bullit et al., 1986). Multiple sclerosis is typically associated with TN (2–4% of patients with TN) (Jensen et al., 1982). Neurophysiological, neuroimaging, and pathological studies indicate that the demyelinating plaque that provokes TN affects the intrapontine presynaptic primary afferents near the root entry zone (Cruccu et al., 1990, 2009; Gass et al., 1997) (Figure 56.1).

As already anticipated, many investigators refute the term "idiopathic TN" because they support the view that, when no lesion affecting the trigeminal system can be demonstrated, TN is due to a vascular compression of the trigeminal nerve root by tortuous or aberrant vessels (Figure 56.2). Microsurgical interventions in the posterior fossa have shown that the compressing vessel is most often the superior cerebellar artery (about 75% of cases). A vein may contribute to compression and can be the only compressing vessel in about 10% of patients (Jannetta, 1967; Barker et al., 1996). Further support to this view comes from magnetic resonance imaging (MRI) studies reporting a frequent contact between vessels and the trigeminal root (Meaney et al., 1995). Consistently, microvascular decompression (MVD) relieves TN pain (Barker et al., 1996). Furthermore, observations during posterior fossa surgery in patients with tumors and TN demonstrated a vessel compressing the nerve at the root entry zone in almost all patients (Barker et al., 1996).

Nevertheless, other investigators do not support the view that a vascular compression is the main factor, because compression of the trigeminal nerve root near the root entry zone is often found (7–12%) during standard autopsy of patients with no history of TN (Klun and Prestor, 1986; Adams, 1989) and on MRI TN patients may have bilateral compressions but no bilateral symptoms. Unfortunately the question cannot be simply solved through MRI screening for neurovascular contact because, according to recent guidelines, no reliable, standardized MRI technique exists to document neurovascular contacts (even if no contact is seen on MRI, neurosurgeons often find one at operation), and because documenting a contact does not prove a causative relationship (MRI scans often show, and neurosurgeons find, contacts with asymptomatic nerves) (Cruccu et al., 2008; Gronseth et al., 2008). Bilateral neurovascular contacts are frequent in patients with unilateral TN (71% according to Anderson et al., 2006), as well as unilateral or bilateral contacts in subjects who do not have TN (75% according to Kress et al., 2006).

Possibly, several factors may contribute to the development of TN. Indeed it is a fairly consistent finding that 25–30% of patients do not experience complete and persistent pain relief after MVD (Cruccu et al., 2008). Neurosurgeons have found that manipulation alone, or even just exposure of the trigeminal nerve, causes a temporary remission of TN (Shelden et al., 1955; Fields and Lemak, 1987). Several investigators believe that the origin of the disease is multifactorial.

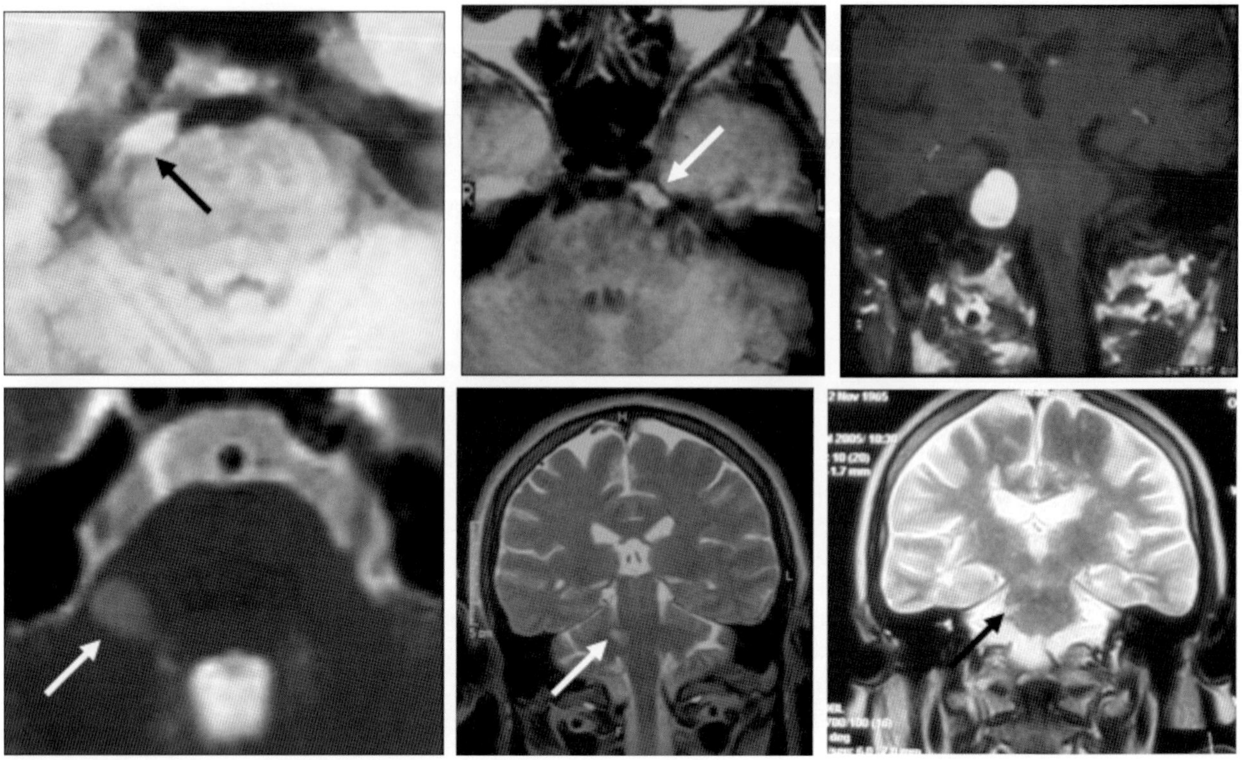

Fig. 56.1. Common causes of symptomatic trigeminal neuralgia. Upper row: benign tumors along the extra-axial course of the trigeminal root. Lower row: demyelinating plaques along the intra-axial course of the trigeminal afferents.

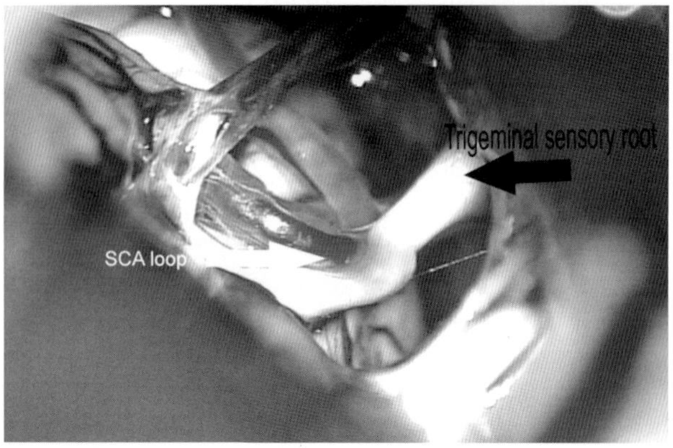

Fig. 56.2. Neurovascular compression. Picture taken during an intervention of microvascular decompression in the posterior fossa: the trigeminal sensory root is distorted by a loop of the superior cerebellar artery (SCA). (Courtesy of Professor Hugh Coakham; reproduced from Zakrzewska, 2006, with permission.)

For TN in multiple sclerosis, a recent study of 139 patients proposed a dual mechanism involving both a demyelinating plaque and a neurovascular contact (Cruccu et al., 2009). These two mechanisms would act on the same primary axons and both would produce demyelination. Indeed, histopathological studies of surgical specimens describe demyelination in the proximal, centrally myelinated part of the trigeminal root both in patients with multiple sclerosis-related TN and in those with classical TN (Love et al., 1998, 2001). This double-crush hypothesis receives further support from neurosurgical studies on the outcome of MVD because patients with multiple sclerosis-related TN, despite experiencing considerable pain relief, benefit less than patients with classical TN (Eldridge et al., 2003; Broggi et al., 2004).

Pathophysiology

As the symptoms of classical and symptomatic TN are identical, and the latter is always secondary to an extra-axial or intra-axial lesion near the root entry zone, the primary site of damage is thought to be peripheral, near the root entry zone. Possibly because the nerve fibers change their myelination (from Schwann cells to oligodendroglia) in this site, this area may represent a *locus minoris resistentiae*.

Demyelination of the primary afferents is necessary (Love and Coakham, 2001). Whether produced by multiple sclerosis or chronic compression exerted by a blood vessel or a benign tumor, demyelination increases the susceptibility of the nerve fibers to ectopic excitation, ephaptic transmission, and high-frequency discharges (Burchiel, 1980). Ephaptic transmission between large myelinated, non-nociceptive afferents and nociceptive afferents may explain how innocuous stimuli can trigger painful paroxysms (Calvin et al., 1982). That the most frequent trigger zones are perioral could be explained by the large number of afferents innervating this area. This theory entails demyelination in Aδ nociceptive afferents, which was only recently demonstrated (Cruccu et al., 2001; Obermann et al., 2007). Paroxysmal bursts of ectopic activity arising from large-diameter, non-nociceptive afferents may induce a secondary central dysfunction: repeated, abnormally high-frequency activity in tactile afferents projecting to WDR neurons in the spinal trigeminal nucleus may increase their excitability and induce a persistent derangement that provokes high-frequency signals from WDR neurons and thus pain. Several instances supporting this hypothesis have been reported. The perioral location of the trigger point would in this case be explained by the large representation of the perioral region in the spinal trigeminal nucleus, which makes it the most likely source of paroxysmal activity (Fromm et al., 1991). In summary, the primary cause of TN must necessarily affect the peripheral afferents, but the pathophysiological mechanism may or may not secondarily involve the brainstem neurons.

Medical therapy

Patients with TN do not respond to conventional analgesic drugs. As the mechanism leading to paroxysmal pain begins in demyelinated fibers, which become hyperexcitable and generate high-frequency discharges, the ideal drugs are those reducing neuronal excitability and in particular those able to limit the discharge frequency, i.e., sodium channel blockers. To this category belong some local anesthetics (lidocaine) and antiepileptic drugs (phenytoin, carbamazepine (CBZ), oxcarbazepine (OXC), lamotrigine).

Currently, the first-choice medical treatments of TN are CBZ and OXC (Attal et al., 2006; Cruccu et al., 2008).

Over 70% of patients respond to CBZ. The starting dose should be 200 mg/day, to be increased by 200 mg every second day, until the patient reaches satisfactory pain relief or encounters unpleasant side-effects. In patients with classical TN, CBZ has a quick and intense antineuralgic effect. Usually 400–800 mg daily is sufficient. A retard formulation can be useful at night. Although in epilepsy CBZ is administered up to 2400 mg/day, its function dose–response is non-linear in TN: the increments in its antineuralgic effects decrease with dose and reach a plateau at about 1200 mg; higher doses of CBZ do not induce further pain relief (Nakata et al., 1991). The most common side-effects of CBZ pertain to the central nervous system (CNS): drowsiness, dizziness, unsteadiness, or difficulty concentrating (less frequently diplopia), which usually subside within a few days or weeks. In some elderly patients, however, the CNS disturbances may cause discontinuation of CBZ. Cutaneous reactions have been reported in about 6% of patients; in most cases these reactions are of minor importance, but rare cases of Stevens–Johnson syndrome have also been reported.

Although very rare (about 1 in 200 000 patients), the most serious complication is aplastic anemia, but mild and transient leukopenia and thrombocytopenia occur in about 10% of patients. A complete blood count should be performed before the first administration of CBZ and every 2 weeks for the first 2 months of treatment; afterwards, two blood counts a year are sufficient. Numerous drug interactions can occur and this is especially important as the majority of patients are elderly and already taking medication.

OXC, a daughter drug of CBZ, was developed in order to minimize the side-effects on the CNS. The number of patients treated with OXC for epilepsy is now large enough to know that the effects on blood cells are low, so blood cell counts are not compulsory. On the other hand OXC may induce a depletion of Na^+ ions (6% of elderly patients), so it is necessary to measure electrolyte concentration in the first month of treatment. This is dose-dependent and at higher dosages (above 1200 mg/day) sodium should be monitored (especially if patients are taking diuretics) (Jensen, 2002; Zakrzewska and Patsalos, 2002; Attal et al., 2006; Cruccu et al., 2008). Several studies have reported that OXC is as effective as CBZ in TN treatment, both drugs yielding at least 50% reduction of the attacks in 88% of patients with classical TN (Beydoun, 2002; Carrazana and Mikoshiba, 2003). Usually the starting dose is 600 mg/day, increasing by 300 mg every few days according to the clinical response. The effective dose ranges between 900 and 1800 mg daily.

According to recent guidelines (Attal et al., 2006; Cruccu et al., 2008), patients who reach effective doses of CBZ or OXC but do not experience enough pain relief become candidates for surgical interventions. Patients who cannot reach effective doses of CBZ and OXC because of contraindications or adverse events should try second-line drugs.

Baclofen has been shown to be possibly effective in treatment of TN. It has the advantage of a synergistic action with CBZ (Fromm et al., 1984), but probably because of the frequent, and sometimes severe, side-effects of this $GABA_B$ agonist, it is currently rarely prescribed.

The new generation of antiepileptic drugs has brought new hope for the treatment of neuropathic pains and many studies are also being carried out in TN.

Although there are case series reporting the efficacy of several new drugs, we are aware of only one randomized controlled trial (RCT), which demonstrates efficacy of lamotrigine as add-on therapy (Zakrzewska et al., 1997).

Oral phenytoin (historically the first antiepileptic drug used for the treatment of TN) is effective in only 25% of patients and its chronic administration has serious adverse effects (Attal et al., 2006). But phenytoin can be administrated intravenously, and thus it is useful in emergency, when extremely frequent TN paroxysms preclude taking anything orally (Cheshire, 2001).

Spontaneous recovery in typical CTN is rare and the condition is cyclical with periods of partial or complete remission and recurrence. It is reasonable to encourage patients to adjust the dosage to the frequency of attacks and some patients may even be able to stop all medication.

There are no placebo-controlled studies regarding medical management of symptomatic TN. The existing studies all deal with TN associated with multiple sclerosis and are small open-label trials. Lamotrigine, gabapentin, topiramate, and misoprostol (a prostaglandin E_1 analog) have been reported to be efficacious in patients with TN and multiple sclerosis (Attal et al., 2006; Cruccu et al., 2008).

Surgical therapy

There is now increasing evidence to suggest that early surgical treatment may be appropriate, especially in patients with classical signs of TN and in whom MRI investigations show evidence of neurovascular compression of the trigeminal nerve. The decision to have surgery is a difficult one and a recent study using a time trade-off methodology suggested that patients prefer surgery to medical management (Spatz et al., 2007). Among surgical treatments patients had preferences for treatments that either yielded longer pain relief periods or had few side-effects. Thus radiofrequency thermocoagulation (RFT) was the treatment least likely to be chosen by patients because the incidence of numbness after this treatment is extremely high. On the other hand, balloon compression (BC) appeared to be a very popular choice as there is currently little in the literature to suggest that patients have complications after this procedure (Spatz et al., 2007). Patients may find further help from support groups which have now been set up in several countries and which also have their own websites and written information (Zakrzewska, 2006).

Surgical treatment divides into two major types of surgery. Many of the procedures could be called ablative or destructive as they aim to reduce sensory transmission along the trigeminal nerve. One procedure, microvascular decompression (MVD), attempts to be curative and aims at removing the presumed cause of TN, i.e., nerve compression by blood vessels. Ablative procedures can be carried out at the peripheral level, at the gasserian ganglion level, or centrally at the root entry zone.

Table 56.1 summarizes benefits and harms of the main surgical procedures.

Peripheral treatments

These are aimed at the discrete trigger points that patients can identify. The procedures involved include cryosurgery, laser, alcohol injection, streptomycin injections, and peripheral radiofrequency treatment. The only RCT in this series of treatments has been of streptomycin injections and this showed no effectiveness (Bittar and Graff-Radford, 1993). The other treatments have only been evaluated in case series and these have shown that, on average, a maximum of 1 year's pain relief is gained and often patients need to remain on small doses of their medication in order to gain complete pain relief. In general, these procedures have few side-effects, although some temporary sensory localized loss can

Table 56.1

Outcomes after surgical management for trigeminal neuralgia yielding 100% pain relief

Procedure	Pain relief period	Complications
Microvascular decompression	High: 70% pain-free at 10 years	0.5% mortality, 4% unilateral hearing loss, minor long-term
Radiofrequency thermocoagulation	Good: 50% pain-free at 5 years	>50% sensory loss of varying degree, anesthesia dolorosa
Percutaneous glycerol rhizotomy	Good: 50% pain-free at 4 years	<50% sensory loss of varying degree
Balloon compression	Good: 50% pain-free at 4 years	Masticatory problems common in first year, <50% sensory loss
Gamma knife	Good: 50% pain-free at 4 years, some partial relief, and can be delayed	7% sensory loss, delayed onset of complications

often be detected. These procedures are now very rarely used and mainly reserved for very frail patients with acute symptoms who want an immediate effect.

Percutaneous gasserian lesions

There are three main procedures that are done at the gasserian ganglion level. These are RFT, percutaneous glycerol rhizotomy (PGR), and BC.

A review of all the literature of surgical managements of TN showed that there were no RCTs of treatments at the gasserian ganglion level. A considerable amount of the evidence is in the form of case series, many of which have not been independently validated and have short follow-ups. Zakrzewska and Lopez (2003) critically reviewed all the published literature and put forward some recommendations for future reporting of trials. It is these recommendations that have been used to assess the current literature. Only data that were validated by an independent observer have been used to provide the following information, which is based on the recent guidelines of the American Academy of Neurology and European Federation of Neurological Sciences (Cruccu et al., 2008; Gronseth et al., 2008).

The gasserian ganglion procedures involve the insertion of a needle under radiographic control through the foramen ovale into the trigeminal cistern. Once the needle is accurately located and checked by the use of radiology then treatment can commence. In RFT an electrical stimulus is passed through the needle tip: this generates a temperature between 60°C and 80°C. This is maintained for 60–300 s. The position of the needle and the area of the lesion can to some extent be predicted by waking the patient at the start of the procedure to test the area that has been affected. Although some believed that the complications would be reduced if RFT were delivered in a more pulsed method, a recent RCT showed that pulsed radiofrequency treatment (although achieving lower temperatures) does not give enough pain relief (Erdine et al., 2007). After undergoing this therapy most patients will report sensory numbness. This can sometimes be confined to only one branch but may extend to all three branches. The level of sensory loss can vary from mild parasthesia through to the rare but extremely debilitating anesthesia dolorosa. RFT should not be aimed at the first division, because of the risk of inducing corneal anesthesia that can lead to corneal damage and subsequent loss of sight.

If the likelihood of sensory loss is to be reduced then either PGR or BC may be better choices. The PGR technique involves first identifying the size of the cistern and then injecting a small volume of glycerol. Altering the patient's head position and adjusting the volume of injected glycerol can produce different areas of sensory loss. The main disadvantage of this technique is that it is relatively imprecise and injection of too much glycerol can cause it to spread more extensively and result in dense sensory loss.

BC involves inflating a small Fogarty catheter within the Meckel's cave to compress the trigeminal nerve and therefore cause decreased sensory transmission. The needle has to be slightly larger to accommodate this Fogarty catheter and this can lead to vasovagal attacks, including arrhythmias and cardiac arrest during penetration of the foramen. There is a much higher incidence of masseteric muscle weakness but this tends to be only temporary. Sensory loss is greatly reduced and there have been no reports of corneal anesthesia.

These procedures are done under heavy sedation or general anesthetic and in most cases patients only need stay in hospital overnight. Overall all these procedures give a pain relief time of around 5 years, with RFT giving the longest pain-free period and PGR the shortest. These procedures are probably best suited to patients who are too frail to undergo major neurosurgery (Figure 56.3).

Posterior fossa surgery

In this area, both an ablative and a reparative procedure can be carried out. MVD is a major neurosurgical procedure which involves access to the posterior fossa. Its goal is to decompress the trigeminal nerve, most frequently near the root entry zone, and so result in pain relief without loss of function. As this is a major neurosurgical procedure, patients need to be medically fit and usually stay in hospital for 5–7 days. Notwithstanding increasing sophistication of MRI it is still difficult to predict the presence of blood vessels compressing the trigeminal root prior to surgery (Cruccu et al., 2008). The most frequently involved vessel is the superior cerebellar artery but other vessels may be involved and there may be more than one compression. Arteries are carefully lifted away from the trigeminal nerve and a material such as Teflon is interposed between the vessel and the nerve. Sometimes a special sling utilizing adjacent veins is made to keep the vessel out of the way. If veins are thought to be compressing the nerve, then these are removed. If no compression is found some surgeons will go on to do a partial sensory rhizotomy which will then lead to sensory loss.

The operation is associated with mortality of around 0.5% and to some extent depends on the expertise of the surgeon. The cause of death is mainly due to hemorrhage and infarcts, although some of them are of the type one would expect after any major operation

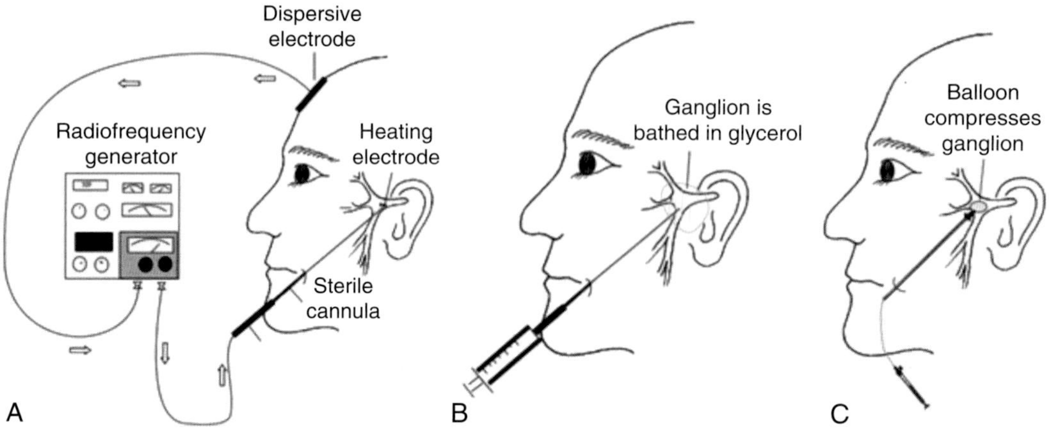

Fig. 56.3. Percutaneous lesions. After a needle is introduced through the foramen ovale under radiographic control into Meckel's cave, a variety of procedures can be carried out. A lesion can be made using currents that will generate temperatures between 60 and 80°C (A), the ganglion can be bathed in glycerol (B), or compressed by a Foley catheter (C). (Courtesy of H. MacParland; modified from Zakrzewska, 2006, with permission.)

such as pulmonary embolus and gastrointestinal hemorrhage. If closure has not been totally secure then a cerebrospinal fluid leak may be encountered; in some cases this will close spontaneously but in other patients it may need reoperation. Meningitis, mainly aseptic, occurs in the perioperative period. Hearing problems are frequent and many of these will resolve with time, but up to 2% of patients may develop ipsilateral hearing loss. Some are due to otitis media whereas others are caused by direct injury to the eighth nerve. Headaches are frequent and may persist for a considerable time postsurgically. Other temporary complications include wound infections and diplopia. Only a very small percentage of patients will notice any sensory changes. The higher-quality data, independent observers' assessed outcomes, and Kaplan–Meier survival data show that the probability of a recurrence of pain after MVD is low and 70% of patients may remain pain-free at 10 years. The highest rate of recurrence is within the first 2 years. Recent independent patient satisfaction surveys have indicated that patients are satisfied with outcomes, especially if these are linked with no complications. They also feel that the operation should have been performed earlier in the disease process (Zakrzewska et al., 2005).

Stereotactic radiosurgery or gamma knife procedure

This is the latest procedure to have been adopted and has been made possible by improvements in MRI scanning. In this procedure, a dose of radiation, 70–90 Gy, is directed towards the trigeminal nerve anywhere between the gasserian ganglion and the root entry zone. Special care is taken to avoid radiation to the brain itself. The major advantage of this procedure is that it is non-invasive and the only surgical procedure is that of fixing the head frame to the patient in four positions. Patients, however, must be able to lie very still within the MRI machine for the duration of the treatment. There is a considerable amount of data being published on this, but a recent systematic review found that there is little information about long-term results (Lopez et al., 2004). There is now one study that has reviewed patients in a prospective way where the assessments postoperatively were made by an independent neurologist (Regis et al., 2006). In their series of 100 patients followed up for a minimum of 12 months, 94% of patients did achieve initial pain relief. However, the medium delay prior to pain relief was 10 days, with a range of 0–25 weeks. By 36 months, the probability of patients remaining pain-free is around 58%. The authors found that 34 patients had reported a recurrence of pain within 1–15 months of initial pain relief. Some of these patients required further surgery. Only 10 adverse events were noted and these were all related to sensory changes. There was no experience of eye problems, masseteric muscle weakness, neuropathic pain, or anesthesia dolorosa. Qualitative sensory testing found no significant change of sensitivity thresholds on the ipsilateral side. No other neurological complications outside the trigeminal nerve territory were found and no systemic complications were reported. Some of the patients had preoperative numbness and therefore these are likely to be the ones who then develop sensory changes. Patient satisfaction was high, with 88% reporting satisfaction with the procedure that they had undergone. Some of these patients had to be on the minimum dosage of medication. In 2008 and 2009, after the publication of the Euro-American guidelines that constitute the basis of our comments about surgical treatment of TN in this chapter (Cruccu et al., 2008; Gronseth et al., 2008), eight studies have been published on gamma knife radiosurgery, largely confirming the rates of success and complications (Broggi et al., 2004; Fariselli et al., 2009).

With the increasing numbers of surgical procedures available, patient choice has increased even further and so decision-making becomes very difficult, as not only are there more drugs available but there are more surgical procedures. However, at the center of management is a clear diagnosis, as it may only be those patients with definitive compression of the trigeminal nerve who really benefit from surgical procedures. The other patients may have other causes for their TN and hence require other forms of therapy.

There is very little in the surgical literature on management of recurrences but in general it appears that patients who have a recurrence either undergo the same procedure they had initially or go on to have another type of procedure. The results are often less effective in terms of outcome measures and if it is a second ablative procedure then the risk of sensory loss rises (Zakrzewska, 2002).

There is very little objective high-quality evidence to direct the management of patients with multiple sclerosis. It has been noted that some patients with multiple sclerosis may also have compression of the trigeminal nerve and if this is found to be the case then surgical treatment can be of benefit, provided there are no plaques of multiple sclerosis present at that point.

OTHER CRANIAL NEURALGIAS

Glossopharyngeal neuralgia

According to the International Headache Society definition, glossopharyngeal neuralgia is a severe transient stabbing pain experienced in the ear, base of the tongue, tonsillar fossa, or beneath the angle of the jaw.

Epidemiology

Glossoparyngeal neuralgia is a rare pain condition which occurs in younger patients than TN (40% of patients are under 50 years). It is more common in female (67%) than male (33%) patients (Patel et al., 2002). Both sides are affected in up to 12% of patients. Trigeminal and glossopharyngeal neuralgia may sometimes be associated in the same patient (Rushton et al., 1981).

Etiology and pathophysiology

Although glossopharyngeal neuralgia usually occurs without any evident lesion affecting the glossopharyngeal nerve, most authors suggest that it is related to a vascular compression of the glossopharyngeal nerve at the root entry zone. According to MRI findings and observations during posterior fossa surgery, the posterior inferior cerebellar artery is the most frequent vessel compressing the glossopharyngeal nerve (Fischbach et al., 2003). Elongated or fractured styloid process, calcified stylohyoid ligament (Eagle's syndrome), cerebellopontine angle tumors, parapharyngeal space lesions, carcinoma of the parapharyngeal space, carcinoma of the pharynx, nasopharyngeal carcinoma, posterior fossa arteriovenous malformation, and multiple sclerosis are causes of symptomatic glossopharyngeal neuralgia (Rushton et al., 1981; Soh, 1999).

The glossopharyngeal nerve innervates the carotid sinus; hyperactivity of the glossopharyngeal afferents can give rise to activation of the dorsal motor nucleus of the vagus nerve, resulting in parasympathetic vagal efferent response, causing severe bradycardia and eventually asystole (Rushton et al., 1981; Soh, 1999).

Clinical features

These are very similar to TN but the major difference is in location of pain. The pain is felt in the back of the throat in the region of the tonsillar fossa and it then radiates to the ear and even down the neck. It may radiate to only one of these areas. It can therefore be mistaken for pain caused by temporomandibular dysfunction. It is also paroxysmal and lasts for seconds to minutes, and remission periods occur. It is commonly provoked by swallowing, especially sharp foods, talking, or coughing, and may remit and relapse in the fashion of TN. Because it is very rare, glossopharyngeal neuralgia is often misdiagnosed (Teixeira et al., 2008).

It is worth emphasizing that pain attacks may lead to cardiac dysrhythmia and syncope. Examination is unremarkable. The symptomatic forms are often secondary to intra- or extracranial compressions near the jugular foramen, where the two nerves lie very close.

As well as MRI a panoramic radiograph is useful to exclude Eagle's syndrome. An electrocardiogram may be useful to rule out cardiac abnormalities.

Management

The first-line medical treatment for glossopharyngeal neuralgia is CBZ, and all the treatment strategies described for TN also apply to glossopharyngeal neuralgia.

The surgical approach for glossopharyngeal neuralgia varies from nerve sectioning to MVD. The nerve section is performed through a posterior fossa approach, through the neck, or with a transtonsillar approach. This is technically more difficult than an

MVD for TN. Currently MVD is the most common surgical treatment of glossopharyngeal neuralgia (Patel et al., 2002; Sampson et al., 2004). Patel et al. (2002) reported on 217 cases managed with MVD; at 10 years over 75% were still pain-free, but only 50 had been followed up long-term. In the series of 47 patients studied by Sampson et al. (2004), 62% of whom were followed up for more than 10 years, there were only two recurrences. The major complications include dysphagia, hoarseness, and facial paresis. Interestingly, some of the surgical procedures for TN often relieve glossopharyngeal neuralgia as well (Teixeira et al., 2008).

Nervus intermedius neuralgia

This is a rare condition characterized by brief paroxysms of pain felt deeply in the ear. Pain paroxysms are intermittent, last for seconds or minutes, and may be triggered by touching the posterior wall of the auditory canal. Pain is sometimes accompanied by disorders of lacrimation, salivation, or taste. There is a common association with herpes zoster (HZ).

Superior laryngeal neuralgia

Again a rare disorder, it is characterized by severe pain in the lateral aspect of the throat, submandibular region, and underneath the ear, precipitated by swallowing, shouting, or turning the head. A trigger point is present on the lateral aspect of the throat overlying the hypothyroid membrane. The condition is relieved by local anesthetic block and cured by section of the superior laryngeal nerve.

Ophthalmic postherpetic neuralgia

HZ is a localized infection caused by the varicella-zoster virus. After remaining dormant in the sensory ganglia since the primary infection, the virus reactivates and spreads along the nerve fibers to the skin, causing a dermatomally distributed painful rash. In the ganglion, the virus causes neuronal death followed by degeneration of spinal and peripheral axons. The main complication of HZ is postherpetic neuralgia (PHN), a neuropathic pain persisting more than 3 months after skin eruption (Dworkin and Portenoy, 1996). Of all patients with HZ, about 10% will develop PHN, with a higher frequency in elderly patients and diabetic patients. Most often PHN involves thoracic dermatomes (about 50% of patients), but the ophthalmic division of the trigeminal nerve is commonly involved (22–25% of patients) (Loeser, 1986; Watson et al., 1988).

Ophthalmic PHN involves the supraorbital region and the eye. In ophthalmic PHN, as well as in non-trigeminal PHN, the areas involved show skin changes such as hyperpigmentation and scarring. The sensory disturbances consist of hypesthesia, involving all sensory modalities, and pain. Pain is both constant (burning, aching, dull) and paroxysmal (stabbing, electric shock-like); most PHN patients also have allodynia, usually of the dynamic mechanical type (Rowbotham and Fields, 1996). Neurophysiological studies confirm damage to both large- and small-size trigeminal afferents (Truini et al., 2003), and suggest that paroxysmal pain is mostly provoked by demyelination of Aβ fibers and constant pain by loss of Aδ and C axons (Truini et al., 2008).

This trigeminal localization of PHN presents special problems because of eye involvement, which strongly limits the use of the various topical agents that are currently used in PHN treatment. Hence medical treatment is the first choice. Although several RCTs have been carried out in PHN, none was dedicated to trigeminal PHN alone. We are unaware, however, of known differences in responsiveness to drugs. Recent European guidelines recommended for first-line treatment are the tricyclic antidepressants, gabapentin/pregabalin, and topical lidocaine (Attal et al., 2006). Amitriptyline is the most widely used tricyclic antidepressant at a 75-mg dose (the optimal dosage is 1 mg/kg), to be titrated very slowly. Unfortunately, since PHN affects elderly patients, amitriptyline is often discontinued because of its adverse effects (dry mouth, constipation, urinary retention), or cannot be initiated at all because of its contraindications (glaucoma, prostatic hypertrophy, heart conduction abnormalities, myocardial infarction). Pregabalin, a daughter drug of gabapentin (similar efficacy and tolerability), has the advantage of linear pharamcokinetics and more rapid onset of pain relief; effective doses range between 150 and 300 mg daily. Topical lidocaine has only been evaluated in patients with allodynia in short-term studies. However, due to excellent tolerability, this treatment may be preferred in the elderly, particularly in patients with allodynia and a small area of pain. Despite established efficacy in PHN, oxycodone, morphine, and methadone were recommended as second choice (Attal et al., 2006).

DIAGNOSTIC TESTS

Trigeminal reflexes

According to recent European and American neurological guidelines on neuropathic pain assessment and TN management (Cruccu et al., 2004, 2008), the neurophysiological recording of trigeminal reflexes represents the most useful and reliable test in the neurophysiological diagnosis of trigeminal pains. The trigeminal reflexes (Figure 56.4) consists of a series of reflex responses (R1 and R2 components of the

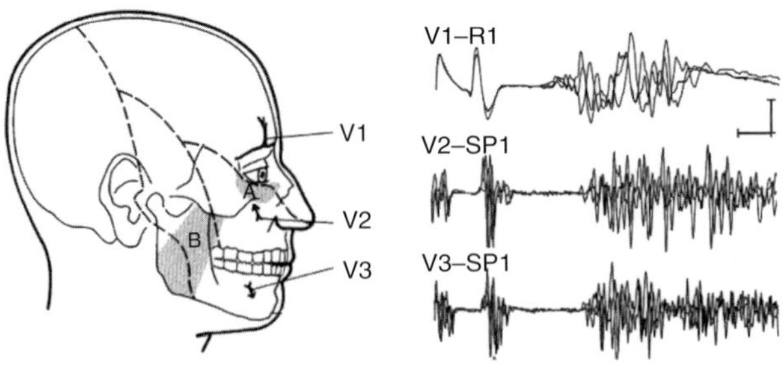

Fig. 56.4. Trigeminal reflexes for diagnosing symptomatic trigeminal neuralgia. One early response is measured for each of the three trigeminal divisions: the R1 blink reflex after stimulation of the supraorbital nerve (V1–R1), the SP1 masseter inhibitory reflex after stimulation of the infraorbital nerve (V2–SP1), and that after stimulation of the mental nerve (V3–SP1). Surface recordings from the orbicularis oculi muscle (for V1) and masseter muscle (for V2 and V3).

blink reflex after electrical stimulation of the ophthalmic division; SP1 and SP2 components of the masseter inhibitory reflex after electrical stimulation of the maxillary or mandibular division; and the jaw jerk to chin taps) that assess function of trigeminal afferents from all trigeminal territories, as well as trigeminal central circuits in the midbrain, pons, and medulla.

In patients reporting pain in the trigeminal territory, trigeminal reflexes offer the clinician useful information. Abnormalities are often discovered in divisions that appear clinically unaffected. An objective demonstration of dysfunction is provided in all patients with pain secondary to a documented disease, such as symptomatic TN, PHN, vascular malformations, benign tumors of the cerebellopontine angle, and multiple sclerosis.

As a tool for disclosing symptomatic TN, neurophysiological testing of trigeminal reflexes provides the same sensitivity (95%) and specificity (93%) as MRI (Cruccu et al., 2006).

Although, like others, we have occasionally seen patients with mild reflex abnormalities, in the majority of patients with classical TN all reflexes are normal. A diagnostic protocol for patients with trigeminal pain should rely primarily on trigeminal reflexes: the technique is easier and less invasive than that for evoked potentials and the finding of any abnormality implies an underlying structural lesion.

Trigeminal evoked potentials

Over recent years continued efforts have been made to find a reliable method to record trigeminal evoked potentials. Several studies have investigated trigeminal evoked potentials elicited by surface stimulation of the lips or gums. Although many investigators have discussed the clinical applicability of these responses, their neural origin has never been proved. Indeed, electrical stimulation of the facial skin unavoidably evokes facial muscle responses, which contaminate or hide the genuine neural signals. A definitive demonstration of this came from a study in curarized subjects, showing that the scalp potentials elicited by surface stimulations consist of myogenic artefacts only (Leandri et al., 1987).

The only certainly genuine and reliable evoked potentials are the very early waves of the scalp potentials described by Leandri and associates (1987), who used two fine needles inserted into the infraorbital foramen (thus avoiding direct stimulation of motor nerve fibers) and recorded from the scalp the far fields generated by trigeminal primary afferents (thus before any reflex could appear). This method, undeniably invasive and technically difficult, is very useful in thermal rhizotomies: the position of the intracranial operating needle can be located, and the severity of the lesion monitored, without awakening the patient from anesthesia (Leandri and Gottlieb, 1996).

Because electrical stimulations unavoidably excite large-diameter afferents, most reflex responses and scalp potentials are mediated by non-nociceptive afferents. To assess nociceptive pathway function, laser stimuli are the best tool. Laser-generated radiant heat pulses selectively excite free nerve endings in the superficial skin layers, activate Aδ and C mechanothermal nociceptors, and evoke scalp potentials generated by the operculoinsular cortex and cingulate gyrus: laser evoked potentials (LEPs) (Garcia-Larrea et al., 2003; Treede et al., 2003). By varying the area of the irradiated spot and the stimulus intensity it is possible to excite preferentially Aδ (evoking pinprick sensations) or C (evoking warmth or burning sensations) receptors (Cruccu et al., 2003).

The short conduction distance and a high receptor density mean that the trigeminal territory is particularly advantageous for LEP recording. Trigeminal LEPs are higher-amplitude and more easily recorded than LEPs after limb stimulations. Trigeminal LEPs have recently been studied in classical and symptomatic TN, trigeminal sensory neuropathy, PHN, Wallenberg syndrome, temporomandibular disorders, and migraine (Cruccu et al., 2001; Truini et al., 2003, 2008).

So far trigeminal LEPs have provided useful pathophysiological information in facial pain syndromes. In the near future they may also be useful as a diagnostic tool. In clinical practice their main limitation is that they are currently available in too few centers.

Recently, a special planar concentric electrode has been developed to preferentially excite nociceptive fibers; because of its concentric design and small anode–cathode distance, this surface stimulating electrode produces high current density at low current intensities, limiting depolarization to the superficial layer of the dermis (Kaube et al., 2000; Katsarava et al., 2006). This electrode proved efficacious in eliciting a nociceptive blink reflex and useful in patients with migraine. The same research group is currently using this electrode to study pain-related evoked potentials in TN (Obermann et al., 2007). If it is confirmed to be selective and devoid of muscle artifacts, this method would have the advantage of being more easily available and thus may become more widespread than laser stimulation.

Neuroimaging and diagnostic process

All patients with a facial pain of unclear origin or suspected of a symptomatic neurological lesion should undergo imaging studies. Currently there are many facial pains of unknown origin, which makes it difficult to determine which patients need imaging. Furthermore computed tomography scans are not sufficiently accurate in conditions such as multiple sclerosis, small tumors, and vascular anomalies.

The following criteria are recommended:

- Always perform, at least once, an MRI or neurophysiological recording of trigeminal reflexes.
- If these are normal, no neuroimaging study is necessary.
- If these are abnormal, perform an MRI to ascertain the nature of the lesion.

Various MRI techniques are used prior to performance of a MVD to demonstrate neurovascular contacts. As already explained, unfortunately no technique is currently considered reliable, both because neurosurgeons may find neurocompression at operation even if the MRI is negative and because of the high frequency of asymptomatic contacts (Cruccu et al., 2008; Gronseth et al., 2008). Hopefully in the future the problem may be solved by the MRI demonstration not only of a contact but also of nerve damage, as suggested by recent findings (Herweh et al., 2007).

Although rare, cranial neuralgias need to be recognized as in many cases effective therapy can be provided through either medical or surgical treatments.

References

Adams CB (1989). Microvascular compression: an alternative view and hypothesis. J Neurosurg 70: 1–12.

Anderson VC, Berryhill PC, Sandquist MA et al. (2006). High-resolution three-dimensional magnetic resonance angiography and three-dimensional spoiled gradient-recalled imaging in the evaluation of neurovascular compression in patients with trigeminal neuralgia: a double-blind pilot study. Neurosurgery 58: 666–673.

Attal N, Cruccu G, Haanpaa M et al. (2006). EFNS guidelines on pharmacological treatment of neuropathic pain. Eur J Neurol 13: 1153–1169.

Barker FG2, Jannetta PJ, Bissonette DJ et al. (1996). The long-term outcome of microvascular decompression for trigeminal neuralgia. N Engl J Med 334: 1077–1083.

Beydoun A (2002). Clinical use of tricyclic anticonvulsants in painful neuropathies and bipolar disorders. Epilepsy Behav 3: S18–S22.

Bittar GT, Graff-Radford SB (1993). The effects of streptomycin/lidocaine block on trigeminal neuralgia: a double blind crossover placebo controlled study. Headache 33: 155–160.

Bowsher D (2000). Trigeminal neuralgia: a symptomatic study of 126 successive patients with and without previous interventions. The Pain Clinic 12: 93–101.

Broggi G, Ferroli P, Franzini A et al. (2004). Operative findings and outcomes of microvascular decompression for trigeminal neuralgia in 35 patients affected by multiple sclerosis. Neurosurgery 55: 830–839.

Bullit E, Tew JM, Boyd J (1986). Intracranial tumors in patients with facial pain. J Neurosurg 64: 865–871.

Burchiel KJ (1980). Ectopic impulse generation in focally demyelinated trigeminal nerve. Exp Neurol 69: 423–429.

Calvin WH, Devor M, Howe JF (1982). Can neuralgias arise from minor demyelination? Spontaneous firing, mechanosensitivity, and afterdischarge from conducting axons. Exp Neurol 75: 755–763.

Carrazana E, Mikoshiba I (2003). Rationale and evidence for the use of oxcarbazepine in neuropathic pain. J Pain Symptom Manage 25: S31–S35.

Cheshire WP (2001). Fosphenytoin: an intravenous option for the management of acute trigeminal neuralgia crisis. J Pain Symptom Manage 21: 506–510.

Cruccu G, Leandri M, Feliciani M et al. (1990). Idiopathic and symptomatic trigeminal pain. J Neurol Neurosurg Psychiatry 53: 1034–1042.

Cruccu G, Leandri M, Iannetti GD et al. (2001). Small-fiber dysfunction in trigeminal neuralgia: carbamazepine effect on laser-evoked potentials. Neurology 56: 1722–1726.

Cruccu G, Pennisi E, Truini A et al. (2003). Unmyelinated trigeminal pathways as assessed by laser stimuli in humans. Brain 126: 2246–2256.

Cruccu G, Anand P, Attal N et al. (2004). EFNS guidelines on neuropathic pain assessment. Eur J Neurol 11: 153–162.

Cruccu G, Biasiotta A, Galeotti F et al. (2006). Diagnostic accuracy of trigeminal reflex testing in trigeminal neuralgia. Neurology 66: 139–141.

Cruccu G, Gronseth G, Alksne J et al. (2008). AAN-EFNS guidelines on trigeminal neuralgia management. Eur J Neurol 15: 1013–1028.

Cruccu G, Biasiotta A, Di Rezze S et al. (2009). Trigeminal neuralgia and pain related to multiple sclerosis. Pain 143: 186–191.

Darian Smith I (1966). Neural mechanism of facial sensation. Int Rev Neurobiol 9: 301–395.

Dubner R (1985). Recent advances in our understanding of pain. In: I Klineberg, B Sessle (Eds.), Oro-Facial Pain and Neuromuscular Dysfunction: Mechanism and Clinical Correlates. Pergamon Press, Oxford, pp. 3–17.

Dworkin RH, Portenoy RK (1996). Pain and its persistence in herpes zoster. Pain 67: 241–251.

Eldridge PR, Sinha AK, Javadpour M et al. (2003). Microvascular decompression for trigeminal neuralgia in patients with multiple sclerosis. Stereotact Funct Neurosurg 81: 57–64.

Erdine S, Ozyalcin NS, Cimen A et al. (2007). Comparison of pulsed radiofrequency with conventional radiofrequency in the treatment of idiopathic trigeminal neuralgia. Eur J Pain 11: 309–313.

Fariselli L, Marras C, De Santis M et al. (2009). Cyberknife radiosurgery as a first treatment for idiopathic trigeminal neuralgia. Neurosurgery 64 (2 Suppl.): A96–A101.

Fields WS, Lemak NA (1987). Trigeminal neuralgia: historical background, etiology and treatment. BNI Q 3: 47–56.

Fischbach F, Lehmann TN, Ricke J et al. (2003). Vascular compression in glossopharyngeal neuralgia: demonstration by high-resolution MRI at 3 Tesla. Neuroradiology 45: 810–811.

Fromm GH, Terrence CF, Chattha AS (1984). Differential effect of antiepileptic and non-antiepileptic drugs on the reticular formation. Life Sci 35: 2665–2673.

Fromm GH, Nakata M, Kondo T (1991). Differential action of amitriptyline on neurons in the trigeminal nucleus. Neurology 41: 1932–1936.

Garcia-Larrea L, Frot M, Valeriani M (2003). Cortical generators of laser-evoked potentials. From dipole modelling to functional significance. Neurophysiol Clin 33: 279–292.

Gass A, Kitchen N, MacManus DG et al. (1997). Trigeminal neuralgia in patients with multiple sclerosis: lesion localization with magnetic resonance imaging. Neurology 49: 1142–1144.

Gobel S, Falls WM, Hockfield S (1977). The division of the dorsal and ventral horns of the mammalian caudal medulla into eight layers using anatomical criteria. In: DJ Andreson, B Matthews (Eds.), Pain in the Trigeminal Region. Elsevier, Amsterdam, pp. 443–453.

Gronseth G, Cruccu G, Alksne J et al. (2008). Practice parameter: the diagnostic evaluation and treatment of trigeminal neuralgia (an evidence-based review): report of the Quality Standards Subcommittee of the American Academy of Neurology and the European Federation of Neurological Societies. Neurology 71: 1183–1190.

Hall GC, Carroll D, Parry D et al. (2006). Epidemiology and treatment of neuropathic pain: the UK primary care perspective. Pain 122: 156–162.

Headache Classification Subcommittee of the International Headache Society (2004). The international classification of headache disorders, second edition. Cephalalgia 24 (Suppl. 1): 1–160.

Herweh C, Kress B, Rasche D et al. (2007). Loss of anisotropy in trigeminal neuralgia revealed by diffusion tensor imaging. Neurology 68: 776–778.

Iannetti GD, Porro CA, Pantano P et al. (2003). Representation of different trigeminal divisions within the primary and secondary human somatosensory cortex. Neuroimage 19: 906–912.

Jannetta PJ (1967). Arterial compression of the trigeminal nerve at the pons in patients with trigeminal neuralgia. J Neurosurg 26: 159–162.

Jensen TS (2002). Anticonvulsants in neuropathic pain: rationale and clinical evidence. Eur J Pain 6 (Suppl. A): 61–68.

Jensen TS, Rasmussen P, Reske-Nielsen E (1982). Association of trigeminal neuralgia with multiple sclerosis: clinical and pathological features. Acta Neurol Scand 65: 182–189.

Johnson LR, Westrum LE, Henry MA (1991). Anatomic organization of the trigeminal system and the effect of deafferentation. In: GH Fromm, BJ Sessle (Eds.), Trigeminal Neuralgia: Current Concepts Regarding Pathogenesis and Treatment. Butterworth-Heinemann, Boston, pp. 27–71.

Katsarava Z, Ayzenberg I, Sack F et al. (2006). A novel method of eliciting pain-related potentials by transcutaneous electrical stimulation. Headache 46: 1511–1517.

Kaube H, Katsarava Z, Kaufer T et al. (2000). A new method to increase nociception specificity of the human blink reflex. Clin Neurophysiol 111: 413–416.

Klun B, Prestor B (1986). Microvascular relations of the trigeminal nerve: an anatomical study. Neurosurgery 19: 535–539.

Kress B, Schindler M, Rasche D et al. (2006). Trigeminal neuralgia: how often are trigeminal nerve-vessel contacts found by MRI in normal volunteers? Rofo 178: 313–315.

Leandri M, Gottlieb A (1996). Trigeminal evoked potential-monitored thermorhizotomy: a novel approach for relief of trigeminal pain. J Neurosurg 84: 929–939.

Leandri M, Parodi CI, Zattoni J et al. (1987). Subcortical and cortical responses following infraorbital nerve stimulation in man. Electroencephalogr Clin Neurophysiol 66: 253–262.

Loeser JD (1986). Herpes zoster and postherpetic neuralgia. Pain 25: 149–164.

Lopez BC, Hamlyn PJ, Zakrzewska JM (2004). Stereotactic radiosurgery for primary trigeminal neuralgia: state of the evidence and recommendations for future reports. J Neurol Neurosurg Psychiatry 75: 1019–1024.

Love S, Coakham HB (2001). Trigeminal neuralgia: pathology and pathogenesis. Brain 124: 2347–2360.

Love S, Hilton DA, Coakham HB (1998). Central demyelination of the Vth nerve root in trigeminal neuralgia associated with vascular compression. Brain Pathol 8: 1–11.

Love S, Gradidge T, Coakham HB (2001). Trigeminal neuralgia due to multiple sclerosis: ultrastructural findings in trigeminal rhizotomy specimens. Neuropathol Appl Neurobiol 27: 238–244.

Meaney JF, Eldridge PR, Dunn LT et al. (1995). Demonstration of neurovascular compression in trigeminal neuralgia with magnetic resonance imaging. Comparison with surgical findings in 52 consecutive operative cases. J Neurosurg 83: 799–805.

Merskey H, Bogduk N (1994). Classification of Chronic Pain. Descriptors of Chronic Pain Syndromes and Definitions of Pain Terms. 2nd edn. IASP Press, Seattle.

Nakamura Y (1980). Brain stem neuronal mechanisms controlling the trigeminal motoneuron activity. In: JE Desmesdt (Ed.), Spinal and Supraspinal Mechanisms of Voluntary Motor Control and Locomotion. Vol. 8. Karger, Basel, pp. 181–202.

Nakata M, Mukawa J, Fromm GH (1991). Why are most GABA agonists not effective antiepileptic drugs? Jpn J Psychiatry Neurol 45: 391–394.

Nurmikko TJ, Eldridge PR (2001). Trigeminal neuralgia – pathophysiology, diagnosis and current treatment. Br J Anaesth 87: 117–132.

Obermann M, Yoon M-S, Ese D et al. (2007). Impaired trigeminal nociceptive processing in patients with trigeminal neuralgia. Neurology 69: 835–841.

Patel A, Kassam A, Horowitz M et al. (2002). Microvascular decompression in the management of glossopharyngeal neuralgia: analysis of 217 cases. Neurosurgery 50: 705–710.

Pennisi E, Cruccu G, Manfredi M et al. (1991). Histometric study of myelinated fibers in the human trigeminal nerve. J Neurol Sci 105: 22–28.

Regis J, Metellus P, Hayashi M et al. (2006). Prospective controlled trial of gamma knife surgery for essential trigeminal neuralgia. J Neurosurg 104: 913–924.

Rowbotham MC, Fields HL (1996). The relationship of pain, allodynia and thermal sensation in post-herpetic neuralgia. Brain 119: 347–354.

Rushton JG, Stevens JC, Miller RH (1981). Glossopharyngeal (vagoglossopharyngeal) neuralgia: a study of 217 cases. Arch Neurol 38: 201–205.

Sampson JH, Grossi PM, Asaoka K et al. (2004). Microvascular decompression for glossopharyngeal neuralgia: long-term effectiveness and complication avoidance. Neurosurgery 54: 884–889.

Sessle BJ (1991). Physiology of the trigeminal system. In: GH Fromm, BJ Sessle (Eds.), Trigeminal Neuralgia: Current Concepts Regarding Pathogenesis and Treatment. Butterworth-Heinemann, Boston, pp. 71–105.

Shelden CH, Pudenz RH, Freshwater DB et al. (1955). Compression rather than decompression for trigeminal neuralgia. J Neurosurg 12: 123–126.

Sinay VJ, Bonamico LH, Dubrovsky A (2003). Subclinical sensory abnormalities in trigeminal neuralgia. Cephalalgia 23: 541–544.

Smyth P, Greenough G, Stommel E (2003). Familial trigeminal neuralgia: case reports and review of the literature. Headache 43: 910–915.

Soh KB (1999). The glossopharyngeal nerve, glossopharyngeal neuralgia and the Eagle's syndrome – current concepts and management. Singapore Med J 40: 659–665.

Spatz AL, Zakrzewska JM, Kay EJ (2007). Decision analysis of medical and surgical treatments for trigeminal neuralgia: how patient evaluations of benefits and risks affect the utility of treatment decisions. Pain 131: 302–310.

Teixeira MJ, de Siqueira SR, Bor-Seng-Shu E (2008). Glossopharyngeal neuralgia: neurosurgical treatment and differential diagnosis. Acta Neurochir (Wien) 150: 471–475.

Tolle T, Dukes E, Sadosky A (2006). Patient burden of trigeminal neuralgia: results from a cross-sectional survey of health state impairment and treatment patterns in six European countries. Pain Pract 6: 153–160.

Treede RD, Lorenz J, Baumgartner U (2003). Clinical usefulness of laser-evoked potentials. Neurophysiol Clin (Paris) 33: 303–314.

Truini A, Haanpaa M, Zucchi R et al. (2003). Laser-evoked potentials in post-herpetic neuralgia. Clin Neurophysiol 114: 702–709.

Truini A, Galeotti F, Haanpaa M et al. (2008). Pathophysiology of pain in postherpetic neuralgia: a clinical and neurophysiological study. Pain 140: 405–410.

Watson CP, Evans RJ, Watt VR et al. (1988). Post-herpetic neuralgia: 208 cases. Pain 35: 289–297.

Zakrzewska JM (2002). Trigeminal neuralgia. In: JM Zakrzewska, SD Harrison (Eds.), Assessment and Management of Orofacial Pain. Elsevier, Amsterdam, pp. 267–370.

Zakrzewska JM (2006). Insights – facts and stories behind trigeminal neuralgia. TNA, Florida.

Zakrzewska JM, Hamlyn P (1999). Epidemiology of facial pain. In: I Crombie et al., (Eds.), Epidemiology of Pain. IASP, Seattle, pp. 171–202.

Zakrzewska JM, Lopez BC (2003). Quality of reporting in evaluations of surgical treatment of trigeminal neuralgia: recommendations for future reports. Neurosurgery 53: 110–122.

Zakrzewska JM, Patsalos PN (2002). Long-term cohort study comparing medical (oxcarbazepine) and surgical management of intractable trigeminal neuralgia. Pain 95: 259–266.

Zakrzewska JM, Chaudhry Z, Nurmikko TJ et al. (1997). Lamotrigine (Lamictal) in refractory trigeminal neuralgia: results from a double-blind placebo controlled crossover trial. Pain 73: 223–230.

Zakrzewska JM, Lopez BC, Kim SE et al. (2005). Patient reports of satisfaction after microvascular decompression and partial sensory rhizotomy for trigeminal neuralgia. Neurosurgery 56: 1304–1311.

Handbook of Clinical Neurology, Vol. 97 (3rd series)
Headache
G. Nappi and M.A. Moskowitz, Editors

Chapter 57

Surgical treatment of cranial neuralgias

ANGELO FRANZINI,* PAOLO FERROLI, GIUSEPPE MESSINA, AND GIOVANNI BROGGI
Department of Neurosurgery, Fondazione IRCCS Istituto Nazionale Neurologico "Carlo Besta", Milan, Italy

TRIGEMINAL NEURALGIA

Introduction

Trigeminal neuralgia (TN) is a relatively uncommon disease, whose incidence is estimated to be about 5/100 000 individuals per year. It is characterized by attacks of recurring, paroxysmal, shock-like pain within the distribution of one or more branches of the trigeminal nerve. Light tactile stimuli, as well as sudden temperature changes perceived at the hemiface, vocalization, chewing, or teeth-brushing, may trigger such attacks. Another feature helping to make the diagnosis of TN is the absence of a significant loss of facial sensation in the cutaneous regions where pain is referred. Even though new drugs have recently been introduced in the treatment of TN (Tew and Keller, 1977; Farago, 1987; Fromm and Terrence, 1987; Lindstrom and Lindblom, 1987; Lechin et al., 1988), about half of all patients eventually require surgery for pain relief. The most common drugs used in such cases are carbamazepine, phenytoin, oxcarbazepine, clonazepam, and gabapentin. Drug resistance or drug intolerance can be commonly observed in patients with a long history of disease.

Since the first description by Fothergill in 1773, from which the clinical features of TN are nowadays well known, many different pharmacological and surgical treatment modalities have been applied. Most of the invasive ones, such as gasserectomy (Rose, 1890), retrogasserian neurotomy, juxtaprotuberantial neurotomy (Dandy, 1929), trigeminal tractotomy (Sjoqvist, 1937), temporal intradural decompression (Taarnhoj, 1952, 1982), gasserian ganglion alchoholization (Taptas, 1911: lateral approach; Hartel, 1911: anterior approach), gasserian ganglion electrocoagulation (Kirschner, 1942), injection of hot water (Jaeger, 1957) or phenol (Jefferson, 1963) or glycerol (Hakanson, 1981) in the trigeminal cistern and gasserian ganglion cryolysis (Fasano, 1976), have only historical value. Nowadays the neurosurgical armamentarium includes more traditional treatment options, either percutaneous (such as radiofrequency thermorhizotomy and balloon microcompression) or open techniques, such as microvascular decompression, along with novel radiosurgical techniques. All of these treatment options seem to have a good success rate with low risk, so that the ideal algorithm of treatment is still far from being established. In this chapter the authors report on their experience in the treatment of this painful condition and discuss the hypothesized etiopathogenesis of the disease.

Microvascular decompression

Surely, a milestone in the management of medically intractable TN is microvascular compression of the trigeminal nerve, a concept that was first described by Dandy in 1934, rediscovered by Gardner and Miklos (1959), and fully recognized and popularized by Jannetta (1967). In the past 30 years thousands of patients have undergone successful microvascular decompression and today it represents one of the most widely used surgical options for TN. Several studies agree on the high rate of long-term success (Table 57.1) and even authors who are against the concept of microvascular compression perform it for its effectiveness (Adams, 1989).

Nevetherless, controversies still exist about the exact role of neurovascular conflict in the pathogenesis of the disorder, about the possible involvement of the same mechanism in patients affected by multiple sclerosis, and about the existence of reliable prognostic factors.

*Correspondence to: Dr. Angelo Franzini, Neurosurgery, Fondazione IRCCS Istituto Nazionale Neurologico "Carlo Besta", Via Celoria 11, 20133 Milan, Italy, Tel: +39-02-23942-411-412, Fax: +39-02-70635017, E-mail: bsvjf@tin.it

Table 57.1

Completely pain-free patients (CPFPs) after microvascular decompression for trigeminal neuralgia

Reference	Number of patients	Number (%) of CPFPs	Significant recurrence (%)	Follow-up (mean)
Taarnhoj (1982)	350	225 (64.3)	113 (32.3)	Up to 11.5 years
Szapiro et al. (1985)	68	56 (82)	2 (3)	1–5 years
Burchiel et al. (1988)	36	19 (53)	11 (30)	7.5–11.5 years (8.5 years)
Bederson and Wilson (1989)	252	189 (75)	44 (17)	0.5–16 years (5 years)
Dahle et al. (1989)	54	43 (79)	11(21)	3–7 years (3.1 years)
Sindou et al. (1990)	60	50 (83)	2 (3)	16 months
Klun (1992)	178	167 (94)	5 (3)	0.5–12 years (5.2 years)
Yamaki et al. (1992)	60	38 (63)	9 (15)	0.5–5.5 years
Sindou and Mertens (1993)	420	–(91)	–(6)	?
Sun et al. (1994)	61	46 (75)	10 (16)	1–10 years (80 months)
Mendoza and Illingworth (1995)	133	95 (71)	18 (13)	0.5–15 years (5.3 years)
Barker et al. (1996)	1185	903 (76)	282 (24)	1–20 years (6.2 years)
Kondo (1997)	281	244 (87)	23 (8)	>5 years
Liao et al. (1997)	80	?	5	0.75–4 years
Coakham and Moss (1998)	>150	?	–(10)	Up to 17 years
Franzini et al. (unpublished data)	563	428 (76)	84 (15)	5–13 years (4.5 years)

Our experience with microvascular decompression started in 1990 and so far 563 patients, including 38 patients affected by multiple sclerosis, have been operated upon. All patients who were drug-resistant or intolerant, who did not want to experience any sensory disturbance, and who were eligible for general anesthesia underwent this kind of surgery as first option. Advanced age was not considered as an absolute contraindication at our institution. All patients had brain magnetic resonance with gadolinium before operation in order to exclude intracranial lesions (such as neoplasms) that could be responsible for the symptomatology. Absence of clear neurovascular conflicts in posterior cranial fossa on neuroradiological studies did not contraindicate surgery, and in fact almost all of the patients who were successfully operated on at our institution did not present such a magnetic resonance imaging (MRI) picture.

Surgical technique and side-effects

Exposure of the cerebellopontine cistern, where trigeminal roots reside, was performed through a small (less than 20 mm in diameter) retromastoid craniectomy, in the supine position with the head rotated to the opposite side of neuralgia and the ipsilateral shoulder slightly elevated. The skin incision was done a few millimeters medial to the mastoid notch (mediolaterally), perpendicular to the inion–zygomatic line, and extending for two-thirds above and for one-third below the mastoid notch. The craniectomy is centered on the astherion, which is the point of convergence of occipitomastoid, lambdoid, and parietomastoid sutures. The margins of the transverse and sigmoid sinuses were exposed; the dura was then opened along the line bisecting their angle. The fifth cranial nerve was exposed through a supracerebellar approach, thus avoiding lateral retraction of cerebellar hemisphere and traction of VII–VIII cranial nerve complex. So as to avoid anatomical modification before dural opening, lumbar cerebrospinal fluid (CSF) draining was not performed, nor was mannitol used. Conversely, CSF outflow following dural opening was useful in reducing the need for retracting the cerebellar hemisphere. In approaching trigeminal nerve, care was taken to spare at least two petrous veins, which drain into the superior petrous sinus.

The trigeminal nerve was then examined microsurgically for vascular (arterial, venous, or both) compression at the root entry zone and along the whole cisternal course (Figure 57.1) A neurovascular contact was graded as a "severe conflict" when there was a clear groove on the trigeminal root. Neurovascular

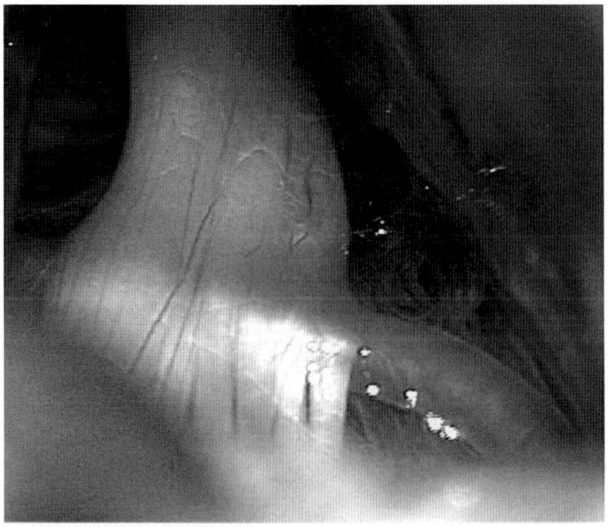

Fig. 57.1. Vascular relationship between trigeminal nerve and the superior cerebellar artery in the cerebellopontine cistern. The distortion of the trigeminal rootlets is evident from this intraoperative microscopic photograph.

contacts without root distortion were graded as "mild conflicts." Sometimes many small venous vessels literally "going through" and distorting the trigeminal sensitive root were seen. In our series the superior cerebellar artery was the vessel most commonly found to be responsible for trigeminal compression, followed by anterior inferior cerebellar artery and basilar artery. The nerve was then cautiously dissected free without unnecessary manipulation. Any compressive arterial vessels were kept away from the nerve as well as from its root entry zone into the brainstem by the use of little pieces of Teflon or fibrillar oxidized cellulose (fibrillar Surgicel). Since in our experience an inflammatory tissue reaction to the Teflon felt was found to be related in some cases to the recurrence of pain, fibrillar absorbable oxidized cellulose has been used since 2002. However, care is taken to avoid, when possible, any contact between the implant and the nerve. Compressive veins were electrocoagulated and divided. Perioperative steroids (dexamethasone) were routinely used.

In our series there was no mortality and no permanent morbidity. Ataxia, disequilibrium, and gait disturbances sometimes found in the early postoperative period generally decreased at hospital discharge (3 days after operation) and fully and spontaneously recovered within 2 weeks without the need for rehabilitation. Collecting data from the literature series on more than 3000 published cases (Table 57.2), the mortality rate is 0.3% (12 of 3033) (Broggi, 2000). Cranial nerve morbidity is reported, but generally diplopia, dysphagia, facial weakness, vertigo, and trigeminal hypoesthesia are all transient. Injury to the acoustic branch of the eighth cranial nerve is the only relevant long-term cranial nerve dysfunction reported in several series, ranging from 0.1% to 3% (Table 57.2). Probably this is the only complication that cannot be prevented in all cases because of the extreme vulnerability of the internal auditory artery and its cochlear branches, as well as its unpredictable intracisternal course. In our hands switching the approach from laterocerebellar to supracerebellar reduced the manipulation of the VII–VIII cranial nerve complex and the incidence of this complication to less than 1%.

Other reported complications, such as CSF leakage, hemotympanum, sigmoid sinus thrombosis, cerebellar infarct, and hematoma can be reduced in incidence with a careful surgical technique and perfect hemostasis.

We did not find any age-related statistically significant difference in the incidence of surgical complications and so we perform microvascular decompression without an absolute age limit. Furthermore, in elderly patients surgical exposure of the cerebellopontine angle was found to be easier because of atrophy and subsequent enlargement of cisternal spaces, and the postoperative course was generally uneventful with early mobilization. Multiple sclerosis (MS) patients tolerate this kind of surgery as well as non-MS patients, and a worsening of MS symptoms related to surgery was never observed, maybe because of the use of perioperative steroids.

Results and prognostic factors

At long-term follow-up (10–17 years) 76% of patients were found to be completely pain-free without medication, 5% were found to be pain-free with a dosage of drugs that was lower than in the preoperative period, and 15% required repeated surgery or high dosage of drugs. We were unable to follow up 4% of patients. The outcome in the MS group was worse. Only 39% of patients were completely pain-free without medication at long-term follow-up; an additional 5% reported no pain with low-dosage, sporadic consumption of drugs.

Despite the high recurrence rate these results show that a generally considered contraindicated surgery can achieve excellent results in some MS patients. Unfortunately, however, as has already been reported (Broggi et al., 1999), we were not able to find any prognostic factor that might allow for a better selection of surgical candidates; this obviously reflects the compartmentalization of knowledge about the pathogenesis of TN in these patients. We utilized a statistical analysis of the essential TN group in order to relate the likelihood of postoperative recurrence of tic to the

Table 57.2

Microvascular decompression: mortality and long-term side-effects

Reference	Patients (*n*)	Mortality	Cerebellar infarct	Def VIII	Def VII	Dipl	Def V	PD
Taarnhoj (1982)	350	2 (1.1%)	0.3%	1.4%	0.6%	0.3%	0	0
Barba and Alksne (1984)	37	0	0	0	0	0	5%	0
Zorman and Wilson (1984)	125	0	0	3%	0	0	0	0
Szapiro et al. (1985)	70	1 (1.43%)	1.4%	0	0	0	0	0
Bederson and Wilson (1989)	252	2 (0.07%)	0	3%	0	0	0	0
Dahle et al. (1989)	57	1 (1.7%)	0	0	0	0	1.7%	1.7%
Sindou et al. (1990)	60	0	0	0	0	0	0	0
Klun (1992)	220	3 (1.3%)	0	0.4%	0	0	0	0
Sun et al. (1994)	61	0	0	1.5%	0	0	1.5%	1.5%
Meneses et al. (1995)	50	0	0	0	0	0	0	0
Pamir et al. (1995)	32	0	3%	0	0	0	0	0
Mendoza and Illingworth (1995)	133	1 (0.7%)	1.4%	0	0	0	0	0
Barker et al. (1996)	1336	2 (0.2%)	0.1%	1%	0	0	0	0
Franzini et al. (unpublished data)	563	1 (0.2%)	1 (0.2%)	0.6%	0	0	0.8%	0

Def VIII: deficit of VIIIth cranial nerve; def VII: deficit of VIIth cranial nerve; Dipl: diplopia; Def V: deficit of Vth cranial nerve; PD: painful dysesthesia.

following variables: patient age and sex; involved side and branch; duration of symptoms; history of previous trigeminal ablative procedures; kind of neurovascular conflict (arterial, venous, or both); postoperative numbness; and arterial hypertension. A long duration of clinical history (>84 months) was the only variable which was found to be statistically associated with a worse outcome ($P < 0.05$). No other statistically significant prognostic factor was identified.

Etiopathogenetic considerations

A peripheral hypothesis (Kerr, 1967; Rappaport and Devor, 1994), central hypothesis (Dubner et al., 1987), and, more recently, theories trying to reconcile central and peripheral hypotheses (Fromm et al., 1984; Pagni, 1993; Scaioli et al., 1996) about the etiopathogenesis of TN have been invoked. Nevertheless it seems to remain a mystery. It seems likely that both trigeminal nerve lesions and central lesions that affect trigeminal pathways (MS, ischemia) (Balestrino and Leandri, 1997) appear to play an etiopathogenetic role in TN. Vascular cross-compression is now increasingly accepted as an important etiological factor. We found a vascular contact in most cases, even in patients with MS. Sometimes the involved vessels are subtle and the root does not seem to be grossly compressed. Our MR data definitively demonstrate that the involvement of trigeminal pathways within the brainstem is very common in TN MS patients. It is possible that demyelination of trigeminal fibers at the level of trigeminal root entry zone in the case of vascular cross-compression (Kerr, 1967; Waxman and Ritchie, 1981; Fromm et al., 1984; Jannetta, 1993; Hilton et al., 1994; Rappaport and Devor, 1994; Love et al., 1998) and demyelination of the trigeminal pathways within the brainstem in the case of MS (Olafson et al., 1966) may result in abnormal ephaptic transmission of impulses. We found that vascular conflict (and possible consequent demyelination) and MS demyelination can coexist and that they may cooperate in the genesis of painful attacks.

The classical distinction between the supposed "all-central" mechanism for MS-associated TN and the "all-peripheral" mechanism for the vascular compression-related TN should therefore come under reconsideration. In its place we offer a unique (TN MS patients are included), mixed central–peripheral mechanism in which abnormal impulses arise from demyelinated axons (MS, vascular compression, and any other possible cause of demyelination along the central and the peripheral course of trigeminal axons) and modulate the nuclear activity. Minimal myelin damage, without any nerve hypofunction, might be involved in the etiopathogenesis of idiopathic TN (Dubner et al., 1987). Major myelin damage may be responsible for MS-associated TN based on the finding of possible clinical signs of trigeminal nerve hypofunction (Vilming et al., 1986), MRI signs of demyelination, and, unfortunately, by the recurrence of pain after MVD. The concept of a central neuromodulatory role of impulses coming from the area of cross-compression also explains the possibility that a long-lasting alteration of discharge modalities of the trigeminal root can cause lowering of the pain threshold, as suggested by reports on extracranial neurovascular conflicts (Rose, 1890; Franzini et al., 1995).

If this mixed peripheral–central hypothesis appears to be compatible with our (Broggi, 2000) and others' (Adams, 1989) apparently contradictory findings in TN, an alternative all-central hypothesis might also be considered. Supporters of this all-central mechanism deny any pathological role for vascular compression. According to this view, microvascular decompression elicits pain relief because it produces a sufficient trauma which then interferes with normal nerve functioning which then dampens the abnormal brainstem activity responsible for TN (Dandy, 1934). Such activity, according to us, could be initialized by nucleus caudalis and then spread to sensory nuclei of thamalus and then to somatosensory, limbic, and associative cortical circuits of cerebral cortex. In our series we were not able to identify any precise prognostic factor. In particular, no statistically significant difference in the outcome between patients with severe versus mild conflicts was found, which we believe adds further emphasis to the major role played by central mechanisms in patients with MS-related TN.

However, microvascular decompression certainly acts on pain modulation by peripheral pathological impulses and, even if it could not be considered as the "definitive etiological cure" (Taarnhoj, 1982), it certainly is the only therapeutic option able to interfere with the peripheral etiological mechanisms of TN without causing any sensory disturbance. Of course, as stated above, the importance of the absence of intracranial (and, in particular, at the cerebellopontine angle) lesions must be kept in mind, such as neoplasms or arteriovenous malformations at preoperative MRI studies, in order to exclude other potential causes of TN.

Percutaneous methods

Hartel's landmarks for cannulation of foramen ovale (Hartel, 1911) are: (1) a point immediately inferior to the medial portion of the ipsilateral pupil in the anterior–posterior plane; (2) a point situated approximately 2.5 cm anterior to the external auditory meatus in a lateral plane; and (3) the cannula's entry point (about 3 cm lateral the ipsilateral side of the oral commissure).

After cannulation, use of lateral fluoroscopic mages is important in order to exclude penetration into the foramina of the skull base, such as inferior orbital fissure (located anterior to the foramen ovale) and the jugular foramen (located posterior to it). Such misplaced cannulation could potentially lead to serious neurovascular injuries. Even punctures of the internal carotid artery, with subsequent catastrophic consequences, have been reported in the literature after percutaneous thermocoagulation (Rish, 1976). Since Hartel introduced this simple and direct percutaneous approach to the foramen ovale and gasserian ganglion in 1911, many different methods of creating therapeutic damage to the trigeminal root and ganglion have arisen.

In order to reduce trigeminal sensory input, chemical agents such as alcohol, phenol, and glycerol (with or without phenol) were used. The possibility of diffusion of more aggressive neurolytic agents (such as alcohol) to untargeted structures and different individual response to chemical neurolysis made the results of the injection of chemicals into the trigeminal cistern and ganglion quite unpredictable. Due to an unfavorable recurrence rate and a high incidence of side-effects these techniques were progressively abandoned in favor of controlled radiofrequency thermal rhizotomy and mechanical balloon microcompression.

Radiofrequency retrogasserian controlled thermorhizotomy

Radiofrequency retrogasserian controlled thermorhizotomy became the widely preferred treatment for TN after Sweet and Wepsic introduced this technique in 1974. The primary objective in such a procedure is generation of a thermal lesion within the trigeminal division whose sensory distribution corresponds to the location of patient's referred pain. The temperature of the electrode for lesioning generally ranges from 65°C to 90°C, and the duration of lesion usually lasts 60–100 s, with sequential increases of 5°C.

Again, with the aid of a fluoroscope it is possible to increase the probability of reaching such a goal, based on the clivus radiological profile in lateral projections. Electrode tips superimposed on the clivus profile will generate lesions within the second trigeminal branch; tips located beyond or beneath the clivus profile will lesion the first and the second branches, respectively. It is also possible to generate lesions in different gasserian locations (Figure 57.2).

Various experimental data supporting the effectiveness of thermorhizotomy for the differential destruction of small-diameter nerve fibers have been reported (Frigyesi et al., 1975; De la Porte and Siegfried, 1983; Broggi and Siegfried, 1997) and its efficacy has been confirmed by many authors in large series of patients (Sheldon et al., 1955; Siegfried and Vosmansky, 1975; Siegfried, 1981, 1984; Apfelbaum,

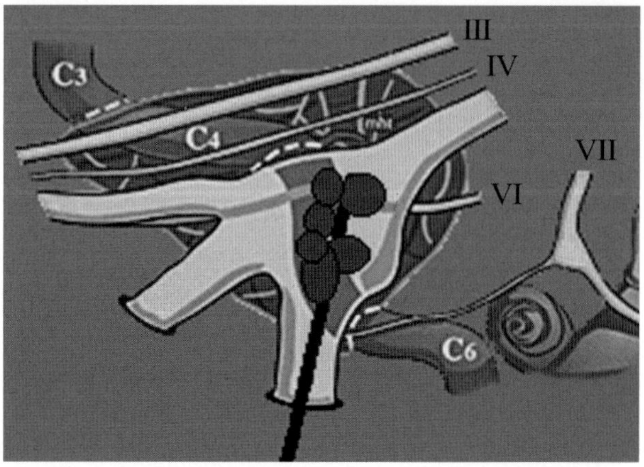

Fig. 57.2. Different possible gasserian ganglion thermoablative sites which can be generated using the lateral clivus profile as a point of reference in lateral fluoroscopic intraoperative views.

1984; Frank et al., 1985; Mittal and Thomas, 1986; Broggi et al., 1990; Taha and Tew, 1996). These experimental and clinical data show that thermorhizotomy allows for sparing of the majority of facial touch sensibility, and hypalgesia or analgesia generally involves only the targeted trigeminal branches.

More than 1700 patients have been treated so far at Istituto Nazionale Neurologico Carlo Besta since 1974. We were able to follow up 97% of patients for a time ranging from 2 to 15 years (mean follow-up 72 months): 71% of patients were found to be completely pain-free without medication, 11% were pain-free with low dosage of antineuralgic drugs, while 15% were still experiencing severe pain requiring a high dosage of drugs or surgery (Table 57.3). Regarding the amount of the inflicted sensory deficit, our data suggest that induced postoperative analgesia prevents the recurrence of pain in most patients. In other words, patients with postoperative hypalgesia have a pain recurrence probability of 41%

Table 57.3

Thermorhizotomy for trigeminal neuralgia: long-term results and side-effects in 1700 cases

Completely pain-free without medication	71%
Pain requiring high dosage of drugs or surgery	15%
Pain-free with low dosage of drugs	11%
Masseter weakness	10%
Dysesthesia requiring medical treatment	5%
Painful anesthesia	1.5%
Ocular palsy and diplopia	0.5%
Corneal reflex impairment without keratitis	19.7%
Corneal reflex impairment with keratitis	0.5%
Cerebral hemorrhage	0%
Death	0%

versus 7.5% for patients with postoperative analgesia. In all patients the sensory deficit tends to diminish with time; nevertheless a high percentage of patients with the more severe sensory postoperative deficit (analgesic patients) complain of dysesthesia. The total percentage of patients who required drugs for severe dysesthesia was 5%, with 1.5% with painful anesthesia that we were never able to alleviate definitively by any of the more advanced surgical antalgic techniques (open or percutaneous trigeminal tractotomy, trigeminal stimulation, cortical stimulation, deep-brain stimulation, CSF direct drug infusion). These complications are clearly related to the technique itself and cannot be completely avoided even with meticulous surgical technique, above all in the cases requiring repeated thermorhizotomy.

By monitoring the corneal reflex during the procedure, however, major ocular deafferentation complications can generally be avoided and keratitis requiring tarsorrhaphy was observed in only 0.5% of patients even if the involvement of the first branch was not considered to be a contraindication to this kind of surgery. Masseter weakness with minor chewing impairment appeared in 10% of patients, ocular palsy and diplopia in 0.5%. Major neurological morbidity due to intracranial bleeding was never observed. Mortality was zero. This method can be proposed to patients accepting the risk of sensory disturbances when previous less aggressive procedures have failed.

Balloon microcompression of the gasserian ganglion

The observation by Sheldon et al. in 1955 that deliberate direct compression of the trigeminal ganglion was able to relieve trigeminal pain led Mullan and Lichtor in 1983 to develop a percutaneous technique for controlled compression of the trigeminal ganglion that could be carried out under short general anesthetic. The results that we were able to obtain using balloon microcompression of the gasserian ganglion in 235 patients operated upon since 1992 are reported in Table 57.4. The end point for compression was the achievement of a pear-shaped balloon in the Meckel's cave (Figure 57.3). The balloon is then maintained inflated for approximately 1 min. A longer compression resulted in a profound hypoesthesia that often led to the complaint of dysesthesias. Results derived from the literature are summarized in Table 57.5. This method appears to have the same limitations that characterize trigeminal surgery whatever the lesional procedure used: the greater the sensorial deficit, the longer the pain-free interval but the higher the rate of severe dysesthesia.

Table 57.4

Percutaneous microcompression for trigeminal neuralgia: long-term results in 235 cases

Completely pain-free without medication	58%
Requiring low dosage of drugs	12%
Requiring high dosage of drugs or surgery	30%
Painful anesthesia	0%
Requiring drugs for dysesthesia	4%
Permanent diplopia	0.4%
Cheratitis	0%

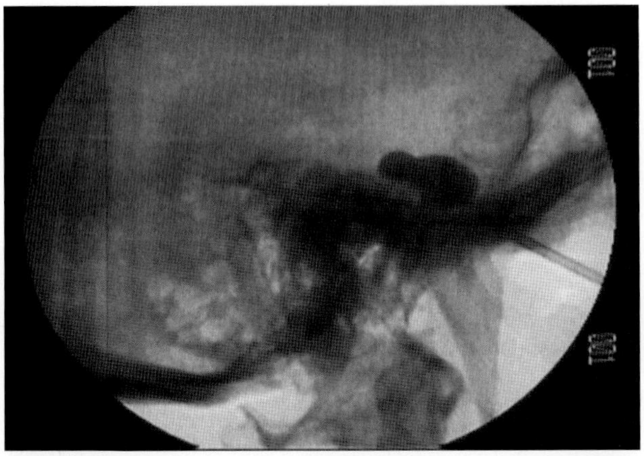

Fig. 57.3. Intraoperative fluoroscopic view of a correctly positioned "pear-shaped" balloon used for percutaneous microcompression of gasserian ganglion.

However, percutaneous microcompression is easy to perform, and the recurrence rate is acceptable with a low rate of complications even in the case of repeated surgery. Diplopia was sometimes observed but it is generally transient. Since in our opinion painful anesthesia and keratitis appear to be too high a price to pay for pain relief, this is at present the method we prefer when microvascular decompression fails or is refused by the patient.

Radiosurgery

Stereotactic gamma knife radiosurgery was first reported for the treatment of TN by Leksell in 1971. Its use, however, remained restricted to few centers until the mid-1990s when it started to become more popular. Radiosurgical treatment of TN has been well investigated with gamma knife devices involving fixed cobalt (^{60}Co) sources. Planning of the target and determination of isodose curves require 2-mm thick (or less) brain MR scans encompassing the course of the trigeminal nerve at its exit from the anterolateral portion of the pons (Figure 57.4), often followed by gadolinium-enhanced images; severely claustrophobic patients can be sedated with oral or endovenous agents, or can undergo brain computed tomography (CT) with or without intracisternal contrast (Worthington et al., 2000).

Indications for gamma knife radiosurgery are substantially the same as for microvascular decompression, except, of course, for the eligibility for general anesthesia and the patient's willingness to undergo surgery. Actual maximal doses, centered on the cisternal trigeminal nerve, are between 75 and 90 Gy (100% isodose). Doses below 70 Gy are unlikely to be effective at ameliorating symptoms (Kondziolka et al., 1996). Few reports exist concerning TN treated using linear accelerator (LINAC)-based devices. In recent years these devices have reached the level of mechanical precision that is required for such functional treatments. The first study to report preliminary data on treatment of TN with Cyberknife was that of Romanelli et al. (2003). In this study the authors reported a response rate of 70% (7 out of 10 patients). Lim et al. (2005) reported an initial pain relief rate of 92.7% after a median of 7 days of treatment, which decreased to 78% at 11-month follow-up. In our institution Cyberknife has been available since March 2004 but our data are too preliminary to be reported. Substantial advantages have been supposed in safety and comfort over other modalities, but so far the evidence is based on

Table 57.5

Trigeminal neuralgia: reported results of percutaneous microcompression

Reference	Recurrence rate	Follow-up	Patients (*n*)
Skirving and Dan (2001)	32%	10.5 years	496
Natarajan (2000)	8%	1 year	40
Abdennebi et al. (1997)	32.5%	51 months	200
Brown and Gouda (1997)	26%		141
Peragut et al. (1991)	20.6%	16.5 months	70
Lobato et al. (1990)	9.7%	10–35 months	144
Mullan and Lichtor (1983)	12%	0.5–4.5 years	50

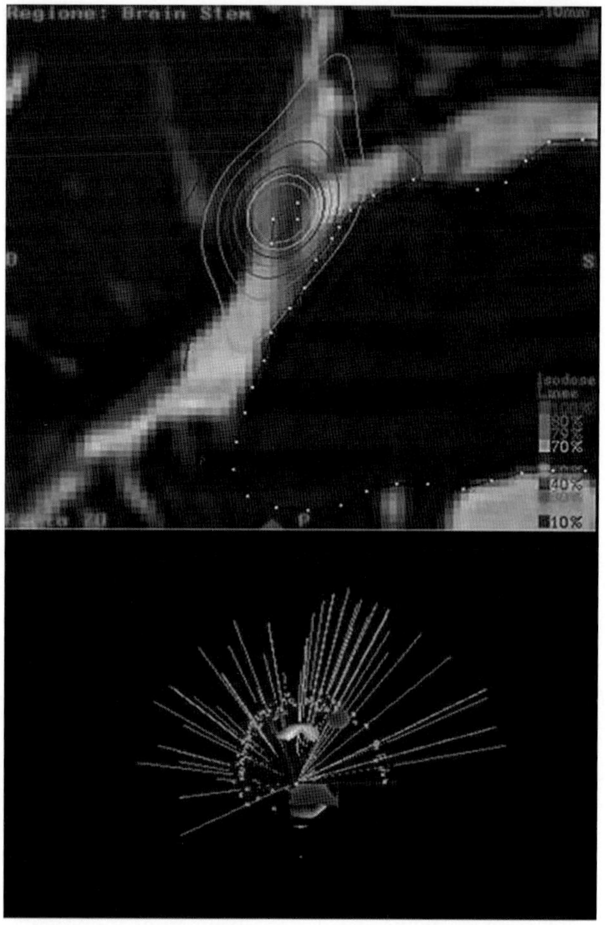

Fig. 57.4. Isodose distribution comprising the entire intracisternal course of the trigeminal nerve. Concentrical isodose lines are also depicted in this T_2-weighted magnetic resonance imaging scan.

case series with a single randomized study comparing two methods of delivery of radiotherapy (Pollock et al., 2001). The results obtained in some of the more significant series are reported in Table 57.6. From an analysis of the literature the following conclusions can be drawn:

1. Radiosurgery should be considered as a lesional procedure.
2. A strong correlation between the development of new facial sensory loss and achievement and maintenance of pain relief after this procedure has been described (Rish, 1976).
3. Quality of data is generally poor: case series have different patient populations, varying doses of radiation and targets, a variety of assessment methods, and differing follow-up.
4. In all, 70–80% of patients are pain-free in the short term, although up to 50% may relapse.
5. Side-effects include facial dysesthesia (up to 12%), corneal irritation (Matsuda et al., 2002), vascular damage, hearing loss, and facial weakness, varying with the dose plan and target area.
6. Follow-up is short and uncertainty persists about possible late complications of radiation therapy.

Summary

Microvascular decompression is the only surgical option that allows for long-term pain relief while avoiding any sensory disturbance. In our opinion it remains the treatment of choice for all patients with drug-resistant typical TN. Old age and central demyelination *per se* do not constitute absolute contraindications to this kind of surgery. No age-related statistically significant difference in incidence of surgical complications has been demonstrated. In addition,

Table 57.6

Results of radiosurgery for idiopathic trigeminal neuralgia

References	Excellent pain relief	Good pain relief	Failures	Follow-up
Shaya et al. (2004)	40%	30%	30%	14 months
Herman et al. (2004)	50%	28%	22%	37.5 months
Goss et al. (2003)	76%	24%	32%	4–13 months
Kanner et al. (2004)	Excellent + good	71.4%	23.2%	
Zheng et al. (2001)	52%	31%	17%	23.7 months
Kondziolka et al. (2002)	55.8% of patients had complete or partial pain relief at 5 years		44.2%	60 months
Matsuda et al. (2002)	52%	29%	19%	13 months
Nicol et al. (2000)	73.8%	21.4%	4.8%	14 months
Han et al. (1999)	42%	35%	23%	9 months
Kondziolka et al. (1996)	58%	36%	6%	18 months

although the results of microvascular decompression in patients affected by MS (as well as the results of percutaneous methods: Broggi et al., 1990) are less satisfactory, about 40% of MS TN patients were found to be pain-free at long-term follow-up. Since sensorial deficits can be far from negligible and are not well tolerated in some patients treated with lesion procedures, our policy is to delay destructive surgery as long as possible. When these procedures cannot be avoided, percutaneous microcompression appears to be the easiest to perform with a low complication rate and good long-term results. In cases requiring more aggressive treatment because of recurrent pain, thermorhizotomy can be performed. The use of radiosurgery is still under investigation and further studies are required to clarify its role in the treatment of TN, and the long-term follow-up rate of responders. Unfortunately, in MS patients both microvascular decompression and lesioning procedures cannot prevent pain recurrence due to MS-related evolving demyelination. Thus, new treatments aiming to modulate the activity of central trigeminal pathways should be investigated to improve the quality of life for these unfortunate patients.

GLOSSOPHARYNGEAL NEURALGIA

Microvascular decompression for glossopharyngeal neuralgia

Idiopathic glossopharyngeal neuralgia (GN) is characterized by severe, paroxysmal episodes of lancinating pain localized to the external ear canal, the base of the tongue, the tonsil, or the area beneath the angle of the jaw. The pain may originate in the external ear canal and then irradiate to the throat, or vice versa, and is similar as regards pattern of recurrence and clinical characteristics to that experienced with TN, except for triggering factors (yawning, swallowing, and coughing in the case of GN). Painful attacks can be associated with hemodynamic instability that can lead to life-threatening syncopal episodes (Ferrante et al., 1995), hypotension (Weinstein et al., 1986), or bradycardia. Females appear to be more affected than males, with a ratio of approximately 2:1 (Patel et al., 2002).

Several surgical approaches to medically intractable GN have been described, but most rely on the destruction of the glossopharyngeal and vagus nerves. In 1936, Lillie and Craig described an anomalous arterial loop in a patient affected by GN. Again, today, microvascular decompression represents one of the most widely used surgical options for GN, though controversies still exist on its role in this kind of neurovascular conflict. Surgery on the lower cranial nerves is in fact generally considered dangerous, and only a few authors have reported on the long-term results of microvascular decompression for GN, due to the rarity of this disease. To bring new insight to this topic we critically reviewed 17 consecutive patients who received microvascular decompression between 1990 and 2007 at our institution. Patients received the diagnosis of typical idiopathic GN if their symptoms met the guidelines of the International Headache Society. Individual symptoms, clinical history, operative findings, and complications were recorded. The most common pain territory distributions were epipharynx, followed by epipharynx and external ear, epipharynx and posterior hemitongue, external ear, and posterior hemitongue. In 3 cases GN was associated with TN and in 1 case with hemifacial spasm.

Duration of preoperative symptoms ranged between 45 days and 12 years (mean 4.6 years). Thirteen patients had GN for more than 4 years. One patient had received section of the stylomastoid ligament.

Operative results were assessed by clinical follow-up and periodic phone surveys. All of these patients had been given previous medical therapy (carbamazepine, diphenylhydantoin, and, more recently, lamotrigine, gabapentin, and pregabalin also) to which they had become refractory or intolerant. Contrast-enhanced CT and MRI were routinely performed to exclude cerebellopontine angle mass lesions and to find signs of demyelinating disease or neurovascular compression. As most cases had had MRI in other hospitals before admission to our institute, sequences varied and specific studies such as magnetic resonance tomographic angiography were used only in some cases.

Surgical technique

Exploration of the cerebellopontine and lateral cerebellomedullary cisterns was performed as for TN, except for the slightly lower skin incision (located half above and half below the mastoid notch). The margin of sigmoid sinuses was exposed from its beginning to the region behind the mastoid tip. A 15–18-mm dural incision parallel to the course of sigmoid sinus was performed. Microsurgical sharp opening of the arachnoid of the cerebellomedullary cistern allowed the course of IX–X cranial nerves to be exposed by using gentle gravity-aided tension on the cerebellum rather than a fixed spatula. Sharp dissection of the arachnoidal adherences around the nerves allowed for the full exposition of glossopharyngeal and vagal nerves, including the root entry zone in the retro-olivar sulcus. The most commonly involved vessel was the posterior inferior cerebellar artery, followed by the vertebral artery. Such compressive arteries were relocated away from the nerves and fixed in the final position far from the nerves themselves using muscle or fibrillar

Surgicel. Compressive veins were electrocoagulated and cut. Great care was taken to identify and respect all the small perforating arteries that could limit artery relocation. Brainstem auditory evoked potentials and endoscopic assistance were sometimes utilized in order to visualize "dark" microscopic areas better (Broggi et al., 1995).

Results

At the first operation a microvascular compression at the vagoglossopharyngeal root entry zone was found in all patients. The stabbing, paroxysmal pain typical of vasoglossopharyngeal neuralgia disappeared immediately after surgery in 15 out of 17 patients (88%) and faded away within 2 weeks in another 2 (12 %). Two patients required repeated surgery after 2 and 5 years for a drug-resistant recurrence of pain. In both incomplete decompression was found at repeated surgery.

A total of 15 out of 17 patients (88%) are pain-free without medication at long-term follow-up (1–17 years, mean 7.5 years). The remaining 2 patients are under medication (low-dose carbamazepine) for pain paroxysms that reappeared after a few weeks and 1 year respectively and that are, however, less frequent and severe than in the preoperative period.

There was neither mortality nor long-term surgical morbidity in this series. No patient had permanent deficits of cranial nerves. Transient function impairment of cranial nerves was observed in almost one-third of cases. The postoperative course was commonly characterized by cephalalgia and nausea due to deliquoration which is always required to expose the cerebellomedullary cistern. Cephalalgia lasted longer (5–7 days) in 4 patients. In 1 of these patients there was a CSF rhinorrhea that ceased after 3 days of external lumbar CSF drainage.

Discussion

Despite the fact that new drugs, such as gabapentin, lamotrigine, levetiracetam, and pregabalin, have been introduced in the treatment of GN (as well as for TN), many patients still require surgery because of refractoriness or intolerance. The diagnosis of GN is clinical and the role of neuroimaging is key only to detect possible causes, including vascular compression, tumors, or demyelinating plaques, as for TN. Again, the absence of an MRI-identified neurovascular compression should not exclude patients with intractable pain from open surgery.

The recognition of an involvement of the vagus nerve in symptoms led to the term "vagoglossopharyngeal neuralgia." In fact, the coexistence of symptoms mediated by ninth and 10th cranial nerves is well explained from an anatomical point of view, since both share the retro-olivar sulcus (the superior portion of the posterior lateral sulcus of medulla oblungata) as the common place of emergence from the brainstem, and where they can be distorted or compressed by a vascular loop or a tumor. The descending trigeminal tract and the nucleus caudalis are also shared as the first station of pain fiber relay coming from both nerves.

Most surgical treatments have historically focused on the lesion of glossopharyngeal and vagal nerve fibers. These lesional surgical procedures include peripheral procedures (extracranial, such as direct surgical neurotomies or percutaneous radiofrequency thermal rhizotomy, or intracranial, such as direct section of glossopharyngeal and vagal nerves in the cerebellopontine angle) and central procedures (percutaneous or open trigeminal tractotomy–nucleotomy, or nucleus caudalis DREZtomy).

As for TN, lesional procedures for pain in general should be avoided when alternative and safer treatments are available. Concerns about safety of microvascular decompression in GN are related to old reports of mortality and morbidity and should be taken into account, since this kind of surgery, along with refinement of microsurgical and anesthesiological techniques, can now be performed with a very low complication rate. In our series there was no mortality and no permanent morbidity. We agree that manipulation of lower cranial nerves can often be associated with morbidity, but our data show that this morbidity can be transient if absolute respect of brainstem vascularization is employed. Cases where the vertebral artery is responsible for root entry zone compression constitute a major challenge and require meticulous attention to avoid any damage to perforating vessels when it is manipulated. When a complete mobilization of the artery away from the retro-olivar sulcus is hampered by short perforators, the simple interposition of some pieces of Surgicel between the artery and the root entry zone should be considered.

Radiosurgery has also been employed with highly variable results that, anyway, are never comparable with the 90% of long-term completely pain-free patients without any medication that microvascular decompression warrants.

Microvascular decompression should therefore be considered as the first choice treatment also in all cases of GN. Old patients should be included since in our experience they do not present a statistically significant increased risk of complications. Peripheral lesional procedures are invariably associated with a deficit of ninth and 10th cranial nerves that is only

Table 57.7

Clinical results of microvascular decompression for glossopharyngeal neuralgia

Reference	Number of patients	Immediate result: number (%) of CPFPs	Long-term result: number (%) of CPFPs	Follow-up
Wakiya et al.(1989)	16	15 (93.75)	15 (93.75)	1–48 months
Resnick et al. (1995)	40	32 (79)	30 (76)	0.5–13 years
Kondo (1997)	17	16 (94)	16 of 17 (1 death)	5–16 years
Patel et al. (2002)	217	145 (67)	121 of 208 (58)	4 years (mean)
Sampson et al. (2004)	47	46 (98)	28 of 29 (96.5) with long-term follow-up	10.5–17.5 years

CPFPs: completely pain-free patients.

Table 57.8

Complication rate in recent surgical series of microvascular decompression for glossopharyngeal neuralgia with more than 10 cases

Reference	Number of patients and years	Mortality	Transient cranial nerve palsy	Permanent cranial nerve palsy	Cerebrospinal fluid leak
Wakiya et. al. (1989)	16	0	1 (6.25%)		0
Resnick et al. (1995)	40	2 (5%)	4 (10%)	3 (8%)	0
Kondo (1997)	20 1980–1995	1 (5%)	6 (30%)	2 of 17 (11.8%)	0
Patel et al. (2002)	217 1973–2000	13 (5.8%)*	/	62 (28.5%)†	25 (11.4%)‡
Sampson et al. (2004)	47 1984–1991	0	16 (34%)	5 of 29 patients (17.2%)	0

*0% mortality after 1987.
†3% after 1995.
‡2% after 1987.

acceptable in desperate cases where all other treatments have failed.

Coming finally to the etiopathogenesis of GN, it is generally considered, because of clinical and pathological similarities, to be the same as that of typical TN.

Conclusions

Tables 57.7 and 57.8 show, respectively, the clinical results and complication rates in microvascular decompression for GN in several series. Even if only few studies report long-term follow-up or patients with GN treated with microvascular decompression in the lateral cerebellomedullary cistern (Resnick et al., 1995; Taha and Tew, 1995; Kondo, 1998; Patel et al., 2002), we think that microvascular decompression is a safe and effective treatment for GN in patients of all ages. Considering that most of patients can withdraw from medication after surgery, it should also be proposed as first-choice treatment for patients who do not tolerate the idea of chronic antiepileptic drug administration.

References

Abdennebi B, Mahfouf L, Nedjahi T (1997). Long-term results of percutaneous compression of the gasserian ganglion in trigeminal neuralgia (series of 200 patients). Stereotact Funct Neurosurg 68: 190–195.

Adams CBT (1989). Microvascular decompression: an alternative view and hypothesis. J Neurosurg 57: 1–12.

Apfelbaum RI (1984). Surgery for tic doloreaux. Clin Neurosurg 31: 351–368.

Balestrino M, Leandri M (1997). Trigeminal neuralgia in pontine ischaemia. J Neurol Neurosurg Psychiatry 62: 297–298.

Barba D, Alksne JF (1984). Success of microvascular decompression with and without prior surgical therapy for trigeminal neuralgia. J Neurosurg 60: 104–107.

Barker FG, Jannetta JJ, Bissonette DJ et al. (1996). The long term outcome of microvascular decompression for trigeminal neuralgia. N Engl J Med 334: 1077–1083.

Bederson JB, Wilson CB (1989). Evaluation of microvascular decompression and partial sensory rhizotomy in 252 cases of trigeminal neuralgia. J Neurosurg 71: 359–367.

Broggi G (2000). Microvascular decompression for trigeminal neuralgia: comments on a series of 250 cases, including 10 patients with multiple sclerosis. J Neurol Neurosurg Psychiatry 68: 59–64.

Broggi G, Siegfried J (1997). The effect of graded thermocoagulation on trigeminal evoked potentials in the cat. Acta Neurochir (Wien) (Suppl 24): 175–178.

Broggi G, Franzini A, Lasio G et al. (1990). Long-term results of percutaneous retrogasserian thermorhizotomy for "essential" trigeminal neuralgia: considerations in 1000 consecutive patients. Neurosurgery 26: 783–787.

Broggi G, Scaioli V, Brock S et al. (1995). Neurophysiological monitoring of cranial nerves during posterior fossa surgery. Acta Neurochir Suppl 64: 35–39.

Broggi G, Ferroli P, Franzini A et al. (1999). Role of microvascular decompression in trigeminal neuralgia and multiple sclerosis. Lancet 354: 1878–1879.

Brown JA, Gouda JJ (1997). Percutaneous balloon compression of the trigeminal nerve. Neurosurg Clin N Am 8 (1): 53–62.

Burchiel KJ, Clarke H, Haglund M et al. (1988). Long term efficacy of microvascular decompression in trigeminal neuralgia. J Neurosurg 69: 35–38.

Coakham HB, Moss T (1998). Microvascular decompression [letter]. J Neurosurg 88: 617–618.

Dahle L, Von Essen C, Kourtopoulos H et al. (1989). Microvascular decompression for trigeminal neuralgia. Acta Neurochir (Wien) 99: 109–112.

Dandy WE (1929). An operation for the cure of tic douloureux: partial section of the sensory root at the pons. Arch Surg 18: 687–734.

Dandy WE (1934). Concerning the cause of trigeminal neuralgia. Am J Surg 24: 447–455.

De la Porte C, Siegfried J (1983). Étude des paramètres de thérmocoagulation à haute fréquence du ganglion de Gasser dans le traitement de la nevralgie du trijumeaux pour l'obtention d'une analgesie sans anésthesie. Neurochirurgie 29: 191–195.

Dubner R, Sharav Y, Gracely RH et al. (1987). Idiopathic trigeminal neuralgia: sensory features and pain mechanisms. Pain 31: 23–33.

Farago F (1987). Trigeminal neuralgia: its treatment with two new carbamazepine analogues. Eur Neurol 26: 73–83.

Fasano VA (1976). Diagnostic and therapeutic studies using the cryoprobe in various forms of facial pain, not of the migraine or trigeminal type. Minerva Med 67 (28): 1845–1849.

Ferrante L, Artico M, Nardacci B et al. (1995). Glossopharyngeal neuralgia with cardiac syncope. Neurosurgery 36: 58–63.

Fothergill J (1773). Observations on the use of herlock. Medical observation and inquires by a society of physicians. London.

Frank F, Gaist T, Fabrizi A et al. (1985). Rèsultats de la thérmocoagulation percutanée sélective du ganglion de Gasser dans la nevralgie faciale essentielle. Synthèse des resultats obtenus chez 939 patients traités. Neurochirurgie 31: 179–182.

Franzini A, Scaioli V, Leocata F et al. (1995). Pain syndrome and focal myokymia due to anterior interosseous neurovascular relationships: report of a case and neurophysiological considerations. J Neurosurg 82: 578–580.

Frigyesi T, Siegfried J, Broggi G (1975). The selective vulnerability of evoked potentials in the trigeminal sensory root to graded thermocoagulation. Exp Neurol 49: 11–21.

Fromm GH, Terrence CF (1987). Comparison of L-baclofen and racemic baclofen in trigeminal neuralgia. Neurology 37: 1725–1728.

Fromm GH, Terrence CF, Maroon JC (1984). Trigeminal neuralgia: current concepts regarding etiology and pathogenesis. Arch Neurol 41: 1204–1207.

Gardner WJ, Miklos MV (1959). Response of trigeminal neuralgia to decompression of sensor y root. Discussion of cause of trigeminal neuralgia. JAMA 170: 1773–1776.

Goss BW, Frighetto L, DeSalles AA et al. (2003). Linear accelerator radiosurgery using 90 gray for essential trigeminal neuralgia: results and dose volume histogram analysis. Neurosurgery 53 (4): 823–828; discussion 828–830.

Hakanson S (1981). Trigeminal neuralgia treated by the injection of glycerol into the trigeminal cistern. Neurosurgery 9: 638–646.

Han PP, Shetter AG, Smith KA et al. (1999). Gamma knife radiosurgery for trigeminal neuralgia: experience at the Barrow Neurological Institute. Stereotact Funct Neurosurg 73: 131–133.

Hartel F (1911). Die Leitungsans thesie und injektions behandlung des Ganglion Gasseri und der Trigem inusstmme langenbecks. Arch Klin Chir 100: 193.

Herman JM, Petit JH, Amin P et al. (2004). Repeat gamma knife radiosurgery for refractory or recurrent trigeminal neuralgia: treatment outcomes and quality-of-life assessment. Int J Radiat Oncol Biol Phys 59 (1): 112–116.

Hilton DA, Love S, Gradidge T et al. (1994). Pathological findings associated with trigeminal neuralgia caused by vascular compression. Neurosurgery 35: 299–303.

Jaeger R (1957). Permanent relief of tic douloureux by Gasserian injection of hot water. Arch Neurol Psychiatry 77: 1–7.

Jannetta PJ (1967). Arterial compression of the trigeminal nerve at the pons in patients with trigeminal neuralgia. J Neurosurg 26: 159–162.

Jannetta PJ (1993). Vascular compression is the cause of trigeminal neuralgia. APS J 2: 217–227.

Jefferson A (1963). Trigeminal root and ganglion injection susing phenol in glicerine for the relief of trigeminal neuralgie. J Neurol Neurosurg Psychiatry 26: 345–352.

Kanner AA, Neyman G, Suh JH et al. (2004). Gamma knife radiosurgery for trigeminal neuralgia: comparing the use of a 4-mm versus concentric 4- and 8-mm collimators. Stereotact Funct Neurosurg 82 (1): 49–57.

Kerr FWL (1967). Evidence for a pheripheral etiology of trigeminal neuralgia. J Neurosurg 26: 168–174.

Kirschner M (1942). Die Behandlung der trigeminusneuralgia. Munchen Med Wschr 89: 235–239.

Klun B (1992). Microvascular decompression and partial sensory rhizotomy in the treatment of trigeminal neuralgia: personal experience with 220 patients. Neurosurgery 30: 49–52.

Kondo A (1997). Follow-up results of microvascular decompression in trigeminal neuralgia and hemifacial spasm. Neurosurgery 40: 46–52.

Kondo A (1998). Follow-up results of using microvascular decompression for treatment of glossopharyngeal neuralgia. J Neurosurg 88: 221–225.

Kondziolka D, Lunsford LD, Flickinger JC et al. (1996). Stereotactic radiosurgery for trigeminal neuralgia: a multiinstitutional study using the gamma unit. J Neurosurg 84 (6): 940–945.

Kondziolka D, Lunsford LD, Flickinger JC (2002). Stereotactic radiosurgery for the treatment of trigeminal neuralgia. Clin J Pain 18 (1): 42–47.

Lechin F, Van Der Dijs B, Amat J (1988). Definite and sustained improvement with pimozide of two patients with severe trigeminal neuralgia. J Med 19: 243–256.

Leksell L (1971). Sterotaxic radiosurgery in trigeminal neuralgia. Acta Chir Scand 137 (4): 311–314.

Liao JJ, Cheng WC, Chang CN et al. (1997). Reoperation for recurrent trigeminal neuralgia after microvascular decompression. Surg Neurol 47: 562–570.

Lillie H, Craig WM (1936). Anomalous vascular lesion in the cerebellopontine angle. Arch Otolaryngol 23: 642–645.

Lim M, Villavicencio A, Burneikiene S et al. (2005). Cyberknife radiosurgery for idiopathic trigeminal neuralgia. Neurosurg Focus 18(5): E9.

Lindstrom P, Lindblom U (1987). The analgesic effect of tocainide in trigeminal neuralgia. Pain 28: 45–50.

Lobato RD, Rivas JJ, Sarabia R et al. (1990). Percutaneous microcompression of the gasserian ganglion for trigeminal neuralgia. J Neurosurg 72: 546–553.

Love S, Hilton DA, Coakham HB (1998). Central demyelination of the Vth nerve root in trigeminal neuralgia associated with vascular compression. Brain Pathol 8: 1–11.

Matsuda S, Serizawa T, Sato M et al. (2002). Gamma knife radiosurgery for trigeminal neuralgia: the dry-eye complication. J Neurosurg 97 (5 Suppl.): 525–528.

Mendoza N, Illingworth RD (1995). Trigeminal neuralgia treated by microvascular decompression: a long term follow-up study. Br J Neurosurg 9: 13–19.

Meneses MS, Clemente R, Russ HHA et al. (1995). Traitment microchirurgical de la névralgie du trijumeau: étude sur 50 cases. Neurochirurgie 41: 349–352.

Mittal B, Thomas DG (1986). Controlled thermocoagulation in trigeminal nuralgia. J Neurol Neurosurg Psychiatry 49: 932–936.

Mullan S, Lichtor T (1983). Percutaneous microcompression of the trigeminal ganglion for trigeminal neuralgia. J Neurosurg 59 (6): 1007–1012.

Natarajan M (2000). Percutaneous trigeminal ganglion balloon compression: experience in 40 patients. Neurol India 48 (4): 330–332.

Nicol B, Regine WF, Courtney C et al. (2000). Gamma knife radiosurgery using 90 Gy for trigeminal neuralgia. J Neurosurg 93 (Suppl. 3): 152–154.

Olafson RA, Rushton JG, Sayre GP (1966). Trigeminal neuralgia in a patient with multiple sclerosis. An autopsy report. J Neurosurg 24: 755–759.

Pagni CA (1993). The origin of tic douloureux: a unified view. J Neurosurg Sci 37: 185–194.

Pamir MN, Zirh TA, Ozer AF et al. (1995). Microvascular decompression in the surgical management of trigeminal neuralgia. Neurosurg Rev 18: 163–167.

Patel A, Kassam A, Horowitz M et al. (2002). Microvascular decompression in the management of glossopharyngeal neuralgia: analysis of 217 cases. Neurosurgery 50: 705–711.

Peragut JC, Gondin-Oliveira J, Fabrizi A et al. (1991). Microcompression of Gasser's ganglion. A treatment of essential facial neuralgia. Apropos of 70 cases. Neurochirurgie 37 (2): 111–114.

Pollock BE, Phuong LK, Foote RL et al. (2001). High-dose trigeminal neuralgia radiosurgery associated with increased risk of trigeminal nerve dysfunction. Neurosurgery 49 (1): 58–62; discussion 62–64.

Rappaport ZH, Devor M (1994). Trigeminal neuralgia: the role of self sustaining discharge in the trigeminal ganglion. Pain 56: 127–138.

Resnick DK, Jannetta PJ, Bissonnette D et al. (1995). Microvascular decompression for glossopharyngeal neuralgia. Neurosurgery 36: 64–69.

Rish BL (1976). Cerebrovascular accident after percutaneous thermocoagulation of the trigeminal ganglion. J Neurosurg 44: 376–377.

Romanelli P, Heit G, Chang SD et al. (2003). Cyberknife radiosurgery for trigeminal neuralgia. Stereotact Funct Neurosurg 81 (1–4): 105–109.

Rose WM (1890). Removal of the Gasserian ganglion for severe neuralgia. Lancet ii: 914.

Sampson JH, Grossi PM, Asaoka K et al. (2004). Microvascular decompression for glossopharyngeal neuralgia: long-term effectiveness and complication avoidance. Neurosurgery 54: 884–889; discussion 889–890.

Scaioli V, Franzini A, Leocata F et al. (1996). Hand dystonia and neuralgic pain due to neurovascular contact to cervical spinal root [letter]. Mov Disord 11: 102–104.

Shaya M, Jawahar A, Caldito G et al. (2004). Gamma knife radiosurgery for trigeminal neuralgia: a study of predictors of success, efficacy, safety, and outcome at LSUHSC. Surg Neurol 61 (6): 529–534; discussion 534–535.

Sheldon CH, Pudenz RH, Freshwater DB et al. (1955). Compression rather than decompression for trigeminal neuralgia. J Neurosurg 12: 123.

Siegfried J (1981). Percutaneous controlled thermocoagulation of Gasserian ganglion in trigeminal neuralgia. Experiences with 1,000 cases. In: M Samii, PJ Jannctta (Eds.), The Cranial Nerves. Springer, Berlin, pp. 322–330.

Siegfried J (1984). La nevralgie typique du trijumeau. Considerations cliniques, étiopatogeniques et therapeutiques. Med Hyg 41: 1753–1757.

Siegfried J, Vosmansky M (1975). Technique of the controlled thermocoagulation of trigeminal ganglion and spinal roots. In: H Krayenbuhl (Ed.), Advances and Technical Standards in Neurosurgery, Vol. 2. Springer, Vienna, pp. 199–209.

Sindou M, Amrani F (1990). Mertens: Decompression vasculaire microchirurgicale pour nèvralgie du trijumeau. Comparaison de deux modalitès techniques et dèduction physiopathologiques. Etude sur 120 cas. Neurochirurgie 36: 16–26.

Sindou M, Mertens P (1993). Microsurgical vascular decompression in trigeminal and glosso-vago-pharyngeal neuralgias. A 20 year experience. Acta Neurochir Suppl 58: 168–170.

Sjoqvist T (1937). Eine neue operations methode bei trigeminus-neuralgie. Durchscheneidung tractus spinalis trigemini. Zbl Neurochir 5: 247.

Skirving DJ, Dan NG (2001). A 20-year review of percutaneous balloon compression of the trigeminal ganglion. J Neurosurg 94 (6): 913–917.

Sun T, Saito S, Nakai O et al. (1994). Long-term results of microvascular decompression for trigeminal neuralgia with reference to probability of recurrence. Acta Neurochir (Wien) 126: 144–148.

Sweet WH, Wepsic JG (1974). Controlled thermocoagulation of trigeminal ganglion and rootlets for differential destruction of pain fibers. J Neurosurg 40: 143–156.

Szapiro J, Sindou M, Szapiro J (1985). Prognostic factors in microvascular decompression for trigeminal neuralgia. Neurosurgery 17: 920–929.

Taarnhoj P (1952). Decompression of the trigeminal root and the posterior part of the ganglion as a treatment in trigeminal neuralgia; preliminary communication. Neurosurgery 9: 288–290.

Taarnhoj P (1982). Decompression of the posterior trigeminal root in trigeminal neuralgia: a 30-year follow-up review. J Neurosurg 57: 14–17.

Taha JM, Tew JM (1996). Comparison of surgical treatments for trigeminal neuralgia: reevaluation of radiofrequency rhizotomy. Neurosurgery 38: 865–871.

Taha JM, Tew JM Jr (1995). Long-term results of surgical treatment of idiopathic neuralgias of the glossopharyngeal and vagal nerves. Neurosurgery 36: 926–931.

Taptas N (1911). Les injections d'alcool dans le ganglion de Gasser travers le trou ovale. Presse Med 19: 798.

Tew JM Jr, Keller JT (1977). The treatment of trigeminal neuralgia by percutaneous radiofrequency technique. Clin Neurosurg 24: 557–578.

Vilming ST, Lyberg T, Lastate X (1986). Tizanidine in the management of trigeminal neuralgia. Cephalalgia 6: 181–182.

Wakiya K, Fukushima T, Miyazaki S (1989). [Results of microvascular decompression in 16 cases of glossopharyngeal neuralgia.] Neurol Med Chir (Tokyo) 29: 1113–1118.

Waxman SG, Ritchie JM (1981). Hyperexcitability of pathologically myelinated axons and positive symptoms in multiple sclerosis. In: G Stephen, SG Waxman, JM Ritchie (Eds.), Demyelinating Diseases, Basic and Clinical Electrophysiology. Raven Press, New York, pp. 289–297.

Weinstein RE, Herec D, Friedman JH (1986). Hypotension due to glossopharyngeal neuralgia. Arch Neurol 43: 90–92.

Worthington C, Hutson K, Boulware R et al. (2000). Computerized tomography cisternography of the trigeminal nerve for stereotactic radiosurgery. Case report. J Neurosurg 93 (Suppl. 3): 169–171.

Yamaki T, Hashi K, Niwa J et al. (1992). Results of reoperation for failed microvascular decompression. Acta Neurochir (Wien) 115: 1–7.

Zheng LG, Xu DS, Kang CS et al. (2001). Stereotactic radiosurgery for primary trigeminal neuralgia using the Leksell gamma unit. Stereotact Funct Neurosurg 76 (1): 29–35.

Zorman G, Wilson CB (1984). Outcome following microvascular decompression or partial sensory rhizotomy in 125 cases of trigeminal neuralgia. Neurology 34: 1362–1365.

Handbook of Clinical Neurology, Vol. 97 (3rd series)
Headache
G. Nappi and M.A. Moskowitz, Editors

Chapter 58

Central pain in the face and head

JÖRGEN BOIVIE *
Department of Neurology, University Hospital, Uppsala, Sweden

INTRODUCTION AND HISTORICAL PERSPECTIVE

Central pain is commonly thought of as being excruciating pain with bizarre character, and covering large areas of the body. This is only part of the truth, however, because central pain can appear in many guises. It can have a trivial character and be restricted to a relatively small area, such as distal pain in one arm, or in the face. It is true, though, that central pain is mostly severe in the sense that it causes the patient much suffering, even though its intensity may be relatively low. This is due to the fact that central pain is commonly irritating and constant.

Central pain has often been overlooked as a possibility in patients with central nervous system (CNS) disease, because of poor knowledge of its characteristics. It may cause puzzling symptoms when several coexisting pains of unusual nature exist. Not infrequently central pain has been thought to be of psychogenic origin. The lack of experimental models for central pain until recently has also contributed to the situation, since this has hampered research into its mechanisms.

Historically central pain appears to have first been knowingly described as early as 1883 by Greiff in a patient who, following cerebrovascular lesions, developed lasting pain ("reissende Schmerzen" – tearing pain). Eight years later Edinger (1891) presented arguments for the existence of central pain. By then it was known that sensory pathways project to the thalamus, which was therefore at an early stage thought to play a crucial role in central pain. Throughout the years thalamic pain, i.e., pain caused by thalamic lesions, has remained the best-known form of central pain, but only a minority of central pains are related to thalamic lesions.

The most cited early description of central pain is Dejerine and Roussy's classic report from 1906. They studied 6 patients with thalamic syndromes including central pain. According to them the syndrome is characterized by: (1) slight hemiplegia; (2) disturbances of superficial and deep sensitivity; (3) hemiataxia and hemiastereognosia; (4) intolerable, persistent, and paroxysmal pain; and (5) choreoathetoid movements.

The cause of the thalamic syndrome is usually a thalamic stroke, but these lesions have often extended lateral to the thalamus to include the posterior part of the internal capsule where the thalamocortical fibers from the ventroposterior thalamic region pass to the cerebral cortex.

Although interest in central pain was mainly focused on thalamic pain for many years, Edinger had already in 1891 introduced the idea that cortical lesions also might cause pain. He also mentioned that the aura of epileptic seizures can include the experience of pain, which has since been reported by several authors. It has now also been demonstrated beyond doubt that lesions above the thalamus can cause central pain (Boivie, 2005), but it is still uncertain whether a lesion strictly limited to the cortex can lead to central pain, because in all published cases the lesions have also included some subcortical white matter.

Evidence showing that lesions in the brainstem can evoke central pain has been accumulating (Boivie, 2005). The most common site of these lesions has been the medulla oblongata, whereas few cases of pontine and midbrain lesions with central pain have been reported. Pontobulbar lesions have been dominated by infarctions in the territory of the posterior–inferior cerebellar artery (PICA), but also syringobulbia, multiple sclerosis, and tumors, as well as spinal cord lesions, can give rise to central pain.

*Correspondence to: Jörgen Boivie, Department of Neurology, University Hospital, SE-781 85 Uppsala, Sweden, Tel: +46 -18 30 01 06, E-mail: jrgen.boivie@telia.com

Many descriptions of the central pain syndrome were published during the first 30 years of the 20th century, showing that the character of this pain can vary considerably from patient to patient and that central pain can be excruciating. Since these case reports vividly illustrate this kind of pain, some of the descriptions given by Head and Holmes (1911) will be cited: crushed feeling, scalding sensation, as if boiling water was being poured down the arm, cramping, aching, soreness, as if the leg was bursting, something crawling under the skin, pain pumping up and down the side, as if the painful region was covered with ulcers, as if pulling a dressing from a wound, as if a log of wood was hanging down from the shoulder, as if little pins were sticking into the fingers, like a wheel running over the arm, cold stinging feeling. In a more recent report of a patient with central poststroke pain (CPSP) with unknown location the following pain components were described: boiling hot, deep as though in the bones, showers of pain like electric shocks or red-hot needles evoked by touch, as though the arm and leg were being twisted, continuous sensation of pins and needles, a strange sensation of the limbs being abnormally full (Loh et al., 1981).

EPIDEMIOLOGY AND TERMINOLOGY

In the World Health Organization diagnostic system (ICD-10; www.who.int) there is no specific code number for central pain in the head and face, but G44.8 (other specified headache syndromes) can be used. In the second edition of the International Classification for Headache Disorders (ICHD-II: Headache Classification Subcommittee of the International Headache Society, 2004) the following codes apply:

- 13.18.1. Central causes of facial pain
- 13.18.1. Anesthesia dolorosa (+code to specify etiology)
- 13.18.12. Central poststroke pain in the head resulting from a cerebrovascular lesion affecting the "quintothalamic (trigeminothalamic) pathway or thalamus"
- 13.18.2. Central poststroke pain
- 13.18.3. Facial pain attributed to multiple sclerosis
- 13.18.4. Persistent idiopathic facial pain
- 13.18.5. Burning-mouth syndrome
- 13.19. Other centrally mediated facial pain (code to specify etiology).

The International Association for the Study of Pain has defined central pain (now named central neuropathic pain in the classification) as pain caused by a lesion or dysfunction in the CNS (Mersky and Bogduk, 1994). Thus, peripherally induced pain with central mechanisms is not central pain, even if the central mechanisms are prominent. Central pain is usually constant and spontaneous, but evoked and paroxysmal pain occur in a minority of patients.

The expression "thalamic pain" has often used in a general sense for all central pain. "Pseudothalamic pain" is then sometimes used for central pain caused by extrathalamic lesions. "Dysesthetic pain" sometimes refers to central pain with a predominantly dysesthetic character but such pain can have either central or peripheral causes.

"Anesthesia dolorosa" denotes pain in a region with decreased sensitivity after lesions in the CNS or peripheral nervous system. The term "deafferentation pain" is used for similar conditions, but it is more commonly used in patients with lesions of spinal nerves.

The prevalence of central pain varies depending on the underlying disorder (Table 58.1). In the absence of large-scale epidemiological studies, only estimates of central pain prevalence can be quoted.

In the only prospective epidemiological study of central pain, 191 patients with CPSP were followed for 12 months after stroke onset (Andersen et al., 1995). Sixteen (8.4%) developed central pain, an unexpectedly high incidence. Among patients with somatosensory deficits (42% of all stroke patients), the incidence of central pain was 18%. These data contrast with figures obtained from a retrospective study of 63 patients with brainstem infarcts (MacGowan et al., 1997); central pain was reported in 44% of those with sensory deficits and in 25% of all patients.

In a recent study of 364 patients with multiple sclerosis a prevalence of 27.5% was found (Österberg et al., 2005). This includes 4.9% who had trigeminal neuralgia, which in this context is considered to be a central pain condition, because it is caused by an inflammatory lesion located in the CNS (Tables 58.1 and 58.2; Figure 58.1). Brain tumors and traumatic

Table 58.1

Causes of central pain

Infarction
Hemorrhage
Vascular malformation
Multiple sclerosis (MS)
Traumatic spinal cord injury
Cordotomy
Traumatic brain injury
Syringomyelia and syringobulbia
Tumor
Abscess
Inflammatory diseases other than MS
Myelitis caused by viruses, syphilis
Epilepsy

Table 58.2

Neurological signs in 27 patients with central poststroke pain (CPSP) and 86 patients with multiple sclerosis (MS)

	Proportion of patients (%)	
	CPSP	MS
Sensory abnormality	100	98
Paresis (moderate/severe)	37/11	48/11
Ataxia	62	38
Choreoathetosis	4	0
Agnosia	17	
Apraxia	17	
Dysphasia (light)	7	
Hemianopia	22	0

(Adapted from Leijon et al., 1989, and Österberg et al., 2005.)

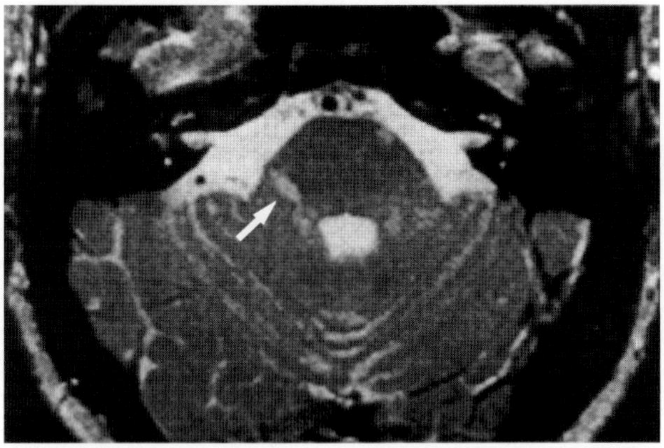

Fig. 58.1. Lesion in the central portion of the trigeminal nerve as shown by magnetic resonance imaging in a patient with trigeminal neuralgia from multiple sclerosis. (Reproduced from Gass et al., 1997, with the permission of the American Academy of Neurology and Lippincott, Williams and Wilkins.)

brain injuries seldom cause central pain. About 3% of patients with spinal anterolateral cordotomy develop late-onset central pain, usually of a dysesthetic nature (Gybels and Sweet, 1989; Pagni, 1998; Tasker, 2001). On the other hand, mesencephalic and pontine tractotomies may carry an even higher risk of central pain (Tasker, 2001).

The highest prevalence of central pain is found in syringomyelia. It appears to be in the order of 50–75% of all patients (Boivie, 2005; Attal and Bouhassira, 2006; Ducreux et al., 2006). It has been suggested that this high incidence depends on the fact that the syrinx directly injures the dorsal horn of the spinal cord, where processes that are of fundamental importance in pain mechanisms reside.

In two studies of CPSP, 33% of 27 patients and 37% of 111 patients, respectively, had facial pain, in addition to pain at other sites (Leijon et al., 1989; Bowsher, 1996). In a mixed material of 73 patients with "central pain of brain origin," 11% had facial pain (Tasker et al., 1991).

PATHOPHYSIOLOGY

Table 58.1 lists diseases and lesions commonly associated with central pain. These include rapidly developing lesions such as parenchymal hemorrhage and the slowly developing inflammatory demyelinating lesions of multiple sclerosis. The incidence of central pain differs in different diseases, suggesting that differences in the lesions are important factors. Unfortunately, little is known about these factors at the cellular level, including what happens to transmitter receptors.

The lesions that cause central pain vary enormously in location, size, and structure. There is no study indicating that a small lesion in the dorsal horn of the spinal cord carries less risk for central pain than a huge infarct involving much of the thalamus and large parts of the white matter lateral and superior to the thalamus. This raises the question whether or not the same pathophysiology underlies all central pain. The fact that the character of the pain also differs widely between patients with the same kind of lesion, and between groups, points in the same direction. However, this does not exclude the possibility that some common pathophysiological factors may be involved in central pain.

Lesion location is an important factor in the genesis of central pain. Central pain only develops if the lesions include part of the spino- and quintothalamic pathways, i.e., pathways that are most important for sensitivity to pain and temperature, including the thalamocortical projections (Leijon et al., 1989; Vestergaard et al., 1995; Bowsher, 1996; Tasker, 2001; Finnerup and Jensen, 2004). This is paradoxical because it means that only patients with decreased pain sensitivity run the risk of developing central pain. However, many patients with such lesions do not develop this pain. The explanation for this is as yet unknown.

Central pain-causing lesions can be located at any level of these pathways along the neuraxis, from the origin of the spinal trigeminal nucleus or the spinal dorsal horn to the cerebral cortex (Bowsher, 1996; Boivie, 2005).

Historically there has been a focus on thalamic lesions as the cause of central pain, particularly following stroke. Thalamic lesions certainly can cause CPSP, but they are not necessary for this pain to occur. Studies with computed tomography and magnetic resonance imaging (MRI) indicate that at most about half of stroke patients with central pain have lesions involving the thalamus (Leijon et al., 1989; Bowsher et al., 1998). Both supra- and infrathalamic lesions, including cortical lesions, can cause central pain. For instance, there is good evidence that lesions involving the parietal cortex, insular and adjacent perisylvian cortex can produce loss of pain and temperature sensitivity (Bassetti et al., 1993). Brainstem strokes of the Wallenberg type, i.e., infarctions in the region of the PICA, are well known to cause central pain in some patients. In one study, such lesions were present in 8 of 27 consecutive patients with CPSP (Leijon et al., 1989). The risk of developing central pain may be higher with brainstem lesions affecting the quintothalamic pathways than with suprathalamic lesions (MacGowan et al., 1997).

Neurosurgical lesions of the trigeminothalamic tract for the treatment of intractable head pain show that lesions of this pathway in the pons and midbrain can lead to central pain (Gybels and Sweet, 1989; Tasker, 2001). Some of these patients develop central pain with a dysesthetic quality several months after the operation.

Other causes of central pain include syringobulbia and multiple sclerosis. Syringobulbia causes central pain by virtue of involvement of the trigeminal nucleus. Central pain is common in multiple sclerosis (Österberg et al., 2005). It is hypothesized that the location of the demyelinating lesion is a crucial factor in the development of pain.

In stroke and multiple sclerosis patients with central pain, pain occurs independently of non-sensory symptoms (Table 58.2; Boivie et al., 1989; Bowsher, 1996; Tasker, 2001). Quantitative sensory tests reveal abnormal temperature and pain sensitivity in all patients and normal thresholds to touch, vibration, and kinesthesia in many.

Two general pathophysiological processes have been hypothesized as possible causes of central pain: (1) an "irritative lesion" hypothesis implying that hyperactive cells at or adjacent to the lesion site produce increased activity in otherwise normal nociceptive pathways; and (2) a "denervation or hypersensitivity" hypothesis suggesting that neurons remote from the lesion, but within nociceptive processing pathways, become hyperactive and hypersensitive because they have lost normal synaptic inputs. These hypothetical mechanisms are not mutually exclusive. Both may participate, to varying degrees, in the pathophysiology of central pain in different patients.

Head and Holmes (1911) hypothesized that pathways mediating tactile sensations normally exert a tonic inhibitory influence on a separate population of pain-mediating neurons, and that central pain is produced when inhibition is removed by a lesion in the lemniscal pathways. Modern research has shown, however, that lesions in the lemniscal pathways are not necessary for central pain to appear.

Craig (1998) has presented a new view of the thalamic disinhibition hypothesis, based on results from experimental studies in cats and monkeys. The hypothesis states that "central pain is due to the disruption of thermosensory integration and the loss of cold inhibition of burning pain." This disruption would be caused by a lesion along the spinothalamic projections to the thalamus, which are activated by cold receptors and delivered to inhibit nociceptive thalamocortical neurons tonically.

Experimental studies of neuropathic pain induced in rodents by lesions of the spinal cord and peripheral nerves indicate that excitatory amino acids, particularly glutamate and its effects on the *N*-methyl-D-aspartate (NMDA) receptors, play an important role in the development of hyperactive and hyperexcitable neuron pools in the CNS (Wiesenfeldt et al., 1997). Willoch and colleagues (2004) used an opioid ligand to estimate the degree of resting availability of opioid receptors in 12 healthy control subjects and 5 patients with hemibody CPSP due to single thalamic, midbrain, or cortical lesions. Despite the focality of the lesion, there was a striking loss of opioid receptor availability in the midbrain periventricular gray and throughout much of the hemisphere contralateral to the pain. The results argue against a focal effect at the lesion site, or a direct or transsynaptic degenerative process. Overall, the observations suggest that there is a reduction or downregulation of the opioid receptors, resulting in reduced effectiveness of endogenous, opioid-mediated analgesic mechanisms (Zubieta et al., 2001). Thus, a single lesion within the spinothalamocortical pathways can produce a functionally and neurochemically specific, yet anatomically extensive, deficit (Bowsher, 1996).

Lenz et al. (1988, 2000) showed that electrical stimulation in a ventroposterior zone deprived of its peripheral input due to a spinal cord lesion or amputation might evoke pain in the deafferented, but painful, region. Stimulation at these thalamic sites in patients without pain did not evoke pain. The fact that the stimulation evoked pain in deafferented regions indicates that there remains a representation in the CNS of the somatic sensitivity for the deafferented region, a kind of long-term memory, which need not necessarily be located in the thalamus. Hypothetically it is possible that such a memory could be activated long after the lesion appeared, which may explain the long delay in the onset of central pain in some patients. Long-term potentiation is thought to be an important aspect in the memory processes. It seems probable that some kind of long-term potentiation is involved in chronic central pain, which is really a long-term process.

NMDA receptors and associated calcium conduction have been implicated in long-term potentiation, thus representing another possible connection with excitatory amino acids (Bear and Molinka, 1994).

It may be possible eventually to prevent central pain with the use of drugs. This will require identifying the patients at risk of developing central pain. Detailed analysis of the sensory abnormalities, including quantitative sensory testing and possibly functional imaging, may be helpful in this identification.

CLINICAL FEATURES

The clinical presentation of patients with central pain is quite variable, sometimes raising difficulties in making a diagnosis. Some patients experience intense pain with or without severe motor and sensory symptoms, while others have only mild pain and minor neurological symptoms. Also, the character and location of the pain vary from one patient to the next. Thus, the diagnosis of central pain rests on the total clinical picture, in which history, symptoms, signs, and the findings of laboratory examinations such as MRI indicate a disease process in the CNS, and with the pain, the characteristics of which are compatible with central pain.

General diagnostic criteria for central pain are suggested in Table 58.3. CPSP can be considered the prototype of central pain syndromes because its characteristics, apart from pain location, seem to be shared by central pain with other diseases (Bowsher, 1996; Tasker, 2001; Boivie, 2005).

In the diagnostic procedure one must consider whether or not the patient has pain due to peripheral neuropathy. Polyneuropathy is not uncommon, for instance in stroke patients, a group with a high incidence of diabetes. Electroneurography and electromyography are therefore indicated in some patients.

Table 58.3

Diagnostic criteria for central pain

Laboratory examinations showing central nervous system disease, including X-ray, magnetic resonance imaging, cerebrospinal fluid assays
Pain starting after the onset of central nervous system disease; onset of pain often delayed
Pain with a regional distribution, rather than corresponding to individual nerves
Pain quality compatible with central pain, mostly burning, aching, pricking, lacerating, or lancinating, often more than one quality
Sensory abnormality, including abnormal sensitivity to temperature and pain, and commonly hyperesthesia and dysesthesia
Non-sensory symptoms and signs may or may not be present

It is usually stated with considerable emphasis that central pain is diffusely located. This notion appears to be largely derived from the fact that central pain often extends over large areas of the body, for instance the whole right or left side, or the lower half of the body. However, central pain can also involve one hand only, or just the ulnar or radial side of the hand, or one side of the face. Even patients with extensive central pain find it relatively easy to describe the extension of the painful regions, as shown in studies of patients with central pain after stroke and multiple sclerosis (Leijon et al., 1989; Österberg et al., 2005). It is therefore more correct to state that most central pain is extensive, than to describe it as diffuse.

CPSP is usually lateralized and includes the face in approximately 33–50% of all patients. Cerebrovascular lesions in the medulla oblongata, i.e., mainly lesions caused by thrombosis in the PICA leading to Wallenberg syndromes, can induce central pain on both sides, the face and head being involved on the lesion side, and the rest of the body on the contralateral side (Leijon et al., 1989; Bowsher et al., 1998). This pattern is due to injury to the ipsilateral incoming trigeminal fasciculus, the spinal trigeminal nucleus, and the crossed spinothalamic tract (Fitzek et al., 2001). A study of sufferers of brainstem infarcts and central pain indicated that all 8 patients had dissociated sensory loss, i.e., severely abnormal sensitivity to temperature and pain and normal or almost normal tactile sensitivity ipsilaterally in the face and contralaterally in the extremities (Boivie et al., 1989). Only 3 had facial pain, which in 1 patient was on the same side as the extremity pain.

The quality of central pain is mostly burning, aching, pricking, lacerating, or lancinating. Most patients, however, experience more than one pain quality (Leijon et al., 1989; Österberg et al., 2005).

The intensity of central pain varies between patients, from excruciating to low-intensity pain. Even low-intensity pain causes much suffering because of its irritating and unpleasant qualities. Central pain is commonly increased by external and internal stimuli, such as light touch, cold, movements, and emotional distress. It is usually constant, but intermittent attacks, spontaneous or evoked, may occur.

The onset of central pain is commonly delayed. In a prospective study of stroke patients it was found that the onset was delayed more than 1 month in 37% of patients (Andersen et al., 1995). Delays as long as several years have been reported (Leijon et al., 1989). The onset of pain often coincides with the return of some sensitivity after a period of deep numbness.

Central pain is a result of CNS disease and, therefore, it should be accompanied by other neurological symptoms. In one study, the only non-painful feature common to all patients with CPSP was abnormal somatic sensitivity (Leijon et al., 1989). The most prominent sensory signs in CPSP are abnormal temperature and pain sensitivity, dysesthesia, and hyperesthesia. Quantitative sensory tests showed that all of 27 patients had abnormal thresholds to temperature and pain, while at most half had abnormal thresholds to touch, vibration, and joint movements (Boivie et al., 1989). This kind of sensory abnormality has also been shown in studies from other centers (Vestergaard et al., 1995; Bowsher, 1996). Such abnormality may not be appreciated with traditional clinical tests, which are less sensitive. However, there are patients with central pain, in whom not even quantitative tests have shown sensory loss (J. Boivie, D. Bowsher, and G. Leijon, unpublished observations).

Many patients with CPSP have hyperesthesia, sometimes of a hyperpathic nature, with painful overreactions to touch, cold (touch and cold allodynia), and pinprick (hyperalgesia: Boivie et al., 1989; Vestergaard et al., 1995; Bowsher, 1996). These hyperesthesias hamper the patients considerably in their activities. Spontaneous dysesthesias are also common.

Syringobulbia can cause central pain in the face, but this condition has not been specifically studied. Syringobulbia is usually present together with syringomyelia, in which central pain is common (Boivie, 2005; Attal and Bouhassira, 2006; Ducreux et al., 2006). In 7 of a series of 25 patients with syringomyelia the syrinx extended into the medulla oblongata (J. Boivie, unpublished observations). Two of these had neck pain that probably formed part of their central pain, but none had facial pain. About half of all patients had central pain. This would appear to be the highest prevalence of central pain reported for any neurological disease. In this group, too, the central pain was accompanied by abnormal temperature and pain sensitivity, which is characteristic of syringomyelia.

Over one-quarter of patients with multiple sclerosis develop central pain, including trigeminal neuralgia in 5% (Figure 58.1; Österberg et al., 2005). Non-trigeminal central pain dominates in the lower and upper extremities (87% and 31%, respectively, of all patients), whereas steady central pain in the face appears to be rare. Four of the 18 multiple sclerosis patients with trigeminal neuralgia also had pain in the legs. The pain in the extremities was not found to be caused by spasticity. It was almost solely constant pain. Multiple sclerosis plaques in the entry zone of the trigeminal nerve in the brainstem have been shown with MRI (Gass et al., 1997).

PROGNOSIS

Central pain is almost always chronic, commonly lasting for many years, and not infrequently for the rest of the sufferer's life. In stable lesions such as those in stroke the pain is usually stable and does not change character with time, but in patients with multiple sclerosis new demyelinating lesions can modify the course of central pain. Central pain can also spontaneously and gradually subside in stroke (Leijon and Boivie, 1996) and multiple sclerosis (Österberg et al., 2005). Apparently central pain can disappear after a second stroke, as reported in 1 patient whose pain disappeared 7 years after the first infarct when he was struck by a second infarct in the internal capsule, ipsilateral to the old thalamic infarct (Soria and Fine, 1991). It is not known whether presently available drug treatments affect the natural course of central pain.

MANAGEMENT

Treating central pain is no easy task, because there is no universally effective treatment. This means that one must often try various treatment modalities to get the best results (Table 58.4). Treatment usually reduces the pain, rather than giving complete relief, but relatively small decreases in pain intensity are often highly valued by patients.

One of the similarities between central pain and peripheral neuropathic pain is treatment. In both pain categories antidepressants and antiepileptic drugs are the most frequently used drugs. These are also the ones

Table 58.4

Treatment modalities used for central pain

Pharmacological
Tricyclic antidepressant drugs
Amitriptyline
Desipramine
Nortriptyline
Serotonin and norepinephrine reuptake inhibitors
Venlafaxine
Duloxetine
Antiepileptic drugs
Carbamazepine/oxcarbamazepine
Lamotrigine
Pregabalin
Gabapentin
Analgesics
Antiarrhythmic drugs, local anesthetic agents
Other drugs (e.g., cannabinoids)
Sensory stimulation
Transcutaneous electrical stimulation
Spinal cord stimulation
Deep-brain stimulation
Motor cortex stimulation
Neurosurgery
Cordotomy
Dorsal root entry zone lesion

with the best-documented effects, and the only ones tested in well-conducted clinical trials. They are the first-line treatments, together with transcutaneous electrical nerve stimulation (TENS).

It is conceivable that treatment affects some aspects of central pain but not others. Therefore it would be desirable to assess the effect of treatment on each pain modality separately, in accordance with ideas about mechanism-based treatments of pain, but no studies have been designed to test this.

Another important, but still largely unanswered, question is whether or not the different central pain conditions and different aspects of central pain respond differently to a particular treatment. This has not been systematically studied, but such differences appear to exist. From the literature and from clinical experience one gets the impression that CPSP responds better to antidepressants than the central pain in spinal cord injury and multiple sclerosis. Conversely, paroxysmal pain in multiple sclerosis seems to respond much better to antiepileptic drugs than other kinds of central pain.

It is still uncertain to what extent patients with central pain benefit from the use of strong analgesics. The conclusion is that some, but only a minority, of the patients experience sufficient relief to continue long-term treatment with analgesics.

Many of the treatments listed in Table 58.4 are more of an experimental character, although some are used quite frequently.

Electrical stimulation of the brain is an exclusive mode of treatment that should be reserved for particularly severe and treatment-resistant pain conditions. The exquisite pain suffered by many central pain patients fulfills this criterion. In recent years the focus has been on surface stimulation of the motor cortex, with several groups reporting good effects, particularly on CPSP (Yamamoto et al., 1997; Mertens et al., 1999).

Many different surgical lesions have been tried to provide relief of central pain, but no particular lesion has been found that reliably results in successful outcome.

Antidepressants

Controlled trials have been done with tricyclic antidepressants only on CPSP (15 patients) and the central pain in spinal cord injury, with conflicting results (Leijon and Boivie, 1989; Cardenas et al., 2002). In the CPSP study there was a statistically significant reduction in pain as compared to placebo. The numbers needed to treat for amitriptyline was 1.7 (CI 1.1–3.0). These results contrast with those from a controlled study of amitriptyline on central pain in 44 patients with spinal cord injury in which no significant effects were found, compared to active placebo, but the doses were relatively low, judging by the plasma concentrations.

Antiepileptic drugs

An effect on central pain has only been demonstrated for lamotrigine in CPSP and for pregabalin in central pain from spinal cord injury (Vestergaard et al., 2001; Siddall et al., 2006). Gabapentin has been recommended for the treatment of neuropathic pain, but the focus is now more on pregabalin, because of the results from the large, well-designed, and well-conducted trial on central pain from spinal cord injury (Siddall et al., 2006).

In trigeminal neuralgia it is clear that the pain-relieving effect of carbamazepine is strongly correlated with the plasma concentration, as in epilepsy. It is not known whether or not this is also the case with antiepileptic drugs in central pain. No such correlation was found in the study on CPSP (Leijon et al., 1989).

Like the antidepressants, the antiepileptic drugs have a tendency to cause troublesome side-effects, and must therefore be managed with caution. It is possible that some groups of patients are more amenable to the side-effects than other patients with neurological diseases, because many neurologists have the impression that carbamazepine, and possibly also other antiepileptic drugs, causes more problems in multiple sclerosis patients than in patients with idiopathic trigeminal neuralgia or epilepsy. This could be explained by the fact that carbamazepine has effects on cerebellar centers for the coordination of movements which are frequently affected by the disease process in multiple sclerosis.

Analgesics, cannabinoids

The question of whether central pain responds to analgesics is still controversial. The results from acute, single-blind tests of opioids, as well as a controlled clinical trial with the potent μ-opioid agonist levorphanol on patients with CPSP, indicate low sensitivity to opioids. This is similar to the experience of many patients with central pain who undergo operations and receive opioids postoperatively, namely that they have a good effect on the pain related to the operation, but no effect on the central pain.

In a study of 5 patients with stroke and 10 with spinal cord injury, intravenous morphine did not give significant pain relief, but there was a strong tendency to better pain suppression by the morphine compared to placebo (Attal et al., 2002). However, in the open posttrial oral medication period, only 3 patients (17%)

continued with morphine for at least 12 weeks. The others stopped before that, because of side-effects and/or poor relief. The conclusion was that opioids may be useful for a minority of patients with central pain, and that the effect is modest in most of these. This is in agreement with common clinical experience.

For many years the use of cannabinoids in neuropathic pain has been discussed. Two controlled clinical trials on central pain in multiple sclerosis have now been reported. A weak but significant pain-relieving effect by oral dronabinol was found in 24 patients during 3 weeks of treatment (Svendsen et al., 2004). In the second study on 64 patients (34 took a whole-plant-based spray for 5 weeks), clear significant pain relief was recorded (Rog et al., 2005).

References

Andersen G, Vestergaard K, Ingeman-Nielsen M et al. (1995). Incidence of central post-stroke pain. Pain 61: 187–193.

Attal N, Bouhassira D (2006). Pain in syringomyelia/bulbia. In: F Cervero, TS Jensen (Eds.), Handbook of Clinical Neurology, Vol. 81. Elsevier, Oxford, pp. 705–713.

Attal N, Guirimand F, Brasseur L et al. (2002). Effects of IV morpine in central pain. A randomized placebo-controlled study. Neurology 58: 554–563.

Bassetti RD, Bogousslavsky J, Regli F (1993). Sensory syndromes in parietal stroke. Neurology 43: 1942–1949.

Bear MS, Molinka RC (1994). Synaptic plasticity: LTP and LTD. Curr Opin Neurobiol 4: 389–399.

Boivie J (2005). Central pain. In: SB McMahon, M Koltzenburg (Eds.), Textbook of Pain. 5th edn. Churchill Livingstone, Edinburgh, pp. 1057–1074.

Boivie J, Leijon G, Johansson I (1989). Central post-stroke pain – a study of the mechanisms through analyses of the sensory abnormalities. Pain 37: 173–185.

Bowsher D (1996). Central pain: clinical and physiological characteristics. J Neurol Neurosurg Psychiatry 61: 62–69.

Bowsher D, Leijon G, Thuomas K-Å (1998). Central post-stroke pain: correlation of MRI with clinical pain characteristics and sensory abnormalities. Neurology 51: 1352–1358.

Cardenas DD, Warms CA, Turner JA et al. (2002). Efficacy of amitriptyline for relief of pain in spinal cord injury: results of a randomized controlled trial. Pain 96: 365–373.

Craig AD (1998). A new version of the thalamic disinhibition hypothesis of central pain. Pain Forum 7: 1–14.

Dejerine J, Roussy G (1906). Le syndrome thalamique. Rev Neurol (Paris) 14: 521–532.

Ducreux D, Attal N, Parker F et al. (2006). Mechanisms of central neuropathic pain: a combined psychophysical and fMRI study in syringomyelia. Brain 129: 963–976.

Edinger L (1891). Giebt es central antstehender Schmerzen. Dtsch Z Nervenheilk 1: 262–282.

Finnerup NB, Jensen TS (2004). Spinal cord injury pain – mechanisms and treatment. Eur J Neurol 11: 73–82.

Fitzek S, Baumgartner U, Fitzek C et al. (2001). Mechanisms and predictors of chronic facial pain in lateral medullary infarction. Ann Neurol 49: 493–500.

Gass A, Kitchen N, MacManus DG et al. (1997). Trigeminal neuralgia in patients with multiple sclerosis: lesion localization with magnetic resonance imaging. Neurology 49: 1142–1144.

Greiff (1883). Zur Localisation der Hemichorea. Arch Psychol Nervenkrankh 14: 598.

Gybels JM, Sweet WH (1989). Neurosurgical Treatment of Persistent Pain. Karger, Basel.

Head H, Holmes G (1911). Sensory disturbances from cerebral lesions. Brain 34: 102–254.

Headache Classification Subcommittee of the International Headache Society (2004). The international classification of headache disorders, 2nd edition. Cephalalgia 24 (Suppl. 1): 9–160.

Leijon G, Boivie J (1989). Central post-stroke pain – a controlled trial of amitriptyline and carbamazepine. Pain 36: 27–36.

Leijon G, Boivie J (1996). Central post-stroke pain (CPSP) – a longterm follow up. Abstracts 8th World Congress on Pain. IASP Press, Seattle, pp. 380.

Leijon G, Boivie J, Johansson I (1989). Central post-stroke pain – neurological symptoms and pain characteristics. Pain 36: 13–25.

Lenz AF, Tasker RR, Dostrovsky JO et al. (1988). Abnormal single-unit activity and response to stimulation in the presumed ventrocandal nucleus of patients with central pain. In: R Dubner, GF Gebhart, MR Bond (Eds.), Pain Research and Clinical Management. Elsevier, Amsterdam, pp. 157–164.

Lenz F, Lee J, Garonzik I et al. (2000). Plasticity of pain-related neuronal activity in the human thalamus. Progr Brain Res Rev 129: 259–273.

Loh L, Nathan PW, Schott GD (1981). Pain due to lesions of central nervous system removed by sympathetic block. BMJ 282: 1026–1028.

MacGowan DJ, Janal MN, Clark WC et al. (1997). Central post-stroke pain and Wallenberg's lateral medullary infarction: frequency, character, and determinants in 63 patients. Neurology 49: 120–125.

Mersky H, Bogduk N (1994). Classification of Chronic Pain. IASP Press, Seattle, pp. 1–222.

Mertens P, Nuti C, Sindou M et al. (1999). Precentral cortex stimulation for the treatment of central neuropathic pain. Stereotact Funct Neurosurg 73: 122–125.

Österberg A, Boivie J, Thuomas K-Å (2005). Central pain in multiple sclerosis – prevalences, clinical characteristics and mechanisms. Eur J Pain 9: 531–542.

Pagni C (1998). Central Pain. A Neurosurgical Challenge. Edizioni Minerva Medica, Torino.

Rog DJ, Nurmikko TJ, Friede T et al. (2005). Randomized, controlled trial of cannabis-based medicine in central pain in multiple sclerosis. Neurology 65: 812–819.

Siddall PJ, Cousins MJ, Otte A et al. (2006). Pregabalin in central neuropathic pain: a placebo-controlled trial in spinal cord injury. Neurology 67: 1792–1800.

Soria ED, Fine EJ (1991). Disappearance of thalamic pain after parietal subcortical stroke. Pain 44: 285–288.

Svendsen K, Jensen T, Bach F (2004). Does the cannabinoid dronabinol reduce central pain in multiple sclerosis? Randomised double blind controlled crossover trial. BMJ 329: 253.

Tasker RR (2001). Central pain states. In: J Loeser (Ed.), Bonica's Management of Pain. Lippincott Williams & Wilkins, Philadelphia, pp. 433–457.

Tasker RR, de Carvalho G, Dostrovsky JO (1991). The history of central pain syndromes, with observations concerning pathophysiology and treatment. In: KL Casey (Ed.), Pain and Central Nervous Disease: The Central Pain Syndromes. Raven Press, New York, pp. 31–58.

Vestergaard K, Nielsen J, Andersen G et al. (1995). Sensory abnormalities in consecutive, unselected patients with central post-stroke pain. Pain 61: 177–186.

Vestergaard K, Andersen G, Gottrup H et al. (2001). Lamotrigine for central post-stroke pain – a randomised controlled trial. Neurology 56: 184–190.

Wiesenfeld-Hallin Z, Hao J-X, Xu X-J (1997). Mechanisms of central pain. In: TS Jensen, TA Turner, Z Wiesenfeld-Hallin (Eds.), Progress in Pain Research and Management. IASP Press, Seattle, pp. 575–588.

Willoch F, Schindler F, Wester HJ et al. (2004). Central poststroke pain and reduced opioid receptor binding within pain processing circuitries: a [^{11}C]diprenorphine PET study. Pain 108: 213–220.

Yamamoto T, Latayama Y, Hirayama T et al. (1997). Pharmacological classification of central post-stroke pain: comparison with the results of chronic motor cortex stimulation therapy. Pain 72: 5–12.

Zubieta JK, Smith YR, Bueller JA et al. (2001). Regional mu opioid receptor regulation of sensory and affective dimensions of pain. Science 203: 311–315.

Section 6

Special issues

Handbook of Clinical Neurology, Vol. 97 (3rd series)
Headache
G. Nappi and M.A. Moskowitz, Editors

Chapter 59

Chronobiological correlates of primary headaches

SARA GORI* AND LUIGI MURRI
University Centre for Adaptive Disorders and Headache, Institute of Neurology, Department of Neuroscience, University of Pisa, Pisa, Italy

A growing body of clinical, biochemical, neurophysiological, and neuroimaging data support the hypothesis that chronobiological disorders may underlie several primary headaches, mainly cluster headache (CH) and, to a lesser extent, migraine, and hypnic headache (HH).

CLUSTER HEADACHE

The periodicity of CH, which includes its relapsing-remitting course, its seasonal variation, and the clockwise regularity of single episodes, strongly suggests involvement of the biological clock, namely the hypothalamus, in the origin of the illness.

A disorder of circadian rhythms and hypothalamic function in CH has, indeed, been widely supported by heterogeneous data coming, as previously reported, from clinical evidence, biochemical (neuroendocrine and metabolic) studies, neurophysiological procedures, neuroimaging techniques, and, even if limited, from genetic data.

Clinical data

It is well known that CH has a remitting course and a "clustering" (Kunkle et al., 1952) of the attacks with symptom-free intervals. In a study of headache charts from 18 patients covering 55 cluster periods and 3276 CH attacks, one-third of the patients had cluster periods at regular intervals or fixed seasons (Trucco and Waldenlind, 1993), suggesting an influence from environmental factors such as length of day and light intensity. In a retrospective study carried out in 404 patients with episodic CH, Kudrow (1987) documented that the frequency of cluster period onset increased with the gradual increase or decrease in daylight throughout the year, with peaks occurring 7–10 days after the longest and the shortest day of the year. The gradual rise of cluster period frequency was interrupted by a significant drop in cluster period onset beginning 7–10 days after the resetting of the clock for daylight saving time in April and standard time in October. The occurrence of headache periods had an opposite trend in the two hemispheres (Costa et al., 1998). These data emphasized the hypothesis that a cluster period may somehow result from an inability to synchronize the internal circannual pacemaker to environmental light clues and, according to this paradigm a cluster period would begin when there is desynchronization and last as long as the time needed for resynchronization of rhythms (Kudrow, 1987; Waldenlind, 1999; Pringsheim, 2002).

CH attacks also showed a clear circadian distribution since they tend to occur with "clockwork" regularity, at least during a part of the cluster period (Horton, 1941; Symonds, 1956), and a preferential timing, since about 75% of them emerge between 2100 and 0010 hours (Russell, 1981).

The association between CH and sleep has long been recognized and Wolff's early observation that the majority of CHs occur always or commonly during sleep with pain so severe that it startles the patient from bed before he or she is fully awake has been confirmed by many authors as a seminal diagnostic feature of this disorder. CH attacks, indeed, tend to occur during sleep in up to two-thirds of patients (Sahota and Dexter, 1990) and this propensity to nocturnal emergence is equivalent in both episodic and chronic CH (Bahra et al., 2002).

The temporal distribution of CH attacks suggests they may be regulated by the circadian clock, but it is also possible that sleep itself may trigger the attacks (Gourineni and Zee, 2005).

Nocturnal attacks usually begin 1–2 h after falling asleep, generally 90 min after the patient falls asleep,

*Correspondence to: Sara Gori, MD, PhD, University Centre for Adaptive Disorders and Headache, Institute of Neurology, Department of Neuroscience, University of Pisa, Via Roma 67, 56126 Pisa, Italy, Tel: 39-050-992443, Fax: 39-050-554808, E-mail: s.gori@med.unipi.it

which coincides with the first rapid eye movement (REM) sleep period. In patients with episodic CH, but not in chronic ones, polysomnographic studies suggest nocturnal cluster attacks are associated with REM sleep (Dexter and Weitzman, 1970; Pfaffenrath et al., 1986). Kudrow et al. (1984) documented that almost 60% of the recorded attacks followed REM sleep, while the REM phase represented only 20% of total sleep time. CH attacks have also been documented to occur in stage 2 and 4 non-REM sleep (Dodick et al., 2003). A possible promoting role of sleep on CH attacks may also be hypothesized since it is possible to postpone attacks while staying awake (Ferrari et al., 1983) and a transient remission of CH may be obtained in some patients by skipping one night's sleep (Nappi et al., 1981).

CH not only exhibits a relationship with normal sleep, mainly REM sleep, but also with sleep disturbances, and the most remarkable data concern the association between CH and sleep-disordered breathing (SDB) in the form of obstructive sleep apnea or upper-airways resistance syndrome. A greater occurrence of obstructive sleep apnea syndrome was documented in CH patients in comparison with the general population (Kudrow et al., 1984; Chervin et al., 2000a, b) and it has been hypothesized that recurrent nocturnal hypoxemia, hypercapnia, excessively negative intrathoracic pressure, increased intracranial pressure, and abrupt changes in sympathetic tone associated with SDB could serve as a trigger for CH attacks (Kudrow et al., 1984; Kudrow and Kudrow, 1990). Oxygen desaturation in patients with obstructive sleep apnea tends to be more frequent, prolonged, and severe in REM sleep (Chervin and Aldrich, 1998) and these data may justify the high occurrence of CH attacks during the first REM sleep phase. However, alternative explanations for a link between CH and REM sleep also exist. During REM sleep oxygenation is often slightly lower than in non-REM sleep, even in the absence of obstructive sleep apnea (Krieger, 1994). Increases in carbon dioxide levels, with apneas or even without apneas during REM sleep (Krieger, 1994), could also conceivably trigger CH, as could abrupt autonomic changes associated with both apneas and REM sleep itself (Somers et al., 1993).

Several data suggest the existence of a relationship not only between CH attack occurrence and the sleep–wake cycle, but also with the activity–relaxation cycle.

Manzoni et al. (1981) found, when plotting the most common hours of onset for all patients, sharp peaks were found between 0100 and 0200, 1300 and 1500 hours, and a final peak reached at around 2100 hours. This study was carried out in Italy and the majority of the patients stopped working between 1300 and 1500 hours, so this social habit may justify the occurrence of the early-afternoon peak of the attacks, which is not seen in Scandinavian countries, where the lunch break is short (Trucco and Waldenlind, 1993). Also data from Russell (1981) emphasize the role of relaxation, since he found that 71% of daytime attacks in his series occurred while patients were physically relaxed.

Experimental data confirmed that the suprachiasmatic nucleus of the hypothalamus controls circadian rhythms not only in neuroendocrine, but also in behavioral and physiological functions; Moore and Danchenko (2002) concluded that pacemaker regulation of the circadian rhythms is mediated by discrete sets of suprachiasmatic nucleus projections, and specifically caudal projections to the subparaventricular zone and hypothalamic arousal system located in the posterior and lateral hypothalamic areas control the rhythm in rest–activity. More recent findings further support the view that the subparaventricular zone is the principal relay nucleus for suprachiasmatic nucleus to the multiple posterior hypothalamic arousal systems involved in the generation of the rest–activity rhythm (Abrahamson and Moore, 2006).

Genetics

Several epidemiological studies have demonstrated that genetic factors may play a role in CH; however the type and the number of genes involved in the disease are still unclear.

Recent molecular genetic studies focused on hypocretin receptor T2 (*HCRT2*) gene involvement in CH with conflicting results; Rainero et al. (2004) documented in an Italian CH sample that the 1246G→A poymorphism of the *HCRT2* gene is significantly associated with CH; these data were replicated in a larger German sample (Schürks et al., 2006), but not confirmed in northern European CH families (Baumber et al., 2006). The *HCRT2* gene involvement is very intriguing from a speculative point of view, since it suggests that the hypocretin system may be involved in the pathogenesis of CH and emphazises the hypothesis that it may represent a chronobiological disorder. Hypocretin-1 and 2 are, indeed, newly discovered neuropeptides processed from a common precursor; prehypocretin and hypocretin-containing cells are located exclusively in the posterolateral hypothalamus, with widespread projections to the entire neuraxis; two known G(q)-coupled receptors HCRTR 1 and HCRTR 2 have been identified. The peptides of the hypocretin system influence a wide range of physiological and behavioral processess in mammals (Siegel, 2004) which include the sleep–wake cycle, neuroendocrine functions, stress reactions, sympathetic functions, and finally pain threshold and nociceptive trasmission modulation (Bartsch et al., 2004). Several of these functions are significantly impaired in patients with CH.

Temperature, blood pressure, and sympathetic dysregulation

Temperature and blood pressure had normal circadian rhythmicity in episodic CH irrespective of active or remission phase (Ferrari et al., 1983). In the same study sleep deprivation for 40 h affected temperature and blood pressure regulation differently; half of the episodic patients, indeed, responded with a reduced attack frequency and the rhythmicity of temperature remained normal. In the other half of patients the attack frequency did not change and the circadian rhythm was lost. After sleep deprivation the circadian blood pressure rhythm disappeared in both responders and non-responders.

Concerning circadian heart rate regulation a phase delay of about 1 h, lowered heart rate variability, and a higher occurrence of arrhythmias was detected in CH during the active period, but not in the remission phase (Micieli et al., 1993).

Studies on catecholamine levels in CH patients are limited and not conclusive. The 24-h variation of norepinephrine was monitored for 3 days in 1 CH patient by means of blood sampling every 4 h. The norepinephrine rhythm was more marked than that in normal controls, maybe because cluster attacks coincided with the diurnal increase of norepinephrine (Igarashi et al., 1985). Strittmatter et al. (1996a) found decreased plasma levels of norepinephrine at 0700 and 2300 hours in CH during the active period, but no significant changes were detected in the corresponding plasma epinephrine levels.

More recently, altered nocturnal lipolysis was shown in CH, affecting not only absolute glycerol levels, but apparently also the circadian lipolysis rhythm (Meyer et al., 2003). Compared with healthy subjects, CH patients in the active period showed lower glycerol concentrations during the entire night, whereas patients in remission demonstrated lower glycerol levels between 0200 and 0600 hours. In addition different temporal glycerol patterns were found in both the active and remission phases in comparison with healthy controls. The authors suggest that a central as well as a peripheral autonomic disturbance could explain the reduced lipolytic activity; however since the hypothalamus regulates the autonomic nervous system as well as the secretion of insulin and growth hormone – both involved in modulating lipolysis – a dysfuncion in this area may exhaustively explain their results. Finally the identification of the altered temporal glycerol pattern in the remission period of CH has been interpreted as an indicator of a disturbance of the internal biological clock related to the pathogenesis of CH rather than changes secondary to pain.

Endocrine rhythms

Several studies have focused on 24-h hormonal secretory patterns in chronic and episodic CH in remission and active periods, and documented alterations in the circadian secretion of hormones, which have provided evidence of deranged hypothalamic function in CH.

Melatonin

The pineal hormone melatonin is of particular interest since its precursor is serotonin and it is considered a marker of circadian system functioning. Its secretion, regulated by an oscillator in the suprachiasmatic nucleus in the hypothalamus, is entrained to environmental light conditions via a noradrenergic retinohypothalamic pathway.

In active CH the characteristic melatonin rhythm, including its nocturnal peak, is altered and blunted compared to that in remission or healthy people (Chazot et al., 1984; Waldenlind et al., 1984, 1987; Leone et al., 1995). It is well known that stress may affect melatonin secretion (Vaughan et al., 1978), but as melatonin levels do not correlate with duration of illness, duration of headache course, time since the last attack, or attack frequency, it is highly improbable that melatonin alteration is only due to pain-induced stress itself in CH (Leone et al., 1995). The reduction in night-time melatonin secretion and loss of melatonin rhythm may reflect a reduced availability of serotonin for melatonin synthesis and/or a dysfunction within the synthetic pathway of melatonin production, including a reduced function of a sympathetic retinohypothalamic pathway, with consequent loss or alteration of its circadian phase-shifting properties.

There are several mechanisms whereby reduced levels of circulating melatonin could be involved in the pathophysiology of CH (Peres, 2005): by means of inhibition of gamma-aminobutyric acid (GABA), probably by interference with $GABA_A$ receptors; by modulation of the cellular distribution of Ca^{2+} through calmodulin binding; by involvement of the melatonin receptors present in the main cerebral arteries; by modulation of the 5-HT_2 receptors involved in the vasoactive responses; and finally by inhibiting the synthesis of prostaglandin E_2 that is involved in activating sterile perivascular inflammation in the trigeminovascular system. A role of deranged melatonin secretion in CH pathophysiology may also be suggested from the evidence that, even if limited, supports oral melatonin efficacy as preventive therapy in CH

(Leone et al., 1996; Peres and Rozen, 2001). It is still debated if the phase-resetting properties of melatonin, i.e., its chronobiotic effect, or the other previously reported properties of melatonin might explain its efficacy as a preventive treatment in some patients with CH.

The hypothalamic–pituitary–adrenal axis

The circadian production of cortisol has been reported to be altered during active episodic and chronic CH (Ferrari et al., 1983; Waldenlind and Gustafsson, 1987; Waldenlind, 1999).

In both chronic and episodic CH during the active period a consistent phase delay of the morning peak (acrophase) and increased 24-h mean and peak levels of cortisol have been observed. These findings suggested hyperactivity of the hypothalamic–pituitary–adrenal axis in this phase of the illness. Increased morning plasma cortisol is also seen in other pain conditions (Strittmatter et al., 1996b); however in episodic CH the morning cortisol levels were also high during the remission phase as compared to healthy controls, indicating that hypothalamic–pituitary–adrenal axis hyperactivity in CH does not simply represent a response to stress. This hypothesis is further supported by the fact that the cortisol response to the ovine corticotropin-releasing hormone (CRH) test is lower than normal in both the remission and cluster periods of CH patients (Leone et al., 1994). This reduced response suggests that pituitary adrenocorticocotropic hormone (ACTH)-secreting cells are downregulated independently of pain stress in CH, i.e., that there is permanent hypothalamic–pituitary–adrenal axis hyperactivity. Similarly, the responses of blood cortisol and ACTH to insulin-induced hypoglycemia are reduced in both phases of CH, suggesting that the hypothalamus of CH patients may be hyporesponsive to hypoglycemia (Strittmatter et al., 1996a). It has been suggested that the hyporesponsiveness of the hypothalamic–pituitary–adrenal axis in CH is mainly due to a serotonergic dysfunction at the level of the hypothalamus since the cortisol response to the administration of *m*-chlorophenylpiperazine – a 5-HT agonist acting on 5-HT$_{1A/2C}$ receptors – is reduced in both phases of CH (Leone et al., 1997).

Other authors emphasized (Pringsheim, 2002) that the abnormal results of the insulin tolerance test point to dysfunction along the hypothalamic–pituitary–adrenal axis in patients with CH, whereas the results of the ovine CRH test suggest an abnormal adrenal response. However this latter finding could also be consistent with hypothalamic dysfunction since there is evidence that the suprachiasmatic nucleus is involved in the setting of sensitivity of the adrenal cortex to ACTH, with experimental demonstration of a polysynaptic suprachiasmatic nucleus–adrenal cortex pathway (Buijs et al., 1999). ACTH and other pro-opiomelanocortin-derived peptides like beta-endorphin and beta-lipotropin also showed a delay of the acrophase during CH periods (Nappi et al., 1985a; Franceschini et al., 1996).

Prolactin

There is heterogeneous evidence with regard to the diurnal rhythm of prolactin in the CH active period since it was found to be normal (Ferrari et al., 1983; Chazot et al., 1984) or altered (Polleri et al., 1982). An impairment in the regulatory mechanisms of prolactin is supported by the evidence of reduced prolactin production over 24 h in both the active and remission phases of illness (Waldenlind and Gustafsson, 1987). The reduction does not seem to be related to sleep alterations or to pain episodes, but to altered central dopaminergic regulation of prolactin levels as supported by a smaller than normal increase in prolactin levels following stimulation by means of D2 antagonist metoclopramide (Klimek, 1985); this latter finding may be related to downregulation of lactotropic cells of hypophysis. A reduced response to thyrotropin-releasing hormone stimulation and a lack of prolactin increase after morphine administration have also been described in CH patients (Waldenlind and Gustafsson, 1987).

Testosterone and luteinizing hormone

Low morning levels of testosterone in CH have been extensively noted in both episodic and chronic CH (Klimek, 1983; Romiti et al., 1983; Facchinetti et al., 1986; Stillman, 2006a). Lowered 24-h production (Facchinetti et al., 1986) and a phase shift of the morning peak (Waldenlind and Gustafsson, 1987) have also been described. Fewer and prolonged luteinizing hormone peaks have been detected in the active period of CH patients (Micieli et al., 1987); however this latter finding is not considered to account for lowered testosterone production, nor can it be explained by an altered sleep–wake cycle, although this mechanism may play a role in some patients with nocturnal pain attacks (Waldenlind and Gustafsson, 1987). Possibly low testosterone levels might be attributed to increased plasma cortisol levels (Facchinetti et al., 1986). The central role of sympathetic impairment in determining both hypercortisolism and low levels of testosterone has also been suggested; it has indeed been hypothesized that sympathetic dysfunction culminates in a syndrome characterized by loss of circadian melatonin rhythm, neuroendocrine dysfunction – in the form of hypothalamic hypercortisolism and hypogonadism – and CH (Stillman, 2006a).

Recently abnormal testosterone levels in patients with episodic or chronic CH refractory to maximal medical management have been identified as a predictive parameter for a positive therapeutic response to testosterone replacement therapy (Stillman, 2006b).

Neuroimaging

Functional imaging studies with both positron emission tomography (PET) and magnetic resonance imaging (MRI) emphasize the importance of the hypothalamus as a key region in the pathophysiological process of CH and the other trigeminal autonomic cephalalgias (TACs), namely sudden unilateral neuralgiform pain with conjunctival injection and tearing (SUNCT) and paroxysmal hemicrania, suggesting its involvement in the pain process in a permissive or triggering manner rather than simply a response to first-division nociception *per se.*

PET studies in CH patients revealed a highly specific activation of the ipsilateral inferior posterior hypothalamus during both nitroglycerine-triggered (May et al., 1998a, 2000) and spontaneous (Sprenger et al., 2004a) attacks. A PET study was also recently performed in paroxysmal hemicrania patients and demonstrated significant activation of the posterior hypothalamus in association with the pain phase (Matharu et al., 2006).

Using blood oxygen-dependent functional MRI (fMRI), three independent case reports investigating 4 patients with spontaneous SUNCT episodes uniformly found an activation next to the hypothalamic spot that was activated in CH (May et al., 1999a; Cohen et al., 2004). The same prominent activation in the hypothalamic gray matter was recently found, using fMRI, in a 68-year-old patient suffering from excruciating trigeminoautonomic headache attacks, in whom frequency, duration, and therapeutic response allowed no clear-cut classification to one of the subtypes of TAC (Sprenger et al., 2004b).

Recently an fMRI study has also been carried out in CH patients and a highly specific activation of the posteroinferior hypothalamic region was documented in six spontaneous attacks of CH patients (personal data, Figure 59.1).

Voxel-based morphometry, a new fully automated whole-brain technique that is sensitive to subtle macroscopic and mesoscopic structural differences between groups of subjects, detected a significant structural difference in gray-matter density, i.e., a "lesion" coinciding with the inferior posterior hypothalamus in CH (May et al., 1999b). Intrinsic structural abnormalities of the posterior hypothalamus were moreover suggested by a proton magnetic resonance spectroscopy study of hypothalamic metabolism that demonstrated reduced *N*-acetylaspartate/creatine ratios in both chronic and episodic CH independently of the attacks (Lodi et al., 2006).

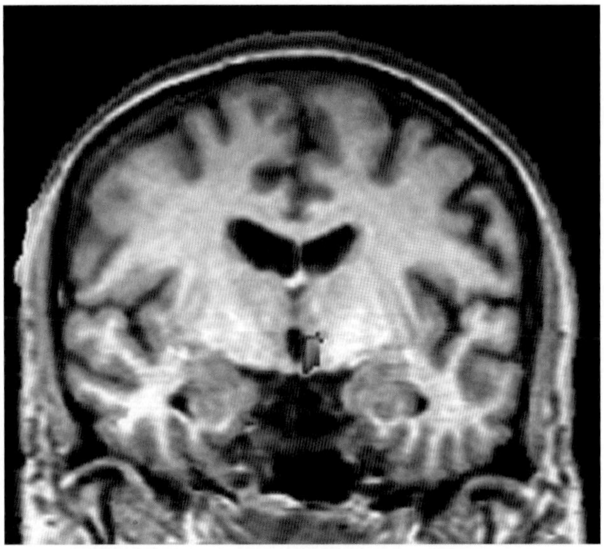

Fig. 59.1. GML multi-study analysis show asymmetric cerebral activation area in the posterior grey hypothalamus, ipsilaterally to the pain side (Bonferoni correction $p < .05$), superimposed on an anatomical reference derived from a T1 weighted MRI scan. Graphic representation of the hypotalamic nuclei.

The posterior hypothalamus is not the only central nervous system region to become activated during attacks of CH or of other TAC. Brain regions associated with the perception of pain such as cingulated areas, frontal cortex, insula, basal ganglia, thalamus, and cerebellum also light up, but in what is thought to be a non-specific way, since these regions are similarly activated upon application of capsaicin to the frontal skin regions to provoke experimental pain (May et al., 1998b). Hypothalamic activation seems not to occur during such experimental pain and has therefore been considered specific to TAC.

The previously reported co-localization of functional and morphometric changes suggesting the precise anatomical location for probable central nervous system lesion in CH prompted the use of deep-brain stimulation (DBS) in the posterior hypothalamic gray matter in intractable CH patients. To date successful operations have been reported in 20 cases, some with a follow-up of more than 4 years (Schoenen et al., 2005; Leone, 2006). Circuits and mechanisms underlying the analgesic effect of DBS are not yet completely understood, even if a recent PET study had shown activation of trigeminal nucleus and ganglion after posterior hypothalamic stimulation, lending support to the hypothesis that hypothalamic stimulation modulates the activity of the trigeminal nucleus caudalis, which in turn controls the brainstem trigeminofacial reflex (May et al., 2006). Since the hypothalamus has been described as a "clock pulse generator," which must oscillate in a non-specific manner over time to modulate distant autonomic and trigeminovascular areas, resulting in unilateral pain and autonomic symptoms, constant depolarization obtained by means of DBS would discontinue the biological clock-like impulses from the distant trigeminal and autonomic "executers" (May, 2005; May et al., 2006).

The chronobiological effect of hypothalamic involvement could be explained by the reciprocal connections between hypothalamic posterior and lateral areas – activated in CH and other TAC attacks and modulated by means of DBS – and the suprachiasmatic nucleus, which has the function of pacemaker and regulates endogenous circadian rhythms (Ralph et al., 1990).

Pain control: neurophysiological and biochemical data

The hypothesis of cyclical failure of pain control in CH is supported by both neurophysiological and biochemical data.

The existence of circadian changes in human pain threshold values has been documented by several studies using psychophysical methods, as well as neurophysiological investigation of nociceptive reflex (Sandrini et al., 1986a).

In episodic CH patients a circadian rhythmicity of the nociceptive reflex threshold was documented, but a clear shift of the phase occurred during the active period, not seen in the remission phase (Nappi et al., 2002). In the same study a complete disruption of the circadian pattern of the lower-limb RIII threshold was, instead, observed in chronic CH patients; these data could indicate a more severe impairment in the circadian pain control system in chronic rather than in episodic CH patients. Both opiatergic and serotonergic control in nociceptive RIII are relevant according to several studies (Sandrini et al., 1986b, c).

Biochemical evidence confirmed a possible cyclic impairment of the pain control system in CH since a lack of beta-endorphin and beta-lipotropin circadian rhythmicity has been observed in episodic CH (Nappi and Sjaastad, 1983; Nappi et al., 1985a, b; 1987; Franceschini et al., 1996). Recently an opioidergic dysfunction in circuitries generating the biological clock was shown in CH by means of a PET study (Sprenger et al., 2006); the authors suggest that the decrease in opioid receptor binding in the pineal gland may in turn be related to pathological melatonin homeostasis in CH.

MIGRAINE

Clinical observations showed that migraine attacks have circadian and circannual timing, suggesting a role for chronobiological mechanisms and of their possible impairment in the disease, and neuroendocrine and neurophysiological investigations have contributed to confirm this.

The menstrual periodicity of migraine without aura is also documented; its epidemiological and clinical aspects and its physiopathological basis and mechanisms are extensively described in Chapter 25.

Clinical data

It is well known that clinical symptoms of migraine may fluctuate; however several patients report their headaches predominantly or specifically during a certain period of the day. A preferential emergence of attacks at nighttime or in the early morning was extensively ascertained. Galego et al. (2002) documented that both episodic (55%) and chronic (62.5%) migraineurs reported waking up in the morning or being woken up during the night by headaches. A more recent study (Kelman and Rains, 2005), carried out in a larger sample of 1283 migraineurs, confirmed that 71% of patients exhibit morning headache on awakening (in 35% of the whole sample it was very frequent or frequent, whereas in 36% it was occasional).

Moreover a chronobiological study by Solomon (1992) indicated the greatest occurrence of attacks in the interval 0400–0600 hours. Successive research by Fox and Davis (1998) that investigated the circadian periodicity observed in the time of onset of 3582 migraine headache attacks experienced by 1698 patients documented the maximum probability of the occurrence of migraine during 0400–0900 hours, with no other time of the day approaching this likelihood. Similar results were confirmed in a selected sample of migraineurs with low monthly frequency attacks; according to clinical diaries referring to the last 3 months, 42% of migraineurs had more than 75% of their attacks at night and in the early morning, especially from 0300 to 0700 hours (Gori et al., 2005).

The preferential occurrence of migraine attack at nighttime and in the early-morning hours might suggest both the existence of a relationship betwen migraine and sleep and possibly an impairment of the circadian rhythm control systems; these hypotheses are not mutually exclusive, since they might simply coexist or also be linked given the role of the hypothalamus in controlling not only circadian rhythms but also sleep (Mistlberger, 2005), especially REM sleep (Suntsova et al., 2000).

The relationship between migraine and sleep is complex and pluridirectional (i.e., excessive sleep causes headache, sleep deprivation causes headache, sleeping will relieve headache, and so on). However, the most relevant data to explain the link between migraine and normal sleep might be that they are intrinsically related by anatomy and physiology.

The limited number of polysomnographic studies performed to date on patients with migraine suggests a relationship between the REM sleep phase, and, to a lesser exent, stage 3 and 4 non-REM sleep, and nocturnal migraine attacks (Dexter and Weitzman, 1970; Dexter, 1979; Sahota and Dexter, 1990).

The anatomical structures involved in both sleep regulation – especially REM sleep – and migraine production are to a larger degree in the brainstem and may be identified in the locus coeruleus (LC) and the dorsal raphe nucleus (DRN). Since these aminergic nuclei represent an important part of the antinociceptive pain-processing network, their strong reduction of firing occurring during the REM sleep phase may contribute to precipitate migraine attack.

Apart from the temporal distribution of the attacks, the evaluation of chronobiological features in migraine also demonstrated the relevancy and effect of sleep schedule changes on migraine clinical pictures. According to Peres et al. (2003), 46.5% of migraine patients reported headache after changing their sleep schedule, mainly in those who experienced a delayed sleep phase and to a lesser extent in advancing it. Data concerning chronotype (Gori et al., 2005) indicated that morning and evening types rather than intermediate ones were better represented among migraineurs in comparison with control group subjects, and differences between actual and preferred times to fall asleep and to awaken were longer than in controls. As morning and evening types showed poor sleep quality and higher disability, at least as assessed by means of the Migraine Disability Assessment Scale, it might be hypothesized that extreme chronotypes and the differences between actual and preferred time to fall asleep and to awaken, experienced because of social rhythms, may worsen the clinical presentation of the disease. In other words chronobiological aspects might interfere with the clinical picture in migraine. Desynchronization between the biological endogenous clock (i.e., hypothalamus) and lifestyle may account for different levels of severity in migraineurs. It is well known that migraine may, indeed, be viewed as a disturbance of the cerebral circuits concerned with adaptive homeostatic mechanisms (Craig, 2003).

A hypothalamic involvement in migraine pathogenesis might also be supported by prodromal symptom analysis: almost 60% of patients with migraine, indeed, report during the 24 h preceding headache elation, irritability, depression, hunger, thirst, or drowsiness, which may account for a hypothalamic site of origin (Blau, 1980).

Finally a dysfunction in biological rhythms generated in the suprachiasmatic nucleus of the hypothalamus may also be suggested from the data concerning seasonal periodicity in migraine: an overrepresentation of attacks during summer months, even if not statistically significant, was documented by Fox and Davis (1998). Moreover migraineurs, especially with aura, as opposed to individuals with other headaches, were more likely to have headache during the bright arctic summer than during the polar night season (Salvesen and Bekkelund, 2000; Alstadhaug et al., 2005).

Endocrine rhythms

Melatonin

Melatonin was first studied in migraine patients by Claustrat et al. (1989). It was shown that patients had lower levels of plasma melatonin in samples drawn at 2300 hours compared with controls; migraine patients without depression had lower levels than controls, but migraineurs also affected by depression exhibited the greatest melatonin deficiency. There is a significant decrease of nocturnal urinary melatonin throughout the ovarian cycle in patients with migraine without aura in comparison with controls. In particular during the luteal phase, when a melatonin level increase was expected according to control data, a less pronounced change was documented in migraine patients and melatonin excretion was further decreased when patients suffered a migraine attack (Murialdo et al., 1994). The study (Brun et al., 1995) of urinary melatonin in women with attacks of migraine without aura that were associated with menses and controls documented that melatonin levels throughout the cycle were significantly lower in migraine patients than in controls. In the control group melatonin excretion increased significantly from the follicular to the luteal phase, whereas no difference was observed in the migraine group. These latest data have supported a hypothesis of a role for melatonin in the pathogenesis of migraine, especially with menstrual preferential occurrence.

Evaluation of plasma melatonin was also carried out in chronic migraine by Peres et al. (2001) by means of collecting samples hourly from 1900 to 0700 hours; a phase delay in the melatonin peak was documented in patients in comparison with controls. Individual plasma profiles were also disturbed in 3 patients affected by status migrainosus, although in a non-homogeneous manner since 2 had a phase delay and the other a phase advance (Claustrat et al., 1997).

Melatonin was also employed as a therapeutic agent in a limited number of studies. Melatonin infusion was associated with headache relief in status migrainosus (Claustrat et al., 1997). Moreover an open-label trial was performed using melatonin 3 mg/day for migraine prevention (Peres et al., 2004): a significant decrease in headache frequency, duration, intensity, and analgesic consumption was observed when baseline data were compared with the last month of treatment.

Melatonin may be implicated in the pathogenesis of migraine, and it might also play a role in migraine comorbid disorders, particularly depression. Several melatonin mechanisms are potentially related to headache disorders, including migraine; for migraine, in the light of recent discoveries it might be hypothesized that melatonin may interfere in cortical spreading depression, probably via its effect on the nitric oxide, GABA, and glutamatergic systems. Moreover it might be involved in the pathophysiology of migraine and psychiatric comorbid conditions through its action on the serotonergic and dopaminergic systems.

Prolactin, cortisol, and growth hormone

Some studies have reported normal prolactin values in episodic migraine (Lara Capellan et al., 1990), whereas a decrease in the prolactin nocturnal peak was documented in chronic migraine patients (Peres et al., 2001). Peres et al. hypothesized that there is a sustained nocturnal inhibition of prolactin by dopamine and therefore an indirect increase in dopamine secretion, so their findings may support the use of antidopaminergic drugs in both acute and preventive therapy of migraine patients. The increase in tumor necrosis factor-alpha 1, a potent proinflammatory cytokine involved in neurogenic inflammation with an inhibitor role on prolactin secretion, may also contribute to suppressing the peak of prolactin in chronic migraine patients.

An increase in cortisol concentration was also found by Peres et al. (2001) in chronic migraine, suggesting that the hypophyseal–adrenal axis is activated in these patients compared with controls.

Secretion of growth hormone did not differ from controls in the same study. Overall the findings by Peres et al. (2001) in chronic migraine patients support the involvement of the hypothalamus in its pathophysiology, as shown by a chronobiological dysregulation and also a possible hyperdopaminergic state.

Blood pressure and heart rate variability studies

The analysis of circadian variation of blood pressure documented that the acrophase amplitude of ambulatory blood pressure decreases in migraineurs, i.e., the amplitudes of systolic, mean, and diastolic blood pressure in the migraine group were significantly lower than those in controls (Takeshima et al., 1997), suggesting that some migraineurs lose or alter their circadian blood pressure rhythm; this abnormality suggests dysfunction of the circadian rhythm generator and the central autonomic nervous system in migraine.

Significant differences in circadian rhythm of different heart rate fluctuation parameters were also documented (Tabata et al., 2000) in migraineurs.

HYPNIC HEADACHE

HH is a rare sleep-associated primary headache disorder, usually affecting older people, first described by Raskin in 1988. Among primary headaches it represents the single entity uniquely associated with sleep; its diagnostic criteria, included in the second edition of the International Classification of Headache Disorders (Headache Classification Subcommittee of the International Headache Society 2004), indeed, require that attacks develop only during sleep and awaken the patient. Attacks usually present themselves at a consistent time each night (therefore HH has also been called clockwise headache or alarm-clock headache), sometimes during a dream, and can recur more than once in one night.

Lithium, melatonin, and caffeine have been effective treatments in several reported cases. Interestingly, 1 patient had a remission for 3 months after traveling across time zones (Montagna, 2006).

Polysomnographic studies indicate that REM sleep, but not SDB, is to be considered a major trigger of HH attacks. According to available literature data (De Simone et al., 2006), an association with REM sleep was found in 15 out of 20 recorded attacks (75%), while 2 attacks occurred in stage 2 non-REM and 3 in stage 3 non-REM sleep. Only 1 attack out of 20 recorded headaches emerged with an occurrence clearly time-related to severe hypoxia.

The pathophysiology of HH is still unclear and available data allow only speculation.

The hypothesis that HH might represent a REM sleep-related disorder caused by a derangement of a brainstem neural network that regulates the sleep–wake rhythm may be supported by the experimental evidence of a physiological marked decrease of DRN (Lydic et al., 1983) and LC (Somers et al., 1993) activities during REM phases of sleep. Since DRN and LC are, together with the periaqueductal gray matter, essential parts of the human antinociceptive system, they could represent an important anatomofunctional intersection between the neural network involved in the regulation of the sleep–wake cycle and in pain processing. Therefore a possible dysfunction of these aminergic nuclei could account for the onset of a headache attack and awakening from sleep.

The onset of HH attacks at a consistent time each night and the efficacy of drugs that can influence circadian rhythms, such as lithium and melatonin,

to demonstrate antinociception induced by this nonapeptide (Berkowitz and Sherman, 1982; Witt et al., 1992; Xu and Wiesenfeld-Hallin, 1994). Whether oxytocin increases the pain threshold through activation of endogenous opioid neurons is also a controversy. In a review, Richard and collaborators (1991) concluded that: "in no case does oxytocin-induced analgesia appear to be opiate-dependent."

The oxytocin perikarya are present largely in the magnocellular nuclei, although fibers are widely distributed in the central nervous system, including the spinal cord, where they end particularly in layers I, II, and X of the gray matter. In the spinal cord, the oxytocin fibers may originate from the paraventricular nucleus (Lang et al., 1983) or from dorsal root ganglia C fibers, using oxytocin as neurotransmitter (Kai-Kai et al., 1986).

Under physiological conditions, pain sensation is mediated by two primary afferent neurons: (1) small-diameter non-myelinated C fibers that transmit slow dull pain; and (2) thinly myelinated Aδ fibers, transmitters of fast sharp pain. Both are referred to as nociceptors that respond to mechanical, thermal, and chemical forms of energy. In this regard, thermal nociceptors are activated by extreme temperatures (>45°C or <5°C). On the other hand, the mechano- and heat-responsive C fibers present heat thresholds ranging from 40°C to 50°C. In humans, rapid immersion of a finger in a hot-water bath (57°C) causes at onset a stinging pain after a time interval of 0.84 s on average. This is followed by a second wave of a burning pain after 2.1 s (Handwerker and Kobal, 1993). The latency between the two forms of pain waves decreases as the stimulus moves up the limbs toward the trunk, and at the trunk level it was not feasible to obtain a double pain sequence. This double pain experience is triggered by fast-rising stimulus (electric shock, pinprick, or heating pulse). Interestingly, opioid substances appear to affect the second pain component more than the first one (Price et al., 1985). In contrast, the first pain component is differentially blocked by compression ischemia (Handwerker and Kobal, 1993).

Previously, we demonstrated that oxytocin caused analgesia in mice (Lins Filho, 2000), an effect abolished by the blockade of opioid receptor with naloxone. The analgesia was evaluated using the tail flick test. The mean latency duration observed, during the tail flick test, in control animals ($n = 80$) before any treatment was 4.8 ± 0.2 s (100%, ranging from 2 to 12 s). Intraperitoneal administration of oxytocin (1 mg/kg; 0.2 ml) induced an analgesic state. It was evident as early as 10 min after oxytocin administration (81.5 ± 6.2% in the saline vehicle-treated group (0.9% NaCl; 0.2 ml) versus 130.0 ± 17.5% in the oxytocin-treated group; $P < 0.01$), which was maximal at 45 min (93.3 ± 6.7% in the saline-treated group versus 205.0 ± 45.3% in the oxytocin-treated group). No significant difference in analgesia was detected after 75 min of oxytocin injection. On the other hand, the previous blockade of opioid receptor by naloxone completely canceled the enhancement in the latencies observed during tail flick test, at all times studied (from 10 to 60 min). This indicates that oxytocin causes analgesia through the involvement of endogenous opioids.

An additional experiment was performed to evaluate the effects of naloxone or the oxytocin antagonist on analgesia induced by immobilization stress (10 min). The mice were treated with the respective receptor blocker 10 min before the beginning of the physical restraint. The analgesia induced by immobilization was amplified by oxytocin administration, which became statistically significant at 40 min. This time is closely correlated with the peak of analgesia occurring at 45 min, when oxytocin was given alone.

The physical restraint stress for a 10-min period caused a strong analgesia, with the latency in the tail flick test increasing from 100.0 ± 6.2% at time 0 min (before intraperitoneal injection) to 197.5 ± 23.3% immediately after the end of the 10 min of immobilization ($P < 0.001$). Oxytocin treatment slightly enhanced the analgesia induced by immobilization (283.2 ± 39.0% at the end of the 10-min period of restraint; $P < 0.05$), although the treatment with oxytocin only modified significantly the increase in latency induced by this type of stress 40 min after the drug injection (124.5 ± 13.2 in saline vehicle-treated animals versus 182.9 ± 21.5% in the oxytocin-treated animals; $P < 0.05$). Naloxone significantly inhibited the analgesia induced by immobilization stress. In contrast, the oxytocin antagonist did not modify the increase in the tail flick test latency induced by this kind of stress. The magnitude of the analgesic response was similar between both analgesic inducers, although immobilization induced a rapid analgesic effect, whereas oxytocin administration caused a delayed (45 min) maximal response in terms of antinociception. Hence, analgesia induced by oxytocin, in mice without restraint stress, is blocked by naloxone, which indicates that the effect of oxytocin is mediated by opioids. But when a restraint stress is applied, the analgesic effect does not involve the oxytocin neurons, suggesting that other circuitries are involved. Indeed, the antinociceptive effects produced by immobilization were mediated by the opioid system, since the blockade of opioid receptors inhibited the analgesia.

In 1982, Berkowitz and Sherman reported that peripheral injection of oxytocin does not have any analgesic effects. In contrast, it was demonstrated that injections of oxytocin intracisternally in mice (Lundeberg et al., 1994) or intrathecally in rats (Yang, 1994) caused analgesia. Lundeberg and collaborators (1993) suggested a central action of oxytocin since intrathecal injection of oxytocin induced a delay in the reaction time in the paw pressure test. Besides, oxytocin levels in plasma and cerebrospinal fluid were found to increase after a 30-min exposure to different non-noxious sensory stimuli, an effect concomitant with the development of analgesia (Uvnas-Moberg et al., 1993b). Immobilization stress also provoked elevation in plasma oxytocin levels (Jezova et al., 1993). The oxytocin antagonist decreased the latency of tail flick test observed after exposure to non-noxious stimuli and reduced the analgesia induced by oxytocin (Uvnas-Moberg et al., 1993a). However, Xu and Wiesenfeld-Hallin (1994) attributed the increase in the latency response in the hot-plate test in rats to the sedative and vasoconstrictive effects of oxytocin, rather than an analgesic phenomenon. Additionally, they also reported that oxytocin antagonist did not influence the latency to heat pain sensitivity in rats.

In humans, acute and chronic low-back pain causes a significant increase of oxytocin concentration within the cerebrospinal fluid and plasma (Yang, 1994). Furthermore, oxytocin administration can alleviate low-back pain (Yang, 1994). In rats, oxytocin had a dose-related analgesic effect. The use of oxytocin antagonists or naloxone can reverse the analgesia induced by oxytocin. It was also shown that oxytocin might increase the levels of endogenous opioid peptides in the spinal cord, whereas oxytocin antagonists caused a decrease (Yang, 1994).

Since during labor the action of oxytocin over the uterus provokes muscle contraction (an event which would trigger pain sensation), it would be expected that the same neuropeptide could exert a dual physiological role – analgesia and uterus contraction during labor. Indeed, parturition and vaginal dilation both cause enhancement in plasma oxytocin concentration and increase in pain threshold (Crowley et al., 1977). Interestingly, vaginal dilation activates oxytocin neurons and induces maternal behavior in ewes, an effect blocked by naltrexone (Kendrick and Keverne, 1989). It was demonstrated that during the first stage of labor the intrathecal administration of sufentanil decreased plasma concentration of oxytocin in women with pain (Stocche et al., 2001). This suggests again a close interaction between endogenous opioid peptides and oxytocin.

The oxytocin present in the systemic blood under physiological conditions does not penetrate into the cerebrospinal fluid or into the brain. In guinea pig, only 2–3% of the intraperitoneally administrated oxytocin was detected in the brain. Hence, the need for high doses of oxytocin, if injected systemically, to induce analgesia, when considering a central site of action (Annat et al., 1986). Two minutes after administration of 1 g [^{3}H]oxytocin, 0.008%/g was found in the brain (Witt et al., 1992). It was reported that the neurohypophyseal hormones or their fragments are transported under normal conditions from blood to brain (van Bree et al., 1989). Furthermore, under either stress condition or injection of epinephrine there is an increased permeability of the blood–brain barrier to peptides (Banks, 2001).

Modifications of the response latencies to the tail flick test due to different temperatures were found with oxytocin antiserum intracerebroventricular injections: no changes at high temperatures, decrease in the latencies at moderate temperature, and increase in latencies at low temperature (analgesia). Similar results were observed with other antisera, such as against vasopressin, met-enkephalin, and beta-endorphin (Bodnar et al., 1984). On the other hand, it has been shown that naloxone, by itself, does not cause pain, but may enhance the perception of pain (Buchsbaum et al., 1983).

The concentration of oxytocin in cerebrospinal fluid of dogs with spinal cord compression was higher than in control dogs, suggesting that during painful conditions oxytocin is released in order to attenuate the unpleasant, hurtful situation (Brown and Perkowski, 1998). Furthermore, analgesia may be caused by different types of stress. The restraint stress-induced analgesia is mediated by endogenous opioid peptides; other kinds of stresses, such as surgical stress, are unaffected by previous opioid receptor blockade (Valença et al., 1999).

It seems that individuals prone to migraine have a genetically determined migraine threshold that renders them susceptible to a migraine attack upon exposure to some or any of a range of patient-specific triggers. Hormonal influences, environmental and physiological stressors, hypoglycemia, and fatigue are all thought to influence this threshold. Associated diseases such as temporomandibular disorders, sinusitis, and obesity may also decrease the pain threshold (Valença et al., 2003). Once the threshold is exceeded, trigeminovascular discharge is thought to be responsible for inducing a migraine.

The physiopathogenic mechanisms involved in the primary headaches are still poorly known. A migraine attack may be the result of nociceptive neuronal activation of the trigeminal vascular system, which would involve the meninges and part of the soft structures of the head. Vasoactive neural peptides are released during migraine crisis, indicating that depolarization of primary afferent neurons, with perivascular release of substance P and calcitonin gene-related peptide (CGRP), occurs at the sensitive terminal. This, in turn,

night or after a missed, delayed, or partial feed, events associated with the beginning of the headache. Afterward, the headaches were relieved by putting the baby to the breast.

Low levels of thyroid hormones (triiodothyronine and thyroxine, hypothyroidism) are the second cause of frequent headaches associated with endocrinological disturbance, after menstrual cephalalgia. Hypothyroidism is very commonly present in people complaining of migraine and tension headaches. Many endocrinological conditions can cause headache, but hypothyroidism should be at the top of the list when evaluating chronic headaches – especially in those patients complaining of fatigue. Moreau and collaborators (1998), studying 102 patients with hypothyroidism, found that 31 (30%) presented with headache 1–2 months after the first symptoms of hypothyroidism. The headache was slight, non-pulsatile, continuous, bilateral, and salicylate-responsive and disappeared with thyroid hormone therapy. They concluded that there is a prevalence of non-specific headache in hypothyroidism and that it has a particular response to thyroid hormone therapy.

As discussed above, headache is one of the neurological manifestations of hypothyroidism but it is unknown whether there is a relationship between hyperthyroidism and chronic headache. In one study, a series of 30 individuals with chronic headache were evaluated in relation to their thyroid function. Six were found to have hyperthyroidism and none had hypothyroidism. The authors concluded that thyroid testing may be beneficial for differential diagnosis of chronic headache, and indicate that headache could be caused by hyperthyroidism (Iwasaki et al., 1991). Recently, an observational study of thyroid function tests performed in patients with headache prior to referral to a neurological clinic found no headache cases attributable to either hypothyroidism or hyperthyroidism. The role of thyroid dysfunction in the etiology of headache remains uncertain (Larner, 2006).

Regarding prolactin influence on headache neurobiology, Strebel et al. (1986) demonstrated that hyperprolactinemia was associated with headache only if a prolactinoma was present and not in the absence of a prolactinoma, in women with non-puerperal hyperprolactinemia. Thus, in women with secondary amenorrhea or galactorrhea, or both, headache may be a practical indicator of the presence of an occult prolactinoma.

MELATONIN AND HEADACHE DISORDERS

Life on Earth is under 24-h rhythmicity, due to the rotation of Earth on its axis. The nervous system evolved over the millennia to meet the demands of environmental conditions, including the light–dark cycle, in order to ensure survival and reproduction of living organisms. A synchronization system to adapt the internal to the external environment is one of the key elements of the central nervous system to maintain life.

The main elements for synchronization between internal biological events and the environment are the pineal gland and its main secretory product, melatonin. Melatonin is absent during the day in humans and its nocturnal secretion is the main biological event signaling what is night to the organism.

Melatonin is a derivative of the essential amino acid tryptophan. The pinealocyte is the principal location for melatonin biosynthesis, After its uptake into cells, tryptophan is first hydroxylated and then decarboxylated, resulting in the formation of 5-HT (Reiter et al., 2000). 5-HT is *N*-acetylated, with the resulting formation of *N*-acetyl-serotonin, which is subsequently *O*-methylated to form melatonin (Reiter et al., 2000). Once melatonin is synthesized in the pineal, it is quickly released, generating a blood melatonin rhythm reminiscent of that seen in the gland.

At present, indications for therapeutic applications for melatonin include sleep disorders, circadian rhythm disorders, insomnia in blind people, insomnia in elderly patients, aging, Alzheimer's disease, and as an adjuvant in cancer therapy (Bubenik et al., 1998). Melatonin has been proposed to be an important element in migraine (Peres, 2005). Its role in headache disorders may have also treatment implications. A potential therapeutic use of melatonin has been considered in several headache disorders, including cluster headaches (the first to be studied), migraines, and indomethacin-responsive headache syndromes.

Sleep is well known to play an important role as a restorative function. In human beings, it has a circadian rhythm, normally occurring at night, usually together with the nocturnal melatonin secretion (Rodenbeck et al., 1999). This has led to the idea that melatonin is an internal sleep facilitator in humans, and therefore useful in the treatment of insomnia and the readjustment of circadian rhythms. There is evidence that administration of melatonin is able to induce sleep when the drive to sleep is insufficient; to inhibit the drive for wakefulness from the suprachiasmatic nucleus; and to induce phase shifts in the circadian clock such that the circadian phase of increased sleep propensity occurs at a new, desired time (Cajochen et al., 2003).

Many neurological disorders occur with a marked rhythmicity, dependent either on the 24-h or the seasonal cycle, thus probably linked to the pineal function and melatonin secretion, including stroke, multiple sclerosis, facial paralysis, and seasonal affective disorder (Checkley et al., 1993; Turek et al., 2001).

The pineal gland is a photoneuroendocrine organ, converting external luminous stimuli into a hormone secretion, being responsible for synchronization between internal homeostasis and the environment; therefore, an altered synchronization system may interfere with all neurological diseases. Sleep and circadian rhythms are often disrupted in people with neurological disorders (Turek et al., 2001). The symptoms associated with neurological diseases may be due in part to disruption of the sleep–wake cycle. In addition, various neurological disorders may themselves disrupt the sleep–wake cycle, resulting in a positive-feedback loop whereby disrupted sleep and wake exacerbate the neurological disorders while the disease itself has a negative effect on the sleep–wake states (Turek et al., 2001).

Symptoms associated with those disorders may fluctuate according to a specific rhythm (circannual, circamenal, circadian) and are often related to either sleep or wake periods. Epilepsy, dementia, movement disorders, multiple sclerosis, cerebrovascular disorders, neuromuscular disorders, and brain tumors have all been linked to an altered chronobiology, melatonin dysfunction, or benefit from melatonin treatment (Turek et al., 2001). Primary headaches also follow this rule. Migraines, cluster headaches, indomethacin-responsive headaches, and hypnic headaches have been related to melatonin.

Melatonin may play a role in headache pathophysiology via several mechanisms. Melatonin has been shown to possess anti-inflammatory effects, among a number of actions. By virtue of its ability to scavenge directly toxic free radicals (Reiter et al., 2000), it reduces macromolecular damage in all organs. Melatonin inhibits the production of adhesion molecules that promote the sticking of leukocytes to endothelial cells, attenuating transendothelial cell migration and edema (Shaikh et al., 1997). Melatonin inhibits the activity of NO synthase (Bettahi et al., 1996), besides acting in membrane stabilization (Garcia et al., 1997).

Inhibition of dopamine release by melatonin has been demonstrated in specific areas of the mammalian central nervous system (hypothalamus, hippocampus, medulla pons, and retina) (Zisapel, 2001). A growing body of biological, pharmacological, and genetic data supports a role for dopamine in the pathophysiology of migraine (Peroutka, 1997).

Melatonin has been related to dopamine, GABA, and glutamate neurotransmission, and to headache pathophysiology (Ramadan, 2003). Melatonin is also involved in cerebrovascular regulation (Ebadi et al., 1998), and modulation of 5-HT neurotransmission (spontaneous efflux and evoked release) (Monnet, 2002).

Melatonin and migraine are linked in several ways. Clinical symptoms may fluctuate; some patients report their headaches predominantly or specifically in a certain period of the day.

Melatonin was first studied in migraine patients by Claustrat and collaborators, in 1989, showing lower plasma levels in patients compared to controls. Migraine patients without depression had lower levels than controls, but migraineurs with superimposed depression exhibited the greatest melatonin deficiency. Murialdo and collaborators (1994) also found nocturnal urinary melatonin to be significantly decreased throughout the ovarian cycle of patients with migraine without aura compared to controls. During the luteal phase, when melatonin levels should normally increase, migraine patients showed a less pronounced change when compared to controls. Melatonin excretion was further decreased when patients suffered a migraine attack.

Brun and collaborators (1995) studied urinary melatonin in women with migraine without aura attacks associated with menses and controls. Melatonin levels throughout the cycle were significantly lower in the migraine patients than in controls. Peres and collaborators (2001a) studied plasma melatonin nocturnal profile, observing lowered melatonin levels in patients with insomnia, suggesting a chronobiological dysfunction in chronic migraineurs.

Some studies showed a benefit in migraine patients from melatonin treatment (Claustrat et al., 1989, 1997; Nagtegaal et al., 1998). An open-label trial has been performed using melatonin 3 mg for migraine prevention (Peres et al., 2004). Thirty-four patients (27 women, 5 men) were included and a significant headache relief was found in 64.7%. Headache response was observed already in the first month of treatment. Complete response was found in 25% of patients. Headache frequency, duration, intensity, and analgesic consumption significantly decreased when baseline was compared to the last month of treatment ($P < 0.001$). The medication was well tolerated; only 2 patients dropped out the study.

It has been suspected that melatonin may be involved in cluster headache genesis, primarily because melatonin is a sensitive marker of endogenous rhythms, which are disrupted in cluster headache (May et al., 1998).

In 1984, Chazot and collaborators identified a decrease in nocturnal melatonin secretion and abolished melatonin rhythm in cluster headache patients. Waldenlind and collaborators (1987) also showed lowered nocturnal melatonin levels during cluster periods than remissions. Determining urinary levels of 6-sulfatoximelatonin throughout the year, Waldenlind and collaborators (1994) found higher melatonin levels in women than men. Swedes had higher melatonin levels than Italians, and smokers lower levels than non-smoking cluster headache patients. Leone and collaborators (1995) observed that melatonin and cortisol acrophases were significantly correlated in controls but not in cluster headache patients, indicating a chronobiological disorder in these patients.

Blau and Engel (1999) found that increases in body temperature from exercise, a hot bath, or elevated environmental temperature triggered cluster headaches in 75 of 200 cluster headache patients. This finding can be explained by a decrease in melatonin secretion caused by an increase in temperature (Peres et al., 2000). Melatonin for cluster headache prevention was then studied in a double-blind, placebo-controlled trial by Leone and collaborators (1996), with a significant decrease in cluster headache attacks in the melatonin-treated group compared with placebo. Twenty patients (2 primary chronic, 18 episodic) received oral melatonin 10 mg ($n = 10$) or placebo ($n = 10$) for 14 days taken in a single evening dose. Five of the 10 treated patients were responders whose attack frequency declined 3–5 days after treatment, and they experienced no further attacks until melatonin was discontinued. No side-effects were observed in either group.

Two patients with chronic cluster headache in Leone and collaborators' (1996) trial did not respond to melatonin therapy, but Peres and Rozen (2001) described 2 chronic cluster headache patients who responded to melatonin 9 mg at bedtime. Melatonin prevented not only nocturnal cluster attacks, but daytime attacks as well. Nagtegaal and collaborators (1998), studying melatonin treatment in delayed-sleep-phase syndrome, identified a patient with episodic cluster headache in whom both disorders improved after melatonin treatment. Melatonin plays an important role in the pathophysiology and treatment of cluster headaches.

Other headache disorders have been linked to melatonin secretion, such as hypnic headaches (Peres et al., 2006), and other trigeminal autonomic cephalalgias. Peres and collaborators (2001b) described a patient with hemicrania continua with seasonal variation, proposing that the chemical structure similarity between melatonin and indomethacin, could be one of the possible mechanisms of action involved in indomethacin-responsive headaches. Rozen (2003) reported a patient with hemicrania continua who responded to melatonin 9 mg, and described 3 idiopathic stabbing headache patients treated with melatonin with excellent clinical response and side-effect profile. A recent study showed hypothalamic activation in paroxysmal hemicranias, a similar mechanism found in cluster headache, which could make the paroxysmal hemicranias potential candidates for melatonin treatment.

FINAL CONSIDERATIONS

We have reviewed the current understanding of how hormones, neurohormones, and neurotransmitters participate in the pain modulation of primary headaches. Stressful conditions and hormones are intimately implicated in the headache neurobiology. With the recent progress in neuroimaging techniques and the development of animal models to study headache mechanisms, the physiopathology of several of the primary headaches is starting to become more evident. Various clinical characteristics of the primary headaches, such as pain, autonomic disturbances, and behavioral changes, are linked to hypothalamic activation and hormonal influence. In summary, primary headaches are under a strong influence of physiological hormonal fluctuation, when nociceptive and non-nociceptive pathways are differentially activated to modulate the perception of pain.

References

Agis-Balboa RC, Pinna G, Zhubi A et al. (2006). Characterization of brain neurons that express enzymes mediating neurosteroid biosynthesis. Proc Natl Acad Sci U S A 103: 14602–14607.

Allen LS, Gorski RA (1990). Sex difference in the bed nucleus of the stria terminalis of the human brain. J Comp Neurol 302: 697–706.

Allen LS, Hines M, Shryne JE et al. (1989). Two sexually dimorphic cell groups in the human brain. J Neurosci 9: 497–506.

Alreja M, Mutalik P, Nayar U et al. (1984). The formalin test: a tonic pain model in the primate. Pain 20: 97–105.

Ambrosini A, Schoenen J (2006). Electrophysiological response patterns of primary sensory cortices in migraine. J Headache Pain 7: 377–388.

Amit Z, Galina ZH (1986). Stress-induced analgesia: adaptive pain suppression. Physiol Rev 66: 1091–1120.

Annat G, Guell A, Gauquelin G et al. (1986). Plasma vasopressin, neurophysin, renin and aldosterone during a 4-day head-down bed rest with and without exercise. Eur J Appl Physiol Occup Physiol 55: 59–63.

Anthony M (1968). Plasma serotonin levels in migraine. Adv Pharmacol 6: 203.

Antunes-Rodrigues J, de Castro M, Elias LL et al. (2004). Neuroendocrine control of body fluid metabolism. Physiol Rev 84: 169–208.

Askmark H, Lundberg PO (1989). Lactation headache – a new form of headache? Cephalalgia 9: 119–122.

Askmark H, Lundberg PO, Olsson S (1989). Drug-related headache. Headache 29: 441–444.

Aygun D, Bildik F (2003). Clinical warning criteria in evaluation by computed tomography the secondary neurological headaches in adults. Eur J Neurol 10: 437–442.

Bahra A, Matharu MS, Buchel C et al. (2001). Brainstem activation specific to migraine headache. Lancet 357: 1016–1017.

Banks WA (2001). Enhanced leptin transport across the blood–brain barrier by alpha 1-adrenergic agents. Brain Res 899: 209–217.

Bardwell A, Trott JA (1987). Stroke in migraine as a consequence of propranolol. Headache 27: 381–383.

Bartolini M, Baruffaldi R, Paolino I et al. (2005). Cerebral blood flow changes in the different phases of migraine. Funct Neurol 20: 209–211.

Baumbach GL, Heistad DD (1983). Effects of sympathetic stimulation and changes in arterial pressure on segmental resistance of cerebral vessels in rabbits and cats. Circ Res 52: 527–533.

Benjamin L, Levy MJ, Lasalandra MP et al. (2004). Hypothalamic activation after stimulation of the superior sagittal sinus in the cat: a Fos study. Neurobiol Dis 16: 500–505.

Berkowitz BA, Sherman S (1982). Characterization of vasopressin analgesia. J Pharmacol Exp Ther 220: 329–334.

Bettahi I, Pozo D, Osuna C et al. (1996). Melatonin reduces nitric oxide synthase activity in rat hypothalamus. J Pineal Res 20: 205–210.

Bigal ME, Lipton RB (2006a). Modifiable risk factors for migraine progression. Headache 46: 1334–1343.

Bigal ME, Lipton RB (2006b). Obesity is a risk factor for transformed migraine but not chronic tension-type headache. Neurology 67: 252–257.

Blau J (2004). Harold G Wolff: the man and his migraine. Cephalalgia 24: 215–222.

Blau JN, Engel HO (1999). A new cluster headache precipitant: increased body heat. Lancet 354: 1001–1002.

Blau JN, Solomon F (1985). Smell and other sensory disturbances in migraine. J Neurol 232: 275–276.

Bodnar RJ, Nilaver G, Wallace MM et al. (1984). Pain threshold changes in rats following central injection of beta-endorphin, met-enkephalin, vasopressin or oxytocin antisera. Int J Neurosci 24: 149–160.

Bolay H, Moskowitz MA (2005). The emerging importance of cortical spreading depression in migraine headache. Rev Neurol (Paris) 161: 655–657.

Brown DC, Perkowski S (1998). Oxytocin content of the cerebrospinal fluid of dogs and its relationship to pain induced by spinal cord compression. Vet Surg 27: 607–611.

Brun J, Claustrat B, Saddier P et al. (1995). Nocturnal melatonin excretion is decreased in patients with migraine without aura attacks associated with menses. Cephalalgia 15: 136–139; discussion 179.

Bubenik GA, Blask DE, Brown GM et al. (1998). Prospects of the clinical utilization of melatonin. Biol Signals Recept 7: 195–219.

Buchsbaum MS, Davis GC, Naber D et al. (1983). Pain enhances naloxone-induced hyperalgesia in humans as assessed by somatosensory evoked potentials. Psychopharmacology (Berl) 79: 99–103.

Burstein R, Yamamura H, Malick A et al. (1998). Chemical stimulation of the intracranial dura induces enhanced responses to facial stimulation in brain stem trigeminal neurons. J Neurophysiol 79: 964–982.

Cajochen C, Krauchi K, Wirz-Justice A (2003). Role of melatonin in the regulation of human circadian rhythms and sleep. J Neuroendocrinol 15: 432–437.

Chazot G, Claustrat B, Brun J et al. (1984). A chronobiological study of melatonin, cortisol growth hormone and prolactin secretion in cluster headache. Cephalalgia 4: 213–220.

Checkley SA, Murphy DG, Abbas M et al. (1993). Melatonin rhythms in seasonal affective disorder. Br J Psychiatry 163: 332–337.

Ching M, Valenca M, Negro-Vilar A (1988). Acute ethanol treatment lowers hypophyseal portal plasma luteinizing hormone-releasing hormone (LH-RH) and systemic plasma LH levels in orchidectomized rats. Brain Res 443: 325–328.

Claustrat B, Loisy C, Brun J et al. (1989). Nocturnal plasma melatonin levels in migraine: a preliminary report. Headache 29: 242–245.

Claustrat B, Brun J, Geoffriau M et al. (1997). Nocturnal plasma melatonin profile and melatonin kinetics during infusion in status migrainosus. Cephalalgia 17: 511–517; discussion 487.

Cooke B, Hegstrom CD, Villeneuve LS et al. (1998). Sexual differentiation of the vertebrate brain: principles and mechanisms. Front Neuroendocrinol 19: 323–362.

Cortelli P, Pierangeli G (2007). Hypothalamus and headaches. Neurol Sci 28 (Suppl. 2): S198–S202.

Cortelli P, Grimaldi D, Guaraldi P et al. (2004). Headache and hypertension. Neurol Sci 25 (Suppl. 3): S132–S134.

Costa-Cruz RR, Amancio-dos-Santos A, Guedes RC (2006). Characterization of cortical spreading depression in adult well-nourished and malnourished rats submitted to the association of pilocarpine-induced epilepsy plus streptozotocin-induced hyperglycemia. Neurosci Lett 401: 271–275.

Crowley WR, Rodriguez-Sierra JF, Komisaruk BR (1977). Analgesia induced by vaginal stimulation in rats is apparently independent of a morphine-sensitive process. Psychopharmacology (Berl) 54: 223–225.

Cutrer FM, Moskowitz MA (1996). Wolff Award 1996. The actions of valproate and neurosteroids in a model of trigeminal pain. Headache 36: 579–585.

Davis EC, Popper P, Gorski RA (1996). The role of apoptosis in sexual differentiation of the rat sexually dimorphic nucleus of the preoptic area. Brain Res 734: 10–18.

Diener HC, May A (1996). New aspects of migraine pathophysiology: lessons learned from positron emission tomography. Curr Opin Neurol 9: 199–201.

Dimitriadou V, Aubineau P, Taxi J et al. (1987). Ultrastructural evidence for a functional unit between nerve fibers and type II cerebral mast cells in the cerebral vascular wall. Neuroscience 22: 621–630.

Dodick D, Silberstein S (2006). Central sensitization theory of migraine: clinical implications. Headache 46 (Suppl. 4): S182–S191.

Eadie MJ (2005). The pathogenesis of migraine – 17th to early 20th century understandings. J Clin Neurosci 12: 383–388.

Ebadi M, Govitrapong P, Phansuwan-Pujito P et al. (1998). Pineal opioid receptors and analgesic action of melatonin. J Pineal Res 24: 193–200.

Ebersberger A, Ringkamp M, Reeh PW et al. (1997). Recordings from brain stem neurons responding to chemical stimulation of the subarachnoid space. J Neurophysiol 77: 3122–3133.

Edvinsson L (2006). Neuronal signal substances as biomarkers of migraine. Headache 46: 1088–1094.

Eggers AE (2001). New neural theory of migraine. Med Hypotheses 56: 360–363.

Eggers AE (2007). Redrawing Papez' circuit: a theory about how acute stress becomes chronic and causes disease. Med Hypotheses 69: 852–857.

Esler M, Jennings G, Lambert G et al. (1990). Overflow of catecholamine neurotransmitters to the circulation: source, fate, and functions. Physiol Rev 70: 963–985.

Farias da Silva W, Sampaio M, Costa Neto J et al. (2005). Migrânea. Sociedade Brasileira de Cefaléia, Rio de Janeiro.

Friedman AP (1972). The headache in history, literature, and legend. Bull N Y Acad Med 48: 661–681.

Gallai V, Sarchielli P, Firenze C et al. (1994). Endothelin 1 in migraine and tension-type headache. Acta Neurol Scand 89: 47–55.

Garcia JJ, Reiter RJ, Guerrero JM et al. (1997). Melatonin prevents changes in microsomal membrane fluidity during induced lipid peroxidation. FEBS Lett 408: 297–300.

Garcia-Segura LM, Chowen JA, Parducz A et al. (1994). Gonadal hormones as promoters of structural synaptic plasticity: cellular mechanisms. Prog Neurobiol 44: 279–307.

Garcia-Segura LM, Naftolin F, Hutchison JB et al. (1999). Role of astroglia in estrogen regulation of synaptic plasticity and brain repair. J Neurobiol 40: 574–584.

Gebhart GF (2004). Descending modulation of pain. Neurosci Biobehav Rev 27: 729–737.

Giffin NJ, Ruggiero L, Lipton RB et al. (2003). Premonitory symptoms in migraine: an electronic diary study. Neurology 60: 935–940.

Goadsby PJ (2007). Recent advances in understanding migraine mechanisms, molecules and therapeutics. Trends Mol Med 13: 39–44.

Goadsby PJ, Duckworth JW (1987). Effect of stimulation of trigeminal ganglion on regional cerebral blood flow in cats. Am J Physiol 253: R270–274.

Goadsby PJ, Zagami AS (1991). Stimulation of the superior sagittal sinus increases metabolic activity and blood flow in certain regions of the brainstem and upper cervical spinal cord of the cat. Brain 114: 1001–1011.

Goldstein JM, Seidman LJ, Horton NJ et al. (2001). Normal sexual dimorphism of the adult human brain assessed by in vivo magnetic resonance imaging. Cereb Cortex 11: 490–497.

Guedes RC (1984). On some conditions that influence cortical spreading depression. An Acad Bras Cienc 56: 445–455.

Guedes RC, Amorim LF, Teodosio NR (1996). Effect of aging on cortical spreading depression. Braz J Med Biol Res 29: 1407–1412.

Guedes RC, Amancio-Dos-Santos A, Manhaes-De-Castro R et al. (2002). Citalopram has an antagonistic action on cortical spreading depression in well-nourished and early-malnourished adult rats. Nutr Neurosci 5: 115–123.

Hagiwara H, Funabashi T, Mitsushima D et al. (2007). Effects of neonatal testosterone treatment on sex differences in formalin-induced nociceptive behavior in rats. Neurosci Lett 412: 264–267.

Handwerker HO, Kobal G (1993). Psychophysiology of experimentally induced pain. Physiol Rev 73: 639–671.

Hasselblatt M, Kohler J, Volles E et al. (1999). Simultaneous monitoring of endothelin-1 and vasopressin plasma levels in migraine. Neuroreport 10: 423–425.

Highley JR, Esiri MM, McDonald B et al. (1999). The size and fibre composition of the corpus callosum with respect to gender and schizophrenia: a post-mortem study. Brain 122: 99–110.

Hoskin KL, Kaube H, Goadsby PJ (1996). Central activation of the trigeminovascular pathway in the cat is inhibited by dihydroergotamine. A c-Fos and electrophysiological study. Brain 119: 249–256.

Hunskaar S, Fasmer OB, Hole K (1985). Formalin test in mice, a useful technique for evaluating mild analgesics. J Neurosci Methods 14: 69–76.

Isler H (1992). The Galenic tradition and migraine. J Hist Neurosci 1: 227–233.

Iwasaki Y, Kinoshita M, Ikeda K et al. (1991). Thyroid function in patients with chronic headache. Int J Neurosci 57: 263–267.

Jansen I, Alafaci C, Uddman R et al. (1990). Evidence that calcitonin gene-related peptide contributes to the capsaicin-induced relaxation of guinea pig cerebral arteries. Regul Pept 31: 167–178.

Jansen I, Alafaci C, McCulloch J et al. (1991). Tachykinins (substance P, neurokinin A, neuropeptide K, and neurokinin B) in the cerebral circulation: vasomotor responses in vitro and in situ. J Cereb Blood Flow Metab 11: 567–575.

Jansen I, Uddman R, Ekman R et al. (1992). Distribution and effects of neuropeptide Y, vasoactive intestinal peptide, substance P, and calcitonin gene-related peptide in human middle meningeal arteries: comparison with cerebral and temporal arteries. Peptides 13: 527–536.

Jezova D, Michajlovskij N, Kvetnansky R et al. (1993). Paraventricular and supraoptic nuclei of the hypothalamus are not equally important for oxytocin release during stress. Neuroendocrinology 57: 776–781.

Kai-Kai MA, Anderton BH, Keen P (1986). A quantitative analysis of the interrelationships between subpopulations of rat sensory neurons containing arginine vasopressin or oxytocin and those containing substance P, fluoride-resistant acid phosphatase or neurofilament protein. Neuroscience 18: 475–486.

Kallela M, Farkkila M, Saijonmaa O et al. (1998). Endothelin in migraine patients. Cephalalgia 18: 329–332.

Kaube H, Keay KA, Hoskin KL et al. (1993). Expression of c-Fos-like immunoreactivity in the caudal medulla and upper cervical spinal cord following stimulation of the superior sagittal sinus in the cat. Brain Res 629: 95–102.

Kelman L (2007). The triggers or precipitants of the acute migraine attack. Cephalalgia 27: 394–402.

Kendrick KM, Keverne EB (1989). Effects of intracerebroventricular infusions of naltrexone and phentolamine on central and peripheral oxytocin release and on maternal behaviour induced by vaginocervical stimulation in the ewe. Brain Res 505: 329–332.

Klein P, Herzog AG (1998). Hormonal effects on epilepsy in women. Epilepsia 39 (Suppl. 8): S9–S16.

Koehler PJ, van de Wiel TW (2001). Aretaeus on migraine and headache. J Hist Neurosci 10: 253–261.

Lagreze HL, Dettmers C, Hartmann A (1988). Abnormalities of interictal cerebral perfusion in classic but not common migraine. Stroke 19: 1108–1111.

Lambert GA, Bogduk N, Goadsby PJ et al. (1984). Decreased carotid arterial resistance in cats in response to trigeminal stimulation. J Neurosurg 61: 307–315.

Lambert GA, Goadsby PJ, Zagami AS et al. (1988). Comparative effects of stimulation of the trigeminal ganglion and the superior sagittal sinus on cerebral blood flow and evoked potentials in the cat. Brain Res 453: 143–149.

Lance JW (1985). The pathophysiology of migraine. Ann Acad Med Singapore 14: 4–11.

Lance JW (1993). Current concepts of migraine pathogenesis. Neurology 43: S11–S15.

Lance JW, Goadsby PJ (1998). Mechanism and Management of Headache. 6th edn. Butterworth-Heinemann, Oxford.

Lang RE, Heil J, Ganten D et al. (1983). Effects of lesions in the paraventricular nucleus of the hypothalamus on vasopressin and oxytocin contents in brainstem and spinal cord of rat. Brain Res 260: 326–329.

Larner AJ (2006). Thyroid dysfunction and headache. J Headache Pain 7: 51–52.

Leone M, Lucini V, D'Amico D et al. (1995). Twenty-four-hour melatonin and cortisol plasma levels in relation to timing of cluster headache. Cephalalgia 15: 224–229.

Leone M, D'Amico D, Moschiano F et al. (1996). Melatonin versus placebo in the prophylaxis of cluster headache: a double-blind pilot study with parallel groups. Cephalalgia 16: 494–496.

Levy MJ, Knight YE, O'Shaughnessy CT et al. (2003). Effect of IL-1beta microinjection into the posterior hypothalamic area on trigeminal nociception in the rat. J Neural Transm 110: 1349–1358.

Lin KC, Huang CC, Wu CC (2007). Association between stress at work and primary headache among nursing staff in Taiwan. Headache 47: 576–584.

Lins Filho R (2000). [Analgesic actions of oxytocin.] In: Physiology, Federal University of Pernambuco, Recife, Brazil, p. 56. MSc thesis.

Loder E (2002). What is the evolutionary advantage of migraine? Cephalalgia 22: 624–632.

Lopez-Jimenez M, Valenca MM, Moreira AC et al. (1989). Ether and immobilization stress effects on pituitary adrenal function in hemidecorticate rats. Braz J Med Biol Res 22: 779–782.

Lundeberg T, Meister B, Bjorkstrand E et al. (1993). Oxytocin modulates the effects of galanin in carrageenan-induced hyperalgesia in rats. Brain Res 608: 181–185.

Lundeberg T, Uvnas-Moberg K, Agren G et al. (1994). Antinociceptive effects of oxytocin in rats and mice. Neurosci Lett 170: 153–157.

Lyngberg AC, Rasmussen BK, Jorgensen T et al. (2005). Incidence of primary headache: a Danish epidemiologic follow-up study. Am J Epidemiol 161: 1066–1073.

Madrazo I, Franco-Bourland RE, Leon-Meza VM et al. (1987). Intraventricular somatostatin-14, arginine vasopressin, and oxytocin: analgesic effect in a patient with intractable cancer pain. Appl Neurophysiol 50: 427–431.

Martin-Araguz A, Bustamante-Martinez C, Emam-Mansour MT et al. (2002). [Neuroscience in ancient Egypt and in the school of Alexandria.] Rev Neurol 34: 1183–1194.

Martin VT, Behbehani M (2006a). Ovarian hormones and migraine headache: understanding mechanisms and pathogenesis – part 2. Headache 46: 365–386.

Martin VT, Behbehani M (2006b). Ovarian hormones and migraine headache: understanding mechanisms and pathogenesis – part I. Headache 46: 3–23.

Matharu MS, Goadsby PJ (2005). Functional brain imaging in hemicrania continua: implications for nosology and pathophysiology. Curr Pain Headache Rep 9: 281–288.

Matharu MS, Cohen AS, McGonigle DJ et al. (2004). Posterior hypothalamic and brainstem activation in hemicrania continua. Headache 44: 747–761.

May A, Bahra A, Buchel C et al. (1998). Hypothalamic activation in cluster headache attacks. Lancet 352: 275–278.

Mendizabal JE, Greiner F, Hamilton WJ et al. (1997). Migrainous stroke causing thalamic infarction and amnesia during treatment with propranolol. Headache 37: 594–596.

Monnet FP (2002). Melatonin modulates [^{3}H]serotonin release in the rat hippocampus: effects of circadian rhythm. J Neuroendocrinol 14: 194–199.

Montagna P (2006). Hypothalamus, sleep and headaches. Neurol Sci 27 (Suppl. 2): S138–S143.

Moreau T, Manceau E, Giroud-Baleydier F et al. (1998). Headache in hypothyroidism. Prevalence and outcome under thyroid hormone therapy. Cephalalgia 18: 687–689.

Moskowitz MA (1984). The neurobiology of vascular head pain. Ann Neurol 16: 157–168.

Moskowitz MA (1990). Basic mechanisms in vascular headache. Neurol Clin 8: 801–815.

Moskowitz MA (1991). The visceral organ brain: implications for the pathophysiology of vascular head pain. Neurology 41: 182–186.

Moskowitz MA, Wei EP, Saito K et al. (1988). Trigeminalectomy modifies pial arteriolar responses to hypertension or norepinephrine. Am J Physiol 255: H1–H6.

Mostallino MC, Mura ML, Maciocco E et al. (2006). Changes in expression of the delta subunit of the GABA (A) receptor and in receptor function induced by progesterone exposure and withdrawal. J Neurochem 99: 321–332.

Mukai H, Takata N, Ishii HT et al. (2006). Hippocampal synthesis of estrogens and androgens which are paracrine modulators of synaptic plasticity: synaptocrinology. Neuroscience 138: 757–764.

Murialdo G, Fonzi S, Costelli P et al. (1994). Urinary melatonin excretion throughout the ovarian cycle in menstrually related migraine. Cephalalgia 14: 205–209.

Naftolin F, Garcia-Segura LM, Keefe D et al. (1990). Estrogen effects on the synaptology and neural membranes of the rat hypothalamic arcuate nucleus. Biol Reprod 42: 21–28.

Nagtegaal JE, Smits MG, Swart AC et al. (1998). Melatonin-responsive headache in delayed sleep phase syndrome: preliminary observations. Headache 38: 303–307.

Negro-Vilar A, Valença MM (1988). Male neuroendocrinology and endocrine evaluation of reproductive disorders. In: JC Lamb 4th, PM Foster (Eds.), Physiology and Toxicology of Male Reproduction. Academic Press, Orlando, pp. 103–136.

Negro-Vilar A, Johnston C, Spinedi E et al. (1987). Physiological role of peptides and amines on the regulation of ACTH secretion. Ann N Y Acad Sci 512: 218–236.

Olesen J (1982). Is ischemia involved in the pathogenesis of migraine? Pathol Biol (Paris) 30: 318–324.

Olesen J, Iversen HK, Thomsen LL (1993). Nitric oxide supersensitivity: a possible molecular mechanism of migraine pain. Neuroreport 4: 1027–1030.

Olsen TS, Friberg L, Lassen NA (1990). [Migraine aura – vascular or neuronal disease?] Ugeskr Laeger 152: 1507–1509.

Pani L, Porcella A, Gessa GL (2000). The role of stress in the pathophysiology of the dopaminergic system. Mol Psychiatry 5: 14–21.

Peres MF (2005). Melatonin, the pineal gland and their implications for headache disorders. Cephalalgia 25: 403–411.

Peres MF, Rozen TD (2001). Melatonin in the preventive treatment of chronic cluster headache. Cephalalgia 21: 993–995.

Peres MF, Seabra ML, Zukerman E et al. (2000). Cluster headache and melatonin. Lancet 355: 147.

Peres MF, Sanchez del Rio M, Seabra ML et al. (2001a). Hypothalamic involvement in chronic migraine. J Neurol Neurosurg Psychiatry 71: 747–751.

Peres MF, Stiles MA, Oshinsky M et al. (2001b). Remitting form of hemicrania continua with seasonal pattern. Headache 41: 592–594.

Peres M, Zukerman E, da Cunha TF et al. (2004). Melatonin, 3 mg, is effective for migraine prevention. Neurology 63: 757.

Peres MF, Masruha MR, Zukerman E et al. (2006). Potential therapeutic use of melatonin in migraine and other headache disorders. Exp Opin Invest Drugs 15: 367–375.

Peroutka SJ (1997). Dopamine and migraine. Neurology 49: 650–656.

Phillips WJ, Ostrovsky O, Galli RL et al. (2006). Relief of acute migraine headache with intravenous oxytocin: report of two cases. J Pain Palliat Care Pharmacother 20: 25–28.

Pietrobon D (2005). Migraine: new molecular mechanisms. Neuroscientist 11: 373–386.

Price DD, Von der Gruen A, Miller J et al. (1985). A psychophysical analysis of morphine analgesia. Pain 22: 261–269.

Prodan CI, Holland NR, Lenaerts ME et al. (2002). Magnetic resonance angiogram evidence of vasospasm in familial hemiplegic migraine. J Child Neurol 17: 470–472.

Rabe A, Fromter E (2000). Micromolar concentrations of steroids and of aldosterone antagonists inhibit the outwardly rectifying chloride channel with different kinetics. Pflugers Arch 439: 559–566.

Raffaelli EJr, Menon AD (1975). Migraine and the limbic system. Headache 15: 69–78.

Ramadan NM (2003). The link between glutamate and migraine. CNS Spectr 8: 446–449.

Raskin NH, Hosobuchi Y, Lamb S (1987). Headache may arise from perturbation of brain. Headache 27: 416–420.

Ray B, Wolff HG (1940). Experimental studies on migraine: pain sensitive structures of the head and their significance in headache. Arch Surg 41: 813–885.

Reiter RJ, Calvo JR, Karbownik M et al. (2000). Melatonin and its relation to the immune system and inflammation. Ann N Y Acad Sci 917: 376–386.

Rhodes ME, Rubin RT (1999). Functional sex differences ('sexual diergism') of central nervous system cholinergic systems, vasopressin, and hypothalamic–pituitary–adrenal axis activity in mammals: a selective review. Brain Res Brain Res Rev 30: 135–152.

Richard P, Moos F, Freund-Mercier MJ (1991). Central effects of oxytocin. Physiol Rev 71: 331–370.

Rodenbeck A, Huether G, Ruther E et al. (1999). Nocturnal melatonin secretion and its modification by treatment in patients with sleep disorders. Adv Exp Med Biol 467: 89–93.

Rose FC (1995). The history of migraine from Mesopotamian to Medieval times. Cephalalgia 15 (Suppl. 15): 1–3.

Rozen TD (2003). Melatonin as treatment for idiopathic stabbing headache. Neurology 61: 865–866.

Rydzewski W (1976). Serotonin (5HT) in migraine: levels in whole blood in and between attacks. Headache 16: 16–19.

Saito K, Liu-Chen LY, Moskowitz MA (1987). Substance P-like immunoreactivity in rat forebrain leptomeninges and cerebral vessels originates from the trigeminal but not sympathetic ganglia. Brain Res 403: 66–71.

Sakai F, Meyer JS (1979). Abnormal cerebrovascular reactivity in patients with migraine and cluster headache. Headache 19: 257–266.

Schmetterer L, Wolzt M, Graselli U et al. (1997). Nitric oxide synthase inhibition in the histamine headache model. Cephalalgia 17: 175–182.

Schwartz-Giblin S, Korotzer A, Pfaff DW (1989). Steroid hormone effects on picrotoxin-induced seizures in female and male rats. Brain Res 476: 240–247.

Selye H (1973). The evolution of the stress concept. Am Sci 61: 692–699.

Shaikh AY, Xu J, Wu Y et al. (1997). Melatonin protects bovine cerebral endothelial cells from hyperoxia-induced DNA damage and death. Neurosci Lett 229: 193–197.

Silberstein SD (1993). Headaches and women: treatment of the pregnant and lactating migraineur. Headache 33: 533–540.

Silberstein SD, Lipton RB, Goadsby PJ (1998). Headache in Clinical Practice. ISIS Medical Media, Oxford.

Sliwka U, Harscher S, Diehl RR et al. (2001). Spontaneous oscillations in cerebral blood flow velocity give evidence of different autonomic dysfunctions in various types of headache. Headache 41: 157–163.

Smith MJ, Adams LF, Schmidt PJ et al. (2002). Effects of ovarian hormones on human cortical excitability. Ann Neurol 51: 599–603.

Solomon GD (1992). Circadian rhythms and migraine. Cleve Clin J Med 59: 326–329.

Spencer CM, Gunasekara NS, Hills C (1999). Zolmitriptan: a review of its use in migraine. Drugs 58: 347–374.

Spierings EL (2004). The aura-headache connection in migraine: a historical analysis. Arch Neurol 61: 794–799.

Stocche RM, Klamt JG, Antunes-Rodrigues J et al. (2001). Effects of intrathecal sufentanil on plasma oxytocin and cortisol concentrations in women during the first stage of labor. Reg Anesth Pain Med 26: 545–550.

Strebel PM, Zacur HA, Gold EB (1986). Headache, hyperprolactinemia, and prolactinomas. Obstet Gynecol 68: 195–199.

Strong AJ, Fabricius M, Boutelle MG et al. (2002). Spreading and synchronous depressions of cortical activity in acutely injured human brain. Stroke 33: 2738–2743.

Suzuki N, Hardebo JE, Owman C (1989). Origins and pathways of cerebrovascular nerves storing substance P and calcitonin gene-related peptide in rat. Neuroscience 31: 427–438.

Suzuki N, Hardebo JE, Kahrstrom J et al. (1990). Selective electrical stimulation of postganglionic cerebrovascular parasympathetic nerve fibers originating from the sphenopalatine ganglion enhances cortical blood flow in the rat. J Cereb Blood Flow Metab 10: 383–391.

Suzuki N, Shimizu T, Takao M et al. (2002). Neurokinin-1 receptors in the cerebrovascular vasoactive intestinal polypeptide-containing nerves in the rat. Auton Neurosci 95: 103–111.

Swica Y (2007). The transdermal patch and the vaginal ring: two novel methods of combined hormonal contraception. Obstet Gynecol Clin North Am 34: 31–42, viii.

Tamaki K, Heistad DD (1986). Response of cerebral arteries to sympathetic stimulation during acute hypertension. Hypertension 8: 911–917.

Taylor BK, Basbaum AI (2003). Systemic morphine-induced release of serotonin in the rostroventral medulla is not mimicked by morphine microinjection into the periaqueductal gray. J Neurochem 86: 1129–1141.

Thomas TD, Harpold GJ, Troost BT (1990). Cerebrovascular reactivity in migraineurs as measured by transcranial Doppler. Cephalalgia 10: 95–99.

Thompson D, Lettich L, Takeshita J (2003). Fibromyalgia: an overview. Curr Psychiatry Rep 5: 211–217.

Thomsen LL, Iversen HK, Brinck TA et al. (1993). Arterial supersensitivity to nitric oxide (nitroglycerin) in migraine sufferers. Cephalalgia 13: 395–399; discussion 376.

Thorley V (1997). Lactational headache: a lactation consultant's diary. J Hum Lact 13: 51–53.

Totaro R, Marini C, De Matteis G et al. (1997). Cerebrovascular reactivity in migraine during headache-free intervals. Cephalalgia 17: 191–194.

Turek FW, Dugovic C, Zee PC (2001). Current understanding of the circadian clock and the clinical implications for neurological disorders. Arch Neurol 58: 1781–1787.

Tzourio C, El Amrani M, Poirier O et al. (2001). Association between migraine and endothelin type A receptor (ETA -231 A/G) gene polymorphism. Neurology 56: 1273–1277.

Uvnas-Moberg K, Petersson M (2005). [Oxytocin, a mediator of anti-stress, well-being, social interaction, growth and healing.] Z Psychosom Med Psychother 51: 57–80.

Uvnas-Moberg K, Bruzelius G, Alster P et al. (1993a). The antinociceptive effect of non-noxious sensory stimulation is mediated partly through oxytocinergic mechanisms. Acta Physiol Scand 149: 199–204.

Uvnas-Moberg K, Lundeberg T, Bruzelius G et al. (1993b). Low doses of ethanol may induce anti-nociceptive effects via an oxytocinergic mechanism. Acta Physiol Scand 149: 117–118.

Valença MM, Ching M, Masotto C et al. (1987a). How does the gonad affect LHRH secretion? Effects of gonadectomy on LHRH release from median eminence nerve terminals incubated in vitro and on LHRH concentration in hypophyseal portal blood. Adv Exp Med Biol 219: 617–621.

Valença MM, Johnston CA, Ching M et al. (1987b). Evidence for a negative ultrashort loop feedback mechanism operating on the luteinizing hormone-releasing hormone neuronal system. Endocrinology 121: 2256–2259.

Valença MM, Dias MH, Araújo AMB et al. (1999). [Analgesia induced by immobilization and surgical stress: participation of the endogenous opioid system.] An Fac de Med UFPE 44: 97–102.

Valença MM, Valenca LP, Menezes TL (2002). Computed tomography scan of the head in patients with migraine or tension-type headache. Arq Neuropsiquiatr 60: 542–547.

Valença MM, Valenca LPAA, Bordini CA et al. (2003). [Poor control headache.] Migrâneas Cefaléias 6: 117–120.

Valença MM, Ferreira AV, Betti KCM et al. (2005). [A new experimental model of headache in rat: evidence of the activation of the analgesic endogenous system by the headache.] Rev Dor 6: 688–695.

Valença MM, Andrade-Valenca LP, da Silva WF et al. (2007). Hemicrania continua secondary to an ipsilateral brainstem lesion. Headache 47: 438–441.

van Bree JB, de Boer AG, Verhoef JC et al. (1989). Transport of vasopressin fragments across the blood–brain barrier: in vitro studies using monolayer cultures of bovine brain endothelial cells. J Pharmacol Exp Ther 249: 901–905.

Velisek L, Veliskova J, Moshe SL et al. (1998). Prenatal morphine exposure alters ovarian steroid hormonal regulation of seizure susceptibility. Brain Res 796: 247–256.

Wahl M, Schilling L (1993). Regulation of cerebral blood flow – a brief review. Acta Neurochir Suppl 59: 3–10.

Waldenlind E, Gustafsson SA, Ekbom K et al. (1987). Circadian secretion of cortisol and melatonin in cluster headache during active cluster periods and remission. J Neurol Neurosurg Psychiatry 50: 207–213.

Waldenlind E, Ekbom K, Wetterberg L et al. (1994). Lowered circannual urinary melatonin concentrations in episodic cluster headache. Cephalalgia 14: 199–204.

Wei EP, Kontos HA, Christman CW et al. (1985). Superoxide generation and reversal of acetylcholine-induced cerebral arteriolar dilation after acute hypertension. Circ Res 57: 781–787.

Witt DM, Winslow JT, Insel TR (1992). Enhanced social interactions in rats following chronic, centrally infused oxytocin. Pharmacol Biochem Behav 43: 855–861.

Wober C, Brannath W, Schmidt K et al. (2007). Prospective analysis of factors related to migraine attacks: the PAMINA study. Cephalalgia 27: 304–314.

Woolley CS, Weiland NG, McEwen BS et al. (1997). Estradiol increases the sensitivity of hippocampal CA1 pyramidal cells to NMDA receptor-mediated synaptic input: correlation with dendritic spine density. J Neurosci 17: 1848–1859.

Xu XJ, Wiesenfeld-Hallin Z (1994). Is systemically administered oxytocin an analgesic in rats? Pain 57: 193–196.

Yang J (1994). Intrathecal administration of oxytocin induces analgesia in low back pain involving the endogenous opiate peptide system. Spine 19: 867–871.

Zagami AS, Goadsby PJ, Edvinsson L (1990). Stimulation of the superior sagittal sinus in the cat causes release of vasoactive peptides. Neuropeptides 16: 69–75.

Zimmermann M, Seifert V (1998). Endothelin and subarachnoid hemorrhage: an overview. Neurosurgery 43: 863–875; discussion 875–866.

Zisapel N (2001). Melatonin–dopamine interactions: from basic neurochemistry to a clinical setting. Cell Mol Neurobiol 21: 605–616.

Handbook of Clinical Neurology, Vol. 97 (3rd series)
Headache
G. Nappi and M.A. Moskowitz, Editors

Chapter 61

Headache in children

VINCENZO GUIDETTI,[1]* FEDERICA GALLI,[1] AND CRISTIANO TERMINE[2]
[1]*Department of Child and Adolescent Neurology, Psychiatry and Rehabilitation, "Sapienza", University of Rome, Rome, Italy*
[2]*Child Neuropsychiatry Unit, Department of Clinical and Biological Sciences, University of Insubria, Varese, Italy*

INTRODUCTION

Headache (migraine and tension-type) is a frequent symptom in the general population and is a notable problem in clinical practice in childhood and adolescence, as it is in adulthood.

The management of headaches with juvenile onset causes several problems related to the specific features distinguishing headache disorders in children and adolescents. The child is not a "little adult": many age-related factors influence the clinical expression of headache, and age-related factors should be taken into account in the diagnosis and treatment of juvenile headache.

Considering the child or the adolescent as a whole in his or her neurobiological and psychological development is the basis of a correct approach.

MIGRAINE

Epidemiology, clinical characteristics, and comorbid disorders of migraine are related to age. Migraine occurs in 2–5% of preschool children, 10% of school-aged children, and 20–30% of adolescent girls (Abu-Arefeh and Russell, 1994). No sex difference is apparent until age 11. Female preponderance begins at about age 12; during adolescence there is a female-to-male ratio of about 2:1 (Aromaa et al., 1997; Sillanpää and Aro, 2000), and this ratio is sustained in the adult population.

Migraine changes clinical characteristics with age, even if differences exist from case to case.

Gastrointestinal symptoms seem to be a more typical expression of childhood migraine than in adults. Preschool children frequently exhibit episodes involving vomiting and abdominal pain, with crying, irritability, and the need to sleep. Schoolchildren may experience bilateral pain, with nausea, vomiting, photophobia, phonophobia, and mood change; the child usually stops activities and sometimes goes to bed in the dark. Older children and adolescents tend to show unilateral location of pain (Wöber-Bingöl et al., 1995). When young children show a stable unilateral location a diagnostic caution is imperative, because of the high risk of secondary headache (Guidetti et al., 1999). The severity of child headache is usually milder than in adults. Furthermore, migraine attacks in children can be shorter and more frequent than in adults (Mack, 2006).

At this time, we do not have a specific system to classify headache in children, even though age-related clinical characteristics have in part been mentioned by the current system of classification of headache (second edition of the International Classification of Headache Disorders-II (ICHD-II): Headache Classification Subcommittee of the International Headache Society, 2004), mainly for migraine without aura. The first edition of ICHD International Headache Society, 1988) gave evidence of limitations of applicability in childhood migraine and some modifications of diagnostic parameters have been discussed (Silberstein, 1990; Guidetti et al., 1991). The changes outlined in the ICHD-I criteria (Headache Classification Committee of the International Headache Society, 1988) referred to shorter duration, not always unilateral localization, photophobia, and phonophobia not always present. ICHD-II provides footnotes stressing differences from adults: attacks in children may last 1–72 h (for adults the minimum is 4 h); attacks are commonly bilateral in young children and an adult pattern of unilateral pain usually emerges in late adolescence or early adult life; occipital headache in children, whether bilateral or unilateral, is rare and calls for diagnostic caution;

*Correspondence to: Professor Vincenzo Guidetti, Department of Child and Adolescent Neurology, Psychiatry and Rehabilitation, "Sapienza", University of Rome, Via dei Sabelli 108, 00185 Rome, Italy, Tel: 0039-06-44712-255, Fax: 0039-06-4957857, E-mail: vincenzo.guidetti@uniroma1.it

in young children phonophobia and photophobia may be inferred from their behavior. Nevertheless it was demonstrated that the ICHD-II criteria, in spite of the notes introduced to take into account the situation of children and adolescents, are poorly applicable to children under the age of 6 years (Balottin et al., 2005). Therefore, the development of "alternative" criteria, better able to take into account the peculiarities of early-onset headache forms (i.e., duration of less than 1 h for migraine without aura), would – as other authors (Arruda et al., 2004) have also pointed out – seem to be useful and opportune. In the ICHD, the criteria to define pain intensity in children are not specified. Studies have shown that pain intensity, together with aggravation of headache by physical symptoms and vomiting, was the most important feature for distinguishing migraine from tension-type headache (TTH) (Wöber-Bingöl et al., 1996). It is very important to bear in mind that the behavior of children (Rossi et al., 2005) during headaches may give elements to rate the "attack intensity." Children may experience different types of migraine and/or headache.

Migraine can be with or without aura. The former occurs in 10–20% of migraine children. The aura usually precedes headache by less than 30 min and lasts for 5–20 min, and may also be present without headache. The visual aura is the most common form as occurs in adults, even though the symptoms are likely difficult for children to describe, and require insistent questioning. Visual disturbances are the most typical symptoms of aura (around 30–50%) in young migraine patients, but also sensory or motor and speech disorders are well recognized.

Variants of migraine

There are few epidemiological data concerning hemiplegic, basilar, and ophthalmoplegic migraine (OM) in childhood, even if case reports suggest that their onset and frequency are more common in children and adolescents than in adults (Hockaday, 1988). Conspicuous and persisting specific neurological symptoms are associated with usual diagnostic criteria for migraine. Hemiplegic migraine is the first form of migraine to be linked to a genetic cause: a point mutation on chromosome 19 found in roughly 50–60% of families experiencing this clinical symptomatology. Basilar migraine occurs most typically in adolescent and preadolescent females, but onset is at an early age. Ophthamoloplegic migraine is the commonest form in children.

Confusional migraine (Evans and Gladstein, 2003), "Alice in Wonderland syndrome" (Evans and Rolak, 2004; Gencoglu et al., 2005), and transient global amnesia (Rami et al., 1986; Riggs and Bodensteiner, 1995) are other variants of migraine characterized by alteration in consciousness and disordered thought process. These aspects open up the differential diagnosis with epilepsy.

To date, the likely relationship between migraine and epilepsy in children is not clarified, as testified by several studies on this topic (Ludvigsson et al., 2006; Piccinelli et al., 2006; Stevenson and Sharon, 2006; Wirrell and Hamiwka, 2006).

Equivalents or precursors of migraine

ICHD-II (Headache Classification Subcommittee of the International Headache Society, 2004) proposes a new diagnostic category: "childhood periodic syndromes that are commonly precursors of migraine."

A precursor of migraine is essentially migraine without headache: abdominal pain, bilious attacks, cyclical vomiting, motion sickness, benign paroxysmal torticollis of infancy, benign paroxysmal vertigo of childhood, and other periodic syndromes in the past have a high incidence in migraine subjects (Lanzi et al., 1997). Traditionally, these disorders have been considered as equivalents or precursors of migraine in children. The new classification recognizes only cyclical vomiting, abdominal migraine, and benign paroxysmal vertigo as precursors of migraine. Benign paroxysmal torticollis and alternating hemiplegia of infancy have been allocated in the appendix of the ICHD-II, because the evidence of a link, either clinical or epidemiological, with migraine is unclear.

However, prudence is necessary: the possibility that abdominal symptoms relate to metabolic disorders (celiac disease, urea cycle disorder, or mitochondrial cytopathy) or epilepsy should be unconditionally tested.

Prognosis

The prognosis is generally thought to be good in the long term (Bille, 1962a, 1981; Congdon and Forsythe, 1979; Dooley and Bagnell, 1995; Guidetti and Galli, 1998). Several studies have recorded a high tendency to improve (around 50% at 5–10-year follow-up) or remit spontaneously (30–40%), at least for several years. The possibility of unchanging or worsening migraine is about 20%.

For males the outcome is better than for females (Guidetti and Galli, 1998). The reason is unknown.

Modifications in the type of headache have been recorded (Dooley and Bagnell, 1995; Guidetti and Galli, 1998). The changes in different subtypes occur mostly from migraine to tension-type (about 25%), but the converse is also true (about 10%). The prognosis is affected by headache type at onset: migraine has a less optimistic outcome, in comparison to episodic tension-type.

The presence of comorbid psychiatric disorders is a negative prognostic factor for all headache subtypes (Guidetti et al., 1998; Galli et al., 2004).

TENSION-TYPE HEADACHE

In contrast to migraine, TTH has been less investigated in both children and adults and there are very few data on the prevalence, features, and prognosis. TTH is considered less severe and disabling than migraine. This may be one of the reasons for the lack of research on TTH. However, TTH is a frequent problem in adulthood, a lot of young patients show comorbidity with migraine, and some patients with episodic TTH become chronic headache patients. It would be important to know the pathogenesis of TTH, the factors involved in triggering, and the chronic trend of the attacks.

ICHD-II (Headache Classification Subcommittee of the International Headache Society, 2004) does not provide specific criteria (or notes) to classify TTH in children, in contrast to migraine. Episodic TTH and migraine without aura may be difficult to distinguish: the mild intensity of pain and absence of nausea are specific for TTH, even if the absence of vomiting is the most sensitive diagnostic criterion for TTH (Wöber-Bingöl et al., 1995).

In ICHD-II, the same diagnostic criteria are used for the diagnosis of TTH in children, adolescents, and adults. These criteria divide TTH into three subtypes: infrequent episodic, frequent episodic, and chronic, and all three subtypes are divided into associated or not with pericranial tenderness.

From an epidemiological point of view the trend is similar to migraine, with boys and girls suffering from TTH equally until age 11–12 years, but after that age female predominance is substantial. The estimates of the prevalence of episodic TTH range from 10% to 25% (Anttila et al., 2002a; Ayatollahi et al., 2002; Ozge et al., 2003; Kaynak et al., 2004; Laurell et al., 2004; Zwart et al., 2004), and increasing with age.

The pathophysiology of TTH is largely unknown. The genetic role seems to be lower in episodic TTH than in chronic TTH (Ostergaard et al., 1997; Russell et al., 1999) and migraine, stressing the role of environmental factors (Ulrich et al., 2004). However, the meaning of "environmental factors" needs to be clarified. If "environmental" means "not genetic," a wide range of different factors may be not only triggers of headache, but causative (etiological) factors. On this topic, we do not have elements to indicate factors clearly "causing" or predisposing to episodic TTH. The smaller genetic effect in TTH than in migraine suggests that the two disorders are distinct. However, many believe that TTH and migraine represent the same pathophysiological spectrum.

In adults, peripheral pain mechanisms are suggested to be important in episodic TTH, while central pain mechanisms are important in chronic TTH (Jensen, 1999). In children, pericranial muscle tenderness does not seem to be associated with episodic TTH (Anttila et al., 2002). However, the presence of increased pericranial muscle tenderness in children with migraine (Anttila et al., 2002b) suggests different mechanisms.

The role of psychological factors in TTH (e.g., life events, psychiatric disorders) has been demonstrated (see below), but it is not specific for TTH compared to any other headache subtype.

CHRONIC DAILY HEADACHE

The diagnosis of chronic daily headache (CDH) is a function of a quantitative parameter (an almost daily frequency of the crises). We do not have clear qualitative parameters (a certain symptomatological characterization of the crises). ICHD-II is an unquestionable advance in classifying CDH, even though no reference is made to pediatric CDH. However, evidence suggests differences compared to adults, even if findings on the clinical characterization of CDH in children and adolescents are unclear.

The application of Silberstein's model (Silberstein, 1993; Silberstein et al., 1994) in the youngest age group does not give us an exhaustive diagnostic framework, leading to the hypothesis of specific symptomatological expression of CDH in children and adolescents. Applying Silberstein's criteria (Silberstein, 1993), Gladstein and Holden (1996) found that 35% of children and adolescents did not fit into these categories. However, the category that they called "comorbid pattern" (migraine crises in comorbid association with TTH) helped the classification of almost all patients (Gladstein and Holden, 1996).

According to Abu-Arefeh's findings (2001), the ICHD-I criteria for classifying chronic headache seem to apply even to the youngest, with all patients meeting the diagnostic parameters (70.6% with chronic TTH (CTTH) and 30.4% with CTTH and migraine without aura). No data support the hypothesis of a probable transformation of migraine or episodic TTH to CDH, as suggested for adults. Hershey et al. (2001) found that 27% of CDH patients could not be classified according to ICHD-I criteria. They underlined the predominance of migrainous characteristics of CDH in children and highlighted a temporal trend of the crises: frequent, daily intermittent, and daily continuous headache. A recent population-based study confirmed the presence of migrainous features of CDH in adolescents (Wang et al., 2006). Migrainous characteristics of CDH in children have been demonstrated, but hypothesized not to be related to the transformation of migraine over time, which is in contrast to adults (Kappler, 1992; Mathew, 1993). According to another study (Galli et al., 2004), CDH with *de novo* onset prevails in the youngest, even if the clinical and differential characteristics need to be clarified with respect to adults and different stages of patient development.

Chronic paroxysmal hemicrania was first described in 1973 (Neubauer et al., 1997), but very few cases have been reported in children (Sjaastad and Dale, 1976). However, many adult patients report onset in childhood. Clinical features are characterized by cyclical and multiple attacks (range 1–30) of excruciating unilateral pain in the ocular, frontal, and temporal areas, both day and night. Lacrimation, nasal stuffiness, and rhinorrhea, sometimes with ptosis, miosis, and upper-lid edema, accompany headache. Nausea and vomiting are rare.

The clinical features are similar to cluster headache, but chronic paroxysmal hemicrania is totally relived by indomethacin, and is much more frequent among females (80–90% of cases).

SECONDARY HEADACHE

About 15–20% of young patients referred to headache centers with may present secondary headache.

The diagnosis of migraine and TTH is by exclusion of the existence of structural lesions or other causes of headache. In most cases (80–85% in our clinical experience), routine and/or more specific examinations rule out symptomatic headache. In the younger age group, the clinical signs of secondary headache may be related to age differences, in contrast to adults. ICHD classification does not provide for these differential age-related symptoms.

In children, adolescents, and young adults, posttraumatic headache has the same symptoms as spontaneous migraine, whereas in over 90% of adults it resembles TTH (Hockaday, 1988). In the younger age, neurological symptoms typically begin after an interval of minutes to hours, even if the symptom-free period is absent. There is not a direct correlation with the gravity of head trauma, and migraine attacks (with or without aura) can be precipitated by minor or mild head trauma. Typical aura with visual, hemiparetic, stuporous, convulsive, or amnesic symptoms, with headache and vomiting, can be present. When sudden onset of headache is present, a posttraumatic cerebrovascular accident must be considered. A slower progressive deterioration indicates posttraumatic bleeding or malignant edema (Hockaday, 1988).

Brain tumor is the second commonest cause of childhood malignancy, after leukemia: 45% of childhood brain tumors lie in the posterior fossa and headache seems mostly to precede neurological and/or ocular signs (Hockaday, 1988). In children, headaches in the occipital region are less common, and may be symptomatic of an organic cause.

Metabolic disorders (urea cycle disorders, aminoacidopathies, mitochondrial cytopathies) or other neurological disorders can start in children with transient neurological symptoms.

Symptoms requiring closely examination because they are related to secondary headache are the following:

- Headache attacks become more severe, more lengthy, or more frequent.
- The child's personality or behavior is changed.
- There is physical or emotional developmental delay.
- Pain is not assuaged by mild painkilling drugs.
- Headache has acute onset and is associated with neck stiffness, lethargy, and vomiting.
- Headache wakes the child in the night and there is morning headache.
- Headache is caused by cough, sneezing, straining, recumbence, or sleep; there are abnormal signs on examination, and visual or neurological symptoms.

A complex bidirectional relationship between migraine, mostly migraine with aura (MA), and ischemic stroke is known. A cerebral infarction can occur during a MA attack, and MA is a risk factor for ischemic stroke, particularly in young women. Conversely, cerebral ischemia can induce MA. Both ischemic stroke and MA may be consequences of many underlying vascular disorders. Despite the relationship between migraine and stroke, migraine as a primary headache disorder is mostly benign (Bousser and Welch, 2005).

In childhood, headache may also be a clinical manifestation of neurofibromatosis (Di Mario and Langshur, 2000), neurocysticercosis (Morales et al., 2000), cerebrovascular hypoplasia (Bojinova et al., 2000), or hypertensive encephalopathy (Pavlakis et al., 1999).

The diagnosis of headache remains principally clinical, and in most cases standard clinical tests suffice to address the differential diagnosis, also when uncommon symptoms occur together with headache (e.g., visual loss in children) (Bain et al., 2000).

COMORBID FACTORS

The recognition of factors associated with headache crises may contribute to advancing our knowledge on the etiology, diagnosis, and therapy of headaches. The high prevalence of headache makes it difficult to recognize a chance co-occurrence of disorders from a true causal relationship. The comorbidity of headache and other disorders (e.g., allergy, oromandibular or eye disorders) has often been hypothesized and the shift to a causal (or syndromic) explanation is intriguing, but not obvious and unquestionable for any such disorder. For some disorders (e.g., epilepsy, sleep and anxiety disorders), more significant evidence supports a causal association, but we are still far from recognizing the common causes and direction of the association.

Epilepsy

To date, the likely relationship between migraine and epilepsy in children is not clarified, as testified by several studies on this topic (Ludvigsson et al., 2006; Piccinelli et al., 2006; Stevenson and Sharon, 2006; Wirrell and Hamiwka, 2006).

The presence of visual phenomena and electroencephalogram (EEG) abnormalities in migraine and occipital lobe epilepsy, as the comorbidity of the two disorders (Guidetti et al., 1987b), may make the differential diagnosis more difficult.

Visual symptoms are almost always present in occipital lobe epilepsy, but in migraine too. The prevalence of visual disturbances in young migraine patients is around 32–56% (Guidetti et al., 1987b), even though several elements markedly distinguish visual seizures from the visual aura of migraine. A study (Brinciotti et al., 2000) on electrical and clinical factors distinguishing epilepsy and migraine with occipital EEG abnormalities showed that a family history of epilepsy, visual symptoms as colored hallucinations and micro/macropsias, unilateral EEG abnormalities, and irregular response to intermittent photic stimulation characterized epilepsy, while a family history of migraine, visual symptoms such as amaurosis and scotomata, bilateral EEG abnormalities, and no changes during intermittent photic stimulation were significantly related to migraine.

Sleep

Clinical observations supported by experimental data suggest that sleep and headache share common anatomical, physiological, and biochemical substrates. Sleep is a precipitating factor for either nocturnal headache (awakening during a usual sleep period with a headache) or as morning arousal with headache (headache present at arousal at the end of a behaviorally defined sleep period).

Headache may cause various degrees of sleep disruption and seems to be associated with several sleep disturbances in either adults or children. Headaches are known to occur during sleep, after sleep, and in relation to various sleep stages. An excess or lack of sleep or a bad quality or inadequate duration of sleep could cause headache. Many chronic headache patients, whatever the type of headache or migraine, may complain of insufficient sleep, lack of restoration in the morning, and severe snoring (Sahota and Dexter, 1990). Different studies proposed a model of interaction between headache and sleep (Paiva et al., 1995). Clinically based studies demonstrated that sleep was efficacious to relieve the head pain or even to terminate the attacks in headache sufferers (Wilkinson et al., 1978; Blau, 1982). However, the power of sleep in terminating the attack is counterbalanced by the ability to precipitate the attack. Although sleep was more commonly referred to as a relieving factor for migraine (70%), migraine attack was also precipitated by sleep deprivation in 24% and by sleep excess in 6% of cases (Inamorato et al., 1993). Indirect evidence for the role of sleep disorders in headache has been given by the improvement of migraine frequency and duration after the application of sleep hygiene guidelines (Bruni et al., 1999).

A study (Bruni et al., 2004) evaluated the sleep–wake cycle in migraine children using the actigraph that allows an activity-based assessment of the sleep–wake cycle. Overall reduced activity was found during the night following the migraine attack. These results supported the hypothesis of a dopaminergic imbalance in migraine children (Dexter, 1986).

From another viewpoint, sleep disorders may be an index of comorbid psychiatric disorders (e.g., shared symptom with anxiety, mood adjustment, or posttraumatic stress disorder). This opens the possibility of a correct approach to comorbid sleep disorders in headache sufferers, stressing the role of a systematic psychological assessment.

HEADACHE AND PSYCHOLOGICAL FACTORS

ICHD-II advances an innovative categorization for headache related to psychological factors. For the first time, there is a recognition of a "direction" ("headache attributed to psychiatric disorders") in this relationship in the main body of the ICHD-II, even though it is related only to somatization and psychotic disorders. If the ICHD-I advanced the role of psychosocial factors only for TTH, the ICHD-II has removed any reference to headache characteristics. Studies on child and adolescent headache suggest no differences between headache subtypes and psychological factors (Guidetti et al., 1998; Karwautz et al., 1999), and more recently between headache and recurrent abdominal pain (Galli et al., 2007). This to say that the role of psychological factors seems related more to the frequency and severity of headaches than to the subtype of headache.

The first studies outlined the relationship between childhood psychological factors and migraine. Vahlquist (1962) recorded neurovegetative instability, ambition and perfectionism, and anxiety among migrainous children. Bille (1962b) described migrainous children as more anxious, sensitive, deliberate, cautious, fearful, vulnerable to frustration, tidy, and less physically enduring than control group children. Among females the differences were stronger. Coch and Melchior (1969) found signs of nervousness, mental instability, and immaturity in migraineurs and non-migraineurs. They suggested "a decreased resistance to psychological stress and conflict situations, rather than overt psychological disorder, or endogenous disease." Maratos and Wilkinson (1982) found higher rates of anxiety and depression associated with conflicting parental relationship. They suggested a disturbed physiological constitution and emotional upset as triggering factors. Guidetti et al. (1986) found feeling of being excluded from the family group, and repressed hostility toward important figures. These findings continue to be of interest, even if they are also relevant for non-migraine headache.

The term "psychiatric comorbidity" has been used to indicate the possible, but unexplained and not casual, relationship between migraine and psychiatric disorders. Population-based studies in young adult samples (Breslau et al., 1991; Merikangas et al., 1993; Merikangas, 1994) have supported the relationship between migraine and specific psychiatric disorders (major depression, anxiety disorder, panic disorder), without significant difference for tension-type compared to headache-free controls. However, further studies demonstrated that the presence of psychiatric disorders is more related to severe and frequent headache (Breslau et al., 2000) than to migraine. The higher prevalence of comorbid psychiatric disorders in CDH than other headache subtypes in both children/adolescents and adults further supports this finding. The burden of childhood adversities on CDH does not differ between chronic migraine and chronic TTH (Juang et al., 2004; population study).

It has been outlined that chronic illness in general explains variations in psychological functioning between chronically ill and healthy children, and not a specific disorder (Cunningham et al., 1987). This is to stress that psychiatric disorders are not specifically related to migraine, but probably to migraine as a kind of disabling and recurrent pain. From a psychological point of view, another aspect to take into consideration is the presence of many subclinical conditions, patients without clear psychopathology, but with psychological distress following life events (e.g., parental divorce) or personality characteristics (e.g., tendency to perfectionism) – all aspects that may contribute to trigger headache. The diagnostic work with headache in children and adolescents should always include a psychological assessment for a complete framing of the clinical situation.

This brief overview shows the consistency of psychological disorders associated with headache, but the nature (genetic, biological, or environmental predisposition? environmental/physical or psychological/emotional stressors?), direction (headache as cause of psychological disorders or vice versa?) and reciprocal correlation of these factors remain unclear. The explanation may have a clarifying role in etiology and pathophysiology, and consequences on treatment of headache.

Distinguishing between biological predisposition (basic vulnerability) and triggering factors (precipitants), and determining the role and the different meaning of personality traits, specific psychological factors (including attentional and cognitive elements, role of stress, and emotional disposition), and psychiatric comorbidity should avoid a confounding overlap among these different elements.

HEADACHE TREATMENT

Taking a careful history in a patient presenting with headache is the prerequisite for further diagnostic and therapeutic management. The family history, the patient's previous history, and the psychosocial, environmental and emotional context (e.g., family, housing conditions, school, leisure activities, and peer relationships) should be explored (Balottin et al., 1989; Wöber and Wöber-Bingöl, 2000; Guidetti and Galli, 2002).

In young children, accurate diagnosis, assessment of the severity of symptoms, and recognition of associated symptoms can be inferred from their behavior. It is essential to ask for factors precipitating, exacerbating, or alleviating the headache. According to a study by Lewis et al. (1996), psychological stress, bright lights, noise, and missed meals are the most important trigger factors in children with idiopathic headache. The child and the parents should be informed of the nature of the migraine and advised to maintain a sound rhythm in daily life, which includes regular meals, sufficient physical exercise, and sleep (Hamalainen, 1998, 2002; Wöber et al., 1998).

The treatment of migraine and TTH overlap. Both require acute and prophylactic treatment. An appropriate treatment requires an individually tailored strategy giving due consideration to both non-pharmacological and pharmacological measures in the context of the degree of disability produced by the headache and/or by the possible comorbidities (e.g., psychiatric).

Considering that few randomized placebo-controlled clinical trials have been conducted in pediatric headache patients for both acute and preventive drugs (see the next paragraph), in clinical practice it is not practicable to rely exclusively on the findings of pharmacological controlled trials, but it is necessary to include further treatment options (Wöber and Wöber-Bingöl, 2000). In a systematic review, Damen et al. (2005) selected controlled trials reporting the effects of non-pharmacological prophylactic treatments in children with migraine. The analysis of the results showed that relaxation, relaxation + biofeedback, and relaxation + biofeedback + cognitive-behavioral treatment were more effective compared with waiting-list controls. The authors concluded that a few non-pharmacological treatments such as relaxation may be effective as prophylactic treatment for migraine in children. Nevertheless, they also suggested that, because of the small number of studies and the methodological shortcomings, conclusions on effectiveness have to be drawn with caution.

Starting from the consideration that children and adolescents with headache show greater indices of psychopathology (Bille, 1962; Maratos and Wilkinson, 1982; Larsson, 1988; Kowal and Pritchard, 1990; Guidetti et al., 1998) and show higher risk of developing psychological disorders in adulthood than healthy controls (Fearon and Hotopf, 2001), different psychotherapeutic approaches are sometimes provided in clinical practice. Relaxation and cognitive-behavioral techniques have been found to reduce the intensity and frequency of headache in children and adolescents (Kazdin, 2002; Eccleston et al., 2003).

Similar conclusions are still lacking in relation to psychodynamic psychotherapy. We think that rigorous studies, conducted in accordance with the principles of evidence-based medicine, should also be performed in this field because, as Fonagy (2003) pointed out, sometimes the lack of evidence could be confused with evidence of lack of efficacy of a treatment.

The parents of headache children often do not consult their physician, but have recourse directly to alternative therapies (e.g., acupuncture, chiropractic manipulation, homeopathy, phytotherapy) which are frequently more economical, seem safer, and whose practitioners often adopt a holistic approach to the care of the patient (Mauskop, 2001). On the basis of a review of the literature on this topic (Termine et al., 2005), we can affirm that scientific proof of their effectiveness is often lacking or obtained in too small studies.

Pharmacological treatment

Few randomized placebo-controlled clinical trials have been conducted in pediatric headache patients for both acute and preventive drugs. Moreover, the few published studies show a high placebo response rate in children (e.g., up to 55% for prophylactic drugs, up to 69% for symptomatic ones) (Table 61.1). The placebo effect is a psychobiological phenomenon that can be attributed to different mechanisms (Benedetti et al., 2005); it should be properly used by the physician, simply bearing in mind that any medical treatment is surrounded by a psychosocial context that affects the therapeutic outcome.

The pharmacological treatment of headache consists of symptomatic and/or prophylactic therapy. The former is aimed at relieving or ameliorating the symptoms of an acute attack, whereas prophylactic therapy, which requires the daily intake of medication for a certain period of time, decreases the frequency of the attacks and the severity of pain.

Acute drug treatment

The risk of medication overuse and the possibility of early self-treatment without parents' control should be kept in mind, thus the frequency of symptomatic drug intake needs to be checked frequently. Although childhood TTH is generally treated with medication, few studies have been published on the efficacy of medication in pediatric TTH. For acute treatment of episodic TTH, acetaminophen and aspirin are effective and inexpensive drugs for those aged 16–65 years (Steiner et al., 2003). Together with aspirin and acetaminophen, non-steroidal anti-inflammatory drugs (NSAIDs) are effective first-line therapy for episodic TTH in adults. In children younger than 15 years, aspirin is not recommended because of the concern of Reye's syndrome. However, acetaminophen is safe even in young children. More studies in children need to be done regarding the treatment of TTH (Anttila, 2006).

At the moment more studies have been conducted regarding the acute treatment of migraine. The available efficacy data about the main drugs are summarized in Table 61.1 and discussed below.

Acetaminophen, ibuprofen, and dihydroergotamine

The comparison of acetaminophen (15 mg/kg) and ibuprofen (10 mg/kg) in a double-blind, placebo-controlled study (Hamalainen et al., 1997a) showed that both drugs were well tolerated and effective in relieving migraine attacks. A more recent study (Lewis et al., 2002) showed that a lower ibuprofen dosage (7.5 mg/kg) is more effective than placebo in reducing headache severity at 2 h. Evers et al. (2006) conducted a trial to investigate the efficacy of oral zolmitriptan and ibuprofen in the treatment of migraine in children and

Table 61.1

Main clinical trials evaluating drugs for migraine treatment

Drugs	Doses	Ages (years)	n	% of responders and/or P-values (*)			Study design	References
Symptomatic drugs								
Ibuprofen	10 mg/kg	4–16	88	68%	37%	<0.05	RCT	Hamalainen et al., 1997a
	7.5 mg/kg	6–12	84	76%	53%	0.006	RCT	Lewis et al., 2002
	200–400 mg	6–18	32	69%	28%	<0.05	RCT	Evers et al., 2006
Acetaminophen	15 mg/kg	4–16	88	54%	37%	<0.05	RCT	Hamalainen et al., 1997a
Dihydroergotamine	20 and 40 μg/kg	5–15	12	58%	16%	NS	RCT	Hamalainen et al., 1997b
Sumatriptan nasal	20 mg	6–10	14	86%	43%	0.03	RCT	Ueberall, 1999
	5–10–20 mg	12–17	510	66%	53%	<0.05	RCT	Winner et al., 2000
	10–20 mg	8–17	83	64%	39%	0.003	RCT	Ahonen et al., 2004
	20 mg	12–17	738	61%	52%	NS	RCT	Winner et al., 2006
Sumatriptan oral	50–100 mg	8–16	23	30%	22%	NS	RCT	Hamalainen et al., 1997c
Sumatriptan subcutaneous	3–6 mg	6–16	17	64%			OT	MacDonald, 1994
	0.06 mg/kg	6–18	50	78%			OT	Linder, 1996
Rizatriptan oral	5 mg	12–17	196	66%	56%	NS	RCT	Winner et al., 2002
	5 mg	12–17	234	68%	69%	NS	RCT	Visser et al., 2004
	5 mg	12–17	686	77%			OT	Visser et al., 2004
Zolmitriptan oral	2.5–5 mg	12–17	38	88–70%			OT	Linder and Dowson, 2000
	2.5 mg	6–18	32	62%	28%	<0.05	RCT	Evers et al., 2006
Almotriptan oral	6.25–12.5 mg	11–17	15	86%			OT	Charles, 2006
Prophylactic drugs								
Propranolol	60–120 mg	7–16	28	82%	14%		RCT	Ludvigsson, 1974
	80 mg	9–15	39	NS			RCT	Forsythe et al., 1984
	3 mg/kg	6–12	28	NS			RCT	Olness et al., 1987
Clonidine	25–50 μg	≤ 15	57	NS			RCT	Sillanpää, 1977
	0.07–0.1 mg	7–14	43	NS			RCT	Sills et al., 1982
Flunarizine	5 mg	10–13	12	66%			OT	Guidetti et al., 1987a
	5 mg	5–11	63	$P < 0.001$ (HA frequency) $P < 0.01$ (HA duration)			RCT	Sorge et al., 1988

Nimodipine	10–20 mg	7–18	37	NS	RCT	Battistella et al., 1990
Pizotifen	1–1.5 mg	7–14	47	NS	RCT	Gillies et al., 1986
Cyproheptadine	2–8 mg	3–12	30	83%	OT	Lewis et al., 2004
Trazodone	1 mg/kg	7–18	35	NS	RCT	Battistella et al., 1990
Amitriptyline	1 mg/kg	9–15	192	80%	OT	Hershey et al., 2000
	10 mg	3–12	73	89%	OT	Lewis et al., 2004
Divalproex sodium	15–45 mg/kg	7–16	42	76%	OT	Caruso et al., 2000
	500–1000 mg	9–17	10	$P = 0.000$ (HA severity) $P = 0.002$ (HA frequency) $P = 0.001$ (HAduration)	OT	Serdaroglu et al,, 2002
Topiramate	1.4 ± 0.7 mg/kg	8–15	75	$P < 0.001$ (HA frequency)	OT	Hershey et al., 2002
	2–3 mg/kg	6–15	162	NS	RCT	Winner et al., 2006
Levetiracetam	250–1500 mg	3–17	19	$P < 0.0001$ (HA frequency)	OT	Miller, 2004
Gabapentin	15 mg/kg	6–17	18	80%	OT	Belman et al.., 2001
Zomisamide	5.8 mg/kg	10–17	12	66%	OT	Pakalnis and Kring, 2006

NS: non-significant difference (active drug versus placebo); HA: headache; RCT: randomized controlled trial; OT: open trial.
*The percentage is expressed as overall percentage of responders (OT) or active drug versus placebo percentage of responders (RCT); *P*-values are referred to active drug versus placebo comparisons (RCT) or pretreatment versus posttreatment comparison of headache characteristics (OT).

adolescents. The authors found that ibuprofen was more effective than placebo at pain relief after 2 h.

The efficacy and safety of other NSAIDs (e.g., acetylsalicylic acid, diclofenac, naproxen, mefenamic acid) in the treatment of migraine in children and adolescents have still not been assessed. Hamalainen et al. (1997a, b, c) conducted a stepwise series of studies: following the first study (Hamalainen et al., 1997a), the children who did not respond to acetaminophen and ibuprofen were entered into two subsequent studies that assessed the effects of dihydroergotamine (Hamalainen et al., 1997b) or sumatriptan (Hamalainen et al., 1997c). In the children with acetaminophen/ibuprofen-resistant migraine, dihydroergotamine was more effective than placebo, but the difference between the treatments was not statistically significant (Hamalainen et al., 1997b).

Triptans

Sumatriptan has been subjected to several clinical trials. The first studies (MacDonald, 1994; Linder, 1996) were non-controlled trials of subcutaneously administered sumatriptan and showed partial relief from migraine in 64% and 78% of patients respectively. The first randomized placebo-controlled trial was conducted to study the effectiveness of oral sumatriptan in children and adolescents with acetaminophen/ibuprofen-resistant migraine. In that study the response rates were lower than those demonstrated in adult studies and oral sumatriptan was no more effective than placebo (Hamalainen et al., 1997c). More recently four prospective, randomized, placebo-controlled trials (Ueberall, 1999; Winner et al., 2000, 2006; Ahonen et al., 2004) assessed both the efficacy and safety of sumatriptan nasal spray in adolescent migraineurs. Ueberall (1999) found significant headache relief at 2 h in 85.7% of treated patients compared with 42.9% in the placebo group ($P = 0.03$). Winner et al. (2000) compared the effectiveness of 5 mg, 10 mg, and 20 mg sumatriptan nasal spray with placebo in 510 adolescents. The 2-h response rate (reduction in headache severity) was 66% for the 5 mg dose ($P < 0.05$), 63% for the 20 mg dose ($P = 0.059$), and 53% for placebo. Ahonen et al. (2004) evaluated the effectiveness of sumatriptan nasal spray in children and adolescents. The primary endpoint (reduction in headache severity at 2 h) was met in 64% of treated patients and in 39% of the placebo group ($P < 0.003$). The fourth trial was conducted by Winner et al. (2006) to compare the efficacy and tolerability of sumatriptan nasal spray (5 and 20 mg) versus placebo in adolescent subjects. The study was conducted because, in the previous randomized, placebo-controlled study of 510 adolescent subjects (Winner et al., 2000), sumatriptan at 5, 10, and 20 mg doses was well tolerated. However, the primary efficacy analysis for headache relief with 20 mg at 2 h did not demonstrate statistical significance. The more recent trial was a randomized (1:1:1), placebo-controlled, double-blind, parallel-group study. A total of 738 adolescent subjects (mean age 14 years) with ≥6-month history of migraine (with or without aura) self-treated a single attack of moderate or severe migraine. The primary endpoints were headache relief at 1 h and sustained relief from 1 to 24 h. The authors found that sumatriptan 20 mg provided greater and significant headache relief than placebo at 30 min and 2 h postdose, but did not reach statistical significance at 1 h (61% versus 52%; $P = 0.087$) or for sustained headache relief from 1 to 24 h ($P = 0.061$). In general, sumatriptan nasal spray 5 mg percentages were slightly higher than placebo but the differences did not reach statistical sgnificance.

Rizatriptan was studied by means of a randomized, placebo-controlled trial that included 296 adolescents (Winner et al., 2002). No difference was found compared to placebo in pain relief at the 2-h primary endpoint. More recently, two studies were conducted in adolescents to examine the short- and long-term efficacy and tolerability of rizatriptan 5 mg (Visser et al., 2004). In the first single-attack study, patients treated a moderate or severe migraine headache and up to two recurrences with rizatriptan 5-mg tablets ($n = 234$) or placebo ($n = 242$). In the second multiple-attack study, patients treated up to six migraine attacks per month with rizatriptan 5-mg tablets ($n = 273$), rizatriptan 5-mg wafers ($n = 281$), or standard care therapy ($n = 132$). In all studies, the primary efficacy measure was pain relief at 2 h postdose. In the single-attack study, the proportion of patients with pain relief at 2 h was not significantly different between rizatriptan 5 mg and placebo. In the multiple-attack study, pain relief at 2 h was achieved in significantly more attacks treated with rizatriptan 5-mg tablet or with rizatriptan 5-mg wafer than with standard care.

Zolmitriptan was assessed in adolescents in a open-labeled multicenter trial (Linder and Dowson, 2000). Doses of 2.5–5 mg were used to treat 276 migraine attacks, reaching an overall response at 2 h of 88% and 70%, respectively. More recently, Evers et al. (2006) conducted a double-blind, placebo-controlled, crossover study to investigate the efficacy of oral zolmitriptan in the treatment of migraine in children and adolescents. Patients received placebo, zolmitriptan 2.5 mg, and ibuprofen 200–400 mg to treat three consecutive migraine attacks. Pain relief rates after 2 h were 28% for placebo, 62% for zolmitriptan, and 69% for ibuprofen (placebo versus zolmitriptan, $P < 0.05$; placebo versus ibuprofen, $P < 0.05$).

Almotriptan was studied in a small open-label pilot study in patients with a history of migraine with or without aura (Charles, 2006). Of the 15 patients, only 2 demonstrated no efficacy without adverse effects. In the other 13 patients almotriptan was effective.

Prophylactic drug treatment

Prophylactic therapy for headache is to be considered: (1) when headache becomes significantly disabling, thus impeding routine activities (e.g., for migraine, when frequency is $\geq$ 4/month, and/or attack duration is $\geq$ 4 h, and/or pain is moderate to severe); (2) when the symptomatic drugs are not effective; (3) when adverse effects from symptomatic treatment are not tolerable. The aim is to reduce the frequency and duration of the attacks, and the severity of pain, thus allowing the patient to resume routine activities and improve quality of life (Lanzi et al., 1996).

In adults, the tricyclic antidepressant amitriptyline has been the only drug with prophylactic efficacy for chronic TTH (Bendsten et al., 1996; Holroyd et al., 2001). Mirtazapine may also be effective in the prophylactic treatment of chronic TTH in adults (Bendsten and Jensen, 2004). For children with frequent TTH, amitriptyline may be beneficial for prophylaxis, although no placebo-controlled studies have been done (Hershey et al., 2000).

More studies have been conducted to investigate the effectiveness of different drugs for migraine prophylaxis. The available efficacy data about the main drugs are summarized in Table 61.1 and discussed below.

Antihypertensive agents

Propranolol has been studied in three trials, with conflicting results. The first study was a double-blind placebo-controlled two-way crossover trial (Ludvigsson, 1974). Twenty-eight children were given propranolol for 13 weeks, followed by a placebo for 13 weeks. The response rate was higher in children after propranolol compared to placebo (82% and 14% respectively). In a second study that started with a 4-week placebo period, after which the children were randomized into propranolol or placebo groups for 12 weeks, there was no difference between groups in the frequency, severity, or duration of migraine attacks (Forsythe et al., 1984). A third trial compared propranolol with self-hypnosis and found no benefit from propranolol but significant improvement with hypnosis (Olness et al., 1987).

Clonidine was evaluated in two studies. The first study (Sillanpää, 1977) compared clonidine to placebo for 2 months and the response rates were not significantly different between groups. The second study (Sills et al., 1982) had two phases: the pilot open-label phase showed headache improvement in 40% of children, but the following double-blind placebo-controlled phase did not show significant difference from placebo (Sillanpää, 1977).

Calcium channel blockers

Flunarizine was studied in an open-label trial of 12 patients, with 8 of 12 showing a 75–100% reduction in headache frequency (Guidetti et al., 1987a). Subsequently, a double-blind, placebo-controlled, crossover trial of flunarizine has been performed in 70 children (Sorge et al., 1988). After 4 weeks of medication-free baseline observation, 35 children received flunarizine and 35 received placebo over a 12-week period. After a 4-week washout they crossed treatments for another 12 weeks. In both groups flunarizine significantly reduced the frequency ($P < 0.001$) and average duration ($P < 0.01$) of headache attacks compared to the placebo group.

Nimodipine was assessed in a double-blind, placebo-controlled crossover trial in 37 patients aged 7–18 years (Battistella et al., 1990). After a 4-week medication-free run-in period, 19 subjects received a placebo while 18 received nimodipine for 12 weeks. After a 4-week washout period, the groups switched therapy for a further 12 weeks. During the first treatment period, there was no difference between active and placebo. During the second period of treatment, nimodipine proved to have a significantly greater effect than placebo with regard to frequency, whereas the response was similar with the placebo as regards duration of attacks.

Serotonergic drugs

Pizotifen was assessed in children with migraine in a double-blind placebo-controlled crossover study. The children received either pizotifen for 3 months followed by placebo or vice versa. Pizotifen was well tolerated. Thirty-nine children completed the trial and there was no significant difference between active and placebo treatment as regards reduction of headache frequency and duration of attacks (Gillies et al., 1986).

Cyproheptadine was evaluated in the ambit of a retrospective study of prophylactic treatment for children and adolescents (Lewis et al., 2004). Thirty patients were administered cyproheptadine, showing an overall positive response rate of 83%.

Antidepressants

Trazodone has been studied in one placebo-controlled crossover study conducted in 35 patients (Battistella et al., 1990). During the first phase of the study the trazodone-treated group did not show a significant headache reduction compared with placebo. During the second phase trazodone was more effective than placebo. However no confirmatory data are available.

Amitriptyline was administered in 192 children with more than three headaches per month (Hershey et al., 2000). A total of 68.5% had migraine (with and without aura), 84.2% of them reported an overall perception of being better, and over 80% reported a significant reduction in headache frequency and severity but no change in headache duration. In a retrospective study amitriptyline showed a positive response rate of 89% (Lewis et al., 2004).

Anticonvulsants

Divalproex sodium has been evaluated as a prophylactic treatment in 42 children (Caruso et al., 2000). Baseline headache frequency was 1–4 headaches per month. Of the 42 patients, 34 (80.9%) successfully discontinued their abortive medications. After 4 months' treatment, 50% headache reduction was seen in 78.5% of patients, 75% reduction in 14.2% of patients, and 9.5% of patients became headache-free. A second study evaluated the efficacy of sodium valproate in 10 children (Serdaroglu et al., 2002). The treatment continued for at least 12 weeks. Both headache severity and frequency were reduced compared to baseline ($P = 0.000$ and $P = 0.002$ respectively). Also the duration of headache was significantly decreased with treatment ($P = 0.001$).

Topiramate was evaluated in terms of safety and efficacy for the prevention of migraine in 75 children (Hershey et al., 2002). All the children were re-evaluated 88.7 ± 35.7 days later and 41 were seen at a second follow-up. The mean headache frequency was reduced from 16.5 ± 10.0 to 11.6 ± 10.2 days per month ($P < 0.001$) with a further reduction to 9.4 ± 8.4 days by the second follow-up ($P < 0.001$). Severity and duration of headache were also reduced. A randomized, double-blind, placebo-controlled trial evaluated the efficacy and tolerability of topiramate in 162 children with migraine (Winner et al., 2006). Topiramate reduced mean monthly migraine days by 2.6 (baseline 5.4 days), compared with 1.9 days for placebo (baseline 5.5 days), which approached statistical significance ($P = 0.065$). A significantly greater percentage of patients with topiramate (32%) had $\geq$75% reduction in mean monthly migraine days compared to patients with placebo (14%, $P = 0.020$).

Levetiracetam was assessed in 19 patients in one retrospective study (Miller, 2004). The mean frequency of headache attacks before treatment was 6.3 per month and, after treatment, fell to 1.7 per month ($P < 0.0001$). Fifty-two percent of patients experienced elimination of migraine attacks during treatment.

Gabapentin was studied in an open trial conducted in 18 children (Belman et al., 2001). Eighty percent of patients experienced a >50% reduction in headache frequency and severity.

Zonisamide was evaluated in 12 patients in a retrospective study (Pakalnis and Kring, 2006). Eight of these patients had a positive response, with greater than 50% reduction in headaches from pretreatment values.

Adverse events

In children younger than 15 years, aspirin is not recommended because of the concern of Reye's syndrome. Acetaminophen is safer and, if used in therapeutic doses, adverse events are extremely rare, although their exact incidence is unknown. Overdoses can occur and are associated with hepatotoxicity and renotoxicity. The potential adverse effects of ibuprofen are similar to those of other NSAIDs. However, gastrointestinal bleeding, renal failure, or anaphylaxis is rare with short-term use in children (Hamalainen, 1998). Sumatriptan is well tolerated and no serious adverse events occurred in clinical trials: taste disturbance was the most common (Ueberall, 1999; Winner et al., 2000, 2006; Ahonen et al., 2004). Propranolol may cause hypoglycemia, bradycardia, and hypotension, and decrease tolerance to physical exercise. Before propranolol therapy, blood pressure should be measured and an electrocardiogram recorded. Drowsiness and weight gain are frequently observed in patients taking flunarizine. Drowsiness is also the most common adverse effect of amitriptyline. Long-term use of valproate may cause weight gain, hair loss, and cytopenia.

CONCLUSIONS

At present, there is a lack of evidence to support pharmacological, psychological, and cognitive-behavioral treatments for TTH and more studies into the treatment of this disorder in pediatric patients are needed.

On the other hand, the available published data about the efficacy and safety of symptomatic drug treatment for migraine in children and adolescents suggest that ibuprofen and acetaminophen are effective and should be considered. Also sumatriptan nasal spray is probably effective but should be considered for the treatment of adolescents only. Insufficient data are currently available to recommend the use of all other NSAIDs and triptans in both children and adolescents. Moreover, the risk of medication overuse and the possibility of self-treatment without parental control should be kept in mind.

With reference to prophylactic drug treatment for migraine, the available data suggest that flunarizine is probably effective for preventive therapy. The efficacy data regarding propranolol, nimodipine, and trazodone are conflicting. Finally, there is insufficient evidence to make any recommendations concerning the use of cyproheptadine, amitriptyline, divalproex sodium, topiramate, levetiracetam, gabapentin, or zonisamide. On the other hand, pizotifen and clonidine are probably ineffective.

There is very good evidence that psychological treatments, principally relaxation and cognitive-behavioral therapy, are effective in reducing the severity and frequency of chronic headache in children and adolescents (Eccleston et al., 2003).

With reference to pharmacological treatment we think that there is a clear and urgent need for controlled, randomized, and masked trials. Lack of evidence should not be confused with evidence of lack of efficacy of a treatment – a risk that is particularly high in the case of treatments not supported by rigorous studies.

In conclusion, it is essential to act directly on factors precipitating or exacerbating the headache. At the same time, the high placebo response rate in childhood migraine and our clinical experience suggest that the clinical approach with the patient and parents should be based on a holistic framing of migraine, taking into consideration that the patient–clinician relationship with children and adolescents is the core of the therapy, thus influencing the course of the disease.

As suggested by Sacks (1992), "if there is one thing that afflicts the migraine patient, other than the headache itself, it is the feeling that he is not really listened to by the doctor, but instead observed, analysed, stuffed with drugs, pressurised . . . but not listened to."

References

Abu-Arafeh I (2001). Chronic tension-type headache in children and adolescents. Cephalalgia 21 (8): 830–836.

Abu-Arefeh I, Russell G (1994). Prevalence of headache and migraine in schoolchildren. BMJ 309: 765–769.

Ahonen K, Hamalainen ML, Rantala H et al. (2004). Nasal sumatriptan is effective in the treatment of migraine attacks in children. Neurology 62: 883–887.

Anttila P (2006). Tension-type headache in childhood and adolescence. Lancet Neurol 5: 268–274.

Anttila P, Metsahonkala L, Aromaa M et al. (2002a). Determinants of tension-type headache in children. Cephalalgia 22: 401–408.

Anttila P, Metsahonkala L, Mikkelsson M et al. (2002b). Muscle tenderness in pericranial and neck-shoulder region in children with headache: a controlled study. Cephalalgia 22: 340–344.

Aromaa M, Silanpää M, Rautava P (1997). Childhood headache at school entry: a controlled clinical study. Neurology 17: 488–491.

Arruda MA, Bordinii CA, Ciciarelli JC et al. (2004). Decreasing the minimal duration of the attack to 1 hour is sufficient to increase the sensitivity of the ICHD-II for migraine in childhood? J Headache Pain 5: 59.

Ayatollahi SM, Moradi F, Ayatollahi SA (2002). Prevalences of migraine and tension-type headache in adolescent girls of Shiraz (Southern Iran). Headache 42: 287–290.

Bain KE, Beatty S, Lloyd C (2000). Non-organic visual loss in children. Eye 14: 770–772.

Balottin U, Borgatti R, Lanzi G (1989). The therapeutic approach to the migraine patient. Headache in children and adolescents. In: G Lanzi, U Balottin, A Cernibori (Eds.), Proceedings of the First International Symposium on Headache in Children and Adolescents. Elsevier Science, Amsterdam.

Balottin U, Termine C, Nicoli F et al. (2005). Idiopathic headache in children under six years of age: a follow up study. Headache 45: 705–715.

Battistella PA, Ruffilli R, Moro R et al. (1990). A placebo-controlled crossover trial of nimodipine in pediatric migraine. Headache 30: 264–268.

Belman AL, Milazo M, Savatic M (2001). Gabapentin for migraine prophylaxis in children. Ann Neurol 50 (Suppl. 1): S109.

Bendsten L, Jensen R (2004). Mirtazapine is effective in the prophylactic treatment of chronic tension-type headache. Neurology 62: 1706–1711.

Bendsten L, Jensen R, Olesen J (1996). A non-selective (amitriptyline), but not a selective (citalopram), serotonin reuptake inhibitor is effective in the prophylactic treatment of chronic tension-type headache. J Neurol Neurosurg Psychiatry 61: 285–290.

Benedetti F, Mayberg HS, Wager TD et al. (2005). Neurobiological mechanisms of the placebo effect. J Neurosci 25: 10390–10402.

Bille B (1962a). Migraine in schoolchildren. Acta Paediatr 51 (Suppl. 136): 1–151.

Bille BS (1962b). Migraine in school children. A study of the incidence and short-term prognosis, and a clinical, psychological and electroencephalographic comparison between children with migraine and matched controls. Acta Paediatr 51 (Suppl. 136): 1–151.

Bille B (1981). Migraine in childhood and its prognosis. Cephalalgia 1: 71–75.

Blau JN (1982). Resolution of migraine attacks: sleep and the recovery phase. J Neurol Neurosurg Psychiatry 45: 223–226.

Bojinova V, Dimova P, Belopitova L (2000). Clinical manifestations of cerebrovascular hypoplasias in childhood. J Child Neurol 15 (3): 166–171.

Bousser MG, Welch KMA (2005). Relation between migraine and stroke. Lancet Neurol 4: 533–542.

Breslau N, Davis GC, Andreski P (1991). Migraine, psychiatric disorders and suicide attempts: an epidemiological study of young adults. Psychiatry Res 37: 11–23.

Breslau N, Schultz LR, Stewart LR (2000). Headache and major depression: Is the association specific to migraine? Neurology 54 (2): 308.

Brinciotti M, Di Sabato ML, Matricardi M et al. (2000). Electroclinical features in children and dolescents with epilepsy and/or migraine, and occipital epileptiform EEG abnormalities. Clin Electroencephalogr 31 (2): 76–82.

Bruni O, Galli F, Guidetti V (1999). Sleep hygiene and migraine in children and adolescents. Cephalalgia 19 (S25): 58–60.

Bruni O, Russo PM, Violani C et al. (2004). Sleep and migraine: an actigraphic study. Cephalalgia 24 (2): 134–139.

Caruso JM, Brown WD, Exil G et al. (2000). The efficacy of divalproex sodium in the prophylactic treatment of children with migraine. Headache 40: 672–676.

Charles JA (2006). Almotriptan in the acute treatment of migraine in patients 11–17 years old: an open-label pilot study of efficacy and safety. J Headache Pain 7: 95–97.

Coch C, Melchior JC (1969). Headache in childhood – a five year material from a pediatric university clinic. Dan Med Bull 16 (4): 109–114.

Congdon PJ, Forsythe WI (1979). Migraine in childhood: a study of 300 children. Develop Med Child Neurol 21: 209–216.

Cunningham SJ, McGrath PJ, Ferguson HB et al. (1987). Personality and behavioral characteristics in pediatric migraine. Headache 27: 16–20.

Damen L, Bruijn J, Koes BW et al. (2005). Prophylactic treatment of migraine in children. Part 1. A systematic review of non-pharmacological trials. Cephalalgia 26: 373–383.

Dexter JD (1986). The relationship between disorders of arousal from sleep and migraine. Headache 26: 322.

Di Mario FJ, Langshur S (2000). Headaches in patients with neurofibromatosis-1. J Child Neurol 15 (4): 235–238.

Dooley J, Bagnell A (1995). The prognosis and treatment of headaches in children – a ten year follow-up. Can J Neurol Sci 22: 47–49.

Eccleston C, Yorke L, Morley S et al. (2003). Psychological therapies for the management of chronic and recurrent pain in children and adolescents. Cochrane Database Syst Rev (1): CD003968.

Evans RW, Gladstein J (2003). Confusional migraine or photoepilepsy? Headache 43: 506–508.

Evans RW, Rolak LA (2004). The Alice in Wonderland syndrome. Headache 44: 624–625.

Evers S, Rahmann A, Kraemer C et al. (2006). Treatment of childhood migraine attacks with oral zolmitriptan and ibuprofen. Neurology 67: 497–499.

Fearon P, Hotopf M (2001). Relation between headache in childhood and physical and psychiatric symptoms in adulthood: national birth cohort study. BMJ 322 (7295): 1145.

Fonagy P (2003). What is the place of psychodynamic psychotherapy and cognitive-behaviour therapy in child and adolescent psychiatry? In: Proceedings of the 12th European Society for Child and Adolescence Psychiatry, Paris, France.

Forsythe WI, Gillies D, Sills MA (1984). Propranolol (Inderal) in the treatment of childhood migraine. Dev Med Child Neurol 26: 737–741.

Galli F, Patron L, Russo PM et al. (2004). Chronic daily headache in childhood and adolescence: clinical aspects and a 4-year follow-up. Cephalalgia 10: 850–859.

Galli F, D'Antuono G, Tarantino S et al. (2007). Headache and recurrent abdominal pain: a controlled study by the means of the Child Behaviour Checklist (CBCL). Cephalalgia 27 (3): 211–219.

Gencoglu EA, Alehan F, Erol I et al. (2005). Brain SPECT findings in a patient with Alice Wonderland syndrome. Clin Nucl Med 30: 758–759.

Gillies D, Sills M, Forsythe I (1986). Pizotifen (Sanomigran) in childhood migraine. A double-blind controlled trial. Eur Neurol 25: 32–35.

Gladstein J, Holden EW (1996). Chronic daily headache in children and adolescents: a 2 year prospective study. Headache 36: 349.

Guidetti V, Galli F (1998). Evolution of headache in childhood and adolescence: an 8-year follow-up. Cephalalgia 18 (7): 434–462.

Guidetti V, Galli F (2002). History taking. In: V Guidetti, G Russell, M Sillanpää et al. (Eds.), Migraine and Headache in Children and Adolescents. Martin Dunitz, London, pp. 51–62.

Guidetti V, Mazzei G, Ottaviano S et al. (1986). The utilization of Rorschach test in childhood migraine: a case controlled study. Cephalalgia 6: 87.

Guidetti V, Moscato D, Ottaviano S et al. (1987a). Flunarizine and migraine in childhood: an evaluation of endocrine function. Cephalalgia 7: 263–266.

Guidetti V, Fornara R, Marchini R et al. (1987b). Headache and epilepsy in childhood: analysis of a series of 620 children. Funct Neurol 2: 323–341.

Guidetti V, Bruni O, Cerutti R et al. (1991). How and why childhood headache and migraine differ from that of the adults. In: V Gallai, V Guidetti (Eds.), Juvenile Headache. Excerpta Medica, Amsterdam p. 27.

Guidetti V, Galli F, Fabrizi P et al. (1998). Headache and psychiatric comorbidity: clinical aspects and outcome in an 8-year follow-up study. Cephalalgia 18 (7): 455–462.

Guidetti V, Fabrizi P, Galli F et al. (1999). Unilateral headache in early and late childhood. Int J Neurol Sci 20: S56–S59.

Hamalainen ML (1998). Migraine in children. Guidelines for treatment. CNS Drugs 10 (2): 105–117.

Hamalainen ML (2002). Medical and dietary management of headache and migraine. In: I Abu-Arafeh (Ed.), Childhood Headache. Mac Keith Press, London.

Hamalainen ML, Hoppu K, Valkeila E et al. (1997a). Ibuprofen or acetaminophen for the acute treatment of migraine in children: a double-blind, randomized, placebo-controlled, crossover study. Neurology 48: 102–107.

Hamalainen ML, Hoppu K, Santavuori PR (1997b). Oral dihydroergotamine for therapy-resistant migraine attacks in children. Pediatr Neurol 16: 114–117.

Hamalainen ML, Hoppu K, Santavuori PR (1997c). Sumatriptan for migraine attacks in children: a randomized placebo-controlled study. Do children with migraine respond to oral sumatriptan differently than adults? Neurology 48: 1100–1103.

Headache Classification Committee of the International Headache Society (1988). Classification and diagnostic criteria for headache disorders, cranial neuralgias and facial pain. Cephalalgia 8 (Suppl. 7): 1–96.

Headache Classification Subcommittee of the International Headache Society (2004). The international classification of headache disorders, second edition. Cephalalgia 24 (Suppl. 1): 1–151.

Hershey AD, Powers SW, Bentti AL et al. (2000). Effectiveness of amitriptyline in the prophylactic management of childhood headaches. Headache 40: 539–549.

Hershey AD, Powers SW, Bentti AL et al. (2001). Characterization of chronic daily headaches in children in a multidisciplinary headache center. Neurology 56: 1032–1037.

Hershey AD, Powers SW, Vockell AL et al. (2002). Effectiveness of topiramate in the prevention of childhood headache. Headache 42: 810–818.

Hockaday JM (1988). Migraine in Childhood and Other Non-epileptic Paroxysmal Disorders. Butterworths, London.

Holroyd KA, O'Donnell FJ, Stensland M et al. (2001). Management of chronic tension-type headache with tricyclic antidepressant medication, stress management therapy, and their combination: a randomized controlled trial. Jama 285: 2208–2215.

Inamorato E, Minatti Hannuch SN, Zukerman E (1993). The role of sleep in migraine attacks. Arq Neuropsiquiatr 51 (4): 429–432.

Jensen R (1999). Pathophysiological mechanisms of tension-type headache: a review of epidemiological and experimental studies. Cephalalgia 19: 602–621.

Juang KD, Wang SJ, Fuh SR et al. (2004). Association between adolescent chronic daily headache and childhood adversity: a community-based study. Cephalalgia 24: 54–59.

Kappler JA (1992). Rebound headache: definition, symptomatology, treatment, and prevention. Headache Quarterly 3: 39–40.

Karwautz A, Wöber C, Lang T et al. (1999). Psychosocial factors in children and adolescents with migraine and tension-type headache: a controlled study and review of the literature. Cephalalgia 19: 32–43.

Kaynak Key FN, Donmez S, Tuzun U (2004). Epidemiological and clinical characteristics with psychosocial aspects of tension-type headache in Turkish college students. Cephalalgia 24: 669–674.

Kazdin AE (2002). The state of child and adolescent psychotherapy research. Child Adolesc Ment Health 2: 53–59.

Kowal A, Pritchard D (1990). Psychological characteristics of children who suffer from headache: a research note. J Child Psychol Psychiatry 31 (4): 637–649.

Lanzi G, Balottin U, Zambrino CA et al. (1996). Guidelines and recommendations for the treatment of migraine in paediatric and adolescent patients. Funct Neurol 11: 269–275.

Lanzi G, Zambrino CA, Balottin U et al. (1997). Periodic syndrome and migraine in children and adolescents. Ital J Neurol Sci 18: 283–288.

Larsson B (1988). The role of psychological, health-behaviour and medical factors in adolescent headache. Dev Med Child Neurol 30 (5): 616–625.

Laurell K, Larsson B, Eeg-Olofsson O (2004). Prevalence of headache in Swedish schoolchildren, with a focus on tension-type headache. Cephalalgia 24: 380–388.

Lewis DW, Middlebrook MT, Mehallick L (1996). Paediatric headaches: what do the children want? Headache 36: 224–230.

Lewis DW, Kellstein D, Burke B et al. (2002). Children's ibuprofen suspension for the acute treatment of pediatric migraine headache. Headache 42 (8): 780–786.

Lewis D, Diamond S, Scott D et al. (2004). Prophylactic treatment of pediatric migraine. Headache 44: 230–237.

Linder SL (1996). Subcutaneous sumatriptan in the clinical setting: the first 50 consecutive patients with acute migraine in the pediatric neurology office practice. Headache 36: 419–422.

Linder SL, Dowson AJ (2000). Zolmitriptan provides effective migraine relief in adolescents. Int J Clin Pract 54: 466–469.

Ludvigsson J (1974). Propranolol used in prophylaxis of migraine in children. Acta Neurol 50: 109–115.

Ludvigsson P, Hesdorffer D, Olafsson E et al. (2006). Migraine with aura is a risk factor for unprovoked seizures in children. Ann Neurol 59 (1): 210–213.

Macdonald JT (1994). Treatment of juvenile migraine with subcutaneous sumatriptan. Headache 34: 581–582.

Mack KJ (2006). Episodic and chronic migraine in children. Semin Neurol 26: 223–231.

Maratos J, Wilkinson M (1982). Migraine in children: a medical and psychiatric study. Cephalalgia 2 (4): 179–187.

Mathew L (1993). Chronic refractory headache. Neurology 43 (Suppl.): 26S–33S.

Mauskop A (2001). Alternative therapies in headache: is there a role? Med Clin North Am 85 (4): 1077–1084.

Merikangas KR (1994). Psychopatology and headache syndromes in the community. Headache 34: S17–S26.

Merikangas KR, Merikangas JR, Angst J (1993). Headache syndromes and psychiatric disorders: association and familial transmission. J Psychiatr Res 2: 197–210.

Miller GS (2004). Efficacy and safety of levetiracetam in pediatric migraine. Headache 44: 238–243.

Morales NM, Agapejev S, Morales RP et al. (2000). Clinical aspects of neurocysticercosis in children. Pediatr Neurol 22 (4): 287–291.

Neubauer D, Kuhar M, Ravnik I (1997). Antihistamine responsive cluster headache in a teenaged girl. Headache 37: 296–298.

Olness K, Macdonald JT, Uden DL (1987). Comparison of self-hypnosis and propranolol in the treatment of juvenile classic migraine. Pediatrics 79: 593–597.

Ostergaard S, Russell MB, Bendtsen L et al. (1997). Comparison of first degree relatives and spouses of people with chronic tension headache. BMJ 314: 1092–1093.

Ozge A, Bugdayci R, Sasmaz T et al. (2003). The sensitivity and specificity of the case definition criteria in diagnosis of headache: a school based epidemiological study of 5562 children in Mersin. Cephalalgia 23: 138–145.

Paiva T, Batista A, Martins P et al. (1995). The relationship between headaches and sleep disturbances. Headache 35: 590–596.

Pakalnis A, Kring D (2006). Zonisamide prophylaxis in refractory pediatric headache. Headache 46 (5): 804–807.

Pavlakis SG, Frank Y, Chusid R (1999). Hypertensive encephalopathy, reversible occipitoparietal encephalopathy, or reversible posterior leukoencephalopathy: three names for an old syndrome. J Child Neurol 14 (5): 277–281.

Piccinelli P, Borgatti R, Nicoli F et al. (2006). Relationship between migraine and epilepsy in pediatric age. Headache 46 (3): 413–421.

Rami A, Shapira Y, Flusser H et al. (1986). Basilar migraine manifesting as transient global amnesia in a 9-year-old child. Headache 26 (1): 17–18.

Riggs SR, Bodensteiner JB (1995). Acute confusional migraine: variant of transient global amnesia. Pediatr Neurol 12 (2): 129–131.

Rossi LN, Cortinovis I, Menegazzo L et al. (2005). Behaviour during attacks and assessment of intensity in primary headaches of children and adolescents. Cephalalgia 26: 107–112.

Russell MB, Ostergaard S, Bendtsen L et al. (1999). Familial occurrence of chronic tension-type headache. Cephalalgia 19: 207–210.

Sacks O (1992). Migraine. Picador, London.

Sahota PK, Dexter JD (1990). Sleep and headache syndromes: a clinical review. Headache 30: 80–84.

Serdaroglu G, Erhan E, Tekgul E et al. (2002). Sodium valproate prophylaxis in childhood migraine. Headache 42: 819–822.

Silberstein SD (1990). Twenty questions about headaches in children and adolescents. Headache 30: 716–724.

Silberstein SD (1993). Tension-type and chronic daily headache. Neurology 43: 1644–1649.

Silberstein SD, Lipton RB, Solomon S et al. (1994). Classification of daily and near-daily headaches: proposed revisions to the IHS criteria. Headache 34: 1–7.

Sillanpää M (1977). Clonidine prophylaxis of childhood migraine and other vascular headache. A double blind study of 57 children. Headache 17: 28–31.

Sillanpää M, Aro H (2000). Headache in teenagers: comorbidity and prognosis. Funct Neurol 15 (Suppl.): 116–121.

Sills M, Congdon P, Forsythe I (1982). Clonidine and childhood migraine. Dev Med Child Neurol 24: 837–841.

Sjaastad O, Dale I (1976). Evidence for a new (?) treatable headache entity. Headache 14: 105–108.

Sorge F, Desimone R, Marano E et al. (1988). Flunarizine in prophylaxis of childhood migraine. A double-blind, placebo-controlled crossover study. Cephalalgia 8: 1–6.

Steiner TJ, Lange R, Voelker M (2003). Aspirin in episodic tension-type headache: placebo-controlled dose-ranging comparison with paracetamol. Cephalalgia 23: 59–66.

Stevenson SB (2006). Epilepsy and migraine headache: is there a connection? J Pediatr Health Care 20 (3): 167–171.

Termine C, Ferrari-Ginevra O, Darrigo S et al. (2005). Alternative therapies in the treatment of headache in childhood, adolescence, and adulthood. Funct Neurol 20 (1): 9–14.

Ueberall MA (1999). Intranasal sumatriptan for the acute treatment of migraine in children. Neurology 52: 1507–1510.

Ulrich V, Gervil M, Olesen J (2004). The relative influence of environment and genes in episodic tension-type headache. Neurology 62: 2065–2069.

Vahlquist B (1962). Migraine in children. International Archives of Allergy 7: 348–352.

Visser Wh, Winner P, Strohmaier K et al. (2004). Rizatriptan Protocol 059 and 061 Study Groups. Rizatriptan 5 mg for the acute treatment of migraine in adolescents: results from a double-blind, single-attack study and two open-label, multiple-attack studies. Headache 44: 891–899.

Wang SJ, Fuh JL, Lu SR et al. (2006). Chronic daily headache in adolescents. Prevalence, impact, and medication overuse. Neurology 66: 193–197.

Wilkinson M, Williams K, Leyton M (1978). Observations on the treatment of an acute attack of migraine. Res Clin Stud Headache 6: 141–146.

Winner P, Rothner Ad, Saper J et al. (2000). A randomized, double-blind, placebo-controlled study of sumatriptan nasal spray in the treatment of acute migraine in adolescents. Pediatrics 106: 989–997.

Winner P, Lewis D, Visser WH et al. (2002). Rizatriptan 5 mg for the acute treatment of migraine in adolescents: a randomized, double-blind placebo-controlled study. Headache 42: 49–55.

Winner P, Rothner Ad, Wooten JD et al. (2006). Sumatriptan nasal spray in adolescent migraineurs: a randomized, double-blind, placebo-controlled, acute study. Headache 46: 212–222.

Wirrell EC, Hamiwka LD (2006). Do children with benign rolandic epilepsy have a higher prevalence of migraine than those with other partial epilepsies or nonepilepsy controls? Epilepsia 47 (10): 1674–1681.

Wöber C, Wöber-Bingöl C (1998). Pediatric migraine and the International Headache Society criteria. Neurology 50 (3): 831–832.

Wöber C, Wöber-Bingöl C (2000). Clinical management of young patients presenting with headache. Funct Neurol 15 (Suppl. 3): 89–105.

Wöber-Bingöl C, Wöber C, Karwautz C et al. (1995). Diagnosis of headache in childhood and adolescence: a study in 437 patients. Cephalalgia 15: 13–21.

Wöber-Bingöl C, Wöber C, Wagner-Ennsgraber C et al. (1996). IHS criteria for migraine and tension-type headache in children and adolescents. Headache 36: 231–238.

Zwart JA, Dyb G, Holmen TL et al. (2004). The prevalence of migraine and tension-type headaches among adolescents in Norway: the Nord-Trondelag Health Study (Head-HUNT-Youth), a large population-based epidemiological study. Cephalalgia 24: 373–379.

Handbook of Clinical Neurology, Vol. 97 (3rd series)
Headache
G. Nappi and M.A. Moskowitz, Editors

Chapter 62

Vestibular migraine

MICHAEL STRUPP,[1]* MAURIZIO VERSINO,[2] AND THOMAS BRANDT[3]

[1]*Department of Neurology and Integrated Center for Research and Treatment of Vertigo, Dizziness and Ocular Motor Disorders, Ludwig-Maximilians University, Münich, Germany*

[2]*University Center for Adaptive Disorders and Headache (UCADH) and Department of Neurology, University of Pavia, Italy; IRCCS National Neurological Institute C. Mondino, Pavia, Italy*

[3]*Institute of Clinical Neurosciences and Integrated Center for Research and Treatment of Vertigo, Dizziness and Ocular Motor Disorders, Ludwig-Maximilians University, Münich, Germany*

Due to the variation of its manifestations, migraine-vertigo/vestibular migraine is the chameleon among the episodic vertigo syndromes. There is even an ongoing debate as to whether it is a separate clinical entity. So far no generally accepted diagnostic criteria have been established. The diagnosis is difficult for several reasons: the duration of attacks may range from minutes to days even in the same patient; the recurrent attacks of vertigo occur in about one-third of the patients without associated headache or phono-/photophobia; and there is a large variation of vestibular and ocular motor dysfunctions during and between the attacks. This, however, does not mean that a diagnosis of migraine-vertigo/vestibular migraine cannot be made. Clinical practice shows that it is easy, if the patient suffers from an already known migraine (with or without aura) and develops recurrent attacks of vertigo with normal hearing.

Migraine-vertigo/vestibular migraine is the most common cause of spontaneous, recurrent vertigo in adults. Differential diagnoses include Menière's disease and episodic ataxia type 2, both of which can mimic migraine-vertigo, vestibular paroxysmia, and non-vestibular dizziness in migraine. Furthermore, transient ischemic attacks have to be excluded, as in typical aura without headache (International Headache Classification of Headache Disorders, second edition (ICHD-II) 1.2.3: Headache Classification Subcommittee of the International Headache Society, 2004).

The question arises as to why there is an ongoing debate on migraine-vertigo/vestibular migraine. The answer is reflected in the vast literature on this topic (according to a PubMed search on "migraine and (vertigo or dizziness or vestibular)" there were 684 papers and 144 reviews). First, a considerable proportion of patients with "migraine with and without aura," namely those with basilar-type migraine, also suffer from migraine-associated dizziness (rarely vertigo), which, however, is not their leading symptom. Second, both migraine and vertigo have a high lifelong prevalence (for migraine about 12%, for vertigo/dizziness about 20–30%) as well as a significant female preponderance. Therefore, they might occur together just by chance. Third, patients with migraine (even without vertigo or dizziness) have a relatively higher rate of (minor) central ocular and/or peripheral and central vestibular dysfunctions, which are again more common in basilar-type migraine. In the past, many of these studies, however, did not differentiate between migraine with or without aura and migraine with aura with or without vertigo/dizziness. This makes a *post hoc* interpretation of the data difficult. Fourth, patients with other vestibular disorders such as benign paroxysmal positional vertigo (BPPV) or Menière's disease also suffer relatively more frequently from migraine. Fifth, as mentioned above, there are no generally accepted diagnostic criteria and no unified term for this entity. It is evident that the absence of diagnostic criteria is a major problem of all studies dealing with the epidemiology, clinical findings, genetics, pathophysiology, and treatment of migraine-vertigo/vestibular migraine. Therefore, an agreement on specific, sensitive, and validated diagnostic criteria is highly warranted for the elaboration of specific findings in this field.

All in all, to write a chapter on migraine-vertigo/vestibular migraine is not only a challenge but also an opportunity. We will not only summarize our current

*Correspondence to: Michael Strupp, MD, Department of Neurology and Integrated Center for Research and Treatment of Vertigo, Dizziness and Ocular Motor Disorders, Ludwig-Maximilians University, Münich, Germany, E-mail: Michael.Strupp@med.uni-muenchen.de

knowledge but also make suggestions on how to improve our future knowledge of this most frequent cause of spontaneous recurrent attacks of vertigo with a lifetime prevalence of about 1%.

This chapter first treats the clinical features and the spectrum of episodic vertigo caused by migraine-vertigo as well as its epidemiology. Then we give current criteria and discuss how to differentiate migraine-vertigo from other causes of recurrent vertigo and motion sickness-like symptoms as well as other forms of headache. Subsequently, we discuss the assumed underlying mechanisms and aspects of the genetics of migraine-vertigo. Finally, a summary is given of its treatment options, which do not differ from the treatment of basilar-type migraine.

DIFFICULTIES WITH THE DEFINITION OF MIGRAINE-VERTIGO/VESTIBULAR MIGRAINE

We have already mentioned the ongoing lively debate as to whether migraine-vertigo/vestibular migraine is a separate entity or just a basilar-type migraine with vertigo as one of its many symptoms (Dieterich and Brandt, 1999; Versino et al., 2003; Brandt, 2004; Neuhauser and Lempert, 2004; Brantberg et al., 2005; Crevits and Bosman, 2005; Lempert and Neuhauser, 2005; Olesen, 2005; Baloh, 2006; Brandt and Strupp, 2006; Eggers, 2007). Further, different diagnostic criteria have been proposed over the years. Problems with a diagnosis are also reflected by the non-uniform terminology: migraine-vertigo, migraine-associated vertigo, migrain(e)ous vertigo, or vestibular migraine. What makes things even worse: none of these terms is included in the ICHD (see below). The background for this debate will be illustrated by a comparison of the similarities and differences between migraine with/without aura, vertigo/dizziness, and migraine-vertigo/vestibular migraine.

Migraine and vertigo/dizziness are both common disorders. More than 70% of patients with known migraine complain of vertigo or dizziness (Kelman and Tanis, 2006). The latter may be caused by disorders other than migraine, and they can be differentiated by a careful patient history and clinical examination. As shown by a meta-analysis on more than 35 461 000 subjects, the prevalence of migraine is about 12% (age 18–65 years) with a male-to-female ratio of 0.4 (Hirtz et al., 2007). The prevalence of vertigo/dizziness is about 20–30% (Yardley et al., 1998; Davis and Moorjani, 2003; Hannaford et al., 2005; Neuhauser, 2007) and also with a female preponderance (male/female ratio 0.37) (Neuhauser et al., 2006; Neuhauser, 2007). Therefore, about 4% of the general population may just by pure coincidence suffer from vertigo/dizziness and migraine. Epidemiological studies in which the prevalence of both symptoms was estimated in different patient groups showed, however, that the correlation between vertigo and migraine is significantly higher and that both do not occur only by chance.

About 60% of patients with migraine-vertigo/vestibular migraine have been reported in several studies to experience dysfunctions of the peripheral and central vestibular and ocular motor system between the attacks (see below). They are, however, not specific, because similar dysfunctions have also been described in a high percentage of patients with migraine without vertigo, such as a unilateral peripheral vestibular dysfunction in 35% of patients with basilar-type migraine (Toglia et al., 1981) or "persisting vestibulocochlear derangements" in 77.5% of another series of patients with migraine (Kayan and Hood, 1984). Two studies reported no difference in the frequency of central ocular dysfunction between migraine patients with or without vertigo (Bir et al., 2003; Furman et al., 2005). This is also true for laboratory examinations in both patient groups. Further studies are, however, necessary to re-evaluate this issue using very strict diagnostic criteria for the different patient groups.

Migraine with aura/basilar-type migraine, migraine-vertigo/vestibular migraine, and vertigo may occur at any age (Cass et al., 1997; Dieterich and Brandt, 1999). For instance, benign paroxysmal vertigo of childhood – the equivalent to migraine-vertigo/vestibular migraine in adults – is the most common cause of vertigo in children (about 2.8% of children) (Russell and Abu-Arafeh, 1999; Erbek et al., 2006). In contrast to migraine, however, the prevalence of vertigo increases with age: it is about 17% and rises to 39% in those over 80 years of age (Davis and Moorjani, 2003). The same is true for migraine-vertigo/vestibular migraine. Migraine begins earlier in life than migraine-vertigo/vestibular migraine, and there is a second peak around the age of 60 (Dieterich and Brandt, 1999; Neuhauser et al., 2001, 2006; Neuhauser, 2007).

To define migraine-vertigo/vestibular migraine, Neuhauser and Lempert (2004) made a thorough survey of what is known about the association of migraine with: (1) vestibular vertigo; (2) motion sickness; (3) cerebellar symptoms; and (4) non-vestibular dizziness. When it is a question of terminology – how to label episodic vertigo that is causally related to migraine – they propose the term "migrainous vertigo," to emphasize the particular etiology of these vertigo attacks. In 15 of 33 patients with migrainous vertigo, vertigo was regularly associated with migrainous headache. In 16 patients, vertigo occurred both with and without headache, and in 2 patients headache and vertigo never occurred together. The duration of attacks varied from minutes to days. These epidemiological data substantiate the association between migraine and vertigo and indicate that migrainous vertigo affects a significant proportion of patients in both dizziness and headache clinics. Others have proposed the term "vestibular migraine" to stress the particular manifestation of migraine with vertigo as the prevailing or sole symptom, often even without associated headache (Dieterich and Brandt, 1999; Brandt, 2004). The latter term is more oriented to the ICHD-II. As mentioned above, none of these terms is included in the ICHD-II. At the end of this chapter the pros and cons of the diagnostic entity will be summarized, conclusions drawn, and suggestions made.

Proposed classification and diagnostic criteria for migrainous vertigo/vestibular migraine

The diagnostic criteria for migraine-vertigo/migrainous vertigo/vestibular migraine have been elaborated (Dieterich and Brandt, 1999; Neuhauser et al., 2001).

Classification of vestibular migraine according to Dieterich and Brandt (1999)

In a retrospective study of 90 patients with episodic vertigo that could be related to migraine as the most probable pathomechanism, the diagnosis was assessed by three means: (1) careful clinical exclusion of relevant differential diagnoses, such as Menière's disease, vestibular paroxysmia, and transient ischemic attacks; (2) the patient's positive response to migraine medication during the attack and/or to prophylactic medication; and (3) follow-up of these patients over 2–7 years (Dieterich and Brandt, 1999). In our experience other causes must often be ruled out first, and in some patients the efficacy of migraine prophylaxis eventually leads to the appropriate diagnosis, but only after frustrating treatment failures with betahistine in suspected cases of Menière's disease, carbamazepine in suspected vestibular paroxysmia, or antiplatelet agents in suspected cases of transient ischemic attacks. In the majority of these patients, however, mild central ocular motor signs such as saccadic pursuit, spontaneous or gaze-evoked nystagmus, and positional nystagmus in the symptom-free interval and normal hearing suggest vestibular migraine (Dieterich and Brandt, 1999). If vestibular or ocular motor dysfunction was the key symptom, the diagnosis of vestibular migraine was based, first, on a history of at least three attacks and, second, on one of the following four typical constellations (A–D), as given in Table 62.1.

This categorization of A–D allows us to define constellations based on a minimum of features necessary to assess the diagnosis. Monosymptomatic audiovestibular attacks (78%) occur without associated headache in 32% of patients. Many patients present with features of more than one category, especially when observed over a longer time. The efficacy of medical treatment of migraine signifies that either acute attacks were suppressed by ergotamines and/or the frequency of the attacks was significantly reduced by preventive medication with beta-receptor blockers (metoprolol) or flunarizine. Others (Furman et al., 2003; Waterston, 2004) have proposed diagnosis on the basis of the effects of treatment (*ex juvantibus*), but such an approach has considerable weaknesses from a methodological viewpoint.

Table 62.1

Diagnostic criteria for vestibular migraine according to Dieterich and Brandt (1999)

Group A
Recurrent attacks of vertigo or dizziness and non-vestibular neurological deficits attributable to a dysfunction in the brainstem
Associated headache during or immediately after vertigo or dizziness ("brainstem aura with headache")
Individual history of migraine
Group B
Recurrent attacks of vestibular and/or ocular motor dysfunction only
Associated headache during or immediately after vertigo or dizziness ("only vestibular or ocular motor aura with headache")
Group C
Recurrent attacks of vestibular and/or ocular motor dysfunction only
Associated headache during or immediately after vertigo or dizziness ("only vestibular or ocular motor aura with headache")
Efficacy of medical (migraine) treatment
Group D
Recurrent attacks of vestibular and/or ocular motor dysfunction only
Without associated headache during or immediately after vertigo or dizziness ("only vestibular or ocular motor aura without headache")
Efficacy of medical (migraine) treatment

Classification of migrainous vertigo according to Neuhauser et al. (2001)

Neuhauser et al. (2001) proposed two separate categories – probable and definite migrainous vertigo. They thus offered a compromise between the requirements of research and of patient care (Stahl and Daroff, 2001). The diagnosis of "definite migrainous vertigo" is based on the criteria given in Table 62.2A. Vestibular symptoms are defined as mild if they do not interfere with daily activities, moderate if they interfere with but do not impede daily activities, and severe if patients cannot continue daily activities. Non-vestibular dizziness, such as

Table 62.2

Diagnostic criteria for definite (A) and probable (B) migrainous vertigo according to Neuhauser et al. (2001)

A. Diagnostic criteria for definite migrainous vertigo
1. Episodic vestibular symptoms of at least moderate severity (rotational vertigo, other illusory self or object motion, positional vertigo, head motion intolerance, i.e., sensation of imbalance or illusory self or object motion that is provoked by head motion)
2. Migraine according to the International Headache Society criteria
3. At least one of the following migrainous symptoms during at least two vertiginous attacks: migrainous headache, photophobia, phonophobia, visual or other auras
4. Other causes ruled out by appropriate investigations

B. Diagnostic criteria for probable migrainous vertigo
1. Episodic vestibular symptoms of at least moderate severity (rotational vertigo, other illusory self or object motion, positional vertigo, head motion intolerance)
2. At least one of the following: migraine according to the International Headache Society criteria; migrainous symptoms during vertigo; migraine-specific precipitants of vertigo, e.g., specific foods, sleep irregularities, hormonal changes; response to antimigraine drugs
3. Other causes ruled out by appropriate investigations

orthostatic hypotension, which frequently occurs during migraine attacks, was not included. The separate diagnostic category of probable migrainous vertigo was chosen for patients who did not entirely fulfill the above criteria for migrainous vertigo but were still considered to have migrainous vertigo as the most likely diagnosis. The diagnostic criteria of "probable migrainous vertigo" are given in Table 62.2B. A diagnosis of migraine was made according to the International Headache Society (IHS) criteria by means of a semistructured face-to-face interview. Migraine with and without aura were considered mutually exclusive. In this study vertigo was not counted as an aura symptom for the diagnosis of migraine with aura (Neuhauser et al., 2001). The application of published criteria for the diagnosis of "migrainous vertigo" or "vestibular migraine" allowed the development of a standardized, structured assessment interview with good test validity and reliability (Furman et al., 2003; Marcus et al., 2004).

How shall we deal with these diagnostic problems in the future? First, diagnostic criteria should be very strict, specific, sensitive, and validated in a uniform group of patients. Those who have probable migrainous vertigo/vestibular migraine should be excluded from clinical trials. This is mandatory in the current state of "certain" uncertainty. Second, many patients will have two diagnoses, such as "vestibular migraine" and "known migraine with visual aura." Third, since the diagnosis is made predominantly on the basis of the patient history, the leading symptom should lead to the diagnosis, i.e., either basilar-type migraine with vertigo if headache dominates or migraine-vertigo/vestibular migraine if vertigo/dizziness is the major complaint of the patient. This is also true for other disorders and by no means unique.

Migraine-vertigo and the ICHD-II

As a first approach, one is tempted to attribute migrainous vestibular vertigo to basilar-type migraine, since vertigo is most often caused by dysfunction of the peripheral (labyrinth, vestibular nerve) or central (brainstem, cerebellum) vestibular circuitry, and both territories are supplied by the basilar artery. Originally the terms "basilar artery migraine" or "basilar migraine" were used, but since it is uncertain that the basilar artery territory is involved (i.e., the disturbance may be bi-hemispheric), the term "basilar-type migraine" is preferred (Headache Classification Subcommittee of the International Headache Society, 2004). The ICHD-II requires an aura with two or more symptoms that originate from the brainstem and/or from both hemispheres simultaneously, usually developing over 5–20 min and lasting no longer than 60 min, to qualify as criteria for basilar-type migraine (Table 62.3).

Table 62.3

Diagnostic criteria for basilar-type migraine according to the second edition of the International Classification of Headache Disorders (ICHD-II 1.2.6: Headache Classification Subcommittee of the International Headache Society, 2004)

Diagnostic criteria

A. At least two attacks fulfilling criteria B–D
B. Aura consisting of at least two of the following fully reversible symptoms, but no motor weakness:
   1. Dysarthria
   2. Vertigo
   3. Tinnitus
   4. Hypacusis
   5. Diplopia
   6. Visual symptoms simultaneously in the temporal and nasal fields of both eyes
   7. Ataxia
   8. Decreased level of consciousness
   9. Simultaneous bilateral paresthesias
C. At least one of the following:
   1. At least one aura symptom developing gradually over $\geq$5 min and/or different aura symptoms occurring in succession over $\geq$5 min
   2. Each aura symptom lasting $\geq$5 and $\leq$60 min
D. Headache fulfilling criteria B–D for migraine without aura beginning during the aura or after aura within 60 min
E. Not attributed to another disorder

There is even an ongoing debate on whether basilar-type migraine is a separate entity or simply a subtype of migraine with aura. This makes the discussion about the term migraine-vertigo/vestibular migraine even more questionable. The Danish Headache Centre (Kirchmann et al., 2006) recruited 105 families comprising 362 patients with migraine with aura or basilar-type migraine. Thirty-eight patients from 29 families had basilar-type migraine. In the 12 families with basilar-type migraine with an apparently dominant inheritance, the authors sequenced all exons of the *CACNA1A* and *ATP1A2* (see below) genes. Basilar-type migraine occurred in 10% of patients with migraine with aura. The basilar-type aura had a median duration of 60 min and vertigo was present in 61%, dysarthria in 53%, tinnitus in 45%, diplopia in 45%, bilateral visual symptoms in 40%, bilateral paresthesias in 24%, decreased level of consciousness in 21%, hypoacusis in 21%, and ataxia in 5%. The relative frequency of the individual basilar-type symptoms was not different from that of patients with hemiplegic migraine from a previous study. The patients with basilar-type migraine were equally distributed among the 105 families with migraine with typical aura ($P = 0.37$). The attacks of migraine with aura were identical in families with or without basilar-type migraine. Neither causative mutations nor a linkage was identified. Kirchmann et al. (2006) concluded from their study that: (1) basilar-type aura may apparently occur at times in any patient with migraine with typical aura; and (2) there seems to be no firm clinical, epidemiological, or genetic evidence that basilar-type migraine is an independent disease entity different from migraine with aura.

Based on the ICHD-II, monosymptomatic attacks with rotational vertigo for seconds to a few minutes or for hours to days cannot be termed basilar-type migraine (Dieterich and Brandt, 1999). If the symptoms, namely vertigo, last longer than 60 min, then they may be classified according to the ICHD-II as "persistent aura without infarction" (ICHD-II 1.5.3). The diagnosis of basilar-type migraine is considered even less appropriate if the attacks are not followed by headache (Dieterich and Brandt, 1999; Neuhauser and Lempert, 2004; Brantberg et al., 2005). This, however, could be classified as "typical aura without headache" (ICHD-II 1.2.3).

"Benign paroxysmal vertigo of childhood," a disorder similar to migraine-vertigo/vestibular migraine (see below), was included in the ICHD-I and II. The term "benign recurrent vertigo in adults" (Slater, 1979; Moretti et al., 1980) is redundant, because its signs and symptoms are sufficiently characterized by migraine-vertigo/vestibular migraine with or without headache (Brandt, 2004).

All in all, there are several reasons why migraine-vertigo/vestibular migraine should be included as an entity in the next version of the ICHD. We would prefer the term "vestibular migraine," because it is similar to other terms like abdominal migraine (ICHD-II 1.3.2), retinal migraine (ICHD-II 1.4), or familial hemiplegic migraine (FHM, ICHD-II 1.2.4), and thus would be very compatible with the ICHD.

CLINICAL FEATURES OF MIGRAINE-VERTIGO/VESTIBULAR MIGRAINE

The basic problems with many studies in this field are that there are: (1) no approved diagnostic criteria and therefore no standardized inclusion and exclusion criteria; (2) no approved protocols considering aspects of the patient history of special relevance; and (3) no approved protocols treating relevant aspects of the clinical examination (namely regarding the peripheral and central vestibular and ocular motor systems), for which laboratory tests (namely electronystagmography, evoked potentials, and audiography) should be used. Therefore, the data from the literature are heterogeneous, and it is often almost impossible to compare the different studies.

Signs and symptoms

Symptoms during the attack

In the study by Dieterich and Brandt (1999) episodic vertigo was classified as vestibular in 84 out of 90 patients; the remaining 6 patients had light-headedness and non-vestibular ocular motor dysfunction causing oscillopsia or double vision (Table 62.4). The prevailing type of vertigo was rotational (70 patients). Fourteen of the patients with episodic rotational vertigo also reported positional vertigo or significant modulation of the intensity of vertigo in certain head positions. Episodic positional vertigo was the sole vestibular symptom in 1 patient. The second most common type was to-and-fro vertigo ($n = 34$). Both sensations were associated with postural imbalance and unsteadiness. Rotational and to-and-fro vertigo occurred in combination ($n = 22$) in single or subsequent attacks. More complex (multisymptomatic) neurological deficits associated with vestibular dysfunction were found in a group of 13 patients (14%). These included dysarthrophonia ($n = 7$); numbness of hand, face, or leg ($n = 7$); double vision; paraparesis; visual field defects; hearing loss; and lack of concentration ($n = 1$ in each). Another group of 7 patients (7.8%) experienced only non-vestibular dizziness (light-headedness) with neurological brainstem deficits due to a combination of ocular motor palsy and

Table 62.4

Characteristics* of vertigo during vestibular migraine attacks in 90 patients

	Rotational vertigo	To-and-fro vertigo
(n = 82)		
Duration of single attacks	70	34
seconds	7	2
<10 min	15	3
10–60 min	8	6
hours	27	14
1–4 days	13	9
Frequency of attacks	62	33
per day	1	4
per week	17	11
per month	26	11
per year	18	7
Positional vertigo	14	9
(n = 8)		
Positional vertigo only		1
Dizziness and gait ataxia only		1
Ocular motor disturbances without vertigo		6

*Patients may report more than one feature in single or subsequent attacks.
(Modified from Dieterich and Brandt, 1999.)

involuntary ocular oscillations (n = 5): dysarthrophonia (n = 3); numbness of the face, hand, or leg (n = 3); disturbance of consciousness (n = 3); and visual field defects (n = 2). These findings are supported by another study (Neuhauser et al., 2006): spontaneous rotational vertigo was reported by 67% of the patients with migraine-vertigo/vestibular migraine, while 24% had positional vertigo. Twenty-four percent always experienced headaches with their vertigo.

Clinical findings during the attack

In a prospective study the clinical spectrum of acute migrainous vertigo attacks was described in 20 patients by von Brevern et al. (2005). Tests included neuro-otological examination, recording of spontaneous and positional nystagmus with three-dimensional video-oculography, and audiometry. Pathological nystagmus was observed in 70% of patients during the attack: 6 had isolated spontaneous nystagmus, 5 had isolated positional nystagmus, and 3 had a combination of the two. Imbalance was observed in all patients except 1. Hearing was not affected in any patient during the attack. The findings during the acute attack pointed to a central vestibular dysfunction in 10 patients and to a peripheral vestibular dysfunction in 3 patients. In the remaining 7 patients the side of involvement could not be determined with certainty. As regards positional vertigo, the same authors evaluated 362 consecutive patients presenting with positional vertigo (von Brevern et al., 2004). Ten of them had migraine-vertigo/vestibular migraine mimicking BPPV. The following factors were suggested to distinguish migrainous positional vertigo from BPPV: short-duration symptomatic episodes, frequent recurrences, manifestation early in life, migrainous symptoms during episodes with positional vertigo, and atypical positional nystagmus. From both studies the authors concluded that migraine-vertigo/vestibular migraine should be considered in the differential diagnosis of vertigo with spontaneous and positional nystagmus; it can present as both a central and a peripheral vestibular disorder.

These data confirm earlier observations on 8 patients who were examined during their migrainous vertigo attacks (Dieterich and Brandt, 1999): all had a transient spontaneous nystagmus (>5°/s), 3 patients had gaze-evoked nystagmus, 3 had a severe positional nystagmus (vertical direction not habituating), 2 had a severe saccadic pursuit, and 1 a directional preponderance in the rotating and caloric tests.

Clinical findings between the attacks

A high incidence (65%) of subtle pathological ocular motor findings of central origin in the symptom-free interval was found in a study of 90 patients (Table 62.5) (Dieterich and Brandt, 1999). As mentioned above, this agrees with a report by Kayan and Hood (1984), who described findings during the attack that indicated a definite dysfunction of the vestibular and/or cochlear systems in 77.5% of their patients; half had a central and half a peripheral pathology (18.8% central, 28.8% peripheral, 30% inconclusive). Their study, however, provided no data on neuro-otological disorders in the symptom-free interval. The frequency (about 20%) of persisting peripheral vestibular deficits in three studies (Cutrer and Baloh, 1992; Celebisoy et al., 2008; Teggi et al., 2009) was larger than in the study by Dieterich and Brandt (1999) (8.3%). Decreased amplitudes of vestibular-evoked myogenic potentials, indicating impaired saccular function, were described more recently (Baier et al., 2009a). Objectively measurable electronystagmographic ocular motor abnormalities (57–80%) were stressed much earlier (Dursteler, 1975; Eviatar, 1981; Toglia et al., 1981).

Are these findings specific for migraine with aura or migraine-vertigo/vestibular migraine? As mentioned above, even patients with migraine (with and without aura) have a relatively high frequency of ocular motor and vestibular dysfunctions. Harno et al. (2003) examined 36 patients with various types of migraine. Neuro-otological

Table 62.5

Vestibular migraine: central ocular motor signs in the symptom-free interval in 90 patients

	n	%
Normal	23	25.6
Congenital strabismus*	5	5.5
Congenital nystagmus	3	3.3
Central ocular motor signs	59	65.6
Saccadic pursuit, vertical	43	48
Saccadic pursuit, horizontal	20	22
Gaze-evoked nystagmus	24	27
Spontaneous nystagmus (>5°/s)†	10	11
Positional nystagmus	10	11
Dissociated gaze-evoked nystagmus	8	9
Downbeat nystagmus	3	3.3
Upbeat nystagmus	2	2.2
Impaired fixation suppression of vestibulo-ocular reflex	3	3.3
Nuclear oculomotor palsy	1	1.1

*Multiple quotations possible.
†In combination with other central ocular motor signs and/or a directional preponderance in caloric testing.
(Modified from Dieterich and Brandt, 1999).

tests were performed between attacks: video-oculography, electronystagmography, static posturography, and audiometry on 12 patients with migraine with aura and 24 patients with migraine without aura. The results were compared to those of test-specific non-migrainous control groups. Only 8 migraineurs (6 with migraine with aura and 2 without aura) had vertigo/dizziness. Despite the absence of clinical neuro-otological symptoms, most of the patients with migraine (83%) showed abnormalities in at least one of these tests. Both migraine types differed significantly from the control group (in video-oculography, saccadic accuracy, and posturography). Vestibular findings tended to be more severe in migraine with aura than without aura. The authors concluded that interictal neuro-otological dysfunction in migraine with and without aura share similar features and that the defective ocular motor function is mostly of vestibulocerebellar origin. Increased body sway in patients with migraine in comparison to patients with episodic tension-type headache has been described by others to indicate dysfunction in the vestibulospinal system (Ishizaki et al., 2002).

In a prospective electronystagmographic study the differences between patients with migraine with and without vertigo were evaluated (Bir et al., 2003). Eighty-four patients with migraine (31 with headache, 53 with headache and vertigo) were included. Patient history, vestibular tests, electronystagmography (ENG), and imaging studies were performed for differential diagnosis. Fifty-three of 84 patients (63%) had episodic vertigo attacks. Vertigo was independent of headache in 24 patients (45%). Vertigo symptoms always appeared later in the history of migraine headache. Headache started at age 27 ± 8.3 years, and vertigo symptoms began 7.7 ± 8.7 years later. The age of manifestation of migraine and the female-to-male ratio were significantly higher in the vertigo group. Fifty-eight of the 84 patients had ENG testing. Fifty-eight percent of the patients with migraine and 55% of the patients with migraine and vertigo had abnormal ENG findings. None of the tests, except the Dix–Hallpike maneuver, revealed a statistically significant difference between the two groups. The authors concluded that the presence of the same ENG abnormalities in patients with headache only shows that the vestibular pathways are also affected in these patients, even when there are no vestibular symptoms (Bir et al., 2003).

From these data one can conclude that the ocular motor and vestibular dysfunctions described in patients with migraine-vertigo/vestibular migraine are not specific. Controlled studies have to be performed with strict inclusion criteria and standardized examination protocols to determine whether these changes are more frequent or severe in patients with migraine-vertigo/vestibular migraine. For the clinical practice this means that at the moment neither clinical nor laboratory examinations are really useful for differentiating migraine-vertigo/vestibular migraine from migraine with or without aura (for further differential diagnoses, see below).

EPIDEMIOLOGY OF MIGRAINE, VERTIGO AND DIZZINESS, AND MIGRAINE-VERTIGO/VESTIBULAR MIGRAINE

As mentioned above, migraine and vertigo/dizziness are both common disorders. According to a meta-analysis on more than 35 461 000 subjects, the prevalence of migraine is about 12% (age 18–65 years) (Hirtz et al., 2007), 5% in men and 15% in women (Stewart et al., 1995) with a male-to-female ratio of 0.4 (Hirtz et al., 2007). Only about 25% of the affected patients have migraine with aura.

The prevalence of vertigo and dizziness is about 20–30% (Kroenke and Price, 1993; Kroenke et al., 1994, 2000; Yardley et al., 1998; Davis and Moorjani, 2003; Hannaford et al., 2005; Neuhauser, 2007; Lempert and Neuhauser, 2009), with a significant increase during lifetime. Based on a more strict neuro-otological survey of 4,869 adults, 1-year prevalence estimates for vertigo (not including dizziness or light-headedness) were 4.9%, with a male-to-female ratio of 0.37

(Neuhauser et al., 2006; Neuhauser, 2007). Therefore, about 4% of the general population may suffer from vertigo/dizziness and migraine just by pure coincidence (see below).

The incidence of vertigo in association with migraine has been reported to range between 25% and 70%, if sensations of dizziness, light-headedness, and unsteadiness are included under the heading of vertigo (Kuritzky et al., 1981b; Kayan and Hood, 1984; Harker and Rassekh, 1987, 1988; Kelman and Tanis, 2006; Vukovic et al., 2007). This high rate does not, however, reflect the clinical importance of vertigo in relation to other more characteristic and distressing symptoms of migraine, since only one-third of these patients report the typical symptoms of "vestibular vertigo." According to others (Kayan and Hood, 1984; Muri and Meienberg, 1993), vertigo appears to be either the major symptom or a severe complication of migraine in only 5–8% of patients.

Several epidemiological studies using different approaches have evaluated the correlation between migraine and vertigo. The prevalence of migraine (according to the IHS criteria) in 200 patients who went to a dizziness clinic was 38% and 24% in 200 age- and sex-matched control patients from an orthopedic clinic ($P < 0.01$) (Neuhauser et al., 2001). These findings were confirmed by a second study: the prevalence of migraine was significantly higher (61.1%) in 72 patients with isolated recurrent vertigo of unknown cause than in a sex- and age-matched control group of orthopedic patients (24%) (Lee et al., 2002). Complementary studies on patients with known migraine showed that episodic vertigo occurs in 25–35% of these patients (Kuritzky et al., 1981a; Kayan and Hood, 1984; Baloh, 2006). A direct comparison of both groups showed that the prevalence of migrainous vertigo was 7% in the dizziness clinic group, and 9% in the migraine clinic group (Neuhauser et al., 2001).

Several other studies have demonstrated that the prevalence of migraine in patients with vertigo is considerably higher than in the general population (Aragones et al., 1993; Savundra et al., 1997), for instance 61% versus 10% (Lee et al., 2002). A different approach showed that only 9 out of 116 patients with tension headache suffered from vertigo (8%), whereas 53 out of 200 patients (27%) with migraine also had vertigo/dizziness. All in all, these epidemiological data provide evidence that there seems to be a causative association between migraine and vertigo/dizziness.

On the basis of the above-mentioned quite strict diagnostic criteria (Neuhauser et al., 2001) (Table 62.2), the 1-year prevalence for migraine-vertigo/vestibular migraine was 0.89% and the lifetime prevalence was 0.98%. In comparison, the 1-year prevalence for BPPV – the most common cause of vertigo – is about 1.6%, and 0.51% for Menière's disease (Neuhauser et al., 2006; Neuhauser, 2007). It is important to note that patients thus afflicted contact dizziness specialists first and foremost and not headache specialists, since their prevailing complaint is distressing vertigo/dizziness. Over the last two decades those who manage dizzy patients have increasingly realized that migraine is an important cause of various forms of episodic vertigo. It is one of the most frequent neurological syndromes and a cause of vertigo (in particular in young females); it is diagnosed in neurological dizziness units with a relative frequency of 9–10% (Table 62.6) (Neuhauser et al., 2001; Brandt et al., 2005). However, migraine-vertigo/vestibular migraine is still underdiagnosed, especially if the attacks of vertigo lack a temporal relationship with typical migraine symptoms (Dieterich and Brandt, 1999; Neuhauser and Lempert, 2004; Brantberg et al., 2005; Brandt and Strupp, 2006). This is also supported by the above-mentioned study (Neuhauser et al., 2006): two-thirds of participants with migraine-vertigo/vestibular migraine had consulted a doctor, but only 20% of these had been correctly diagnosed.

The initial manifestation may occur at any time of life (Dieterich and Brandt, 1999; Neuhauser et al., 2001; Brantberg et al., 2005). Two studies showed that migraine often begins earlier than migraine-vertigo/vestibular migraine headache (Dieterich and Brandt, 1999; Neuhauser et al., 2001). A typical course in many patients is that their migraine headache becomes better and subsequently they develop migraine-vertigo/vestibular migraine without headache (Dieterich and Brandt,

Table 62.6

The frequency of different vertigo/dizziness syndromes in 8,546 patients seen in a neurological dizziness unit

Diagnosis	Frequency	
	n	%
BPPV	1583	18.5
Phobic postural vertigo	1335	15.6
Central-vestibular vertigo	999	11.7
Vestibular migraine	904	10.6
Menière's disease	803	9.4
Neuritis vestibularis	625	7.3
Bilateral vestibulopathy	538	6.3
Vestibular paroxysmia	342	4.0
Psychogenic vertigo	267	3.1
Perilymph fistula	54	0.6
Unknown vertigo syndromes	255	3.0
Other disorders	841	9.8

1999; Neuhauser et al., 2001). As is the case for migraine, females are more frequently affected than males (1.5–5:1) (Cass et al., 1997; Johnson, 1998; Dieterich and Brandt, 1999; Neuhauser et al., 2001).

DIFFERENTIAL DIAGNOSIS

The differential diagnosis does not primarily cover only headache syndromes but also different vestibular disorders. When recurrent vertigo attacks are associated with headache and other migrainous symptoms in a patient with known migraine and normal hearing, the diagnosis is easy. In many patients, however, other causes must be ruled out, namely Menière's disease and episodic ataxia type 2, both of which can mimic migraine-vertigo (Strupp et al., 2007), vestibular paroxysmia (caused by neurovascular cross-compression of the eighth nerve: Brandt and Dieterich, 1994), and non-vestibular dizziness in migraine. Furthermore, as in typical aura without headache (ICHD-II 1.2.3), a distinction from more serious diagnoses such as transient ischemic attack has to be made (Rathore et al., 2002; Kerber et al., 2006; Murray et al., 2007). In a large retrospective study it was shown that only 3% of "dizzy patients" presenting to an emergency department were diagnosed to have stroke (Kerber et al., 2006). Transient pure vertigo was even more rarely caused by cerebrovascular ischemia: only 0.7% (9 of 1,297) of those with isolated dizziness/vertigo had had a stroke/transient ischemic attack (Kerber et al., 2006).

Benign paroxysmal vertigo of childhood and benign recurrent vertigo in adults

In contrast to migraine-vertigo/vestibular migraine, "benign paroxysmal vertigo of childhood" is included in the ICHD-II. The diagnostic criteria are given in Table 62.7.

Table 62.7

Diagnostic criteria of benign paroxysmal vertigo of childhood according to the second edition of the International Classification of Headache Disorders (Headache Classification Subcommittee of the International Headache Society, 2004)

A. At least five attacks fulfilling criterion B
B. Multiple episodes of severe vertigo,* occurring without warning and resolving spontaneously after minutes to hours
C. Normal neurological examination and audiometric and vestibular functions between attacks
D. Normal electroencephalogram

*Often associated with nystagmus or vomiting; unilateral throbbing headache may occur in some attacks.

The prevalence of vertigo in children, in particular "benign paroxysmal vertigo of childhood," was evaluated in several studies. In a questionnaire designed to determine the prevalence of migraine and migraine equivalents in children of school age, they included an item on "attacks of dizziness in the past year" (Abu-Arafeh and Russell, 1995; Russell and Abu-Arafeh, 1999). This questionnaire was administered to 2,165 children. A total of 314 children had experienced at least one episode of dizziness in the year before examination; this remained unexplained in 44%. A total of 57 children with three attacks (either unexplained or attributed to migraine) were interviewed and examined. Forty-five fulfilled the criteria for benign paroxysmal vertigo of childhood (prevalence rate 2.6%, 95% confidence interval 1.9–3.4). Other symptoms suggestive of migraine were found in a small majority, but in 47% paroxysmal vertigo was an isolated symptom. The age of onset peaked at 12 years, but it was seen in all age groups. Paroxysmal vertigo was commonly accompanied by other features of migraine and migraine was twice as common in first-degree relatives compared to controls (24% versus 10.6%). The authors concluded that "benign paroxysmal vertigo of childhood" is indeed common in children but seldom diagnosed (Abu-Arafeh and Russell, 1995; Russell and Abu-Arafeh, 1999). This is supported by other studies (Weisleder and Fife, 2001; Al-Twaijri and Shevell, 2002; Wiener-Vacher, 2004; Niemensivu et al., 2007). For instance, in a survey of 5,848 children, 1,106 of whom were migraineurs, 108 patients (1.8% of total, 9.8% of migraineurs) were identified to have "benign paroxysmal vertigo of childhood" (Al-Twaijri and Shevell, 2002). In the migraineurs benign paroxysmal vertigo was the most frequent equivalent of migraine: 41 patients (38%). Further, Weisleder and Fife (2001) reviewed the charts of all children and adolescents referred for vestibular function testing in a specialized center. The most common reason for vestibular testing referral was the combination of dizziness and headache. The final diagnoses were vestibular migraine ($n = 11$), benign paroxysmal vertigo of childhood ($n = 6$), anxiety attacks ($n = 3$), and Menière's disease ($n = 2$). The stereotypical patient with vestibular migraine was a teenage female with repeated episodes of headache and dizziness, a past history of carsickness, a family history of migraine, and a normal neurological examination. The author pointed out that patients who fit this profile are likely to have migrainous vertigo. During a long-term follow-up of 7 cases of benign paroxysmal vertigo, it was found that the benign paroxysmal vertigo of 5 of 7 patients spontaneously resolved and 6 of 7 patients later developed migraine and other migraine-related symptoms (Lanzi et al., 1994). This course differed from that described for migraine-vertigo only in the age of onset of headache and in the chronological relationship with vertigo. All these authors suggested that benign paroxysmal vertigo is closely related to migraine and can be interpreted as a precursor of migraine.

This view is not supported by other studies, namely long-term studies. For instance, according to a follow-up in 19 children (13–20 years after diagnosis) in whom attacks of vertigo had begun 5 months to 8 years before, the symptoms disappeared between the age of 3 months and 8 years (Lindskog et al., 1999). Twenty-one percent developed migraine, i.e., more than the normal population of this age, and 39% had a family history of migraine, i.e., less than in a migraine population. None suffered from vertigo or a balance disorder. The authors concluded that benign paroxysmal vertigo has a favorable outcome, and may not be a general precursor of migraine. These data are still controversial. Long-term follow-up studies with strict inclusion criteria are necessary to resolve this controversy.

Nevertheless, since there are basically no differences between this entity and migraine-vertigo/vestibular migraine except for the age of manifestation, one might consider classifying these patients as migraine-vertigo/vestibular migraine in analogy with other forms of migraine with aura, in which age is also a criterion. This is also true for the term "benign recurrent vertigo in adults," because its signs and symptoms are sufficiently characterized by migraine-vertigo/vestibular migraine with/or without accompanying headache. Further, almost 90% of patients with "benign recurrent vertigo" meet the diagnostic criteria for migraine and the onset of migraine precedes the onset of vertigo attacks by an average of 14 years (Cha et al., 2009).

Menière's disease

The American Academy of Ophthalmology and Otolaryngology, Head and Neck Surgery formulated the diagnostic criteria for Menière's disease in 1995 which are given in Table 62.8. In several patients it is difficult to differentiate migraine-vertigo/vestibular migraine from Menière's disease, especially at the beginning of the course of the disease: it is well known in dizziness units that an acute single attack in some patients with episodic vertigo cannot be attributed to either migraine or Menière's disease with certainty (Cutrer and Baloh, 1992; Brandt, 1999; Dieterich and Brandt, 1999; Radtke et al., 2002; Neuhauser and Lempert, 2004). Further, there is an overlap between both disorders, i.e., a considerable number of patients suffer from both at the same time. A positive link between migraine and Menière's disease was already mentioned by Menière himself (Menière, 1861). Later others published support

Table 62.8

Diagnostic criteria of Menière's disease according to the American Academy of Ophthalmology and Otolaryngology, Head and Neck Surgery, 1995

Certain Menière's disease
Histopathological confirmation of endolymphatic hydrops
Symptoms as in criteria for definite Menière's disease

Definite Menière's disease
Two or more attacks of vertigo, each lasting more than 20 min
Audiometrically documented hearing loss in at least one examination
Tinnitus or aural fullness in the affected ear
Other causes excluded

Probable Menière's disease
At least one vertigo episode
Audiometrically documented hearing loss in at least one examination
Tinnitus or aural fullness in the affected ear
Other causes excluded

Possible Menière's disease
Episodic vertigo but without documented hearing loss
Sensorineural hearing loss, fluctuating or fixed, with disequilibrium, but without definite episodes of vertigo
Other causes excluded

for this view (Atkinson, 1962; Kayan and Hood, 1984). A controlled study provided well-documented evidence for such an association (Radtke et al., 2002): 72 patients with idiopathic unilateral and bilateral Menière's disease, according to the above-mentioned criteria (Neuhauser et al., 2001), were compared with age- and sex-matched controls (Radtke et al., 2002). The lifetime prevalence of migraine with and without aura was higher in the group with Menière's disease (56%) compared to controls (25%; $P < 0.001$); in other studies the prevalence ranged between 22% and 76% (Baloh, 2006; Perez et al., 2006). Further, 45% of patients with Menière's disease experienced at least one migrainous symptom (migrainous headache, photophobia, aura symptoms) with Menière attacks. The authors concluded that the frequent occurrence of migrainous symptoms during Menière attacks suggests a pathophysiological link between the two diseases. There might be, for instance, a common neurotransmitter imbalance or ion channel dysfunction (see below) (Neuhauser and Lempert, 2004; Minor, 2005).

Alternatively, since migraine itself is a frequent cause of audiovestibular symptoms, current diagnostic criteria may not differentiate between Menière's disease and migraine-vertigo/vestibular migraine. One hallmark of Menière's disease is impairment of hearing, which may help to differentiate both entities. Therefore, hearing function was compared in 76 patients with migraine-associated dizziness and 34 with Menière's disease (Battista, 2004). Pure-tone average and low-frequency pure-tone average were significantly worse for patients with Menière's disease. Only 3 patients in the migraine-associated dizziness group had an elevated pure-tone average ($\geq$26 dB) and/or low-frequency pure-tone average. In contrast, in the Menière's disease group only 2 patients had normal hearing. Therefore, audiometric findings may help to distinguish migraine-associated dizziness from late Menière's disease.

Regarding treatment, patients thus afflicted often have to be treated for both disorders simultaneously.

Episodic ataxia type 2

Often episodic ataxia 2 and vestibular migraine cannot be differentiated solely by clinical presentation. Both disorders are characterized by a combination of episodic vertigo or ataxia as well as ocular motor disturbances in the spell-free interval. Monosymptomatic presentations of vestibular migraine without headaches occur in up to 30% of cases. In a subgroup of patients with a familial hemiplegic migraine there is a genetic linkage to the *CACNA1A* gene, which is most often the mutated gene locus in episodic ataxia 2. The frequency of *CACNA1A* gene mutations in migraine-vertigo/vestibular migraine is not known (Table 62.9).

Vestibular paroxysmia

Vestibular paroxysmia is suspected if a patient suffers from brief and frequent attacks of vertigo. This form of disorder is most likely caused by a neurovascular cross-compression in the root entry zone of the eighth cranial nerve, analogous to trigeminal neuralgia (Brandt and Dieterich, 1994). Clinical criteria are given in Table 62.10.

Motion sickness-like symptoms

Episodic vestibular vertigo, as described above, must be distinguished from longer-lasting motion sickness-like symptoms. It is striking that patients with both vestibular migraine and migraine without aura complain of motion sickness (up to 50%), i.e., normal body motion provokes dizziness and nausea during the attack. Therefore it was speculated that the pathomechanism of migraine and motion sickness may involve the hyperexcitability of vestibular receptors (Cutrer and Baloh, 1992). Susceptibility to motion sickness is higher in migraineurs than in controls with tension headache or headache-free subjects (Kuritzky et al., 1981b; Neuhauser and Lempert, 2004); this is especially true in children (Barabas et al., 1983). To prevent motion sickness, migraineurs should avoid vigorous head motion and large-field visual motion stimulation during the attack.

Association of migraine with other vertigo disorders

BPPV was reported to be frequently associated with migraine (Kayan and Hood, 1984; Ishiyama et al., 2000; Lempert et al., 2000). Migraine was twice as common in patients with idiopathic BPPV than in age- and sex-matched controls (Lempert et al., 2000) and three times as common in patients with idiopathic

Table 62.9

Similarities between episodic ataxia type 2 and migraine-vertigo/vestibular migraine

	Episodic ataxia type 2	Migraine-vertigo/vestibular migraine
Clinical features	Recurrent attacks of vertigo imbalance and ataxia (minutes to hours)	Spontaneous recurrent attacks of vertigo/ dizziness (minutes to hours)
	Migraine headaches (>50%)	Associated with headache or other migrainous symptoms (60–70%)
	In the majority, familial history	In the majority an individual or familial history of migraine
Examination findings during attacks	Pathological positional nystagmus (70%)	Pathological spontaneous or positional nystagmus (70%)
	Ataxia/postural imbalance (>90%)	Postural imbalance (90%)
During attack-free interval	Central ocular motor signs (>90%)	Central ocular motor signs (>60%)
		Peripheral vestibular deficit (10–20%)
Genetic background	*CACNA1A* mutations (60%)	*CACNA1A* mutations in familial hemiplegic migraine, none found in vestibular migraine yet
Treatment of choice	Acetazolamide, 4-aminopyridine	Beta-blockers, valproic acid, topiramate

(Modified from Strupp et al., 2007; data adapted from Jen et al., 2004; Brandt and Strupp, 2006.)

Table 62.10

Clinical criteria of vestibular paroxysmia

Short attacks of rotatory or to-and-fro vertigo last for seconds to minutes with instability of posture and gait
Attacks most often occur spontaneously but may be triggered in some patients by particular head positions, hyperventilation, or the attack may be influenced by changing the head position
Rarely transient unilateral hypacusis or tinnitus during the attack
In some patients in the course of the disease, measurable vestibular and/or cochlear deficits increase during the attack, but they are less pronounced during the attack-free interval (neurophysiological function tests used include audiogram, acoustic evoked potentials, caloric testing, test for subjective visual vertical)
Attacks are improved or lessened by administering carbamazepine (even low dosage is effective)
No central vestibula/ocular motor disorders or brainstem signs

(Modified from Brandt and Dieterich, 1994; Brandt et al., 2005.)

BPPV than in patients with posttraumatic BPPV (Ishiyama et al., 2000); up to almost 60% of patients with BPPV suffer from migraine (Uneri, 2004). It was also shown that patients with migraine-vertigo/vestibular migraine as well as patients with Menière's disease show a high psychiatric comorbidity, even though vestibular tests were normal (Best et al., 2006). Furman et al. (2005) hypothesized the existence of a new disorder called migraine-anxiety-related dizziness, in which the different symptoms share the same pathophysiological mechanism.

PATHOPHYSIOLOGY, MECHANISMS, AND GENETICS

As in migraine with aura, several underlying mechanisms are discussed, namely, vasospasm, spreading depression associated with a dysfunction of voltage-sensitive ion channels or neurotransmitters.

As regards the specific aspects of the pathophysiology of migraine-vertigo/vestibular migraine, a vasospasm within the vestibular and/or auditory labyrinth may explain: (1) the acute onset of vertigo and/or hearing problems; (2) the observed peripheral vestibular spontaneous nystagmus in some patients, which indicates a central or peripheral vestibular tone imbalance; (3) the persisting vestibular and (rare) auditory deficits (Viirre and Baloh, 1996; Cass et al., 1997; Lee et al., 2000; Baloh, 2006; Jen, 2008); and (4) the association between migraine-vertigo/vestibular migraine and Menière's disease. The latter is caused by endolymphatic hydrops, which can develop due to labyrinthine ischemia (Lee et al., 2000).

Several neurotransmitters and neuromodulators are involved in neurotransmission in the inner ear, such as glutamate, acetylcholine, or calcitonin gene-related peptide. It is speculated that they may be involved in the pathophysiology of the aura, which may arise in migraine-vertigo/vestibular migraine from the brainstem as well as the inner ear. No substantial progress, however, has been achieved in the last decade. An interesting hypothesis is that there is a simultaneous involvement of the vestibular nuclei, the trigeminal system, and the thalamocortical pathways (Furman et al., 2003). This may well explain why patients with migraine-vertigo/vestibular migraine have central and peripheral vestibular as well as central ocular motor disturbances during the attack and in the attack-free interval.

These hypotheses are supported by experiments in animals and humans. Studies in the mouse showed that the intravenous administration of serotonin induced plasma extravasation in the murine inner ear, namely in the apical spiral ganglion, modiolus, and intralabyrinthine superior and inferior vestibular nerve. In contrast, there was no significant serotonin-induced plasma extravasation in the brain parenchyma, Scarpa's ganglion, basal spiral ganglion and modiolus, or the central vestibular nerve segment. This seems to be a possible mechanism of migraine-associated inner-ear dysfunction with vertigo and sound sensitivity (Koo and Balaban, 2006). Another candidate is capsaicin and capsaicin-induced permeability changes in the basilar and cochlear vascular bed with release of substance P via the trigeminal fibers (Vass et al., 2001, 2004). The authors proposed that vertigo, tinnitus, and hearing deficits associated with migraine may arise from perturbations of capsaicin-sensitive trigeminal sensory ganglion neurons projecting to the cochlea.

In an elegant study in humans it was demonstrated that trigeminal stimulation elicits nystagmus, indicating a peripheral vestibular tone imbalance in migraine patients but not in healthy controls. Two electrodes for electrical stimulation were applied on the supraorbital point of one side of the head and the intensity of stimulation corresponding to pain threshold was calculated. Supraorbital painful electrical stimulation was able to modify or to evoke nystagmus in 8 of 10 migraineurs but in none of the 10 volunteers. It was concluded that painful trigeminal stimulation can induce an imbalance of the vestibular system in migraine patients and this possibly explains their predisposition to vertigo (Marano et al., 2005).

Details of the genetics of migraine with aura are described in Chapter 6 (Wessman et al., 2004, 2007; Colson et al., 2007). Migraine-vertigo/vestibular migraine is a genetically heterogeneous disorder. Several loci were identified in different families, for instance 1q31 (Lea et al., 2002), 4q24 (Wessman et al., 2002), 5q21 ((Nyholt et al., 2005), or 11q (Baloh, 2006; Lee et al., 2008). The locus 19p13 and thereby the *CACNA1A* gene, which encodes the PQ-calcium channel, is of special interest. Mutations of this gene cause FHM, spinocerebellar ataxia 6, and episodic ataxia type 2 (see above), and thus it seems to be of particular interest. However, despite intensive work in this field by many groups, no mutations have been found in patients with migraine-vertigo/vestibular migraine (Kim et al., 1998; Baloh, 2006; von Brevern et al., 2006). This is also true for "benign recurrent vertigo" (Lee et al., 2006). However, the number of patients examined so far is quite small; for instance, in the study by von Brevern et al. (2006), only 14 patients were examined with a mutation analysis of the coding exons and exon/intron junctions of *CACNA1A*, *ATP1A2*, *SCN1A*, and *CACNB4*. There is an ongoing genome-wide search for candidate genes in these patients which may elucidate this open question.

TREATMENT

The treatment of migraine with aura is described in Chapter 26. Theoretically, the treatment of migraine-vertigo/vestibular migraine should not differ from these treatment regimens. The evidence published so far, however, for medical treatment of the acute attacks and prevention of the attacks (Kayan and Hood, 1984; Dieterich and Brandt, 1999; Maione, 2006; Strupp and Brandt, 2006; Baier et al., 2009b; Fotuhi et al., 2009) is weak, since it is only based on case reports and observational studies. In our management of more than 500 patients with vestibular migraine over the last two decades, we have had the clinical experience that both acute and prophylactic medication (with beta-blockers, valproic acid, and now more often with topiramate) effectively suppresses the acute attacks and reduces the frequency of attacks. For migraine-vertigo/vestibular migraine there are no controlled, double-blind studies so far. Observational studies on the treatment of migraine-related dizziness and vertigo recommend physical therapy and exercise programs (Whitney et al., 2000) as well as dietary changes (Johnson, 1998; Reploeg and Goebel, 2002) as prophylactic treatment. For treatment of the acute attack the following substances have been reported anecdotally: ergotamines (Dieterich and Brandt, 1999), sumatriptan (Bikhazi et al., 1997; Evans and Baloh, 2001), and for prophylactic treatment: lamotrigine (Bisdorff, 2004) and topiramate (Carmona and Settecase, 2005; Olesen et al., 2005), which is well tolerated (Silberstein et al., 2006). The only controlled study on the efficacy of oral triptans (zolmitriptan) was conducted in fewer than 20 patients and remained inconclusive due to its limited power (Neuhauser et al., 2003). In an observational trial with a systematic diagnostic approach but without a control group or a masked design, 53 patients with migraine-related vertigo were selected from a cohort of 652 vertiginous patients. Inclusion criteria were at least five vertigo attacks occurring in any period of time or dizziness and/or positional vertigo for at least 6 months; migraine, past or present; a family history of migraine and/or motion intolerance; and exclusion of other causes. Patients were submitted to migraine pharmacological prophylaxis on the basis of their characteristics and of the drug side-effects. The efficacy of the treatment was evaluated after 6 months by a questionnaire with five outcome categories (resolution, substantial control, moderate control, minimal control, and no improvement or worsening) and, for patients with recurrent vertiginous attacks, it also reported the percentage reduction of the attack frequency. Thirty-six patients completed the study: 10 reported complete resolution of symptoms, 15 substantial control, 7 moderate control, 1 minimal control, and 3 no improvement. Thirty-three of them had recurrent vertigo: 19 reported complete disappearance of the attacks, 8 reduction of the frequency >50%, 5 reduction <50%, and 1 no reduction. The authors concluded that migraine prophylactic treatment shows encouraging results in patients with migraine-related vertigo who had been selected with our inclusion criteria: 69.3% reported satisfactory control of symptoms and 81.8% had at least a 50% reduction of the vertiginous episode frequency.

A multicenter approach with a controlled, double-masked design is imperative for studies on the acute and prophylactic treatment of migraine-vertigo/vestibular migraine in which the differential effects on vertigo and/or headache should also be evaluated in order to screen a large number of patients for inclusion; to apply nasal, sublingual, subcutaneous, or rectal application routes, which may offer faster relief of vertigo, thus allowing the inclusion of patients with nausea and with attacks lasting less than 2 h; and to include a conservative power estimation that takes a drop-out rate of about 50% into consideration (Neuhauser et al., 2003).

CONCLUDING COMMENTS

Migraine-vertigo/vestibular migraine is a disease entity that accounts for approximately 10% of all patients presenting at a dizziness unit and is the most frequent cause of spontaneous episodic vertigo in children and adults. We advocate its inclusion in the next edition of the ICHD.

Olesen (2005), in contrast, has published some arguments against treating "migrainous vertigo" as a specific subtype similar to hemiplegic migraine or basilar-type migraine. He argues that, if vertiginous symptoms are regarded as just one of more manifestations of migraine, then it follows logically that no specific subcategory of migraine is needed. Further, he stresses that the treatment efficacy cited is very weak and the response to prophylactic agents is a useless criterion as these drugs have multiple actions that affect other symptoms than migraine (Olesen, 2005). Finally, he considers the category of probable migrainous vertigo meaningless, if it only requires recurrent episodic vestibular symptoms plus one of a range of migraine symptoms, as previously proposed (Neuhauser and Lempert, 2004). These points sound logical; however, benign paroxysmal vertigo of childhood and "typical aura without headache" have been included in ICHD-I and II, and these conditions mostly occur without associated headache.

In our opinion vestibular migraine requires a place as a specific subcategory of migraine in the ICHD. This category should be separate and distinct from basilar-type migraine. Benign paroxysmal vertigo of childhood should be subsumed under the category, especially since it manifests as monosymptomatic episodic vertigo in two-thirds and without associated headache in one-third of attacks. This entity is clinically highly relevant: many neurologists are not yet aware that migraine is the most common cause of spontaneous episodic vertigo, even if patients do not fulfill the current criteria of the IHS. We have seen numerous patients with frequent distressing attacks of vertigo who had contacted many doctors before receiving the beneficial prophylactic treatment for migraine. We prefer the term "vestibular migraine" rather than "migraine-vertigo" or "migrainous vertigo," since the latter could be understood as one heterogeneous symptom among others of migraine and could refer to vestibular dysfunction, orthostatic hypotension, motion sickness, or drug-induced dizziness. Thus, vestibular migraine is characterized by features summarized in Table 62.11. For clinical trials, however, more restrictive criteria should now be used and, for instance, only patients with recurrent attacks of vertigo accompanied by headache or other migrainous symptoms should be included.

Table 62.11

Clinical characteristics of migraine-vertigo/vestibular migraine

Clinical features
Spontaneous recurrent attacks of vertigo/dizziness (prevailing type rotational) most often lasting minutes to hours
Associated with headache or other migrainous symptoms (60–70%)
In the majority an individual history of migraine according to the International Headache Society criteria
Examination findings
During the attack
Pathological spontaneous or positional nystagmus (about 70%)
Postural imbalance (about 90%)
During the attack-free interval
Central ocular motor signs (>60%) less severe than in the attack
Peripheral vestibular deficit (10–20%)
Diagnostic tests and procedures to exclude other entities
Basic tests for migraine-vertigo/vestibular migraine
Neuro-ophthalmological and neuro-otological examinations
Tests for Menière's disease
Auditory testing
Oculography with caloric irrigation
Tests for transient ischemic attacks
Magnetic resonance imaging (MRI)
Doppler sonography
Tests for vestibular paroxysmia
MRI (constructive interference in steady state (CISS) sequence) of the eighth nerve and treatment with carbamazepine

Acknowledgment

The authors thank Judy Benson and Katie Ogston for critically reading the manuscript.

References

Abu-Arafeh I, Russell G (1995). Paroxysmal vertigo as a migraine equivalent in children: a population-based study. Cephalalgia 15: 22–25.

Al-Twaijri WA, Shevell MI (2002). Pediatric migraine equivalents: occurrence and clinical features in practice. Pediatr Neurol 26: 365–368.

American Academy of Ophthalmology and Otolaryngology (1995). Committee on Hearing and Equilibrium guidelines for diagnosis and evaluation of therapy in Menière's disease. Otolaryngol Head Neck Surg 113: 181–185.

Aragones JM, Fortes-Rego J, Fuste J et al. (1993). Migraine: an alternative in the diagnosis of unclassified vertigo. Headache 33: 125–128.

Atkinson M (1962). Migraine and Meniere's disease. Arch Otolaryngol 75: 220–225.

Baier B, Stieber N, Dieterich M (2009a). Vestibular-evoked myogenic potentials in vestibular migraine. J Neurol 256: 436–442.

Baier B, Winkenwerder E, Dieterich M (2009b). "Vestibular migraine": effects of prophylactic therapy with various drugs. A retrospective study. J Neurol 256: 436–442.

Baloh RW (2006). Migraine and vertigo: epidemiology, genetics, and mechanisms. Headache Currents 3: 1–7.

Barabas G, Matthews WS, Ferrari M (1983). Childhood migraine and motion sickness. Pediatrics 72: 188–190.

Battista RA (2004). Audiometric findings of patients with migraine-associated dizziness. Otol Neurotol 25: 987–992.

Best C, Eckhardt-Henn A, Diener G et al. (2006). Interaction of somatoform and vestibular disorders. J Neurol Neurosurg Psychiatry 77: 658–664.

Bikhazi P, Jackson C, Ruckenstein MJ (1997). Efficacy of antimigrainous therapy in the treatment of migraine-associated dizziness. Am J Otol 18: 350–354.

Bir LS, Ardic FN, Kara CO et al. (2003). Migraine patients with or without vertigo: comparison of clinical and electronystagmographic findings. J Otolaryngol 32: 234–238.

Bisdorff AR (2004). Treatment of migraine related vertigo with lamotrigine an observational study. Bull Soc Sci Med Grand Duche Luxemb 2: 103–108.

Brandt T (1999). Vertigo; Its Multisensory Syndromes. 2nd edn. Springer, London.

Brandt T (2004). A chameleon among the episodic vertigo syndromes: "migrainous vertigo" or "vestibular migraine". Cephalalgia 24: 81–82.

Brandt T, Dieterich M (1994). Vestibular paroxysmia: vascular compression of the eighth nerve? Lancet 343: 798–799.

Brandt T, Strupp M (2006). Migraine and vertigo: classification, clinical features, and special treatment considerations. Headache Currents 3: 12–19.

Brandt T, Dieterich M, Strupp M (2005). Vertigo and Dizziness – Common Complaints. Springer, London.

Brantberg K, Trees N, Baloh RW (2005). Migraine-associated vertigo. Acta Otolaryngol 125: 276–279.

Carmona S, Settecase N (2005). Use of topiramate (Topamax) in a subgroup of migraine-vertigo patients with auditory symptoms. Ann N Y Acad Sci 1039: 517–520.

Cass SP, Furman JM, Ankerstjerne K et al. (1997). Migraine-related vestibulopathy. Ann Otol Rhinol Laryngol 106: 182–189.

Celebisoy N, Gokcay F, Sirin H et al. (2008). Migrainous vertigo: clinical, oculographic and posturographic findings. Cephalalgia 28: 72–77.

Cha YH, Lee H, Santell LS et al. (2009). Association of benign recurrent vertigo and migraine in 208 patients. Cephalalgia 29: 550–555.

Colson NJ, Fernandez F, Lea RA et al. (2007). The search for migraine genes: an overview of current knowledge. Cell Mol Life Sci 64: 331–344.

Crevits L, Bosman T (2005). Migraine-related vertigo: towards a distinctive entity. Clin Neurol Neurosurg 107: 82–87.

Cutrer FM, Baloh RW (1992). Migraine-associated dizziness. Headache 32: 300–304.

Davis A, Moorjani P (2003). The epidemiology of hearing and balance disorders. In: LM Luxon, JM Furman, A Martini et al. (Eds.), Textbook of Audiological Medicine. Martin Dunitz, London, pp. 89–99.

Dieterich M, Brandt T (1999). Episodic vertigo related to migraine (90 cases): vestibular migraine? J Neurol 246: 883–892.

Dursteler MR (1975). [Migraine and the vestibular apparatus (author's transl.)]. J Neurol 210: 253–269.

Eggers SD (2007). Migraine-related vertigo: diagnosis and treatment. Curr Pain Headache Rep 11: 217–226.

Erbek SH, Erbek SS, Yilmaz I et al. (2006). Vertigo in childhood: a clinical experience. Int J Pediatr Otorhinolaryngol 70: 1547–1554.

Evans RW, Baloh RW (2001). Episodic vertigo and migraine. Headache 41: 604–605.

Eviatar L (1981). Vestibular testing in basilar artery migraine. Ann Neurol 9: 126–130.

Fotuhi M, Glaun B, Quan SY et al. (2009). Vestibular migraine: a critical review of treatment trials. J Neurol 256: 711–716.

Furman JM, Marcus DA, Balaban CD (2003). Migrainous vertigo: development of a pathogenetic model and structured diagnostic interview. Curr Opin Neurol 16: 5–13.

Furman JM, Sparto PJ, Soso M et al. (2005). Vestibular function in migraine-related dizziness: a pilot study. J Vestib Res 15: 327–332.

Hannaford PC, Simpson JA, Bisset AF et al. (2005). The prevalence of ear, nose and throat problems in the community: results from a national cross-sectional postal survey in Scotland. Fam Pract 22: 227–233.

Harker LA, Rassekh CH (1987). Episodic vertigo in basilar artery migraine. Otolaryngol Head Neck Surg 96: 239–250.

Harker LA, Rassekh C (1988). Migraine equivalent as a cause of episodic vertigo. Laryngoscope 98: 160–164.

Harno H, Hirvonen T, Kaunisto MA et al. (2003). Subclinical vestibulocerebellar dysfunction in migraine with and without aura. Neurology 61: 1748–1752.

Headache Classification Subcommittee of the International Headache Society (2004). The international classification of headache disorders, 2nd edn. Cephalalgia 24: 1–160.

Hirtz D, Thurman DJ, Gwinn-Hardy K et al. (2007). How common are the "common" neurologic disorders? Neurology 68: 326–337.

Ishiyama A, Jacobson KM, Baloh RW (2000). Migraine and benign positional vertigo. Ann Otol Rhinol Laryngol 109: 377–380.

Ishizaki K, Mori N, Takeshima T et al. (2002). Static stabilometry in patients with migraine and tension-type headache during a headache-free period. Psychiatry Clin Neurosci 56: 85–90.

Jen JC (2008). Recent advances in the genetics of recurrent vertigo and vestibulopathy. Curr Opin Neurol 21: 3–7.

Jen J, Kim GW, Baloh RW (2004). Clinical spectrum of episodic ataxia type 2. Neurology 62: 17–22.

Johnson GD (1998). Medical management of migraine-related dizziness and vertigo. Laryngoscope 108: 1–28.

Kayan A, Hood JD (1984). Neuro-otological manifestations of migraine. Brain 107: 1123–1142.

Kelman L, Tanis D (2006). The relationship between migraine pain and other associated symptoms. Cephalalgia 26: 548–553.

Kerber KA, Brown DL, Lisabeth LD et al. (2006). Stroke among patients with dizziness, vertigo, and imbalance in the emergency department: a population-based study. Stroke 37: 2484–2487.

Kim JS, Yue Q, Jen JC, Nelson SF et al. (1998). Familial migraine with vertigo: no mutations found in CACNA1A. Am J Med Genet 79: 148–151.

Kirchmann M, Thomsen LL, Olesen J (2006). Basilar-type migraine: clinical, epidemiologic, and genetic features. Neurology 66: 880–886.

Koo JW, Balaban CD (2006). Serotonin-induced plasma extravasation in the murine inner ear: possible mechanism of migraine-associated inner ear dysfunction. Cephalalgia 26: 1310–1319.

Kroenke K, Price RK (1993). Symptoms in the community. Prevalence, classification, and psychiatric comorbidity. Arch Intern Med 153: 2474–2480.

Kroenke K, Lucas C, Rosenberg ML et al. (1994). One-year outcome for patients with a chief complaint of dizziness. J Gen Intern Med 9: 684–689.

Kroenke K, Hoffman RM, Einstadter D (2000). How common are various causes of dizziness? A critical review. South Med J 93: 160–167.

Kuritzky A, Toglia UJ, Thomas D (1981a). Vestibular function in migraine. Headache 21: 110–112.

Kuritzky A, Ziegler DK, Hassanein R (1981b). Vertigo, motion sickness and migraine. Headache 21: 227–231.

Lanzi G, Balottin U, Fazzi ET et al. (1994). Benign paroxysmal vertigo of childhood: a long-term follow-up. Cephalalgia 14: 458–460.

Lea RA, Shepherd AG, Curtain RP et al. (2002). A typical migraine susceptibility region localizes to chromosome 1q31. Neurogenetics 4: 17–22.

Lee H, Lopez I, Ishiyama A et al. (2000). Can migraine damage the inner ear? Arch Neurol 57: 1631–1634.

Lee H, Sohn SI, Jung DK et al. (2002). Migraine and isolated recurrent vertigo of unknown cause. Neurol Res 24: 663–665.

Lee H, Jen JC, Wang H et al. (2006). A genome-wide linkage scan of familial benign recurrent vertigo: linkage to 22q12 with evidence of heterogeneity. Hum Mol Genet 15: 251–258.

Lee H, Jen JC, Cha YH et al. (2008). Phenotypic and genetic analysis of a large family with migraine-associated vertigo. Headache 48: 1460–1467.

Lempert T, Neuhauser H (2005). Migrainous vertigo. Neurol Clin 23: 715–730,vi.

Lempert T, Neuhauser H (2009). Epidemiology of vertigo, migraine and vestibular migraine. J Neurol 256: 333–338.

Lempert T, Leopold M, von Brevern M et al. (2000). Migraine and benign positional vertigo. Ann Otol Rhinol Laryngol 109: 1176.

Lindskog U, Odkvist L, Noaksson L et al. (1999). Benign paroxysmal vertigo in childhood: a long-term follow-up. Headache 39: 33–37.

Maione A (2006). Migraine-related vertigo: diagnostic criteria and prophylactic treatment. Laryngoscope 116: 1782–1786.

Marano E, Marcelli V, Di SE et al. (2005). Trigeminal stimulation elicits a peripheral vestibular imbalance in migraine patients. Headache 45: 325–331.

Marcus DA, Kapelewski C, Rudy TE et al. (2004). Diagnosis of migrainous vertigo: validity of a structured interview. Med Sci Monit 10: CR197–CR201.

Menière P (1861). Mémoire sur les lésions de l'oreille interne donnant lieu a des symptomes de congestion cérébrale apoplectiforme. Gaz Med Paris Sér 3: 597–601.

Minor LB (2005). Meniere's disease and migraine. Arch Otolaryngol Head Neck Surg 131: 460.

Moretti G, Manzoni GC, Caffarra P et al. (1980). "Benign recurrent vertigo" and its connection with migraine. Headache 20: 344–346.

Muri RM, Meienberg O (1993). [Vertigo and migraine.] Schweiz Med Wochenschr 123: 1331–1336.

Murray S, Bashir K, Lees KR et al. (2007). Epidemiological aspects of referral to TIA clinics in Glasgow. Scott Med J 52: 4–8.

Neuhauser HK (2007). Epidemiology of vertigo. Curr Opin Neurol 20: 40–46.

Neuhauser H, Lempert T (2004). Vertigo and dizziness related to migraine: a diagnostic challenge. Cephalalgia 24: 83–91.

Neuhauser H, Leopold M, von Brevern M et al. (2001). The interrelations of migraine, vertigo, and migrainous vertigo. Neurology 56: 436–441.

Neuhauser H, Radtke A, von Brevern M et al. (2003). Zolmitriptan for treatment of migrainous vertigo: a pilot randomized placebo-controlled trial. Neurology 60: 882–883.

Neuhauser HK, Radtke A, von BM et al. (2006). Migrainous vertigo: prevalence and impact on quality of life. Neurology 67: 1028–1033.

Niemensivu R, Kentala E, Wiener-Vacher S et al. (2007). Evaluation of vertiginous children. Eur Arch Otorhinolaryngol 264: 1129–1135.

Nyholt DR, Morley KI, Ferreira MA et al. (2005). Genome-wide significant linkage to migrainous headache on chromosome 5q21. Am J Hum Genet 77: 500–512.

Olesen J (2005). Vertigo and dizziness related to migraine: a diagnostic challenge. Cephalalgia 25: 761–762.

Olesen J, Carmona S, Settecase N et al. (2005). Vertigo and dizziness related to migraine: a diagnostic challenge. Cephalalgia 25: 761–762.

Perez LL, Belinchon de DA, Bermell CA et al. (2006). [Meniere's disease and migraine.] Acta Otorrinolaringol Esp 57: 126–129.

Radtke A, Lempert T, Gresty MA et al. (2002). Migraine and Meniere's disease: is there a link? Neurology 59: 1700–1704.

Rathore SS, Hinn AR, Cooper LS et al. (2002). Characterization of incident stroke signs and symptoms: findings from the atherosclerosis risk in communities study. Stroke 33: 2718–2721.

Reploeg MD, Goebel JA (2002). Migraine-associated dizziness: patient characteristics and management options. Otol Neurotol 23: 364–371.

Russell G, Abu-Arafeh I (1999). Paroxysmal vertigo in children – an epidemiological study. Int J Pediatr Otorhinolaryngol 49 (Suppl. 1): S105–S107.

Savundra PA, Carroll JD, Davies RA et al. (1997). Migraine-associated vertigo. Cephalalgia 17: 505–510.

Silberstein SD, Hulihan J, Karim MR et al. (2006). Efficacy and tolerability of topiramate 200 mg/d in the prevention of migraine with/without aura in adults: a randomized, placebo-controlled, double-blind, 12-week pilot study. Clin Ther 28: 1002–1011.

Slater R (1979). Benign recurrent vertigo. J Neurol Neurosurg Psychiatry 2: 363–367.

Stahl JS, Daroff RB (2001). Time for more attention to migrainous vertigo? Neurology 56: 428–429.

Stewart W, Simon D, Shechter A et al. (1995). Population variation in migraine prevalence: a meta-analysis. J Clin Epidemiol 153: 2474–2480.

Strupp M, Brandt T (2006). Pharmacological advances in the treatment of neuro-otological and eye movement disorders. Curr Opin Neurol 19: 33–40.

Strupp M, Zwergal A, Brandt T (2007). Episodic ataxia type 2. Neurotherapeutics 4: 267–273.

Teggi R, Colombo B, Bernasconi L et al. (2009). Migrainous vertigo: results of caloric testing and stabilometric findings. Headache 49: 435–444.

Toglia JU, Thomas D, Kuritzky A (1981). Common migraine and vestibular function. Electronystagmographic study and pathogenesis. Ann Otol Rhinol Laryngol 90: 267–271.

Uneri A (2004). Migraine and benign paroxysmal positional vertigo: an outcome study of 476 patients. Ear Nose Throat J 83: 814–815.

Vass Z, Steyger PS, Hordichok AJ et al. (2001). Capsaicin stimulation of the cochlea and electric stimulation of the trigeminal ganglion mediate vascular permeability in cochlear and vertebro-basilar arteries: a potential cause of inner ear dysfunction in headache. Neuroscience 103: 189–201.

Vass Z, Dai CF, Steyger PS et al. (2004). Co-localization of the vanilloid capsaicin receptor and substance P in sensory nerve fibers innervating cochlear and vertebro-basilar arteries. Neuroscience 124: 919–927.

Versino M, Sances G, Anghileri E et al. (2003). Dizziness and migraine: a causal relationship? Funct Neurol 18: 97–101.

Viirre ES, Baloh RW (1996). Migraine as a cause of sudden hearing loss. Headache 36: 24–28.

von Brevern M, Radtke A, Clarke AH et al. (2004). Migrainous vertigo presenting as episodic positional vertigo. Neurology 62: 469–472.

von Brevern M, Zeise D, Neuhauser H et al. (2005). Acute migrainous vertigo: clinical and oculographic findings. Brain 128: 365–374.

von Brevern M, Ta N, Shankar A et al. (2006). Migrainous vertigo: mutation analysis of the candidate genes CACNA1A, ATP1A2, SCN1A, and CACNB4. Headache 46: 1136–1141.

Vukovic V, Plavec D, Galinovic I et al. (2007). Prevalence of vertigo, dizziness, and migrainous vertigo in patients with migraine. Headache 47: 1427–1435.

Waterston J (2004). Chronic migrainous vertigo. J Clin Neurosci 11: 384–388.

Weisleder P, Fife TD (2001). Dizziness and headache: a common association in children and adolescents. J Child Neurol 16: 727–730.

Wessman M, Kallela M, Kaunisto MA et al. (2002). A susceptibility locus for migraine with aura, on chromosome 4q24. Am J Hum Genet 70: 652–662.

Wessman M, Kaunisto MA, Kallela M et al. (2004). The molecular genetics of migraine. Ann Med 36: 462–473.

Wessman M, Terwindt GM, Kaunisto MA et al. (2007). Migraine: a complex genetic disorder. Lancet Neurol 6: 521–532.

Whitney SL, Wrisley DM, Brown KE et al. (2000). Physical therapy for migraine-related vestibulopathy and vestibular dysfunction with history of migraine. Laryngoscope 110: 1528–1534.

Wiener-Vacher SR (2004). [Vertigo in children.] Arch Pediatr 11: 1542–1545.

Yardley L, Owen N, Nazareth I et al. (1998). Prevalence and presentation of dizziness in a general practice community sample of working age people. Br J Gen Pract 48: 1131–1135.

Handbook of Clinical Neurology, Vol. 97 (3rd series)
Headache
G. Nappi and M.A. Moskowitz, Editors

Chapter 63

Pharmacological migraine provocation: a human model of migraine

MESSOUD ASHINA * AND JAKOB MØLLER HANSEN
Danish Headache Center and Department of Neurology, Glostrup Hospital, Faculty of Health Sciences, University of Copenhagen, Copenhagen, Denmark

INTRODUCTION

The last two decades of migraine research have shown that translational research is crucial in drug development. Animal experiments are necessary to separate and analyze different components of the migraine attack such as the transmission of nociceptive impulses, vascular reactions, and the role of inflammatory mechanisms (Reuter et al., 2001). However, an animal model that is identical or almost identical to human migraine has not yet been developed, and eventually all predictions from animal studies need to be confirmed in a suitable human model. Human experimental models of migraine allow the study of the pathophysiological events during an attack. This is not always possible during spontaneous migraine attacks because disability inhibits migraineurs from traveling to the hospital. Furthermore, experimental models allow migraine attacks to be studied under carefully controlled and monitored conditions, which is a definitive advantage from a scientific viewpoint. In the present chapter the most important experimental human models of migraine will be outlined and discussed.

GLYCERYL TRINITRATE-INDUCED MIGRAINE

Nitric oxide (NO) involvement in migraine has been analyzed in a series of provocation experiments using nitroglycerine, glyceryl trinitrate (GTN) as an NO donor (Iversen et al., 1989). It has for many years been known that GTN induces headache (Hering, 1849). Patients with a migraine history may, also experience a delayed migraine attack after administration of GTN. However, many important details of GTN-induced headache, such as headache time profile, pain characteristics, and accompanying symptoms, were not previously recorded. This has been investigated in placebo-controlled studies. Olesen et al. (1993) demonstrated that patients with migraine were hypersensitive to NO, i.e. migraineurs developed significantly stronger headache after GTN infusion than healthy subjects. Furthermore, Thomsen et al. (1994) reported that patients with migraine without aura developed an immediate headache during GTN infusion and that 80% of patients developed a delayed headache, fulfilling International Headache Society (IHS) criteria for migraine several hours after the infusion was stopped. This study has clearly shown that GTN may trigger a genuine migraine attack in migraine sufferers and that NO may play a crucial role in migraine pathogenesis. The next question was whether NO was involved throughout the duration of a migraine attack. To test this hypothesis Lassen et al. (1997) examined the antimigraine action of the non-selective NO synthase (NOS) inhibitor, N^{G}-monomethyl-L-arginine (L-NMMA). This proof-of-concept study demonstrated that NOS inhibition was effective in treating spontaneous migraine attacks. These data have greatly stimulated the pharmaceutical industry to develop selective NOS inhibitors, which have already entered clinical phase II trials (Bart Van der Schueren et al., 2007; www.clinicaltrials.gov, 2008).

Neurobiological mechanisms of GTN-induced migraine-like attacks are not fully clarified. An immediate headache after GTN infusion may originate from NO-induced activation and/or sensitization of sensory nerves around extra- and intracranial arteries

*Correspondence to: Messoud Ashina, MD, PhD, DrSci, Danish Headache Center and Department of Neurology, Glostrup Hospital, Faculty of Health Sciences, University of Copenhagen, DK-2600 Glostrup, Copenhagen, Denmark, E-mail: ashina@dadlnet.dk

(Holthusen and Arndt, 1995) or from NO-induced arterial dilation (Tegeler et al., 1996), or both. In support, GTN induces a 23–30% increase in the cross-sectional area of the middle cerebral artery (MCA) during immediate headache in healthy subjects (Hansen et al., 2007). However, mechanisms of delayed migraine are complex and cannot be explained by dilation of the cerebral arteries (Schoonman et al., 2008). Reuter et al. (2001) reported macrophage inducible NOS (iNOS) up-regulation and dural mast cell granular changes consistent with secretion 4 and 6 h after GTN infusion. These data suggest a possible antimigraine action of iNOS inhibitors. However, other mechanisms, such as GTN induced liberation of calcitonin gene-related peptide (CGRP) (Bellamy et al., 2006) or brainstem activation (Afridi et al., 2005), should also be considered.

In summary, experimental studies have clearly shown that NO plays a crucial role in the initiation of migraine attacks and that the delayed headache phase may reflect pathophysiological events that occur during spontaneous migraine attack. Furthermore, human models suggest a possible antimigraine action of NOS inhibitors.

HISTAMINE-INDUCED MIGRAINE

In 1957, Sicuteri et al. reported that intravenous or subcutaneous injection of histamine may induce a short-lasting throbbing headache (Sicuteri et al., 1957). Krabbe and Olesen (1980) infused increasing doses of histamine to patients with migraine without aura, patients with chronic tension-type headache, and healthy controls. In a dose-dependent fashion, migraine patients developed more severe and more pulsating headache than healthy subjects. There was no report on either accompanying symptoms or observation of delayed headache in this short study. These important data were collected systematically in a study by Lassen et al. (1995). In this double-blind study patients with migraine without aura were randomized to receive either mepyramine (H_1-receptor blocker) or placebo before histamine infusion. Patients who received both histamine and pretreatment with placebo developed a biphasic nociceptive response with a headache peak during infusion (immediate headache), a reduction in headache intensity for approximately 2 h (intermediate phase), and a second headache peak several hours later (delayed headache). Seventy percent of patients experienced a migraine-like attack fulfilling the diagnostic criteria for migraine without aura (Lassen et al., 1995). Interestingly, the time profile of the histamine-induced headache in patients is strikingly similar to the time profile of GTN-induced headache in patients with migraine without aura (Thomsen et al., 1994). The histamine-induced headache was also accompanied by a prolonged decrease in MCA blood flow velocity throughout a 3-h observation. Interestingly, mepyramine blocked not only the histamine-induced headache but also the histamine-induced decrease in MCA velocity (Lassen et al., 1995). Given that activation of endothelial H_1-receptors induces the endogenous formation of NO, it is possible that histamine-induced migraine is caused by hypersensitivity to activation of the NO pathway. However, NOS inhibitor in the highest possible dose did not block the histamine-induced headache response or arterial dilation (Lassen et al., 2003). This suggests that histamine dilates arteries and causes headache via NO-independent mechanisms.

PHOSPHODIESTERASE INHIBITION AND MIGRAINE

NO activates intracellular soluble guanylate cyclase and thus catalyzes the formation of cyclic guanosine monophosphate (cGMP). Sildenafil (Viagra), a highly selective inhibitor of phosphodiesterase 5 (PDE5), is the major enzyme responsible for the breakdown of cGMP. Inhibition of this enzyme results in accumulation of cGMP, and the effect of sildenafil could therefore mimic the effects of NO, such as activation of soluble guanylate cyclase and increased cGMP formation. To test this hypothesis Kruuse and colleagues (2003) included 12 patients with migraine without aura in a double-blind, placebo-controlled, crossover study, in which placebo or sildenafil 100 mg was administered orally on two separate days. Migraine-like attack was induced by sildenafil in 10 of 12 migraine patients and by placebo in 2 of 12 patients. The authors also found that blood flow velocity in the MCA, regional cerebral blood flow in the territory of the MCA, and diameters of radial and temporal artery were unaffected by sildenafil (Kruuse et al., 2003). Thus, it appears that sildenafil-triggered experimental migraine is induced via a cGMP-dependent mechanism, and that this occurs without initial dilation of the MCA. The authors proposed that triggering mechanisms might reside within the perivascular sensory nerve terminals or the brainstem (Kruuse et al., 2003). However, future studies are needed to explore the molecular sites of action responsible for sildenafil-induced experimental migraine. Another important outcome of this study is that patients using sildenafil should also be informed about the risk of migraine attacks.

The migraine and headache-eliciting effect of the PDE5 inhibitor dipyridamole was examined in a single-blind study, including 10 migraineurs and 10 healthy controls (Kruuse et al., 2006). This study showed that dipyridamole induced headache in all patients and migraine attack in 50% of patients.

The headache-generating effect of cilostazol, an inhibitor of PDE3, has been studied in healthy subjects (Birk et al., 2006). The participants received either cilostazol 200 mg or placebo. The authors reported that cilostazol induced moderate headache in 11 of 12 participants with no family history of migraine. The headache had migraine-like features such as pulsating pain quality and aggravation by physical activity. In two participants, the symptoms fulfilled the criteria for migraine without aura. Interestingly, cilostazol is one of the most important cyclic adenosine monophosphate (cAMP)-degrading enzymes in cerebral arteries and it has been suggested that not only cGMP- but also cAMP-dependent pathways may be involved in the pathogenesis of head pain (Birk et al., 2006). Whether cilostazol may induce migraine pain should be examined in future studies.

CGRP-INDUCED MIGRAINE

McCulloch et al. (1986) demonstrated that a dense supply of CGRP-containing fibers originated in the trigeminal ganglion around the cerebral vessels. This was the first report of CGRP involvement in the trigeminovascular reflex. In 1988 Goadsby et al. reported that CGRP was released into the extracerebral circulation of humans during thermocoagulation of the trigeminal ganglion. Studies in migraine patients showed elevation of CGRP during (Goadsby et al., 1990) and outwith migraine attacks (Ashina et al., 2000). However, a recent study challenged these reports, showing no changes in plasma CGRP during migraine attacks compared to outwith attacks (Tvedskov et al., 2005).

Despite this controversy, the importance of CGRP in migraine pathogenesis became firmly established using the experimental migraine model. Lassen et al. (2002) conducted a double-blind crossover study, where human α-CGRP (2 μg/min) or placebo was infused for 20 min in 12 patients suffering from migraine without aura. During the following 11 h all patients experienced headaches after human α-CGRP and only 1 patient after placebo. In 3 patients after human α-CGRP, but in no patients after placebo, the delayed headache fulfilled the IHS criteria for migraine without aura (Lassen et al., 2002).

Mechanisms responsible for CGRP-induced migraine attacks are unknown. Using the mean velocity of blood flow in the middle cerebral artery (V_{MCA}) and the corresponding cerebral blood flow values, the CGRP infusion caused a modest 7.5% increase in MCA diameter, which makes it unlikely that vasodilation is the mechanism of CGRP-induced migraine (Lassen et al., 2008). CGRP receptor activation leads to increased cAMP levels (Jansen et al., 1992; Jansen-Olesen et al., 1996). Cilostazol, an inhibitor of cAMP degradation, may induce pronounced headache and migraine-like pain in healthy subjects (Birk et al., 2006), which suggests that increased levels of cAMP may contribute to CGRP-induced headache and migraine.

Findings of increased ictal levels of CGRP and hypersensitivity to CGRP infusion in migraineurs triggered interest in CGRP antagonism as a potential target for antimigraine drugs. This has now been confirmed in a phase II clinical trial showing that olcegepant (BIBN 4096), a selective CGRP antagonist, was effective in treating acute migraine attacks (Olesen et al., 2004). Recently an oral CGRP receptor antagonist, telcagepant, was shown to be effective in a phase II trial (Ho et al., 2008) and this drug is now in phase III.

Collectively, the CGRP model of migraine predicted a key role of CGRP in migraine pathogenesis and confirmed the antimigraine action of CGRP antagonists.

VASOACTIVE INTESTINAL PEPTIDE AND PITUITARY ADENYLATE CYCLASE ACTIVATING POLYPEPTIDE-INDUCED MIGRAINE

Release of vasoactive peptides during attacks could be the result of activation of a brainstem reflex (Edvinsson and Petersen, 2007), where activation of trigeminal nerves and subsequent nociceptive signaling to the central nervous system mediates a parasympathetic reflex arc during migraine, leading to the release of neuropeptides, NO, and acetylcholine (Burstein and Jakubowski, 2005).

Vasoactive intestinal peptide (VIP) and pituitary adenylate cyclase activating polypeptide (PACAP) are found in perivascular parasympathetic nerve fibers (Jansen-Olesen et al., 2004), and PACAP is also found in trigeminal nerve fibers surrounding cerebral blood vessels (Baeres and Moller, 2004). Their release regulates cerebrovascular tone and hemodynamics of the brain (Gulbenkian et al., 2001). Two receptors, $VPAC_1$ (Hosoya et al., 1993) and $VPAC_2$ (Lutz et al., 1993), are activated with equal affinity by PACAP and VIP, but a third receptor, PAC_1, is selectively activated by PACAP (Harmar et al., 1998).

The headache-eliciting effect of VIP and its effect on brain hemodynamics have been systematically studied in both healthy volunteers (Hansen et al., 2006) and in patients with migraine without aura (Rahmann et al., 2008). The systemic administration of VIP induces only a very mild and short-lasting headache, and no migraine attacks. VIP does not seem to be a trigger factor for headache and migraine, and VIP is probably not critically involved in migraine pathogenesis.

The headache/migraine-provoking effects of PACAP38 were studied in double-blind placebo-controlled crossover studies in both healthy subjects

Table 63.1

Percentages of patients who reported migraine-like attacks in experimental studies

Compound		Dose	Migraine-like attacks	Reference
Glyceryl trinitrate	Migraine with aura	Intravenous 0.5 μg/kg/min	50–67%	Christiansen et al., 1999; Afridi et al., 2004
		Sublingual 0.9 mg	40.9%	Sances et al., 2004
	Migraine without aura	Intravenous 0.5 μg/kg/min	80–83%	Thomsen et al., 1994; Afridi et al., 2004
		Sublingual 0.9 mg	82.1%	Sances et al., 2004
Histamine		Intravenous 0.5 μg/kg/min	70%	Lassen et al., 1995
Sildenafil		100 mg per os	83%	Kruuse et al., 2003
Dipyridamole		Intravenous 0.142 mg/kg/min	50%	Kruuse et al., 2006
Calcitonin gene-related peptide	Migraine without aura	Intravenous 2 μg/min	33%	Lassen et al., 2002
	Hemiplegic migraine	Intravenous 1.5 μg/min	22%	Hansen et al., 2008b
Vasoactive intestinal peptide		Intravenous 8 pmol/kg/min	0%	Rahmann et al., 2008
Pituitary adenylate cyclase activating polypeptide		Intravenous 10 pmol/ kg/min	66%	Schytz et al., 2009

and migraine patients. Infusion of the most predominant form, PACAP38, in healthy subjects induced vasodilation of a similar magnitude to VIP but longer lasting (Birk et al., 2007). Furthermore, PACAP38 was found to induce sustained cephalic vasodilation and migraine attacks in migraine patients without aura (Schytz et al., 2009). Given that VIP infusion does not cause migraine, the shared VIP/PACAP receptors are unlikely to be causal for induction of migraine after PACAP38 infusion. The migraine induction by PACAP38, in contrast to VIP, might be due to active transport across the blood–brain barrier or to the action of PACAP38 on the selective PAC_1 receptor. Further studies are warranted to investigate the pronociceptive mechanisms of PACAP and its receptors (Table 63.1).

CAN WE USE EXPERIMENTAL MODELS TO STUDY FUNCTIONAL CONSEQUENCES OF MIGRAINE MUTATIONS?

Familial hemiplegic migraine (FHM) is a rare, dominantly inherited subtype of migraine with aura, where hemiplegia occurs during the aura phase (Headache Classification Subcommittee of the International Headache Society, 2004).

The identification of the mutated FHM genes (Ophoff et al., 1996; De Fusco et al., 2003; Dichgans et al., 2005) stimulated interest in the link between genotype and phenotype using both molecular studies and animal models. Thus, FHM knock-in mice showed increased susceptibility to cortical spreading depression (van den Maagdenberg et al., 2004). The functional consequences of the FHM mutations in humans, however, are unknown, and the potential species differences should be considered. Genotyped FHM patients offer us the chance to study the interplay between genotype and phenotype and may be regarded as a valuable genetic migraine model (van de Ven et al., 2007). A series of experiments using the human experimental model examined whether the FHM mutations were associated with hypersensitivity to the migraine triggers NO and CGRP. It was shown that both GTN and CGRP failed to induce more migraine aura or migraine headache in FHM patients than in healthy controls (Hansen et al., 2008a, b, c). These data indicate that the FHM genotype does not confer hypersensitivity to migraine triggers such as GTN and CGRP. Moreover, these findings raise the question whether FHM shares neurobiological background with common types of migraine.

CAN WE USE EXPERIMENTAL MODELS TO TEST ACUTE AND PREVENTIVE ANTIMIGRAINE DRUGS?

Experimental headache models may help us to explore molecular mechanisms of action of existing antimigraine drugs. The effect of sumatriptan on GTN-induced headache has been examined in several studies (Iversen and Olesen, 1996; Schmetterer et al., 1996; Fullerton et al., 1999). In a double-blind cross-over study Iversen and Olesen (1996) injected subcutaneously sumatriptan 6 mg or placebo in 10 healthy subjects, followed by GTN infusion. This study demonstrated that sumatriptan significantly reduced the GTN-induced immediate headache and the temporal and radial artery diameter. Another study by Schmetterer et al. (1996) confirmed the efficacy of sumatriptan in GTN-induced headache and in addition demonstrated that sumatriptan also prevents GTN-induced dilation of the MCA.

Tvedskov and colleagues (2004a) introduced for the first time the GTN model of migraine to test the effect of a prophylactic drug, valproate. This study showed that pretreatment with valproate was better than placebo in preventing migraine. In another study (Tvedskov et al., 2004b), the authors observed no effect of propranolol on GTN-induced headache and migraine.

In summary, these interesting data suggest that the GTN model of experimental headache may represent a powerful tool for testing antimigraine drugs and thereby contribute to understanding better the mechanism of action of existing and future migraine therapies (Figure 63.1).

CONCLUSION AND FUTURE PERSPECTIVES

Human models of migraine offer unique possibilities to study mechanisms responsible for migraine and to explore the mechanisms of action of existing and future antimigraine drugs. Furthermore, these models have played an important role in the translational migraine research, leading to the identification of three new, principally different, targets in the treatment of acute migraine attacks (Lassen et al., 1997; Read et al., 2001; Olesen et al., 2004). New additions to the model, such as advanced magnetic resonance imaging methods (Borsook et al., 2006; Schoonman et al., 2008), may lead to a better understanding of the complex events that constitute a migraine attack, and better and more targeted methods of intervention.

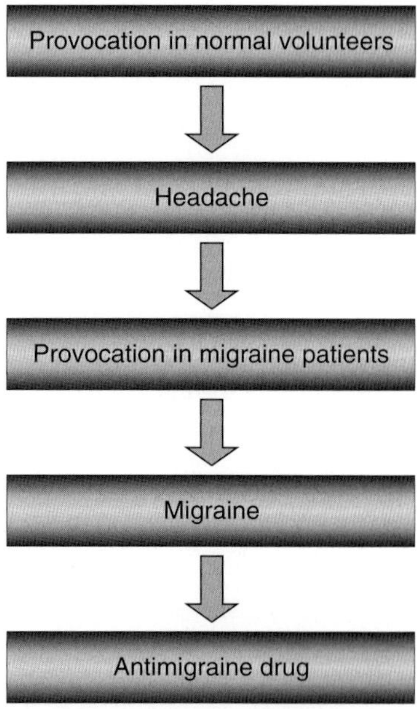

Fig. 63.1. Proposed target identification for antimigraine drug. A human provocation model has been validated and extensively used in normal volunteers and in migraine sufferers. The present experience is that normal volunteers should be used in the first instance. Only substances that produce substantial headache in healthy volunteers have the potential to induce migraine in migraine sufferers and only such substances should therefore be tested in migraine sufferers.

References

Afridi SK, Kaube H, Goadsby PJ (2004). Glyceryl trinitrate triggers premonitory symptoms in migraineurs. Pain 110: 675–680.

Afridi SK, Matharu MS, Lee L et al. (2005). A PET study exploring the laterality of brainstem activation in migraine using glyceryl trinitrate. Brain 128: 932–939.

Ashina M, Bendtsen L, Jensen R et al. (2000). Evidence for increased plasma levels of calcitonin gene-related peptide in migraine outside of attacks. Pain 86: 133–138.

Baeres FM, Moller M (2004). Origin of PACAP-immunoreactive nerve fibers innervating the subarachnoidal blood vessels of the rat brain. J Cereb Blood Flow Metab 24: 628–635.

Bart Van der Schueren MWL, Laurijssens B, Guillard F et al. (2007). iNOS inhibition in acute migraine: pharmacokinetic characteristics, safety and tolerability of GW273629. Paper presented at the International Headache Congress, Stockholm.

Bellamy J, Bowen EJ, Russo AF et al. (2006). Nitric oxide regulation of calcitonin gene-related peptide gene expression in rat trigeminal ganglia neurons. Eur J Neurosci 23: 2057–2066.

Birk S, Kruuse C, Petersen KA et al. (2006). The headache-inducing effect of cilostazol in human volunteers. Cephalalgia 26: 1304–1309.

Birk S, Sitarz JT, Petersen KA et al. (2007). The effect of intravenous PACAP38 on cerebral hemodynamics in healthy volunteers. Regul Pept 140: 185–191.

Borsook D, Burstein R, Moulton E et al. (2006). Functional imaging of the trigeminal system: applications to migraine pathophysiology. Headache 46 (Suppl. 1): S32–S38.

Burstein R, Jakubowski M (2005). Unitary hypothesis for multiple triggers of the pain and strain of migraine. J Comp Neurol 493: 9–14.

Christiansen I, Thomsen LL, Daugaard D et al. (1999). Glyceryl trinitrate induces attacks of migraine without aura in sufferers of migraine with aura. Cephalalgia 19: 660–667; discussion 626.

De Fusco M, Marconi R, Silvestri L et al. (2003). Haploinsufficiency of ATP1A2 encoding the Na^+/K^+ pump alpha2 subunit associated with familial hemiplegic migraine type 2. Nat Genet 33: 192–196.

Dichgans M, Freilinger T, Eckstein G et al. (2005). Mutation in the neuronal voltage-gated sodium channel SCN1A in familial hemiplegic migraine. Lancet 366: 371–377.

Edvinsson L, Petersen KA (2007). CGRP-receptor antagonism in migraine treatment. CNS Neurol Disord Drug Targets 6: 240–246.

Fullerton T, Komorowski-Swiatek D, Forrest A et al. (1999). The pharmacodynamics of sumatriptan in nitroglycerin-induced headache. J Clin Pharmacol 39: 17–29.

Goadsby PJ, Edvinsson L, Ekman R (1988). Release of vasoactive peptides in the extracerebral circulation of humans and the cat during activation of the trigeminovascular system. Ann Neurol 23: 193–196.

Goadsby PJ, Edvinsson L, Ekman R (1990). Vasoactive peptide release in the extracerebral circulation of humans during migraine headache. Ann Neurol 28: 183–187.

Gulbenkian S, Uddman R, Edvinsson L (2001). Neuronal messengers in the human cerebral circulation. Peptides 22: 995–1007.

Hansen J, Sitarz J, Birk S et al. (2006). Vasoactive intestinal polypeptide evokes only a minimal headache in healthy volunteers. Cephalalgia 26: 992–1003.

Hansen J, Pedersen D, Larsen VA et al. (2007). Magnetic resonance angiography shows dilatation of the middle cerebral artery after infusion of glyceryl trinitrate in healthy volunteers. Cephalalgia 27: 118–127.

Hansen J, Thomsen L, Marconi R et al. (2008a). Familial hemiplegic migraine type 2 does not share hypersensitivity to nitric oxide with common types of migraine. Cephalalgia 28: 367–375.

Hansen J, Thomsen L, Olesen J et al. (2008b). Calcitonin gene-related peptide does not cause the familial hemiplegic migraine phenotype. Neurology 71: 841–847.

Hansen J, Thomsen L, Olesen J et al. (2008c). Familial hemiplegic migraine type 1 shows no hypersensitivity to nitric oxide. Cephalalgia 28: 496–505.

Harmar AJ, Arimura A, Gozes I et al. (1998). International Union of Pharmacology. XVIII. Nomenclature of receptors for vasoactive intestinal peptide and pituitary adenylate cyclase-activating polypeptide. Pharmacol Rev 50: 265–270.

Headache Classification Subcommittee of the International Headache Society (2004). The international classification of headache disorders, 2nd edn. Cephalalgia 24: 1–160.

Hering C (1849). Glonoine, a new medicine for headache etc. Am J Homeopathy 4: 3.

Ho TW, Mannix LK, Fan X et al. (2008). Randomized controlled trial of an oral CGRP receptor antagonist, MK-0974, in acute treatment of migraine. Neurology 70: 1304–1312.

Holthusen H, Arndt JO (1995). Nitric oxide evokes pain at nociceptors of the paravascular tissue and veins in humans. J Physiol 487: 253–258.

Hosoya M, Onda H, Ogi K et al. (1993). Molecular cloning and functional expression of rat cDNAs encoding the receptor for pituitary adenylate cyclase activating polypeptide (PACAP). Biochem Biophys Res Commun 194: 133–143.

Iversen HK, Olesen J (1996). Headache induced by a nitric oxide donor (nitroglycerin) responds to sumatriptan. A human model for development of migraine drugs. Cephalalgia 16: 412–418.

Iversen HK, Olesen J, Tfelt-Hansen P (1989). Intravenous nitroglycerin as an experimental model of vascular headache. Basic characteristics. Pain 38: 17–24.

Jansen I, Mortensen A, Edvinsson L (1992). Characterization of calcitonin gene-related peptide receptors in human cerebral vessels. Vasomotor responses and cAMP accumulation. Ann N Y Acad Sci 657: 435–440.

Jansen-Olesen I, Mortensen A, Edvinsson L (1996). Calcitonin gene-related peptide is released from capsaicin-sensitive nerve fibres and induces vasodilatation of human cerebral arteries concomitant with activation of adenylyl cyclase. Cephalalgia 16: 310–316.

Jansen-Olesen I, Gulbenkian S, Engel U et al. (2004). Peptidergic and non-peptidergic innervation and vasomotor responses of human lenticulostriate and posterior cerebral arteries. Peptides 25: 2105–2114.

Krabbe AA, Olesen J (1980). Headache provocation by continuous intravenous infusion of histamine. Clinical results and receptor mechanisms. Pain 8: 253–259.

Kruuse C, Thomsen LL, Birk S et al. (2003). Migraine can be induced by sildenafil without changes in middle cerebral artery diameter. Brain 126: 241–247.

Kruuse C, Lassen LH, Iversen HK et al. (2006). Dipyridamole may induce migraine in patients with migraine without aura. Cephalalgia 26: 925–933.

Lassen LH, Thomsen LL, Olesen J (1995). Histamine induces migraine via the H1-receptor. Support for the NO hypothesis of migraine. Neuroreport 6: 1475–1479.

Lassen LH, Ashina M, Christiansen I et al. (1997). Nitric oxide synthase inhibition in migraine. Lancet 349: 401–402.

Lassen LH, Haderslev PA, Jacobsen VB et al. (2002). CGRP may play a causative role in migraine. Cephalalgia 22: 54–61.

Lassen LH, Christiansen I, Iversen HK et al. (2003). The effect of nitric oxide synthase inhibition on histamine induced headache and arterial dilatation in migraineurs. Cephalalgia 23: 877–886.

Lassen LH, Jacobsen VB, Haderslev PA et al. (2008). Involvement of calcitonin gene-related peptide in migraine: regional cerebral blood flow and blood flow velocity in migraine patients. J Headache Pain 9: 151–157.

Lutz EM, Sheward WJ, West KM et al. (1993). The VIP2 receptor: molecular characterisation of a cDNA encoding a novel receptor for vasoactive intestinal peptide. FEBS Lett 334: 3–8.

McCulloch J, Uddman R, Kingman TA et al. (1986). Calcitonin gene-related peptide: functional role in cerebrovascular regulation. Proc Natl Acad Sci U S A 83: 5731–5735.

Olesen J, Iversen HK, Thomsen LL (1993). Nitric oxide supersensitivity: a possible molecular mechanism of migraine pain. Neuroreport 4: 1027–1030.

Olesen J, Diener HC, Husstedt IW et al. (2004). Calcitonin gene-related peptide receptor antagonist BIBN 4096 BS for the acute treatment of migraine. N Engl J Med 350: 1104–1110.

Ophoff RA, Terwindt GM, Vergouwe MN et al. (1996). Familial hemiplegic migraine and episodic ataxia type-2 are caused by mutations in the Ca^{2+} channel gene CACNL1A4. Cell 87: 543–552.

Rahmann A, Wienecke T, Hansen JM et al. (2008). Vasoactive intestinal peptide causes marked cephalic vasodilation, but does not induce migraine. Cephalalgia 28: 226–236.

Read SJ, Hirst WD, Upton N et al. (2001). Cortical spreading depression produces increased cGMP levels in cortex and brain stem that is inhibited by tonabersat (SB-220453) but not sumatriptan. Brain Res 891: 69–77.

Reuter U, Bolay H, Jansen-Olesen I et al. (2001). Delayed inflammation in rat meninges: implications for migraine pathophysiology. Brain 124: 2490–2502.

Sances G, Tassorelli C, Pucci E et al. (2004). Reliability of the nitroglycerin provocative test in the diagnosis of neurovascular headaches. Cephalalgia 24: 110–119.

Schmetterer L, Wolzt M, Krejcy K et al. (1996). Cerebral and ocular hemodynamic effects of sumatriptan in the nitroglycerin headache model. Clin Pharmacol Ther 60: 199–205.

Schoonman GG, van der Grond J, Kortmann C et al. (2008). Migraine headache is not associated with cerebral or meningeal vasodilatation – a 3T magnetic resonance angiography study. Brain 131: 2192–2200.

Schytz H, Birk S, Wienecke T et al. (2009). PACAP38 induces migraine and vasodilatation in migraine without aura — a causative role in migraine pathogenesis? Brain 132: 16–25.

Sicuteri F, Ricci M, Monfardini R et al. (1957). Experimental headache with endogeneous histamine; first results obtained by 48/80, a histamine-liberator drug, in the cephalic and peripheral circulatory systems of man. Acta Allergol 11: 188–192.

Tegeler CH, Davidai G, Gengo FM et al. (1996). Middle cerebral artery velocity correlates with nitroglycerin-induced headache onset. J Neuroimaging 6: 81–86.

Thomsen LL, Kruuse C, Iversen HK et al. (1994). A nitric oxide donor (nitroglycerin) triggers genuine migraine attacks. Eur J Neurol 1: 73–80.

Tvedskov JF, Thomsen LL, Iversen HK et al. (2004a). The prophylactic effect of valproate on glyceryltrinitrate induced migraine. Cephalalgia 24: 576–585.

Tvedskov JF, Thomsen LL, Iversen HK et al. (2004b). The effect of propranolol on glyceryltrinitrate-induced headache and arterial response. Cephalalgia 24: 1076–1087.

Tvedskov JF, Lipka K, Ashina M et al. (2005). No increase of calcitonin gene-related peptide in jugular blood during migraine. Ann Neurol 58: 561–568.

van den Maagdenberg AM, Pietrobon D, Pizzorusso T et al. (2004). A Cacna1a knockin migraine mouse model with increased susceptibility to cortical spreading depression. Neuron 41: 701–710.

van de Ven RC, Kaja S, Plomp JJ et al. (2007). Genetic models of migraine. Arch Neurol 64: 643–646.

www.clinicaltrials.gov (2008). An Adaptive Design Trial of GW274150 in the Treatment of Acute Migraine. Available from http://www.clinicaltrials.gov/ct/show/NCT00319137?order = 1.

Handbook of Clinical Neurology, Vol. 97 (3rd series)
Headache
G. Nappi and M.A. Moskowitz, Editors

Chapter 64

Neuroimaging in headache

MARGARITA SÁNCHEZ DEL RIO [1]* AND JUAN ALVAREZ-LINERA [2]
[1]*Neurology Department, Hospital Ruber Internacional, Madrid, Spain*
[2]*Neuroradiology Department, Hospital Ruber Internacional, Madrid, Spain*

INTRODUCTION

Until the late 1990s, the pathophysiology of primary headache disorders was attributed to a dysfunction of the cerebrovascular regulation. Evidence from tomographic studies showing cortical hypoperfusion during the migraine aura seemed to support this hypothesis. However, more recent studies using advanced imaging technology have modified the previous theory in two major ways: (1) they clarified that the vascular changes represent an epiphenomenon of the neuronal cortical activation; and (2) they revealed the participation of subcortical structures in the modulation of the pain signal in multiple primary headache disorders.

These findings have enriched the knowledge of the complex mechanism involved in the pathogenesis of primary headache disorders.

FUNCTIONAL NEUROIMAGING OF HEADACHE

Migraine aura

The initial groundbreaking work was done by Olesen and colleagues (1981). These investigators, using xenon blood flow measurements, reported reductions in cerebral blood flow during migraine aura in posterior regions of the brain that ranged from 17% to 35% (Lauritzen and Olesen, 1984). The hypoperfusion spread towards anterior cortical regions at a rate of 2–3 mm/min, across neurovascular boundaries. Decreased blood flow persisted from 30 min to 6 h, slowly returning to baseline or even increasing above baseline. The measured cortical hypoperfusion never reached ischemic levels, although it has been argued that the values may be underestimated due to the artifact of scattered radiation, the so-called "Compton scatter effect."

Subsequent perfusion-weighted magnetic resonance imaging (MRI) studies, which are not susceptible to radiation artifacts, have corroborated that blood flow reductions observed during migraine visual aura (maximum 37%) remain well above the threshold associated with ischemic injury (>50%) (Sanchez del Rio et al., 1999). Furthermore, the use of high-field functional MRI with near-continuous recording during visual aura has revealed multiple neurovascular events in the occipital cortex within a single attack that closely resemble cortical spreading depression (CSD): (1) an initial hyperemia lasting 3–4.5 min, spreading at a rate of 3.5 mm/min; (2) followed by mild hypoperfusion lasting 1–2 h; (3) an attenuated response to visual activation; and (4) like CSD, in migraine aura, the first affected area is the first to recover (Figure 64.1) (Hadjikhani et al., 2001). In this study, the initial cortical changes were mapped to a specific visual area (V3A). V3A is known to possess a unique retinotopic representation of the visual hemifield and is an area that is motion- and contrast-sensitive.

Interestingly, a recent study has revealed increased cortical thickness bilaterally in V3A in migraineurs compared to controls (see below) (Granziera et al., 2006). Among the possible explanations for these findings is the presence of a focal dysplasia leading to exaggerated excitability of regional neurons. Alternatively, the changes observed may also develop as a consequence of repetitive migraine attacks leading to repeated glial activation following CSD. These findings, together with concomitant increased thickness in motion-sensitive area MT (middle temporal visual area), may well explain the

*Correspondence to: Margarita Sánchez del Río, Director of Headache Program, Neurology Department, Hospital Ruber Internacional, C/La Masó 38, 28034 Mirasierra, Madrid, Spain, Tel: +34 91 387 52 50, Fax: +34 91 387 53 33, E-mail: msanchezdelrio@ruberinternacional.es

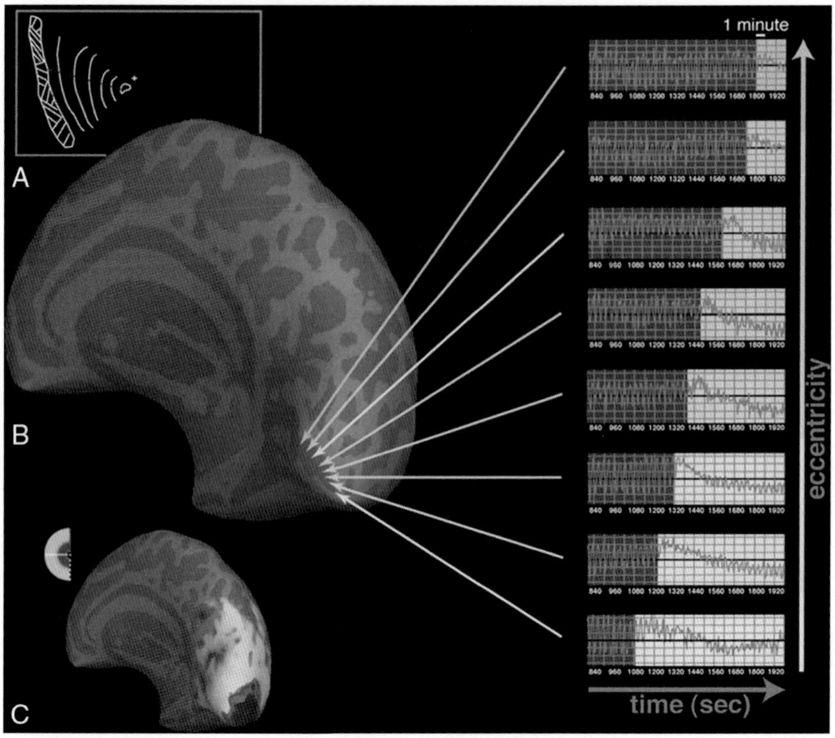

Fig. 64.1. Spreading suppression of cortical activation during migraine aura. (A) A drawing showing the progression over 20 min of the scintillations and the visual field defect affecting the left hemifield, as described by the patient. (B) A reconstruction of the same patient's brain, based on anatomical magnetic resonance (MR) data. The posterior medial aspect of occipital lobe is shown in an inflated cortex format. In this format, the cortical sulci and gyri appear in darker and lighter gray, respectively, on a computationally inflated surface. MR signal changes over time are shown to the right. Each time course was recorded from one in a sequence of voxels that were sampled along the calcarine sulcus, in the primary visual cortex (V1), from the posterior pole to a more anterior location, as indicated by arrowheads. A similar (blood oxygenation level-dependent or BOLD) response was found within all of the extrastriate areas, differing only in the time of onset of the MR perturbation. The MR perturbations developed earlier in the foveal representation, compared with more eccentric representations of retinotopic visual cortex. This finding was consistent with the progression of the aura from central to peripheral eccentricities in the corresponding visual field (A and C). (C) The MR maps of retinotopic eccentricity from this same subject, acquired during interictal scans. As shown in the logo in the upper left, voxels that show retinotopically specific activation in the fovea are coded in red (centered at 1.5° eccentricity). Parafoveal eccentricities are shown in blue, and more peripheral eccentricities are shown in green (centered at 3.8° and 10.3°, respectively). (Reproduced from Hadjikhani et al., 2001: © 2001 National Academy of Sciences, USA.)

abnormalities in motion processing frequently exhibited by migraineurs and the vulnerability of this region to facilitate migraine aura. Even though these specific visual areas have been identified so far, it is plausible that blood flow changes could also begin in other cortical areas.

Studies performed with magnetoencephalography, measuring changes in cortical magnetic fields, have shown that migraine visual aura is associated with shifts in direct current neuromagnetic field potentials, similar to those observed during CSD (Bowyer et al., 1999, 2001). These findings, together with direct evidence of an adequate local oxygen supply, support the concept of migraine as a primarily neuronal disorder, whereas vascular changes represent an epiphenomenon (Cao et al., 1999; Sanchez del Rio et al., 1999; Bowyer et al., 2001).

Migraine without aura

Silent cortical spreading depression?

The interpretation of neuroimaging findings in migraine without aura is a continuous source of debate. Studies performed during recent decades point to the possibility of a clinically silent CSD in migraine without aura.

The first positron emission tomography (PET) study during a single case of spontaneous migraine without aura attack revealed a bilateral cortical spreading hypoperfusion (Woods et al., 1994). The drop in blood flow was estimated to be 40%, starting in the visual associative cortex and progressing with time across vascular and anatomical boundaries. This cortical hypoperfusion resembled closely that observed in migraine with aura, suggesting that CSD might also occur in migraine without aura.

It took more than a decade for Geraud and colleagues (2005) to replicate this observation. In this study, 7 patients with spontaneous migraine without aura were imaged with PET within 6 h of attack onset. In all cases, a bilateral cortical hypoperfusion (10–12% reduction) was observed together with increased blood flow in the hypothalamus and rostral brainstem. Thus, once more, cortical hypoperfusion points to the presence of CSD in migraine without aura, without evident clinical correlate. Yet it has been also argued that this decreased blood flow may be secondary to the activation of brainstem noradrenergic nuclei that project to the cortex (Adams et al., 1989).

The second source of evidence is provided by the Cerebral Abnormalities in Migraine, an Epidemiological Risk Analysis (CAMERA) study (Kruit et al., 2004, 2005). This MRI study found a high prevalence of silent lesions resembling small infarcts in the posterior circulation of migraineurs. Most lesions were located in the cerebellum, more prevalent in migraine with aura (7.5%), but also present in migraine without aura (2.2%), as compared to controls (0.7%) (Kruit et al., 2005). Interestingly, there were no cardiovascular risk factors other than age. The location of these silent infarcts does not seem fortuitous: first, there is clinical evidence of cerebellar dysfunction in migraine with and without aura in up to 83% of patients (Harno et al., 2003). Second, in cases of hemiplegic migraine (mostly type I but also recently in type II), cerebellar atrophy and hypoperfusion have been documented (Crawford and Konkol, 1997; Spadaro et al., 2004). Third, proton MR spectroscopy (^{1}H-MRS) performed in cases of familial hemiplegic migraine has documented distinct metabolic abnormalities, consistent with decreased glutamate and *N*-acetyl aspartate (NAA) and elevated myoinositol in the cerebellum (Dichgans et al., 2005). These findings are consistent with neuronal impairment and glial proliferation. Therefore clinical and imaging data support a special vulnerability of the cerebellum in different types of migraine.

Based on this evidence one might speculate that repeated waves of CSD lead to silent infarcts in migraine patients in vulnerable regions such as the cerebellum versus supratentorial areas.

Subcortical structures

PET studies during migraine without aura have provided valuable information about the participation of subcortical structures in migraine pathogenesis (Figure 64.2).

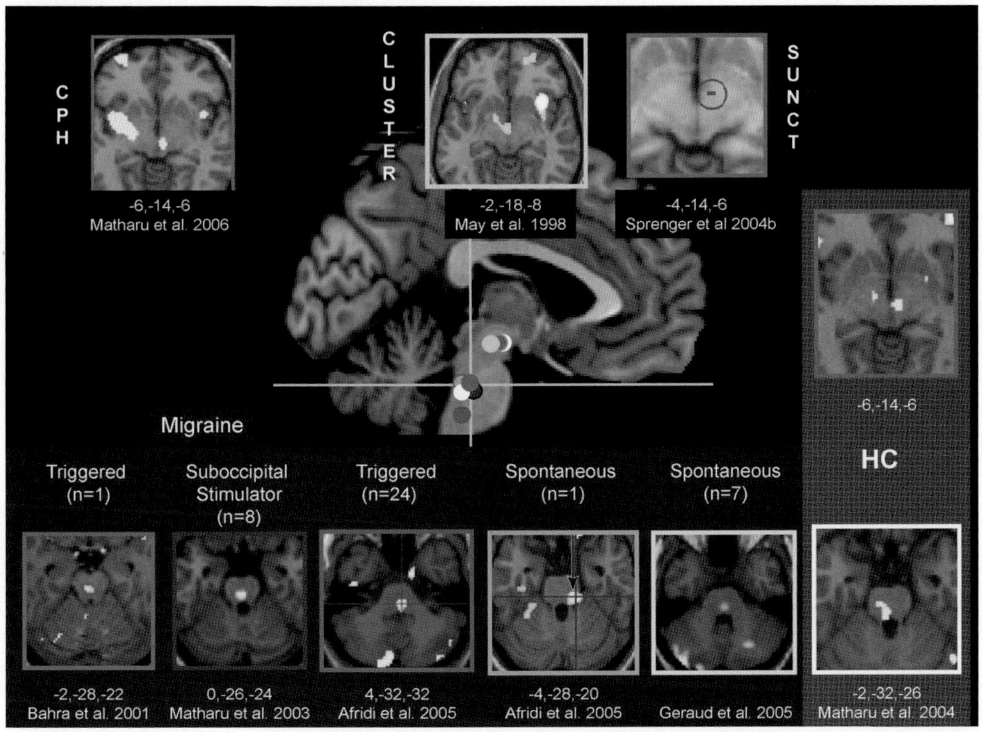

Fig. 64.2. Summary of subcortical activation in primary headache disorders. In the sagittal and axial view of the brain is represented the activation reported in multiple studies in the dorsal rostral pons for migraine and hemicrania continua. Activation in midbrain tegmentum has been reported for cluster headache, short-lasting unilateral neuralgiform paroxysms with conjunctival injection and tearing (SUNCT), hemicrania continua (HC), and chronic paroxysmal hemicrania (CPH). The numbers correspond to the Talairach coordinates. The color code framing the images corresponds to the color of the points plotted in the brain.

Weiller and colleagues (1995) studied 9 cases of spontaneous migraine without aura within 6 h of onset of pain. During the attacks, a significant increase in blood flow was found in cingulate, auditory, and visual association cortices. In addition, an increase in regional cerebral blood flow (rCBF) (+11%) was observed in medial brainstem structures, slightly contralateral to the headache side. Brainstem activation persisted after an injection of sumatriptan that induced complete relief of headache and associated symptoms. The pattern of activation in the brainstem took place in a region important for nociceptive and vascular control (locus coeruleus and dorsal raphe nucleus). The persistent increase in rCBF even after relief of symptoms reveals the importance of these structures in the pathophysiology of migraine. Subsequent PET studies during both spontaneous and glyceryl trinitrate (GTN)-triggered migraine attacks have shown activation in the brainstem in its rostral portion as well as in other brain structures related to pain processing not specific to migraine (Bahra et al., 2001; Afridi et al., 2005).

In order to determine the laterality of brainstem activation, Afridi et al. (2005) studied 24 migraine patients (8 right-sided pain, 8 left-sided pain, and 8 with bilateral pain) during a migraine attack induced using a GTN infusion. Significant activation was seen in the ipsilateral dorsal pons in the lateralized groups, and bilaterally in the bilateral headache group, with a left-side preponderance. Activation in similar areas was also observed in 8 chronic migraine patients treated with a suboccipital stimulator (Matharu et al., 2004a).

The findings of a common brainstem activation have been used as the main argument for attributing a *primun movens* role to this pontine locus in migraine pathogenesis. But further clarification is needed to establish whether these brainstem nuclei: (1) serve as migraine generator; (2) participate in modifying the threshold for neuronal activation; (3) are part of the neuronal system that terminates an attack; or (4) are required to avoid recurrence of pain.

In the study by Geraud and colleagues (2005), besides the above-mentioned cortical blood flow changes, activation was observed in the midbrain, pons, and hypothalamus. For the first time in migraine patients, activation was observed in the hypothalamus in addition to midbrain activation and cortical hypoperfusion. Unfortunately the design of the study and the timing of the imaging did not allow the authors to glimpse at the sequence of activation in different structures.

Evidence of participation of other subcortical structures such as periaqueductal gray matter has been provided by measurement of the transverse relaxation rates. This MRI method is able to quantify brain iron levels (non-heme iron). In episodic migraine and chronic daily headache a positive correlation was found between the transverse relaxation rate in the periaqueductal gray matter and duration of illness (Welch et al., 2001). This was interpreted as a selective and persistent impairment in iron homeostasis in the periaqueductal gray matter, most likely resulting from repeated migraine attacks, and hence might be a marker of the transformation from episodic to chronic daily pain.

Medication overuse headache

Glucose metabolism was investigated in 16 patients suffering from medication overuse headache (MOH) using 18-FDG PET. Studies were performed before and 3 weeks after medication withdrawal, and compared to a control population (Fumal et al., 2006). MOH patients showed hypometabolim in the thalamus (bilateral), orbifrontal cortex, anterior cingulate gyrus, insula/ventral striatum, and the right inferior parietal lobule. The cerebellar vermis was hypermetabolic. Three weeks after withdrawal and returning to an episodic migraine pattern, all areas returned to a normal metabolic pattern except the orbitofrontal cortex, where metabolic decrease was still present. The orbitofrontal cortex is known to be involved in drug dependence, thus a logical assumption is that this brain region may be involved in predisposing migraine patients to recurrent analgesics overuse.

Cluster headache

PET scans using flow measurements during cluster headache attacks have provided evidence that regions close to the hypothalamus participate in cluster headache pathogenesis (Goadsby and May, 1999). In 9 patients studied during a GTN-induced attack, significant increases in blood flow were found in the ipsilateral inferior hypothalamus and basal ganglia, contralateral posterior thalamus, bilateral cavernous sinus, cingulate, and insulae. Hypothalamic activation was also observed during a spontaneous cluster headache attack and in 10 operated chronic cluster headache patients, while switching off the hypothalamic stimulator (Sprenger et al., 2004a; May et al., 2006). Increased blood flow in the cavernous sinus was secondary to internal carotid artery vasodilation, as confirmed by MR angiography (May et al., 1999a). Hypothalamic activation was present only in cluster patients during the induced attack. The specificity of rCBF increase in the hypothalamus was confirmed by the lack of rCBF changes when experimental pain in the distribution of the first division of the trigeminal nerve was induced by applying capsaicin to the forehead. Further evidence for hypothalamic involvement has been provided by anatomical MRI of cluster patients and voxel-based morphometry analysis. This technique allows an objective and automated method of analyzing changes in brain structure (May et al., 1999b). An increase in gray-matter volume in the hypothalamus ipsilateral to the side of cluster pain was identified.

Although the true nature of this volume change is yet to be determined, measurements of the ^{1}H-MRS metabolite ratios in the hypothalamus have revealed a dysfunction or loss of neurons and myelin (Wang et al., 2006). Forty-seven episodic cluster headache patients were imaged during a cluster period as well as during the remission phase and compared to 21 controls and 16 chronic migraineurs. Due to spatial resolution and in order to increase the signal-to-noise ratio, measurements were performed bilaterally in the hypothalamus. NAA/creatine and choline/creatine ratios were significantly reduced in cluster headache compared to controls and migraineurs. No difference was found between cluster headache in the remission period and the symptomatic phase, arguing in favor of a primary abnormality rather than a secondary finding.

Short-lasting unilateral neuralgiform headache attacks with conjunctival injection and tearing (SUNCT)

A single case of SUNCT has been studied with blood oxygenation level-dependent (BOLD: May et al., 1999c). Significant activation was seen in the region of the ipsilateral hypothalamic gray, similar to what was reported in cluster headache. A second case has also revealed activation close to this same site (Sprenger et al., 2004b) (Figure 64.2).

Hemicrania continua and hemicrania paroxistica

Hemicrania continua (HC) and hemicrania paroxistica (HP) are two syndromes where a complete response to indomethacin is required for the diagnosis. The absence of pain in response to indomethacin facilitates the design of imaging studies.

To date, only one study investigated the pathogenesis of HC using PET (Matharu et al., 2004b). Seven patients were studied under three conditions: (1) during pain; (2) after treatment with indomethacin (while the patients were completely pain-free); and (3) after administration of placebo. A significant activation of the contralateral posterior hypothalamus and ipsilateral dorsal rostral pons in association with the headache was reported (Matharu et al., 2004b). In addition there was activation of the ipsilateral ventrolateral midbrain, which extended over the red nucleus and substantia nigra and bilateral pontomedullary junction. Seeing these results, one is tempted to attribute the migraine phenotype of HC to the brainstem activation, whereas the more rostral midbrain activation could be responsible for the cluster-like phenotype of HC (Figure 64.2).

Seven cases of HP were also studied using PET. Each patient was scanned in three states: (1) acute PH attack, off indomethacin; (2) pain-free, off indomethacin; and (3) pain-free after administration of intramuscular indomethacin 100 mg (Matharu et al., 2006). Authors identified activations in the contralateral posterior hypothalamic and ventral midbrain regions, besides activation in other structures of the pain neuromatrix. These areas were activated when comparing the pain state versus pain-free after administration of indomethacin. These results were not observed when the comparison was made between the pain state and pain-free state off indomethacin (stopped 24–48 h before scanning). These data point to a modulatory effect of indomethacin on the pain matrix.

STRUCTURAL IMAGING OF HEADACHE

Until quite recently the only structural abnormality reported in migraineurs compared to non-headache patients was an increased incidence of white-matter abnormalities (Figure 64.3), located mostly in the posterior circulation (Kruit et al., 2005).

Initial attempts to detect volumetric differences in gray-matter structures, similar to those observed in cluster headache, showed negative results (Matharu et al., 2003). In this study volumetric measurements using voxel-based morphometry in 11 patients with migraine with aura, 17 patients with migraine without aura, and 17 controls did not show any global or regional macroscopic structural difference between migraineurs and controls. A second attempt was performed by Rocca and colleagues (2006) using a higher-field MRI scanner in 16 migraine patients with T_2-visible

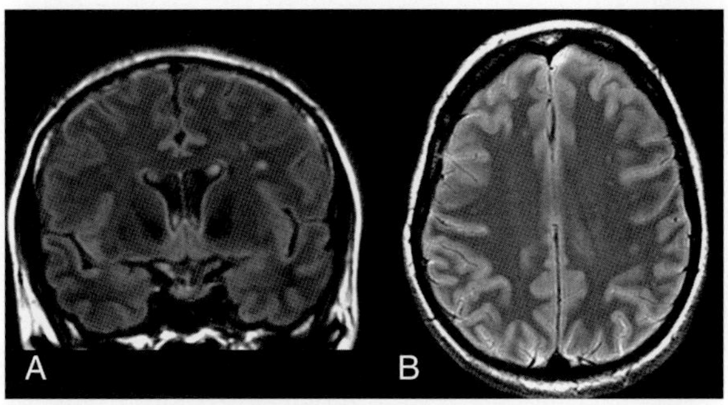

Fig. 64.3. Typical white-matter lesions observed in migraine patients. Coronal fluid-attenuated inversion recovery (A) and axial T_2-weighted image (B) showing subcortical hyperintense white-matter abnormalities in both frontal lobes.

abnormalities and 15 matched controls. Migraine patients with and without aura showed increased periacqueductal gray-matter density, while migraine with aura patients also showed increased density of the dorsolateral pons. These sites closely match the areas with increased blood flow during attacks of migraine without aura in PET studies.

In addition, quite recently an increased cortical thickness in visual areas and in the somatosensory cortex (SSC) in migraineurs has been identified (Granziera et al., 2006; DaSilva et al., 2007a, b). High-resolution cortical thickness measurement and diffusion tensor imaging (DTI) were used to examine the motion-processing network and SSC in 24 migraine patients (12 with migraine with aura and 12 with migraine without aura) and 15 age-matched controls. An increased cortical thickness of motion-processing visual areas MT+, V3A, and SSC was observed in migraineurs compared to controls. Cortical thickness increases were accompanied by abnormalities of the subjacent white matter, as measured with DTI. In addition, DTI revealed that migraineurs have alterations in the superior colliculus and lateral geniculate nucleus, which are also involved in visual processing, and along the thalamocortical tract.

In summary, recent imaging studies have provided evidence of both abnormal brain functioning and structural changes in migraineurs. In migraine aura, blood flow changes have been observed initially to occur in V3A, an area also showing morphometric abnormalities in migraine with and without aura. Pontine activation is also associated with increased volumetric changes. Similar findings are observed in the hypothalamic region in cluster headache. Thus, further studies are required in order to determine whether these changes are the cause or the consequence of the progression of the disease.

References

Adams RW, Lambert GA, Lance JW (1989). Stimulation of brainstem nuclei in the cat: effect on neuronal activity in the primary visual cortex of relevance to cerebral blood flow and migraine. Cephalalgia 9: 107–118.

Afridi SK, Giffin NJ, Kaube H et al. (2005). A positron emission tomographic study in spontaneous migraine. Arch Neurol 62: 1270–1275.

Bahra A, Matharu MS, Buchel C et al. (2001). Brainstem activation specific to migraine headache. Lancet 357: 1016–1017.

Bowyer SM, Tepley N, Papuashvili N et al. (1999). Analysis of MEG signals of spreading cortical depression with propagation constrained to a rectangular cortical strip. II. Gyrencephalic swine model. Brain Res 843: 79–86.

Bowyer SM, Aurora KS, Moran JE et al. (2001). Magnetoencephalographic fields from patients with spontaneous and induced migraine aura. Ann Neurol 50: 582–587.

Cao Y, Welch KM, Aurora S et al. (1999). Functional MRI-BOLD of visually triggered headache in patients with migraine. Arch Neurol 56: 548–554.

Crawford JS, Konkol RJ (1997). Familial hemiplegic migraine with crossed cerebellar diaschisis and unilateral meningeal enhancement. Headache 37: 590–593.

DaSilva AF, Granziera C, Snyder J et al. (2007a). Thickening in the somatosensory cortex of migraine patients. Neurology 69: 1990–1995.

DaSilva AF, Granziera C, Snyder J et al. (2007b). Interictal alterations of the trigeminal somatosensory pathway and PAG in migraine. Neuroreport 18 (4): 301–305.

Dichgans M, Herzog J, Freilinger T et al. (2005). 1H-MRS alterations in the cerebellum of patients with familial hemiplegic migraine type 1. Neurology 64: 608–613.

Fumal A, Laureys S, Di Clemente L et al. (2006). Orbitofrontal cortex involvement in chronic analgesic-overuse headache evolving from episodic migraine. Brain 129: 543–550.

Geraud G, Denuelle M, Fabre N et al. (2005). Positron emission tomographic studies of migraine. Rev Neurol (Paris) 161: 666–670.

Goadsby PJ, May A (1999). PET demonstration of hypothalamic activation in cluster headache. Neurology 52: 1522.

Granziera C, DaSilva AF, Snyder J et al. (2006). Anatomical alterations of the visual motion processing network in migraine with and without aura. PLoS Med 3: e402.

Hadjikhani N, Sanchez del Rio M, Wu O et al. (2001). Mechanisms of migraine aura revealed by functional MRI in human visual cortex. Proc Natl Acad Sci U S A 98: 4687–4692.

Harno H, Hirvonen T, Kaunisto MA et al. (2003). Subclinical vestibulocerebellar dysfunction in migraine with and without aura. Neurology 61: 1748–1752.

Kruit MC, van Buchem MA, Hofman PA et al. (2004). Migraine as a risk factor for subclinical brain lesions. JAMA 291: 427–434.

Kruit MC, Launer LJ, Ferrari MD et al. (2005). Infarcts in the posterior circulation territory in migraine. The population-based MRI CAMERA study. Brain 128: 2068–2077.

Lauritzen M, Olesen J (1984). Regional cerebral blood flow during migraine attacks by xenon-133 inhalation and emission tomography. Brain 107: 447–461.

Matharu MS, Good CD, May A et al. (2003). No change in the structure of the brain in migraine: a voxel-based morphometric study. Eur J Neurol 10: 53–57.

Matharu MS, Bartsch T, Ward N et al. (2004a). Central neuromodulation in chronic migraine patients with suboccipital stimulators: a PET study. Brain 127: 220–230.

Matharu MS, Cohen AS, McGonigle DJ et al. (2004b). Posterior hypothalamic and brainstem activation in hemicrania continua. Headache 44: 747–761.

Matharu MS, Cohen AS, Frackowiak RS et al. (2006). Posterior hypothalamic activation in paroxysmal hemicrania. Ann Neurol 59: 535–545.

May A, Buchel C, Bahra A et al. (1999a). Intracranial vessels in trigeminal transmitted pain: a PET study. Neuroimage 9: 453–460.

May A, Ashburner J, Buchel C et al. (1999b). Correlation between structural and functional changes in brain in an idiopathic headache syndrome. Nat Med 5: 836–838.

May A, Bahra A, Buchel C et al. (1999c). Functional magnetic resonance imaging in spontaneous attacks of SUNCT: short-lasting neuralgiform headache with conjunctival injection and tearing. Ann Neurol 46: 791–794.

May A, Leone M, Boecker H et al. (2006). Hypothalamic deep brain stimulation in positron emission tomography. J Neurosci 26: 3589–3593.

Olesen J, Larsen B, Lauritzen M (1981). Focal hyperemia followed by spreading oligemia and impaired activation of rCBF in classic migraine. Ann Neurol 9: 344–352.

Rocca MA, Ceccarelli A, Falini A et al. (2006). Brain gray matter changes in migraine patients with T2-visible lesions: a 3-T MRI study. Stroke 37: 1765–1770.

Sanchez del Rio M, Bakker D, Wu O et al. (1999). Perfusion weighted imaging during migraine: spontaneous visual aura and headache. Cephalalgia 19: 701–707.

Spadaro M, Ursu S, Lehmann-Horn F et al. (2004). A G301R Na^+/K^+-ATPase mutation causes familial hemiplegic migraine type 2 with cerebellar signs. Neurogenetics 5: 177–185.

Sprenger T, Boecker H, Tolle TR et al. (2004a). Specific hypothalamic activation during a spontaneous cluster headache attack. Neurology 62: 516–517.

Sprenger T, Valet M, Hammes M et al. (2004b). Hypothalamic activation in trigeminal autonomic cephalgia: functional imaging of an atypical case. Cephalalgia 24: 753–757.

Wang SJ, Lirng JF, Fuh JL et al. (2006). Reduction in hypothalamic 1H-MRS metabolite ratios in patients with cluster headache. J Neurol Neurosurg Psychiatry 77: 622–625.

Weiller C, May A, Limmroth V et al. (1995). Brain stem activation in spontaneous human migraine attacks. Nat Med 1: 658–660.

Welch KM, Nagesh V, Aurora SK et al. (2001). Periaqueductal gray matter dysfunction in migraine: cause or the burden of illness? Headache 41: 629–637.

Woods RP, Iacoboni M, Mazziotta JC (1994). Brief report: bilateral spreading cerebral hypoperfusion during spontaneous migraine headache. N Engl J Med 331: 1689–1692.

Handbook of Clinical Neurology, Vol. 97 (3rd series)
Headache
G. Nappi and M.A. Moskowitz, Editors

Chapter 65

Current and emerging therapies for migraine prevention and treatment

CHRISTIAN WAEBER [1]* AND RICHARD HARGREAVES [2]
[1]*Massachusetts General Hospital, Charlestown, MA, USA*
[2]*Merck Research Laboratories, West Point, PA, USA*

Discoveries in the field of migraine genetics, functional imaging, trigeminovascular pharmacology and physiology, and the biochemistry of events preceding and during migraine headache have become interwoven into a sophisticated integrated hypothesis that provides a framework for the understanding of antimigraine agents and the generation of new hypotheses to fuel the discovery of the next generation of acute and prophylactic antimigraine therapeutics (Ayata et al., 2006). This chapter considers current and emerging strategies for migraine prevention and treatment in the light of our understanding of migraine pathophysiology.

MIGRAINE PROPHYLAXIS AGENTS

According to the US Headache Consortium Guidelines, prophylactic therapy is indicated for patients with 3 or more days of headache-related disability per month, or with headaches refractory to acute treatment (Silberstein, 2000; Silberstein et al., 2000). In contrast to the effectiveness of acute antimigraine therapies, there is still, however, a significant unmet medical need for migraine prophylactics, and choice of therapy remains a matter of trial and error (Tfelt-Hansen et al., 2000). Although physicians can select from a considerable number of agents, the efficacy of most of them has been discovered serendipitously. This is probably due to the fact that, while the pathophysiology of the late phase of a migraine headache is now reasonably understood, the mechanisms leading to an attack are still mostly unknown.

It is beyond the scope of this chapter to examine the criteria for initiating preventive medication, or what particular medication to use or avoid in given patients. Often, the choice of a specific class of preventive therapy is based more on the presence of coexisting conditions and its tolerability than on an understanding of the mechanism of action of these drugs and the subtle differences in the pathology of each patient (Cutrer et al., 1998). While the efficacy of current prophylactic medications has been established based on serendipity more than rational drug design, recent research has focused on the characterization of pathophysiological events leading to a migraine attack. This research has followed three main directions: (1) the study of biochemical and physiological processes leading to the development of neurogenic dural inflammation in animal models; (2) imaging studies of migraine patients during the aura phase of "classic" migraine; and (3) analysis of the genetic traits associated with different migraine subtypes. The next section will summarize some of these findings and examine their clinical implications for emerging drug treatments.

Nitric oxide and the delayed inflammation hypothesis

Nitric oxide (NO), a short-lived vasodilator and weak oxygen radical, has been implicated in the genesis of migraine headache beginning with the observations of Wolff (1929). Headache is a well-known side-effect of NO donors such as nitroglycerine (glyceryl trinitrate or GTN) or sodium nitroprusside. A controlled study in humans linked NO with migraine headaches by showing that intravenous infusion of nitroglycerine caused two-thirds of migraineurs, but not control subjects, to

*Correspondence to: Christian Waeber, PhD, Massachusetts General Hospital, Charlestown, MA 02129, USA, E-mail: waeber@helix.mgh.harvard.edu

develop a delayed migraine attack (Olesen et al., 1993). The non-isoform-selective NO synthase inhibitor L-N^G-methylarginine (L-NMMA) effectively improved spontaneous migraine headaches and associated symptoms such as phono- and photophobia (Lassen et al., 1998). Other studies have shown that platelet levels of cyclic guanosine monophosphate (cGMP), the second messenger of NO, as well as NO metabolites such as nitrate/nitrite are increased in migraineurs and rise further during attacks (Stepien and Chalimoniuk, 1998; Shimomura et al., 1999). Interestingly, *m*-chlorophenylpiperazine (*m*-CPP), a major metabolite of the antidepressant trazodone, causes delayed migraine-like headaches in humans, presumably by activating 5-HT_{2B} receptors and leading to increased NO production by cerebral vessels (Leone et al., 2000). Finally, animal models have provided abundant evidence about the role of NO in nociception (Luo and Cizkova, 2000).

A 30-min infusion of GTN has been shown to cause the appearance of interleukin-1β in the dura mater, followed by mast cell degranulation, interleukin-6 expression, delayed expression of inducible NO synthase (iNOS) in rat meningeal macrophages and plasma protein extravasation (Reuter et al., 2001) (blocked by administration of an iNOS inhibitor), indicating the occurrence of GTN-induced inflammatory events in the meninges. In another study, bolus injection of a high dose of GTN caused delayed c-fos expression in rat trigeminal nucleus caudalis (TNC), reflecting activation of the trigeminovascular system (Tassorelli and Joseph, 1995).

Understanding the signaling pathways involved in the action of NO or NO donors in these animal models will be crucial to gain insight into the early pathophysiological events leading to migraine headache in humans, and is likely to identify new therapeutic targets for prophylactic drugs. In this context, it is worth mentioning that a multicenter, double-blind, placebo-controlled trial is currently under way to evaluate the tolerability, pharmacokinetics, and antimigraine efficacy of the iNOS inhibitor GW274150.

Cortical spreading depression and the hyperexcitability hypothesis

Exogenous agents such as NO donors might induce an attack (see above), and it is possible that other precipitants, found in air, water, food, or drugs, activate similar pathways in susceptible individuals. Several lines of evidence suggest that migraine could also be caused by endogenous factors. Migraine patients have been postulated to have an increased cortical hyperexcitability based on the results of transcranial magnetic stimulation experiments (Aurora et al., 1998; Battelli et al., 2002). An enhanced neuronal excitation, coupled with firing in a localized region of the cortex, can result in the local build-up of extracellular K^+, which depolarizes adjacent neurons, causing the phenomenon to spread. If diffusion, reuptake, and transport processes cannot contain the glutamate release and change in ionic concentrations, a wave of spreading depression is generated (Somjen, 2001).

A link between cortical spreading depression (CSD) and migraine pathogenesis has been hypothesized for more than 20 years (Lauritzen et al., 1982; Kunkler and Kraig, 2003). Recent evidence has strengthened the concept that the neurological symptoms that can precede or accompany an attack (e.g., aura) arise from CSD, whereas migraine headache results from the ensuing trigeminal-induced meningeal inflammation and central activation. Using high-field functional magnetic resonance imaging (fMRI) to map the progression of blood oxygenation level-dependent (BOLD) signal during spontaneous migraine aura, Hadjikhani et al. (2001) discovered at least eight neurovascular events in the occipital cortex that resembled CSD, expanding the results of a previous fMRI study of visually triggered migraine, which showed a suppression of BOLD response propagating into contiguous occipital cortical areas at a rate of 3–6 mm/min (Cao et al., 1999).

Data from animal studies suggest that CSD can activate the trigeminal sensory system leading to migraine headache. In rats, KCl-induced CSDs in the parietal cortex activate ipsilateral ventrolateral TNC (Moskowitz et al., 1993). Chronic transection of meningeal afferents, or pretreatment with intravenous sumatriptan, prevents this activation, but not the ability of KCl to induce CSD. In addition, CSD causes a long-lasting blood flow increase in the middle meningeal artery (Bolay et al., 2002), an effect which is abolished after transection of either the trigeminal branch innervating the meninges (nasociliary nerve) or postganglionic parasympathetic fibers projecting from the sphenopalatine ganglion. Dural plasma protein leakage is also observed ipsilaterally following CSD in control rats and in rats with chronic parasympathetic denervation, but is not seen in rats after trigeminal rhizotomy or after pretreatment with a neurokinin-1 (NK-1) receptor antagonist. Taken together, these studies suggest that blockade of CSD and or reducing the putative cortical hyperexcitability of migraineurs are potential targets for the development of prophylactic agents.

Migraine genetics and voltage-gated calcium channels

Studies with subtype-selective channel blockers show that N-, and P/Q-type voltage-gated Ca^{2+} channels play a major role in the generation of KCl-induced CSD

(Richter et al., 2002). P/Q-type Ca^{2+} channels are predominantly found in presynaptic terminals (Westenbroek et al., 1995) and play a major role in the control of neurotransmitter release (Dunlap et al., 1995). Several genetic diseases, collectively called "channelopathies," result from small but critical alterations in ion channel genes. The gene encoding the α1 subunit of the P/Q-type Ca^{2+} ($Ca_v2.1$) channel is mutated in half the familial hemiplegic migraine families (FHM-1) studied. Point mutations linked to FHM-1 lead to channel kinetics that favor increased Ca^{2+} influx through single $Ca_v2.1$ channels (Tottene et al., 2002). This may lead to a larger action potential-evoked Ca^{2+} influx at the presynaptic active zone, channel opening at lower levels of depolarization, and to increased neurotransmitter release.

Because the control of transmitter release by $Ca_v2.1$ channels is more prevalent in excitatory than inhibitory synapses (Caddick et al., 1999; Ayata et al., 2000), FHM-1 gain-of-function mutations may increase neuronal excitability and lower CSD threshold. Indeed, knock-in mice expressing the precise human mutations (R192Q or S218L) exhibit enhanced CSD susceptibility (van den Maagdenberg et al., 2004; van de Ven et al., 2007). Interestingly, a gain-of-function mutation in neurons (FHM-1) and a loss-of-function mutation in glia (FHM-2, which results from a point mutation in the α2 subunit of Na^+/K^+ ATPase) result in a nearly identical phenotype (e.g., hemiplegia and other auras) and both may render the brain more susceptible to CSD (Moskowitz et al., 2004). CSD spread may be facilitated by excessive glutamate accumulation in the extracellular space caused by the combination of increased calcium influx to the presynaptic terminal (the FHM-1 $Ca_v2.1$ channelopathy), resulting in increased glutamate release, and decreased clearance of glutamate from the synaptic cleft by adjacent astrocytes (the FHM-2 sodium channelopathy). A third FHM mutation (FHM-3) has been found in the *SCN1A* gene, encoding the pore-forming α1 subunit of voltage-gated neuronal $Na_v1.1$ sodium channels. This mutation causes a more rapid recovery from fast inactivation of neuronal $Na_v1.1$ sodium channels after depolarization (Dichgans et al., 2005). Because these channels play a key role in the generation and propagation of action potentials, the overall effects of FHM-3 mutations are most likely increased frequency of neuronal firing and enhanced neuronal excitability and neurotransmitter release.

Taken together, these studies are consistent with the notion that CSD blockade and reducing the putative cortical hyperexcitabilility of migraineurs are potential targets for the development of prophylactic agents. In support of this idea, a series of antimigraine prophylactic agents have the common property of inhibiting CSD after protracted administration (Ayata et al., 2006). These drugs belong to various classes of therapeutic agent and, importantly, the antimigraine efficacy of these agents does not appear to be a class effect. For instance, clinical trials have shown the efficacy of some, but not other, β-adrenergic antagonists in migraine therapy (Cutrer et al., 1998). Similarly, the antimigraine efficacy of amitriptyline has not convincingly been shown for other tricyclic antidepressants (Cutrer et al., 1998). Therefore developing novel agents based only on the known pharmacological profile of known drugs is a poor strategy for migraine drug discovery.

A relevant model proposed for the effects of psychotropic drugs (e.g., antidepressants) must account for the fact that their therapeutic effects require several weeks and are generally not immediately reversed upon drug discontinuation. This temporal profile is consistent with mechanisms involving gene regulation. While the episodic nature of migraine makes it difficult to determine the onset of therapeutic efficacy, a recent study showed that the mean change from baseline in monthly migraine frequency in patients treated with topiramate increased with treatment time (Silberstein et al., 2004). Similar results were reported for valproate (Silberstein and Collins, 1999). It is tempting to speculate that chronic treatment with antimigraine agents induces consistent changes in the expression of genes involved in the control of neuronal excitability and/or CSD propagation (e.g., glutamate receptor signaling, transporters, Ca^{2+} and K^+ channels, gap junctions, or energy metabolism). Modulating directly the function of the products of these genes might lead to the development of novel migraine prophylactic strategies.

ANTIEPILEPTIC DRUGS

Both epilepsy and migraine are likely to be disorders of neuronal hyperexcitability. Although this concept has long been accepted in epilepsy, for migraine the hyperexcitability hypothesis has garnered increasing support mostly over the past two decades. Various causes for hyperexcitability of the migrainous brain have been suggested. These include low concentrations of γ-aminobutyric acid (GABA) and magnesium, high concentrations of glutamate, mitochondrial abnormalities, dysfunctions related to NO, or various channelopathies. It is therefore not surprising that antiepileptic drugs are used for both disorders. Robust evidence supports the use of sodium valproate/divalproex and of topiramate in the prophylaxis of migraine. In addition to these two drugs, other antiepileptic drugs reported to show migraine efficacy include gabapentin, levetiracetam, tiagabine, and zonisamide, but large-scale double-blind placebo-controlled studies have yet to be reported. Antiepileptic drugs comprise only one class of effective treatment for migraine prophylaxis. While this was once thought to imply the existence of migraine mechanisms that might not be present in epilepsy, recent findings indicate that even agents not used in the treatment of epilepsy (propranolol, amitriptyline, and methysergide) can increase the threshold for the generation of CSD, and hence, putatively, neuronal excitability (Ayata et al., 2006).

Topiramate

The sulfamate-substituted monosaccharide topiramate (2,3:4,5-bis-*O*-(1-ethylethylidene)-β-D-fructopyranose sulfamate) is a structurally novel agent currently used as a broad-spectrum antiepileptic drug. Electrophysiological studies have shown effects of topiramate on various ion channels, including negative modulatory effects on voltage-gated Na^+, K^+, and Ca^{2+} channels, blockade of kainate-evoked inward current and modulation of GABAergic current. In addition, topiramate is able to depress sustained repetitive firing mediated by Na^+ currents. Although the exact mechanism of action of topiramate at a molecular level is not well understood, various studies suggest that the phosphorylation state of target receptors/channels can affect its activity (Curia et al., 2007).

There are contradicting data regarding the role of voltage-sensitive sodium channel blockade in the mechanism of action of topiramate. For instance, topiramate only exerts a modest inhibition of glutamate release induced by the sodium channel opener veratridine, at variance with other antiepileptic drugs such as carbamazepine, phenytoin, lamotrigine, and oxcarbazepine (Sitges et al., 2007). This suggests that topiramate possesses a different mechanism of action, which might be related to the fact that the antimigraine efficacy of topiramate has been established in various clinical trials, whereas the efficacy of carbamazepine, phenytoin, lamotrigine, and oxcarbazepine is less clear.

Topiramate has also been reported to exert negative modulatory effects on AMPA (alpha-amino-3-hydroxy-5-methyl-4-isoxazolepropionic acid) and kainate subtypes of glutamate receptors by binding to these receptors in their dephosphorylated state, and selective antagonism of GluR5 kainate receptor-mediated currents was put forward as a novel anticonvulsant mechanism of action of topiramate (Gryder and Rogawski, 2003). Topiramate has also been shown to inhibit carbonic anhydrase, to interact with the glycine receptor, and to influence mitochondrial permeability.

The role of the substantia nigra in gating and control of seizure activity has been studied extensively. Most compounds that exert an anticonvulsant effect when administered intranigrally are agonists of, or have potentiating effects on, $GABA_A$ receptors. Topiramate is also known to potentiate $GABA_A$-mediated Cl^- currents, and it resembles other known antiepileptic drugs (including phenobarbital, midazolam, and levetiracetam) in that it exerts anticonvulsant effects when injected into the substantia nigra (Meurs et al., 2006). The neuronal circuitry involved in the control of limbic seizures by the substantia nigra is only partly understood, and might be related to the brainstem generator for migraine that has been postulated on the basis of positron emission tomography studies during and between attacks (Diener and May, 1996).

Which of the pleiotropic actions of topiramate contributes to its efficacy in migraine and/or to its anticonvulsant effect remains unclear. To make matters worse, it should be repeated that only chronic, not acute, treatment with topiramate increases CSD threshold in rodents. Similarly, in humans the mean change from baseline in migraine frequency (per month) was –1.00, –1.52, –1.72, and –2.11 in patients treated with 100 mg/day topiramate for 1, 2, 3, and 6 months, respectively (Silberstein et al., 2004). Taken together, these data obtained in an animal model and in humans strongly suggest that alteration of common sets of genes underlies the therapeutic efficacy of diverse antimigraine drugs. Chronic treatment with antimigraine agents might induce consistent changes in the expression of genes involved in the control of neuronal excitability and/or CSD propagation (e.g., glutamate receptor signaling, transporters, Ca^{2+} and K^+ channels, gap junctions, or energy metabolism). Therefore, the effects of topiramate and other prophylactic drugs may be mediated by modulation of gene expression, and not necessarily via a direct effect on the known targets mentioned in the previous paragraphs.

Zonisamide

The benzisoxazole derivative zonisamide shares a sulfonamide moiety with topiramate, but is structurally distinct from other antiepileptic drugs. It has efficacy in a number of experimental seizure models (Baulac, 2006) and produces centrally mediated analgesic effects on thermal and mechanical hypersensitivity developing in mice after peripheral nerve injury (Tanabe et al., 2007). Several studies have shown that zonisamide may be effective in migraine prevention (Ashkenazi et al., 2006), but the drug failed to show a statistically significant beneficial effect in a population of refractory patients who had failed multiple migraine-preventive drugs (Ashkenazi et al., 2006). Because of its bioavailability approaching 100% and very long half-life, zonisamide has a favorable pharmacokinetic profile, which permits a once- or twice-daily dosing regimen (Ashkenazi et al., 2006). Current evidence suggests that zonisamide exerts its pharmacological effects by blockade of neuronal voltage-gated sodium channels (as carbamazepine and phenytoin) and low-voltage-activated (T-type) calcium channels (as ethosuximide) (Rogawski and Loscher, 2004). Zonisamide has also been reported to scavenge free radicals (Mori et al., 1998) and inhibits the formation of NO (Noda et al., 1999). The latter effects may be therapeutically relevant if NO synthase induction and delayed meningeal inflammation underlie migraine pathophysiology (Reuter et al., 2001).

Carbonic anhydrase inhibition

Zonisamide, as well as topiramate, inhibit the isoenzymes I–VI of carbonic anhydrase at therapeutically relevant concentration. While there is some doubt regarding the significance of this action to the antiepileptic effects of these drugs (Masuda et al., 1994), other studies suggest that the apparent decrease of steady-state intracellular neuronal pH (via a combined effect on Na^+-independent Cl^-/HCO_3^- exchange and carbonic anhydrase) contributes to their anticonvulsive properties (Leniger et al., 2004). Other carbonic anhydrase inhibitors (such as sulthiame and acetazolamide) have also been shown to lower neuronal intracellular pH, thereby effectively reducing the epileptiform activity in *in vitro* epilepsy models. Rapid shifts in extracellular (interstitial) pH are known to accompany neuronal discharge. Because these changes can affect neuronal function by modulating both the conductance and gating properties of voltage-gated ion channels (Tombaugh and Somjen, 1996) and intravenous administration of the carbonic anhydrase inhibitor acetazolamide is known to cause extracellular acidosis (Heuser et al., 1975), carbonic anhydrase inhibitors might modulate neuronal excitability by shifting firing threshold, altering the probability of multiple spikes and burst firing, or by modifying the degree of synaptic integration during periods of multiple or high-frequency synaptic input. Hypercarbia has been shown to inhibit spreading depression (Gardner-Medwin, 1981), and hypoxic spreading depression can be delayed by mild acidosis (Tombaugh, 1994); acidosis produced by administration of carbonic anhydrase inhibitors may be expected to reduce the frequency or impair the propagation of spreading depression.

Acetazolamide has been reported as effective in migraine aura status, familial hemiplegic migraine, and in migraine with aura episodes in cerebral autosomal-dominant arteriopathy with subcortical infarcts and leukoencephalopathy (CADASIL), whereas it was ineffective and poorly tolerated in migraine without aura patients. More recently, it was shown to reduce the frequency of migraine with aura and, to a lesser degree, of migraine without aura attacks in a uncontrolled pilot trial involving 22 patients (De Simone et al., 2005). These results are at odds with the negative outcome of a multicenter, double-blind, randomized trial involving 53 patients. Although this study was prematurely stopped because of a high number of withdrawals, no difference in efficacy appeared between the placebo and *verum* groups at the last trial period of 4 weeks (Vahedi et al., 2002). Although the relatively small sample size and early termination do not allow firm conclusions about efficacy, acetazolamide did not seem to have a prophylactic effect. These results may not apply to FHM or to migraine with aura and they clearly contrast with the remarkable efficacy and tolerance of this drug in episodic ataxia type 2. Interestingly, abnormally elevated cerebellar intracellular pH has been demonstrated between attacks in the cerebellum of episodic ataxia type 2 patients, returning to normal after acetazolamide administration (Bain et al., 1992), but similar studies in migraine patients have failed to show abnormal intracellular pH even in prolonged attacks of migraine with aura or hemiplegic migraine (Welch et al., 1989; Uncini et al., 1995).

Levetiracetam

Levetiracetam ((*S*)-α-ethyl-2-oxo-pyrrolidine acetamide) is chemically related to piracetam, a cyclic derivative of GABA. In animal models, it is effective for neuropathic, but not acute, pain (Ardid et al., 2003). Limited open-label studies suggest that it is a safe and effective treatment for migraine with (Brighina et al., 2006) and without (Gallai et al., 2003) aura.

Animal models for the development of antiepileptic drugs indicate that levetiracetam may work differently than other anticonvulsants (Klitgaard et al., 1998). It does not seem to modulate voltage-dependent ion channels, inhibit excitatory neurotransmission, or enhance GABA activity. Binding studies have shown that levetiracetam binds to brain cell membranes in a reversible, saturable, and stereoselective manner. Its precise binding site has not been elucidated, although a specific vesicular presynaptic membrane protein, SV2A, has been identified (Fuks et al., 2003). Studies in neurons from SV2 knock-out mice suggest that SV2 proteins enhance synaptic currents and increase the probability of transmitter release by maintaining the size of the readily releasable pool of vesicles (Custer et al., 2006). A recent report showed that brief levetiracetam exposure had no effect on transmission in rat hippocampal slices, and that longer exposures significantly altered paired pulse responses and reduced late synaptic potentials delivered in an 80-Hz train, possibly because levetiracetam antagonized the effect of the SV2 proteins (Yang et al., 2007).

Interestingly, SV2 is the receptor for botulinum neurotoxin A, an agent shown in some studies to be effective in migraine prophylaxis (Dong et al., 2006). After binding to SV2, botulinum neurotoxin A is internalized by endocytosis into clathrin-coated vesicles. Endocytotic vesicles acidify, which triggers membrane insertion of the B chains and translocation of the A chains across the membrane into the cytoplasm. The A chain of botulinum neurotoxin A cleaves SNAP-25 (synaptosome-associated protein of 25 kDa), preventing the formation of stable SNARE complexes that are required for exocytotic fusion of synaptic vesicles with the plasma membrane. Preventing the function of SV2 proteins may therefore be a novel target for prophylactic drugs. It will be interesting to examine the antimigraine potential of several levetiracetam congeners (e.g., seletracetam, brivaracetam) that were recently discovered because of their high binding affinity to SV2A.

Gabapentin and pregabalin

These two compounds have proven clinical efficacy in neuropathic pain and are effective in other disorders of the nervous system, including epilepsy and anxiety (Ettinger and Argoff, 2007). Pregabalin seems to possess a better potency and pharmacokinetic profile than gabapentin (Guay, 2005). Gabapentin was shown in several controlled studies to reduce the frequency and intensity of migraine attacks (Calabresi et al., 2007), and clinical trials to test the efficacy of pregabalin in the prevention of migraine are currently ongoing (Puppe and Limmroth, 2007).

Although gabapentin and pregabalin are similar in structure to the neurotransmitter GABA, they are not believed to act on the same receptors, nor do they interact with GABA uptake transporters. Their exact mechanism of action is unknown, but they bind to the $\alpha2\delta$ subunit of the voltage-dependent calcium channel in the central nervous system (CNS). $\alpha2\delta$ is one of three regulatory subunits, along with β and γ, that configure around the pore-forming $\alpha1$ subunit to form the complete channel complex. Several studies have shown that $\alpha2\delta$ subunits increase the expression of different $\alpha1$ and β subunit combinations, and all $\alpha2\delta$ subunits seem to increase peak Ca^{2+} current amplitude, probably by associating with $\alpha1$ subunits in the endoplasmic reticulum and altering their trafficking to the plasma membrane (Davies et al., 2007).

Knock-in mice, whose R217A-mutated $\alpha2\delta$-1 binds gabapentin and pregabalin with a much lower affinity than wild-type $\alpha2\delta$-1, have been shown to have a neuropathic pain response that is not sensitive to these drugs, indicating that $\alpha2\delta$-1 is the therapeutic target of these agents in neuropathic pain (Field et al., 2006). Because the pain response is still sensitive to morphine and amitriptyline, this observation indicates that gabapentin and pregabalin act specifically at their $\alpha2\delta$-1-binding site. In addition, the anticonvulsant effects of pregabalin are seen at higher doses in the R217A $\alpha2\delta$-1 knock-in mouse than in wild-type strains, consistent with the idea that both $\alpha2\delta$-1 and $\alpha2\delta$-2 play a role in the anticonvulsant action of this drug. There is also preliminary evidence that the R217A mutation prevents the anxiolytic-like action of pregabalin (Davies et al., 2007).

Interestingly, pregabalin and gabapentin reduce the release of substance P and calcitonin gene-related peptide (CGRP) from rat spinal tissues only after inflammation or activation of protein kinase C (Fehrenbacher et al., 2003). Similarly, the effect of gabapentin on glutamate release from the trigeminal nucleus is minimal under basal conditions, but is observed after induction of diabetic neuropathy or after activation of protein kinase C or adenylyl cyclase (Maneuf et al., 2004). Gabapentin was recently shown to inhibit Ca^{2+} currents in dorsal root ganglia from mice overexpressing $\alpha2\delta$-1, but not wild-type mice (Li et al., 2006). Based on these findings, it is tempting to speculate that $\alpha2\delta$ subunits might have little acute influence on native Ca^{2+} currents under normal physiological conditions, unless $\alpha2\delta$ is overexpressed or some second-messenger pathways are activated.

γ Amino acid derivatives other than gabapentin and pregabalin, as well as α- and β-amino acids and non-amino acid structures, have been identified as $\alpha2\delta$ ligands and show potency in various models in neuropathic pain models (Field et al., 2007). Because allodynia and hyperalgesia, with underlying hyperexcitability and central sensitization, characterize migraine as well as neuropathic pain, efficacy in these models may predict efficacy in migraine prophylaxis. It is therefore likely that more $\alpha2\delta$ ligands will soon be introduced in migraine prevention.

OTHER THERAPEUTIC CLASSES

Memantine

A recent retrospective study of 60 cases suggested that memantine was an effective preventive therapy for patients with frequent migraine (Charles et al., 2007). *N*-methyl-D-aspartate (NMDA) receptor antagonists are known to inhibit CSD, which is believed to be a fundamental mechanism of migraine. But potent NMDA receptor channel blockers and competitive NMDA receptor antagonists produce phencyclidine-like psychotropic symptoms in humans and rodents, indicating that such uncompetitive antagonism of NMDA receptors is not a promising therapeutic approach. Attempts have been made to circumvent these side-effects by targeting modulatory sites of the NMDA receptor such as the strychnine-insensitive glycine and NR2B-selective polyamine sites (Parsons, 2001).

Alternatively, recent data indicate that non-competitive antagonists with moderate affinity such as memantine (1-amino-3,5-dimethyl-adamantane) and neramexane (1-amino-1,3,3,5,5-pentamethyl-cyclohexane, MRZ 2/579) could be useful therapeutics due to their strong voltage-dependency and rapid unblocking kinetics (Parsons et al., 1999). Indeed, memantine is registered in Europe and the USA for the treatment of moderate to severe Alzheimer's disease.

It is unclear whether the mechanism of action of memantine in the context of this disease (Parsons et al., 2007) is similar to its possible mode of action in migraine. Because memantine has been found to modulate CSD (Peeters et al., 2007), it is possible that it could reduce the increased cortical excitability thought to underlie migraine. This potential mechanism is supported by observations that memantine reduces the frequency of aura as well as headache (Charles et al., 2007). Besides its activity at NMDA receptors, memantine blocks $\alpha9/\alpha10$ nicotinic receptors with similar affinity to NMDA receptors (Oliver et al., 2002), but these receptors show a very discrete, non-CNS, distribution, i.e., in cochlear hair cells, and this action is therefore highly unlikely to be responsible for the therapeutic effects of memantine. It also blocks $\alpha7$ and $\alpha4/\beta2$ receptors, but with an affinity too low to be of real therapeutic significance. Finally, memantine blocks murine and human 5-HT_3 receptors with similar or somewhat lower affinity to NMDA receptors *in vitro*, but in a non-use, non-voltage-dependent manner. The possibility nevertheless remains that memantine could have multiple mechanisms of action that may modulate migraine.

Tonabersat, and its congener carabersat, are benzopyrans structurally related to the adenosine triphosphate (ATP)-sensitive potassium channel opener cromakalim. However, their site of action is distinct from potassium channels or from the target of other anticonvulsants. Tritiated tonabersat (SB-220453) binds with stereospecificity and high affinity to a unique CNS binding site, in mouse, rat, cat, marmoset, and human brains with particularly high levels in the cerebral cortex, hippocampus, and cerebellum. Tonabersat has shown activity in various animal models of migraine, where it inhibits CSD and neurogenic inflammation, induces carotid dilatation, and decreases cortical NO concentrations during CSD. However, it showed no significant pre-emptive antimigraine activity compared with placebo in a human model of migraine (Tvedskov et al., 2004).

Carabersat does, however, show activity in some, but not all, models predictive for antiepileptic activity (Hovinga, 2002). In a recent double-blind placebo-controlled trial, the responder rate (defined as a 50% reduction in migraine attacks) was 62% and 45% for tonabersat and placebo, respectively (Goadsby et al., 2007). Although tonabersat failed to meet its primary endpoint (possibly due to the large placebo response), these results support further exploration of this compound in larger controlled trials.

ACUTE ANTIMIGRAINE AGENTS

In the earlier sections of this chapter, we reviewed migraine prophylaxis therapy in the context of the potential predisposition and initiating events in migraine. In this section we consider the mechanisms of action of current and future acute antimigraine therapies in the context of the processes that could evoke trigeminal sensory activation and headache pain during an attack.

Trigeminal system

In the late 1970s the Moskowitz laboratory proposed that the trigeminal nerve was a critical player in the pathogenesis of migraine pain (Moskowitz et al., 1979; Moskowitz, 1984, 1991). Over the following three decades the neuroanatomy and neuropharmacology of the trigeminal sensory nerves have been revealed and the term "trigeminovascular system" introduced to describe the systems involved in headache pain (Goadsby, 2005a, 2007; Moskowitz, 2007). The innervation of the trigeminovascular system has been mapped immunohistochemically. In the trigeminal ganglion CGRP-immunoreactive neurons predominate (40%), with substance P-containing neurons (18%) the next most prevalent. Sensory, parasympathetic, and sympathetic nerves clearly decorate the meningeal blood vessels with fibers that contain vasoactive and proinflammatory mediators such as substance P (typical of sensory C fibers), CGRP (in C and A δ sensory fibers), vasoactive intestinal polypeptide (VIP colocalized with acetylcholine in parasympathetic nerves) and neuropeptide Y (colocalized with norepinephrine) in sympathetic fibers (Edvinsson, 2001).

Emerging concepts propose that migraine may result from activation and sensitization of sensory trigeminal afferent nerves triggered by a CSD arising from neuronal hyperexcitability in the cerebral cortex of migraineurs (Olesen et al., 1981; Lauritzen and Hansen, 1992; Moskowitz et al., 1993; Bolay et al.,

2002; Berger et al., 2008). In this scenario, the extracellular environmental changes (ionic and increased glutamate levels) (Chen et al., 2001) resulting from spreading depression are proposed to activate sensory fibers in the meninges initiating retrograde impulse transmission centrally via the trigeminal ganglion to second-order pain relay neurons in the TNC. Activation of the TNC in turn produces vasodilation of meningeal blood vessels via a parasympathetic pathway originating in the superior salivatory nucleus and that reaches the vessels via the sphenopalatine ganglion. This vasodilation, even if brief, has the potential to activate perivascular trigeminal sensory fibers and provoke the release of vasodilator proinflammatory neuropeptides (CGRP and substance P). It has been proposed that this could set up a vicious cycle that amplifies pain signal transmission to the sensory cortex through second-order sensory neurons in the brainstem TNC and third-order neurons in the thalamus (Iadacola, 2002).

An alternative hypothesis is that it could be the hypothalamus that is triggered at the outset of a migraine attack. The hypothalamus is involved, amongst a multitude of functions, in setting biological rhythms, cardiovascular regulation, thermoregulation, feeding, emotional behaviors, arousal, and stress responses. The hypothalamus is widely connected throughout the CNS to cortex, thalamus, amygdala, and brainstem nuclei, including direct connectivity with sensory processing centers in the trigeminal and spinal dorsal horn where it can affect descending pain control pathways and modulate nociceptive processing (Holland and Goadsby, 2007) and indirect linkage through parasympathetic nuclei such as the superior salivatory nucleus. Hypothalamic activation could explain migraine triggers (e.g., barometric pressure, reduction in stress, odor, sleep) and cortical phenomena such as CSD and visual and auditory disturbances early in an attack. Activation of brainstem nuclei involved in pain processing (thalamus, TNC, periaqueductal gray) could lead to headache pain with associated symptoms of migraine such as nausea and emesis (e.g., nucleus tractus solitarius, dorsal vagomotor nuclei) being driven from brainstem nuclei linked to the TNC (Burstein and Jakubowski, 2005a). Activation of the autonomic loop involving the parasympathetic system may explain the etiology of autonomic symptoms during a migraine attack (prominent during cluster headache) and misdiagnosis of some migraineurs as having sinus headache.

Once migraine pain starts and the TNC is activated conceptually, these two hypotheses on migraine pathogenesis converge. The big question has always surrounded the role of meningeal vasodilation and mechanical activation of perivascular trigeminal sensory fibers in migraine headache pain and the contribution of neurogenic inflammation mediated by concomitant sensory neuropeptide release. Early imaging studies in migraine with aura suggested that pain could start when cerebral blood flow was actually decreased and that pain could subside whilst flow was increased (Olesen et al., 1990). Most recently clinical experimental pharmacological studies have shown that migraine can be induced by sildenafil without changes in middle cerebral artery diameter (Kruuse et al., 2003) and that cephalic vasodilation induced by VIP does not induce migraine (Rahman et al., 2008). In humans neurogenic inflammation during migraine has not been clearly demonstrated (Pietrobon and Striessnig, 2003;Pietrobon, 2005) and in clinical trials drugs that prevent trigeminally evoked neurogenic inflammation in preclinical models have not been universally active (Goadsby, 2005a). This suggests that, although meningeal neurogenic vasodilation and inflammation may occur in migraine, they are markers of trigeminal activation and alone are insufficient to produce pain. These observations suggest that the pain of migraine is a central rather than peripheral phenomenon and that it may not be necessary for antimigraine drugs to affect the status of the meningeal vasculature (Goadsby, 2007).

As the attack ensues, primary (trigeminal ganglion), second- (TNC), and third-order (thalamic) sensory neurons may become sensitized, intensifying the headache attack and cutaneous allodynia. Preclinical models of migraine pathophysiology (Strassman et al., 1996; Burstein et al., 1998; Burstein and Jakubowski, 2004; Levy et al., 2004) and clinical migraine studies (Burstein et al., 2000, 2004, 2005; Goadsby, 2005b) have shown compelling evidence linking trigeminal sensitization to allodynia and drug responsivity during migraine attacks (Burstein and Jakubowski, 2005b; Dodick and Silberstein, 2006; Lipton et al., 2008).

It is also noteworthy that the reactivity of the TNC may be modulated by other brainstem circuits and centers (such as the hypothalamus, periaqueductal gray, dorsal raphe nucleus, and locus coeruleus) that could initiate activity, impair descending inhibition of pain signal processing, or lower the threshold for TNC activation. In addition to its role in the pathogenesis of migraine pain, interconnected brainstem nuclei (locus coeruleus, nucleus tractus solitarius, dorsal vagal complex) may also be involved in many of the associated symptoms of migraine such as sensory gating abnormalities (phonophobia, photophobia), nausea, emesis, and gastrointestinal stasis.

Receptor pharmacology of the trigeminovascular system

Understanding the pharmacology of the trigeminovascular system using known active antimigraine agents has been central to therapeutic advances. Using methysergide (Lance et al., 1963), Saxena and Ferrari (1992) identified a novel atypical cerebrovascular vasoconstrictor 5-HT receptor that was initially called the 5HT$_1$-like receptor and then labeled the 5-HT$_{1B}$ receptor (Hoyer et al., 1994).

Immunohistochemical studies using highly selective antibodies revealed the distribution of serotonin receptors in the human trigeminovascular system. The vasoconstrictor 5-HT$_{1B}$ receptors were shown to be located on the smooth muscle of meningeal blood vessels (Longmore et al., 1998) with inhibitory 5-HT$_{1D}$ receptors on the peripheral and central terminals of the trigeminal sensory nerves where they could modulate neuropeptide release and central trigeminal pain signal transmission (Longmore et al., 1997a). Autoradiographic studies also showed the presence of these serotonin receptors together with 5-HT$_{1F}$ receptors in the trigeminal dorsal horn (Pascual et al., 1996; Castro et al., 1997). 5-HT$_{1F}$ receptors are absent from meningeal blood vessels (Razzaque et al., 1999). 5-HT$_{1B}$ and 5-HT$_{1D}$ receptors have also been shown to be present in human trigeminal sensory ganglion (Hou et al., 2001) and 5-HT$_{1D}$ receptors are colocalized with CGRP and substance P on sensory nerve fibers (Ma et al., 2001; Smith et al., 2002) peripherally and centrally, suggesting potential for an interaction between the serotonergic and sensory peptidergic systems that are altered in migraine. 5-HT$_{1B/1D/1F}$ receptors also colocalize with glutamate on sensory trigeminal ganglion neurons (Ma, 2001), suggesting that they could also have a role to modulate release of this primary sensory neurotransmitter and that this could contribute to their therapeutic effect.

Sensory neuropeptide receptors have also been mapped in the trigeminovascular system. Substance P is present in the sensory C fibers of the trigeminal nerves and exerts its effects through neurokinin NK1 receptors (Longmore et al., 1997b; Saria, 1999) that are present on the endothelium of blood vessels where they mediate vasodilation and increased blood vessel permeability (extravasation). NK1 receptors are also present on second-order sensory neurons throughout pain relay nuclei in the dorsal horn and brainstem. CGRP is found within C and Aδ nerve fibers throughout the trigeminovascular sensory nervous system. Only one receptor has been defined molecularly for CGRP, calcitonin receptor-like receptor (CLR), and it is a member of the G-protein-coupled receptor B family. CLR forms a heterodimer with a transmembrane protein that has been termed a receptor activity-modifying protein (RAMP). There are three different RAMPs, 1, 2, and 3, that, when coupled with the CLR, define the agonist receptor pharmacology of the complex and the selectivity of CLR for different peptides of the CGRP/calcitonin family (McLatchie et al., 1998; Christopoulos et al., 1999; Foord and Marshall, 1999; Poyner et al., 2002; Hay et al., 2006). RAMP1 plus CLR form the CGRP receptor whereas CLR plus RAMP2 form the adrenomedullin receptor. It should be noted that another intracellular protein may be required for the coupling of the CLR–RAMP1 heterodimer to intracellular second-messenger systems such as cyclic adenosine monophosphate (cAMP) (Evans et al., 2000). There is also evidence that responses to CGRP could be mediated through cGMP, NO, with an involvement of K^+ channels (Brain and Grat, 2004).

Oliver et al. (2002) showed the distribution of CGRP receptors in the meningeal blood vessels that are thought to be involved in migraine pain. CLR and RAMP1 proteins and mRNA (Edvinsson et al., 1997) were highly expressed in human meningeal blood vessels and this correlated well with high binding site density, revealed by autoradiography with [^{125}I]CGRP and the functional dilator effects of CGRP on meningeal blood vessels *in vitro* (Edvinsson et al., 2002; Edvinsson and Hargreaves, 2005) and *in vivo* (Williamson et al., 1997a). CGRP itself and CLR and RAMP1 have also been mapped immunohistochemically within the brainstem, showing clearly that the transmitter and its receptors are highly expressed in sensory nerve terminals and on central sensory pain relay neurons throughout the trigeminal nuclei in primate and human brain (K. Oliver, unpublished observations). In addition it is thought that the RAMPs enable expression of CLR on the cell surface and influence drug binding. In a study with potential relevance to migraine, RAMP1 has been suggested to be functionally rate-limiting for CGRP activity in the trigeminal ganglion, giving rise to the hypothesis that RAMP1 levels may modulate activity in the trigeminal neurons and modulate susceptibility to migraine (Zhang et al., 2007).

Studying and targeting CGRP receptors is complicated as cross-species differences are seen in the structure of RAMP1. Mallee et al. (2002) found in a mutagenesis study that a single amino-acid difference in the RAMP protein, lysine residue at amino acid position 74 in the rat RAMP1 to tryptophan in the human, could drive large differences in the affinity of drug molecules between humans, primates, and rats. This finding indicates that cell surface drug binding involves RAMP1 and not just CLR and, importantly, raises a cautionary flag for pharmacological studies that do not use the appropriately matched species and compounds for investigation of CGRP physiology and pharmacology *in vivo* (Hershey et al., 2005).

Glutamate receptors

Glutamate is the main excitatory transmitter in the brain. It normally fulfills important sensorimotor and protective functions. Excess or underproduction of glutamate through injury or disease can have pathophysiological effects. The glutamate hypothesis for migraine has been discussed by Ramadan (2003) and reviewed recently by Vikelis and Mitsikostas (2007). Ionotropic glutamate receptors (NMDA, non-NMDA (AMPA), and kainate (KA)) and metabotropic glutamate (mGlu) receptors are widely distributed throughout the brain and trigeminal system where they can modulate sensory processing. The ionotropic receptors are ligand-gated ion channels whilst the metabotropic receptors are G-protein-coupled to intracellular second-messenger systems. In migraine the most studied receptor subtypes are the ionotropic AMPA GluR2/GluR5 subtypes that are present on trigeminal neurons (Sahara et al., 1997) where they could modulate trigeminal activation (Bleakman and Lodge, 1998; Quartu et al., 2002). The metabotropic mGluR5 subtype (Jaeschke et al., 2008) is widely expressed at postsynaptic excitatory synapses throughout the brain and nervous system, including cortex, thalamus, dorsal horn (trigeminal and spinal), and peripherally on C fibers. Thus, mGluR5 receptors are well located to modulate pain signaling at several distinct levels in the nervous system. Immunohistochemical studies have shown colocalization of 5-HT_{1B}, 5-HT_{1D}, and 5-HT_{1F} receptors on glutamate-positive trigeminal neurons (Ma, 2001), where agonists at these 5-HT receptors could reduce glutamate release contributing to their therapeutic effect.

Orexinergic systems

In recent reviews (Holland and Goadsby, 2007; Raniero et al., 2008) it has been suggested that the hypothalamic orexinergic system may be involved in the pathogenesis of primary headaches such as migraine, chronic migraine, and cluster headaches. This hypocretin orexinergic system has been the subject of recent reviews (Saper et al., 2005; Nishino, 2007) for its role in sleep disorders. The hypocretin/orexin system projects widely across the CNS and is involved in the regulation of sleep, circadian, autonomic, and metabolic functions with the potential to trigger and modulate trigeminal nociceptive processing directly and indirectly (see above). The orexin neuropeptides (orexin A and orexin B) are derived from a common precursor pre-pro-orexin and act via the G-protein-coupled receptors OX1 (Gq-coupled) and OX2 (Gq or Gi/Go-coupled). Orexin A is the preferred agonist at the OX1 receptor whereas orexin A and orexin B can signal through the OX2 receptor. Preclinical studies and mouse genetic studies have demonstrated the potential for orexin antagonists to be antinociceptive, although it is not yet clear whether OX1 or OX2 receptors are the most important mediators of this effect, as both are found in central pain pathways, nor whether the effects of orexin agonists and antagonists are dependent on their activation state. The role of poor sleep hygiene in triggering migraine versus the beneficial effects of darkness and sleep in its non-pharmacological resolution (Dodick et al., 2003) makes this system an interesting target for future drug discovery. Currently there is no direct clinical evidence for the role of orexinergic systems in primary headaches and it is unknown whether orexin agonists or antagonists could have value in therapy. The neuroanatomical, preclinical, and circumstantial evidence is however compelling to investigate the orexinergic system further in headache using the orexin drug candidates (almorexant: dual orexin receptor antagonist for OX1 and OX2 receptors: http://www.actelion.com) that are known to be effective sleep-promoting agents and are currently in clinical development for the treatment of sleep disorders.

Antimigraine therapeutics

It is useful to consider the actions of effective acute antimigraine treatments in the context of the trigeminovascular system. To date, strategies targeting the autonomic systems (anticholinergic muscarinic antagonists preventing dilation and adrenergic agonists causing constriction) that are thought to be involved early in the initiation of a migraine headache attack have not proven beneficial in the treatment of migraine. Anecdotal reports have indicated that in some early clinical experimental studies the administration of serotonin caused palpable temporal artery vasoconstriction and gave transient migraine headache relief. The ergot alkaloids and the triptan agents are highly effective antimigraine agents (Silberstein and Hargreaves, 2000; Ferrari et al., 2002; Tfelt-Hansen, 2006; Pascual et al., 2007) but both classes have the potential for cardiovascular side-effects (reviewed by Dodick et al., 2004). The discovery and development efforts for the next generation of antimigraine agents therefore targeted: (1) the inhibition of sensory neuropeptide release to curtail inflammation in pain-producing meningeal blood vessels and inhibit nociceptive transmission within central pain relay nuclei in the brainstem; (2) antagonism of the sensory transmitters that are released peripherally and centrally from activated trigeminal sensory nerves; (3) modulation of central nociceptive pathways (glutamatergic) that could be involved in the trigeminal nociceptive processing during migraine; and (4) novel approaches through hypothalamic orexinergic systems.

Triptan $5\text{-}HT_{1B/1D}$ and $5\text{-}HT_{1F}$ agonists

The triptans as a class have generally similar receptor profiles and selectively target serotonin $5\text{-}HT_{1B}$ receptors and $5\text{-}HT_{1D}$ receptors with varying activity at $5\text{-}HT_{1F}$ receptors (Goadsby and Hargreaves, 2000; Hargreaves and Beer, 2001, 2002; Hargreaves, 2007). One view of the triptans is that they are next-generation ergot alkaloids – known effective antimigraine agents – as they have focused activity on the "antimigraine" serotonin receptors but eliminated activity at other monoamine receptors that mediate the unwanted side-effects of the ergots (Silberstein and Hargreaves, 2000). Within the conceptual framework for the generation of headache pain during a migraine attack it seems the triptans are almost ideal antimigraine agents (Hargreaves and Shepheard, 1999). Triptans acting at $5\text{-}HT_{1B}$ receptors constrict dilated meningeal blood vessels (Friberg et al., 1991) and their simultaneous action at $5\text{-}HT_{1D}$ receptors on perivascular nerve terminals inhibits release of vasoactive proinflammatory neuropeptides such as substance P and CGRP peptides, so breaking the vicious cycle (Goadsby and Edvinsson, 1993; Williamson et al., 1997b; Edvinsson and Goadsby, 1998; Williamson and Hargreaves, 2001). The triptans may also act centrally within the TNC at $5\text{-}HT_{1D}$ receptors on the terminals of incoming trigeminal sensory fibers (Goadsby and Hoskin, 1996; Cumberbatch et al., 1997, 1998a, b; Potrebic et al., 2003; Ahn et al., 2004; Levy et al., 2004; Ahn and Basbaum, 2005) where they can interrupt pain signal transmission and, it is hypothesized, if given early in the attack can prevent the central sensitization that leads to cutaneous allodynia in some patients (Goadsby, 2005b). Finally, there is a potential for triptans to act at $5\text{-}HT_{1B}$ receptors that are widespread on neuronal cell bodies throughout the brain, including regions involved in the modulation of pain such as the periaqueductal gray (Castro et al., 1997; Bartsch et al., 2004) and it is possible that this too may be involved in their therapeutic effects.

The triptans were developed initially (Humphrey, 2007) on the basis of a selective reversal of meningeal vasoconstriction in migraine through their action at the atypical cerebrovascular $5\text{-}HT_{1B}$ receptor (Humphrey et al., 1998) and on their ability to prevent meningeal inflammation (Buzzi and Moskowitz, 1990), but the importance of these peripheral versus trigeminal central effects has now been questioned (Humphrey and Goadsby, 1994; Goadsby, 2005a). Moreover the triptan activity at $5\text{-}HT_{1B}$ receptors produced a potential side-effect liability. $5\text{-}HT_{1B}$ receptors, preferentially expressed on smooth muscle in the trigeminovasculature (Nilsson et al., 1999), were also present, albeit at much lower densities, in the coronary vasculature (Nilsson et al., 1999) making them contraindicated in patients with cardiovascular disease. It is worth mentioning however that the primary constrictor serotonin receptor in the coronary circulation is the $5\text{-}HT_{2A}$ receptor at which the triptans have no activity and this may underlie their safety profile (Longmore et al., 1997c, 1998; Razzaque et al., 1999, 2002). The need for an improved real and perceived safety profile and the questionable role of vasoconstriction in the antimigraine action of the triptans set the goal for subsequent drug discovery efforts to find antimigraine efficacy without cardiovascular liability.

The first targets pursued were $5\text{-}HT_{1D}$ and $5\text{-}HT_{1F}$ receptors, which are localized on the terminals of the trigeminal nerves, in the hope that this mechanism could provide migraine headache relief by preventing proinflammatory neuropeptide release and interrupting pain signal transmission without vasoconstriction. The trials with a selective $5\text{-}HT_{1D}$ receptor agonist (Ferrari, 2001; Gomez-Mancilla et al., 2001), PNU 142663 by the Pharmacia-Upjohn company, probably failed because there was insufficient pharmacological efficacy of the molecule, developed using gorilla receptors, that went into the studies (Pregenzer et al., 1999; Alberts et al., 2000). It was hypothesized on the basis of the pharmacology of sumatriptan that $5\text{-}HT_{1F}$ receptors (Castro et al., 1997; Shepheard et al., 1999) may also contribute to the clinical effectiveness of the triptans. Triptans such as rizatriptan lacked activity at this receptor subtype but were still effective antimigraine agents, indicating that $5\text{-}HT_{1F}$ activity was not essential for antimigraine actions, but leaving open the possibility that it may contribute to the action of sumatriptan. The $5\text{-}HT_{1F}$ hypothesis (Ramadan et al., 2003) was substantiated clinically using a $5\text{-}HT_{1F}$ receptor-selective agonist LY334370 (Goldstein et al., 2001). Preclinical studies (Mitsikostas et al., 1999b; Shepheard et al., 1999; Goadsby and Classey, 2003) suggested that the $5\text{-}HT_{1F}$ mechanism was likely to be centrally mediated through inhibition of pain signal transmission in the TNC, in line with the central distribution of this receptor in the brainstem. Importantly, $5\text{-}HT_{1F}$ agonists were devoid of vasoconstrictor activity, as this receptor is not present in blood vessels (Razzaque et al., 1999). Development of LY334370 was discontinued due to animal toxicity. Subsequent $5\text{-}HT_{1F}$ receptor selective agonist back-up molecules from these series (LY573144) are still being pursued in the biotechnology sector (Colucid COL144: http://www.colucid.com).

Substance P NK1 receptor antagonists

On the basis of a preclinical trigeminal extravasation model of migraine in which the dihydroergotamine, triptans, and NK1 receptor antagonists were active, it was hypothesized that blockade of the proinflammatory effects of the substance P released from perivascular sensory nerves during a migraine attack may produce headache relief without having frank vasoconstrictor activity (Markowitz et al., 1987, 1988; Buzzi and Moskowitz, 1990; Buzzi et al., 1991; Shepheard et al., 1993; Saito et al., 1998). In addition to blocking neurogenic inflammation, NK1 receptor antagonists inhibited c-fos expression in the TNC after mechanical, electrical, or chemical stimulation of the trigeminal system (Shepheard et al., 1995; Mitsikostas and Sanchez-del-Rio, 2001). Clinically Nicolodi and Del Bianco (1990) found elevated levels of substance P in the saliva of migraineurs during an attack and Goadsby and colleagues (1988) found increased substance P in jugular blood of humans and animals after trigeminal stimulation, but this did not replicate in migraineurs during an attack (Goadsby and Edvinsson, 1993). Unfortunately several different structural classes of NK1 receptor antagonists (Fosaprepitant (Merck), GR205171 (GlaxoSmithKline), RPR 100893 (Rhône Poulenc) LY303870 (Lilly)) that were highly effective in preclinical assays of trigeminal inflammation failed when they were tested for the acute treatment of migraine. The only full paper published on these was for LY303870 lanepitant (Goldstein et al., 1997). The possibility that NK1 receptor antagonists may be valuable for migraine prophylaxis was also tested, but results were negative (Goldstein et al., 2001). Interestingly, NK1 receptor antagonists have failed in all clinical pain treatment trials in which they have been tested, despite the obvious receptor localization and pharmacology in the TNC, spinal dorsal horn, and much preclinical evidence suggesting that they might be effective (Salt et al., 1983; Hill, 2000).

Calcitonin gene-related peptide – CGRP1 receptor antagonists

CGRP is one of the most potent long-lived endogenous vasodilators in the human body yet is minimally, if at all, involved in the maintenance of normal major vascular tone (Brain, 2004). CGRP antagonism holds promise as a novel strategy to relieve migraine headache pain without overt vasoconstriction (Olesen et al., 2004; Doods et al., 2007; Goadsby, 2008; Ho et al., 2008).

Preclinical studies have examined the effects of CGRP antagonists in experimental assays of trigeminal activation that mimicked some aspects of the physiology of a migraine attack. The prototypic CGRP receptor antagonist BIBN4096 (Doods et al., 2000; Doods, 2001) blocked increases in facial blood flow caused by peripheral trigeminal ganglion stimulation (Escott et al., 1995) and cephalic vasodilation induced by CGRP or transcranial electrical stimulation (Petersen et al., 2004). Intravital microscope studies showed that electrical stimulation of the dural sensory nerves caused a pronounced vasodilation of the meningeal vessels as a result of release of CGRP as the responses were blocked by the peptide CGRP antagonist CGRP8-37 and BIBN4096. In these intravital assays the triptans are active but they work by preventing the release of CGRP as they block electrically stimulated vasodilation but not that evoked by exogenous CGRP. In this intravital model, as in the clinic, substance P NK1 receptor antagonists were inactive (Williamson et al, 1997a, b; Williamson and Hargreaves, 2001). Using intravital microscopy with simultaneous central electrophysiological recording from single trigeminal neurons it was also shown that CGRP not only induced meningeal vasodilation but also appeared to sensitize TNC second-order sensory neurons to non-nociceptive stimuli (Cumberbatch et al., 1999). It was speculated that there may be a link between the vasodilation and sensitization that could explain migraine pain and associated allodynia. However, it has recently been suggested that the site of action for CGRP-induced sensitization is central within the TNC rather than peripheral in nature (Levy et al., 2005), as CGRP did not excite or sensitize peripheral nociceptors directly, nor did meningeal vasodilation caused by CGRP increase firing in trigeminal pathways. Moreover, Jenkins et al. (2004) showed *in vitro* that CGRP could be released from TNC slices and Storer and colleagues (2004) showed direct activation ionophoretic application of CGRP caused excitation of second-order central sensory neurons receiving meningeal input. Importantly, Fischer et al. (2005) showed that the CGRP antagonist BIBN4096BS only reduced the activity of central trigeminovascular neurons after central administration. Most recently spinal CGRP receptors have been shown to contribute to supraspinally organized pain behavior and pain-related sensitization of amygdala neurons (Adwanikar et al., 2007). Taken together these preclinical and clinical findings suggest that the involvement of CGRP in migraine depends on its role as a central pain transmitter rather than through vasodilation and activation of meningeal nociceptors. The current view is therefore that the site of antimigraine action of CGRP antagonists could be central (Levy et al., 2005; Strassman and Levy, 2006), perhaps through an action at central trigeminal nerve terminals (Marvizon et al., 2007; Lennerz et al., 2008) or at second- or third-order sensory neurons that process nociceptive information from the meninges (Fischer et al., 2005).

In nitroglycerine-induced migraine attacks CRGP is released (Fanciullaci et al., 1995) and the 5-$HT_{IB}/_{ID}$ agonist sumatriptan has been shown to cause a parallel decrease in plasma CGRP and headache (Juhasz et al., 2005). In primary headache studies, CGRP levels in external jugular venous blood have been shown to be elevated in migraine and cluster headache attacks and, as in animal models of trigeminal stimulation (Buzzi et al., 1991), to be normalized by successful antimigraine drug therapy with sumatriptan (Edvinsson and Goadsby, 1998). These findings were replicated in patients during a migraine attack after administration of rizatriptan (Stepien, 2003) and it has been suggested that this may be predictive of a positive response (Sarchielli, 2005). Interestingly Ashina and colleagues (2000) showed that CGRP levels may be elevated in migraineurs compared to non-migraineurs out with attacks predisposing to the disorder. Whilst it was previously thought that CGRP in the meningeal vasculature could be involved in trigeminovascular activation, it is interesting to speculate that it is actually a fluid biomarker or "barometer" that reflects trigeminal activation during a migraine attack (Edvinsson, 2006) since focused preclinical studies have indicated that the key sites of action of CGRP and its antagonists are central rather than peripheral in nature (Strassman and Levy, 2006).

Animal and human studies with CGRP receptor antagonists show that they prevent vasodilation caused by CGRP but lack direct vasoconstrictor activity, suggesting that they may be relatively free of cardiovascular side-effect liability (Doods, 2001; Edvinsson et al., 2002; Shen et al., 2003; Edvinsson and Hargreaves, 2005). In clinical studies, BIBN4096 was shown to have no effect on cerebral blood flow or on flow in the middle meningeal artery (Petersen et al., 2005a). In experimental medicine provocation studies human αCGRP is capable of inducing in volunteers headache and extracerebral vasodilation that can be blocked by the CGRP antagonist BIBN4096 (Lassen et al., 2002; Petersen et al., 2005b). Care should be taken with these studies not to infer that the site of action of CGRP in producing head pain is vascular, as the two effects may be parallel phenomena since evidence is accumulating that the site of CGRP-induced head pain is central in origin.

For many years the only pharmacological agent available to block the effects of CGRP was a fragment of the full-length peptide containing amino acids 8–37 (CGRP8–37). The field of CGRP receptor antagonism was opened with the discovery of the high-affinity antagonist BIBN4096 (Doods et al., 2007). This molecule provided a unique opportunity to examine whether CGRP antagonism could treat migraine but, due to its "peptidic" nature, had to be administered by the intravenous route. Positive proof of concept in spontaneous migraine was reported using an innovative adaptive trial design (Olesen et al., 2004). More recently new classes of CGRP antagonist have been described (Goadsby, 2005c; Salvatore et al., 2008). MK-0974 (Wang, 2008), an orally active CGRP antagonist, has now been developed and shown in an adaptive clinical trial design to be generally well tolerated and active acutely against migraine with a similar efficacy profile to the 5-$HT_{1B/1D}$ agonist rizatriptan (Goadsby, 2008; Ho et al., 2008).

Glutamatergic modulators

The therapeutic potential of glutamate receptor antagonists in migraine has recently been comprehensively reviewed by Andreou and Goadsby (2009). Preclinical pharmacological studies *in vivo* have shown that glutamate can activate trigeminal systems (Mitsikostas et al., 1998, 1999a; Goadsby and Classey, 2000; Classey et al., 2001) and excess glutamate production, resulting perhaps from CSD, has the potential to activate these pathways in migraine. Storer and Goadsby (1999) showed electrophysiologically *in vivo* that trigeminovascular nociceptive transmission involves NMDA and non-NMDA glutamate receptors. Some support for the involvement of glutamate early in migraine is given by a small study by Kaube et al. (2000) in familial hemiplegic migraine patients that showed that the NMDA antagonist ketamine prevented migraine in 5 of 11 patients but interestingly had no effect on the headache pain itself. Elevated plasma levels of excitatory amino acids, including glutamine and glutamate, have been shown in some studies in migraineurs interictally and during a migraine headache attack (Ferrari et al., 1990; Alam et al., 1998). The relationship of these plasma changes to extracellular and synaptic glutamate is difficult to predict, especially since there is good evidence that even cerebrospinal fluid and brain extracellular glutamate do not reflect synaptic glutamate. The allodynia observed during migraine reflects central sensory sensitization, which is a known consequence of glutamate receptor activation (Woolf and Salter, 2000; Chizh, 2002).

LY466195 has shown clinical activity against migraine when given intravenously (Johnson et al., 2008). LY466195 is an iGluR5 antagonist and was active against neurogenic extravasation and c-fos expression in the trigeminal nucleus caudalis after trigeminal stimulation (Weis et al., 2006) but was inactive versus CGRP-mediated dural neurogenic vasal dilatation (Andreou et al., 2009), suggesting that it may exert its effects centrally. LY293558 (tezampanel: NGX424) is an AMPA/KA (Glur2/GluR5) antagonist which is active in clinical and preclinical pain models (Sang et al., 1998). It is also active in the trigeminal plasma protein extravasation model and inhibits c-fos expression in the trigeminal dorsal horn after trigeminal nerve activation. LY293558 does not have vasoconstrictor properties. Early proof-of-concept studies showed that intravenous LY293558, an AMPA/kainate antagonist, was effective acutely against migraine, providing another non-vasoactive approach to treating migraine (Ramadan, 2003; Sang et al., 2005; Ramadan and Buchanan, 2006). Subsequent studies with this intravenous formulation have confirmed this activity. Most recently NGX426 (TorreyPines Therapeutics), an orally active prodrug of tezampanel, has been introduced into clinical trials and is currently being studied for the treatment of migraine and pain (http://www.torreypinestherapeutics.com). The relative roles of AMPA and kainate receptor agonism and antagonism in the modulation of trigeminal nociceptive transmission is an active area of research.

ADX10059 is a potent selective negative allosteric modulator of the mGluR5 metabotropic glutamate receptor. Recent studies have shown it to be effective in the acute treatment of migraine (Goadsby and Keywood, 2009), providing another non-vasoactive approach to therapy. Addex Pharmaceuticals have announced that they will also pursue this mechanism for migraine prevention in phase IIB clinical studies (http://www.addexpharma.com).

CONCLUSIONS

This review has selected several of many targets that are currently being followed for the prevention and treatment of migraine. The targets appear to have face validity within what we know and have theorized about migraine predisposition, the initiation of the attack, and the pain and associated symptoms of the disorder. Recent advances in neuroimaging (Da Silva et al., 2002; Sanchez del Rio and Alvarez-Linera, 2004; Borsook et al., 2005) together with the development of pharmacological tools studied in astute clinical trials will undoubtedly help inform us further about the neurobiology and neuropharmacology of the systems involved in primary headache disorders. These discoveries should lead to novel safe and effective therapeutic strategies for improving migraine prevention and building forward from the triptan antimigraine agents that, over the last two decades, have brought such enormous benefits to the clinical care of migraineurs.

References

Adwanikar H, Guangchen J, Weidong L et al. (2007). Spinal CGRP receptors contribute to supraspinally organized pain behaviour and pain related sensitization of amygdala neurons. Pain 132: 53–66.

Ahn A, Basbaum A (2005). Where do triptans act in the treatment of migraine? Pain 115: 1–4.

Ahn AH, Fields HL, Basbaum AI (2004). The triptan receptor 5-HT1D is dynamically regulated in the central terminals of primary afferents in models of pain. Neurology 62: A440–A441.

Alam Z, Coombes N, Waring RH et al. (1998). Plasma levels of neuroexcitatory amino acids in patients with migraine or tension headache. J Neurol Sci 156: 102–106.

Alberts GL, Pregenzer JF, Im WB et al. (2000). Cloning of serotonin 5-HT_1 receptor subtypes from the chimpanzee, gorilla and Rhesus monkey and their agonist-induced guanosine 5′ gamma ^{35}S triphosphate binding. Neurosci Lett 280: 223–227.

Andreou AP, Goadsby PJ (2009). Therapeutic potential of novel glutamate receptor antagonists in migraine. Expert Opin Investig Drugs 18: 789–803.

Andreou AP, Holland AR, Goadsby PJ (2009). Activation of iGluR5 kainate receptors inhibits neurogenic dural vasodilatation in an animal model of trigeminovascular activation. Br J Pharmacol 157: 464–473.

Ardid DY, Lamberty A, Alloui MA et al. (2003). Antihyperalgesic effect of levetiracetam in neuropathic pain models in rats. Eur J Pharmacol 473: 27–33.

Ashina M, Bendtsen L, Jensen R et al. (2000). Evidence for increased plasma levels of calcitonin gene related peptide in migraine outside of attacks. Pain 86: 133–138.

Ashkenazi A, Benlifer A, Korenblit J et al. (2006). Zonisamide for migraine prophylaxis in refractory patients. Cephalalgia 26: 1199–1202.

Aurora SK, Ahmad BK, Welch KM et al. (1998). Transcranial magnetic stimulation confirms hyperexcitability of occipital cortex in migraine. Neurology 50: 1111–1114.

Ayata C, Shimizu-Sasamata M, Lo EH et al. (2000). Impaired neurotransmitter release and elevated threshold for cortical spreading depression in mice with mutations in the alpha1a subunit of P/Q type calcium channels. Neuroscience 95: 639–645.

Ayata C, Jin H, Kudo C et al. (2006). Suppression of cortical spreading depression in migraine prophylaxis. Ann Neurol 59: 652–661.

Bain PG, O'Brien MD, Keevil SF et al. (1992). Familial periodic cerebellar ataxia: a problem of cerebellar intracellular pH homeostasis. Ann Neurol 31: 147–154.

Bartsch T, Knight YE, Goadsby PJ (2004). Activation of 5-HT1B/1D receptors in the periaqueductal gray inhibits meningeal nociception. Ann Neurol 56: 371–381.

Battelli L, Black KR, Wray SH (2002). Transcranial magnetic stimulation of visual area V5 in migraine. Neurology 58: 1066–1069.

Baulac M (2006). Introduction to zonisamide. Epilepsy Res 68 (Suppl. 2): S3–S9.

Berger M, Speckmann EJ, Pape HC et al. (2008). Spreading depression enhances human neocortical excitability in vitro. Cephalalgia 28: 558–562.

Bleakman D, Lodge D (1998). Neurophramacology of AMPA and Kainate receptors. Neuropharmacology 37: 1187–1204.

Bolay H, Reuter U, Dunn AK et al. (2002). Intrinsic brain activity triggers trigeminal meningeal afferents in a migraine model. Nat Med 8: 136–142.

Borsook Burstein R, Becerra L (2005). Functional imaging of the human trigeminal system: opportunities for new insights into pain processing in health and disease. J Neurobiol 61: 107–125.

Brain SD (2004). Calcitonin gene related peptide (CGRP) antagonists: blockers of neuronal transmission in migraine. Br J Pharmacol 142: 1053–1054.

Brain SD, Grat AD (2004). Vascular actions of calcitonin gen-related peptide and adrenomedullin. Physiol Rev 84: 903–934.

Brighina F, Palermo A, Aloisio A et al. (2006). Levetiracetam in the prophylaxis of migraine with aura: a 6-month open-label study. Clin Neuropharmacol 29: 338–342.

Burstein R, Jakubowski M (2004). Analgesic triptan action in an animal model of cranial pain: a race against the development of sensitization. Ann Neurol 55: 27–36.

Burstein R, Jakubowski M (2005a). Unitary hypothesis for multiple triggers of the pain and strain of migraine. J Comp Neurol 493: 9–14.

Burstein R, Jakubowski M (2005b). Implications of multimechanism therapy: when to treat? Neurology 64: S16–S20.

Burstein R, Yamamura H, Malick A et al. (1998). Chemical stimulation of the intracranial dura induces enhanced responses to facial stimulation in brainstem trigeminal neurons. J Neurophysiol 79: 964–970.

Burstein R, Yarnitsky D, Goor-Aryeh I et al. (2000). An association between migraine and cutaneous allodynia. Ann Neurol 47: 614–624.

Burstein R, Collins B, Jakubowski M (2004). Defeating migraine pain with the triptans: a race against the development of cutaneous allodynia. Ann Neurol 55: 19–26.

Burstein R, Jakubowski M, Levy D (2005). Anti-migraine action of triptans is preceded by transient aggravation of headache caused by activation of meningeal nociceptors. Pain 115: 21–28.

Buzzi MG, Moskowitz MA (1990). The antimigraine drug sumatriptan GR 43175 selectively blocks neurogenic plasma extravasation from blood vessels in the dura mater. Br J Pharmacol 99: 202–206.

Buzzi MG, Carter WB, Shimizu T et al. (1991). Dihydroergotamine and sumatriptan attenuate levels of CGRP in plasma in rat superior sagittal sinus during electrical stimulation of the trigeminal ganglion. Neuropharmacology 30: 1193–1200.

Caddick SJ, Wang C, Fletcher CF et al. (1999). Excitatory but not inhibitory synaptic transmission is reduced in lethargic (Cacnb4(lh)) and tottering (Cacna1atg) mouse thalami. J Neurophysiol 81: 2066–2074.

Calabresi P, Galletti F, Rossi C et al. (2007). Antiepileptic drugs in migraine: from clinical aspects to cellular mechanisms. Trends Pharmacol Sci 28: 188–195.

Cao Y, Welch KM, Aurora S et al. (1999). Functional MRI-BOLD of visually triggered headache in patients with migraine. Arch Neurol 56: 548–554.

Castro ME, Pascual J, Romon T et al. (1997). Differential distribution of [^{3}H]sumatriptan binding sites (5-HT1B, 5-HT1D and 5-HT1F receptors) in human brain: focus on brainstem and spinal cord. Neuropharmacology 36: 535–542.

Charles A, Flippen C, Romero Reyes M et al. (2007). Memantine for prevention of migraine: a retrospective study of 60 cases. J Headache Pain 8: 248–250.

Chen G, Dunbar RL, Gao W et al. (2001). Role of calcium, glutamate neurotransmission and nitric oxide in spreading acidification and depression in the cerebellar cortex. J Neurosci 21: 9877–9887.

Chizh BA (2002). Novel approaches to targeting glutamate receptors for the treatment of chronic pain: review article. Amino Acids 23: 169–176.

Christopoulos G, Perry KJ, Morfis M et al. (1999). Multiple amylin receptors arise from receptor activity-modifying protein interaction with the calcitonin receptor gene product. Mol Pharmacol 56: 235–242.

Classey JD, Knight YE, Goadsby PJ (2001). The NMDA receptor antagonist MK-801 reduces Fos-like immunoreactivty within the trigeminocervical complex following superior sagittal sinus stimulation in the cat. Brain Res 907: 117–124.

Cumberbatch MJ, Hill RG, Hargreaves RJ (1997). Rizatriptan has central antinociceptive effects against durally evoked responses. Eur J Pharmacol 328: 37–40.

Cumberbatch MJ, Hill RG, Hargreaves RJ (1998a). Differential effects of naratriptan on trigeminal versus spinal nociceptive processing. Cephalalgia 18: 659–663.

Cumberbatch MJ, Hill RG, Hargreaves RJ (1998b). The role of $5HT_{1A}$, $5HT_{1B}$ and $5HT_{1D}$ receptors in trigeminal nociceptive neurotransmission in anaesthetized rats. Eur J Pharmacol 362: 43–46.

Cumberbatch MJ, Williamson DJ, Mason GS et al. (1999). Dural vasodilatation causes sensitization of rat caudal trigeminal neurons in vivo that is blocked by a 5-HT1B/1D agonist. Br J Pharmacol 126: 1478–1486.

Curia G, Aracri P, Colombo E et al. (2007). Phosphorylation of sodium channels mediated by protein kinase-C modulates inhibition by topiramate of tetrodotoxin-sensitive transient sodium current. Br J Pharmacol 150: 792–797.

Custer KL, Austin NS, Sullivan JM et al. (2006). Synaptic vesicle protein 2 enhances release probability at quiescent synapses. J Neurosci 26: 1303–1313.

Cutrer FM, Waeber C, Moskowitz MA (1998). Headache. In: S Enna, J Coyle (Eds.), Pharmacological Management of Neurological and Psychiatric Disorders. McGraw-Hill, New York.

Da Silva AF, Becerra L, Makris N et al. (2002). Somatotopic activation in the human trigeminal pain pathway. J Neurosci 22: 8183–8192.

Davies A, Hendrich J, Van Minh AT et al. (2007). Functional biology of the alpha(2)delta subunits of voltage-gated calcium channels. Trends Pharmacol Sci 28: 220–228.

De Simone R, Marano E, Di Stasio E et al. (2005). Acetazolamide efficacy and tolerability in migraine with aura: a pilot study. Headache 45: 385–386.

Dichgans M, Freilinger T, Eckstein G et al. (2005). Mutation in the neuronal voltage-gated sodium channel SCN1A in familial hemiplegic migraine. Lancet 366: 371–377.

Diener HC, May A (1996). New aspects of migraine pathophysiology: lessons learned from positron emission tomography. Curr Opin Neurol 9: 199–201.

Dodick DW, Silberstein S (2006). Central sensitization theory of migraine: clinical implications. Headache 46 (Suppl. 4): S182–S191.

Dodick DW, Eross EJ, Parish JM (2003). Clinical, anatomical and physiologic relationship between sleep and headache. Headache 43: 282–292.

Dodick D, Lipton RB, Martin V et al. (2004). Consensus statement: cardiovascular safety profile of triptans (5-HT agonists) in the acute treatment of migraine. Headache 44: 414–425.

Dong M, Yeh F, Tepp WH et al. (2006). SV2 is the protein receptor for botulinum neurotoxin A. Science 312: 592–596.

Doods H (2001). Development of CGRP antagonists for the treatment of migraine. Curr Opin Invest Drugs 2: 1261–1268.

Doods H, Hallermayer G, Wu D et al. (2000). Pharmacological profile of BIBN4096BS, the first selective small molecule CGRP antagonist. Br J Pharmacol 129: 420–423.

Doods H, Arndt K, Rudolf K et al. (2007). CGRP antagonists: unravelling the role of CGRP in migraine. Trends Pharmacol Sci 28: 580–587.

Dunlap K, Luebke JI, Turner TJ (1995). Exocytotic Ca^{2+} channels in mammalian central neurons. Trends Neurosci 18: 89–98.

Edvinsson L (2001). Sensory nerves in man and their role in primary headaches. Cephalagia 21: 761–764.

Edvinsson L (2006). Neuronal signal substances as biomarkers of migraine. Headache 46: 1088–1094.

Edvinsson L, Goadsby PJ (1998). Neuropeptides in headache. Eur J Neurol 5: 329–341.

Edvinsson L, Hargreaves R (2005). CGRP receptors: a new target for the treatment of headache? In: J Olesen (Ed.), The Headaches. 3rd edn. Lippincott Williams & Wilkins, Philadelphia.

Edvinsson L, Cantera L, Jansen Olesen I et al. (1997). Expression of calcitonin gene-related peptide 1 receptor mRNA in human trigeminal ganglia and cerebral arteries. Neurosci Lett 229: 209–211.

Edvinsson L, Alm R, Shaw D et al. (2002). Effect of the CGRP receptor antagonist BIBN4096BS in human cerebral, coronary and omental arteries and in SK-N-MC cells. Eur J Pharmacol 434: 49–53.

Escott KJ, Beattie DJ, Connor HE et al. (1995). Trigeminal ganglion stimulation increases facial blood flow in the rat: a role for calcitonin gene-related peptide. Brain Res 669: 93–99.

Ettinger AB, Argoff CE (2007). Use of antiepileptic drugs for nonepileptic conditions: psychiatric disorders and chronic pain. Neurotherapeutics 4: 75–83.

Evans BN, Rosenblatt MI, Mnayer LO et al. (2000). CGRP-RCP, a novel protein required for signal transduction at calcitonin gene-related peptide and adrenomedullin receptors. J Biol Chem 275: 31438–31443.

Fanciullacci M, Alessandri M, Figin M et al. (1995). Increase in plasma calcitonin gene-related peptide from the extracerebral circulation during nitroglycerine-induced cluster headache attack. Pain 60: 119–123.

Fehrenbacher JC, Taylor CP, Vasko MR (2003). Pregabalin and gabapentin reduce release of substance P and CGRP from rat spinal tissues only after inflammation or activation of protein kinase C. Pain 105: 133–141.

Ferrari M (2001). Editorial commentary on PNU 142633: Gomez-Mancilla et al. Cephalalgia 21: 727–732.

Ferrari MD, Odink K, Bos KD et al. (1990). Neuroexcitatory plasma aminoacids are elevated in migraine. Neurology 40: 1582–1586.

Ferrari MD, Goadsby PJ, Roon KI et al. (2002). Triptan (serotonin 5-HT1B/1D agonists) in migraine: detailed results and methods of a metaanalysis of 53 trials. Cephalalgia 22: 633–658.

Field MJ, Cox PJ, Stott E et al. (2006). Identification of the alpha2-delta-1 subunit of voltage-dependent calcium channels as a molecular target for pain mediating the analgesic actions of pregabalin. Proc Natl Acad Sci U S A 103: 17537–17542.

Field MJ, Li Z, Schwarz JB (2007). Ca^{2+} channel alpha2-delta ligands for the treatment of neuropathic pain. J Med Chem 50: 2569–2575.

Fischer MJM, Koulchitsky S, Messlinger K et al. (2005). The non-peptide calcitonin gene-related peptide receptor antagonist BIBN4096BS lowers the activity of neurons with meningeal input in the rat spinal trigeminal nucleus. J Neurosci 25: 5877–5883.

Foord SM, Marshall FH (1999). RAMPs: accessory proteins for seven transmembrane domain receptors. Trends Pharmacol Sci 20: 184–187.

Friberg L, Olesen J, Iversen HK et al. (1991). Migraine pain associated with middle cerebral artery dilatation: reversal by sumatriptan. Lancet 338: 13–17.

Fuks B, Gillard M, Michel P et al. (2003). Localization and photoaffinity labelling of the levetiracetam binding site in rat brain and certain cell lines. Eur J Pharmacol 478: 11–19.

Gallai V, Alberti A, Rossi C et al. (2003). An open-label pilot study on the efficacy and tolerability of levetiracetam in the prophylaxis of migraine. J Headache Pain 4: 92–96.

Gardner-Medwin AR (1981). Possible roles of vertebrate neuroglia in potassium dynamics, spreading depression and migraine. J Exp Biol 95: 111–127.

Goadsby P (2005a). Can we develop neurally acting drugs for the treatment of migraine? Nat Rev Drug Discov 4: 741–750.

Goadsby PJ (2005b). Migraine, allodynia sensitization and all of that. Eur Neurol 53 (Suppl. 1): 10–16.

Goadsby PJ (2005c). Calcitonin gene-related peptide antagonists as treatments of migraine and other primary headaches. Drugs 65: 2557–2567.

Goadsby PJ (2007). Recent advances in understanding migraine mechanism molecules and therapeutics. Trends Mol Med 13: 39–44.

Goadsby PJ (2008). Calcitonin gene related peptide (CGRP) and migraine. Is this a new era? Neurology 70: 1300–1301.

Goadsby PJ, Classey JD (2000). Glutamatergic transmission in the trigeminal nucleus assessed with local blood flow. Brain Res 875: 119–124.

Goadsby PJ, Classey JD (2003). Evidence for 5-HT1B, 5-HT1D and 5-HT1F receptor inhibitory effects on trigeminal neurons with craniovascular input. Neuroscience 122: 491–498.

Goadsby PJ, Edvinsson L (1993). The trigeminovascular system and migraine: studies characterizing cerebrovascular and neuropeptide changes seen in humans and cats. Ann Neurol 33: 48–56.

Goadsby PJ, Hargreaves RJ (2000). Mechanisms of action of serotonin 5-$HT_{1B/1D}$ agonists: insights into migraine pathophysiology using rizatriptan. Neurology 55: S8–S14.

Goadsby PJ, Hoskin KL (1996). Inhibition of trigeminal neurons by intravenous administration of the serotonin (5HT)1B/D receptor agonist zolmitriptan (311C90): are brain stem sites therapeutic target in migraine? Pain 67: 355–359.

Goadsby PJ, Evinsson L, Ekman R (1988). Release of vasoactive peptides in the extracerebral circulation of humans and cats during activation of the trigeminovascular system. Ann Neurol 23: 193–196.

Goadsby PJ, Keywood C (2009). Investigation of the role of mGluR5 inhibition in migraine: a proof of concept study of ADX10059 in acute treatment of migraine. Cephalalgia 29 (Suppl 1): abstract MPS01.

Goadsby PJ, Ferrari M, Mills JG et al. (2007). Double-blind placebo-controlled trial of tonabersat in the preventive management of migraine. Paper read at the 13th International Headache Congress, Stockholm.

Goldstein DJ, Wang O, Saper JR et al. (1997). Ineffectiveness of the neurokinin-1 antagonist in migraine. Cephalalgia 17: 785–790.

Goldstein DJ, Roon KI, Offen WW et al. (2001). Selective serotonin 1F (5-HT1F) receptor agonist LY334370 for acute migraine: a randomized controlled clinical trial. Lancet 358: 1230–1234.

Gomez-Mancilla B, Cutler NR, Leibowitz MT et al. (2001). Safety and efficacy of PNU-142633, a selective 5-HT1D agonist, in patients with acute migraine. Cephalagia 21: 727–732.

Gryder DS, Rogawski MA (2003). Selective antagonism of GluR5 kainate-receptor-mediated synaptic currents by topiramate in rat basolateral amygdala neurons. J Neurosci 23: 7069–7074.

Guay DR (2005). Pregabalin in neuropathic pain: a more "pharmaceutically elegant" gabapentin? Am J Geriatr Pharmacother 3: 274–287.

Hadjikhani N, Sanchez Del Rio M, Wu O et al. (2001). Mechanisms of migraine aura revealed by functional MRI in human visual cortex. Proc Natl Acad Sci U S A 98: 4687–4692.

Hargreaves RJ (2007). New migraine and pain research. Headache 47: S26–S43.

Hargreaves RJ, Beer M (2001). 5-HT receptors in brain and vasculature. In: J Olesen, M Ferrari, PPA Humphrey (Eds.), Frontiers in Headache Research, Vol. 10. The Triptans: Novel Drugs for Migraine. Oxford University Press, New York, pp. 11–22.

Hargreaves RJ, Beer M (2002). 5-Hydroxytryptamine and its receptors. In: L Edvinsson, DN Krause (Eds.), Cerebral Blood Flow and Metabolism. Lippincott, Williams and Wilkins, Philadelphia, pp. 283–294.

Hargreaves RJ, Shepheard SL (1999). Pathophysiology of migraine: new insights. Can J Neurol Sci 26 (Suppl 3): 12–19.

Hay DL, Poyner DR, Sexton PM (2006). GPCR modulation by RAMPs. Pharmacol Ther 109: 173–197.

Hershey JC, Corcoran HA, Baskin EP et al. (2005). Investigation of the species selectivity of a non peptide CGRP receptor antagonist using a novel pharmacodynamic assay. Regul Pept 127: 71–77.

Heuser D, Astrup J, Lassen NA et al. (1975). Brain carbonic acid acidosis after acetazolamide. Acta Physiol Scand 93: 385–390.

Hill RG (2000). NK1 (substance P) receptor antagonists – why are they not analgesic in humans? Trends Pharmacol Sci 21: 244–246.

Holland P, Goadsby PJ (2007). The hypothalamic orexinergic system: pain and primary headaches. Headache Currents 47: 951–962.

Ho TW, Mannix LK, Fan X et al. (2008). Randomized control trial of an oral CGRP receptor antagonist MK-0974 in acute treatment of migraine. Neurology 70: 1304–1312.

Hou M, Kanje M, Longmore J et al. (2001). 5-HT1B and 5-HT1D receptors in the human trigeminal ganglion: colocalization with calcitonin gene related peptide, substance P and nitric oxide synthase. Brain Res 909: 112–120.

Hovinga CA (2002). Novel anticonvulsant medications in development. Expert Opin Investig Drugs 11: 1387–1406.

Hoyer D, Clarke DE, Fozard JR et al. (1994). International Union of Pharmacology classification of receptors for 5-hydroxytryptamine (serotonin). Pharmacol Rev 46: 157–203.

Humphrey PPA (2007). The discovery of a new drug class for the acute treatment of migraine. Headache 47: S10–S19.

Humphrey PP, Goadsby PJ (1994). Controversies in headache. The mode of action of sumatriptan is vascular? A debate. Cephalalgia 14: 401–410.

Humphrey PPA, Fenuik W, Perren MJ et al. (1988). GR43175, a selective agents for the 5-HT1-like receptor in the dog isolated saphenous vein. Br J Pharmacol 94: 1123–1132.

Iadacola C (2002). From CSD to headache: a long and winding road. Nat Med 8: 110–112.

Jaeschke G, Wettstein JG, Nordquist RE et al. (2008). mGluR5 receptor antagonists and their therapeutic potential. Expert Opin Ther Patents 18: 123–142.

Jenkins DW, Langmead CJ, Parsons AA et al. (2004). Regulation of calcitonin-gene related peptide release from rat trigeminal caudalis slices in vitro. Neurosci Lett 366: 241–244.

Johnson KW, Niesenbaum ES, Johnson MP et al. (2008). Innovative drug development for headache disorders: glutamate. In: J Olesen, N Ramadan (Eds.), Frontiers in Headache Research, Vol. 16. Oxford University Press, Oxford, pp. 185–194.

Juhasz G, Zsombok T, Jakab B et al. (2005). Sumatriptan causes parallel decrease in plasma calcitonin gene-related peptide (CGRP) concentration and migraine headache during nitroglycerin induced migraine attack. Cephalalgia 25: 179–183.

Kaube H, Herzog J, Kaufer T et al. (2000). Aura in some patients with familial hemiplegic migraine can be stopped with intranasal ketamine. Neurology 55: 139–141.

Klitgaard H, Matagne A, Gobert J et al. (1998). Evidence for a unique profile of levetiracetam in rodent models of seizures and epilepsy. Eur J Pharmacol 353: 191–206.

Kruuse C, Thomsen LL, Birk S et al. (2003). Migraine can be induced by sildenafil without changes in middle cerebral artery diameter. Brain 126: 241–247.

Kunkler PE, Kraig RP (2003). Hippocampal spreading depression bilaterally activates the caudal trigeminal nucleus in rodents. Hippocampus 13: 835–844.

Lance JW, Fine RD, Curran DA (1963). An evaluation of methysergide in the prevention of migraine and other vascular headaches. Med J Austr 1: 814–818.

Lassen LH, Ashina M, Christiansen I et al. (1998). Nitric oxide synthase inhibition: a new principle in the treatment of migraine attacks. Cephalalgia 18: 27–32.

Lassen LH, Haderslev PA, Jacobsen VB et al. (2002). CGRP may play a causative role in migraine. Cephalalgia 22: 54–61.

Lauritzen M, Hansen AJ (1992). The effect of glutamate recptor blockade on anoxic depolarization and cortical spreading depression. J Cereb Blood Flow Metab 12: 223–229.

Lauritzen M, Jorgensen MB, Diemer NH et al. (1982). Persistent oligemia of rat cerebral cortex in the wake of spreading depression. Ann Neurol 12: 469–474.

Leniger T, Thone J, Wiemann M (2004). Topiramate modulates pH of hippocampal CA3 neurons by combined effects on carbonic anhydrase and Cl^-/HCO_3^- exchange. Br J Pharmacol 142: 831–842.

Lennerz JK, Ruhle V, Ceppe EP et al. (2008). Calcitonin receptor like receptor (CLR), receptor activity modifying protein 1 (RAMP1), and calcitonin gene related peptide (CGRP) immunoreactivity in the rat trigeminovascular system. Differences between central and peripheral CGRP receptor distribution. J Comp Neurol 507: 1277–1299.

Leone M, Attanasio A, Croci D et al. (2000). The serotonergic agent m-chlorophenylpiperazine induces migraine attacks: a controlled study. Neurology 55: 136–139.

Levy D, Jakubowski M, Burstein R (2004). Disruption of communication between peripheral and central trigeminovascular neurons mediates the anti-migraine action of 5-HT1B/1D agonists. Proc Natl Acad Sci U S A 101: 4274–4279.

Levy D, Burstein R, Strassman AM (2005). Calcitonin gene-related peptide does not excite or sensitize meningeal nociceptors: implications for the pathophysiology of migraine. Ann Neurol 55: 698–705.

Li CY, Zhang XL, Matthews EA et al. (2006). Calcium channel alpha2delta1 subunit mediates spinal hyperexcitability in pain modulation. Pain 125: 20–34.

Lipton RB, Bigal ME, Ashina S et al. (2008). Cutaneous allodynia in the migraine population. Ann Neurol 63: 148–158.

Longmore J, Shaw D, Smith D et al. (1997a). Differential distribution of 5-HT1D- and 5-HT1B-immunoreactivity within the human trigemino-cerebrovascular system: implication for the discovery of new antimigraine drugs. Cephalalgia 17: 833–842.

Longmore J, Hill RG, Hargreaves RJ (1997b). Neurokinin receptor antagonists: pharmacological tools and therapeutic drugs. Can J Pharmacol 75: 612–621.

Longmore J, Hargreaves RJ, Boulanger CM et al. (1997c). Comparison of the vasoconstrictor properties of the 5-HT1D receptor agonists rizatriptan (MK-462) and sumatriptan in human isolated coronary artery: outcome of two independent studies using different experimental protocols. Funct Neurol 12: 3–9.

Longmore J, Razzaque Z, Shaw D et al. (1998). Comparison of the vasoconstrictor effects of rizatriptan and sumatriptan in human isolated cranial arteries: immunohistochemical demonstration of the involvement of 5-HT1B receptors. Br J Clin Pharmacol 46: 577–582.

Luo ZD, Cizkova D (2000). The role of nitric oxide in nociception. Curr Rev Pain 4: 459–466.

Mallee JJ, Salvatore CA, LeBourdelles B et al. (2002). Receptor activity-modifying protein 1 determines the species selectivity of non-peptide CGRP receptor antagonists. J Biol Chem 277: 14294–14298.

Ma QP (2001). Co-localization of 5-HT (1B/1D/1F) receptors and glutamate in trigeminal ganglia in rats. Neuroreport 12: 1589–1591.

Ma QP, Hill R, Sirinathsinghji D (2001). Co-localization of CGRP with 5-HT1B/1D receptors and substance P in trigeminal ganglion neurons in rats. Eur J Neurosci 13: 2099–2104.

Maneuf YP, Blake R, Andrews NA et al. (2004). Reduction by gabapentin of K^+-evoked release of $[^3H]$-glutamate from the caudal trigeminal nucleus of the streptozotocin-treated rat. Br J Pharmacol 141: 574–579.

Markowitz S, Saito K, Moskowitz MA (1987). Neurogenically mediated leakage of plasma protein occurs from blood vessels in dura mater but not brain. J Neurosci 7: 4129–4136.

Markowitz S, Saito K, Moskowitz MA (1988). Neurogenically mediated plasma extravasation in the dura mater: effect of ergot alkaloids. A possible mechanism of action in vascular headache. Cephalagia 8: 83–91.

Marvizon JCG, Perez OA, Song B et al. (2007). Calcitonin receptor-like receptor activity and receptor activity modifying protein 1 in the rat dorsal horn. Localization in presynaptic terminals containing opioids and adrenergic alpha 2c receptors. Neuroscience 148: 250–265.

Masuda Y, Noguchi H, Karasawa T (1994). Evidence against a significant implication of carbonic anhydrase inhibitory activity of zonisamide in its anticonvulsive effects. Arzneimittelforschung 44: 267–269.

McLatchie LM, Fraser NJ, Main MJ et al. (1998). RAMPs regulate the transport and ligand specificity of the calcitonin-receptor-like receptor. Nature 393: 333–339.

Meurs A, Clinckers R, Ebinger G et al. (2006). Substantia nigra is an anticonvulsant site of action of topiramate in the focal pilocarpine model of limbic seizures. Epilepsia 47: 1519–1535.

Mitsikostas DD, Sanchez del Rio DD (2001). Receptor systems mediating c-fos expression within trigeminal nucleus caudalis in animal models of migraine. Brain Res Rev 35: 20–35.

Mitsikostas DD, Sanchez del Rio M, Waeber C et al. (1998). The NMDA receptor antagonist MK-801 reduces capsaicin-induced c-fos expression within rat trigeminal nucleus caudalis. Pain 76: 239–248.

Mitsikostas DD, Sanchez del Rio M, Waeber C et al. (1999a). Non-NMDA glutamate receptors modulate capsaicin induced c-fos expression within trigeminal nucleus caudalis. Br J Pharmacol 127: 623–630.

Mitsikostas DD, Sanchez-del-Rio M, Moskowitz MA et al. (1999b). Both 5-HT1B and 5-HT1F receptors modulate c-fos expression within rat trigeminal nucleus caudalis. Eur J Pharmacol 369: 271–277.

Mori A, Noda Y, Packer L (1998). The anticonvulsant zonisamide scavenges free radicals. Epilepsy Res 30: 153–158.

Moskowitz MA (1984). The neurobiology of vascular head pain. Ann Neurol 16: 157–168.

Moskowitz MA (1991). The visceral organ brain; implications for the pathophysiology of vascular head pain. Neurology 41: 182–186.

Moskowitz MA (2007). Pathophysiology of headache – past and present. Headache 47 (Suppl. 1): S58–S63.

Moskowitz MA, Reinhard JF, Romero J et al. (1979). Neurotransmitters and the fifth cranial nerve: Is there a relation to the headache phase of migraine? Lancet 2: 883–885.

Moskowitz MA, Nozaki K, Kraig RP (1993). Neocortical spreading depression provokes the expression of c-fos protein-like immunoreactivity within trigeminal nucleus caudalis via trigeminovascular mechanisms. J Neurosci 13: 1167–1177.

Nicolodi M, Del Bianco E (1990). Sensory neuropeptides (substance P, calcitonin gene-related peptide) and vasoactive intestinal polypeptide in human saliva. Their pattern in migraine and cluster headache. Cephalalgia 10: 39–50.

Nilsson T, Longmore J, Shaw D et al. (1999). Characterisation of 5-HT receptors in human coronary arteries by molecular and pharmacological techniques. Eur J Pharmacol 372: 49–56.

Nishino S (2007). The hypocretin/orexin receptor: therapeutic prospect in sleep disorders. Expert Opin Investig Drugs 16: 1785–1797.

Noda Y, Mori A, Packer L (1999). Zonisamide inhibits nitric oxide synthase activity induced by *N*-methyl-D-aspartate and buthionine sulfoximine in the rat hippocampus. Res Commun Mol Pathol Pharmacol 105: 23–33.

Olesen J, Larsen B, Lauritzen M (1981). Focal hyperemia followed by spreading oligemia and impaired activation of rCBF in classic migraine. Ann Neurol 9: 344–352.

Olesen J, Friberg L, Olsen TS et al. (1990). Timing and topography of cerebral blood flow aura and headache during migraine attacks. Ann Neurol 28: 791–798.

Olesen J, Iversen HK, Thomsen LL (1993). Nitric oxide supersensitivity: a possible molecular mechanism of migraine pain. Neuroreport 4: 1027–1030.

Olesen J, Diener HC, Husstedt IW et al. (2004). Calcitonin gene related peptide antagonist BIBN 4096BS for the acute treatment of migraine. N Engl J Med 350: 1104–1110.

Oliver KR, Wainwright A, Edvinsson L et al. (2002). Immunohistochemical localization of calcitonin receptor-like receptor and receptor activity-modifying proteins in the human cerebral vasculature. J Cereb Blood Flow Metab 22: 620–629.

Parsons CG (2001). NMDA receptors as targets for drug action in neuropathic pain. Eur J Pharmacol 429: 71–78.

Parsons CG, Danysz W, Bartmann A et al. (1999). Amino-alkyl-cyclohexanes are novel uncompetitive NMDA receptor antagonists with strong voltage-dependency and fast blocking kinetics: in vitro and in vivo characterization. Neuropharmacology 38: 85–108.

Parsons CG, Stoffler A, Danysz W (2007). Memantine: a NMDA receptor antagonist that improves memory by restoration of homeostasis in the glutamatergic system – too little activation is bad, too much is even worse. Neuropharmacology 53: 699–723.

Pascual J, Arco CD, Romon T et al. (1996). [^{3}H]sumatriptan binding sites in human brain: regional dependent labeling of 5-HT1D and 5-HT1F receptors. Eur J Pharmacol 295: 271–274.

Pascual J, Mateos V, Roig C et al. (2007). Marketed oral triptans in the acute treatement of migraine: a systematic review on efficacy and tolerability. Headache 47: 1152–1168.

Peeters M, Gunthorpe MJ, Strijbos PJ et al. (2007). Effects of pan- and subtype-selective N-methyl-D-aspartate receptor antagonists on cortical spreading depression in the rat: therapeutic potential for migraine. J Pharmacol Exp Ther 321: 564–572.

Petersen KA, Birk S, Doods H et al. (2004). Inhibitory effect of BIBN4096BS on cephalic vasodilatation induced by CGRP or by transcranial electrical stimulation in the rat. Br J Pharmacol 143: 697–704.

Petersen KA, Birk S, Lassen LH et al. (2005a). The novel CGRP-antagonist, BIBN4096BS does not affect cerebral or systemic hemodynamics in healthy volunteers. Cephalalgia 25: 139–147.

Petersen KA, Lassen LH, Birk S et al. (2005b). BIBN4096BS antagonizes human alpha-calcitonin gene-related peptide-induced headache and extracerebral artery dilatation. Clin Pharmacol Ther 77: 202–213.

Pietrobon D (2005). Migraine: new molecular mechanisms. Neuroscientist 11: 373–386.

Pietrobon D, Striessnig J (2003). Neurobiology of migraine. Nat Rev Neurosci 4: 386–398.

Potrebic S, Ahn AH, Skinner K et al. (2003). Peptidergic nociceptors of both trigeminal and dorsal root ganglia express serotonin 1D receptors: implications for the selective anti-migraine action of the triptans. J Neurosci 23: 10988–10997.

Poyner DR, Sexton PM, Marshall I et al. (2002). The mammalian calcitonin gene-related peptides, adrenomedullin, amylin and calcitonin receptors. Pharmacol Rev 54: 233–246.

Pregenzer JF, Alberts GL, Im WB et al. (1999). Differential pharmacology between the guinea-pig and the gorilla 5-HT1D receptor as probed with isochromans (5-HT1D-selective ligands). Br J Pharmacol 127: 468–472.

Puppe A, Limmroth V (2007). GABAergic drugs for the treatment of migraine. CNS Neurol Disord Drug Targets 6: 247–250.

Quartu M, Serra MP, Ambu R et al. (2002). AMPA- type glutamate receptor subunits 2/3 in the human trigeminal sensory ganglion and subnucleus caudalis from prenatal ages to adulthood. Mech Ageing Dev 123: 463–471.

Rahman A, Wienecke T, Hansen JM et al. (2008). Vasoactive intestinal polypeptide causes marked cephalic vasodilation but does not induce migraine. Cephalalgia 28: 226–236.

Ramadan NM (2003). The link between glutamate and migraine. CNS Spectr 8: 446–449.

Ramadan N, Buchanan TM (2006). New and future migraine therapy. Pharmacol Ther 112: 199–212.

Ramadan NM, Skljarevski V, Phebus LA et al. (2003). 5-HT1F receptor agonists in acute migraine treatment: a hypothesis. Cephalalgia 23: 776–785.

Raniero I, de Martino P, Pinessi A (2008). Hypocretins and primary headaches; neurobiology and clinical implications. Exp Rev Neurother 8: 409–416.

Razzaque Z, Heald MA, Pickard JD et al. (1999). Vasoconstriction in human isolated middle meningeal arteries: determining the contribution of 5-HT1B and 5-HT1F receptor activation. Br J Clin Pharmacol 47: 75–82.

Razzaque Z, Pickard JD, Ma Q-P et al. (2002). 5-HT1B receptors and vascular reactivity in human isolated blood vessels: assessment of the potential craniovascular selectivity of sumatriptan. Br J Clin Pharmacol 53: 266–274.

Reuter U, Bolay H, Jansen-Olesen I et al. (2001). Delayed inflammation in rat meninges: implications for migraine pathophysiology. Brain 124: 2490–2502.

Richter F, Ebersberger A, Schaible HG (2002). Blockade of voltage-gated calcium channels in rat inhibits repetitive cortical spreading depression. Neurosci Lett 334: 123–126.

Rogawski MA, Loscher W (2004). The neurobiology of anti-epileptic drugs. Nat Rev Neurosci 5: 553–564.

Sahara Y, Noro N, Iida Y et al. (1997). Glutamate receptor subuits GluR5 and KA-2 are co-expressed in rat trigeminal ganglion neurons. J Neurosci 17: 6611–6620.

Saito K, Markowitz S, Moskowitz MA (1998). Ergot alkaloids block neurogenic extravasation in dura mater: proposed action in vascular headaches. Ann Neurol 24: 732–737.

Salt TE, Morris R, Hill RG (1983). Distribution of substance P-responsive and nociceptive neurones in relation to substanceP-immunoreactivity within the caudal trigeminal nucleus of the rat. Brain Res 273: 217–228.

Salvatore CA, Hershey JC, Corcoran HA et al. (2008). Pharmacological chnaracterization of MK-0974 [N-[(3R,6S)-6-(2,3-difluorophenyl)-2-oxo-1-(2,2,2-trifluoroethyl) azepan-3-yl]-4-(2-oxo-2,3-dihydro-1H-imidazo[4,5-b] pyridine-1-yl)piperidine-1-carboxamide], a potent and orally active calcitonin gene-related peptide receptor antagonist for the treatment of migraine. J Pharmacol Exp Ther 324: 416–421.

Sanchez del Rio M, Alvarez-Linera J (2004). Functional neuroimaging of headaches. Lancet Neurol 3: 645–651.

Sang CN, Hostetter MP, Gracely RH et al. (1998). AMPA/kainate antagonist LY293558 reduces capsaicin-evoked hyperalgesia but not pain in normal skin in humans. Anesthesiology 89: 1060–1067.

Sang CN, Ramadan NM, Wallihan RG et al. (2005). LY293558, a novel AMPA/GluR5 antagonist, is efficacious and well-tolerated in acute migraine. Cephalalgia 24: 596–602.

Saper CB, Scammell TE, Lu J (2005). Hypothalamic regulation of sleep and circadian rhythms. Nature 437: 1257–1263.

Sarchielli P (2005). Clinical biochemical correlates of migraine attacks in rizatriptan responders and non-responders. Cephalalgia 26: 257–265.

Saria A (1999). The tachykinin NK1 receptor in the brain: pharmacology and putative functions. Eur J Pharmacol 375: 51–60.

Saxena P, Ferrari M (1992). From receptor classification to the antimigraine drug sumatriptan. Cephalalgia 12: 187–196.

Shen Y, Hong X, Malleee JJ et al. (2003). Effects of inhibition of alpha CGRP receptors on cardiac and peripheral vascular dynamics in conscious dogs with chronic heart failure. J Cardiovasc Pharmacol 42: 656–661.

Shepheard SL, Williamson DJ, Hill RG et al. (1993). The non-peptide neurokinin1 receptor antagonist RP 67580, blocks neurogenic plasma extravasation in the dura mater of rats. Br J Pharmacol 108: 11–12.

Shepheard SL, Williamson DJ, Williams J et al. (1995). Comparison of the effects of sumatriptan and the NK_1 antagonist CP99,994 on plasma extravasation in dura mater and c-fos mRNA expression in trigeminal nucleus caudalis of rats. Neuropharmacology 34: 255–261.

Shepheard S, Edvinsson L, Cumberbatch M et al. (1999). Possible anti-migraine mechanisms of action of the 5-HT1F receptor agonist LY334370. Cephalagia 19: 851–858.

Shimomura T, Murakami F, Kotani K et al. (1999). Platelet nitric oxide metabolites in migraine. Cephalalgia 19: 218–222.

Silberstein SD (2000). Practice parameter: evidence-based guidelines for migraine headache (an evidence-based review): report of the Quality Standards Subcommittee of the American Academy of Neurology. Neurology 55: 754–762.

Silberstein SD, Collins SD (1999). Safety of divalproex sodium in migraine prophylaxis: an open-label, long-term study. Long-term Safety of Depakote in Headache Prophylaxis Study Group. Headache 39: 633–643.

Silberstein SD, Hargreaves RJ (2000). History and pharmacology of ergotamine and dihydroergotamine. In: HC Diener (Ed.), Monographs in Clinical Neuroscience; Drug Treatment of Migraine and Other Headaches. Karger, Basel, pp. 52–65.

Silberstein SD, Goadsby PJ, Lipton RB (2000). Management of migraine: an algorithmic approach. Neurology 55 (Suppl. 2): S46–S52.

Silberstein SD, Neto W, Schmitt J et al. (2004). Topiramate in migraine prevention: results of a large controlled trial. Arch Neurol 61: 490–495.

Sitges M, Chiu LM, Guarneros A et al. (2007). Effects of carbamazepine, phenytoin, lamotrigine, oxcarbazepine, topiramate and vinpocetine on Na^+ channel-mediated release of [^{3}H]glutamate in hippocampal nerve endings. Neuropharmacology 52: 598–605.

Smith D, Hill RG, Edvinsson L et al. (2002). An immunocytochemical investigation of human trigeminal nucleus caudalis: CGRP, substance P and 5-HT1D receptor immunoreactivities are expressed by trigeminal sensory fibers. Cephalagia 22: 424–431.

Somjen GG (2001). Mechanisms of spreading depression and hypoxic spreading depression-like depolarization. Physiol Rev 81: 1065–1096.

Stepien A (2003). [Suppressing effect of the serotonin 5-HT1B/1D receptor agonist rizatriptan on calcitonin gene-related peptide (CGRP) concentration in migraine attacks.] Neurol Neurochir Pol 37: 1013–1023.

Stepien A, Chalimoniuk M (1998). Level of nitric oxide-dependent cGMP in patients with migraine. Cephalalgia 18: 631–634.

Storer RJ, Goadsby PJ (1999). Trigeminovascular nociceptive transmission involves N-methyl-D-aspartate and non-N-methyl-D-aspartate receptors. Neuroscience 90: 1371–1376.

Storer RJ, Akerman S, Goadsby PJ (2004). Calcitonin gene-related peptide (CGRP) modulates nociceptive trigeminovascular transmission in the cat. Br J Pharmacol 142: 1171–1181.

Strassman AM, Levy D (2006). Response properties of dural nociceptors in relation to headache. J Neurophysiol 95: 1298–1306.

Strassman AM, Raymond SA, Burstein R (1996). Sensitization of meningeal sensory neurons and the origin of headaches. Nature 384: 560–564.

Tanabe M, Takeuchi Y, Ono H (2007). The supraspinally mediated analgesic effects of zonisamide in mice after peripheral nerve injury are independent of the descending monoaminergic system. J Pharmacol Sci 104: 335–340.

Tassorelli C, Joseph SA (1995). NADPH-diaphorase activity and Fos expression in brain nuclei following nitroglycerin administration. Brain Res 695: 37–44.

Tfelt-Hansen P (2006). A review of evidence-based medicine and meta-analytic reviews in migraine. Cephalagia 26: 1265–1274.

Tfelt-Hansen P, Block G, Dahlof C et al. (2000). Guidelines for controlled trials of drugs in migraine: second edition. Cephalalgia 20: 765–786.

Tombaugh GC (1994). Mild acidosis delays hypoxic spreading depression and improves neuronal recovery in hippocampal slices. J Neurosci 14: 5635–5643.

Tombaugh GC, Somjen GG (1996). Effects of extracellular pH on voltage-gated Na^+, K^+ and Ca^{2+} currents in isolated rat CA1 neurons. J Physiol 493: 719–732.

Tottene A, Fellin T, Pagnutti S et al. (2002). Familial hemiplegic migraine mutations increase Ca(2+) influx through single human $Ca_v2.1$ channels and decrease maximal cav2.1 current density in neurons. Proc Natl Acad Sci U S A 99: 13284–13289.

Tvedskov JF, Iversen HK, Olesen J (2004). A double-blind study of SB-220453 (Tonerbasat) in the glyceryltrinitrate (GTN) model of migraine. Cephalalgia 24: 875–882.

Uncini A, Lodi R, Di Muzio A et al. (1995). Abnormal brain and muscle energy metabolism shown by ^{31}P-MRS in familial hemiplegic migraine. J Neurol Sci 129: 214–222.

Vahedi K, Taupin P, Djomby R et al. (2002). Efficacy and tolerability of acetazolamide in migraine prophylaxis: a randomised placebo-controlled trial. J Neurol 249: 206–211.

van de Ven RC, Kaja S, Plomp JJ et al. (2007). Genetic models of migraine. Arch Neurol 64: 643–646.

van den Maagdenberg AM, Pietrobon D, Pizzorusso T et al. (2004). A Cacna1a knockin migraine mouse model with increased susceptibility to cortical spreading depression. Neuron 41: 701–710.

Vikelis M, Mitsikostas DD (2007). The role of glutamate and its receptors in migraine. CNS Neurol Disord Drug Targets 6: 251–257.

Wang Y (2008). MK-0974. Drugs of the Future 33: 116–122.

Weiss B, Alt A, Ogden AM et al. (2006). Pharamcological characterization of the competitive Gluk5 receptor antagonist decahydroisoquinoline LY466195 in vitro and in vivo. J Pharmacol Exp Ther 318: 772–781.

Welch KM, Levine SR, D'Andrea G et al. (1989). Preliminary observations on brain energy metabolism in migraine studied by in vivo phosphorus 31 NMR spectroscopy. Neurology 39: 538–541.

Westenbroek RE, Sakurai T, Elliott EM et al. (1995). Immunochemical identification and subcellular distribution of the alpha 1A subunits of brain calcium channels. J Neurosci 15: 6403–6418.

Williamson DJ, Hargreaves RJ (2001). Neurogenic inflammation in the context of migraine. Microsc Res Tech 53: 167–178.

Williamson DJ, Hargreaves RJ, Hill R et al. (1997a). Intravital microscope studies on the effects of neurokinin agonists and calcitonin gene-related peptide on dural blood vessel diameter in anaesthetized rat. Cephalalgia 17: 518–524.

Williamson DJ, Shepheard SL, Hill RG et al. (1997b). The novel anti-migraine agent rizatriptan inhibits neurogenic dural vasodilation and extravasation. Eur J Pharmacol 328: 61–64.

Wolff HG (1929). The cerebral circulation. Arch Neurol Psychiatry 22: 686–699.

Woolf CJ, Salter MW (2000). Neuronal plasticity: increasing the gain in pain. Science 288: 1765–1768.

Yang XFA, Weisenfeld S, Rothman SM (2007). Prolonged exposure to levetiracetam reveals a presynaptic effect on neurotransmission. Epilepsia 48: 1861–1869.

Zhang Z, Winborn CS, Marquez de Prado B et al. (2007). Sensitization of calcitonin gene related peptide receptors by receptor activity modifying protein-1 in the trigeminal ganglion. J Neurosci 27: 2693–2703.

Subject Index

NB: Page numbers in **bold** refer to figures and tables

D

E

Q

R

T